MICHAEL J. HOGAN, M.D.

Professor and Chairman, Department of Ophthalmology, and Research Associate, Francis I. Proctor Foundation for Research in Ophthalmology, University of California, San Francisco, California

JORGE A. ALVARADO, A.B.

Francis I. Proctor Foundation for Research in Ophthalmology; 2nd Year Medical Student, University of California School of Medicine, San Francisco, California

JOAN ESPERSON WEDDELL

Medical Illustrator, Department of Ophthalmology and the Francis I. Proctor Foundation for Research in Ophthalmology

HISTOLOGY of the HUMAN EYE

An Atlas and Textbook

W. B. SAUNDERS COMPANY

Philadelphia London Toronto Mexico City Rio de Janeiro Sydney Tokyo

W. B. Saunders Company: West Washington Square
Philadelphia, PA 19105

1 St. Anne's Road
Eastbourne, East Sussex BN21 3UN, England

1 Goldthorne Avenue
Toronto, Ontario M8Z 5T9, Canada

Apartado 26370 – Cedro 512
Mexico 4, D.F., Mexico

Rua Coronel Cabrita, 8
Sao Cristovao Caixa Postal 21176
Rio de Janeiro, Brazil

9 Waltham Street
Artarmon, N.S.W. 2064, Australia

Ichibancho, Central Bldg., 22-1 Ichibancho
Chiyoda-Ku, Tokyo 102, Japan

Histology of the Human Eye ISBN 0-7216-4720-0

 Made in the United States of America. Press of W. B. Saunders Company. Library of Congress catalog card number 78-135327.

Print No.: 9 8 7

A set of 35 mm. teaching slides of drawings and photographs from this book is available through the publisher.

ACKNOWLEDGMENTS

Many individuals have contributed in some way to the completion of this textbook. Mrs. Irmgard Wood has been identified with it almost from the beginning. Her very fine technical work in preparation, viewing and photographing the tissues, as well as in organizing the final prints for each chapter, has been a major contribution, and we are grateful for her association. Dr. Manfred Spitznas of the Eye Clinic, Essen, Germany, made a major contribution to the Retina chapter. Almost all the prints used in this chapter were made from his plates, and we are grateful also for the time he spent reviewing the manuscript. His work was done during a fellowship year in San Francisco, and we look forward to his future publication of a book on the retina. Dr. Lynette Feeney spent several months with us after obtaining her doctoral degree and produced many of the plates that have been used in the Lens chapter. She also has reviewed the Lens chapter and made contributions to the legends accompanying the photographs; we thank her for her assistance. Miss Nanette Carroll, University of Melbourne, Australia, spent many hours working on the Iris chapter, and her fine technical work on the iris tissues is greatly appreciated. The National Society for the Prevention of Blindness supported her work. We thank Dr. Douglas Anderson of the University of Miami, who kindly allowed us to use his manuscripts and some photographs and drawings of the Optic Nerve in this chapter of our text. Without his pioneering work in electron microscopy of the optic nerve, our task would have been much more difficult. We would like to thank Professor Giambattista Bietti and Dr. Giovanni Moschini for their great assistance in collecting a bibliography for this book in the Library of the Clinica Oculistica, University of Rome and also Dr. Jose Pecori Giraldi for her help in translation of foreign articles.

Dr. David Maurice, Division of Ophthalmology, Stanford Medical School, very kindly spent many hours working with us on the Cornea chapter, and we acknowledge that his careful study and revision have contributed greatly to the value of this chapter. We are grateful to Dr. William McEwen of our department and the Francis I. Proctor Foundation for Research in Ophthalmology for his reviews and changes in the chapters on the Limbus, Sclera and Vitreous; his suggestions in these areas have been of great value. We are indebted to Dr. Fraser Muirhead for his evaluation and suggestions on the physiology section of the Retina chapter. Dr. Brooks Crawford of our department reviewed the chapter on the Eyeball and made some valuable suggestions. Drs. Paul Henkind and Robert Foos are thanked for their photographic contributions to the Retina chapter. Miss Jeremy Hewes, editor, worked long and hard to make the manuscript clear and readable, as well as checking all bibliographic references. Mrs. Betty Hart freely donated her time to a review of the scientific aspects of many chapters, and we appreciate her many fine revisions. Mrs. Mary Helen Stull did a careful and conscientious job of mounting and lettering all the microphotographs used in this book. We are grateful to Mrs. Sue Allen for all the hours she spent typing and retyping the chapters of this text.

We especially wish to thank Drs. Phillips Thygeson and G. Richard O'Connor for their cooperation and encouragement in the preparation and completion of this book. Without the use of the fine facilities of the Francis I. Proctor Foundation for Research in Ophthalmology we would not have been able to complete the work. We also want to thank the members of our Department of Ophthalmology and the Francis I. Proctor Foundation for their long forebearance in relinquishing valuable art time so that the book could be completed.

Research to Prevent Blindness, New York, made an unrestricted grant for use in the Department of Ophthalmology. These funds were used to provide technical assistance in preparing the book. Laboratory and technical help on this book also was supported by the National Eye Institute Program, Project Grant #USPHS EY-00310.

M.J.H.

J.A.A.

J.E.W.

CONTENTS

Chapter One

THE CELL

Recent studies using the electron microscope and the techniques of cell fractionation, centrifugation and autoradiography are largely responsible for our present understanding of the relationship between structure and physiologic properties of the cell (Palade, 1966, Fawcett, 1966, DuPraw, 1968). The membrane which bounds the surface of all cells is complex, exerting a strong influence on cell metabolism and retention of the cellular contents. The cell contains a number of compartments, or organelles, which are equipped with enzyme systems that carry out specific metabolic functions. The organelles generally are oriented around the nucleus, which is the repository for genetic information and the site of the highest level of control of cellular activity by means of gene activation.

This chapter discusses the major morphologic features of the cell and offers a brief description of cell function.

THE CELL MEMBRANE (Figs. 1–1 to 1–3)

Visual demonstration of a limiting layer around all cells is a recent development in biology. Previously, the existence and composition of such a layer had only been inferred from physiologic data regarding the exchange of water and solutes between the cells and their extracellular fluid environment. Muscle physiologists, for example, assumed the existence of a cell membrane because of the difference in ionic concentration between the interior of the muscle cells and their surrounding fluid.

More than a century ago Overton (1845) showed that the cells he was studying were more easily penetrated by lipid-soluble substances than by water-soluble ones. He postulated that the cell membrane contains a lipid material that is responsible for cellular permeability. Early in this century Langmuir (1917) described the orientation of lipids along an air-water interface. He demonstrated that the polar ends of an amphophilic lipid dispersed in an air-water interface were oriented toward the water side, and the nonpolar fatty acid ends were on the air side. Gorter and Grendel (1925) measured the amount of lipid in a known volume of erythrocytes. Because the solvent they used to extract erythrocyte lipid was inadequate, these investigators could measure only a portion of the total lipid present. Their calculation of the surface area of the extracted cells, however, was less than the actual surface area so that the two errors partially cancelled each other out. These authors arrived at the conclusion that sufficient lipid was present to form a double layer over the erythrocyte surface. These calculations have been confirmed and are generally accepted today. Gorter and Grendel then postulated that the limiting cell membrane of the erythrocyte consists of a continuous bimolecular layer of lipid with the hydrophobic nonpolar ends facing each other, and that one of the polar hydrophilic ends faces the extracellular space and the other faces the interior of the cell (Fig 1–1 *A*).

The next major development in the understanding of the organization of the cell membrane came about through studies on the elastic and surface tension properties of the sea urchin egg. It was shown that the surface tension was less than might be expected from the lipid layer described by Gorter and Grendel. In 1935 Danielli and Davson modified the Gorter-Grendel model in an effort to explain the surface tension properties of the cell. Danielli previously had studied the changes in surface tension of an oil droplet after the addition of various substances. He observed that adding protein lessened the surface tension of the oil droplet. The model proposed by Danielli and Davson includes a layer of protein on both sides of the bimolecular lipid layer; according to them, this arrangement accounts for the low surface tension of the membrane (Fig. 1–1 *B*). The Danielli-Davson model received experimental support from the studies of Schmitt and coworkers (1936), who showed that erythrocyte cell membranes possess a positive, radial birefringence when studied with polarized light. Later Schmidt (1937) showed this birefringence to be sensitive to lipid solvents. By the time the electron microscope was finally used to visualize the cell

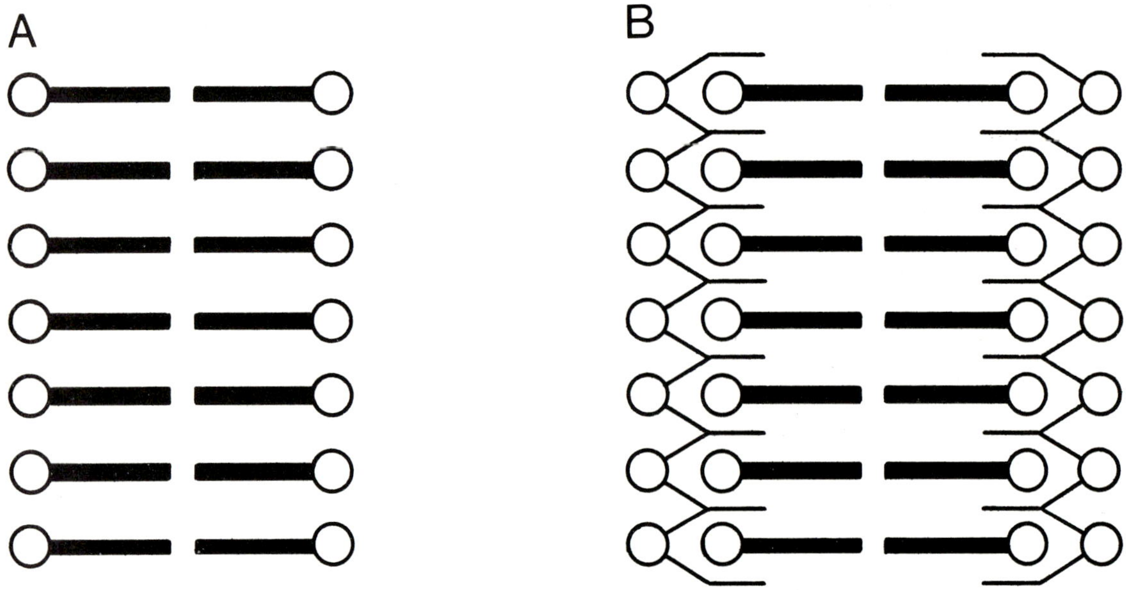

Figure 1–1. *A*, Gorter and Grendel's representation of the cell membrane. *B*, The Danielli-Davson scheme for the cell membrane adds a protein layer to the bimolecular lipid layer shown in the model of Gorter and Grendel.

membrane, the Danielli-Davson model was accepted and the results were well anticipated. It was not expected, however, that similar membranes would be found in the interior of the cell, enclosing the nucleus, mitochondria, Golgi complex and endoplasmic reticulum.

Robertson (1959) subsequently investigated the ultrastructure of the membranes of several types of cells and of myelin with OSO_4 and $KMnO_4$; he showed that the cell membrane could be resolved into two dark lines measuring 25 A. thick and separated by a clear space approximately 50 A. wide. He showed that this arrangement was present not only in the cell membrane but also in the membranes around the intracellular organelles, and he proposed the term "unit membrane" for such a trilaminar structure (Fig. 1–2). Stoeckenius (1962) suggested that the two dark lines of the unit membrane seen in electron micrographs are visible because of the reduction of OSO_4 by the protein layer and the polar hydrophilic ends of the lipid molecule. Recent electron microscopic studies with freeze-etching preparations, which do not depend on chemical fixation, have produced pictures of the cell membrane that closely resemble those shown by conventional electron microscopic methods.

The size and chemical composition of the surface and intracellular membranes vary from cell to cell as well as within the cells. The thickness of the cell membrane usually is slightly greater than that of the intracellular ones. Sjostrand (1968) measured the surface and intracellular membranes in the proximal tubular cells of the mouse kidney and found the following:

Plasma or cell membrane	93–96 A.
Smooth-surfaced membranes	72–77 A.
Mitochondrial membranes	51–62 A.

Studies of the chemical composition of the cell membrane constitute a very active area of research today. At present more is known about the lipid than about the protein component of the membrane. The lipids consist mainly of phospholipids, glycolipids and a sterol, usually cholesterol. Rouser and co-workers (1968) have made extensive studies of the lipid composition of surface, mitochondria, endoplasmic reticulum and nuclear membranes, and have found the lipid composition of these membranes to vary both qualitatively and quantitatively. Glycolipids, for instance, are found almost exclusively in myelin and the cell membrane, while diphosphatidyl glycerol usually is found only in the mitochondrial membranes. The membranes of the nucleus and the endoplasmic reticulum contain the same lipid classes, but the lipid is present in different proportions. The composition of the cell membrane varies among cell types, whereas that of the nuclear membrane is quite consistent from organ to organ and among various species. The composition of the mitochondrial membrane shows only slight differences when one organ is compared to another.

The total weight of the protein component of the cell membrane is one to two times that of the lipid. Some of the proteins are mainly structural in nature, such as lipoproteins, whereas others have an enzymatic function. Outstanding examples of the latter are a sodium potassium-activated triphosphatase and an acetylcholinesterase identified in erythrocytes (Stein, 1967).

The permeability properties of the cell membrane generally depend on the lipid solubility, the size and the ionic charge of the solute. There are a number of membranes which exhibit permeability properties, however, that are not explained by the above criteria. For example, most cell mem-

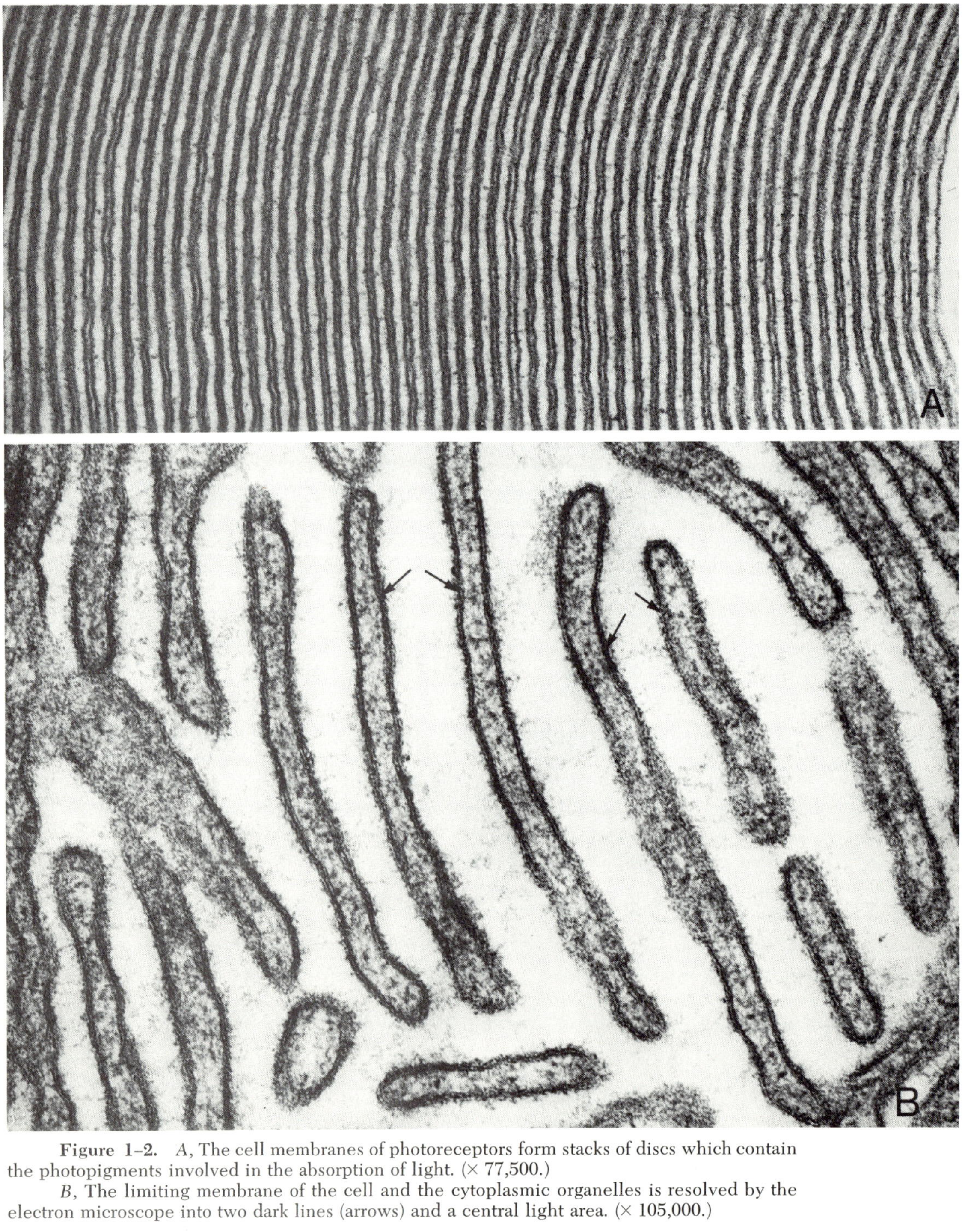

Figure 1–2. *A*, The cell membranes of photoreceptors form stacks of discs which contain the photopigments involved in the absorption of light. (× 77,500.)

B, The limiting membrane of the cell and the cytoplasmic organelles is resolved by the electron microscope into two dark lines (arrows) and a central light area. (× 105,000.)

branes offer no resistance to the flow of water, but the cells of the ascending limb of the loop of Henle are relatively impermeable, while those of the collecting duct can alter their permeability to water. Similarly, the red blood cell has been found to be more permeable to anions than to cations under certain conditions.

Most cells are more permeable to lipid-soluble than to water-soluble molecules. Molecules smaller than urea penetrate the cell membrane with relative ease, whereas those larger than urea molecules penetrate the membrane with great difficulty. In general, cells are less permeable to electrolytes than to nonelectrolytes of similar size. The ability of monovalent cations to penetrate the cell membrane correlates well with the hydrated size of the cations, so that hydrated potassium ions, which are smaller than hydrated sodium ions, penetrate the membrane more readily than sodium. Divalent cations and anions penetrate the cell membrane less easily than monovalent ions. Nonionized weak electrolytes usually enter the cells much more readily than the ionized forms of weak electrolytes.

The cell membrane also is equipped with ion pumps which can move water against chemical and electrical concentration gradients; for example, the eye has special cell layers that are believed to be involved in the active transport of salts. This mechanism is probably very important in the production of aqueous humor by the ciliary epithelium and in the maintenance of the clarity and thickness of the cornea by its endothelium. In addition to the pumping of ions, large molecules also may be moved across cell membranes by an active carrier mechanism or by the process of *pinocytosis*.

Recently a great deal of attention has been directed toward other models of the cell membrane that may improve our understanding of its permeability properties, its structural and chemical differences, and the mechanism of membrane synthesis. For example, in the *subunit model* the cell membrane is depicted as formed by small subunits which are polymerized or bound together to form the larger unit membrane as bricks form a wall. The cell membrane subunits are both structural and functional, measuring 40 to 50 A. in diameter, and are arranged in a hexagonal or mosaic pattern. The proponents of this model believe that it best explains most membrane phenomena. Stoeckenius and Engelman (1969) have recently reviewed all the proposed models and conclude that the Danielli-Davson model adequately explains all of the physiologic and biochemical data presently known about the cell membrane.

THE NUCLEUS (Figs. 1–4 to 1–7)

The morphology of the nucleus is specific for each stage in the cell cycle. During mitosis the chromosomes become easily visible, the nuclear envelope disappears, the mitotic apparatus is formed, and a set of chromosomes is distributed to each daughter cell. The interphase nucleus between divisions shows no distinct chromosomes; the chromatin is dispersed throughout the nucleus, which is enclosed by the nuclear membrane (Fig. 1–4). The chromatin stains with basic dyes such as hematoxylin and it also stains positively for the Feulgen reaction for nucleic acids. It is accepted today that the genetic material of eukaryotic cells is located in the nuclear chromatin. The chromatin itself consists of deoxyribonucleic acid (DNA) and some basic proteins, called histones, that form salt linkages with the nucleic acids.

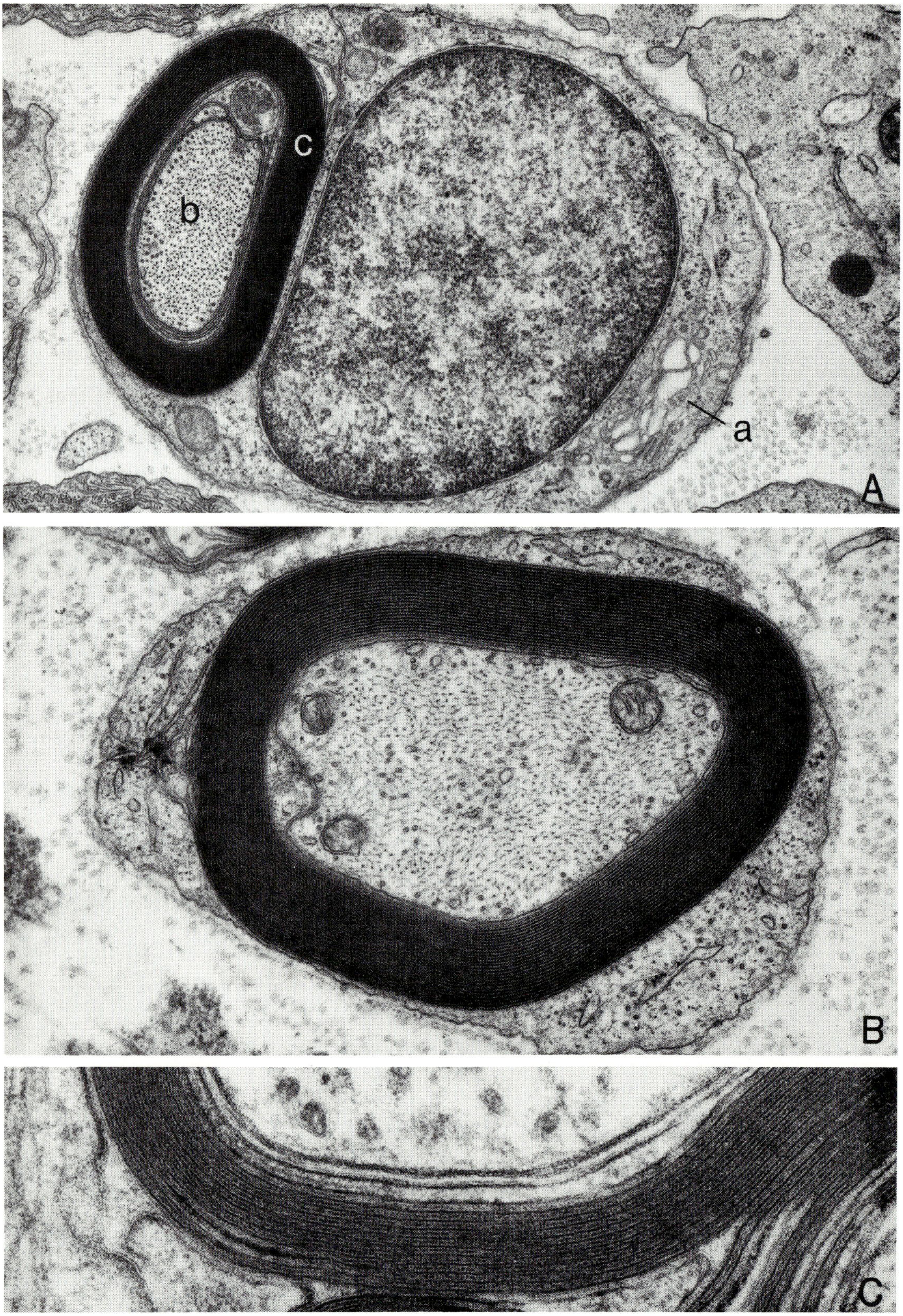

Figure 1–3. *See legend on opposite page.*

When viewed with the electron microscope, the nuclear chromatin is seen to exist in two interchangeable states of condensation. The basophilic chromatin that is seen with the light microscope appears as a very electron-dense clumped material when examined with the electron microscope. The lighter, less basophilic areas of the nucleus seen with the light microscope contain a finely granular, dispersed chromatin when examined with the electron microscope. The latter form of chromatin is not stainable with ordinary dyes, but it is Feulgen-positive. The condensed basophilic chromatin is called heterochromatin; the less condensed, finely granular, dispersed chromatin is called euchromatin or "true" chromatin (Fig. 1–5). The genetic material of the heterochromatin is tightly packed and so linked with the histones that it is relatively inactive or inaccessible for gene duplication and activation. Euchromatin, on the other hand, represents the portion of the chromosome where genes are being transcribed to be used as a template for the synthesis of proteins in the cytoplasm. The ratio of histone to nucleic acid in both types of chromatin is similar, but the histones in the euchromatic portion are acetylated. In this form, the histones do not interfere with the transcription of the genetic material. Metabolically active cells, like the fibroblasts of healing wounds, have a greater proportion of their chromatin in the dispersed, nonstainable euchromatin form; less active cells show a great portion of their chromatin in the condensed or heterochromatic state.

DNA is composed of chains of nucleotides containing one of four types of nitrogenous bases attached to a sugar by a glycosidic linkage. The sugars of adjacent nucleotides are linked to each other by phosphate diester groups. The nitrogenous bases are the purines *adenine* and *guanine* and the pyrimidines *cytosine* and *thymine*; the sugar is a pentose, *deoxyribose*. The DNA molecule consists of two chains of nucleotides that form a double helix (Watson and Crick, 1953). The specific sequence of nucleotide coding for each of the amino acids has been worked out and appears to be the same for most organisms. A sequence of three nucleotides or triplets consitutes a code word, and the message formed by a series of these is known as a gene. The gene concept is actually more complicated than this and is not completely understood for mammalian cells. In bacterial systems, however, a distinction is made between a *structural* gene, which has the nucleotide coding sequence for a specific polypeptide or protein, and the *control* genes, which control the activity of the structural genes. Within the control genes are *regulator* and *operator* components. The regulator gene contains the code sequence for the production of a *repressor*, which inactivates or represses the activity of the operator. When the operator is combined with the repressor, the structural gene is not transcribed. When the repressor substance, however, combines with a specific metabolite usually formed in the cytoplasm, it

---

Figure 1–3. The cell membranes of Schwann cells and oligodendroglia become wrapped around the axons of neurons forming myelin sheaths. The myelin sheath insulates the axons from each other and facilitates the conduction of nerve impulses.

A, A Schwann cell (a) and an axon (b) surrounded by a myelin sheath (c) are shown. (× 21,000.)

B, Electron micrograph showing the concentric arrangement of membranes forming the myelin sheath. (× 39,200.)

C, View of the myelin sheath at higher magnification. (× 97,500.)

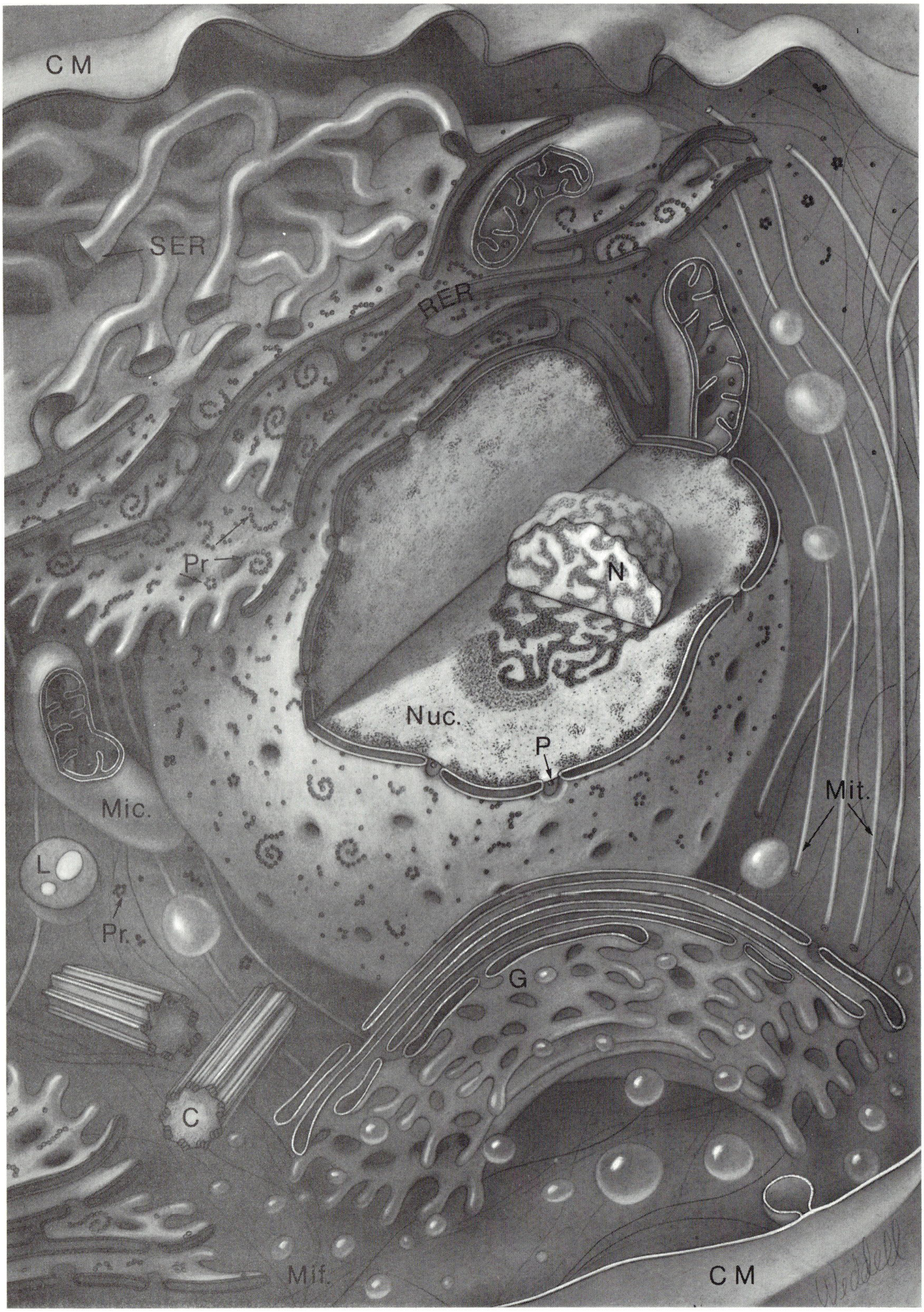

Figure 1–4. *See legend on opposite page.*

loses its ability to bind the operator site so that the structural gene can then be transcribed. Since structural genes commonly provide the code for enzymes, the metabolite reacting with the repressor usually is formed as a by-product of the enzyme action. Such interaction between the genetic material and the metabolic system of the cells also exists in mammalian cells.

Upon transcription of the genes, another nucleic acid is formed, ribonucleic acid (RNA), known as messenger RNA. RNA differs from DNA in having the pyrimidine *uracyl* instead of *thymine* and the pentose *ribose*, instead of *deoxyribose*. The messenger RNA (mRNA) subsequently passes from the nucleus into the cytoplasm, where its base sequence is "translated" into a given sequence of amino acids to form a polypeptide or protein.

Another prominent structure of the interphase nucleus is the nucleolus (Fig. 1–6). There is usually one nucleolus for each haploid set of chromosomes, so that most cells contain two nucleoli. At times, however, one to four nucleoli are observed that have been produced either by fusion or by polyploidy. The nucleolus of living cells is visible with the light and phase-contrast microscopes and usually occupies an eccentric position in the nucleus. It is associated with a specific region of the chromosome known as the nucleolar organizer, and there is one nucleolar organizer per haploid set of chromosomes. The nucleolus of fixed cells stains with both basic and acid dyes. The basophilic material has been shown by spectrophotometric and enzymatic digestion studies to be rich in RNA. In electron micrographs the nucleolus is composed of a coarse, prominent electron-dense strand, known as the *nucleolonema,* that is coiled into a three-dimensional network. The remainder of the nucleolus is composed of a less dense, finely granular material known as the *pars amorpha* (Fig. 1–6).

Many studies show that RNA is present in both the nucleolonema and the pars amorpha, but ribonucleoprotein particles are not present throughout the nucleolus. This difference in appearance and density between the nucleolonema and pars amorpha probably is related to the stage in the synthesis

---

Figure 1–4. Three-dimensional drawing of an "idealized" cell containing the most common cell organelles. The cell or plasma membrane (CM) is seen at the top and bottom of the drawing. In the centrally located nucleus a greater proportion of the chromatin is in the dispersed, finely granular form known as euchromatin. A smaller amount of chromatin in the periphery of the nucleus is in a dense, clumped state known as heterochromatin. The nucleolus (N) is composed of a dense band, the nucleolonema, which forms a network that encloses an electron-lucent material known as the pars amorpha. A group of electron-dense nuclear ribonucleoprotein particles is adjacent to the nucleolus. The double membrane of the nuclear envelope contains nuclear pores (P) that are composed of a thin diaphragm and a centrally located hole that has a diameter of around 150 A. The rough-surfaced or granular endoplasmic reticulum (RER) is composed of stacks of cisternae. Polyribosomes (Pr) on the surface of this endoplasmic reticulum form groups of five, known as pentasomes, as well as rows of 10, or spiralling forms containing 15 or more particles. Continuous with the granular reticulum is the second component of the endoplasmic reticulum known as the smooth-surfaced or agranular reticulum (SER). The Golgi (G) apparatus is formed of flattened, closely stacked cisternae and a number of adjacent vesicles and vacuoles. The mitochondria (Mic) are enclosed by a double membrane, the inner of which forms shelves known as cristae mitochondriales. A number of round particles are seen within the mitochondrion; these are crystals of divalent cations such as calcium or magnesium. Several lysosomes (L) are shown, one containing two round bodies that are undergoing hydrolytic digestion. Other cell components shown are centrioles (C), microtubules (Mit), microfilaments (Mif) and clusters of unattached, or free, polyribosomes (Pr). The remainder of the cytoplasm includes the cell sap, or cytosol, which contains the enzymes of the Embden-Meyerhof glycolytic pathway.

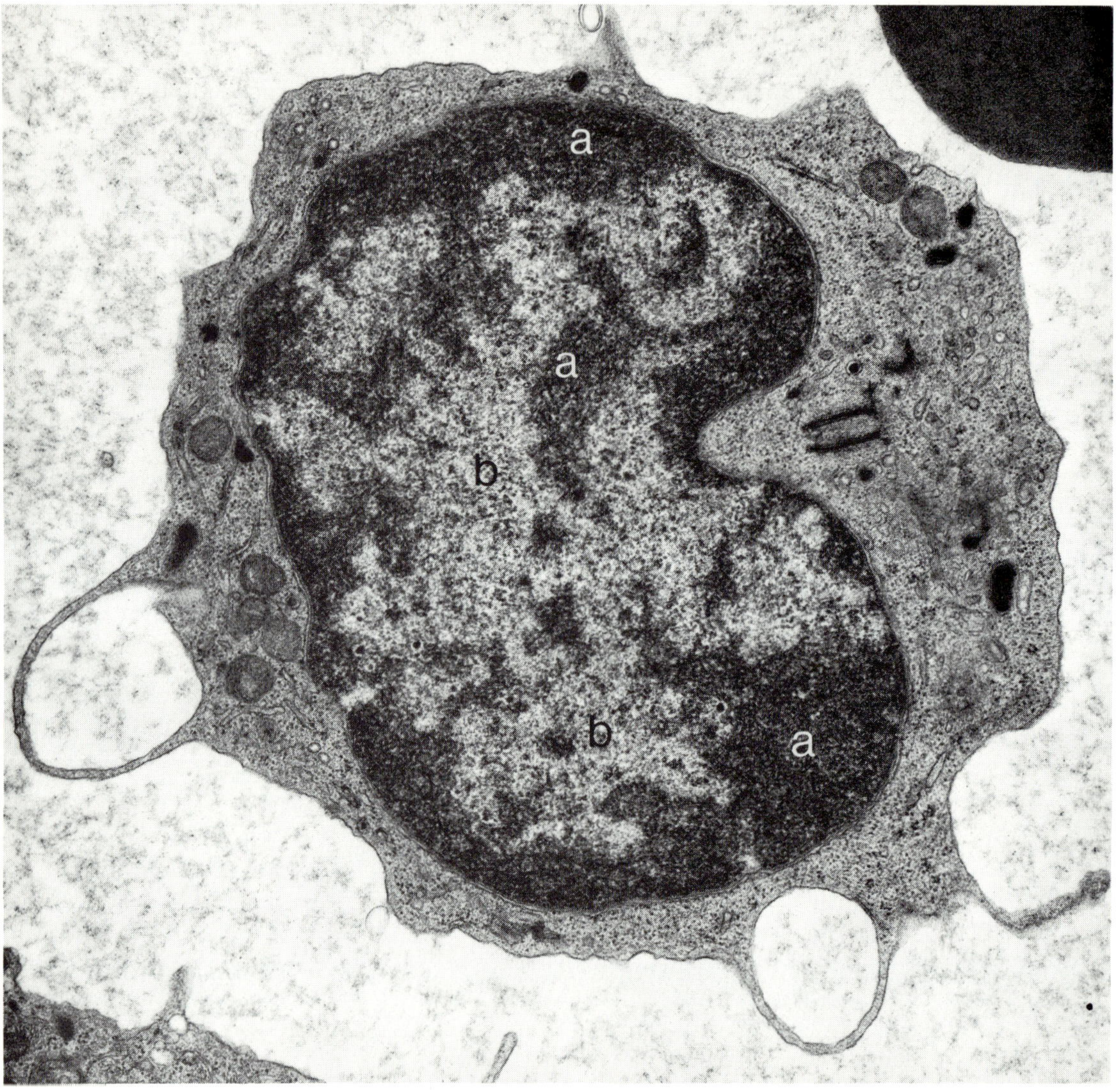

Figure 1–5. Nucleus of a choroidal intravascular lymphocyte. The nuclear chromatin is composed of an electron-dense, coarse granular material known as heterochromatin (a), and a light, fine granular material called euchromatin (b). (× 18,000.)

of ribonucleoprotein particles. These particles measure 150 A. in diameter and are believed to be ribosomes that are formed within the nucleolus. The ribosomes subsequently move to the cytoplasm, where they function in the synthesis of proteins. They are spherical and contain a number of basic proteins and RNA. Two other types of nucleic acids function in concert with the ribosomes to synthesize proteins: the mRNA containing the information for the sequence of amino acids, and transfer RNA (tRNA), which is involved in bringing the amino acids in contact with the ribosome. The nucleolus also contains DNA, which is believed to contain the genes or cistrons that code for the ribosomal RNA, as well as the proteins found in the ribosomes. Thus, one function of the nucleolus is specifically concerned with the synthesis of the ribosomal RNA (rRNA). The RNA strand is tortuously folded within the spherical ribosome, where it plays a very important part in the assembly of

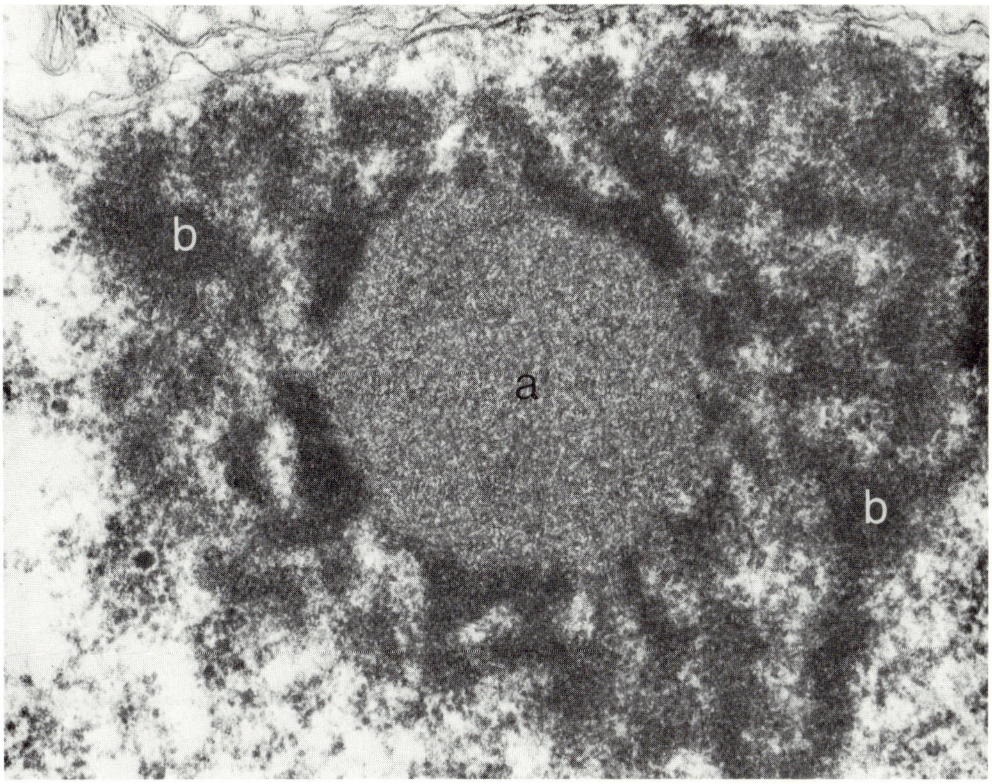

Figure 1–6. Nucleolus of a prelaminar astrocyte in the optic nerve. The astrocytes of this portion of the optic nerve characteristically exhibit prominent nucleoli. The nucleolus is composed of a *pars amorpha* (a) and the *nucleolonema* (b). (× 32,000.)

polypeptide chains. It is probable that transfer RNA is likewise synthesized by the nucleolus. The appearance of prominent nucleoli in metabolically active cells is to be expected because of its functions, and the size and prominence of the nucleolus provides a reliable indicator that the cell is actively synthesizing protein.

In addition to the chromatin and the nucleolus, the nucleus also contains a number of proteins, metabolites and enzymatic systems. The nuclear dry mass is mostly protein, which may be either soluble, such as that forming part of the hexose monophosphate shunt (pentose sugar formation), or insoluble, such as the histones or basic proteins which form salt linkages with the nucleic acids. The insoluble nonhistone proteins include the DNA and RNA polymerases involved in the reduplication of DNA and the formation of mRNA.

The nucleus is enclosed by a double membrane known as the *nuclear envelope,* which measures 75 A. in thickness (Fig. 1–7). Each unit membrane of this envelope is slightly thinner than the cell membrane. It has the same thickness as the membranes of the endoplasmic reticulum, with which it is continuous. The two unit membranes of the nuclear envelope are separated by a space measuring between 400 and 800 A. The inner unit membrane is in contact with a dense, finely granular material in the nucleus; the outer membrane is continuous with the endoplasmic reticulum, and in some cells it has ribosomes attached to its outer surface. The two membranes of the

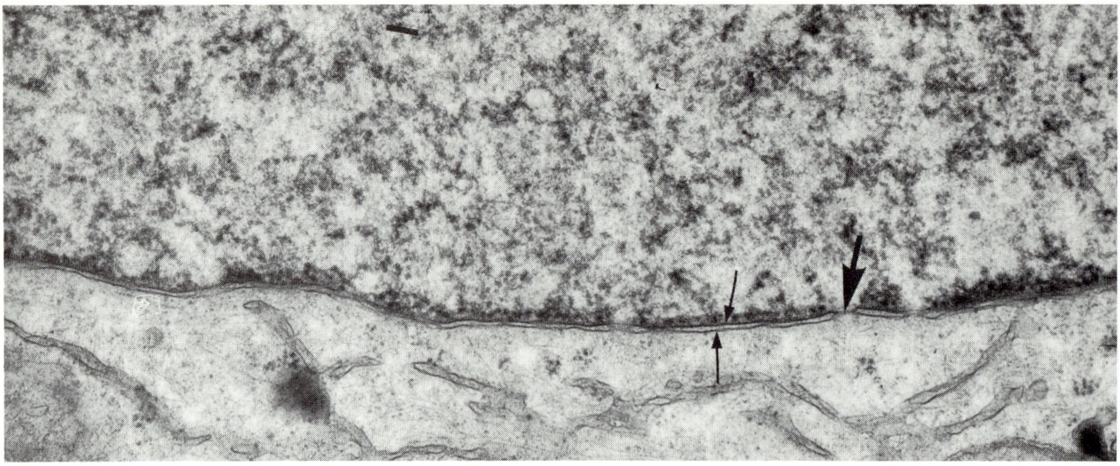

Figure 1–7. Nuclear envelope in an unpigmented epithelial cell of the ciliary body. The karyoplasm is above the nuclear envelope and the cytoplasm is below it. The envelope is composed of inner and outer membranes (arrows) and exhibits pores (heavy arrow). (× 33,000.)

nuclear envelope frequently fuse to form nuclear pores. These pores are between 400 and 500 A. in diameter and have an annular diaphragm that covers most of the pore except a very small central hole, which is probably large enough to permit passage of ribosomes and such macromolecules as messenger RNA (Fig. 1–4).

THE CYTOPLASM (Figs. 1–4; 1–8 to 1–10)

A large portion of the cytoplasm is liquid, and if the cell membrane is ruptured the cytoplasmic contents leak out through the opened area. When large cells are centrifuged, the granular contents of the cytoplasm move toward the centrifugal pole, and the nucleus and fat droplets move toward the centripetal pole. When nickel particles are introduced into the cell and moved with a magnet, the particles are seen to move quickly and easily. When the magnetic force is removed, the nickel particles are not seen to move back to their former positions, indicating an absence of elastic recoil. These facts indicate that the cytoplasm is probably a very dilute gel containing about 70 to 80 per cent water and a fibrillar cytoskeleton that gives it rigidity. With the use of differential centrifugation, the cytoplasm of the cell can be separated into three components: mitochondria, microsomes and a supernatant which fails to sediment under high centrifugal forces. The microsomal portion contains all the cytoplasmic membranes, the endoplasmic reticulum and ribosomes.

ENDOPLASMIC RETICULUM (Fig. 1–4)

The endoplasmic reticulum forms a system of interconnecting channels that freely anastomose in the cytoplasm and are joined to the outer

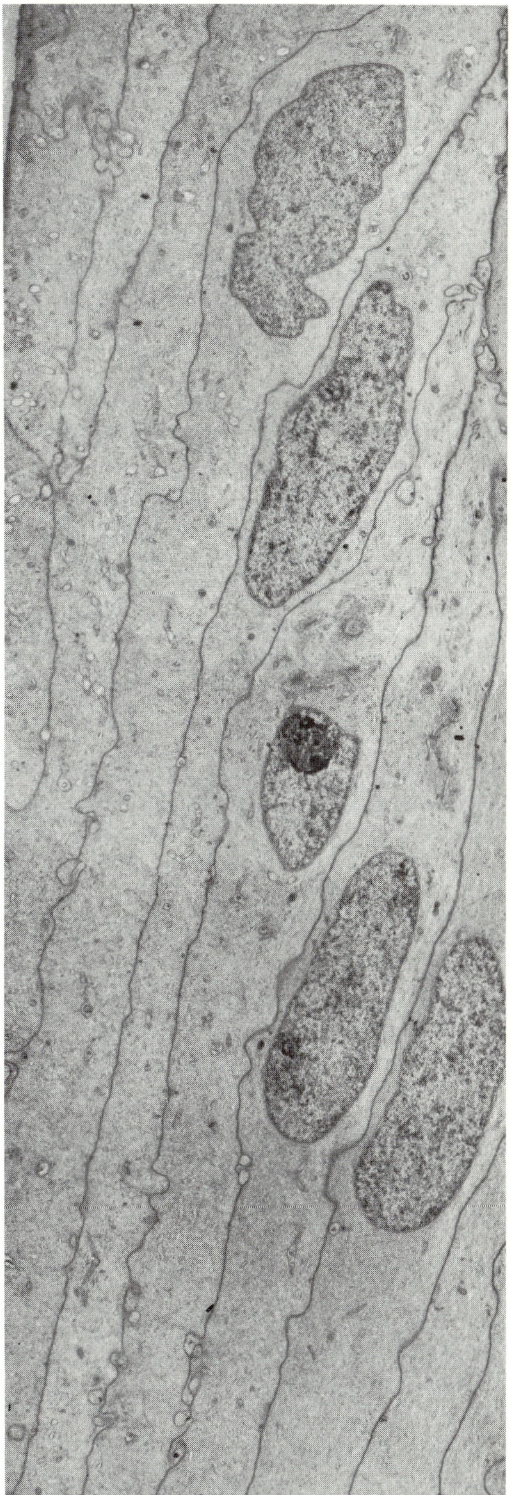

Figure 1–8. The cytoplasm of the lens cells is unusual, being several millimeters in length and having only a few cytoplasmic organelles. These cells in the deeper lens and erythrocytes are the only cells in the human body lacking a nucleus. The nucleated lens cells seen in this photograph are found in the lens equator, where the lens epithelial cells divide and extend posteriorly to form the lens sutures. (× 2800.)

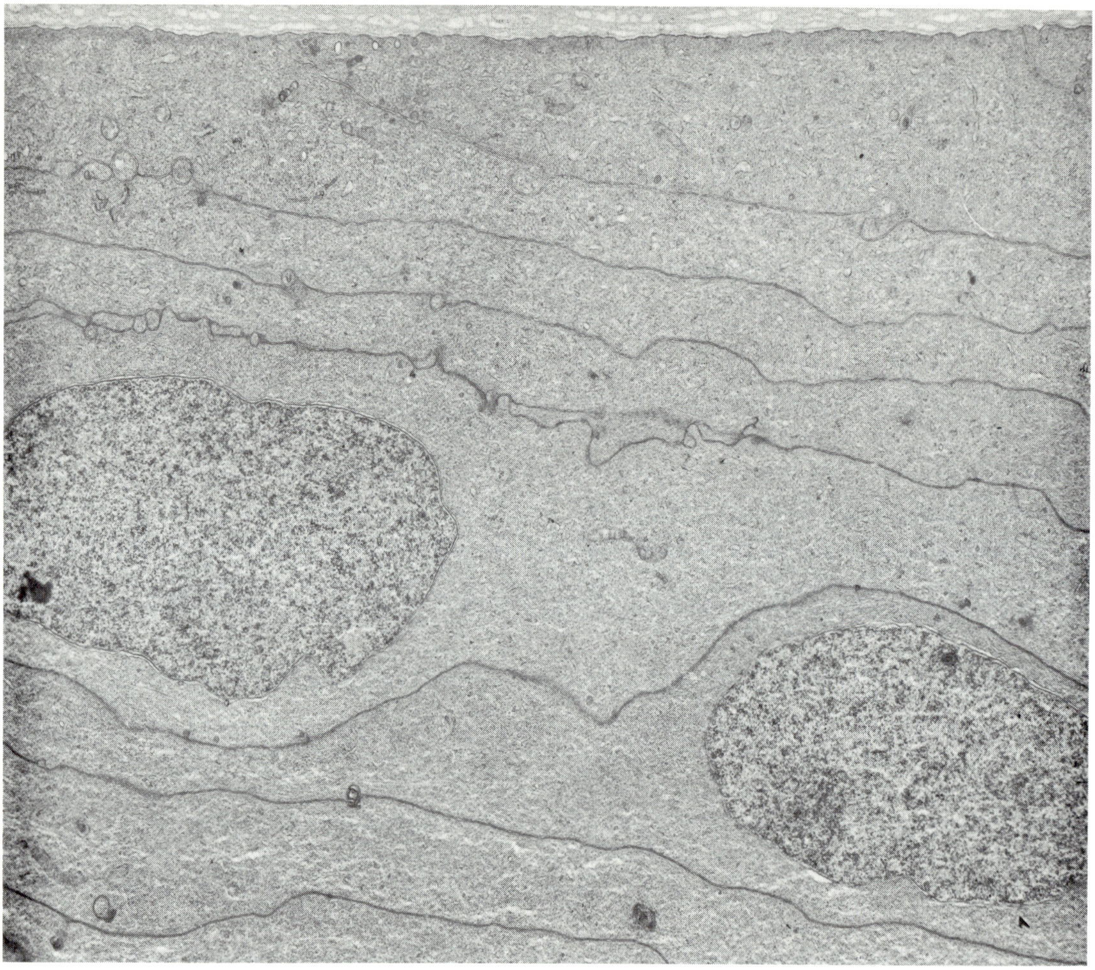

Figure 1–9. Higher magnification of the cytoplasm of the lens cell showing its granular composition and paucity of cell organelles. (× 5600.)

membranes of the nuclear envelope. Figure 1–4 shows the channels of the endoplasmic reticulum to be arranged in two ways: one consisting of tubular channels, and the other composed of flattened interconnecting cisternae which are stacked on each other. These flattened cisternae have numerous ribosomes on their outer surfaces and for this reason form a subdivision of the endoplasmic reticulum known as the *rough-surfaced* or *granular* endoplasmic reticulum. The tubular system does not contain ribosomes and constitutes the *smooth-surfaced* or *agranular* endoplasmic reticulum. These two types of reticulum vary in amount in different types of cells. Plasma cells contain a large amount of rough-surfaced endoplasmic reticulum, liver cells contain both types, and the retinal pigment epithelium and the Müller cells contain mostly smooth-surfaced endoplasmic reticulum. As shown in Figure 1–4, these two types of endoplasmic reticulum are in communication with each other, and they form a cytoplasmic canalicular system for the intracellular transport of many substances.

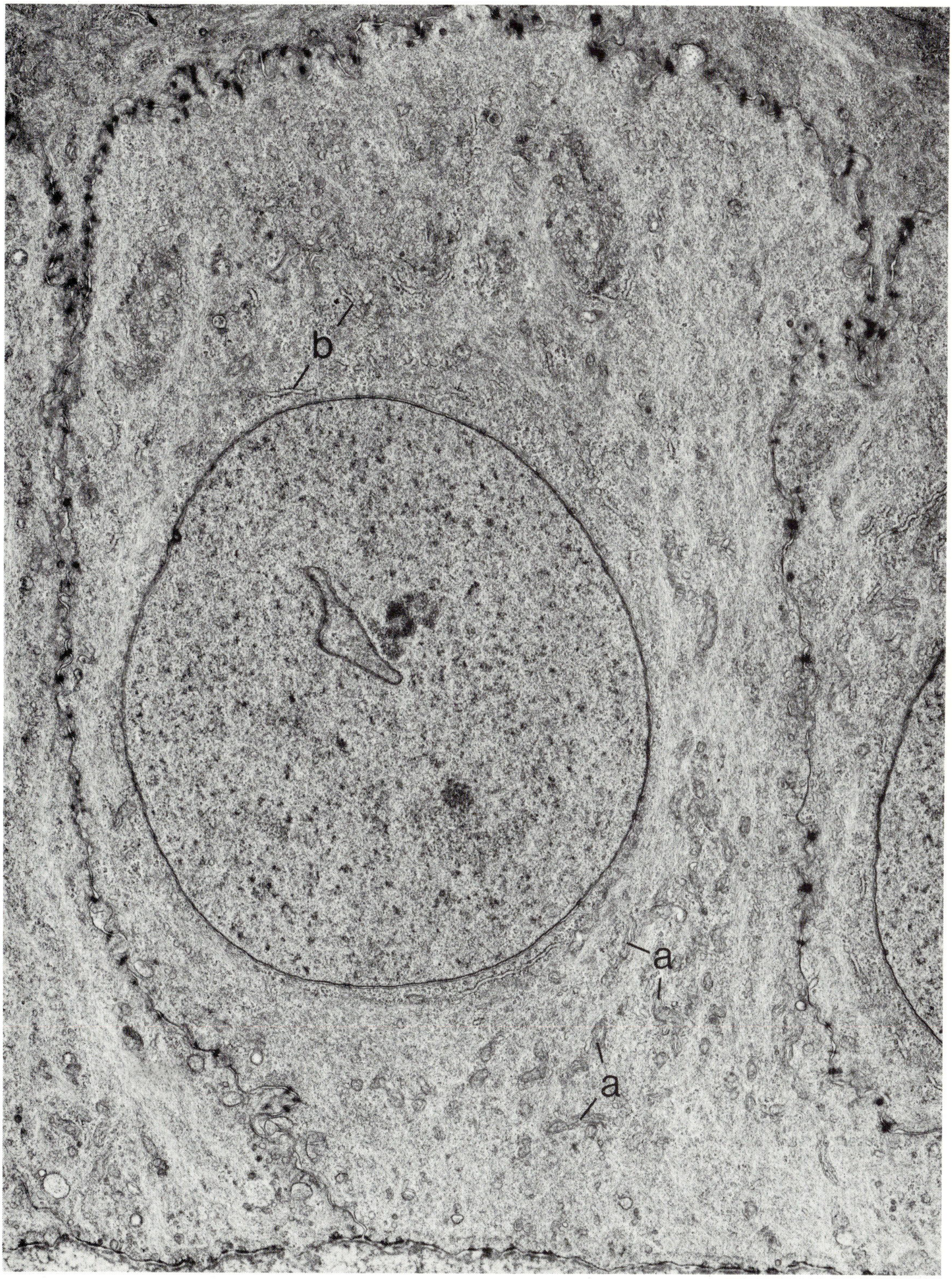

Figure 1–10. The cytoplasm of the cells of the corneal epithelium is also unusual in having few cytoplasmic organelles, such as mitochondria (a) and cisternae of the endoplasmic reticulum (b). Fine filaments occupy a great portion of the cytoplasm. (× 11,200.)

Rough-surfaced Endoplasmic Reticulum (Figs. 1–11 to 1–14)

This reticulum stains with basic dyes because of its ribosomal content, and it can be identified with the light microscope, especially in cells having a well developed granular endoplasmic reticulum, such as the pancreatic acinar cells. Almost all cells have at least one or two cisternae of the rough-surfaced endoplasmic reticulum, but it is found in abundance in cells elaborating protein for export or secretion. The ribosomes found in mammalian cells are much larger than bacterial ribosomes; they have a sedimentation coefficient of 80 S. and measure 150 A. in diameter. Each ribosome is formed by two particles of unequal size. These particles are mainly held together by

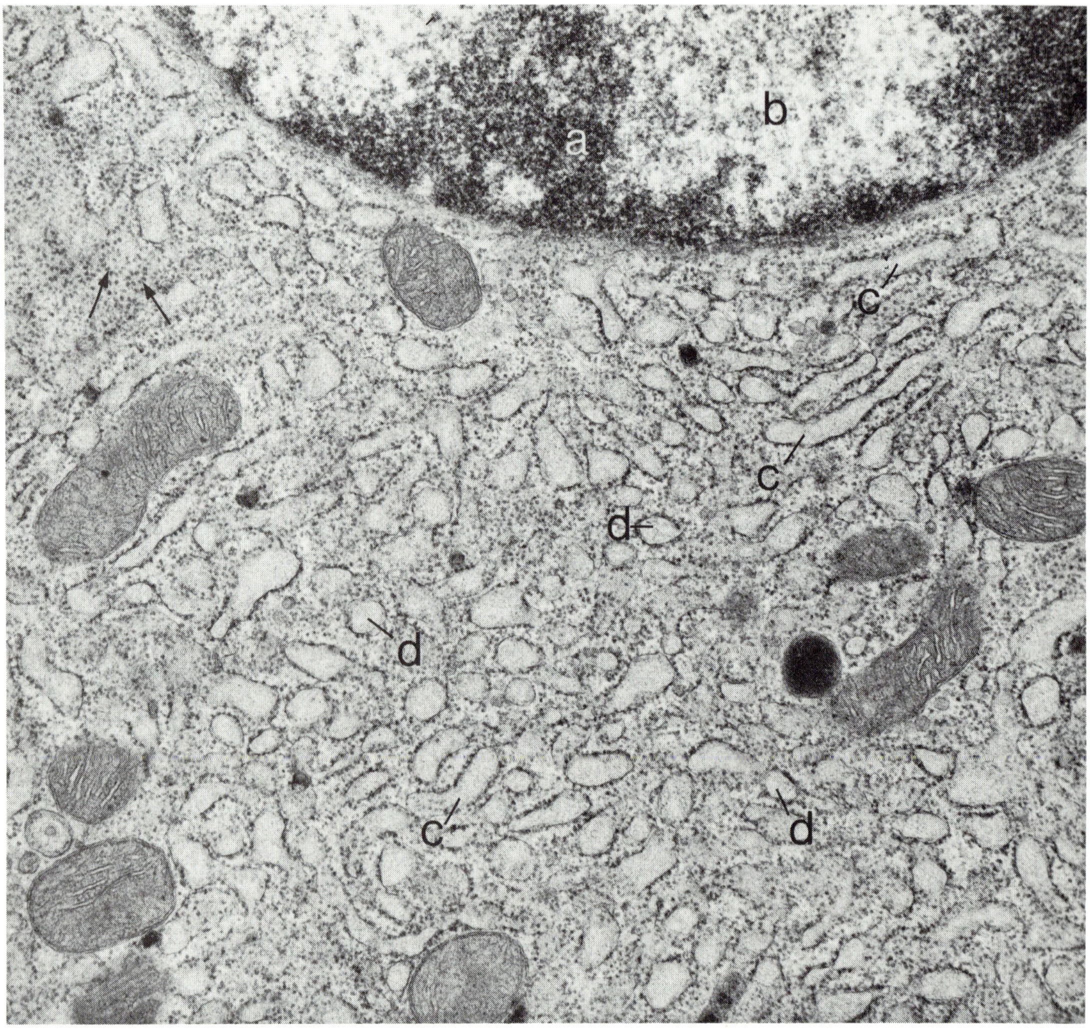

Figure 1–11. Rough-surfaced endoplasmic reticulum in a choroidal plasma cell. The nuclear chromatin has only a small amount of heterochromatin (a) and a larger amount of euchromatin (b), a characteristic of cells actively synthesizing protein. The cytoplasm contains numerous cisternae of rough-surfaced endoplasmic reticulum that is sectioned both longitudinally (c) and in cross-section (d). Ribosomes are attached to the membranes of the cisternae, where they are arranged in a linear pattern. This arrangement can be seen at the upper left, where the cisternae are sectioned tangentially (arrow). (× 23,600.)

magnesium (Mg^{++}); they separate into the component particles when they are suspended in a solution having a low Mg^{++} concentration. The larger particle sediments with a Svedberg coefficient of 60 S. and the smaller particle has a sedimentation coefficient of 40 S. Each ribosome is composed of RNA and proteins. The RNA of the smaller ribosomal particle has a sedimentation coefficient of 16 S., while the RNA of the larger particles has a Svedberg coefficient of 28 S. Recent evidence indicates that the larger particle contains a 5 S. RNA, present in an equimolar amount with the 28 S. component. The protein content of mammalian ribosomes accounts for 50 or more per cent of the dry mass of the ribosome. There may be as many as 10 different types of proteins, one of which contains a considerable number of basic groups similar to the histones of the nucleus.

The ribosomes function as the units where polypeptide chains are assembled. The whole assembly process is complicated and is not completely understood, but it can be generally described as follows: Three different

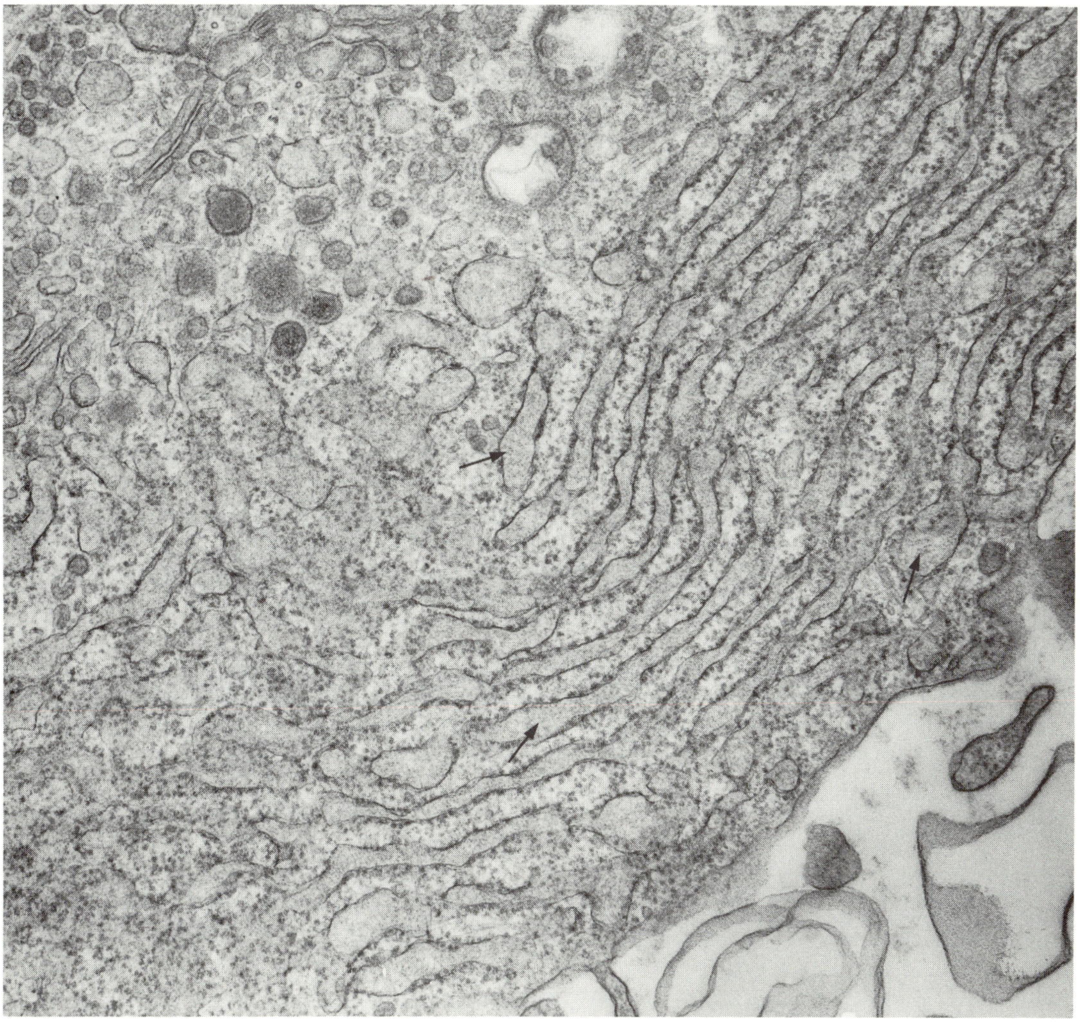

Figure 1–12. Rough-surfaced endoplasmic reticulum in a choroidal plasma cell. The lumina of the cisternae of the endoplasmic reticulum are distended by protein (arrows). (×33,700.)

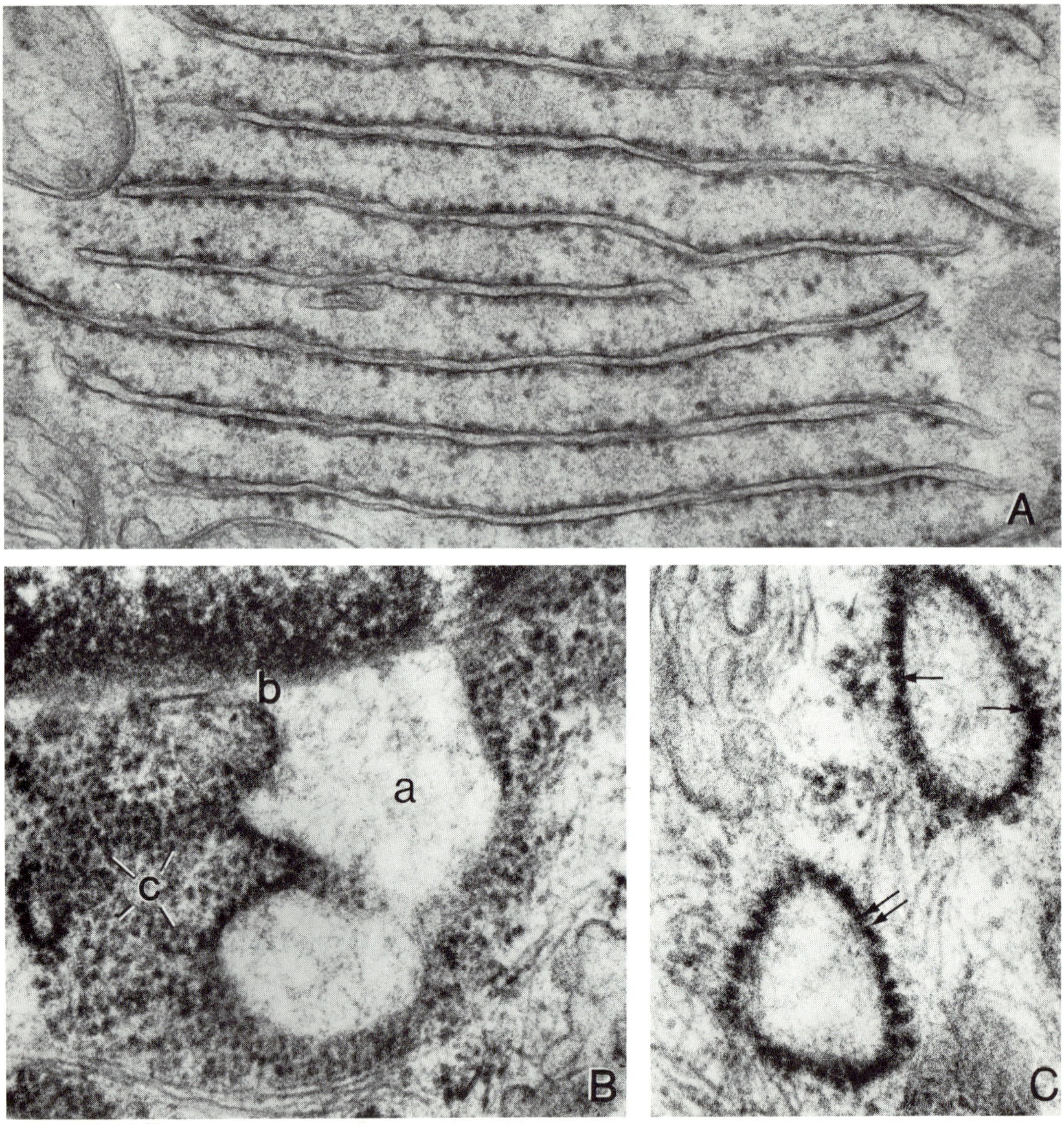

Figure 1–13. *A*, Rough-surfaced endoplasmic reticulum in the unpigmented epithelium of the ciliary body. The cisternae of these cells commonly are arranged in stacks as shown here. (× 35,000.)

B, This section is through a cisterna of the rough-surfaced endoplasmic reticulum (a) that is continuous with the nuclear envelope (b). Ribosomes presumably attached to the membrane of a cisternae are shown at (c). (× 72,000.)

C, Cross-section of a cisterna of the endoplasmic reticulum to show the ribosomes (arrow) attached to its membrane. (× 80,000.)

RNA components, transfer or soluble RNA (tRNA), ribosomes and a template RNA or mRNA are involved. In addition, a set of specific enzymes participates in the activation of the amino acids that are to be polymerized into a given polypeptide chain or protein. The activated amino acids become associated with specific tRNA. The template or messenger RNA attaches to the smaller ribosomal particle (40 S.), and the transfer RNA somehow recognizes a specific nucleotide triplet or *codon* in the mRNA by means of a complimentary triplet or *anticodon*. The amino acid borne by this transfer RNA becomes associated with the larger 60 S. ribosomal particle, which is attached to the membrane of the endoplasmic reticulum. Subsequently other transfer RNA associates with messenger RNA and their amino acids become linked by peptide bonds to the preceding amino acids to form nascent protein (Fig. 1–14). The protein eventually appears in the lumen of the cisternae of the endoplasmic reticulum, where it is transported toward the Golgi apparatus for packaging and concentration into zymogen granules (Palade, 1966).

The ribosomes do not appear to be randomly distributed on the surface of the endoplasmic reticulum but, as shown in Figure 1–4, they are grouped into clusters of five ribosomes known as pentasomes, or in a linear spiraling chain containing 30 or more ribosomes. During protein synthesis 80 or more per cent of the ribosomes exist in clusters or spirals (Redman, 1969). It is believed that this ribosomal disposition permits a strand of mRNA of sufficient length to be used as a template by several ribosomes at

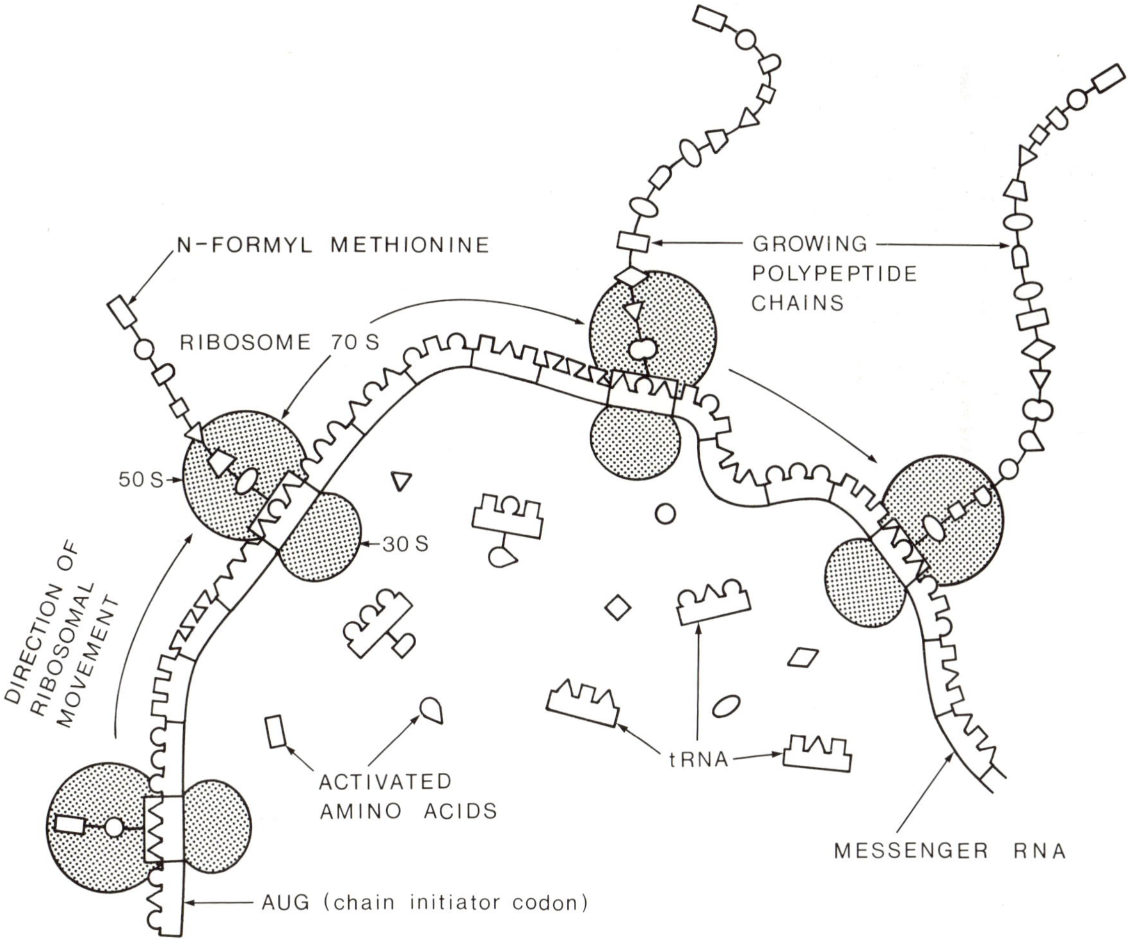

Figure 1–14. Relationship of messenger RNA to ribosomes in protein synthesis. This figure is reproduced with the permission of the author and publisher from Review of Physiological Chemistry, Lange Medical Publications, 1969, page 70.

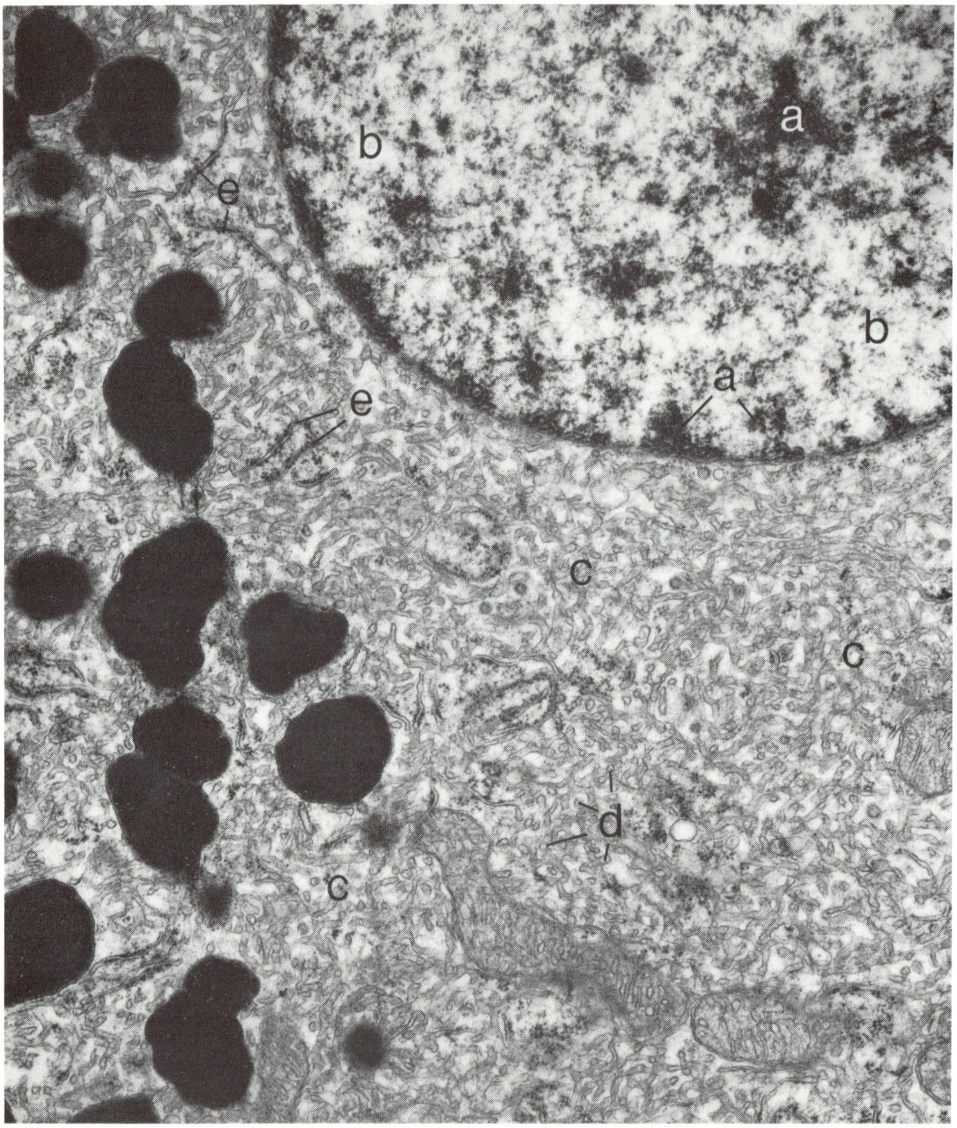

Figure 1–15. The smooth-surfaced endoplasmic reticulum of the retinal pigment epithelium. The nucleus of this cell characteristically shows a few small patches of heterochromatin (a) along the periphery of the nucleus and throughout the karyoplasm, most of which is occupied by euchromatin (b). The cytoplasm of this cell contains a voluminous smooth-surfaced endoplasmic reticulum (c). There are short, branching interconnecting tubules that are seen mainly in longitudinal section; a few cross-sectional views are shown at (d). Cisternae of the rough-surfaced endoplasmic reticulum are shown at (e). These two systems of the endoplasmic reticulum are continuous with each other. (× 18,900.)

once. Those ribosomes not associated with membranes and which are floating freely in the cytoplasm also form clusters during protein synthesis.

The observation that cells primarily engaged in the production of protein for secretion, such as the pancreatic acinar cells and plasma cells, have an extraordinarily developed rough-surfaced endoplasmic reticulum led to the notion that granular reticulum is specifically involved in the production of protein for export (Palade, 1966). Redman (1969) recently studied the relations between protein synthesis of attached and unattached ribosomes and the production of exportable and nonexportable proteins by the rat liver. He analyzed production of serum proteins as an example of secretory proteins and ferritin as an example of a nonexportable protein. He found that about 80 per cent of the newly formed serum protein was synthesized by attached ribosomes, while ferritin was synthesized mainly by the free ribosomes.

SMOOTH-SURFACED ENDOPLASMIC RETICULUM (Figs. 1–4; 1–15 to 1–19)

This reticulum has no attached ribosomes and usually does not form cisternae but is composed of intercommunicating tubules of varying size and shape (Fig. 1–4). Unlike the rough-surfaced endoplasmic reticulum, it is not in contact with the nuclear membrane, but it usually is found in the region of the Golgi apparatus. The smooth-surfaced differs functionally from the rough-surfaced endoplasmic reticulum in that its membranes have specific enzyme systems which are involved in such activities as detoxification of drugs, inactivation of hormones and lipid synthesis. It is prominent in cells of the adrenal gland, testis and ovaries, which are involved in the synthesis

Text continued on page 25

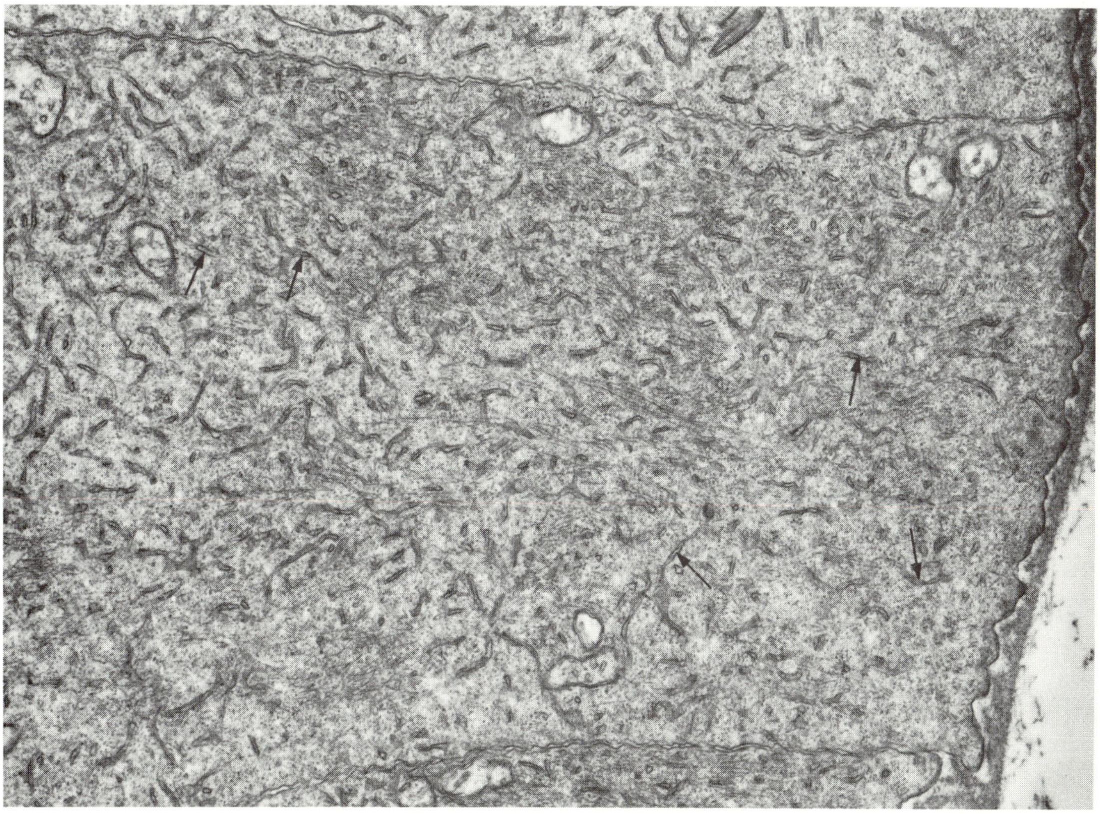

Figure 1–16. Smooth-surfaced endoplasmic reticulum of the Müller cells of the retina. Aside from the retinal pigment epithelium, the Müller cells possess the largest amount of smooth-surfaced endoplasmic reticulum in the ocular tissues. This low-power electron micrograph shows the tubules (arrows) to be evenly dispersed throughout the cytoplasm. (× 16,500.)

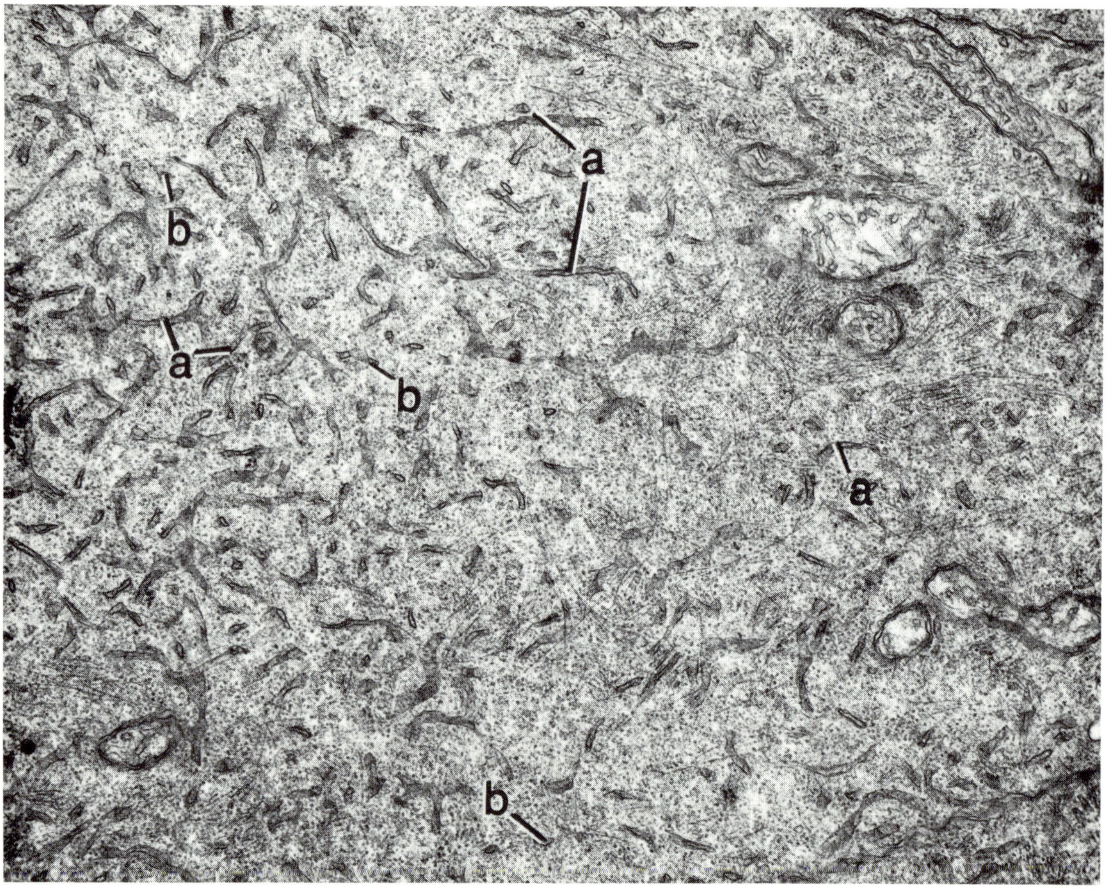

Figure 1–17. Müller cell of the retina. The elements of the smooth-surfaced endoplasmic reticulum (a) interconnect with each other and bend at sharp angles; in cross-section (b) they are seen to be narrow and triangular. (× 22,500.)

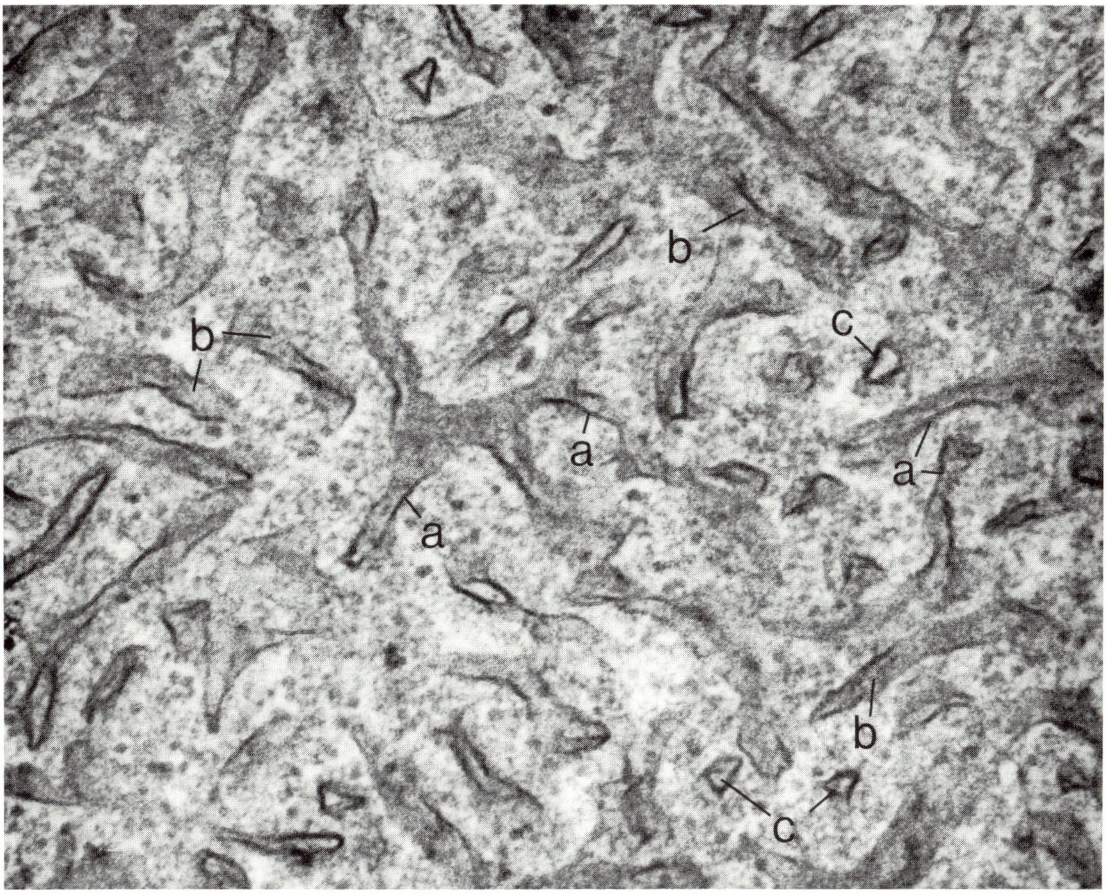

Figure 1–18. Müller cell of the retina. Higher magnification to show the trilaminar structure of the membrane enclosing the tubules of smooth endoplasmic reticulum (a), the osmiophilic contents of the twisting, interconnecting tubules (b), and their shape in cross-section (c). (× 90,000.)

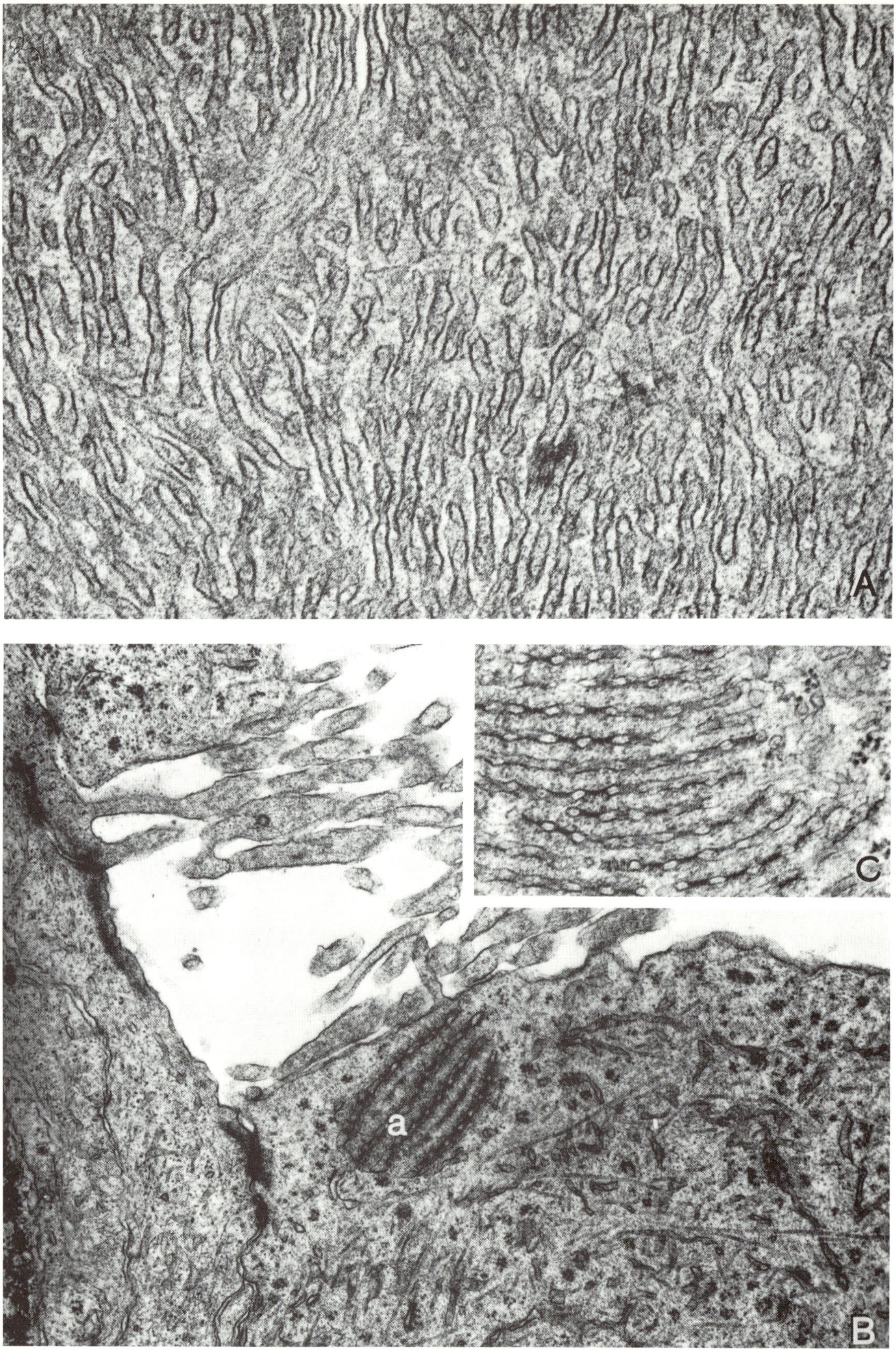

Figure 1–19. *See legend on opposite page.*

of steroid hormones, and in the liver, which is involved in detoxification of drugs, alcohol and other substances.

THE GOLGI COMPLEX (Figs. 1–4; 1–20; 1–21)

This organelle was first described by Camilo Golgi (1898), who observed it after using a special silver stain he had developed. It was not completely accepted as a component of all cells until the electron microscope was used to study cells. The Golgi complex generally is found near the nucleus, as shown in Figure 1–4. Its morphology varies in different cells as well as in individual cells under different functional states. It can be brought out consistently in most cells after osmium fixation or by incubating with glycerophosphate followed by precipitation with cobalt sulfide. By electron microscopy the Golgi apparatus is seen to consist of four to eight flattened saccules or cisternae arranged concentrically in the form of an open circle or C-shape. The cisternae are arranged as shown in Figure 1–4, so that the convex surface lies near the nuclear envelope and the concave surface faces the cell cytoplasm and is associated with a number of vesicles. Unlike the cisternae of the granular endoplasmic reticulum, the Golgi cisternae are closely apposed, being separated from each other by an intercisternal space measuring 200 to 300 A. wide. A second component of the Golgi complex consists of a number of small vesicles that are commonly located adjacent to the concave surface of the Golgi cisternae, and less numerous but larger vacuoles that are usually located near their convex surfaces. These vacuoles are prominent in protein-secreting cells, where they appear to be filled with protein in various degrees of condensation.

The polypeptides or proteins synthesized by the ribosomes of endoplasmic reticulum are deposited in their cisternae and then pass into the Golgi apparatus. The endoplasmic reticulum in the vicinity of the Golgi complex is of a transitional type and its contents are believed to be transferred into the Golgi by vesicles which are formed by the endoplasmic reticulum. These vesicles somehow come into functional contact with the Golgi complex; subsequently a larger vacuole is formed in which the protein is condensed into zymogen granules (Beams and Kessel, 1968). Because of its role in the formation of zymogen granules in protein-secreting cells, the Golgi apparatus often is referred to as the "packaging plant" of cells. This organelle also plays an important role in the synthesis of glycoproteins, such as those of the ground substance of the cornea and those synthesized by the intestinal goblet cells. These glycoproteins are composed of a protein core to which a number of mucopolysaccharides or glycosaminoglycan side chains are covalently linked. The initial coupling of the sugar probably occurs in

---

Figure 1–19. *A*, Smooth-surfaced endoplasmic reticulum of the prelaminar astrocytes of the optic nerve. Compare the close packing and alignment of the tubules of the reticulum of this cell with that of the retinal pigment epithelium and the Müller cell. (× 66,000.)

B, Annulate lamellae (a), cone ellipsoid. This is a specialized form of the smooth-surfaced endoplasmic reticulum occasionally found in cones. (× 22,000.)

C, Annulate lamellae are consistently found in the pigment epithelium of the retina; their function is not known. (× 58,200.)

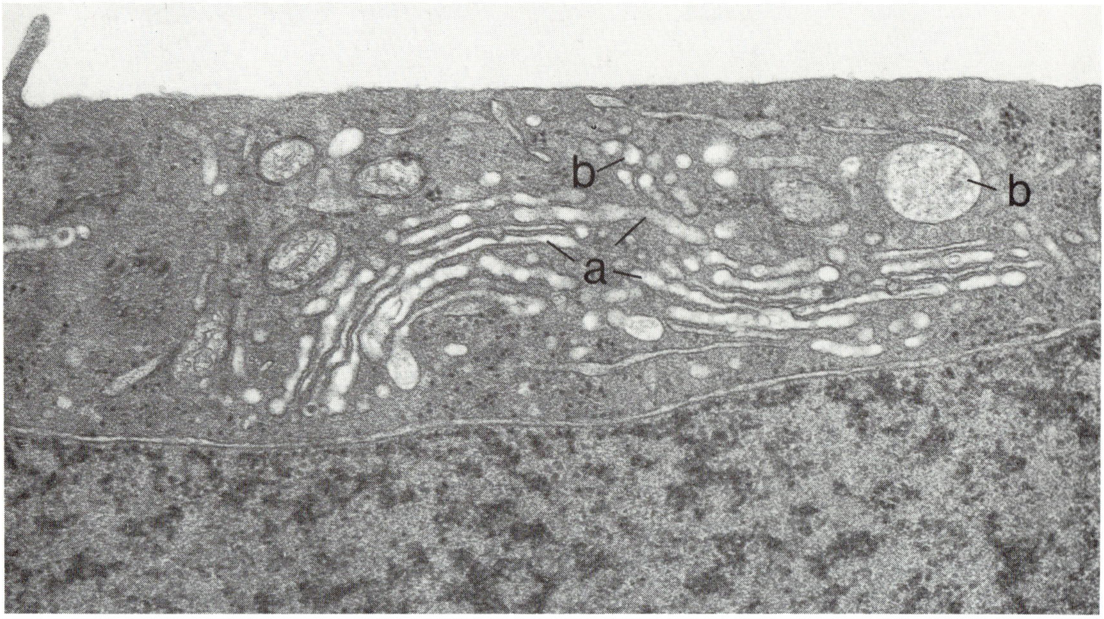

Figure 1–20. The Golgi apparatus in the corneal endothelium. Few cells in the ocular tissues have such a highly developed Golgi apparatus. The vitreous cells have a prominent Golgi apparatus and the prelaminar astrocytes (see Fig. 10–18, Optic Nerve) have an unusual Golgi consisting of short, membrane-bound, tubular structures that are tightly packed within another membrane. The Golgi apparatus of the corneal endothelium is usually located near the anterior chamber; it is composed of 6 to 10 lamellae (a) and vesicles (b) of various sizes. (× 27,500.)

the cisternae of the endoplasmic reticulum, perhaps at the same time as the polypeptide is being polymerized. There is increasing evidence that the final polymerization of the sugar moiety and the sulfation of the polysaccharide occurs in the Golgi apparatus (Neutra and Leblond, 1969). The Golgi complex also participates in the formation of a number of vacuolar or globular structures such as lysosomes, melanin granules and mast cell granules.

It should be observed that the Golgi complex is not an obligatory pathway for the secretion of protein. Some cells, such as plasma cells and fibroblasts, may circumvent the Golgi apparatus and secrete protein directly from the cisternae of the rough-surfaced endoplasmic reticulum.

MITOCHONDRIA (Figs. 1–4; 1–22 to 1–26)

Mitochondria can be seen after staining with alizarin and crystal violet in fixed tissues, and by phase-contrast microscopy in living tissues. They have also been studied by cinematography; films show that they are constantly in motion within the cytoplasm and that they frequently fuse or divide. The mitochondria vary considerably in size, measuring from 0.2 to 1.0 μm. in diameter and 3 to 5 μm. in length; they may be even longer. They are present in large numbers in very active cells, such as those of the liver, where the cells may contain 1000 or more, but in general there are 100 to 200 mitochondria per cell. By electron microscopy, the mitochondrion is seen to have a double membrane, as shown in Figure 1–4. The mitochondrial unit

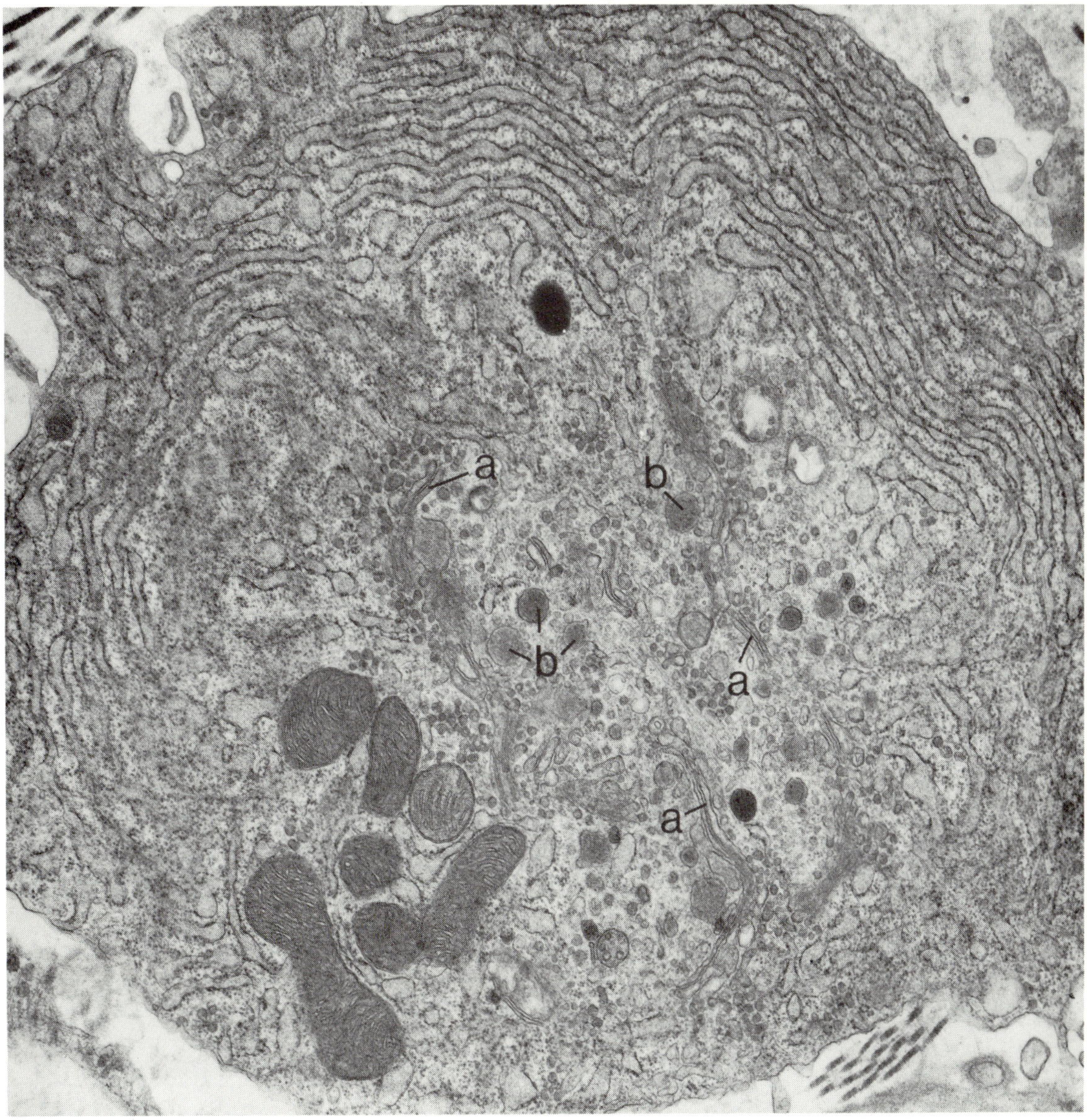

Figure 1-21. The Golgi apparatus in a plasma cell of the choroid. The Golgi apparatus occupies a large area of the cytoplasm in this portion of the cell; the lamellae are not prominent, forming strands (a) that are associated with a large number of vesicles (b) of various sizes. (× 14,000.)

membrane is thinner than the unit membrane of the other intracytoplasmic organelles, measuring around 60 A. in thickness. The outer membrane is smooth; the inner membrane forms a number of infoldings that produce shelf-like structures across the cavity of the mitochondrion. These shelves are known as cristae mitochondriales. Michaelis (1900) observed that mitochondria could be stained in vivo with the dye Janus green. This dye is an oxidation-reduction indicator; it is colorless in its reduced state and green when oxidized. This early observation indicated the high oxygen content of the mitochondria and the role of this organelle in respiration of the cell. With the advent of fractionation studies, it was shown that the enzymes of

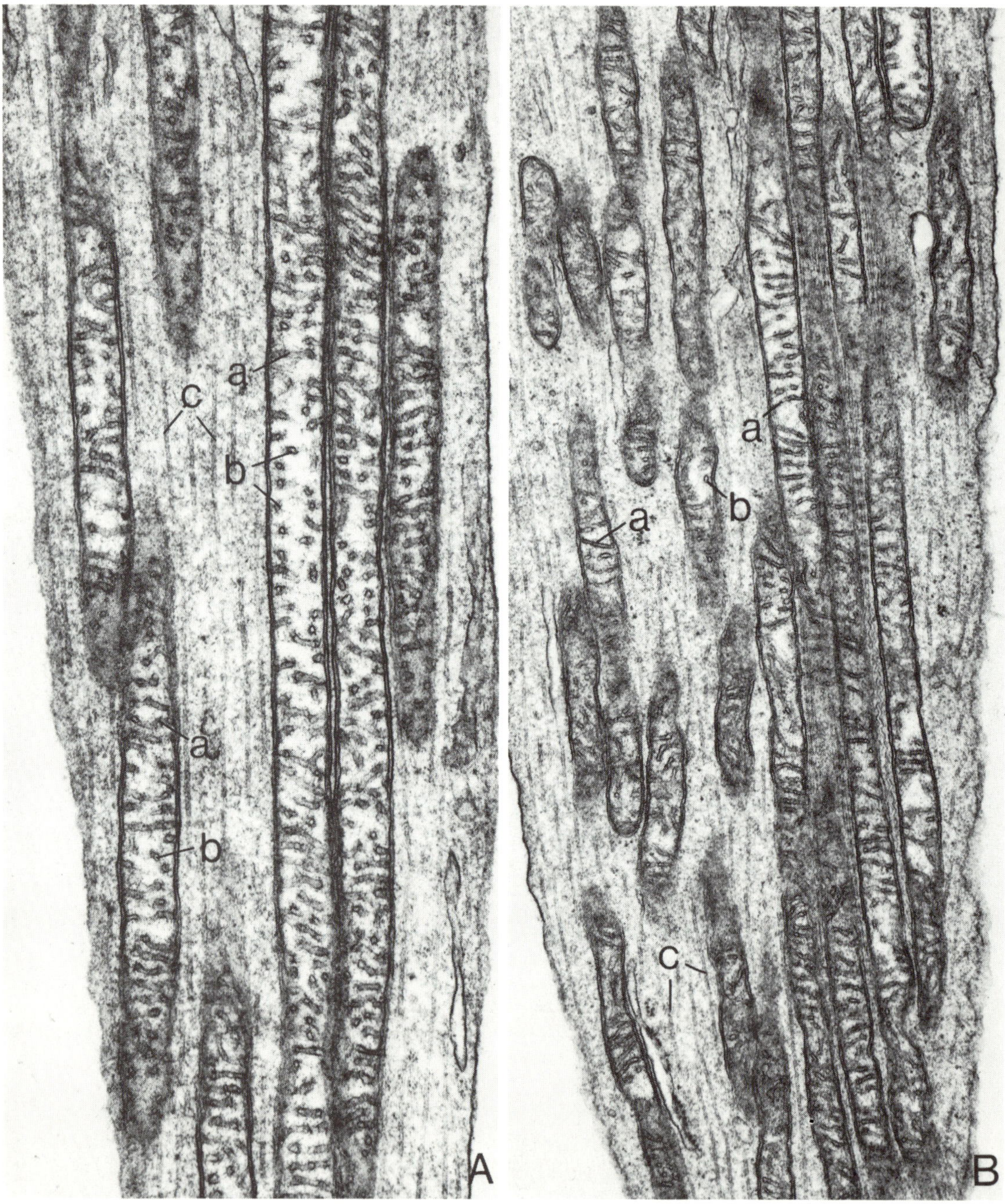

Figure 1–22. Mitochondria of the rod ellipsoid. The rod ellipsoid contains very long, thin mitochondria that may measure 20 μm. or more in length. The cristae (a) are short, shelf-like, tubular structures formed by the inner membrane of the mitochondria; they extend across the short axis of the mitochondrion. The cristae are shown in cross-section (b). Numerous microtubules (c) run parallel to each other among the mitochondria. (× 30,000.)

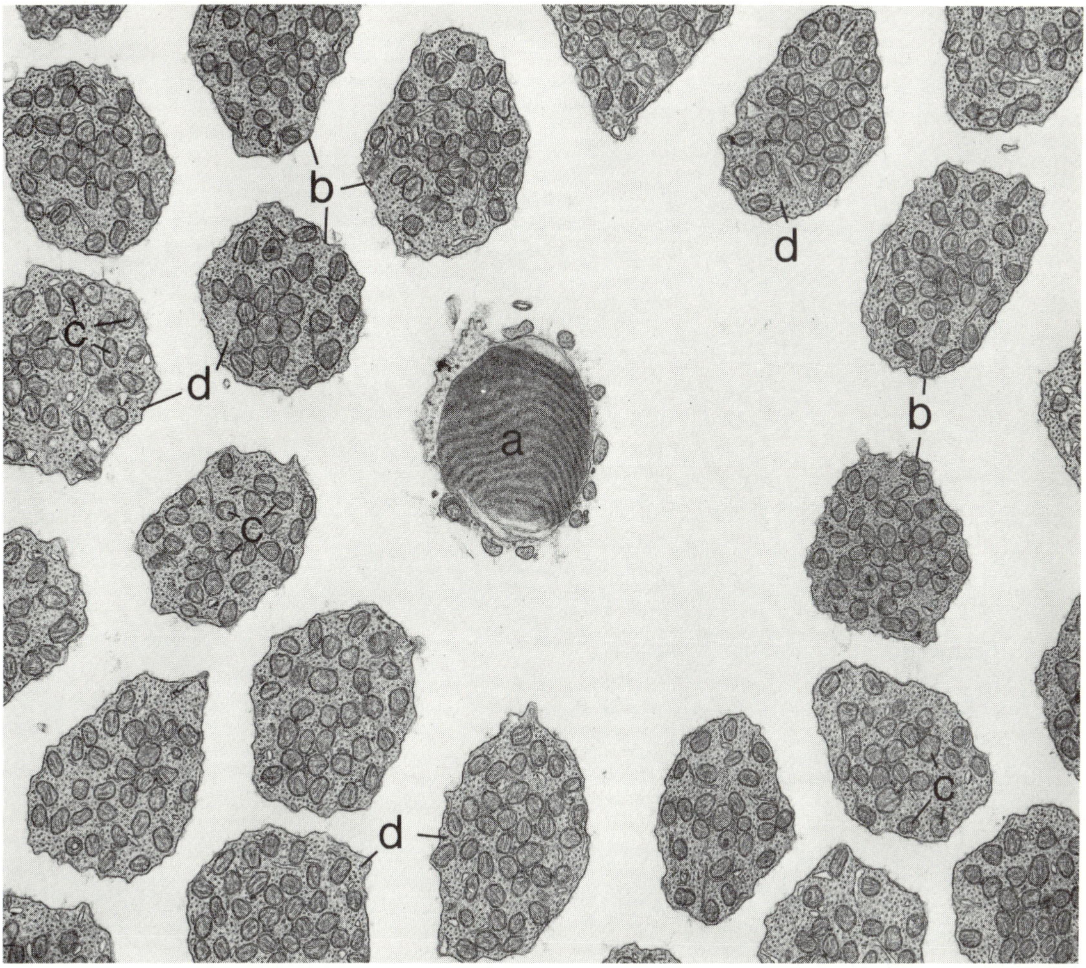

Figure 1-23. Mitochondria of the rod ellipsoid shown in cross-section. The outer segment (a) of a cone is surrounded by the ellipsoids (b) of several rods; there are about 30 to 35 mitochondria (c) per cross-sectional view of a rod ellipsoid. Microtubules (d) are uniformly distributed among the mitochondria (× 11,200.)

the glycolytic pathways could not be sedimented and that they were located in the cytoplasmic matrix. The Krebs cycle enzymes, electron-transport enzymes, those involved in coupled oxidative phosphorylation, and those in fatty acid β oxidation are found in the mitochondrion. The electron-transport and oxidative phosphorylation systems have been found to be associated with the cristae mitochondriales, while the Krebs cycle enzymes and those involved in fatty acid oxidation occur in the matrix of the mitochondrion. Mitochondria are therefore capable of utilizing all the useful energy formed during the oxidation of fatty acids, amino acids and carbohydrates by channeling the metabolites through the final common metabolic pathway in Krebs cycle. The metabolic products of the Krebs cycle are further broken down to yield H_2O and CO_2 and adenosine triphosphate (ATP) by the membrane-bound enzymes of the electron-transport chain and by oxidative phosphorylation. Since the mitochondria provide most of the ATP used by energy-requiring cell processes, coupling energy-yielding with energy-re-

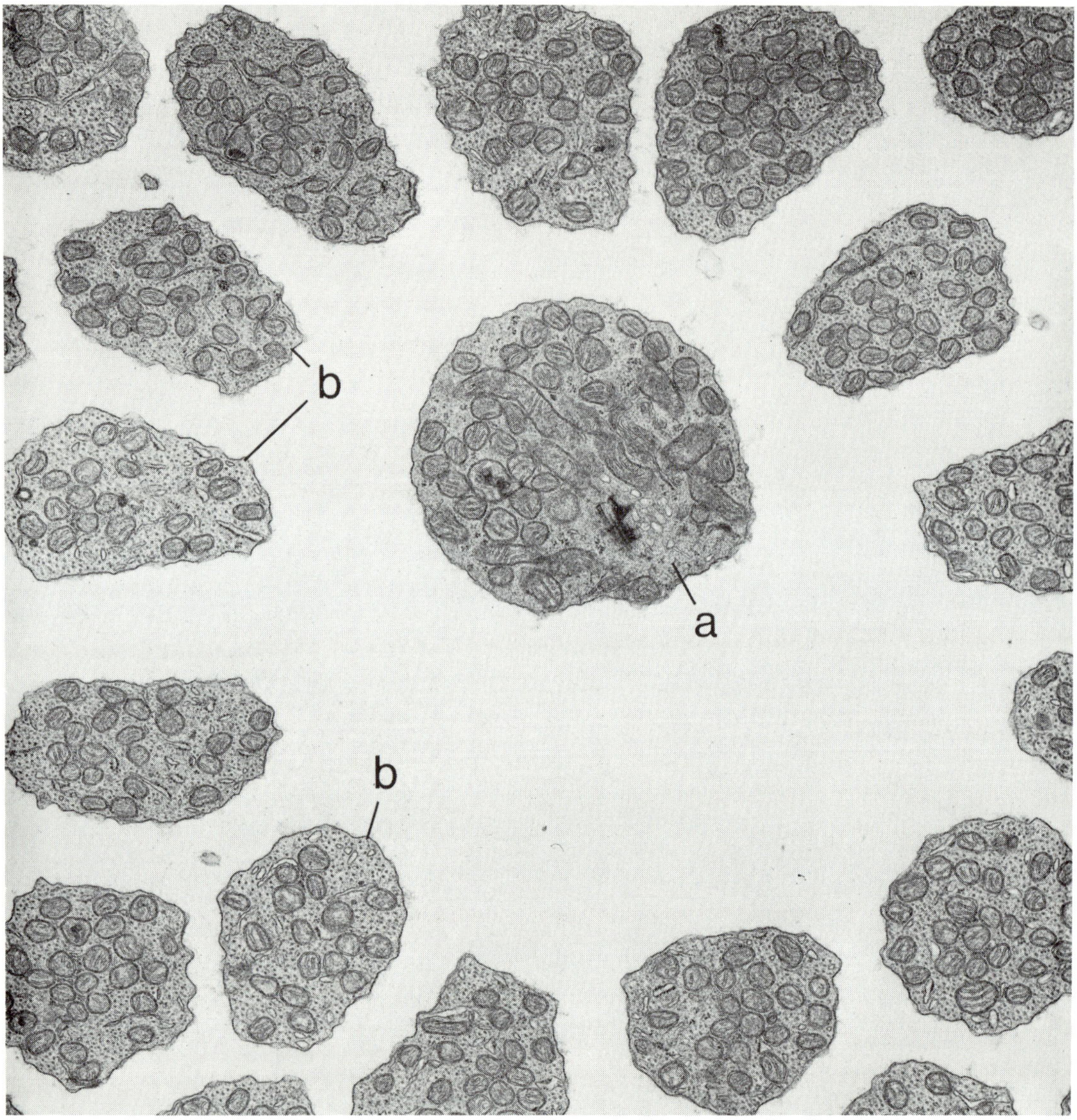

Figure 1–24. A cone ellipsoid (a) containing numerous mitochondria is surrounded by rod ellipsoids (b) containing slightly fewer mitochondria. (× 12,800.)

quiring reactions, the mitochondria are known as the power houses of the cell.

The mitochondria are unique because they are independent genetic units of the cell (Nass, 1969). Mitochondria contain their own DNA, which is similar to bacterial DNA in that it exists in a circular or ring form and not in the chromosomal form of eukaryotic or nucleated cells. They also contain ribosomes, which are smaller than those of the cytoplasm, and they have tRNA and amino acid activating enzymes. Mitochondria indeed possess all the protein synthetic apparatus, but it is not likely that the mitochondrial DNA is sufficiently large to code for all the proteins necessary to synthesize a mitochondrion. It is more probable that only certain structural lipoproteins

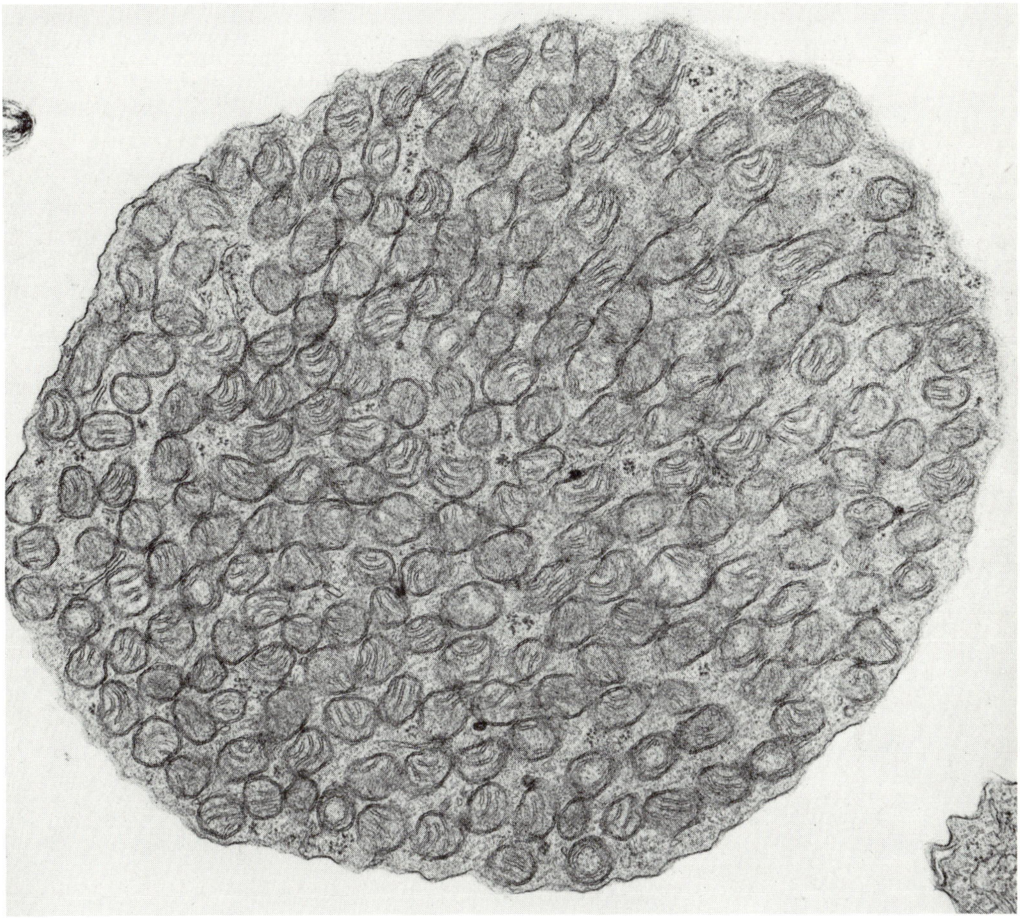

Figure 1-25. Cone ellipsoid showing the extreme concentration of numerous closely packed mitochondria, characteristic of this portion of the cone; there are more than 200 mitochondria per cross-section. The mitochondria of the cones are not as long as those of the rods, but they are much more numerous. (× 19,500.)

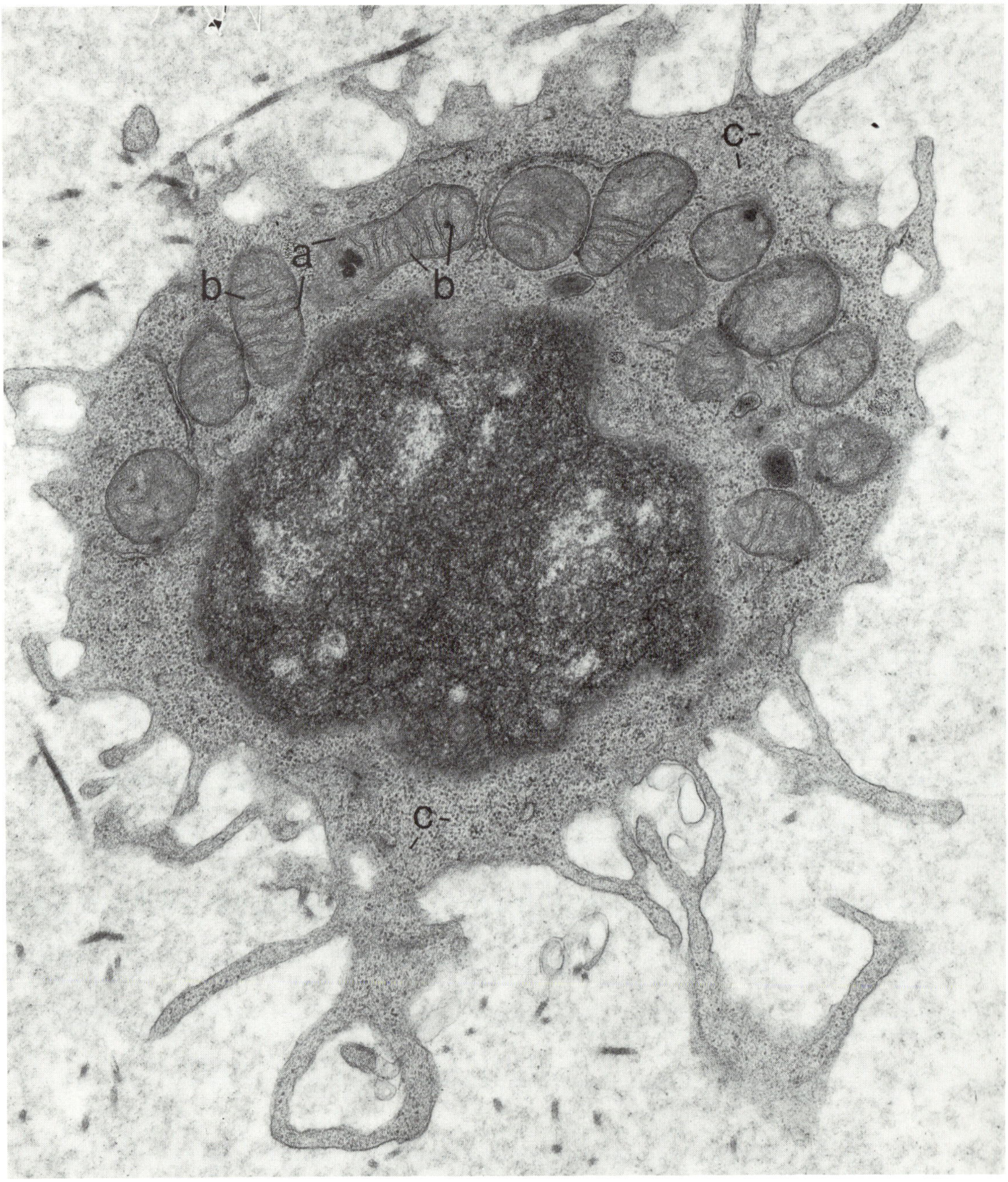

Figure 1–26. Extravascular lymphocyte in the choroidal stroma. The mitochondria (a) in these cells are shorter and rounder than those shown in the photoreceptor. The cristae (b) are oriented across the short axis and the cytoplasm is filled with free unattached ribosomes (c). (× 20,800.)

required to make a mitochondrion are coded and synthesized in the mitochondrion and that the rest are transferred from the cytoplasm.

LYSOSOMES (Fig. 1–4)

Within the mitochondrial fraction obtained by ultracentrifugation of broken-up cells, a fluffy layer is found that has been shown by de Duve (1963) to possess acid phosphatase activity. This layer contains particles that are smaller in size than those of mitochondria; because of their high content of hydrolytic enzymes they have been identified as lysosomes, which are capable of breaking down and solubilizing nucleic acids, proteins, glycogen and mucopolysaccharides. They have little effect on lipids, however. Although lysosomes are present in most, if not all, cells, they are very heterogeneous in shape and cannot be definitely identified as lysosomes solely on morphologic grounds. Stains for acid phosphatases are used regularly, however, to show lysosomal activity at the light and electron microscopic levels. As shown in Figure 1–4, lysosomes are vacuoles measuring between 0.25 and 0.5 μm. and bound by a single membrane. Since the hydrolytic enzymes of the lysosomes are proteins, they are probably first synthesized in the endoplasmic reticulum, and subsequently the Golgi complex participates in the segregation and concentration of the enzymes in the mature or *primary lysosome*. During the process of phagocytosis, ingested particles such as bacteria are segregated into membrane-bound vacuoles known as *phagosomes*, which then join the primary lysosomes by fusion of the membranes of these two structures. Such a vacuole is now designated as a *secondary lysosome*; within it the bacterium is killed and digested by the acid hydrolases of the lysosome. After a period of time only undigestable materials remain within the lysosomal vacuole, and it is not then possible to demonstrate further hydrolytic activity; the vacuole then becomes known as a *residual body*. These residual bodies are frequently electron-dense, possibly because of their high content of undigested lipids. Lysosomes engaged in the destruction of exogenous substances are said to be engaged in *heterophagy*, and when they participate in the breakdown of endogenous substances such as glycogen, or organelles like mitochondria, they are said to be engaged in *autophagy*. The lipofuscin granules of neurons in the retina, central nervous system and cardiac muscle, as well as those in the retinal pigment epithelium, probably represent residual bodies formed by autophagy.

FILAMENTS (Figs. 1–27 to 1–29)

Almost all cells contain filaments measuring 40 to 50 A. in diameter and of variable or indeterminate length. Filaments are a prominent feature of the cytoplasm of stratified squamous epithelia. Because of their density in skin epithelium they have been called tonofibrils; they are involved in the process of keratinization. Filaments are found in nonkeratinizing cells throughout the body, however, such as endothelium, epithelial cells of mucous membranes and the cornea, neural and neuroglial cells and many others. Since the actin filaments of striated muscle have a diameter of 60 A., like the filaments of other cells, it has been suggested that the cytoplasmic filaments of cells may also be contractile.

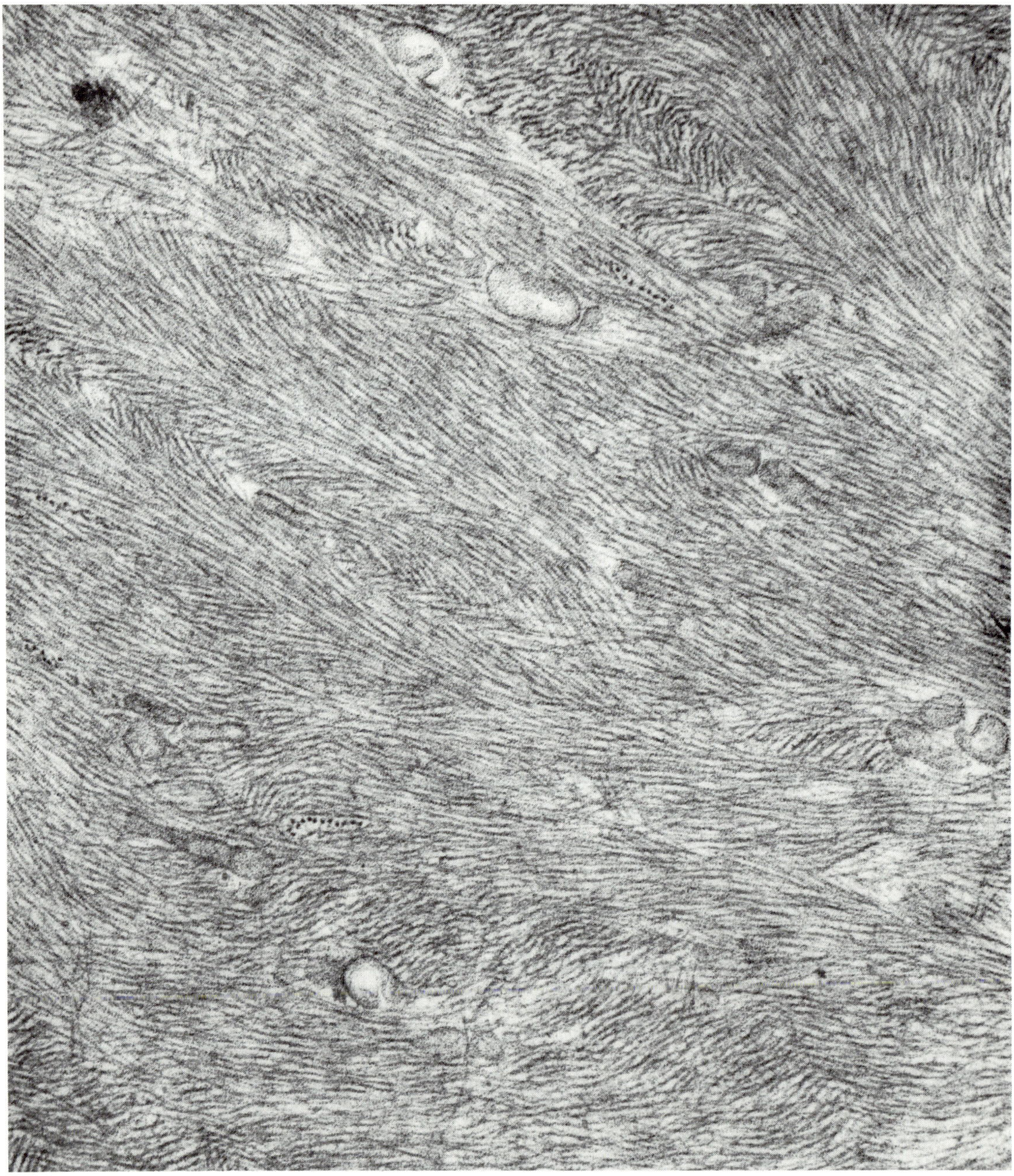

Figure 1–27. Cytoplasmic filaments in a prelaminar astrocyte of the optic nerve. The astrocytes of the optic nerve, the Müller cells of the retina, the unpigmented epithelium of the ciliary body, the endothelium of the trabecular meshwork and the corneal and conjunctival epithelium contain large quantities of microfilaments. These filaments are uniform in size and measure between 80 and 100 A. in diameter; their length is undetermined. (× 50,000.)

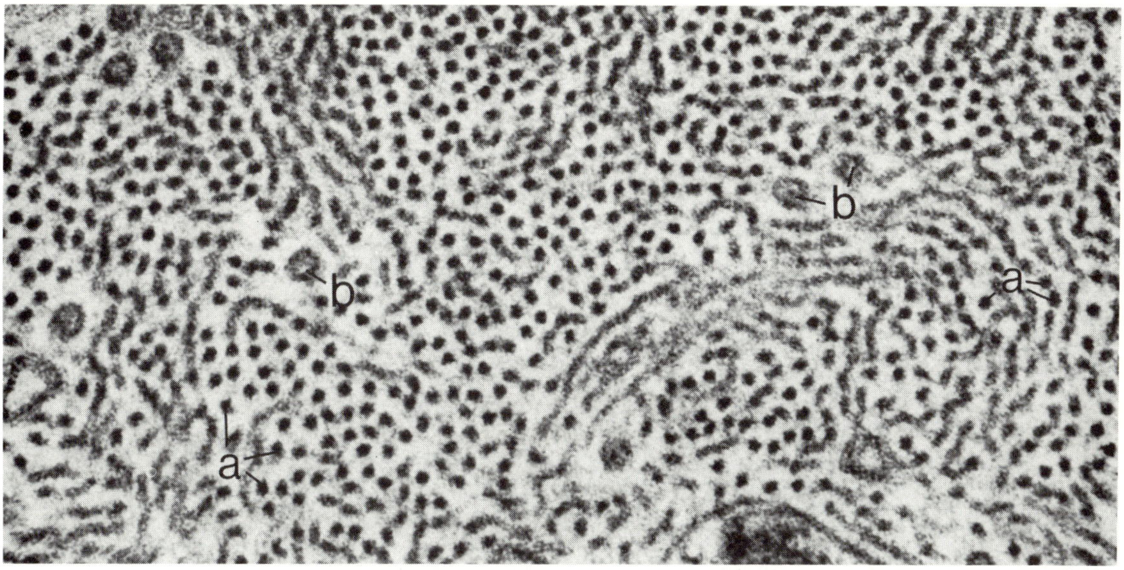

Figure 1–28. Cross-section of a prelaminar astrocyte showing filaments (a) and microtubules (b). The latter measure 330 A. in diameter and possess a central dense core. (× 150,000.)

MICROTUBULES (Figs. 1–4; 1–28)

Microtubules are found in the cytoplasm of a wide variety of cells, sometimes arranged in regular patterns, sometimes in a random fashion. They are straight structures with an outside diameter of 200 to 270 A. and are of variable length (Fig. 1–4). Their walls are quite dense and measure about 50 to 70 A. thick. Between the two walls is an area of lesser density that has no specific content. With high magnification and special techniques, each microtubule is seen to be composed of 13 longitudinal filamentous subunits.

Microtubules form the spindle apparatus of dividing cells; they are prominent in neural cells. They probably play a role in maintenance of the rigidity of the cell, and in the motion of cilia and flagella.

CENTRIOLES (Figs. 1–4; 1–30)

Almost every cell in the body contains a pair of centrioles, which are located near the nucleus at the apical end of the cell in glandular epithelial cells, and in varying positions in other cells (Fig. 1–4). The pair of centrioles are closely related to each other, the long axis of one centriole being oriented perpendicular to the long axis of its fellow. The centrioles are located in a specially differentiated region of the cytoplasm called the centrosome. They are concerned with cell reproduction, separating in the beginning stages of division and migrating to opposite poles of the elongating nucleus. Some cells, such as the polyploid cells of the liver and the megakaryocytes of the bone marrow, contain more than one pair of centrioles. The cilia of ciliated cells are formed from *basal bodies* which arise from the division of centrioles.

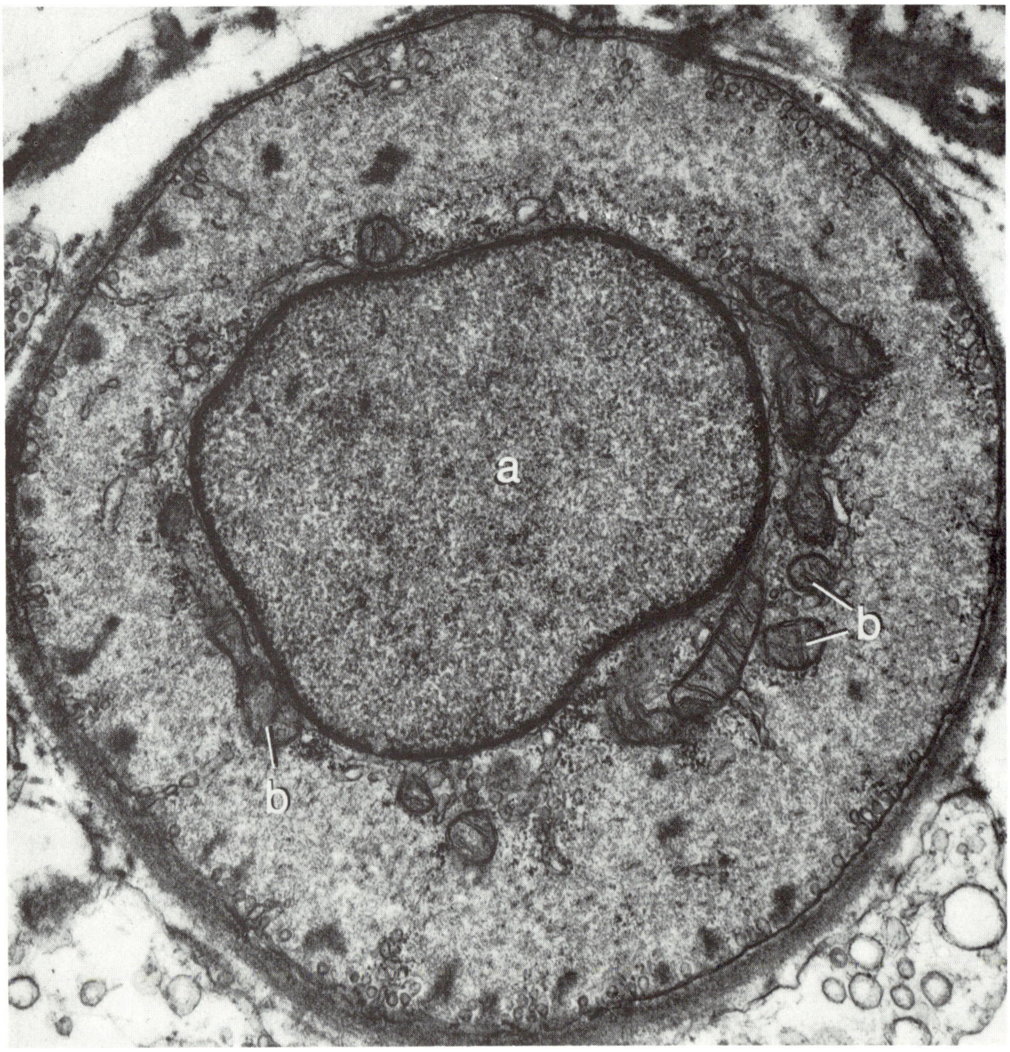

Figure 1–29. Cytoplasmic filaments that are considerably finer than those shown in the preceding figures are found in the smooth muscles of the iris and the blood vessels of the eye. This smooth muscle cell has a centrally located nucleus (a), surrounded by several mitochondria (b). The cytoplasm is filled with very fine actin and myosin filaments that give it a ground-glass appearance. (× 21,000.)

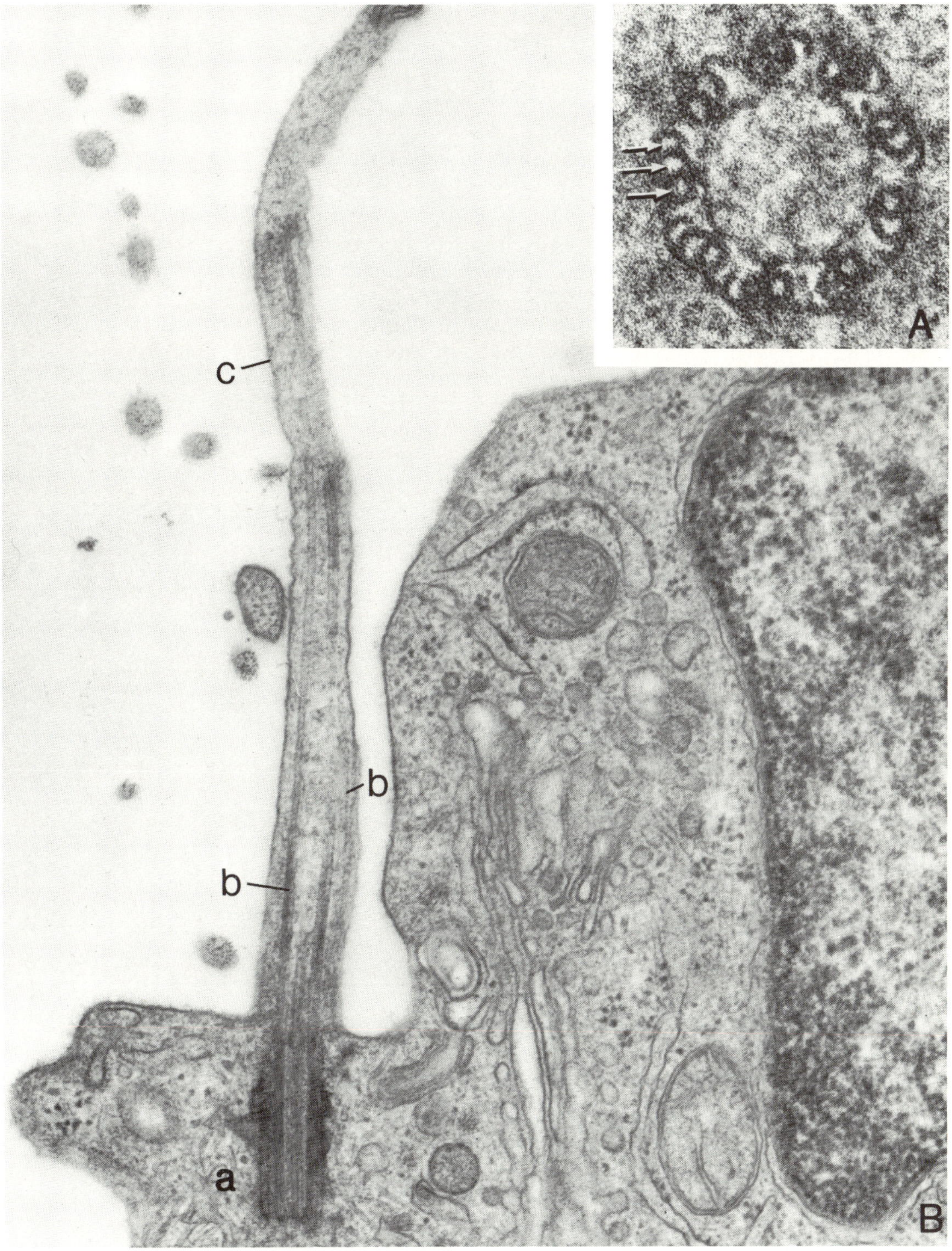

Figure 1–30. A centriole, basal body and cilium in an iris melanocyte and a fibroblast.

A, The nine triplets (arrows) forming the centriole. (× 100,000.)

B, The basal body (a) has a structure similar to that of the centriole shown in the insert. It gives rise to nine microtubules (b) that extend outward from the cell to form the cilium (c). (× 41,600.)

When viewed with the electron microscope, each centriole measures 300 to 500 μm. in length and 150 μm. in diameter and is seen as a hollow tube composed of nine evenly spaced triplet filaments embedded in a matrix (Stubblefield and Brinkley, 1967).

PIGMENT (Fig. 1–31)

Lipofuscin. Wear and tear pigment is found in many cells of older persons. It occurs extensively in the neurons of the nervous system and becomes more prominent in the retinal pigment epithelial cells with increasing age. These granules are sudanophilic and have a brown color; they are resistant to acid, alkali and fat solvents. They probably represent wear and tear products formed within individual cells, perhaps arising from degeneration of pre-existing organelles. By electron microscopy, lipofuscin pigments have a variable morphology and are enclosed by a very fine membrane. The

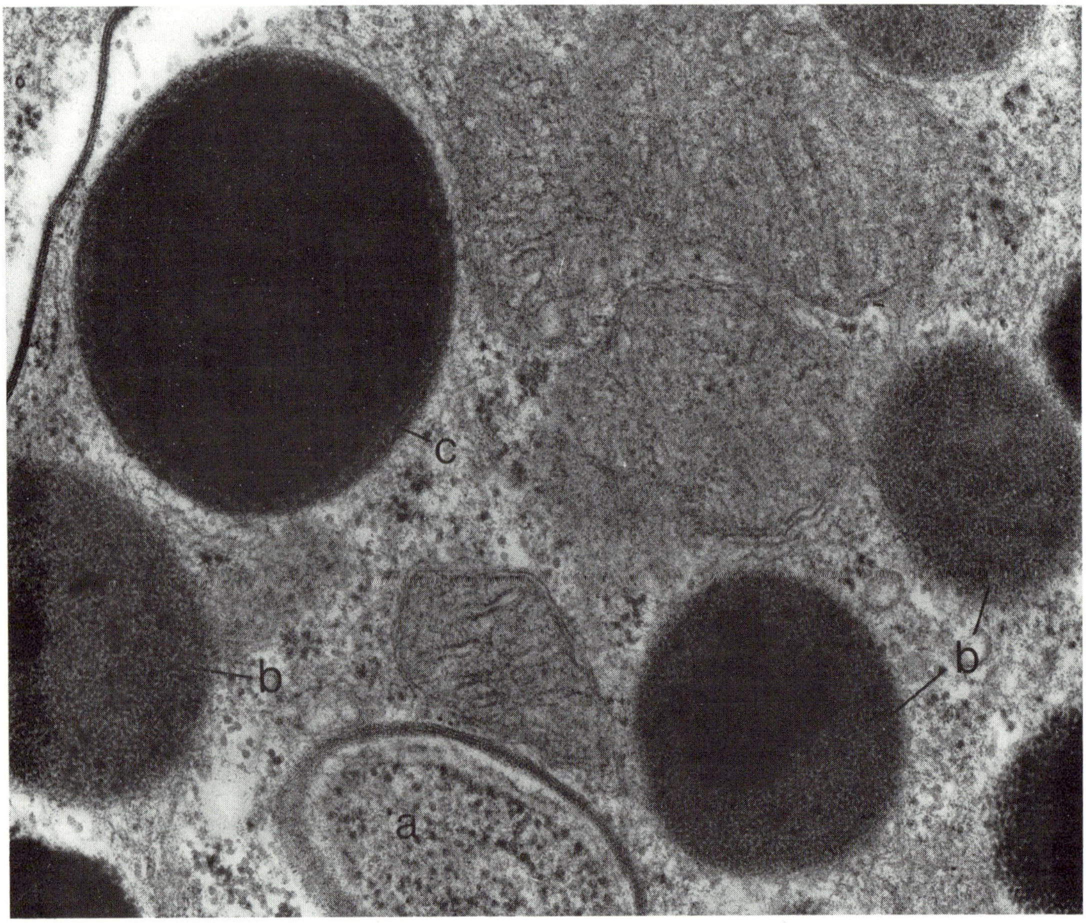

Figure 1–31. Pigment epithelium of the iris. A premelanosome is shown at (a). Several melanosomes exhibiting various degrees of melanization are shown at (b) and an almost completely melanized granule is at (c). (× 50,000.)

contents are usually osmiophilic; the osmiophilia varies in intensity, some areas being very dense and others more granular.

Melanin. The size and shape of melanin granules will be discussed in more detail in the chapters covering the uveal tract. Melanin is found in the skin, hair, uveal tract, mucosal surfaces and leptomeninges. Some melanin is found as a storage product in epithelial cells and as an ingested material in endothelial cells, as well as a variety of other cells in the vicinity of pigment-producing cells. Melanogenesis occurs only in melanocytes, which are widely distributed in the tissues mentioned. They are derived from the neural crest and migrate into the various tissues during embryonic life. The melanin itself is formed in the cytoplasm of pigment-producing cells, probably within the vesicles of the Golgi apparatus, or as a result of manufacture of precursors in the endoplasmic reticulum which are then concentrated in the Golgi apparatus. The melanin of cells is actually a complex of melanin and a protein. The melanin is a product of enzymatic activity involving the amino acid tyrosine, which is polymerized with protein to form melanoprotein. The melanoprotein is deposited on filaments in tyrosinase-positive cytoplasmic vesicles called *premelanosomes*. The mature vesicles are completely filled with melanin, are tyrosinase-negative and are known as *melanosomes*.

Melanoprotein is extremely resistant to solvents and other chemical agents, but it can be bleached by oxidation with hydrogen peroxide and potassium permanganate. The melanosomes have a varying shape and size, depending on the cell; those within the cells derived from neuroectoderm are much larger than those of the melanocytes of the uveal tract and skin. Mature melanocytes have melanin granules throughout their cytoplasm and into the processes. Immature ones have melanin mainly in the region of the cell body.

Glycogen. The polysaccharide glycogen is synthesized from glucose through the enzymatic activity of glycogen synthetase. Glycogen is stored mainly in the liver and other parts of the body for later use. When needed it is again broken down to glucose, which is then utilized for energy. Significant amounts of glycogen are found in tissues having an active metabolism, however, such as the superficial layers of the corneal epithelium and the retinal Müller cells, which store it to provide energy for adjacent neurons. The method of fixation and preparation of the cell causes much extraction of glycogen granules, but by using phosphate buffers the granules may be preserved. They are located in various parts of the cytoplasm, without preference for a given location. The granules measure 150 to 200 A. in diameter and have a slightly irregular outline. They may be single or rosette in form; the rosettes vary in size, but may be up to 0.1 μm. in diameter. The glycogen found in the liver is most often found in the alpha particle or rosette form. In Müller cells of the retina, corneal epithelium and cardiac muscle, the glycogen particles most often are found singly, in the beta form (Fig. 1–32).

Lipid. Lipids of various types are found in many cells, sometimes as part of a regular metabolic process such as occurs in the intestinal epithelium. At other times lipid is found in lysosomes, where it is being degraded. Triglycerides of fatty acids are most commonly seen, especially in adipose cells. Lipids of this type can be used for synthesis of such components as the membranes of endoplasmic reticulum and cell membranes. They also can be used in the manufacture of specific secretory products. Most lipids are

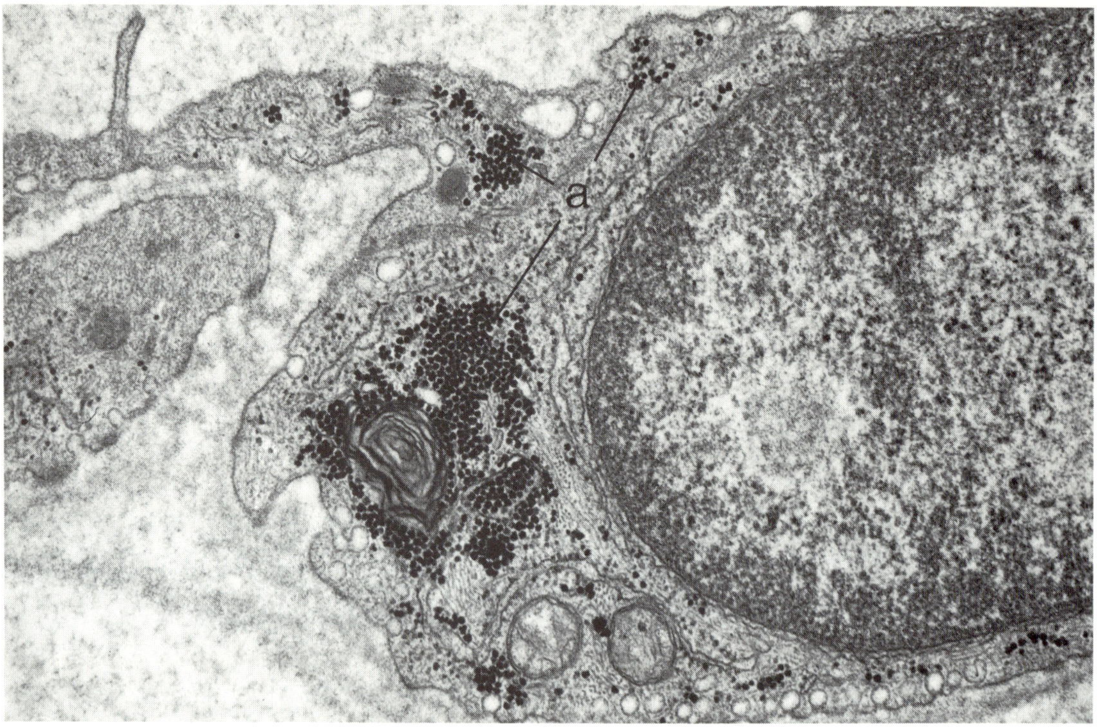

Figure 1–32. Glycogen granules (a) in the cytoplasm of a choroidal fibroblast. (× 19,100.)

rendered insoluble with osmium, and more saturated lipids stain less densely with osmium than unsaturated lipids.

The cytoplasmic lipid deposits appear in the form of vacuoles which are not membrane-bound except for the lipid in the intestinal epithelium, which is being transported across the epithelium in pinocytotic vesicles.

SURFACE COAT

The surface coating of many cells is composed of mucoprotein and may be specialized, like that of plant cells and the cuticle of insect cells. A similar mucoprotein surface coat exists over the outermost layer of corneal epithelial cells; it is likely that most cells have a mucopolysaccharide-protein coat associated with the cell membrane. One of the most studied surface coats is that found in the intestinal epithelium, which measures between 0.1 and 0.5 μm. thick.

BASEMENT MEMBRANE OR BASAL LAMINA

Basement membranes adjacent to the basal surface of epithelial cells have been described for many years. This distinct layer lies close to the cell surface and is periodic acid-Schiff (PAS) positive. Most basement membranes are rather thin, but two tissues of the eye possess the thickest basement membranes known. Descemet's membrane is the basement membrane of the corneal epithelium, and the lens capsule is the basement membrane of the lens epithelium; these membranes are actually thicker than the cells resting upon them. It is probable that the components of the basement membrane are produced by the overlying cells.

Electron microscopists prefer to use the term basal lamina rather than basement membrane, because the latter term was used by light microscopists to describe a structure containing not only the basement membrane as seen by electron microscopy but some of the adjacent collagenous elements of the tissues as well. The word lamina is preferred because use of the term membrane causes confusion with the descriptions of cell or plasma membranes. The basement membrane is formed by an electron-lucent zone measuring 400 A. in thickness and an electron-dense layer measuring 500 to 700 A. in thickness.

CELL JUNCTIONS (Fig. 1–33)

A number of specialized structures exist for the attachment of cells to each other. These structures exist as well to provide communication between cells and to provide electrical coupling between cells (Pappas and Bennett, 1966, Bennett et al., 1967, Lowenstein and Kanno, 1967). A very important function is to join the lateral cell membranes to provide a barrier to passage of fluids, electrolytes and macromolecules along the intercellular space.

The intercellular junctions usually are classified as *occluding* or *tight* when the cell membranes physically fuse with each other to completely obliterate the intercellular space. The junctions are classified as *adhering* when they produce cellular attachments to each other by means of an intercellular substance. In such a case the space which separates the cells is of uniform thickness and the cell membranes are parallel to each other. All these junctions can be further classified according to the size and shape of the intercellular contacts. Among these are focal junctions or *maculae*, *bands* or *fasciae*, and *belts* or *zonulae* which surround the entire cell (Fig. 1–33) (Farquhar and Palade, 1963, 1965). Recent high-resolution electron microscopic studies have shown that many junctions which formerly were believed to be tight junctions do not exhibit fusion of the two cell membranes. The cell membranes, instead, have been found to be separated by a space measuring only a few A.; such junctions have come to be known as "gap" junctions and are common between smooth muscle cells and in the cells of the central nervous system (Brightman and Reese, 1969). The commonest types of junctions will be described here to avoid repetition in subsequent chapters.

Zonula Occludens. This tight junction is characterized by fusion of the cell membranes, so that there is complete closure of the intercellular space. This junction is of the belt type and encircles the entire cell, binding it firmly to neighboring cells. The most important function of junctions of this type is believed to be prevention of diffusion of substances between the cells into underlying tissues, for example, from the lumen of a capillary between the endothelial cells into the tissues surrounding them. These junctions are characteristically found in many epithelia, such as the kidney tubular epithelium where transepithelial potentials exist, and in the capillaries of the central nervous system, where they are important in maintaining the blood-brain barrier. The corneal endothelium is another example, for it

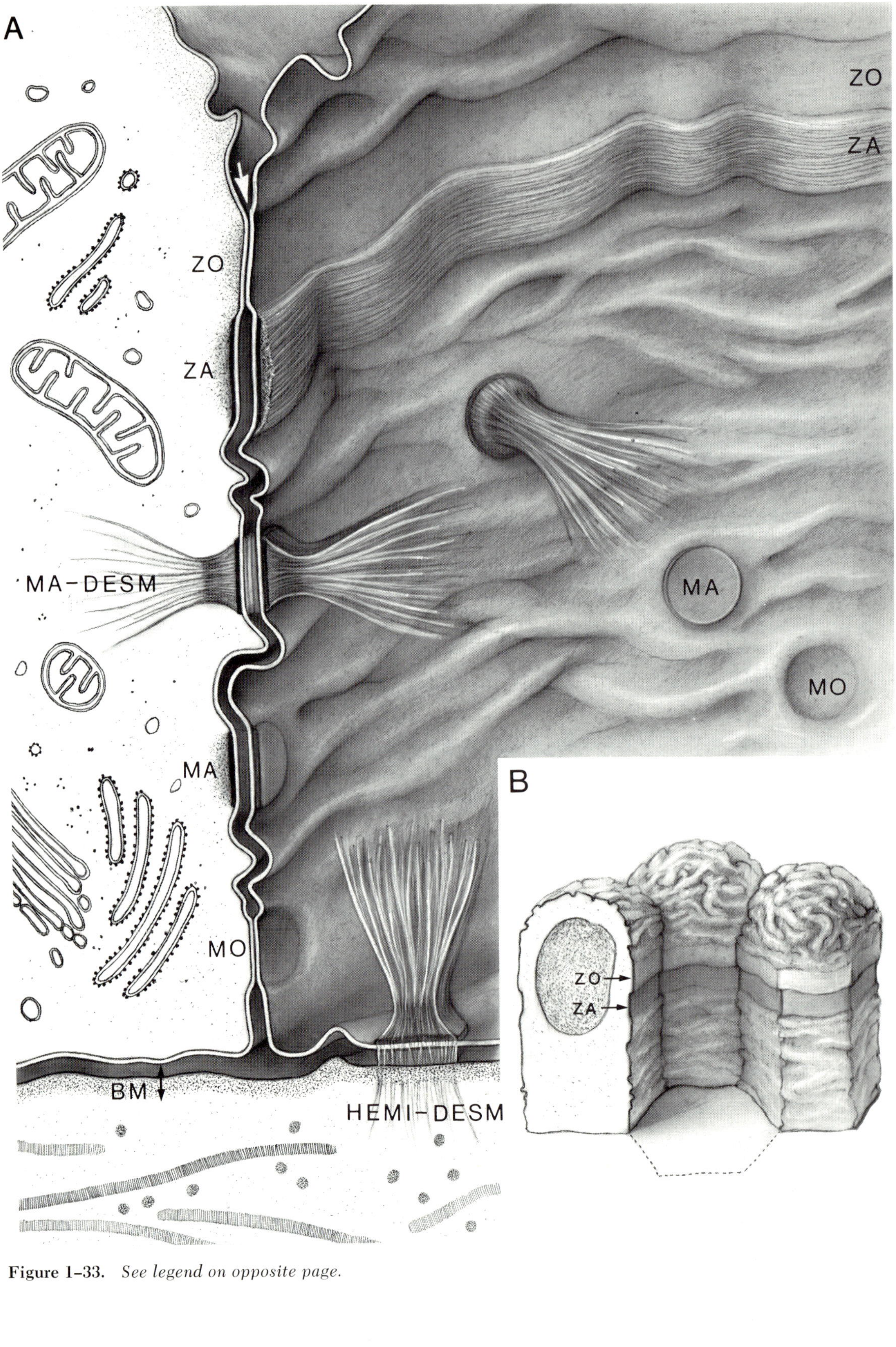

Figure 1–33. *See legend on opposite page.*

is an important cell layer possessing a zonula occludens. This zonula is believed to play a vital part in regulating flow of fluids into the corneal stroma.

Zonula Adherens. This type of junction also forms an encircling band around the circumference of the cell, binding it to the adjacent cell. The intercellular space of these junctions is narrowed to about 200 A. but it is preserved. Along the junction the cytoplasm close to the cell membrane is slightly more dense. This type of junction, shown in Figure 1–33, is usually found adjacent to a zonula occludens. The two junctions, along with a macula adherens, form the so-called "junctional complex" or terminal bar. The intercellular junctions of the retinal pigment epithelium include a zonula adherens near their apical portions, as do the junctions between the Müller cells and myoids of the retinal receptors to form the outer limiting membrane of the retina.

Macula Adherens. This junction is characterized by a localized or button-like attachment between two cells (Fig. 1–33). The cytoplasm adjacent to the junction is finely granular and denser. This increased density is helpful in identifying the macula adherens. Junctions of this type form the third component of the "junctional complex" found in the epithelia of glands and the intestinal tract.

Macula Adherens, Desmosomal Type. This junction is the equivalent of "cellular bridges" that have been described in the epidermis by light microscopy. The term desmosome is more commonly used to describe these adhesions; they are usually present in those epithelia of man which are derived from ectoderm, such as the epidermis and corneal epithelium and the epithelial layers of the optic cup and central nervous system. Desmosomes show two distinctive features: the arrangement of an electron-dense intercellular material parallel to the cell membranes that form a line, and the orientation of numerous tonofilaments in the cytoplasm at a right angle to the junction in the cytoplasm (Kelly, 1966). The bundles of tonofilaments terminate in an electron-dense cytoplasmic bar that is oriented parallel to the cell membrane.

Hemidesmosome or Half-desmosome. The half-desmosome is a special type of desmosome found at the base of epithelial cells. This structure probably fastens the epithelium to the underlying basement membrane.

Figure 1–33. Intercellular junctions. *A*, View of the intercellular junctions as seen from the interior of the cell. Two belt-like junctions appear near the apex of the cells. One is a zonula occludens (ZO) that completely obliterates the intercellular space, characterized by fusion of the outer leaflets of the two contiguous cells (arrow). The second is a zonula adherens (ZA), in which the intercellular space is unchanged and the contiguous cell membranes are strictly parallel. Cytoplasmic fibrils are found along this junction. A macula adherens, desmosomal-type (MA-DESM), contains an intercellular cement substance; numerous tonofilaments are attached to an electron-dense, plate-like structure that is closely apposed to the cell membrane. These three junctions are arranged in the epithelia of many glands to form a terminal-bar or junctional complex. A macula adherens (MA) is shown in cross-section and in a "head-on" view. Fine fibrils are associated with it, and it has a button-like shape. A macula occludens (MO) appears toward the bottom of the intercellular space, and since this is a tight junction, the adjacent cell membranes are fused. In a "head-on" view the macula occludens appears as a round, button-like depression. A hemi-desmosome (HEMI-DESM) is seen along the basal portion of the cell. Fine fibrils appear to attach the hemi-desmosome to the underlying basement membrane (BM). The basement membrane, or basal lamina, is composed of an electron-lucent layer immediately adjacent to the cell membrane, as well as an electron-dense layer consisting of fine filaments. The basement membrane filaments continue into the underlying connective tissue.

B, This insert shows that the zonula occludens and the zonula adherens actually form a continuous structure around the circumferences of two cells.

REFERENCES

Beams, H. W., and Kessel, R. G.: The Golgi apparatus: Structure and function. Int. Rev. Cytol. *23*:209, 1968.

Bennett, M. V. L., Pappas, G. D., Aljure, E., and Nakajima, Y.: Physiology and ultrastructure of electrotonic junctions. II. Spinal and medullary electromotor nuclei in mormyrid fish. J. Neurophys. *30*:180, 1967.

Brightman, M. V., and Reese, T. S.: Junctions between intimately apposed cell membranes in the vertebrate brain. J. Cell Biol. *40*:648, 1969.

Danielli, J. F., and Davson, H.: A contribution to the theory of permeability of thin films. J. Cell Comp. Physiol. *5*:495, 1935.

de Duve, C.: The lysosome. Sci. Amer. *208*:64, 1963.

DuPraw, E. J.: Cell and Molecular Biology. New York, Academic Press, Inc., 1968.

Farquhar, M. G., and Palade, G. E.: Junctional complexes in various epithelia. J. Cell Biol. *17*:375, 1963.

Farquhar, M. G., and Palade, G. E.: Cell junctions in Amphibian skin. J. Cell Biol. *26*:263, 1965.

Fawcett, D. W.: The Cell: Its Organelles and Inclusions. Philadelphia, W. B. Saunders Company, 1966.

Golgi, C.: Sulla struttura delle cellule nervose dei gangli spinali. Arch. Ital. Biol. *30*:60, 1898.

Gorter, E., and Grendel, F.: Bimolecular layers of lipoids on chromocytes of blood. J. Exp. Med. *41*:439, 1925.

Kelly, D. E.: Fine structure of desmosomes, hemidesmosomes, and an adepidermal globular layer in developing new epidermis. J. Cell Biol. *28*:51, 1966.

Langmuir, I.: The constitution and fundamental properties of solids and liquids. II. Liquids. J. Amer. Chem. Soc. *39*:1848, 1917.

Lowenstein, W. R., and Kanno, T.: Intercellular communication and tissue growth. I. Cancerous growth. J. Cell Biol. *33*:225, 1967.

Michaelis, L.: Die vitale eine darstellungsnephode der zellgranule. Arch. Mikroskop. Anat. *55*:558, 1900.

Nass, S.: The significance of the structural and functional similarities of bacteria and mitochondria. Int. Rev. Cytol. *25*:55, 1969.

Neutra, M., and Leblond, C. P.: The Golgi apparatus. Sci. Amer. *200*:100, 1969.

Overton, E.: Vierteljahresscher, Naturforsch. Ges. Zurich *40*:159, 1845.

Palade, G. E.: Structure and function at the cellular level. J.A.M.A. *198*:815, 1966.

Pappas, G. D., and Bennett, M. V. L.: Specialized junctions involved in electrical transmission between neurons. Ann. N. Y. Acad. Sci. *136*:495, 1966.

Redman, C. M.: Biosynthesis of serum proteins and ferritin by free and attached ribosomes of rat liver. J. Biol. Chem. *22*:4308, 1969.

Robertson, J. D.: The ultrastructure of cell membranes and their derivatives. In Crook, E. M. (ed.): The Structure and Function of Subcellular Components. Biochemical Society Symposium No. 16. New York, Cambridge University Press, 1959, pp. 3–43.

Rouser, G., Nelson, G. J., Fleischer, S., and Simon, G.: Lipid composition of animal cell membranes, organelles, and organs. *In* Chapman, D. (ed.): Biological Membranes, Physical Fact and Function. New York, Academic Press, Inc., 1968, pp. 5–70.

Schmidt, W. T. Z.: Über die Formdoppelbrechung der osmierten Markscheide des Nerven. Wiss. Mikroskopic *54*:159, 1937.

Schmitt, F. O., Bear, R. S., and Ponder, E.: Optical properties of red cell membrane. J. Cell. Comp. Phys. *9*:89, 1936.

Sjostrand, F. S.: Ultrastructure in biological systems. *In* Dalton, A. J., and Haguenau, A. (eds.): The Membranes. Vol. IV. London, Academic Press, 1968.

Stein, W. D.: Movement of molecules across cell membranes. New York, Academic Press, Inc., 1967.

Stoeckenius, W.: Some electron microscopical observations on liquid crystalline phases in lipid-water systems. J. Cell Biol. *12*:220, 1962.

Stoeckenius, W., and Engelman, D. M.: Current models for the structure of biological membranes. J. Cell Biol. *42*:613, 1969.

Stubblefield, E., and Brinkley, B. R.: Architecture and function of the mammalian centriole. *In* Warren, K. (ed.): Formation and Fate of Cell Organelles. Symposia of the International Society for Cell Biology. Vol. 6. New York, Academic Press, Inc., 1967, pp. 1–392.

Watson, J. D., and Crick, F. H. C.: The Watson-Crick model for DNA and replication hypothesis. Nature *171*:737, 1953.

Chapter Two

EYEBALL

GENERAL ANATOMY

The eyeball is placed in the orbit so that it is closer to the lateral than to the medial wall and slightly nearer the superior orbital margin than to the inferior. The anteroposterior axis of the eyeball is parallel to the medial bony wall of the orbit, but makes about a 45 degree angle with the lateral wall. The eye can be displaced easily in most directions by pressure with the fingers, the amount of displacement being dependent on the size of the orbit, the density of the orbital fat and the development of the orbital muscles and check ligaments. The anterior orbital margin slopes backward toward the temporal side, its plane oblique to that of the face. For this reason, when the eye looks directly forward, the anterior sclera is more exposed on the temporal side and is more susceptible to injury. Considerable variation exists in the degree of prominence of the eyes, depending on the volume of the orbital cavity, the amount of orbital fat, the structure of the eyelids and conjunctiva, and the size of the eye itself. A slight difference in the prominence of the two eyes is common.

The anterior surface of the eyeball is in contact with the eyelids. During the periods when the eyelids are open the cornea is exposed to air, but it is protected from drying by frequent blinking of the eyelids and by the precorneal tear film, which is composed of lacrimal fluid, mucus and lipid (see pages 56 and 80). The anterior part of the scleral coat of the eye is visible through the semitransparent conjunctiva, episclera and Tenon's capsule. Tenon's capsule surrounds the eye like a glove; it originates anteriorly in the limbus and terminates posteriorly where it joins the dura mater of the optic nerve. Tenon's capsule also is reflected backward onto the rectus muscle tendons at their insertions to form a perimuscular sheath which is continuous to their origins at the orbital apex, where it then merges with the orbital periosteum.

The eyeball is composed of three tissue layers, which enclose the anterior and posterior chambers, the lens and the vitreous humor. The anterior and posterior chambers are almost completely separated from each other by the iris and lens, and from the vitreous humor by the lens and its zonular attachments. The outermost coat of the eyeball is known as the *fibrous tunic* and is composed of the clear, transparent cornea and the white, opaque sclera (Fig. 2-1). These two collagenous tissues provide a slightly elastic envelope which maintains the shape of the eye.

The *cornea* is a clear, transparent tissue which readily transmits light and has the strongest refracting surface of the eye. These properties make it one of the most important parts of the optical system. The *sclera* is opaque and tough; it is a viscoelastic tissue whose elasticity diminishes with age because of changes in its collagen. This change in elasticity is important for

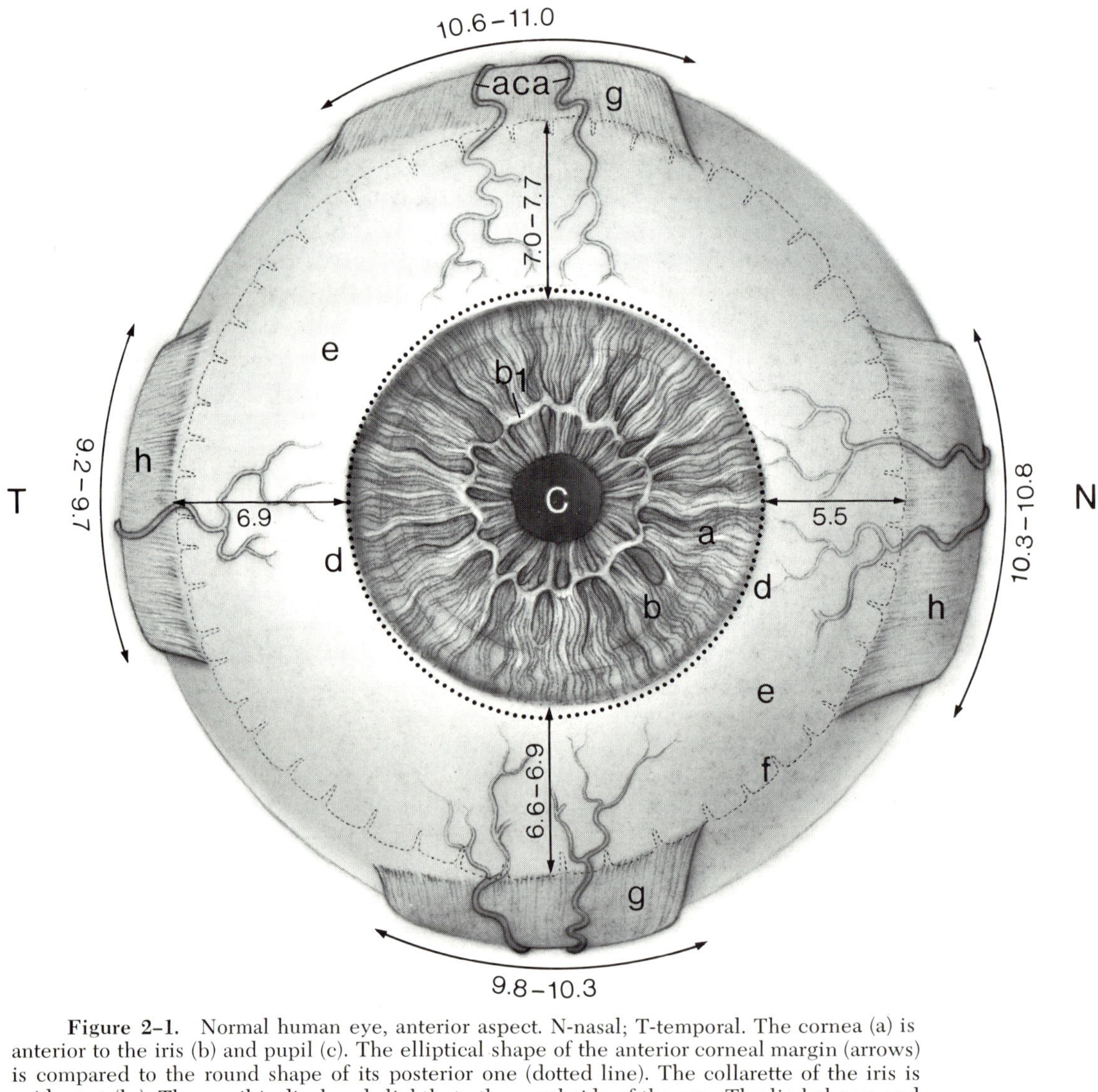

Figure 2–1. Normal human eye, anterior aspect. N-nasal; T-temporal. The cornea (a) is anterior to the iris (b) and pupil (c). The elliptical shape of the anterior corneal margin (arrows) is compared to the round shape of its posterior one (dotted line). The collarette of the iris is evident at (b_1). The pupil is displaced slightly to the nasal side of the eye. The limbal area and external scleral sulcus surround the margin of the cornea (d). The sclera (e) is peripheral to the limbus. The sclera has been made artificially transparent to show the ora serrata (f), which is farther posterior on the temporal than on the nasal side. The superior and inferior rectus tendons (g) are curved and are inserted obliquely to the axis of the eye. The tendons of the medial and lateral recti (h) also have curved insertions which are not oblique to the horizontal meridian. Each rectus muscle has two anterior ciliary arteries (ACA) except the lateral rectus, which has one. The measurements of all these structures are given in the illustration.

the measurement of intraocular pressure with the impression tonometer because it may cause false high readings. The inherent strength of the intricately arranged collagen of the cornea and sclera protects the ocular contents from injury. If the contents of the eye are removed, the cornea and sclera retain most of their normal shape as a result of their inherent rigidity. The cornea and sclera meet each other in a transition zone with respect to the corneal and scleral curvature, producing a circular depression known as the external scleral sulcus.

The middle layer of the eye is known as the *uveal tract* and is composed of the iris anteriorly, the choroid posteriorly and an intermediate part, the ciliary body. The uveal tract is attached to the internal sclera anteriorly at a collagenous protuberance known as the scleral spur. Posteriorly the choroidal portion ends at the edge of the optic nerve. Along its outer side it is loosely attached to the sclera by bands of pigmented collagenous tissue, the suprachoroidea and the supraciliaris. The large uveal blood vessels and nerves which penetrate the sclera also bind the uvea to the sclera. The uveal tract carries the principal blood vessels and nerves of the eye, and its function is largely nutritive. The anterior part of the ciliary body, the pars plicata, forms most of the aqueous humor, and the ciliary muscle is important in the act of accommodation (Fig. 2-2). The posterior part of the ciliary body, the pars plana, is lined by epithelial layers that may form some of the vitreous mucopolysaccharide. The iris arises from the anteromedial ciliary body and extends across the anterior eye as a diaphragm to improve its optical qualities. Because of its great vascularity, the choroid has been compared to an erectile tissue. The caliber of the choroidal vessels depends partly on the intraocular pressure; they dilate when the intraocular pressure is reduced and assume their usual caliber when it returns to normal. The change in blood volume in these vessels probably plays some part in maintaining a uniform intraocular pressure.

The innermost layer of the eye is the *retina*, which because of its embryologic origin and histologic structure is an extension of the central nervous system. The retina extends from the optic nerve forward to its termination at the ora serrata. Beyond the ora serrata it is continuous over the ciliary body with a layer of unpigmented epithelium, and onto the posterior iris, with a layer of pigmented epithelium. The retinal rods and cones or photoreceptors occupy the external part of the retina. Information exciting these receptors is transformed into some type of energy which recent studies show to be electrical initially, although photochemical changes are principally involved in the generation of the final visual response. The retinal receptors are precisely oriented with respect to the retinal pigment epithelium, and they are held in relatively fixed positions by a cementing mucopolysaccharide and by their interdigitation with the retinal pigment epithelium. This solid support is important for the production of undistorted retinal images.

The *optic nerve* is found in the posterior eye just nasal to the posterior pole of the eye. At its entrance into the interior of the eye it forms the optic disc. The disc edge is located an average of 3.42 ± 0.34 mm. from the foveola; the disc itself has an average vertical diameter of 1.86 ± 0.21 mm. and an average horizontal diameter of 1.75 ± 0.19 mm. (Straatsma et al., 1969).

The transparent and gel-like *vitreous* has a volume of about 4 cu. ml.

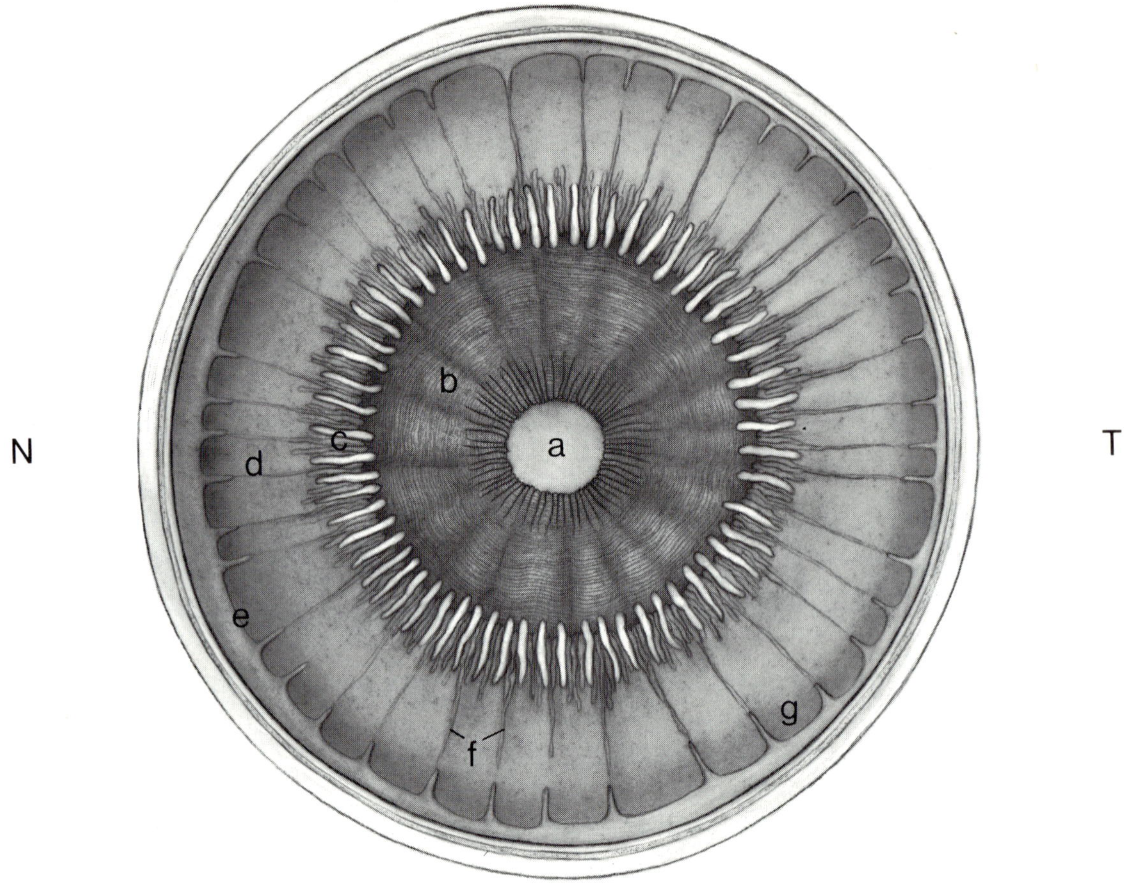

Figure 2–2. Interior view of the anterior half of the eye. The lens has been removed. N-nasal; T-temporal. The pupil (a) is slightly displaced nasally. The radial folds of the posterior iris (b) extend outward from the pupil. More peripherally are the radial and circular contraction furrows of the ciliary portion of the iris. Approximately 60 ciliary processes (c) form the pars plicata of the ciliary body, and posterior to the ciliary processes is the pars plana (d), which ends at the ora serrata (e). Dentate processes (f) extend from the ora serrata through the pars plana toward the pars plicata. Between them are the bays of the ora serrata (g). The ciliary body is narrower on the nasal than it is on the temporal side.

At its periphery it is intimate with the inner retina, and it is tightly fixed to the tissues around the ora serrata and adjacent ciliary body in an area known as the vitreous *base.* The vitreous is anchored posteriorly around the edge of the optic disc, but it is not adherent to the disc surface. Anteriorly, where it is in contact with the posterior surface of the lens, it exhibits a concavity, the patellar fossa. The vitreous plays some part in maintenance of the intraocular pressure, and its transparency is important for vision.

The posterior *lens* occupies the patellar fossa, and the zonules or suspensory ligament of the lens are attached to its equatorial region (see Figs. 11–2, Vitreous; 12–3, Lens) and to the epithelial cells of the pars plicata and pars plana of the ciliary body. The tension on the zonular fibrils is controlled by the ciliary muscle, the amount of tension controlling the shape and, therefore, the accommodation of the lens. The anterior lens capsule is free in the pupillary region, and peripheral to the pupil it is in contact with the central third of the iris.

The *posterior chamber* is not a large, open chamber like the anterior chamber. It is an irregular, thin space which lies behind the iris and extends as thin slit-like spaces between the ciliary processes and the lens. It contains aqueous humor which is produced by the ciliary body. The aqueous humor flows from this space through the pupil into the anterior chamber, where it leaves the eye through the trabecular meshwork, canal of Schlemm and scleral veins. The dynamics of aqueous humor circulation is the most important determinant of the intraocular pressure.

The *anterior chamber* lies in front of the iris and behind the cornea. Laterally it is bordered by the ciliary body and the corneoscleral tissues which form the trabecular meshwork.

GENERAL TOPOGRAPHY

The *anterior pole* of the eyeball is at the corneal center, and the *posterior pole* is located posteriorly at the center of the scleral curve. A line joining the two poles describes the *geometric axis* of the eye. The *visual axis* is a line joining the fixation point, the nodal point near the posterior surface of the lens, and the fovea. The *optic axis* of the eye is a theoretical line through the center of the principal refracting surfaces of the eye.

The equator is the *greatest circle* of the eye, transverse to the geometric axis. Because of the nasally eccentric position of the optic nerve in the sclera, the temporal sclera is longer than the nasal portion. For this reason the great circle of the eye is farther posterior temporally than nasally, and this anatomic equator is oblique with respect to the geometric axis. All the points on the sclera equidistant from the anterior and posterior poles form the *geometric* equator, which is perpendicular to the geometric axis.

A *meridian* (and therefore a meridional histologic section) is a line passing through the two poles and crossing the anatomic and geometric equators of the eye. The vertical meridian divides the eye into nasal and temporal portions, and the horizontal meridian into upper and lower sections.

Histologic sections thus can be made in meridional (vertical, horizontal, oblique) and transverse (frontal) directions, and tangential to the surface. Frontal sections tilted at a right angle to the surfaces of some tissues, such as the limbus and trabecular meshwork, are very useful for study of the anatomic details of those tissues.

Shape. The shape of the eye is determined by the structure of its layers, the ocular contents and the attachments of the rectus muscles. It is approximately round, but actually can be subdivided into two partial spheres. The anterior corneal one is more curved and comprises one sixth of the circumference of the eye; its radius of curvature is close to 8.0 mm. The posterior scleral curve is flatter, its radius of curvature being about 12.0 mm., and it comprises about five sixths of the ocular circumference. The cornea has an elliptical shape because the vertical diameter is less than the horizontal.

A consistent asymmetry is found in all eyes, the three layers being shorter nasally than temporally. This asymmetry is caused by displacement of the optic nerve center 3 mm. nasally and 1 mm. inferior to the posterior pole of the eye. On the nasal side of the eye the ciliary body and its muscle are about a millimeter shorter, so that the ora serrata is correspondingly closer to the limbus. The pupil and lens also are displaced slightly to the nasal side, causing the anterior chamber angle to be slightly narrower on this side. The anatomic asymmetry may be exaggerated in myopic eyes, especially if there is a temporal staphyloma.

Dimensions. There is a good deal of variation in the dimensions of an adult human eye, but on the average it is about 24 mm. in the anteroposterior, transverse and vertical diameters. The anteroposterior diameter may vary the most, being 21 to 26 mm. in the normal eye. It may be as small as 20 mm. in hypermetropia and as large as 29 mm. in myopia (Stenström, 1946). The transverse and vertical diameters vary less, the extremes being 23 to 25 mm. At birth the anteroposterior diameter is about 16 to 17 mm. There is an increase to 22.5 or 23 mm. by three years of age, and the final increase occurs by age 13 (Sorsby and Sheridan, 1960).

The weight of the eye is about 7.5 gm., and its volume is 6.5 cc.

Surface Anatomy. Anteriorly the external scleral sulcus indicates the junction of the cornea and sclera in an area known as the limbus. Small vessels frequently can be seen to emerge from the sclera in this region. In the region of the pars plana of the ciliary body about 4 mm. posterior to the limbus, an intrascleral nerve loop accompanied by pigmented melanocytes may be seen in one or another quadrant of the eye. This branch of the long posterior ciliary nerve emerges from the sclera and then returns to the ciliary body. Anterior to the rectus muscle insertions, the channels of the anterior ciliary arteries and veins can be seen piercing the sclera. There are two arteries for each rectus muscle, except the lateral rectus, which has only one. The arteries often branch before entering the sclera. The rectus muscle tendons insert into the sclera as follows:

	DISTANCE OF MIDPOINT OF INSERTION FROM CORNEA (MM.)	DISTANCE FROM NEAREST POINT OF INSERTION TO CORNEA (MM.)	DISTANCE FROM FARTHEST POINT OF INSERTION TO CORNEA (MM.)	WIDTH OF TENDON (MM.)
Medial rectus	5.5	5.5	6.0	10.3–10.8
Lateral rectus	6.9	6.7	7.0	9.2– 9.7
Superior rectus	7.0–7.7	6.5–6.7	9.0–11.0	10.6–11.0
Inferior rectus	6.6–6.9	5.5	8.0	9.8–10.3

The insertions of the medial and lateral recti form a fairly straight line, while those of the superior and inferior recti are curved slightly forward and obliquely, with the nasal ends being closer to the cornea than the temporal.

A view of the posterior eye shows the optic nerve with its surrounding meningeal sheaths (Fig. 2–3). Twenty short posterior ciliary arteries and about ten short posterior ciliary nerves all pierce the sclera in a ring around the optic nerve, with those on the nasal side closer to the nerve and those on the temporal side farther away. Two long ciliary arteries and nerves enter the sclera on either side of the nerve close to the horizontal meridian, the nasal ones 3.6 mm. and the temporal 3.9 mm. from the nerve. Their courses can be traced forward beneath the sclera along the horizontal meridian for a considerable distance as they remain in the suprachoroidal space. Additional long ciliary arteries and nerves may be located in different positions, most commonly on the inferior half of the eye where they pierce the sclera more anteriorly than the horizontal ones.

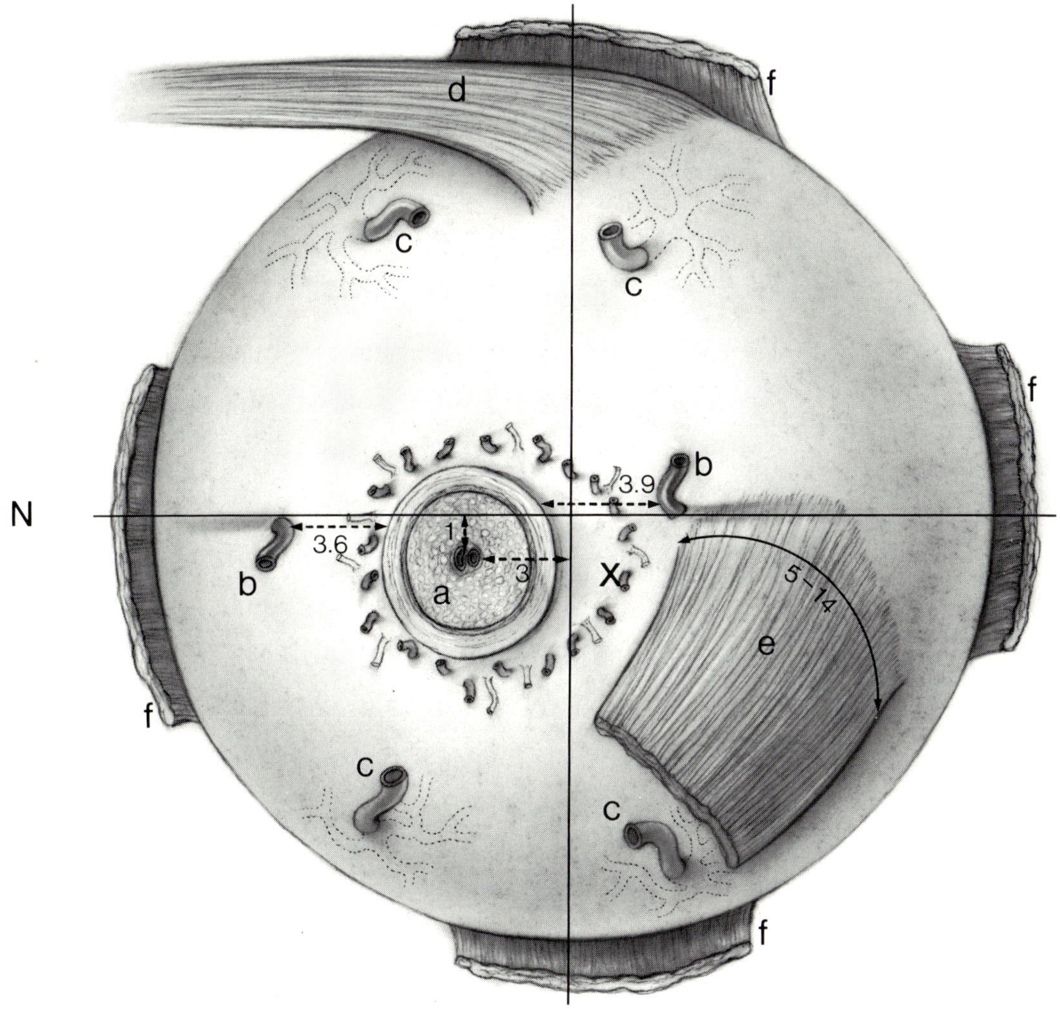

Figure 2–3. Drawing of the posterior eye. T-temporal; N-nasal. The optic nerve (a) with its central vessels and surrounding meningeal sheaths is seen. Its center is located 3 mm. nasal and 1 mm. inferior to the posterior pole of the eye. Surrounding it are the short posterior ciliary arteries and nerves. The approximate position of the macula is at (x). Along the horizontal meridian which bisects the eye are the long posterior ciliary arteries and nerves (b). The exits of four vortex veins are shown, one for each quadrant (c). The curved, oblique insertions of the superior oblique (d) and inferior oblique (e) muscles are seen. The cut ends of the four rectus muscles are at (f).

The vortex veins can be seen from the posterior side. These veins drain the venous system of the choroid, ciliary body and iris. Vortex veins were studied ophthalmoscopically by Rutnin (1967), who found 1478 of these veins in the choroid of 200 normal eyes. He discussed the presence or absence of the main trunk of the vortex vein within the choroid. If the vein was absent, only its branches were found in the choroid and entered the scleral canal directly. If the vein was incomplete, some tributaries were found to enter the scleral canal along with the vortex vein. His findings are as follows:

TYPES	MAIN TRUNK VORTEX VEIN ABSENT	TWO INCOMPLETE	THREE INCOMPLETE	FOUR COMPLETE WITH AMPULLA	TOTAL
Number	177	17	640	644	1478
Percentage	12.0	1.13	43.30	43.57	100

It is seen that each eye contains about seven vortex veins. Among these veins, more were found nasally than temporally. The internal scleral opening of the vortices varied in position from a location at the equator to 6.36 mm. posterior to the equator. The most common location was 3.0 mm. posterior to the equator. Rutnin compared his findings with those of Fuchs (1884) and furnished the arc distances between scleral exits of the vortex veins and the limbus in the following table:

		UPPER HALF		LOWER HALF		OVERALL
		Temporal	*Nasal*	*Temporal*	*Nasal*	
Present survey	Range (mm.)	20–25	17–22.25	13.75–22.5	14.75–25.0	13.75–25.0
	Avg. (mm.)	22.75	20.52	18.12	18.47	19.86
Fuchs	Avg. (mm.)	20.2	19.3	17.4	18.0	

The oblique muscle insertions can also be seen from the posterior side of the eye. The *superior oblique* muscle inserts temporal to the vertical meridian of the eye. It has a long, oblique, curved insertion with its concavity anterior. The length of the insertion varies between 7 and 18 mm. and most of it is behind the equator (Fig. 2–4). The obliquity of the insertion causes the anterior edge of the insertion to be about 12 to 14 mm. and the posterior edge 17 to 19 mm. from the limbus. The anterior edge may be close to the lateral insertion of the superior rectus, whereas the posterior edge may be as much as 14 mm. posterior to the medial insertion of the superior rectus.

The *inferior oblique* muscle either has a very short tendon, or the muscle itself inserts directly into the sclera. The line of insertion varies between 5 and 14 mm. in length; it is oblique and curved, with its concavity anterior. The posterior insertional margin is 3 to 6 mm. anterior to the edge of the optic nerve, about 1 mm. inferior to it, and 1 to 2 mm. from the fovea. The lower temporal vortex vein may lie close to the posterior edge of the muscle near its insertion.

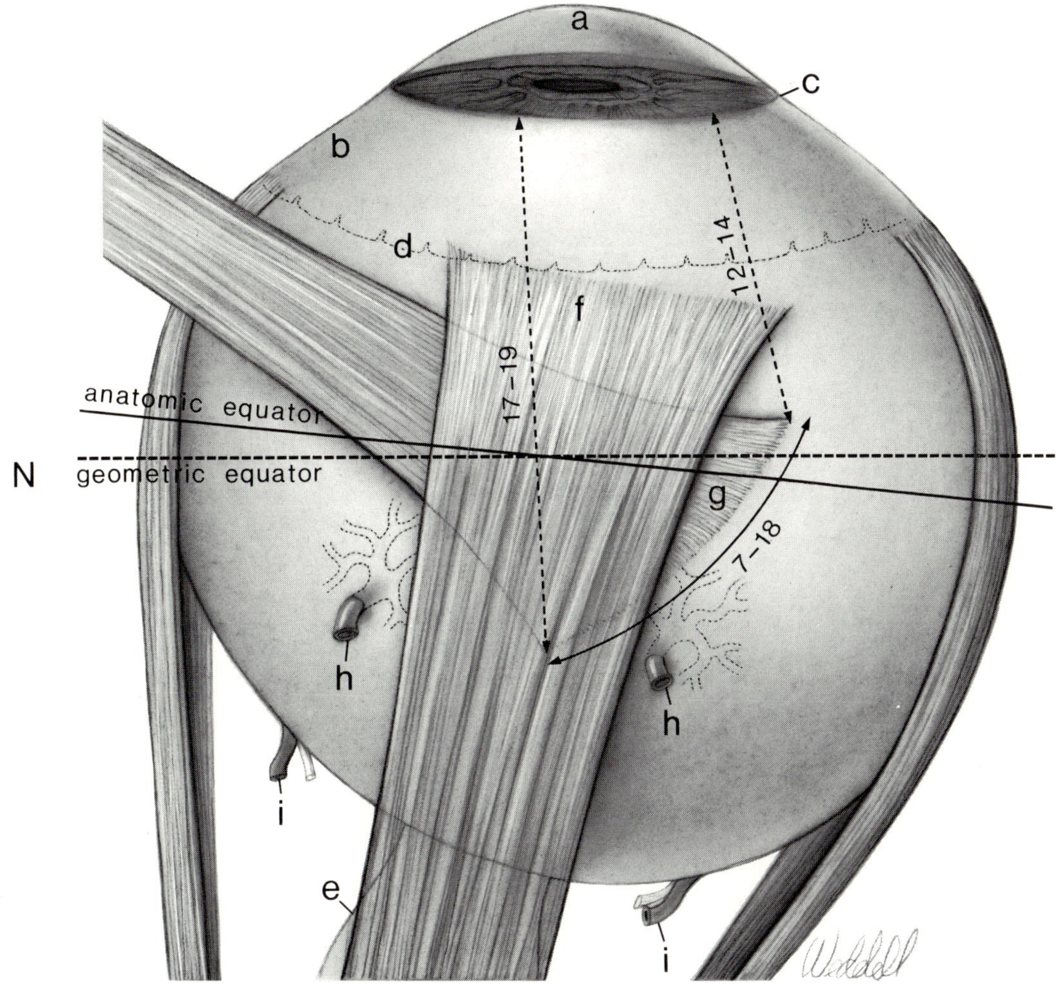

Figure 2–4. Drawing of the upper half of the eye. T-temporal; N-nasal. The contrasting degree of curvature of the cornea (a) and sclera (b) are evident. At the limbus (c), where they join, is the external scleral sulcus. The relation of the ora serrata (d) to the surface is shown. The nasal displacement of the optic nerve (e) with respect to the posterior pole of the eye makes the three layers of the temporal eye longer than those on the nasal side. The slightly curved oblique insertion of the superior rectus muscle is at (f), and the tendinous oblique insertion of the superior oblique muscle is at (g). Two vortex veins are seen (h), and the long posterior ciliary arteries and nerves are at (i).

Some surface measurements are important for histologic as well as surgical procedures. The conjunctiva at the limbus terminates at Bowman's layer of the cornea, which is the anteriormost extension of the limbus. The most posterior extension of the angle of the anterior chamber is 2.0 mm. posterior to the limbus. The iris root lies just in front of the angle. The ora serrata is closer to the limbus on the nasal than the temporal side and can be located by measuring backward 6 mm. on the nasal and 7 mm. on the temporal sides. From the ora serrata to the equator is 6 to 8 mm., and from the equator to the macula is 18 to 20 mm. The average distances from the ora serrata to the disc is 32.5 mm. on the temporal side, 27 mm. nasally, and 31 mm. superiorly and inferiorly. The macula is 2.2 mm. above and to the nasal side of the medial border of the insertion of the inferior oblique muscle (Stallard, 1950).

REFERENCES

Fuchs, E.: Studies on the normal anatomy of the eye. Graefe's Arch. Ophthal. *30*:1, 1884.

Rutnin, U.: Fundus appearance in normal eye. I. The choroid. Amer. J. Ophthal. *64*:821, 1967.

Sorsby, A., and Sheridan, M.: The eye at birth: Measurement of the principal diameters in forty-eight cadavers. J. Anat. *94*:192, 1960.

Stallard, H. B.: Eye Surgery. Baltimore, The Williams & Wilkins Co., 1950, p. 499.

Stenström, S.: Untersuchungen über die Variation und Kovariation der optischen Elemente des menshlichen Auges. Acta Ophthal. *26*:1, 1946.

Straatsma, B. R., Foos, R. Y., and Spencer, L. M.: The retina-topography and clinical correlations. Symposium on the Retina and Retinal Surgery. Trans. New Orleans Acad. Ophthal., 1969, p. 1.

Chapter Three

THE CORNEA

The cornea and sclera form a tough protective envelope which encloses the ocular tissues. The optical property of the cornea, however, is its main function, for the interface between the air and the corneal surface is the principal refracting surface of the dioptric system of the eye. The cornea is transparent, avascular, viscoelastic and quite resistant to deformation. Since it is one of the large avascular tissues of the body, its nutrition is of keen interest to the physiologist and biochemist. The processes which maintain the transparency of the cornea have been studied for many years by individuals working in diverse fields, yet these mechanisms are incompletely understood. In view of its histologic appearance, it is remarkable that the cornea is so clear when examined clinically. The refractive index of this tissue changes very little with increasing age, and its shape also remains quite constant.

Because of its exposed position the cornea commonly sustains injury from foreign bodies and sharp objects. It has a good inherent resistance to infection, however, and in spite of its avascularity has a remarkable ability to heal penetrating wounds. The collagen fibrils of Bowman's layer in the superficial stroma are randomly distributed and form a tightly packed meshwork. For this reason Bowman's layer is very resistant to the effect of shearing forces, and it offers considerable protection against the penetration of foreign bodies and the spread of epithelial infections into the corneal stroma.

PHYSIOLOGY AND BIOCHEMISTRY

The cornea must be quite transparent in order for the eye to have good vision. For this reason rather strict limitations exist as to the structural composition, organization and nutrition of this tissue. Several factors contribute to the corneal transparency and to its maintenance: (1) the regularity and smoothness of the epithelium; (2) the absence of blood vessels; and (3) the organization of the corneal collagen, ground substance, and cells. This depends on (a) the chemical composition and hydration of the tissues, which is a function of (b) their metabolism and nutrition.

Epithelium of Cornea. The corneal epithelium differs from the surrounding conjunctival epithelium in a number of ways. First, the corneal epithelium is uniform in thickness and is quite regular in the arrangement of the cells; second, it is unpigmented, except in the extreme periphery in dark races; and third, its cells are arranged to provide an orderly replacement of the surface cells as they desquamate. Any slight epithelial irregularity in the cornea is compensated for by an overlying complex fluid layer, the *precorneal tear film*.

The thickness of the precorneal tear film has been reported to range from 6 to 20 μm., depending on the eye and the technique used to measure it. The most recent and probably most accurate measurements, however, show it to be around 7 μm. in thickness. The exact physical structure of the precorneal tear film is not entirely clear. It is believed to exist as a two-layer or two-phase fluid, whose outermost layer is composed of a lipid produced by the sebaceous glands of the eyelids and caruncle. Beneath this lipid is a second layer which is composed mostly of water derived from the lacrimal fluid and some mucoprotein from the conjunctival goblet cells. These two layers are not affected significantly by the forces of gravity, and for this reason the layers can correctly be called a film. The replacement of this film depends on the forces generated by the movement of the eyelids. Recent studies suggest that the precorneal film is held in position against the surface epithelial cells by a structural specialization of their surfaces in the form of microplicae.

An additional structural specialization of the surface epithelial cells which is probably related to the tear film has been described by Blümcke and associates (1967). They studied these cells with the electron microscope and found an osmiophilic lipid layer measuring 30 A. in thickness in and upon the outer leaflet of the anterior cell membrane. The integrity of this lipid layer was maintained in tissue cultures of corneal epithelium, indicating that the epithelial cells are probably responsible for its synthesis.

Avascularity. The normal cornea is avascular, and new vessels invade it only if there is a disturbance of the corneal nutrition. This absence of vessels allows the cornea to maintain its remarkable degree of transparency.

Organization of Tissues. The special organization of the collagen, ground substance and cells of the corneal stroma provides the single most important factor responsible for the clarity of the cornea. The collagen fibrils are organized into sheets or lamellae averaging 2 μm. in thickness; within these lamellae the fibrils are parallel and run the diameter of the cornea. The fibrils differ from ordinary collagen in thinness and uniformity in diameter; they also are uniformly spaced.

The mucoprotein and glycoprotein in the ground substance of the stroma are believed to be responsible for maintaining the very even separation of the collagen fibrils. The refractive index of the ground substance has been calculated to be 1.34 and that of the collagen 1.47 (Maurice, 1957). Such a difference in refractive index should result in an undesirable scattering of light; the cornea, however, scatters less than 1 per cent of light impinging upon it. Maurice (1957) offers an explanation for the high degree of transmittance of the stroma based on the arrangement of the collagen fibrils (Fig. 3–26). If the collagen fibrils are uniformly separated so that they form an orderly structure resembling a three-dimensional array of diffraction gratings, the rays scattered by the system will interact with each other in an organized way. The result of this interaction is the elimination of scattered light by destructive interference. Thus, as long as the fibrils are properly oriented within the lattice and separated from each other by less than one half wavelength of light, the cornea remains transparent. Some evidence for this theory is found by observing that pressure exerted on the cornea makes it opaque; when the pressure is released, the corneal transparency is immediately restored.

Maurice's theory, as originally stated, is based upon the absolute regularity in the disposition of the collagen fibrils within the lamellae. There are some species, however, which have rather transparent corneas even though Bowman's layer, with its irregularly oriented collagen fibrils, occupies the larger portion of the cornea. According to Maurice (1969), the degree of irregularity permitted by his theory is as yet undefined; it is possible that sufficient regularity may remain in Bowman's layer for his theory to hold true. The sclera, on the other hand, has collagen fibrils which show considerable variation in size as well as orientation, yet when its water content is changed, the sclera becomes transparent. Some investigators (Schwarz and Keyserlink, 1966; Smith, 1969) believe that the corneal transparency results from the distribution of water between the ground substance and collagen in such a way that their refractive indices have a similar value. This suggestion, according to Maurice (1969), is not compatible with the electron microscopic appearance of the collagen fibrils in the cornea at various degrees of hydration, or the birefringence and x-ray diffraction studies of the corneal collagen fibrils.

The corneal stromal cells are thin, flattened and elongated, and their location between the corneal lamellae does not disturb the lamellae or collagen fibrils or alter the corneal transparency significantly. These cells, however, are responsible for much of the 1 per cent of light normally scattered by the cornea.

Chemical Composition and Hydration of Tissues. The organization of the corneal stroma depends on its chemical composition and hydration.

Most analyses of the chemical composition of the cornea have been made on whole cornea, but there are significant differences between the epithelium and endothelium, as compared to the corneal stroma. The lipid content of the epithelium and endothelium is about 100 times that of the stroma; such a difference is to be expected because of the lipid content of the cell membranes. The transfer of substances through the intact cornea is largely determined by phase solubility; epithelium and endothelium are most permeable to those substances possessing a fat soluble phase, and the stroma is permeable to those having a water soluble phase (Adler, 1965).

The chemical composition of the cornea is roughly as follows (Maurice and Riley, 1968):

Substance	*Per Cent*
Water	78.0
Collagen	15.0
Other proteins	5.0
Keratin sulfates	0.7
Chondroitin sulfates	0.3
Salts	1.0

Two types of glycosaminoglycans (mucopolysaccharide) chains composed of (1) keratosulfate, (2) chondroitin sulfate and chondroitin are contained in the ground substance of the cornea, and it appears from recent studies that there is a great deal of heterogeneity among these compounds (Maurice and Riley, 1968). Their degree of sulfation varies, depending upon the relative amounts of chondroitin or chondroitin sulfate present. Laurent and Anseth (1961) have suggested a molecular weight of 40,000 for the chondroitin polymers, while the smaller keratosulfates vary from 4000 to 14,000 in molecular weight. The keratosulfates may account for as much as 70 per cent of the total mucopolysaccharides.

The cornea has a distinct affinity for water, so that if excised corneal tissue is placed in water or even in physiologic solutions it becomes swollen or turgesced; at the same time the stroma becomes less transparent. For a variety of reasons it is believed that the ground substance rather than the collagen takes up most of the water, since it has been shown that the collagen fibrils themselves are not altered during the swelling process. Some mechanism must exist to maintain corneal thickness by counteracting its tendency to imbibe water and to swell. Removal of the corneal epithelium leads to stromal edema and swelling in the area of the defect. As soon as the epithelium regenerates, the edema disappears. Removal of corneal endothelium also results in edema and stromal swelling, but because of the poorer recuperative powers of the endothelium the resulting edema may be more prolonged and severe. Small areas of endothelial loss lead only to localized edema, and the surrounding endothelial cells usually spread out to fill the gap, after which the edema and swelling disappear. The epithelium and endothelium, therefore, are important for the maintenance of corneal thickness and detergescence.

The movement of fluid into the stroma must result from internal forces within the tissue that manifest themselves as the *swelling pressure* of the cornea. The swelling pressure has been measured in various ways, either by balancing it with a concentration of any nonpenetrating solute whose osmotic pressure equals the swelling pressure, or more directly by determining the mechanical force necessary to prevent the entrance of fluid and swelling. Mechanical pressures of 60 mm. Hg must be applied to pieces of corneal stroma immersed in saline to maintain normal corneal transparency and hydration. Therefore, the swelling pressure of the cornea exceeds the colloidal osmotic pressure of the blood plasma by at least 40 mm. Hg.

Metabolism and Nutrition. Evidence has accumulated that aerobic glycolysis plays an important role in the metabolic mechanism for removal of water. Oxygen is important because, if it is lacking, the cornea will absorb water. The cornea will become hydrated if its temperature is reduced, but in the presence of oxygen the process is reversed after warming. Metabolic inhibitors such as ouabain will also lead to corneal swelling. It is fairly clear that the epithelium and endothelium as limiting membranes are involved in the active maintenance of the corneal thickness, and that metabolic energy is required for this purpose. The exact mechanism employed by these cell layers to maintain detergescence is not known. The presence of a metabolic pump which can move certain ions out of the stroma has been investigated. According to some investigators the epithelium transports sodium, while according to others it transports chloride. These ions are, however, moved toward the stroma and should then bring water into rather than out of the stroma. An endothelial pump is not well characterized as yet, and there is no evidence that any ion is selectively transported there.

Most of the corneal nutrients are received from the aqueous humor and the tear film. Some nutrients enter the peripheral cornea from the pericorneal vessels, but they supply only the peripheral cornea. Glucose and oxygen are of primary significance for the metabolism of the cornea, and they pass into the cornea across both the epithelium and the endothelium, the glucose coming almost entirely from the aqueous humor. The corneal oxygen is derived from the air across the tear fluid and epithelium and from the aqueous humor across the endothelium.

Kinoshita (1962) has shown that the cornea exhibits a high rate of aerobic glycolysis (in common with the brain, retina and lens). Even in the presence of a high oxygen tension more glucose is broken down to lactic acid than to carbon dioxide. The hexose-monophosphate shunt is active in accounting for the breakdown of as much as 35 per cent of the glucose utilized, the remainder following the Embden-Meyerhoff glycolytic pathways (Kinoshita et al., 1955; Kinoshita and Masurat, 1959).

EMBRYOLOGY

During the fifth week of pregnancy (5 to 8 mm. stage) the cells of the associated mesoderm extend into the optic cup beyond its anterior margin to become aligned beneath and in close relation to the single layer of surface ectoderm. A matrix exists beneath the epithelium, and it becomes infiltrated by fibrillary processes which are formed by the mesodermal cells. By the end of the sixth week (10 to 14 mm. stage), the early corneal endothelium has appeared, originating near the surface ectoderm from the deepest layer of mesoderm. It first appears as a single layer of cells which differentiates from the periphery toward the center of the future cornea. The ectoderm covering this developing mesoderm now consists of two layers of cells that will eventually differentiate into the corneal epithelium. During this period of gestation a second wave of mesoderm extends in to form the primitive corneal substantia propria; this activity is restricted initially to the periphery, but by the early part of the seventh week (17 to 22 mm.) it is possible to stain fine collagen fibers in this tissue. Near the end of the seventh week the mesodermal cells have extended across the entire cornea, and numerous collagen fibrils can be identified in the matrix of the cornea. During the eighth week (28 to 30 mm. stage), the primitive cornea and the sclera can be distinguished from each other as collagen fibers become more abundant in the corneal matrix than in that of the sclera. Continued development of the epithelium and stroma during the twelfth week (50 to 70 mm. stage) causes the cornea to become thicker than the sclera, and the limbal region becomes apparent as a result of differentiation of the outer sclera.

During the fourth month (70 to 110 mm. stage) Bowman's layer and Descemet's membrane appear, the latter at about the 60 to 75 mm. stage and the former at about 103 mm., but Descemet's membrane may be evident as early as the 50 mm. stage (third month). The shorter radius of curvature of the cornea compared to that of the sclera becomes evident at this time. The corneal collagen fibrils have reached their full thickness by the 85 mm. stage (Schwarz, 1961). Further differentiation of the two-layered epithelium commences during the sixth month (160 to 200 mm. stage) with the formation of a layer of polyhedral cells between the two layers. At this time the horizontal diameter of the cornea is around 5.0 mm. It increases to 6.5 mm. during the seventh month (200 to 240 mm.), when the corneal curvature has reached its final dimensions. During the final months of pregnancy there is a slight increase in corneal thickness and diameter, so that at birth the cornea measures 10.0 mm. in diameter. After birth it continues to develop, reaching its full dimensions by the end of the first year.

GROSS ANATOMY

Anteriorly in the interpalpebral fissure the corneal epithelium is in contact with the air, being separated from it by the precorneal film, and with the mucous membrane of the upper and lower lids. *Posteriorly* the corneal endothelium is bathed by the aqueous humor. *Peripherally* the cornea blends with the conjunctiva, the episclera and the sclera in a transition zone, the limbus. At the limbal junction there is a gradual change in the arrangement, size and direction of the corneal collagen, an increase in thickness of the epithelium, development of a vascular conjunctival connective tissue and the disappearance of Descemet's membrane and Bowman's layer. At the limbus there is a gradual transition of clear cornea to opaque sclera, the superficial third becoming opaque earlier than the deeper two thirds.

The shape of the cornea is that of an elliptical meniscus when viewed from the front, with the horizontal diameter slightly greater than the vertical (Fig. 3–1 *A*). The elliptical shape of the anterior corneal surface is produced by the greater extension of the more opaque limbal tissue onto the cornea in the superior and inferior portion, making the vertical part of the cornea shorter (10.6 mm.) than the horizontal (11.7 mm.) These measurements are approximately 0.1 mm. less in the female. When viewed from behind, the corneal contour is circular and its diameter is 11.7 mm. The superficial area of the cornea is 1.3 $cm.^2$ or one fourteenth of the total area of the globe (Maurice, 1969).

If the eyeball is viewed from the side, the cornea is seen to have a greater curvature than that of the sclera; however, the corneal surface does not protrude much above that of the sclera because of the flattening of the tissues at the junction between the cornea and sclera (the external scleral sulcus) (Fig. 3–1 *B*). Although the anterior and posterior surfaces of the cornea are not exactly parallel throughout the whole cornea, there is an optically important region in the central cornea measuring approximately 4 mm. in diameter (Fig. 3–1 *C*) where the two surfaces are fairly parallel. In this zone the shape of the cornea is perfectly spherical, while peripheral to it the cornea is slightly flattened. The radius of curvature of the anterior corneal surface in the central area in the adult male is 7.8 mm. Depending on the method of measurement, the radius of the posterior surface is 6.2 to 6.8 mm., the accepted average measurement being 6.5 mm.

The central cornea has a thickness of 0.52 mm. when measured optically (Maurice, 1969), with little difference in thickness between males and females. Toward the periphery the cornea increases in thickness up to 0.67 mm. near the limbus (Fig. 3–1 *C*). Martola and Baum (1968) have shown that the limbal thickness is reduced from 0.67 mm. in the fourth decade to 0.63 mm. in the sixth decade of life. A plane can be drawn through the base of the cornea across the limbus to measure the corneal height, which is approximately 2.6 mm. (Fig. 3–1 *C*). There is some variation in height depending on the radius of curvature; corneas with shorter radii are greater in height. In

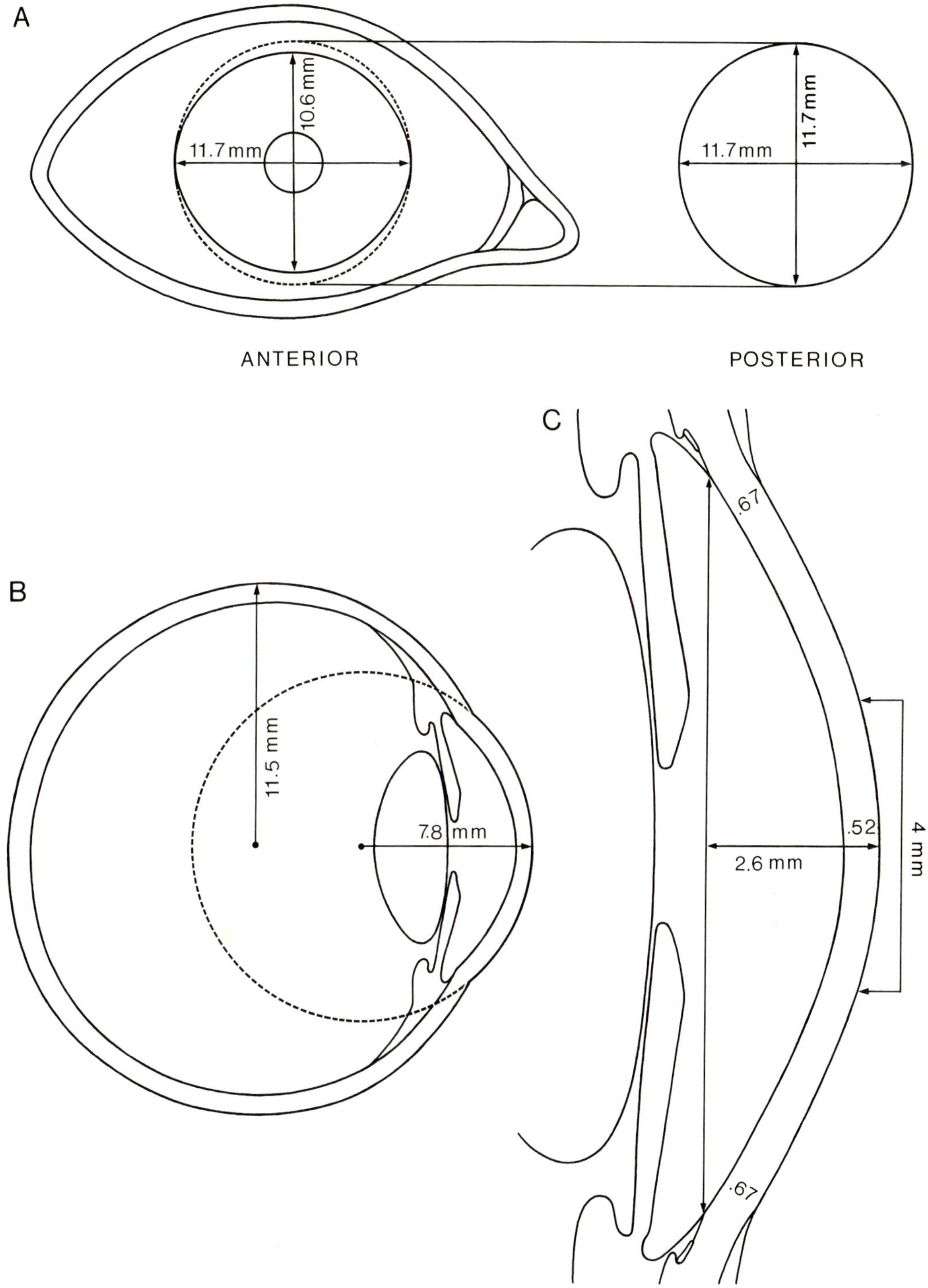

Figure 3-1. These three diagrams show: *A*, The elliptical shape of the anterior and the round shape of the posterior corneal edges; also the vertical and horizontal diameters of the anterior and the posterior cornea.

B, The radius of curvature of the cornea and of the sclera.

C, The corneal height and the central 4 mm. of the cornea which is optically important; also the comparative thickness of the central and peripheral cornea.

keratoconus the central cornea becomes ectatic, increasing the central height only, whereas in keratoglobus the entire cornea protrudes forward, noticeably increasing the total corneal height.

INNERVATION

The cornea has one of the richest sensory nerve supplies of any eye tissue. Most of the nerves are derived from the ophthalmic division of the fifth cranial nerve (Mawas, 1951). Some superficial nerve branches enter the peripheral cornea from the subconjunctival and episcleral region, but the principal nerves enter through the sclera. The long ciliary nerves provide the principal nerve supply, and they branch in the outer part of the choroid near the ora serrata region. The branches extend forward in the ciliary body and supraciliary space to the region of the anterior sclera (Zander and Weddell, 1951). Some nerve branches enter the sclera and are widely distributed to the anterior sclera all around the limbus, but most of them pass into the middle third of the peripheral cornea as myelinated nerve bundles of varying size, their branches interconnecting with adjacent nerves. Eventually 70 to 80 large nerves are formed, and most of these lose their myelin sheaths in the peripheral 2 to 3 mm. of the cornea (Fig. 3–2).

In many eyes a few small myelinated branches may continue into the cornea for some distance. Those bundles which become unmyelinated continue to have a sheath of Schwann for long distances. Considerable dichotomous and trichotomous branching occurs throughout the stroma; and many branches interconnect as they traverse the stroma. With the use of silver stains nerves are found in all layers of the cornea, but they are sparse in the posterior third, and it is probable that the region of Descemet's membrane does not contain nerves in the human (Mawas, 1951). Wolter (1957) has demonstrated a nerve supply into the region of Descemet's membrane in the rabbit. The nerves become smaller and smaller as they extend into the central cornea, eventually losing their sheath of Schwann and terminating as "bare" filaments in the corneal stromal collagen and around the cells. These filaments are beaded for some distance prior to their termination.

A particularly well developed plexus of nerves congregates in the region of Bowman's layer, finally penetrating this layer to form the epithelial plexus. After entering the epithelium, filaments are distributed under and into the basal layer, lying between the cells, surrounding them, and then extending forward to the more superficial layers. Finally, all the epithelial layers are innervated up to the two surface layers of cells. The nerves end in the epithelium as fine beaded filaments, but there are no specialized nerve endings (Whitear, 1960; Abraham, 1955; Toussaint, 1958). The question of nerve endings within the epithelial cytoplasm was debated for many years, but electron microscopy shows that the nerves terminate between cells. Electron microscopic study shows the tiny bundles and single axones to be enfolded in or surrounded by the epithelial cell membranes (Fig. 3–3).

By electron microscopy we have encountered corneal nerves frequently in the epithelium, Bowman's layer and anterior stroma. All have been unmyelinated and are wrapped by Schwann cells in the stroma but not in the corneal epithelium. The Schwann cell wrapping ceases at the level of Bowman's layer.

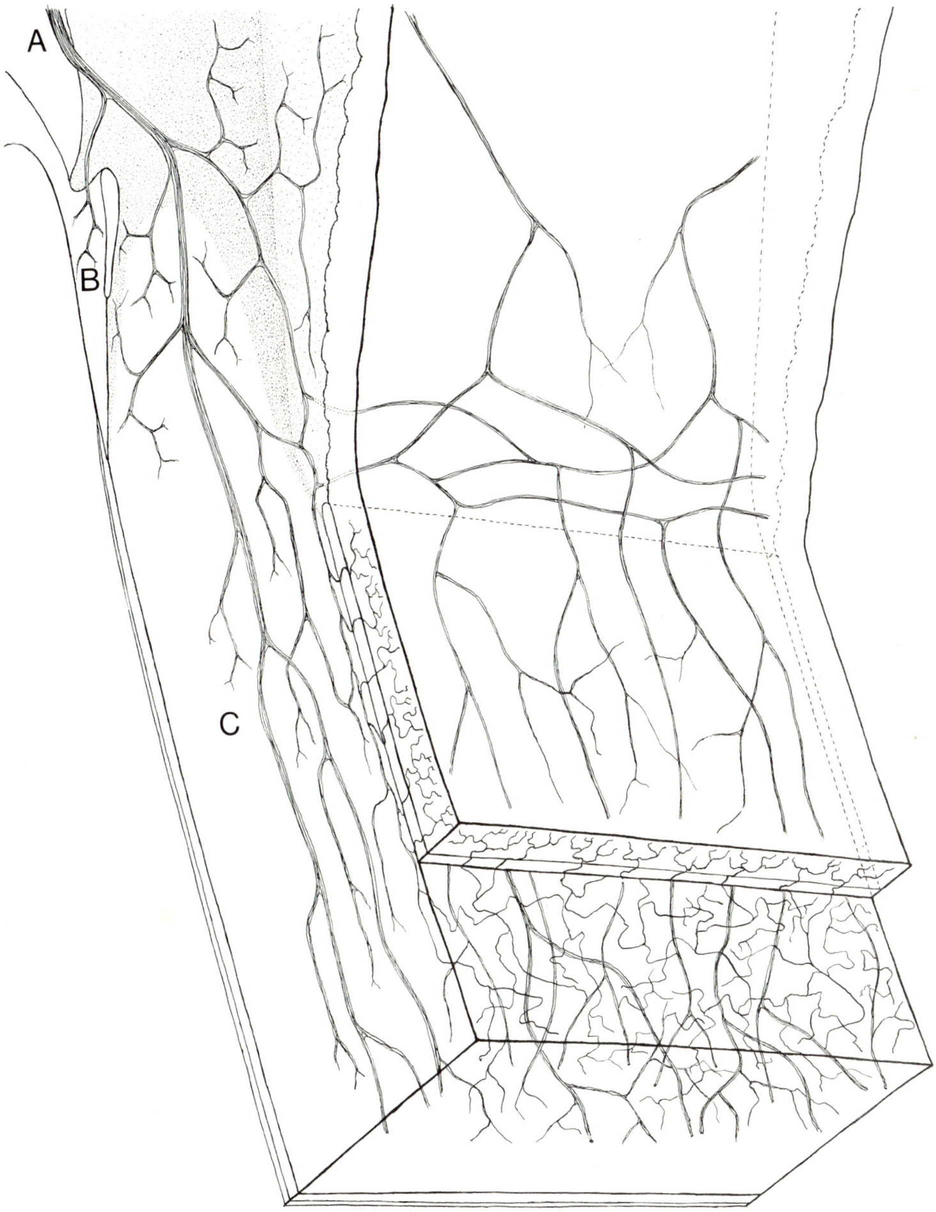

Figure 3-2. Schematic representation of the innervation of the limbus and cornea. The long ciliary nerve (A) supplies the limbal region, then sends branches into the cornea. Nerves also supply the trabecular meshwork (B) and the region of the canal of Schlemm. Note the paucity of nerves in the deep cornea (C), and their absence in the region of Descemet's membrane.

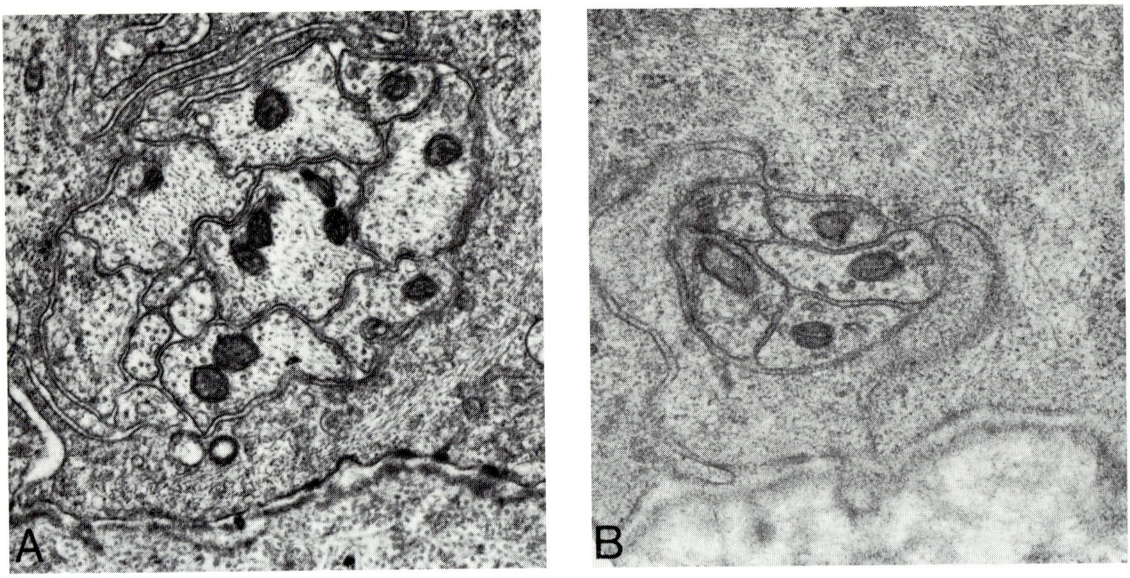

Figure 3–3. Corneal epithelium. Nerves between two basal epithelial cells. *A*, Eleven nerves in a bundle. (× 54,000.)

B, A bundle containing five nerves. There is no sheath of Schwann around any of these nerves. The nerves can be differentiated from the adjacent epithelial cells by their denser mitochondria and fewer cytoplasmic filaments. (× 45,000.)

The nerve axones have a cross-sectional diameter varying between 1000 and 2500 A. In the basal epithelial layer the nerves are easy to recognize because of their mitochondrial type, which is longer and denser than that of the adjacent epithelial cells. Within the epithelium the nerves become single axons and are quite difficult to distinguish from the epithelial cytoplasm in the region of the epithelial interdigitations. We have not as yet encountered nerves in the deeper central stroma.

Blood Supply

The peripheral cornea is supplied by conjunctival, episcleral and scleral vessels (Fig. 4–2). These vessels are terminal branches of the circumcorneal vessels. They ramify at different levels in the limbus. Most of them supply the sclera in the region of the canal of Schlemm. These vessels play a small part in the corneal nutrition and metabolism, since it has been shown that some constituents of plasma are present in the outer corneal stroma.

MICROSCOPIC ANATOMY

The cornea is composed of five layers (Fig. 3–4): (1) epithelium, (2) Bowman's layer, (3) stroma, (4) Descemet's membrane, and (5) endothelium.

Most textbooks include the limbus in any discussion of the cornea. Because of the importance of the limbus in the removal of aqueous humor and as a transition zone between the cornea and sclera, this area is considered separately in the next chapter.

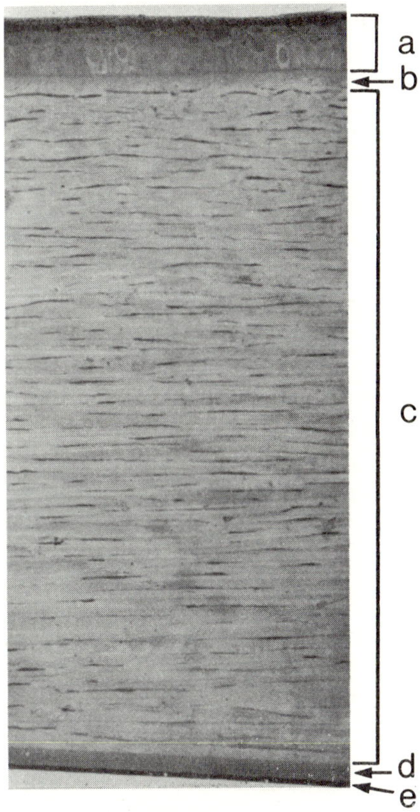

Figure 3-4. Light micrograph of a complete section of the cornea showing its five principal parts: (a) epithelium; (b) Bowman's layer; (c) stroma; (d) Descemet's layer; and (e) endothelium. Note the relative thickness of the various portions, especially that of Descemet's membrane and the endothelium. (× 200.)

EPITHELIUM (Figs. 3–4 to 3–20)

The epithelium occupies about 10 per cent of the total corneal thickness. It is composed of five to six superimposed layers of cells which have a total thickness of about 50 μm. (Fig. 3–4). The turnover time for this epithelium has been estimated to be seven days (Hanna et al., 1961). Near the termination of Bowman's layer at the corneal periphery the epithelium becomes thicker because the number of cell layers increases to eight or ten. Beneath the epithelium and closely related to the basal layer of cells is a thin basement membrane which can be demonstrated easily with special staining techniques such as the periodic acid-Schiff reaction. The basement membrane has a uniform thickness across the cornea and becomes continuous with the basement membrane of the limbal epithelium beyond the corneal periphery. In carefully prepared specimens a thin layer of granular material is found on the surface of the most superficial epithelium. It is faintly eosinophilic, strongly osmiophilic, and is probably formed by the lipid and mucoprotein of the precorneal tear film. It is continuous with a similar material over the limbal epithelium.

The epithelium has a very smooth anterior surface and is quite uniform in its thickness and cellular arrangement. Three groups of cells are identified in the epithelium: (1) a single row of basal cells; (2) the wing or polygonal cell layer, an intermediate zone two or three cells thick; and (3) two layers of flattened plate-like surface cells (Figs. 3–5 and 3–6). Lymphocytes and occasional macrophages are seen in the basal and wing cell layers.

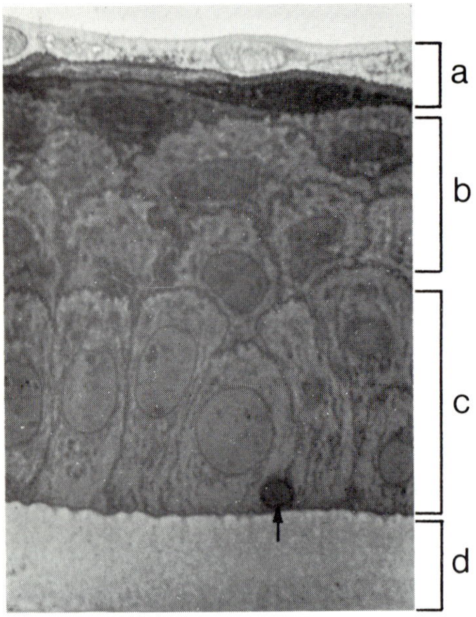

Figure 3–5. Light microphotograph of the corneal epithelium showing its cell layers: (a) surface cells; (b) wing cells; (c) basal cells. There is a lymphocyte in the basal cell layer (arrow). Bowman's layer is seen at (d). (× 1000.)

BASAL LAYER (Figs. 3–7 to 3–11)

Several varieties of cells have been described in the basal layer by use of light and electron microscopy, but except for an occasional lymphocyte the cells of the basal layer are entirely basal epithelial cells. We have not identified the dendritic, dark or other specialized cells which have been described. The basal cells are articulated with each other at their edges and rest on a fine basement membrane.

This single layer of epithelium extends across the cornea without significant variation in size or shape and becomes continuous with the same layer in the conjunctiva. The cells are tall and polygonal in shape and measure 18 μm. in height by 10 μm. in breadth. With most histologic stains the cytoplasm in these cells stains less intensely than that of the other epithelial layers. The slightly oval nucleus is about 5.7 μm. in diameter and is oriented at a right angle to the surface of the cornea. It is displaced toward the apex of the cell in the cytoplasm. Mitoses are frequently seen in this layer.

Redslob (1935) studied embryo chicken and fetal human cornea and showed for the first time that there is a basement membrane under the corneal epithelium. Loewenstein (1940) and Busacca (1949) later confirmed its presence in adult human eyes. Since that time the basement membrane has been demonstrated in almost all vertebrate corneas. The studies of Teng and Katzin (1953), LaTessa and associates (1954), and Calmettes and co-workers (1956) elucidated the histochemical and microscopic aspects of this membrane. It is periodic acid-Schiff positive, not metachromatic and stains positively with silver, behaving like reticulin. This membrane also can be dissolved by trypsin and chymotrypsin (LaTessa et al., 1954).

The epithelial cell membrane on the basal side is about 80 A. thick (Kayes and Holmberg, 1960). It is separated from the adjacent basement membrane by a very narrow space measuring 110 A. Scattered along this basal cell membrane are numerous half-desmosomes. Fine osmiophilic fib-

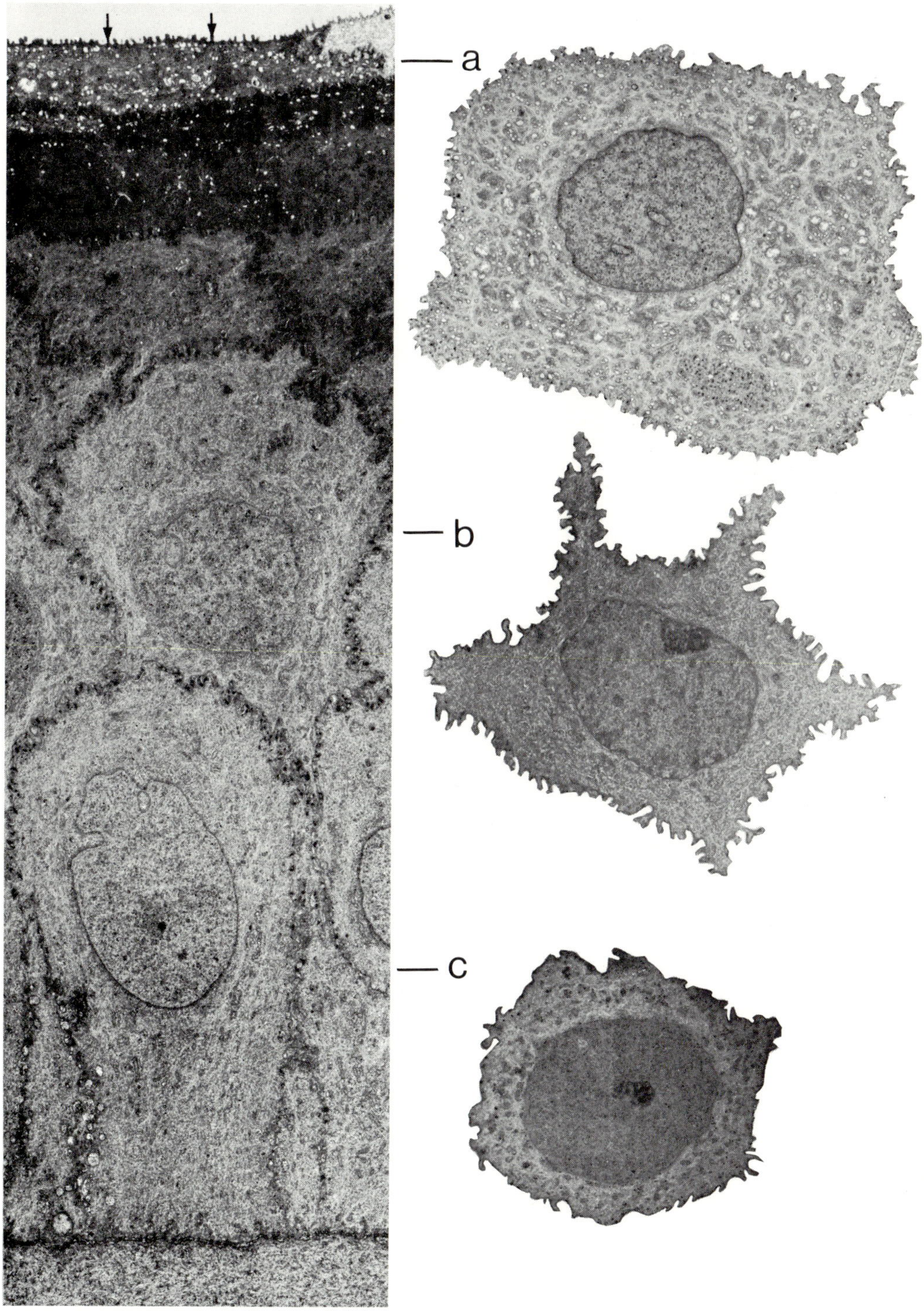

Figure 3-6. Corneal epithelium, electron micrograph. Note the surface microplicae and microvilli (arrows), and the vesicular structures in the cytoplasm of the outermost wing and surface cells. Desmosomal attachments between cells are seen as dark spots around the periphery of the cells. At the right are tangential sections of a surface (a), a wing (b), and a basal cell (c). Note their polygonal shape, the comparative size, and the cytoplasmic differences, especially the vesiculation in the surface layers. The cell borders show extensive interdigitations and a high density at the sites of desmosomes. (× 4250.)

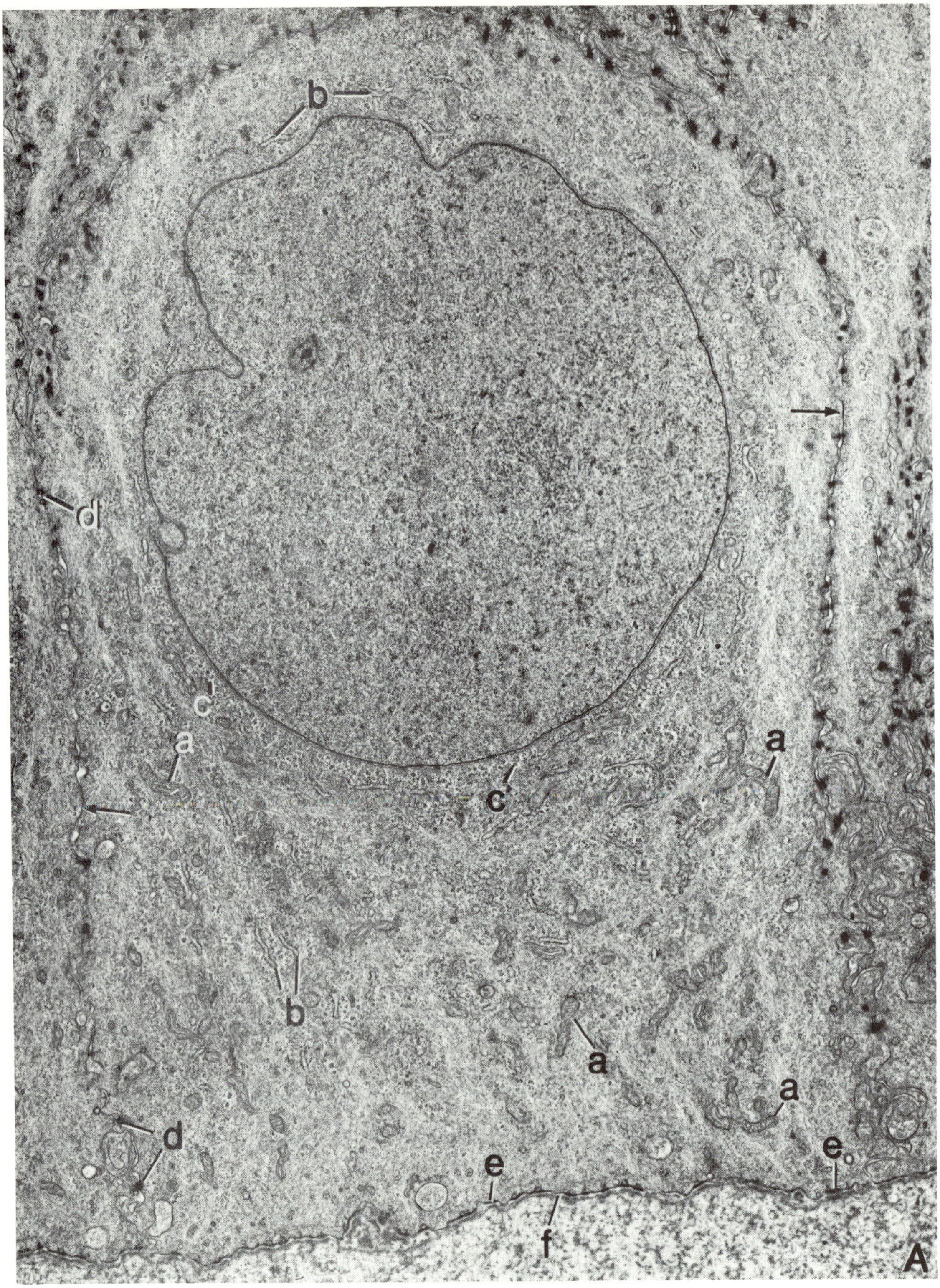

Figure 3-7. *A* and *B*, Corneal epithelium. Electron micrographs of two basal cells showing the general configuration, intercellular relations, and cytoplasmic organelles. The dense cytoplasm contains a large number of dispersed tonofilaments. The mitochondria are sparse and very small (a). The cisternae of the rough-surfaced endoplasmic reticulum are perinuclear in location and occur singly rather than in stacks (b). Free ribosomes are abundant around the

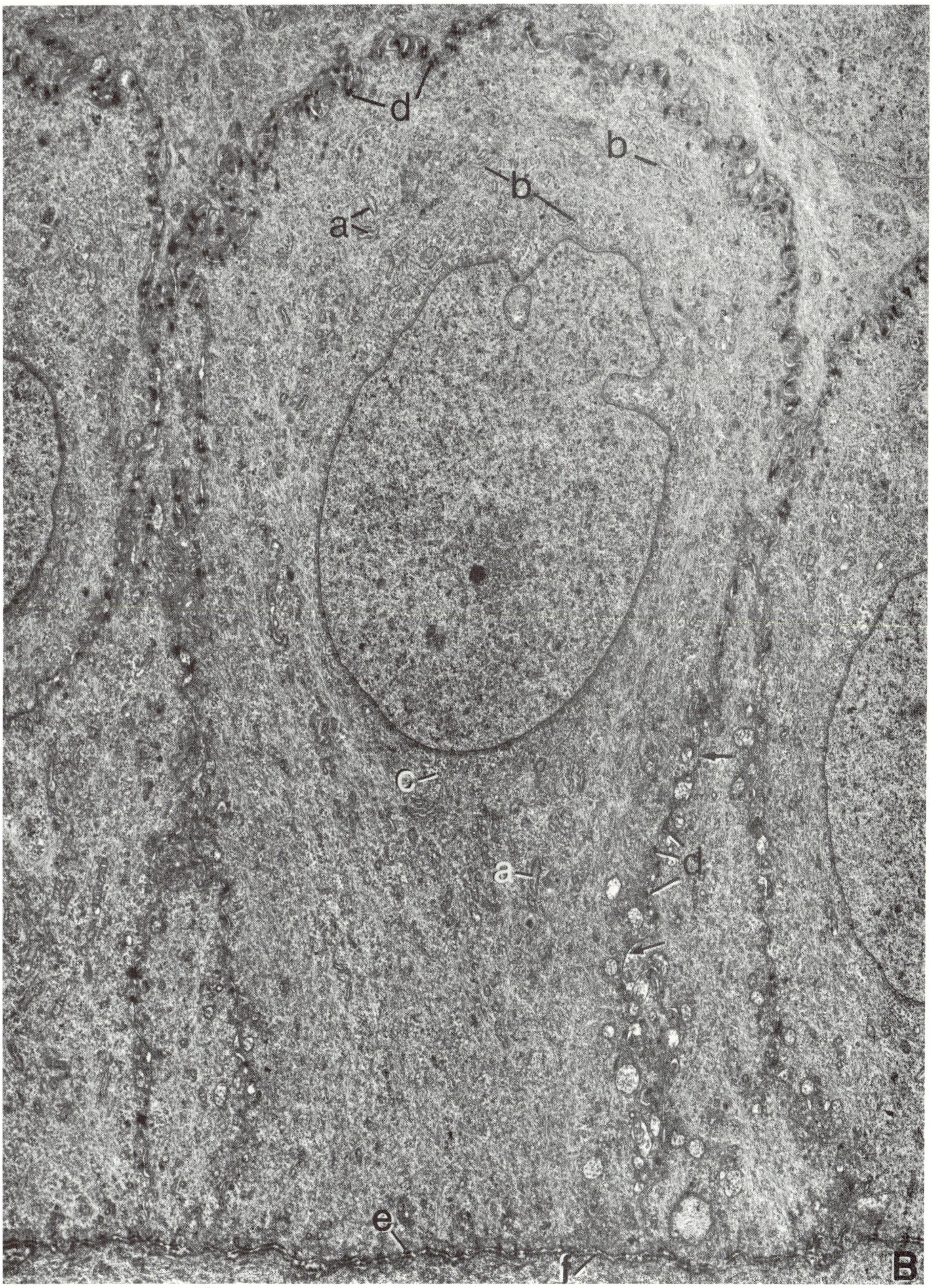

Figure 3–7. *Continued.*

nucleus (c). The Golgi apparatus is not observed in these cells. Desmosomes (d) articulate adjacent cells laterally and anteriorly, while half-desmosomes (e) are seen along the basal cell membrane. The basement membrane is clearly seen at (f). Arrows show areas of close apposition of the cell membranes. ($A = \times 8000$; $B = \times 7500$.)

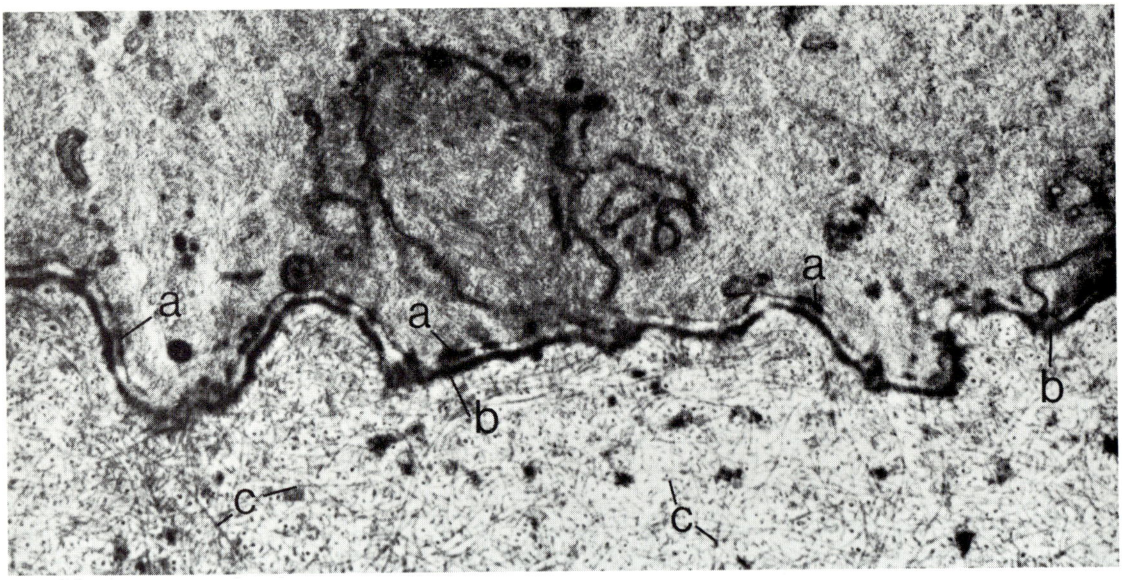

Figure 3–8. Corneal epithelium. A basal cell, its basement membrane, and Bowman's layer. Half-desmosomes (a) are seen along the basal cell membrane, with filaments extending from them to the basement membrane (b). The basement membrane is a dark osmiophilic line which is separated from the cell membrane by a less dense zone. The collagen of Bowman's layer (c) has a random disposition. (× 42,800.)

rils radiate from the half-desmosomes across the space between the cell membrane and the basement membrane to join the latter, and even extend beyond it a short distance into Bowman's layer.

Electron microscopy shows the basement membrane as a well defined osmiophilic layer measuring 480 A. in thickness beneath the basal layer of epithelium, and separated from it by a more lucent zone 230 A. in width which contains a faintly granular material, especially in the region of the half-desmosomes. Like most basement membranes it contains fine fibrils and a mucoprotein matrix.

The basement membrane is said to vary in thickness in different parts of the cornea, being thinner in the central area and thicker peripherally. However, we have not been able to detect much difference in thickness in various parts of the membrane. The membrane blends with Bowman's layer posteriorly in a very indistinct way; its anterior surface is irregular, especially opposite the half-desmosomes of the basal epithelial cell membranes. Opposite the half-desmosomes the membrane is thickened and there is a tongue-shaped extension of dense filaments from the membrane for a short

---

Figure 3–9. Corneal epithelium. Basal cell membrane specialization. *A*, A macula occludens along the lateral cell membrane (arrow). (× 162,000.)

B, Desmosomes along the lateral and anterior cell membranes (a); cytoplasmic density at the desmosome (b). The arrow indicates the intercellular space. (× 42,800.)

C, Half-desmosomes (a) along the basal cell membrane. Filaments (arrows) extend from the cell membrane to the basement membrane (b). (× 32,000.)

D, Two half-desmosomes (a). The fine filaments extend beyond the basement membrane (b) into Bowman's layer (arrows). The half-desmosomes are linked to the basement membrane by similar filaments. (× 52,000.)

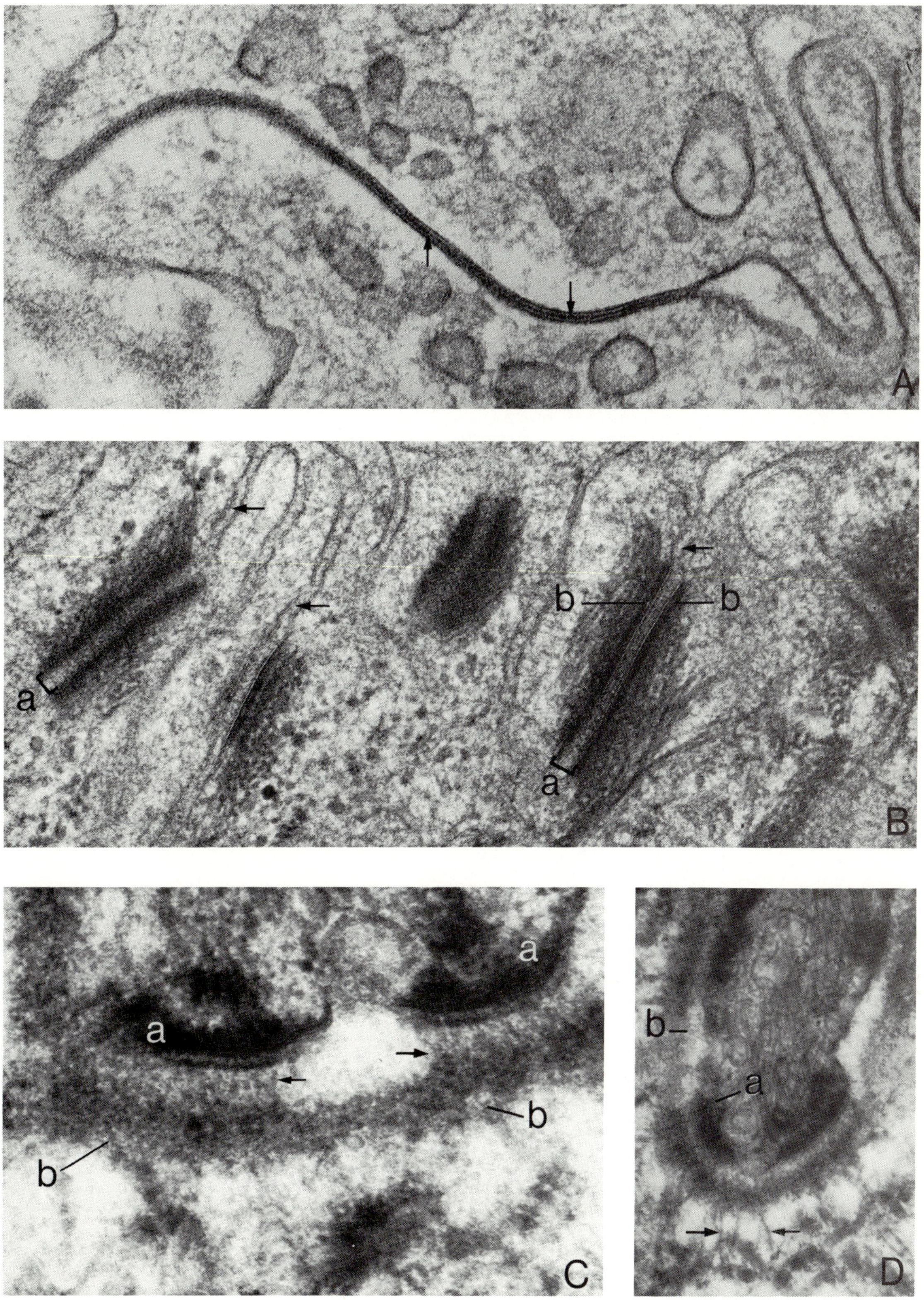

Figure 3–9. *See legend on opposite page.*

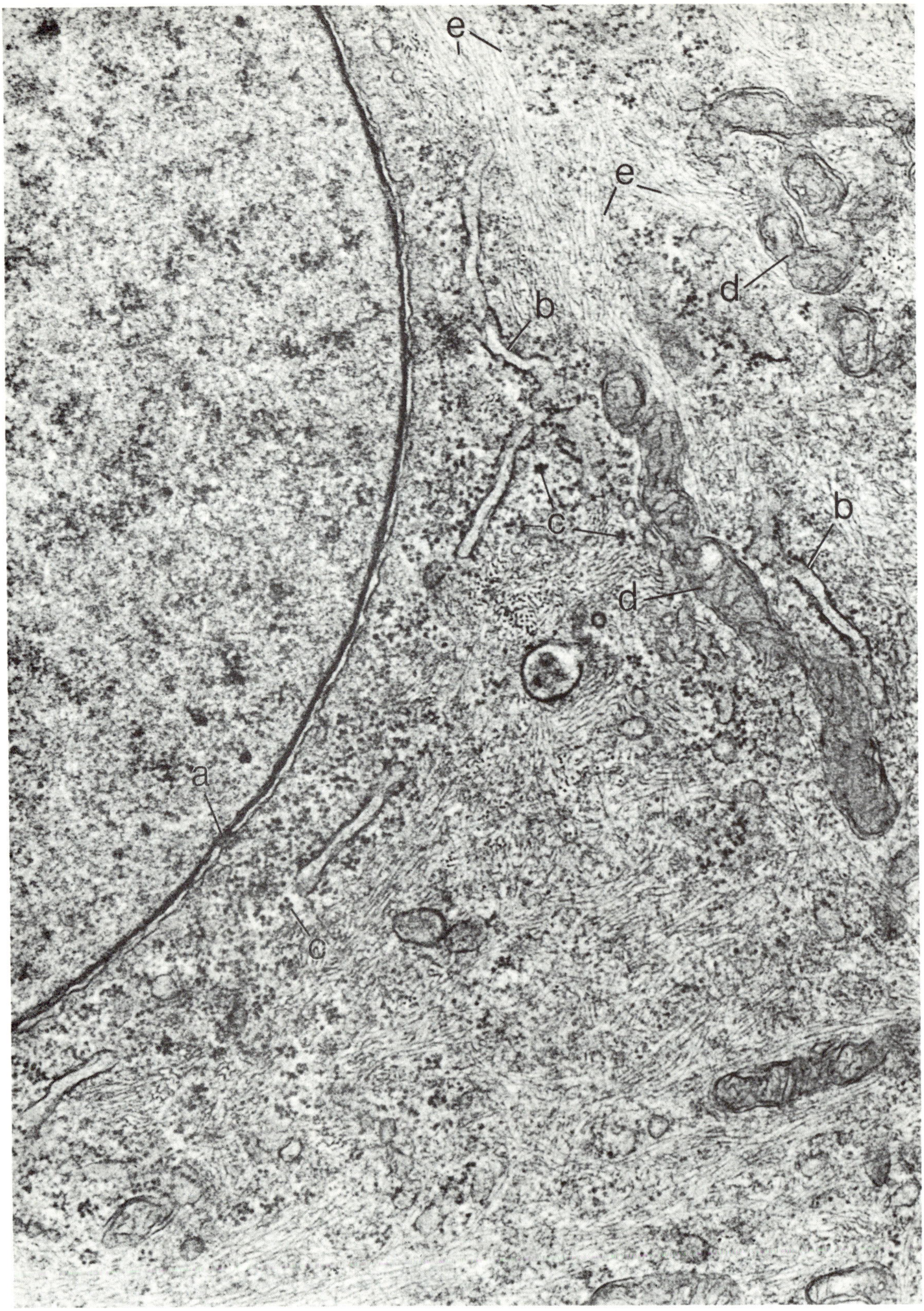

Figure 3-10. Corneal epithelium. Perinuclear cytoplasm of a basal cell. The nuclear chromatin is dispersed and the nuclear envelope has a dense inner membrane. A pore is seen in the nuclear membrane at (a). A few cisternae of rough-surfaced endoplasmic reticulum (b), free ribosomes (c) and mitochondria (d) are seen. The tonofibrils are uniformly distributed and do not form bundles (e). (× 37,500.)

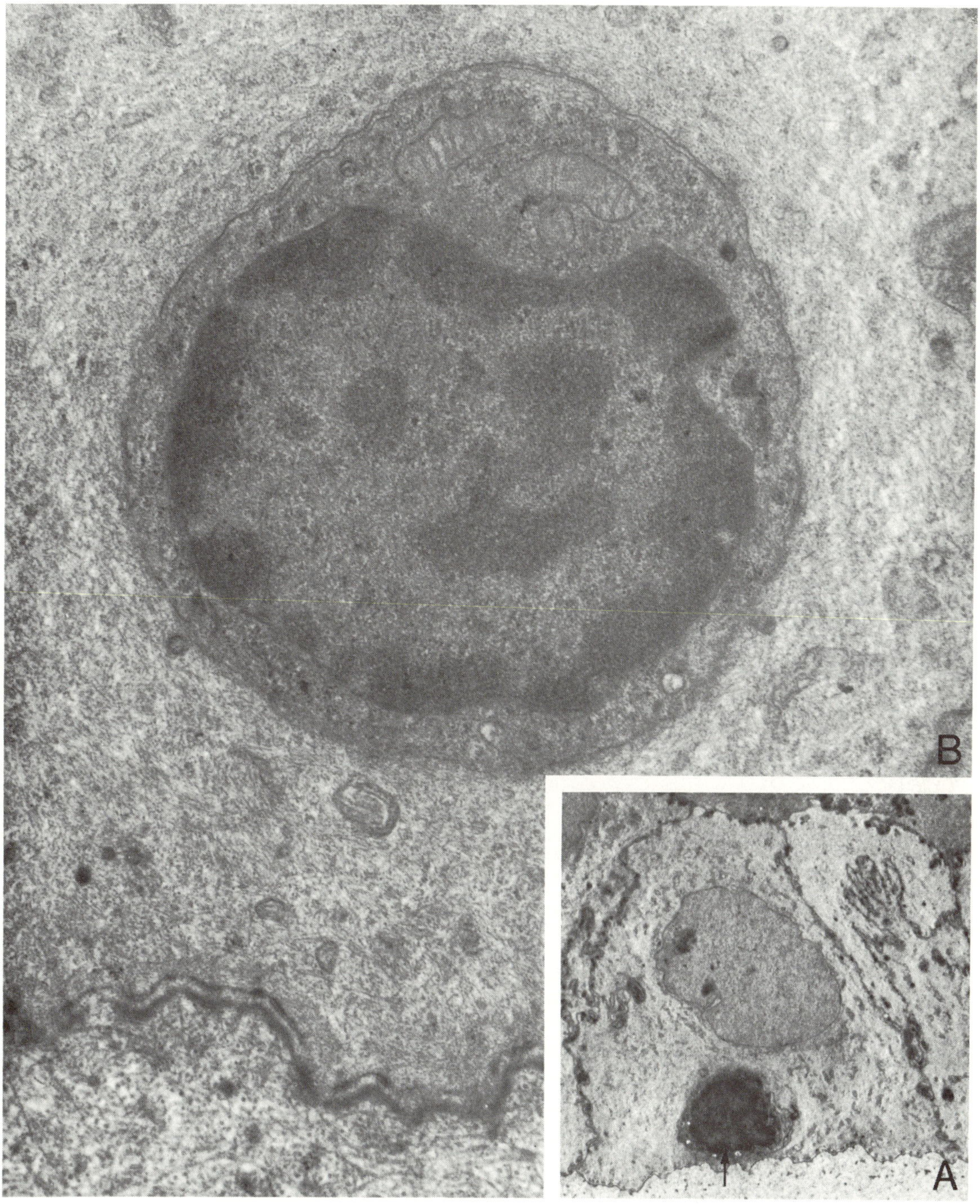

Figure 3-11. Corneal epithelium. *A*, A lymphocyte (arrow) in the basal epithelial layer near Bowman's layer. The comparative size of the epithelial cell and the lymphocyte are evident. (× 2,400.)

B, A lymphocyte invaginates the basal cell surface. At first glance this lymphocyte may be taken for the nucleus of a basal cell, but it is surrounded by its own cell membrane which encloses a scanty dense cytoplasm containing a few large mitochondria. There are no intercellular junctions between the lymphocyte and the basal cell. (× 29,700.)

distance into Bowman's layer. These extensions increase in depth toward the peripheral cornea (Ishida, 1958).

The lateral cell membranes of the basal cells show much less pronounced infoldings than are seen in the wing and surface layers of cells. Here the cells are joined by desmosomes and maculae occludentes. The desmosomal attachments are fewer than in other cell layers and the maculae occludentes are so uncommon here that they have not been noticed by previous investigators. Unmyelinated nerves containing single or multiple axones are found between the basal cells.

On the anterior side these cells are in contact with the layer of wing cells through desmosomes and occasional maculae occludentes. On this surface there are numerous interdigitations between the basal and wing cells, interlocking the cells like a zipper.

The cytoplasm of the basal cell is characterized by the presence of diffusely distributed tonofilaments and the paucity of the common cell organelles. These filaments measure less than 80 A. in diameter, and while they are randomly distributed, they are mostly oriented perpendicular to the surface of the cornea. A considerable number of free ribosomes are found in the cytoplasm around the nucleus. A few profiles of rough-surfaced endoplasmic reticulum are located mainly in a narrow perinuclear zone. The mitochondria are few in number and are very small, measuring 0.324 μm. in length by 0.162 μm. in width. The cristae are disposed along the long axis of the mitochondrion. The Golgi apparatus is seldom seen in the basal cells, possibly because of its small size, but when it is observed it occupies a position near the nucelus in the apical portion of the cell. Centrioles are seen here more frequently than in the other epithelial layers, probably because cell division is frequent in this layer. The nucleus is almost spherical, being somewhat oval in meridional sections and round in tangential sections. It contains uniformly dispersed chromatin and a nucleolus.

Nonepithelial Cells in the Basal Layer. Some nonepithelial cells have been found in the corneal epithelium in the eyes of humans and other species, especially in the basal cell layer. Dendritic cells with long branching processes extending from the basal layer into the wing cell layer have been described. Originally seen with the light microscope, they were believed to be wandering histiocytes. Later observers believed that these dendritic cells were like those in the basal layer of the epidermis because of their shape and staining properties. Others suggested they might be Schwann cells or even Langerhans' cells. Henkind (1965), however, found that pigmented melanocytes were found only at the corneal periphery, and our studies confirm his finding.

Lymphocytes are seen frequently in the corneal epithelium and mainly in the basal cell layer. Their cell bodies are smaller and denser than the epithelial cells, measuring 5 to 7 μm. in diameter, and their cytoplasm contains scattered osmiophilic granules and abundant cytoplasmic organelles. They have no dendritic processes and show no desmosomal attachments to other cells. The mitochondria of these cells are larger than those of the epithelial cells and their cristae run transversely rather than longitudinally. There is a Golgi apparatus, rough-surfaced endoplasmic reticulum, and a rather dark nucleus which has a large part of its chromatin in the form of heterochromatin. We have not seen the tall deep-staining cells in this layer which have been described by other observers.

Wing Cells (Figs. 3–12 and 3–13). The wing cells comprise two to three layers of polygonal-shaped cells which are closely interlocked. The anterior surfaces of these cells are convex and their posterior surfaces are concave. Their lateral extensions are thin and wing-like, joining the adjacent wing cells as well as the basal cells. The basal cells retain their polygonal shape and gradually become thinner as they divide and migrate anteriorly into the wing cell layer (Hanna and O'Brien, 1960). The nuclei also become flattened parallel to the surface of the cornea and the cytoplasm appears denser. In the peripheral cornea the number of wing cells increases to four or five layers.

The cell membranes of this layer show deep interdigitations; desmosomal junctions join these cells to each other and to the basal cells. The desmosomes in the wing cell layer are more numerous than in the basal layer and they increase in number in the superficial layer of wing cells. Maculae occludentes are more common in the wing cell layer than in the basal layer.

The cytoplasm of the wing cells, especially the deepest layer, contains many diffusely distributed tonofibrils that measure around 80 A. in diameter. Otherwise the cytoplasm contains only moderate numbers of small thin mitochondria, which are widely dispersed. The Golgi apparatus is more apparent than in the basal cell layer.

Vesicles are a prominent finding in the cytoplasm of the surface and wing cell layers. They first appear in the cytoplasm of the middle layer of wing cells and increase in size and number in the outer layer; they become even more prominent in the cytoplasm of the surface cells. These vesicles are most frequent in the region of the Golgi apparatus and probably arise from its cisternae. The wing cell nuclei are long and oval and the nucleoplasm is dense.

Superficial Cells (Figs. 3–14 to 3–19). The two layers of surface cells are long and thin, measuring up to 45 μm. in length by about 4 μm. in thickness. Their flattened nuclei measure about 25 μm. in length and both nuclei and cytoplasm stain well with Giemsa and hematoxylin and eosin.

The desmosomal attachments and maculae occludentes become more numerous in the wing and surface cell layers. The surface cells are the only epithelial cells having a zonula occludens; this zonula is found along the lateral walls of the cells near the surface, adjacent to the precorneal tear film.

If the superficial layer of cells is preserved well, the anterior cell membrane of this layer shows many small microplicae and microvilli similar to those seen on the surfaces of cells grown in tissue culture. The studies of Blümcke and Morgenroth (1967) suggest that microplicae and microvilli are a normal part of the structure of these cells. These authors studied the epithelium with the scanning and transmission electron microscopes and found the most superficial epithelial cells to have rather straight lateral borders and slightly curved anterior surfaces. Most of these cells were found to have a length of 20 to 30 μm. Surface views with the scanning electron microscope showed a dense arrangement of microvilli and microplicae, the former being 0.5 to 1.0 μm. high and up to 0.5 μm. thick. The microplicae measured 0.5 μm. high, 0.5 μm. thick and 1.0 to 3.0 μm. long. These authors found the osmiophilic outer leaflet of the cell membrane to differ from others of this type in that it measured 60 to 70 A. in thickness, instead of the usual 30 A. Because of this increased thickness, the unit membrane of the outer portion of the surface cells measures around 100 A. in thickness rather

Text continued on page 80

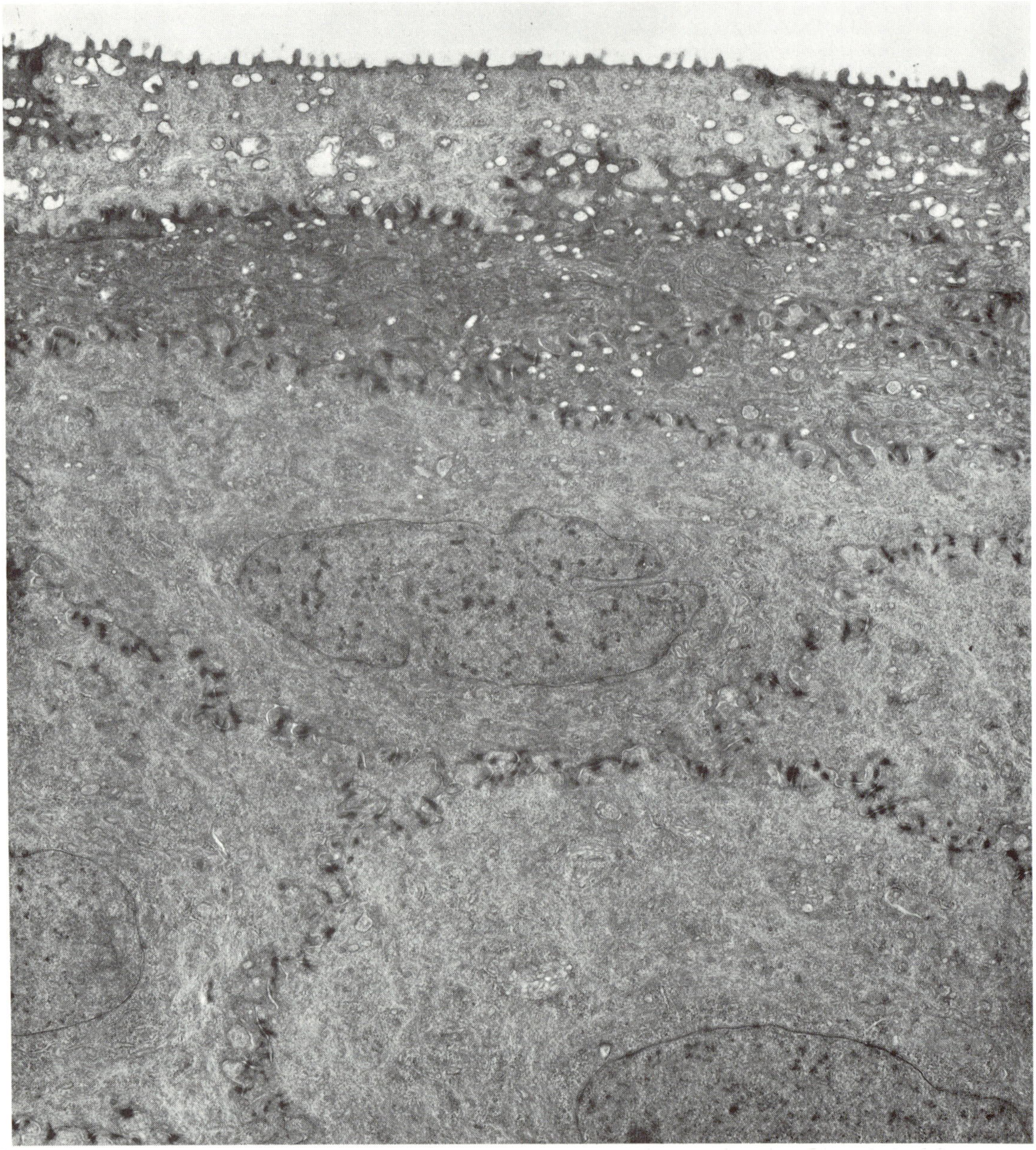

Figure 3-12. Corneal epithelium. Wing cell and superficial cell layers. Dense desmosomal connections join all these cells. The indented nuclei are oriented parallel to the surface of the cornea. The cytoplasm of the surface cells and the most superficial layer of wing cells contains many vesicles. Microplicae and microvilli are evident on the surface of the cornea. (× 12,180.)

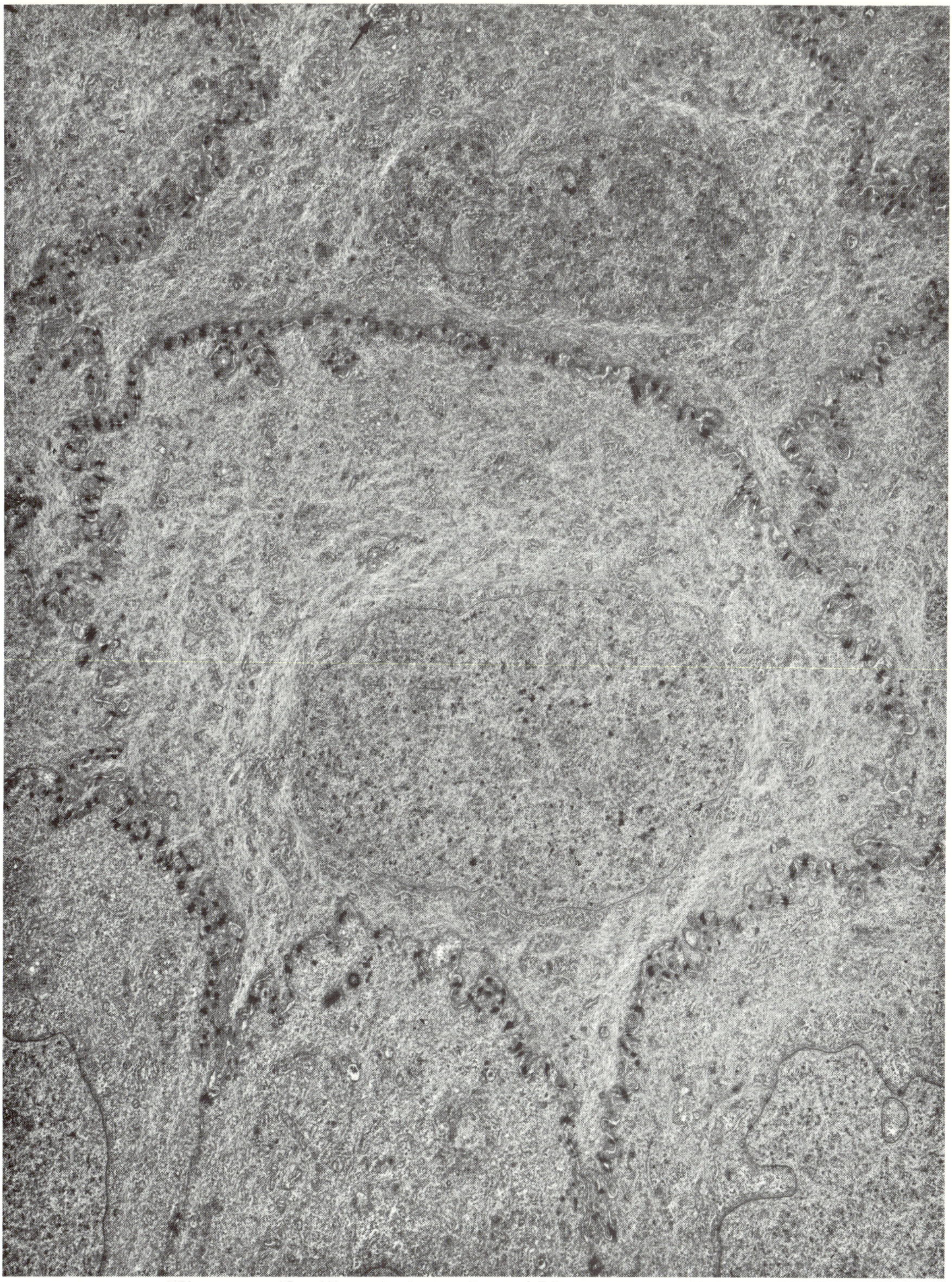

Figure 3-13. Corneal epithelium, wing cell. This cell differs from the basal cell mainly in its configuration. Note the wing-like processes which extend between the basal cells. Numerous interdigitations and desmosomes articulate this cell with its neighbors. The cytoplasm is filled with dispersed tonofilaments, small mitochondria, a few cisternae of rough-surfaced endoplasmic reticulum and many free ribosomes. A small Golgi apparatus is marked by an arrow (top). (× 14,520.)

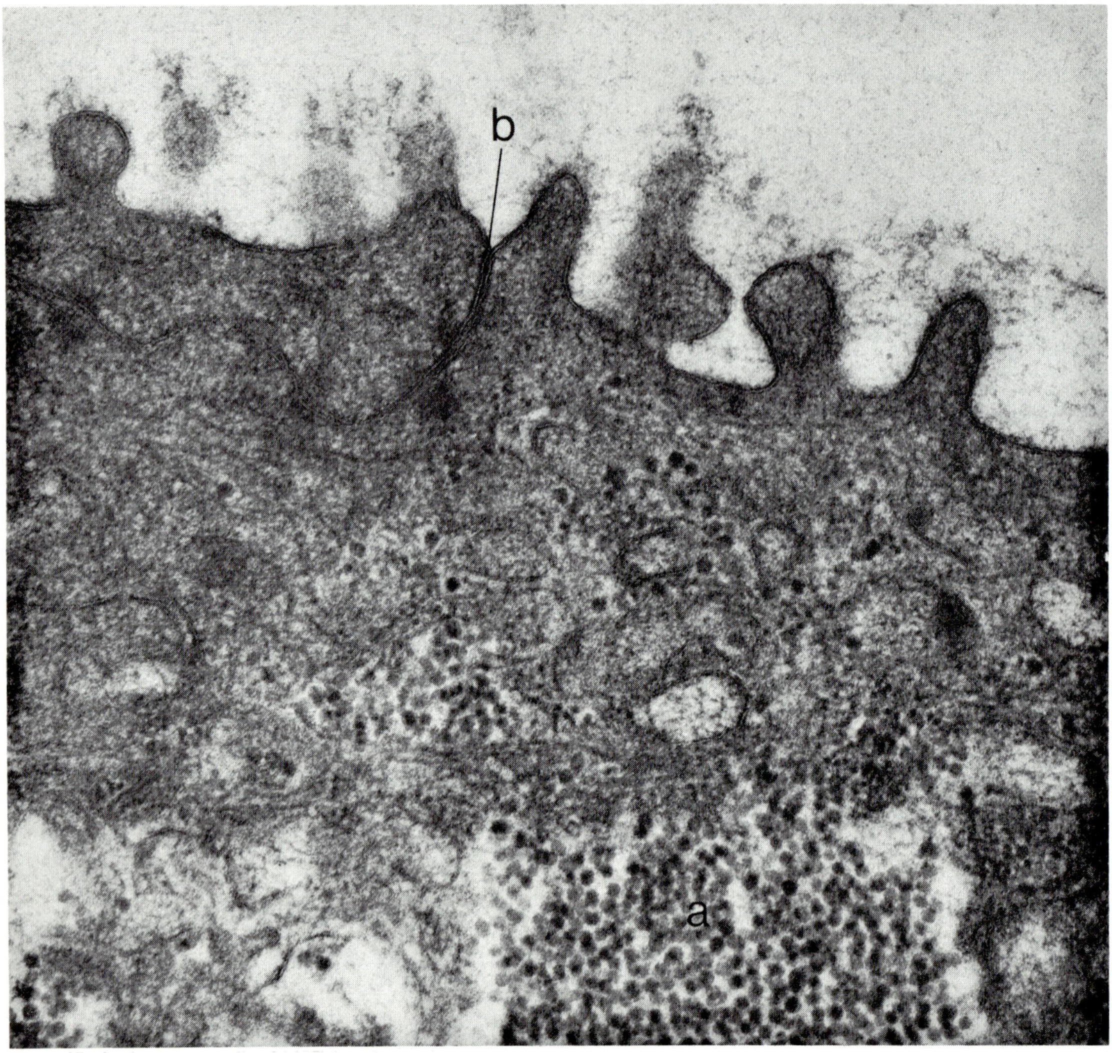

Figure 3-14. Corneal epithelium, surface cell. This cell differs in many respects from the basal epithelium. Two distinguishing features are the aggregations of glycogen granules (a), which are encountered in the surface cells exclusively, and a zonula occludens (b), which is found only along the lateral intercellular space of surface cells. (× 90,000.)

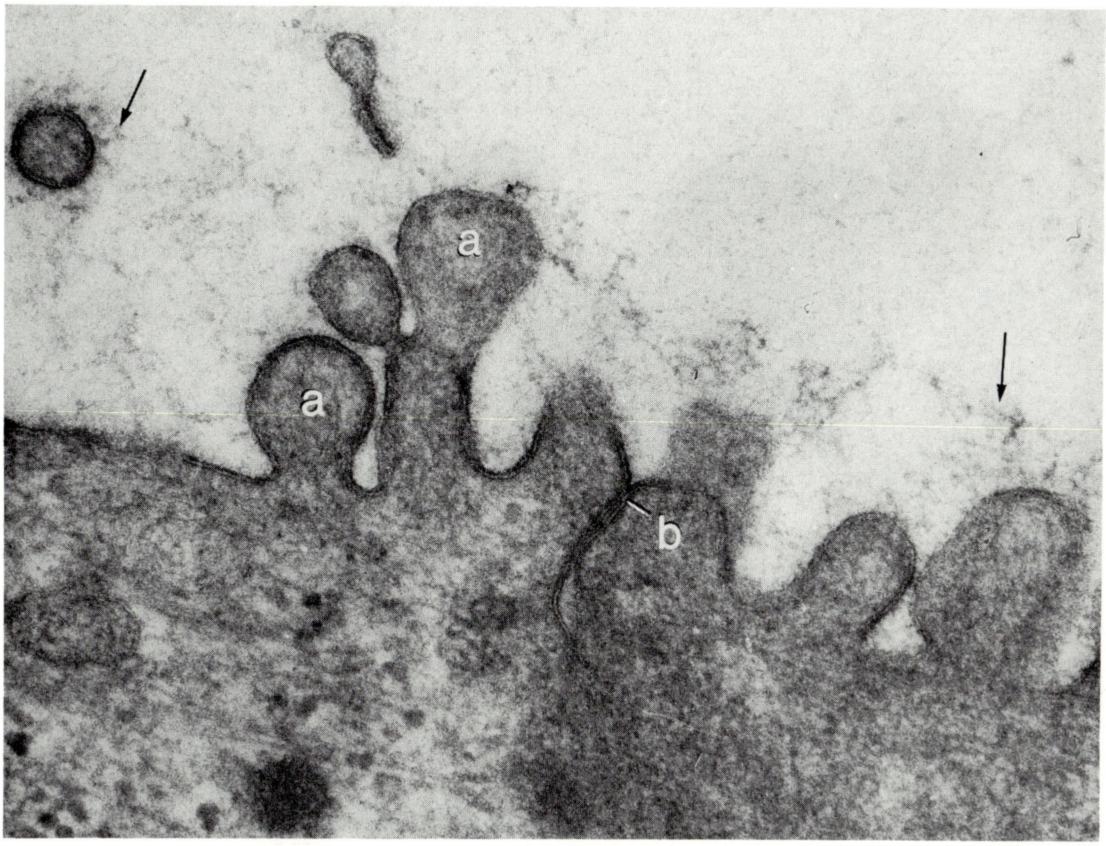

Figure 3-15. Corneal epithelium, surface cell. Microplicae and microvilli (a) protrude from the cell surface into the space occupied by the precorneal tear film. Fine filamentous strands are observed (arrows) within this space. A zonula occludens (b) is constantly found in this position. It probably extends for 360 degrees around the intercellular space. (× 105,000.)

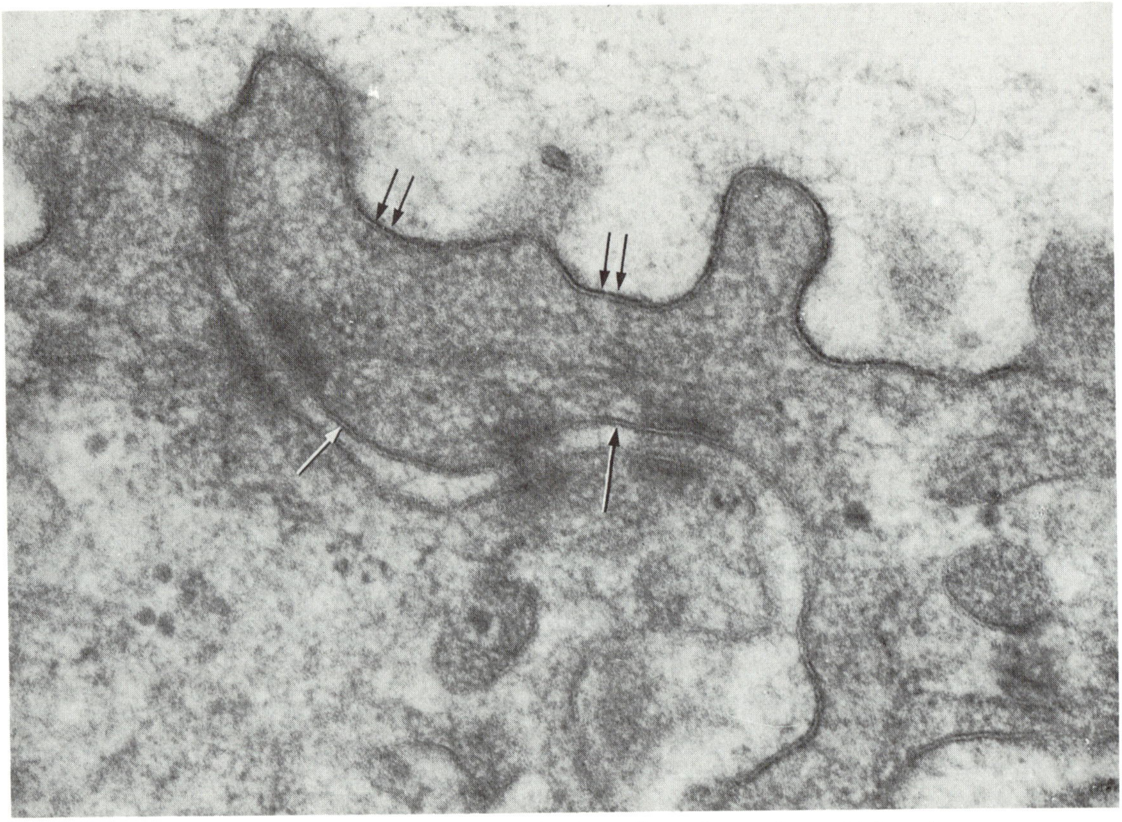

Figure 3–16. Corneal epithelium, surface cell. The cell membrane shows thickened outer leaflets facing the precorneal tear film (double arrows). Compare this with the normal leaflets of the intercellular membrane between adjacent epithelial cells (single arrows). (× 156,000.)

than the normal 75 A. This thick outer layer of the membrane may be the osmiophilic and PAS-positive layer of phospholipid described by Ehlers (1965). Pedler (1962) believed the microplicae might be the remnants of desmosomal attachments after desquamation of the most superficial cells. We have not observed desmosomal placque-like thickenings of the outer cell membranes of the anterior layer, however, so that this idea probably is not correct. Microplicae and microvilli have been demonstrated by a number of observers in well fixed tissue and it seems likely that they are a normal anatomic configuration of these cells. It has been suggested that the microplicae and microvilli may be important for retention of the precorneal film, but Maurice and Riley (1968) expressed doubt about this theory because of their small size in comparison to the 6 μm. reported for the thickness of this film by Mishima (1965).

The cytoplasm of the surface cells is filled with membrane-bound vesicles which increase in size toward the surface of the cornea. They all seem to be associated with the Golgi apparatus, which is highly developed in these cells. The vesicles measure between 1800 and 3600 A. in size; they frequently are observed to be fused with the cell membrane and to open into the intercellular spaces. They more often open into the lateral and posterior

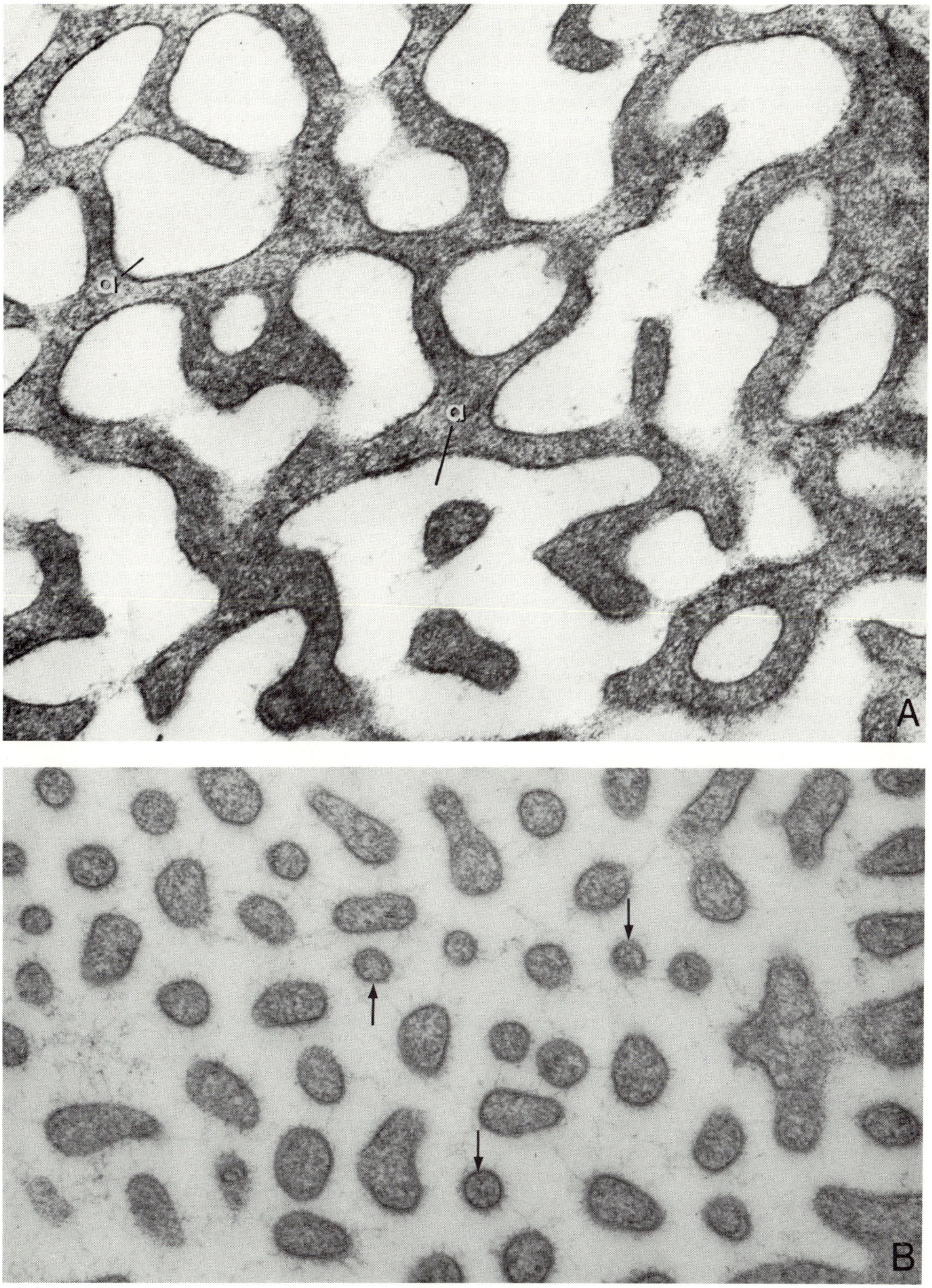

Figure 3-17. Corneal epithelium, surface cell. *A*, Tangential sections of microplicae are seen forming interconnecting ridges which, according to some authors, are involved in the retention of the precorneal film (a). (× 76,500.)

B, Some microvilli (arrows) appear among the microplicae. A filamentous material possibly related to the tear film is seen on the corneal surface between the villi. (× 72,000.)

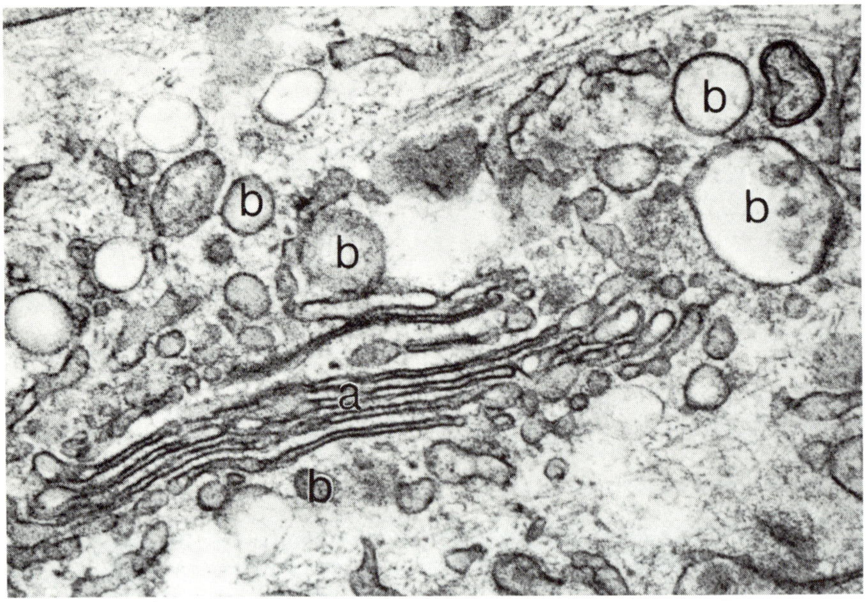

Figure 3-18. Corneal epithelium, surface cell. A prominent Golgi complex (a) which is surrounded by numerous vesicles (b) is commonly seen in these cells, in contrast to the cytoplasm of basal epithelial cells. The lumina of some of the vesicles contains a granular material while others are electron lucent. (× 56,000.)

intercellular spaces than onto the external surface. A granular material can often be seen in the lumina of these vesicles. Glycogen deposits exist only in these cells, and usually they are lost during the processing of the tissues. Figure 3–20 summarizes the structure of the corneal epithelial layers.

Bowman's Layer (Figs. 3–21 and 3–22)

This layer formerly was considered to be a special corneal membrane, but electron microscopic study has shown it to be composed mainly of collagen. For this region the term "layer" rather than membrane is preferred (McTigue, 1967). This layer exists in a few vertebrates besides humans and primates and it also is found in some birds and reptiles, as well as in Elasmobranches (Payrau et al., 1967; Goldman and Benedek, 1968). Its thickness varies in all these species; in the chameleon, for example, Bowman's layer and the epithelium have a thickness greater than the stroma (Payrau et al., 1967).

Bowman's layer measures 8 to 14 μm. in thickness, being somewhat thicker in the peripheral third. It is composed almost entirely of collagen and ground substance but contains no cells, except for the fine extensions of Schwann cells along the canals of the perforating nerves to the corneal epithelium. The anterior surface of Bowman's layer is smooth where it faces the basement membrane of the corneal epithelium, but the posterior surface blends less distinctly with the corneal stroma. Posteriorly the collagen of some of the anterior stromal lamellae arcs forward to blend with the collagen

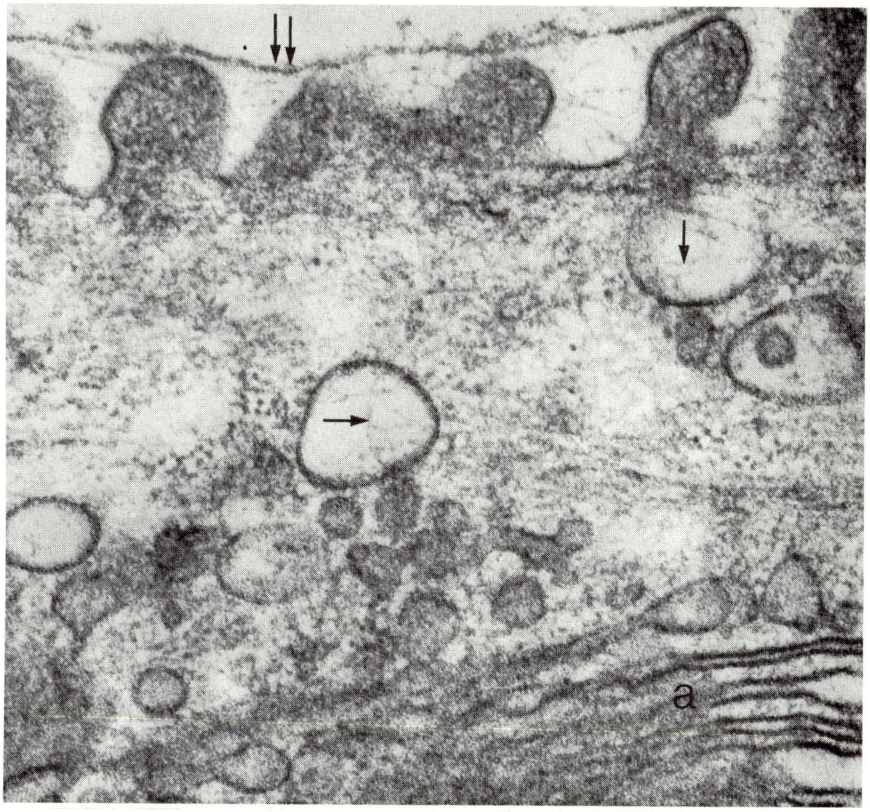

Figure 3-19. Corneal epithelium, surface cell. A small portion of the Golgi apparatus is seen at the lower right cornea (a). Small and large vesicles are prominent in the cytoplasm of these cells. Note the presence of a filamentous material within the lumina of the large vesicles (arrow). The surface cell membrane shows microplicae and between these folds is a filamentous material. On top of this material is an osmiophilic (lipid) layer (double arrows). (× 44,000.)

of the membrane. Toward the periphery Bowman's layer becomes thinner and less dense, and in this zone cells and even capillaries may appear in its meshes. The layer stains poorly with mucopolysaccharide stains, its tinctorial properties being like those of the corneal stroma. It is somewhat metachromatic, but less so than the corneal stroma (Wislocki et al., 1952).

The collagen fibrils in Bowman's layer are quite randomly dispersed and are smaller in diameter and less tightly packed than in the corneal stroma. Its collagen fibrils are quite uniform in thickness; according to Jakus (1961), they measure 140 to 160 A. in thickness, while Kayes and Holmberg (1960) found them to measure 260 to 360 A. Most of our specimens fixed with glutaraldehyde show them to measure between 240 and 270 A. The interstices surrounding the fibrils in the membrane are filled with a mucoprotein ground substance, probably of the same composition as that of the corneal stroma. In the periphery of Bowman's layer the arrangement of the fibers is even looser, and the collagen gradually merges with that of the conjunctiva. The tapering of the peripheral membrane is produced by a gradual loss of some of the posterior collagen.

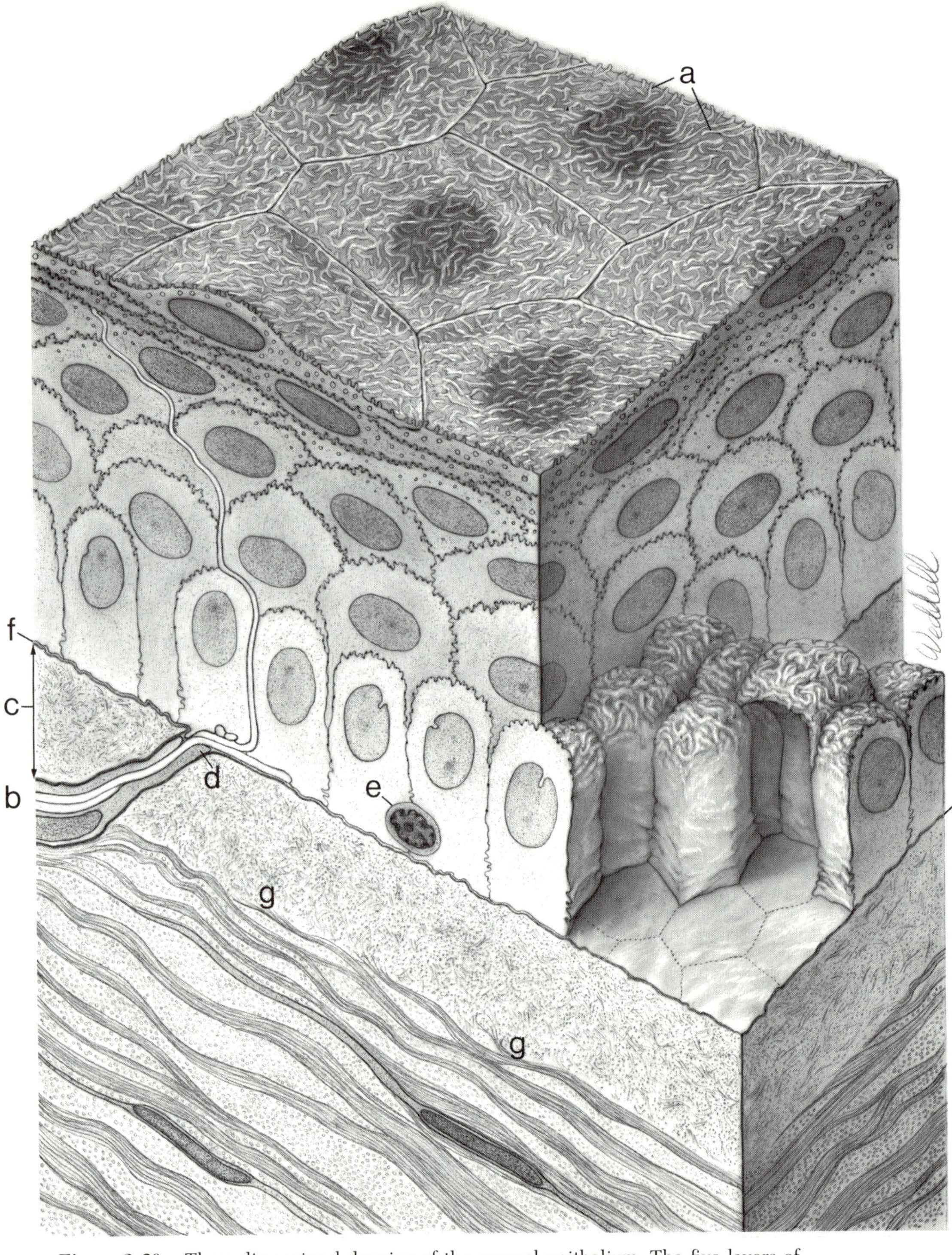

Figure 3-20. Three dimensional drawing of the corneal epithelium. The five layers of cells forming this epithelium are shown. The drawing brings out the polygonal shape of the basal and surface cells and their relative size. The wing cell processes fill the spaces formed by the dome-shaped apical surface of the basal cells. The turnover time for these cells is seven days, and during this time the columnar basal cell is gradually transformed into a wing cell, then into a thin flat surface cell. During this transition the cytoplasm changes and the Golgi apparatus becomes more prominent. Numerous vesicles develop in the superficial wing and surface layers and glycogen appears in the surface cells. The intercellular space separating the

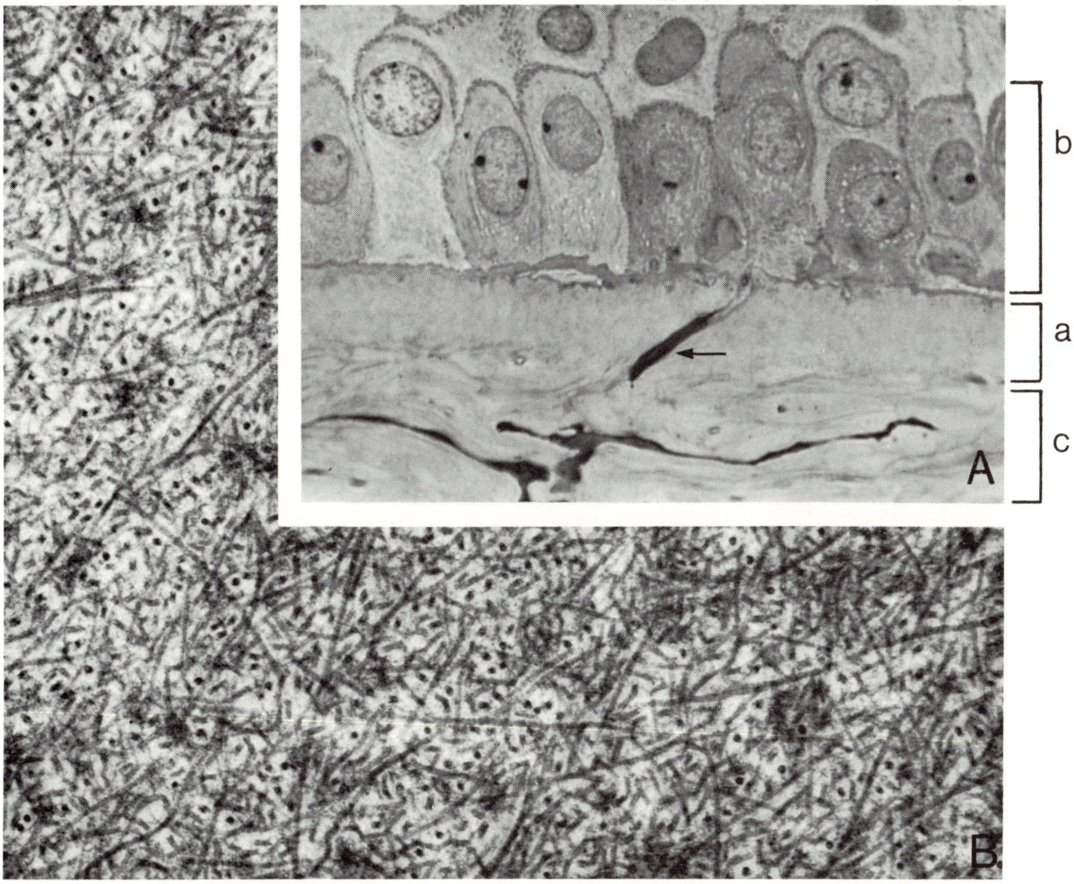

Figure 3-21. Bowman's layer. *A*, Light micrograph of Bowman's layer (a), the basal epithelium (b) and the anterior stroma (c). Bowman's layer is about 8 μm. in thickness and lacks cells except for an occasional nerve bundle with its Schwann cell (arrow). (× 1200.)

B, Long, fine collagen fibrils are randomly dispersed to form Bowman's layer. These fibrils measure 250 A. in diameter, and are smaller than the collagen fibrils of the corneal stromal lamellae. (× 41,800.)

Figure 3-20. *Continued.*
outermost surface cells is closed by a zonula occludens forming a barrier which prevents ingress of the precorneal tear film into the corneal stroma. The cell surface shows an extensive net of microplicae (a) and microvilli which may be involved in the retention of the precorneal film.

A corneal nerve (b) passes through Bowman's layer (c); it loses its Schwann sheath near the basement membrane (d) of the basal epithelium. The nerve then passes between the epithelial cells toward the superficial layers as a naked nerve. A lymphocyte (e) is seen between two basal epithelial cells. The basement membrane is seen at (f). Some of the most superficial corneal stromal lamellae (g) are seen curving forward to merge with Bowman's layer. The regular arrangement of the corneal stromal collagen differs from the random disposition of that in Bowman's layer.

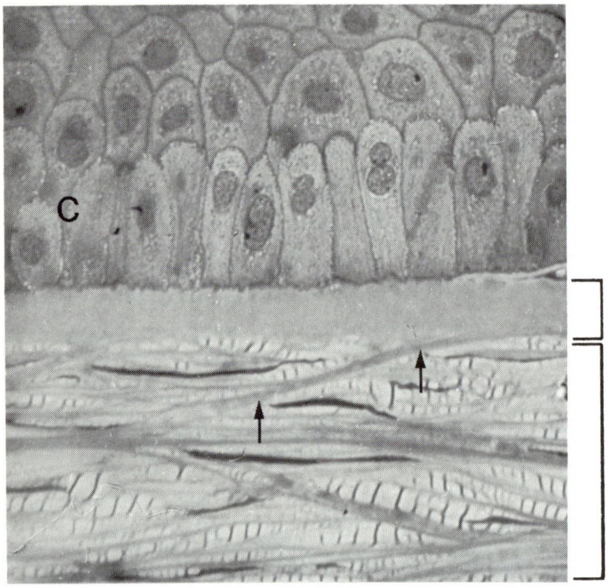

Figure 3-22. Bowman's layer. Light micrograph of Bowman's layer (a), the anterior stroma (b) and the corneal epithelium (c). There is a change in the direction of the superficial lamellae as they curve forward to merge with Bowman's layer (arrows). (× 800.)

STROMA (Figs. 3–23 to 3–26)

The corneal stroma measures approximately 500 μm. in thickness, and it constitutes nine tenths of the thickness of the entire cornea in man (Fig. 3–4). It is composed almost entirely of collagenous lamellae, in which are fibroblasts (keratocytes) and ground substance. The turnover time for the stromal collagen is rather long, and Smelser and co-workers (1965) showed that there was little turnover in a period of 12 months. Except for the Schwann cells around the corneal nerves, the only other cells found are occasional lymphocytes, scattered macrophages and a rare polymorphonuclear leukocyte. The latter cells are occasionally seen among the lamellae, being short and flattened, recognizable by their lobulated nuclei (Virchow, 1910; Weimar, 1960). Clinical analyses suggest that the corneal fibroblasts occupy about 5 per cent of the volume of the stroma (Davson, 1949; Langham and Taylor, 1956). Otori (1967), using direct measurements, found

---

Figure 3-23. Corneal stroma. *A*, Low power electron micrograph. The stromal collagen varies in density and has a lamellar arrangement. Dark bands are created when the stromal lamellae are cut longitudinally, whereas the lighter bands result when they are sectioned obliquely or in cross-section. The lamellae have a regular arrangement except in the most anterior stroma, as shown in Figure 3-22. Several very long thin fibroblasts lie between the lamellae (arrows). (× 2390.)

B, Higher magnification of the lamellae and cells. One lamella measuring around 6 μm. in thickness is cut longitudinally (brackets). Other lamellae are sectioned obliquely (a) or in cross-section (b). Two long, thin fibroblasts (keratocytes) are seen in the upper and lower part of the photograph. (× 3360.)

C, Collagen fibrils cut in longitudinal section. Four fibrils measuring 360 A. in width are separated by an interfibrillar space measuring between 120 and 180 A. A granular material occupies the interfibrillar space. The fibrils show fine striations, each of which is separated by an interval of 60 A. (microperiodicity). Arrows indicate the positions of darker striations which are separated from each other by 620 to 640 A. (× 160,000.)

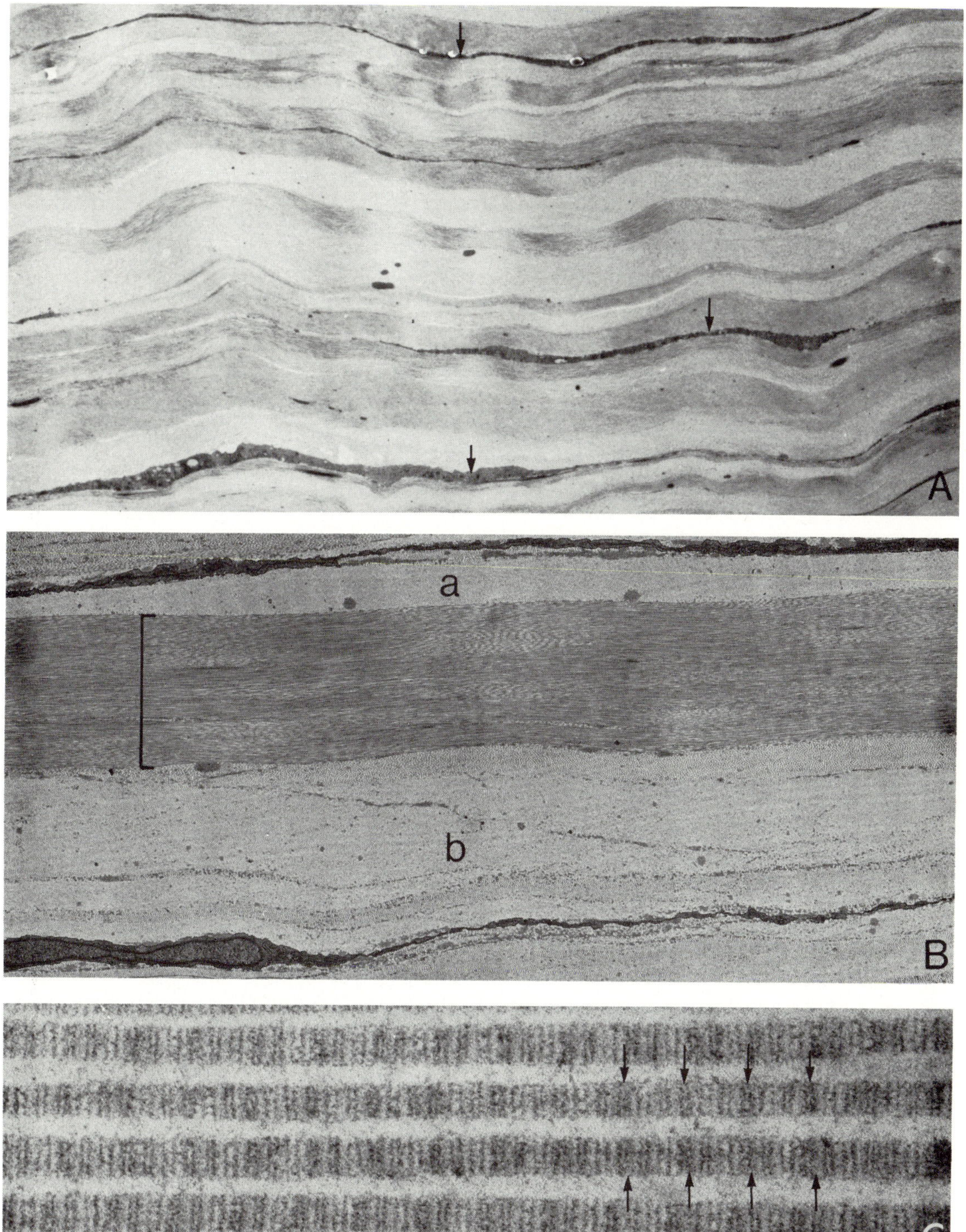

Figure 3–23. *See legend on opposite page.*

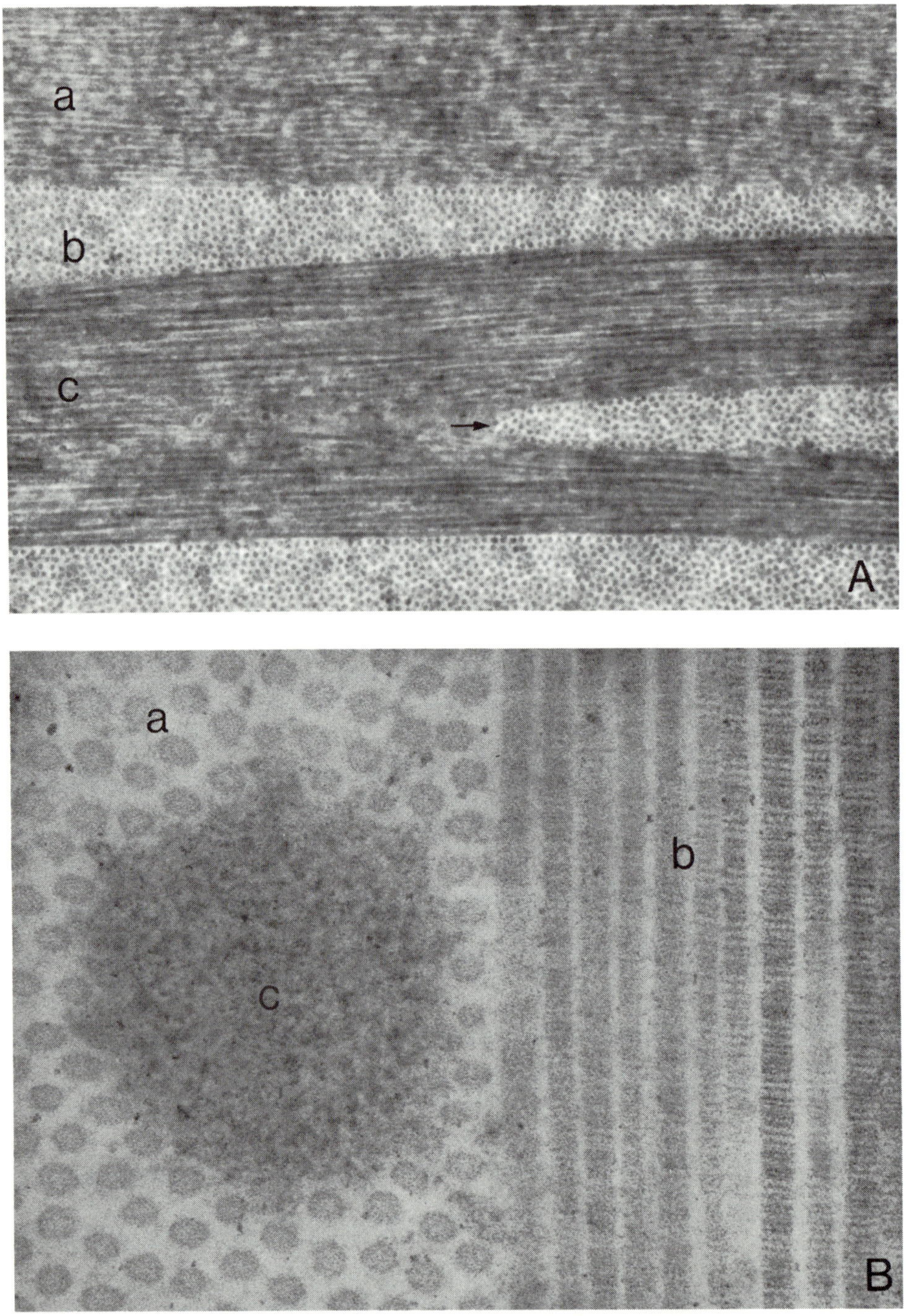

Figure 3-24. Corneal stroma. *A*, A view of lamellae which are cut in three planes. The upper lamella (a) is cut obliquely, the next below it (b) is cut in cross-section, and the third (c) is cut longitudinally. This lamella splits into two lamellae (arrow). (× 28,000.)

B, Cross (a) and longitudinal (b) views of two lamellae. The fibrils measure 340 to 400 A. in diameter and are separated from each other by a space measuring 200 to 500 A. A large, round granular mass (c) is observed within the lamella cut in cross-section. Such masses are seen in most of the collagenous tissues of the eye and they may represent a stage in the formation of the mature fiber. (× 104,000.)

them to occupy 2 to 3 per cent of the rabbit corneal stroma. Maurice and Riley (1968) confirmed this finding in man, with a figure of 2.4 per cent.

Lamellae. The cornea contains about 200 to 250 lamellae which are superimposed on each other, each having a thickness of 2.0 μm. and a width of 9 to 260 μm.; their length encompasses the entire cornea. The lamellae are parallel to each other and to the surface of the cornea, and within each lamella the collagen fibrils are all parallel. McTigue (1967) found the superficial one third of the corneal stroma to contain lamellae arranged in a less orderly way than in the deeper two thirds, so that the superficial third could be separated as a layer from the deeper portion more easily than it is possible to separate the deeper layers from each other. It was presumed by McTigue that this arrangement in the superficial third of the cornea is possibly related to the continuation of the conjunctival and episcleral collagen into the cornea, although by electron microscopy the diameters of these corneal fibrils are the same as those of the deeper layers and not like those of the conjunctiva and episclera. This superficial zone of the corneal stroma does stain less intensely than the deeper two thirds.

If sections are made through the cornea perpendicular to its surface in any meridian of the clock, the sections always show a regular layering of the lamellae. The fibrils within the lamellae in any one plane of the cornea apparently never change direction to join a neighboring plane. Kokott (1934, 1938) found a tendency for the fibrils in the superficial lamellae to run vertically in the cornea, while those in the middle layers most often are oriented toward the four rectus muscles. He also found the fibrils in the deep periphery of the cornea to be oriented circularly. Polack (1961) studied the corneas of the rabbit, dog and human and found considerable interweaving and branchings at various levels within the lamellae of the outer cornea. Some of the superficial bundles of collagen were found to end in the region of the epithelium.

The branching of the lamellae is easily seen by electron microscopy, especially in the central cornea. In any one section the bundles may be cut in longitudinal, oblique or cross-section, depending on the direction of the fibrils. The fibrils within the bundles are parallel to each other and are uniform in size and spacing. They are coated and separated from each other by a cementing ground substance. At the periphery the corneal lamellae and their constituent fibrils are not so regularly oriented and their structure gradually approaches the form seen in the sclera. Larger fibrils that measure 600 to 700 A. in diameter appear, and the regular spacing between the fibrils is lost. Typical elastic fibers have not been seen in the corneal stroma.

In contrast to the scleral fibrils, the corneal collagen fibrils are embedded in a more abundant matrix, and they are characterized by their remarkably uniform size. Each fibril probably extends across the diameter of the cornea; otherwise; fibrils with tapering ends indicating their termination would be seen frequently in the stroma, and they do not occur. The scleral collagen fibrils, on the other hand, do exhibit tapering ends. Reported diameters of the corneal fibrils range from 210 to 650 A. Kayes and Holmberg (1960) found them to be 330 to 416 A., and Jakus (1961) gave figures of 240 to 280 A. in the midstroma and 275 to 400 A. near Descemet's membrane. We find them to be around 320 to 360 A. in diameter in most corneas studied. Most observers agree that the stromal collagen fibrils are at least one third larger than those of Bowman's layer. The macroperiodicity of the fibrils is in the vicinity of 620 to 640 A., with a microperiodicity of 60 A. In the posterior

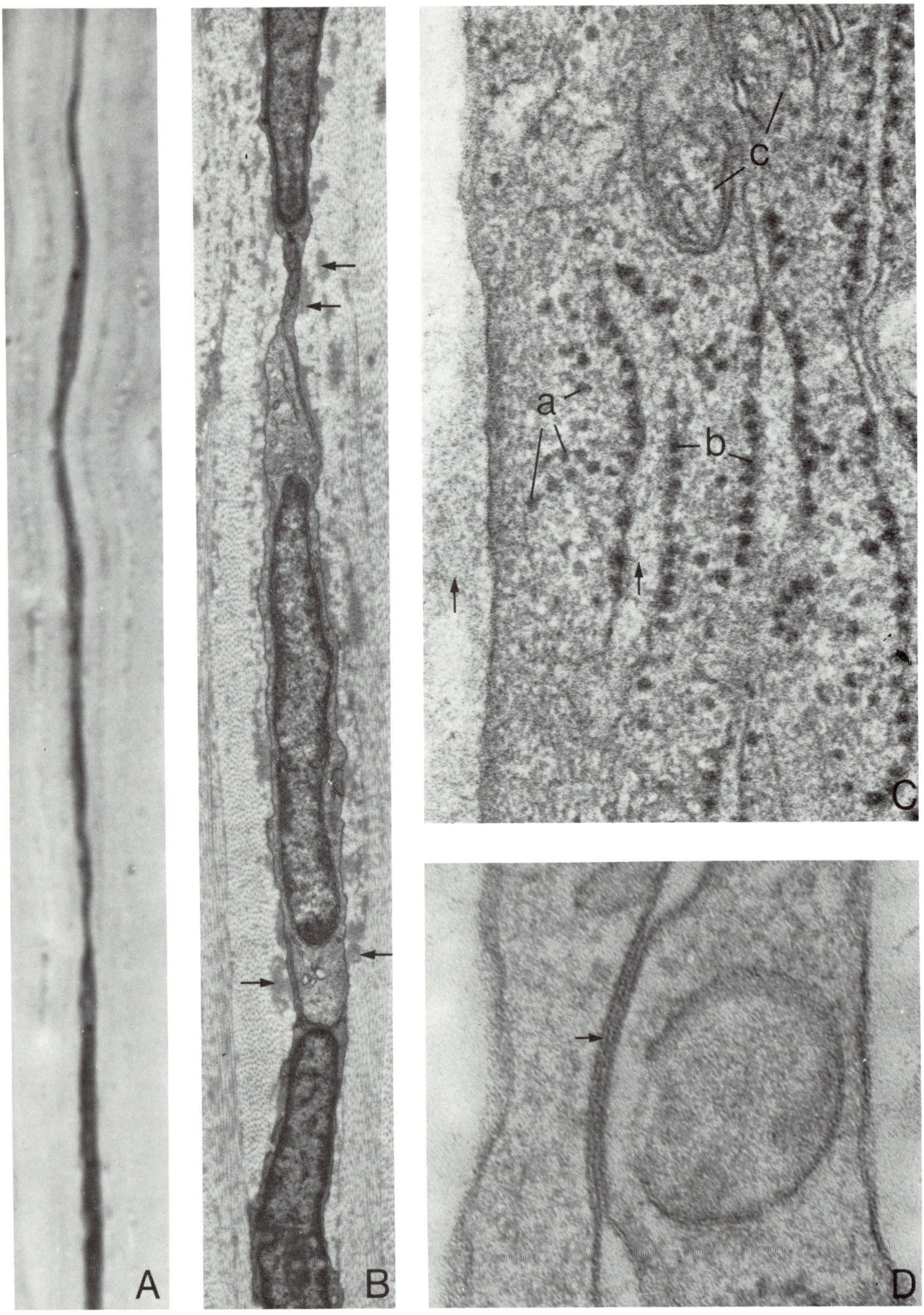

Figure 3–25. *See legend on opposite page.*

cornea adjacent to Descemet's membrane there is a thin transition zone containing fibrils with a diameter of 100 A. These fibrils are like the tropocollagen or immature collagen fibrils seen in the region of the scleral spur. The uniformity and size of the adult human corneal collagen fibrils is like that of embryonal collagen (Garzino, 1955). After the healing of corneal wounds the diameter of the regenerated collagen fibrils is greater, being similar to that of the scleral collagen.

Ground Substance. The ground substance of the cornea consists of mucoprotein and glycoprotein plus other substances exclusive of collagen. It fills all the space not occupied by the fibrils and cells, forms a coating for each fibril, and is responsible for the exact spacing of the corneal fibrils.

Cells. Fibroblasts are found throughout the corneal stroma, but in ordinary light microscopic sections it is not possible to determine whether they are more often interlamellar or intralamellar. Virchow (1910) showed that the cells are interlamellar because the spaces within which the cells lie extend across the cornea and do not unite with each other. Electron microscopic studies show that the cells do lie between the lamellae, but that they occasionally extend into the lamellae. Under the light microscope the corneal cells are thin, their extensive processes paralleling the corneal lamellae. Their cytoplasm is rarely thicker than 2 μm. around the nucleus. Flat sections of the cornea show the fibroblasts to have long branching processes which extend in many directions from the cell body. In embryonic human corneas and in newborn animals the structure of these cells indicates that they are synthesizing collagen and mucoprotein (Schwarz, 1961).

With the electron microscope the corneal cells show most of the characteristic features of fibroblasts. Their processes can be traced for extraordinary distances, and frequent contacts are made with other fibroblasts. A 200 A. space usually separates the cells where they contact each other, but occasionally the cells are joined by a tight junction. Junctions of this type have been seen at all levels of the cornea in both osmium and glutaralde-

---

Figure 3-25. Corneal stroma, showing fibroblasts. *A*, Light micrograph showing fibroblasts occupying a space between the lamellae. These cells are characteristically long and thin. (× 2400.)

B, Three fibroblasts lying partly within and partly between the stromal lamellae. Each cell is wider in the nuclear region, where it measures between 1 and 2 μm. in diameter. The cytoplasm is scanty around the nucleus and may be as thin as a 0.1 μm. Arrows point to masses of a homogeneous electron-dense material lying in the vicinity of the cells. This material is similar to that shown in Figure 3-24 *B*. (× 16,500.)

C, Higher magnification of a portion of a fibroblast. The cytoplasmic structures and organelles involved in protein synthesis are prominent in these cells. Free ribosomes (a) which are responsible for the synthesis of structural proteins and enzymes are found. Granular endoplasmic reticulum is abundant, its associated ribosomes being concerned with synthesis of proteins for secretion or excretion into the extracellular space (b). The Golgi apparatus which is not seen in this photograph participates in the packaging of the proteins produced by the granular endoplasmic reticulum by segregating them in vesicles which move to the cell membrane and empty their contents into the extracellular space. Arrows point to a fine, granular material inside the cisternae of the rough-surfaced endoplasmic reticulum and in the extracellular substance. Material of this type may be either a collagen precursor, or mucoprotein and glycoproteins. Two mitochondria are indicated at (c). (× 123,000.)

D, Area of contact between two fibroblasts of an adult human cornea (arrow). The intercellular space separating these fibroblasts is the usual 200 A., except for some areas where it is closed by a macula occludens. Such areas of close contact between fibroblasts are normally observed only in embryonic tissues. (× 147,000.)

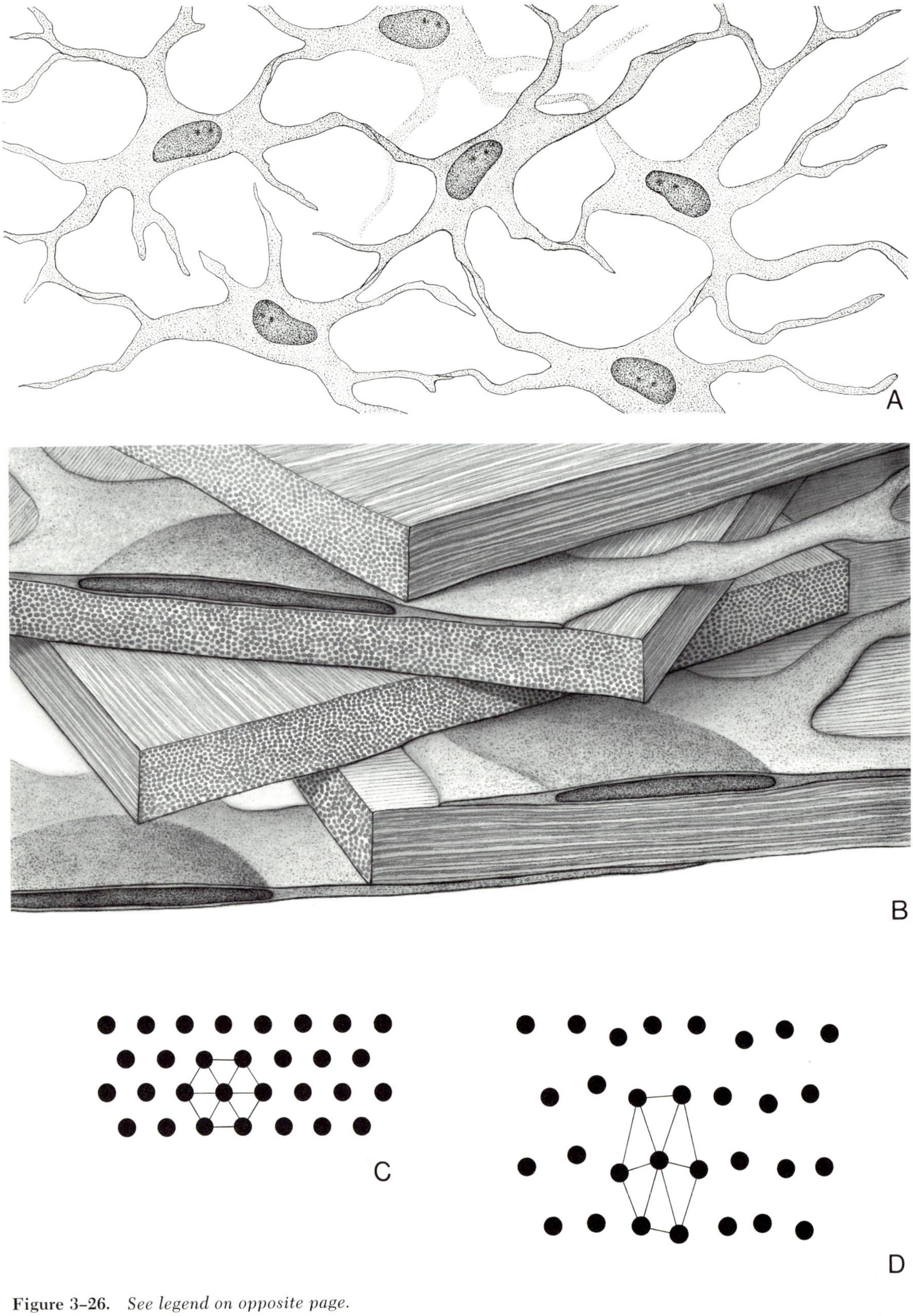

Figure 3–26. *See legend on opposite page.*

hyde fixed tissue, and are an unusual finding in mesenchymal tissues. Connective tissue cells have been observed to be joined by tight junctions during embryonic development, and the existence of these junctions has been linked with contact inhibition during this stage of rapid growth.

Organelles are not numerous in the cytoplasm of the fibroblasts, but all the common organelles are present. In flat sections a prominent feature is an extensive rough-surfaced endoplasmic reticulum. The Golgi apparatus is seen in the nuclear region, and the mitochondria are small and not too numerous. An amorphous jelly-like material and a granular material are found in the vicinity of the corneal fibroblasts. These materials probably represent an early form of the ground substances and collagen fibrils. A summary of the structure of the corneal stroma is given in Figure 3–26.

DESCEMET'S MEMBRANE (Figs. 3–27 to 3–35)

This membrane has always been considered to be a true "glass" membrane because it apparently has no substructure. Descemet's membrane is the basement membrane of the corneal endothelial cells. It is quite unusual because of its thickness and structure, and it is PAS-positive. It can be separated easily from the adjacent stroma as well as from the endothelium. If it is incised or torn in a small area so that a gap forms between the two edges, the corneal endothelial cells will form a new layer to fill the defect. If the incision is sufficiently large, the cut edges tend to curl backward into the anterior chamber, indicating some elasticity in this layer.

During fetal life Descemet's membrane is thinner than the endothelium, but after birth the membrane has approximately the same thickness as that of the endothelial cells. Thereafter Descemet's membrane gradually

---

Figure 3–26. Summary diagram of the corneal stroma. *A*, Fibroblasts. This diagram shows six fibroblasts lying between the stromal lamallae. The cells are thin and flat with long processes which contact fibroblast processes of other cells lying in the same plane. These cells were believed to form a true syncytium, but electron microscopy has disproved this idea. There is almost always a 200 A. wide intercellular space which separates the cells. Unlike fibroblasts elsewhere, these cells occasionally join each other at a macula occludens.

B, Lamellae. The cornea is composed of a very orderly, dense, fibrous connective tissue. Its collagen, which is a very stable protein having a half-life estimated at 100 days, forms many lamellae. The collagen fibrils within a lamella are parallel to each other and run the full length of the cornea. Successive lamellae run across the cornea at an angle to each other. Three fibroblasts are seen between the lamellae.

C, Diagram to show the theoretical orientation of the corneal collagen fibrils. Each of the fibrils is separated from its fellows by an equal distance. Maurice has explained the transparency of the cornea on the basis of this very exact equidistant separation. As a result of this arrangement the stromal lamellae form a three-dimensional array of diffraction gratings. Scattered-rays of light passing through such a system interact with each other in an organized way, resulting in the elimination of scattered light by destructive interference. The mucoproteins, glycoproteins and other components of the ground substance are responsible for maintaing the proper position of the fibrils.

D, Orientation of the collagen fibrils in an opaque cornea. The diagram shows the orderly positions of the fibrils to have been disturbed. Because of this disarrangement, scattered light is not eliminated by destructive interference and the cornea becomes hazy. Edema fluid in the ground substance also produces clouding of the cornea by disturbing the interfibrillar distance.

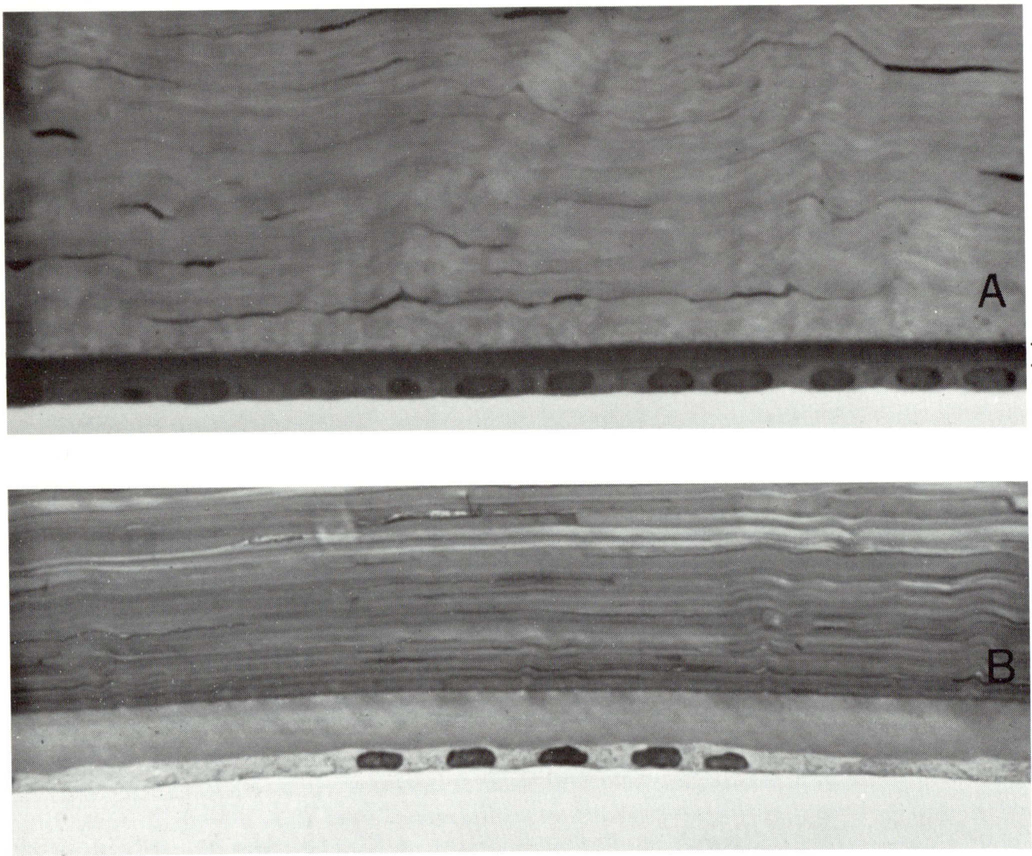

Figure 3–27. Descemet's membrane. *A*, The thickness of Descemet's membrane changes with increasing age. Eye of a one and a half year old child. Light micrograph showing the endothelium (e) and Descemet's membrane (d). They have approximately the same thickness. (× 500.)

B, Eye of a 50 year old person. Descemet's membrane (d) is a little more than double the thickness of the endothelium (e). (× 800.)

increases in thickness so that it is approximately two to three times that of the endothelium. At birth it is 3 to 4 μm. thick, and by adult life it has increased in thickness to 10 to 12 μm. At the corneal edge the membrane frays out into the trabecular sheets.

Ultramicroscopy with dark ground illumination (Peschell, 1905; Grignolo, 1954) and with polarization microscopy (Kohler and Tobgy, 1929; Baud and Balavoine, 1953) has shown Descemet's membrane to be composed of stratified layers. Electron microscopy has confirmed this observation and shown that the membrane is formed of a number of very regularly arranged stratified layers (Bairati and Grignolo, 1954; Jakus, 1956, 1961; Feeney and Garron, 1961; Kaye and Pappas, 1962).

Just inside the periphery, in persons over age 20, the membrane regularly shows periodic thickenings which bulge into the anterior chamber; these protrusions are known as Hassall-Henle warts. The warts are dome-shaped thickenings of the periphery of Descemet's membrane which protrude into the anterior chamber and are covered by a distinctly altered corneal endothelium. Thin sections show the warts to contain numerous

Text continued on page 102

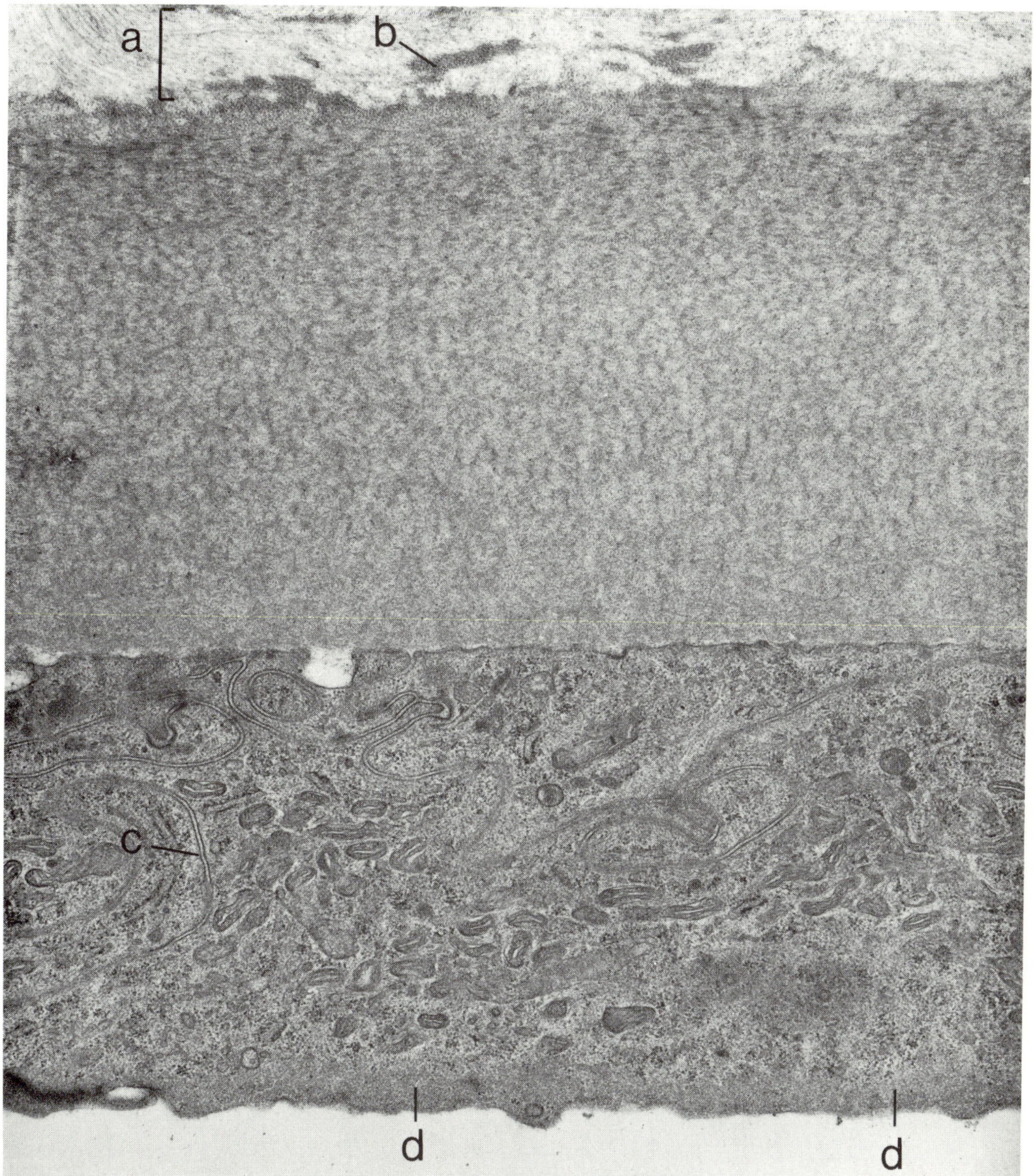

Figure 3–28. Descemet's membrane and endothelium in a young eye. At (a) the deep corneal lamellae are seen to be curving backward to merge with Descemet's membrane. Collections of fine filaments (b) almost identical to those composing Descemet's membrane are seen in the collagen anterior to the membrane. The periodic structure of the fibrils in the meridional section extends throughout the whole thickness of Descemet's membrane. Only the anterior third of the membrane shows this periodic structure in older eyes. Two endothelial cells show the characteristic marked interdigitations of their lateral cell membranes (c). The endothelial cytoplasm contains a notable number of mitochondria. The terminal web (d) is found in the cytoplasm near the anterior chamber; it contains no organelles. (× 18,200.)

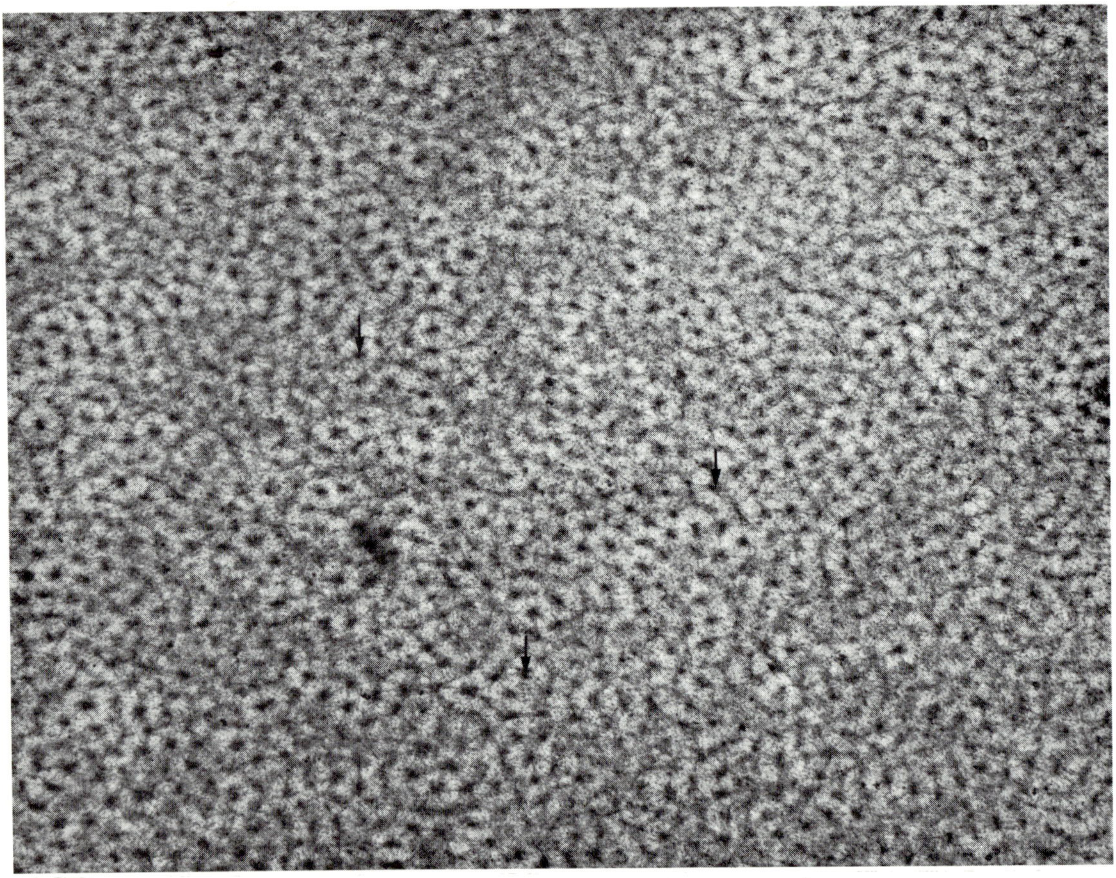

Figure 3–29. Descemet's membrane, tangential section. Descemet's membrane is composed of extremely fine collagenous filaments which have a very uniform distribution and join each other at nodular thickenings. The three-dimensional lattice pattern can be seen throughout the membrane of the young eye, but is seen only in the anterior one third of the membrane of adult eyes. (× 27,000.)

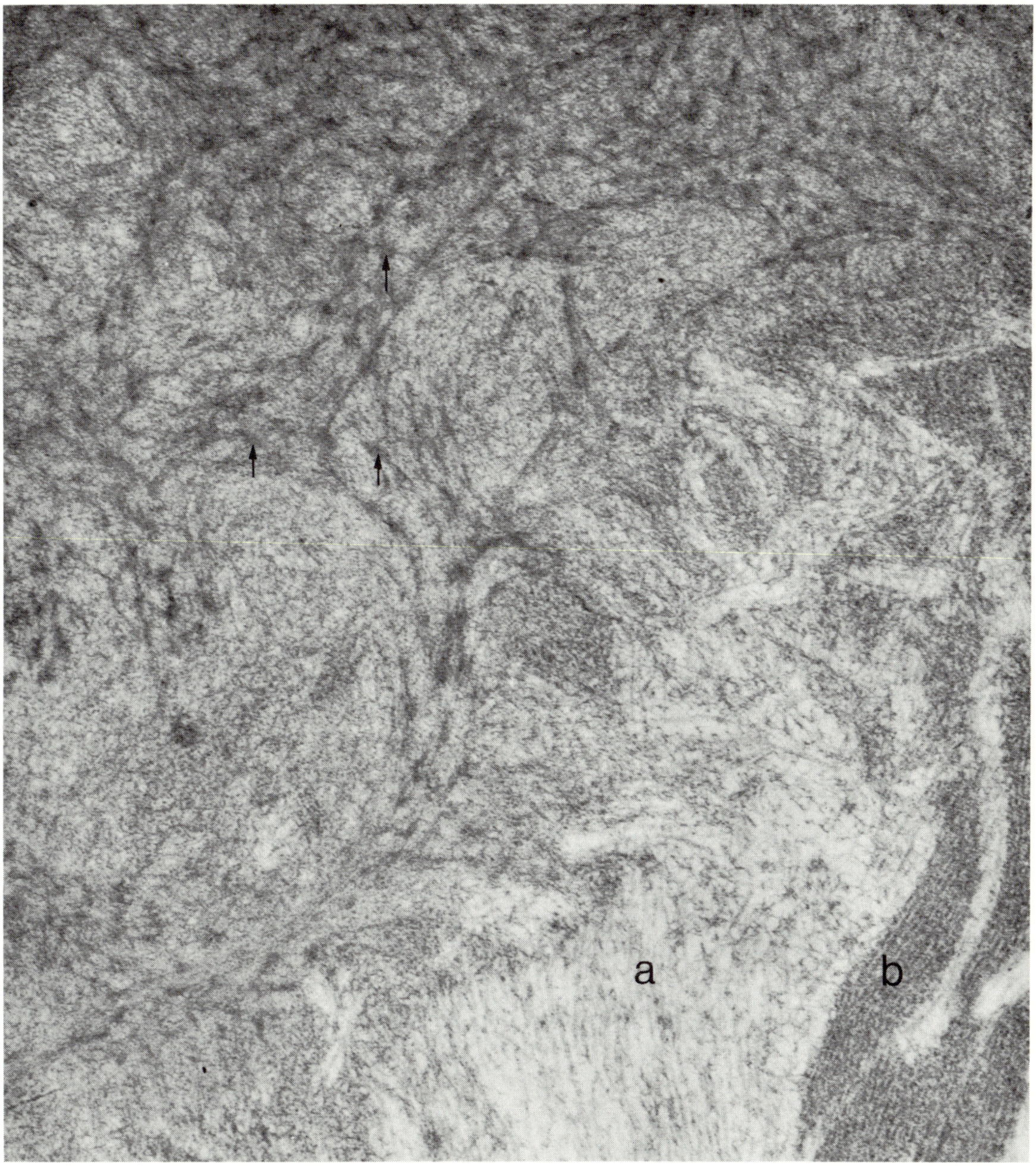

Figure 3–30. Descemet's membrane, oblique section at the junction of the membrane with the deepest lamella. The filaments and nodes are indicated by arrows. Collagen fibrils (a) and denser aggregations of finer fibrils (b) are seen to merge with the membrane. (× 37,000.)

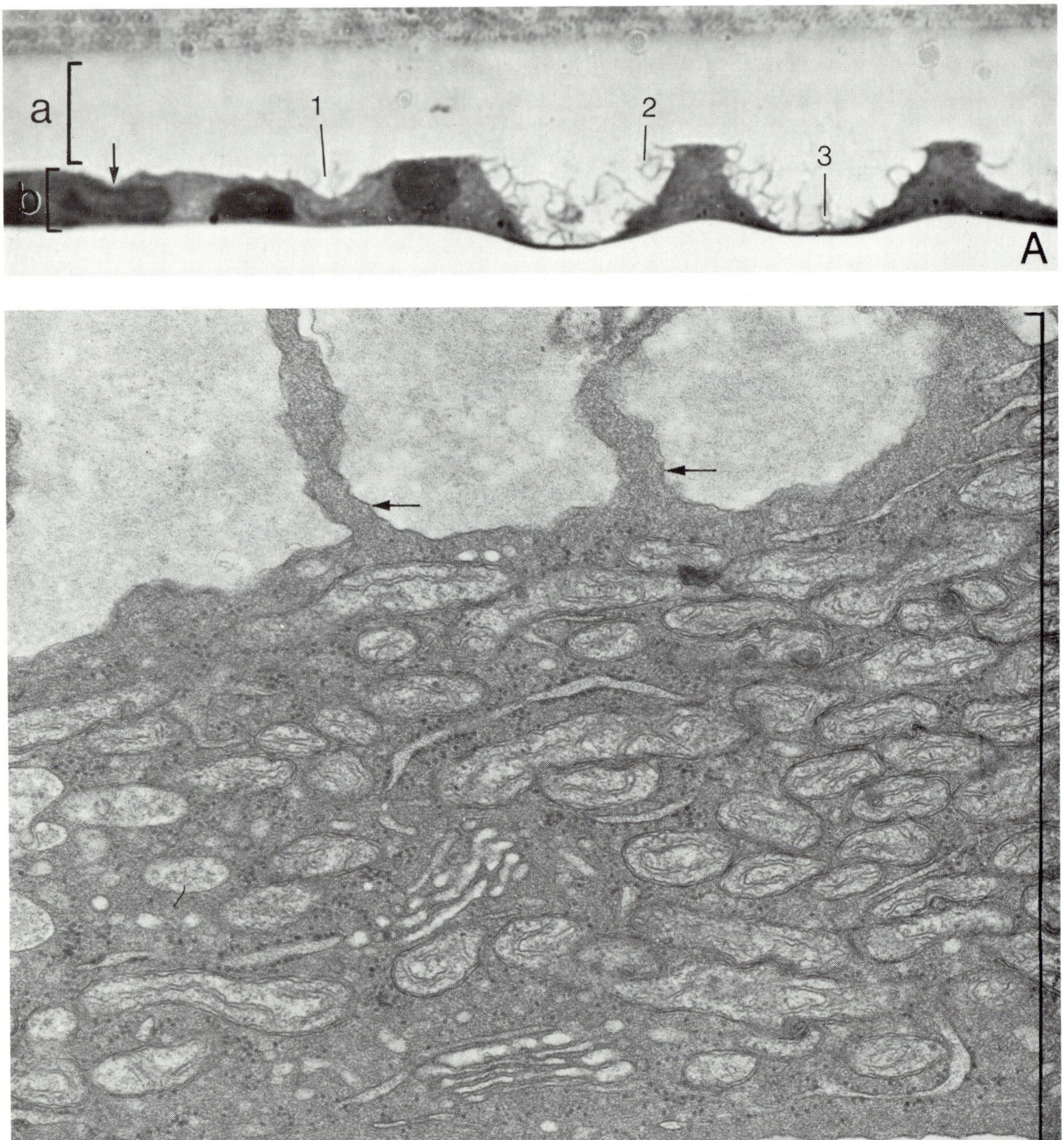

Figure 3-31. *A*, Light microphotograph of Descemet's membrane and the corneal endothelium in the corneal periphery of an older person. The normal appearance and relative size of Descemet's membrane (a) and the endothelium (b) are seen on the extreme left. Different stages in the formation of Hassall-Henle warts are seen on the right. An arrow points to a small depression in the anterior surface of the endothelium and probably represents an early stage in the formation of a wart. At (1) endothelial cytoplasmic processes extend into a fissure in Descemet's membrane; the processes do not extend into Descemet's membrane beyond the area formerly occupied by an intact endothelium. (2) and (3) represent further stages in the formation of the warts. There is extreme thinning of the endothelial cell at (3). Equivalent areas are illustrated in Figures 3-32 and 3-33. (× 760.)

B, Electron micrograph of area labeled (1) in *A*. The bracket indicates the usual thickness of the endothelium in corneal areas which are free of warts. The endothelial mitochondria appear to be tightly grouped, and other cytoplasmic organelles are present. Arrows point to cytoplasmic extensions of the corneal endothelium into Descemet's membrane. (× 30,800.)

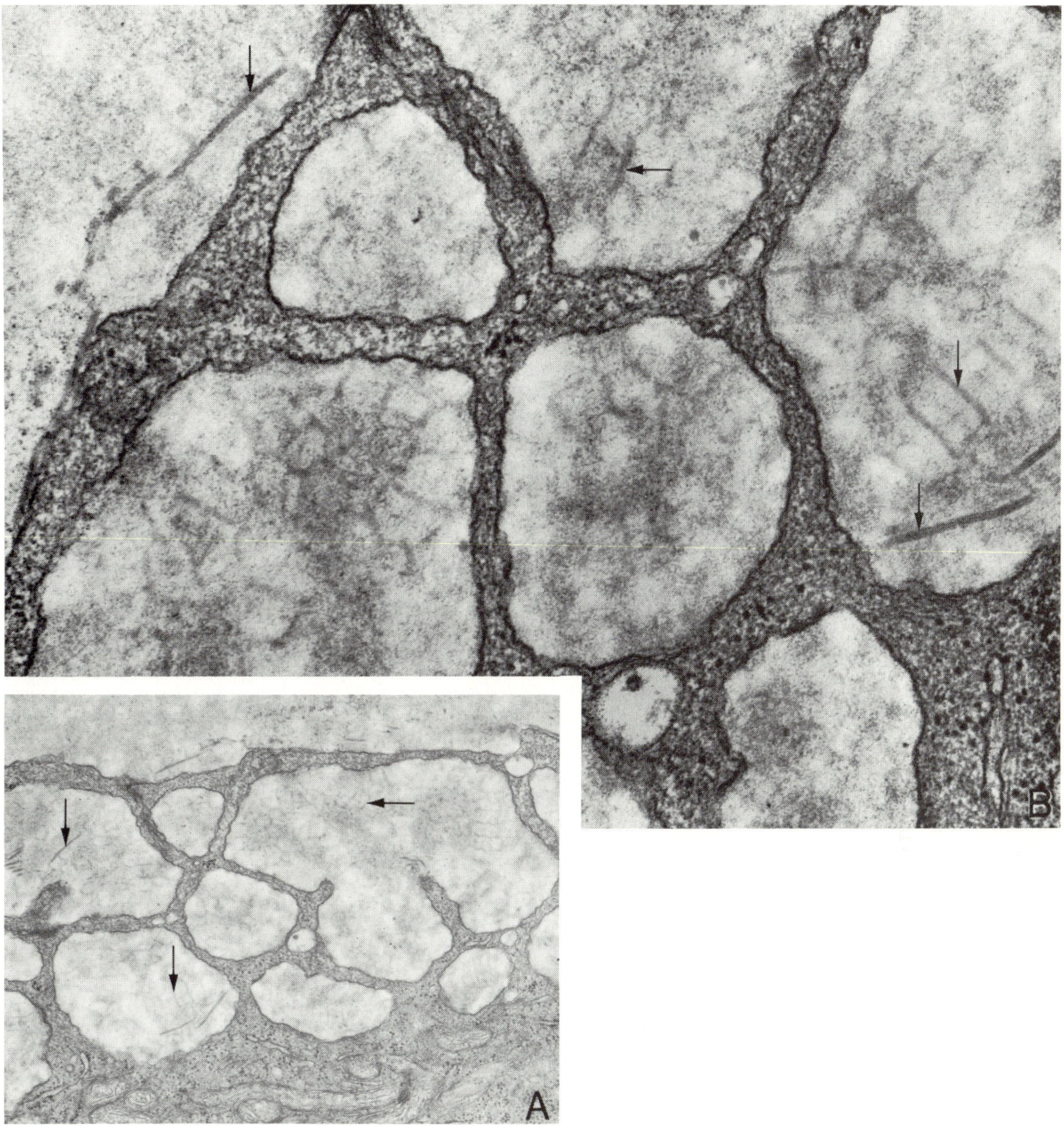

Figure 3–32. *A*, Low-magnification electron microscopic photograph of area labeled (2) in Figure 3-31 *A*. The cytoplasmic extensions of endothelium into Descemet's membrane enclose a network which contains numerous fibrils (arrows). (× 13,200.) *B*, Higher magnification of area seen in *A*. A finely granular material and fibrils are seen to be surrounded by the cytoplasmic extensions. (× 50,000.)

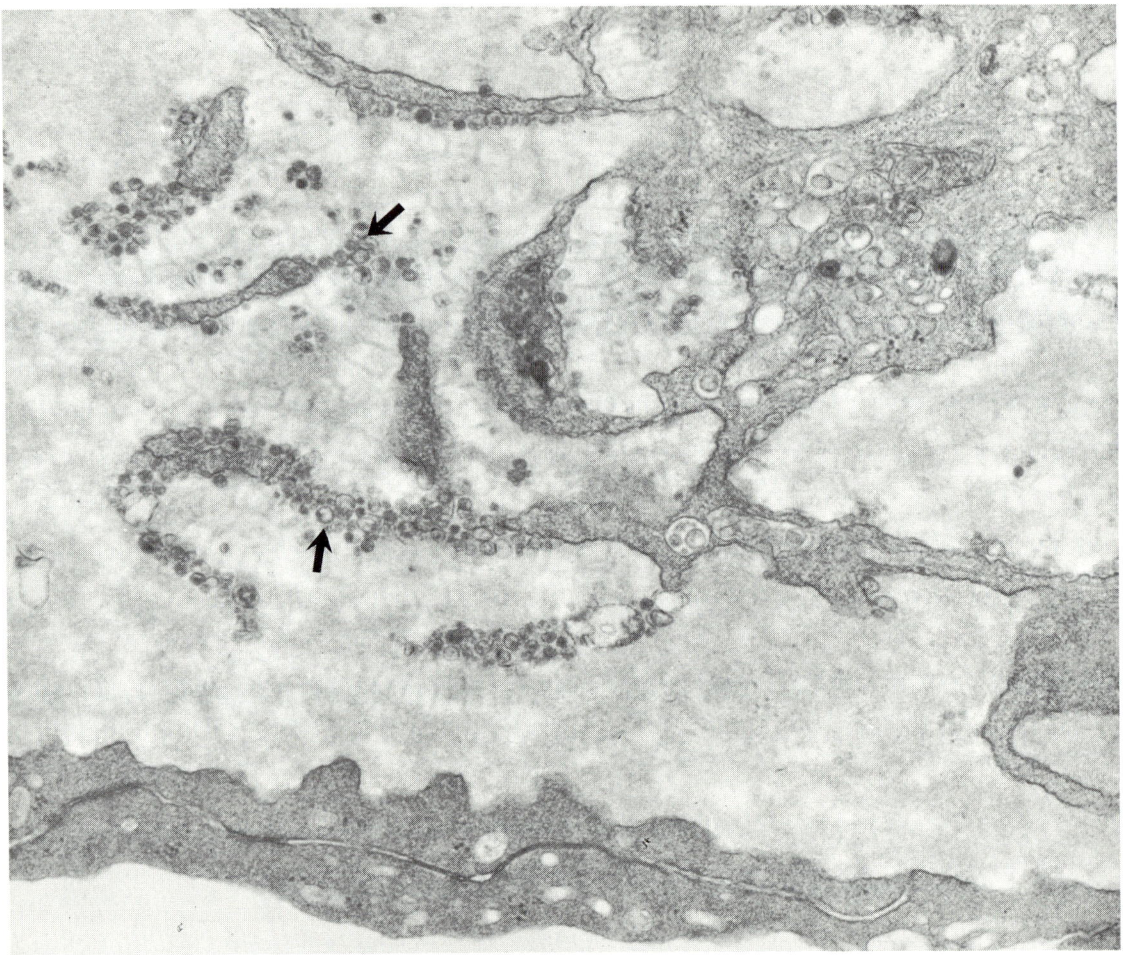

Figure 3-33. Electron micrograph of area labeled (3) in Figure 3-31 A. The endothelium has become very thin and the cytoplasmic processes have degenerated into small round fragments (arrows). The cell processes eventually disappear, leaving fissures in Descemet's membrane which are occupied only by cellular debris. (× 26,400.)

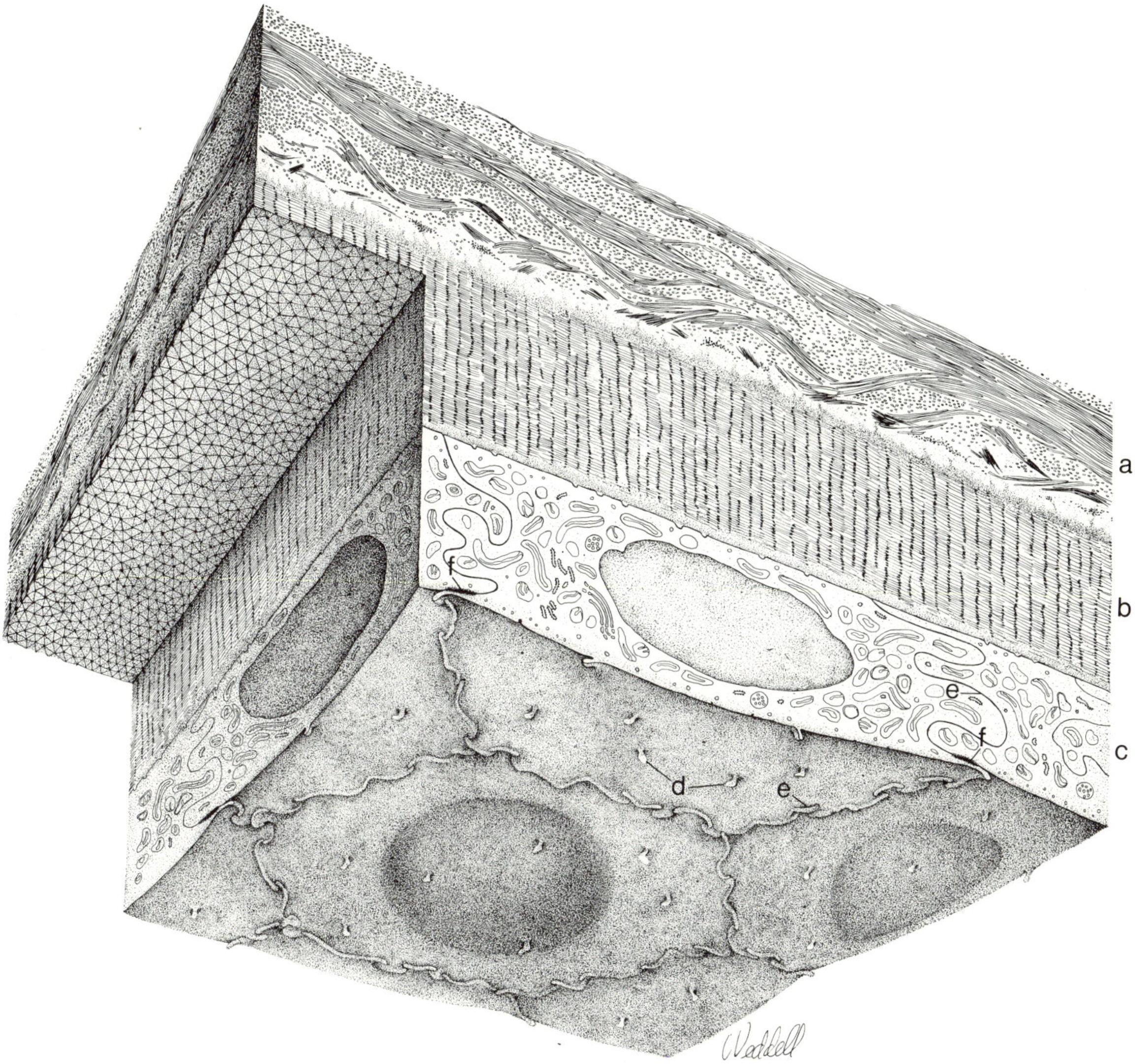

Figure 3–34. Three-dimensional drawing of the deep cornea showing the deepest corneal lamellae (a), Descemet's membrane (b) and the endothelium (c). The deeper stromal lamellae split and some branches curve posteriorly to merge with Descemet's membrane. Descemet's membrane is seen in meridional and tangential planes. The collagenous lattice of this membrane has intersecting filaments which form nodes. The nodes are separated from each other by 1100 A. and are quite exactly superimposed on each other to form a linear pattern in meridional sections. The endothelial cells are polygonal in shape, measuring approximately 3.5 μm. in thickness and 7 to 10 μm. in length. Microvilli (d) protrude into the anterior chamber from the posterior cell, and the marginal folds (e) at intercellular junctions project into the anterior chamber. The intercellular space near the anterior chamber is closed by a zonula occludens (f). The cytoplasm contains an abundance of rod-shaped mitochondria. The nucleus is round and flattened in the anteroposterior axis.

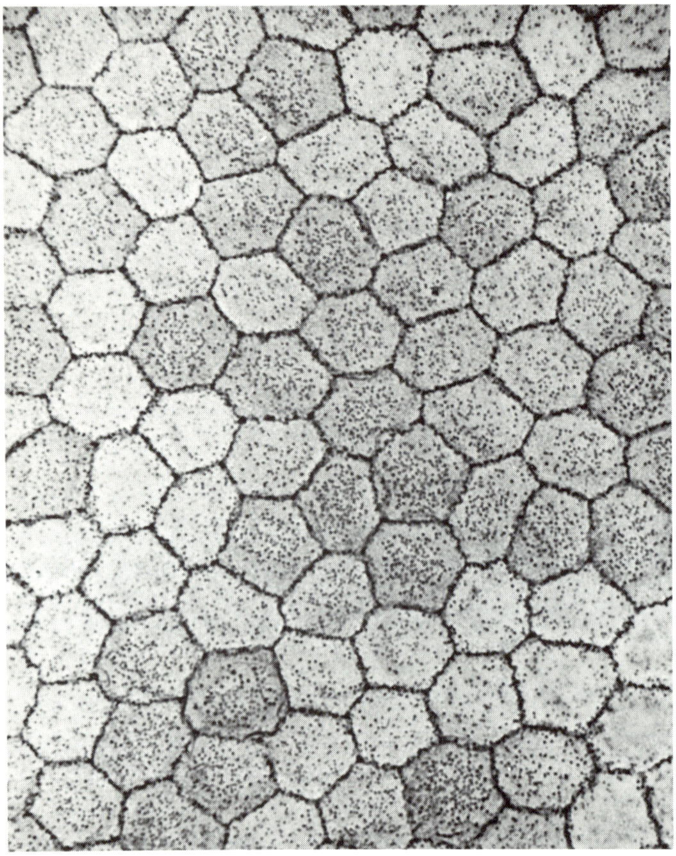

Figure 3–35. Flat, whole mount of the corneal endothelium seen by phase contrast micrography. The polygonal endothelial cells form a mosaic. The polygonal pattern of the peripheral endothelial cells is less regular than that in the central endothelium. The serrated lateral borders at the cell junctions can be seen clearly. (× 656.)

fissures and channels. In the young eye (third and fourth decade) the fissures are filled with endothelial cell cytoplasm that is coarsely granular, whereas in older eyes they contain only cellular debris. Figure 3–34 is a diagram which summarizes the relation of Descemet's membrane to the deep cornea and to the endothelium.

ENDOTHELIUM (Figs. 3–28 and 3–36 to 3–41)

The corneal endothelium comprises a single layer of approximately 500,000 thin polygonal (mostly hexagonal) cells measuring 5 μm. in height and 18 to 20 μm. in width. The nucleus is oval and measures about 7 μm. in diameter; it is located centrally in the cell. Early in life these nuclei are regularly spaced across the cornea, but they become less regular with increasing age due to endothelial cell degeneration and a coincident failure of replacement. Mitoses occur in the young endothelial cell but are extremely rare in adult cells, and its seems that multiplication occurs only by amitosis in adult life. In the adult eye loss of endothelial cells in the central two thirds of the cornea leads to replacement by thinning and spreading out of the surrounding cells rather than by division of adjacent cells. The reduced regularity of spacing of the nuclei in the adult eye and the decreased height of these cells is probably due to the infrequency of mitosis of cells in

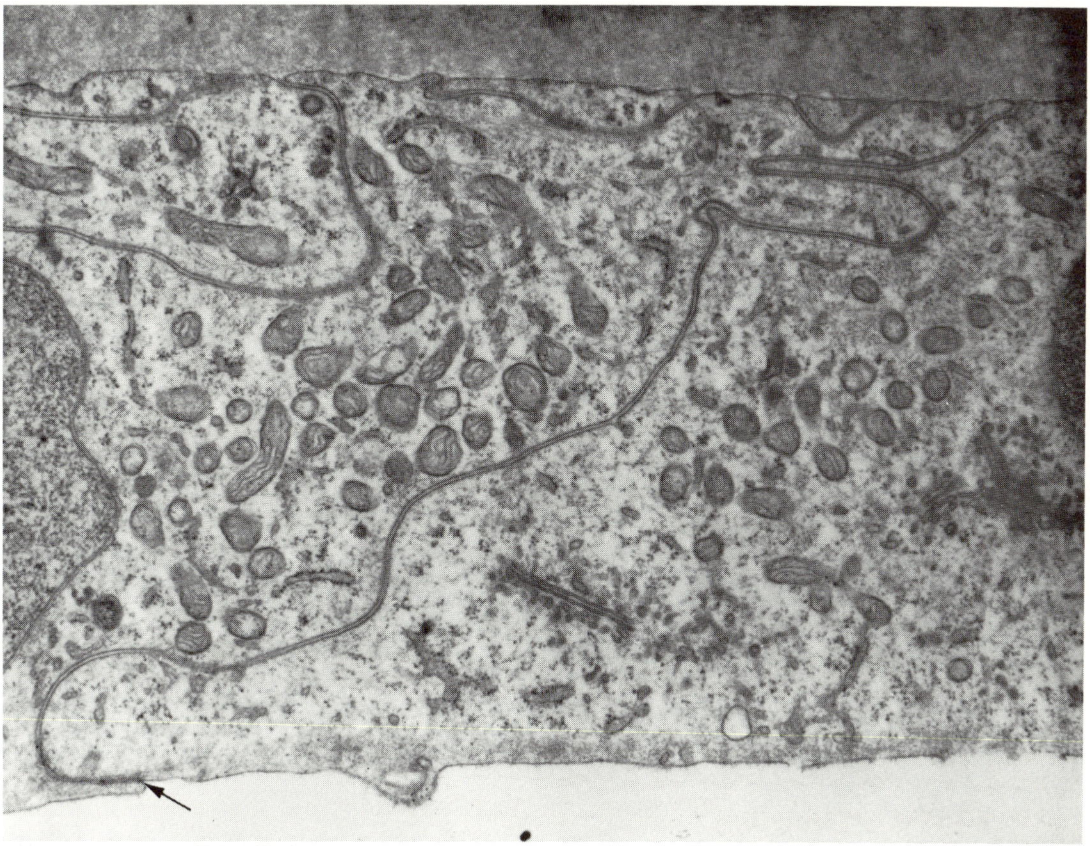

Figure 3–36. Endothelial cells. Intercellular space and lateral walls. The entire intercellular space from the anterior chamber to Descemet's membrane is shown. The space is 200 A. wide along most of the lateral wall, except for an area near the anterior chamber where it is closed by a zonula occludens (arrow). Occasionally along the lateral edge the intercellular space may become narrower at the site of a macula adherens, and maculae occludentes have also been observed. (× 20,000.)

different portions of the adult cornea, as well as in different age groups (Irvine and Irvine, 1953).

Electron microscopic, biochemical and radioisotopic studies have accomplished a great deal toward explaining the structure and function of the corneal endothelium. These cells possess the organelles characteristic of cells engaged in active transport and protein synthesis for secretion. They appear to be engaged in the movement of osmotically active substances and also synthesize some components of Descemet's membrane.

The cell membrane of the endothelium is a typical unit membrane, having numerous pinocytotic vesicles on the anterior and posterior sides. The surface of the posterior cell membrane shows 20 to 30 microvilli per cell measuring and projecting into the anterior chamber 0.1 to 0.2 μm. in width and 0.5 to 0.6 μm. in height. These endothelial microvilli are a constant feature of all the endothelial cells. Wolf (1969) showed these microvilli in the peripheral endothelia of the corneas of mammals with the use of replication methods, and Blümcke and Morgenroth (1967) demonstrated them with the scanning electron microscope.

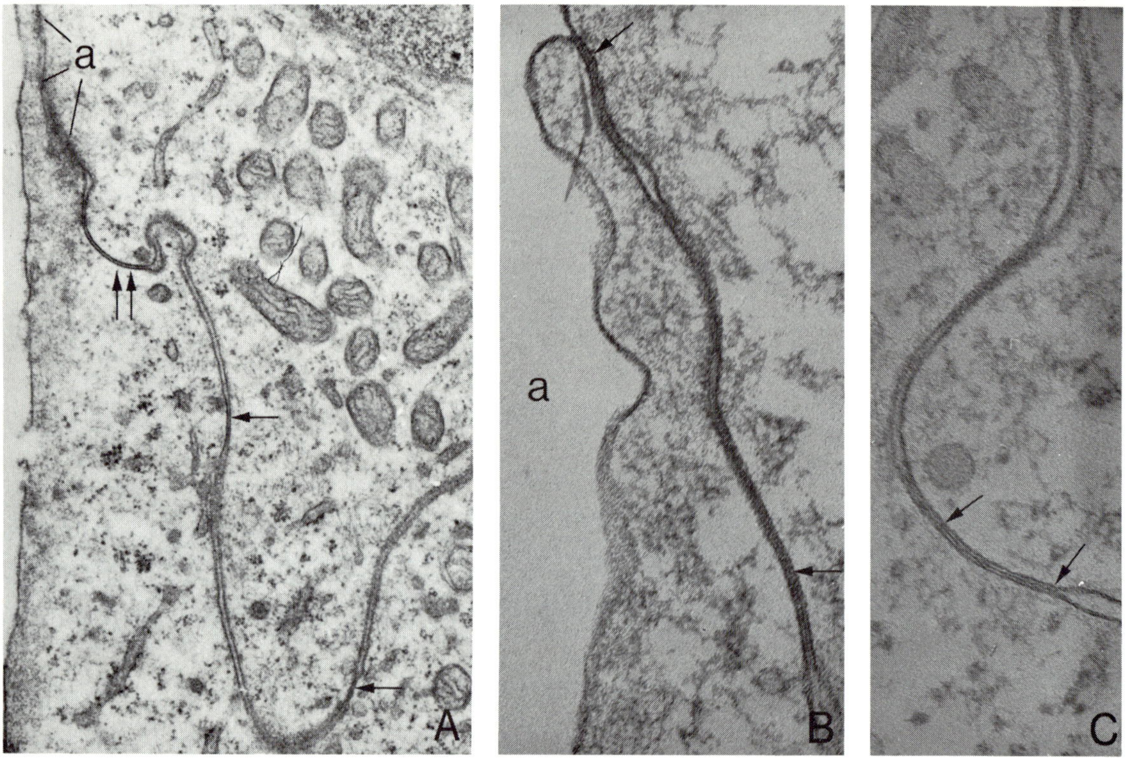

Figure 3–37. Endothelial junctions. *A*, Low magnification electron micrograph showing a zonula occludens (a) near the anterior chamber, a macula occludens (double arrows), and two areas of narrowing of the intercellular space produced by a macula adherens (single arrows). (× 31,500.)

B, Higher magnification view of a zonula occludens. The anterior chamber is located at (a) and the arrows show the area of membrane fusion. (× 82,000.)

C, Enlarged view of a macula occludens. The arrows indicate the site of membrane fusion. (× 107,000.)

The lateral cell membranes between adjacent cells show interesting modifications. The endothelial cells are joined to each other by zonulae occludentes, maculae occludentes and maculae adhaerentes, but no desmosomes. The zonula occludens joins the cells in their posterior one third, most often near the anterior chamber. The macula occludens is uncommon, appearing along the anterior two thirds of the lateral membranes. The macula adherens is also uncommon, being located along the anterior two thirds of the membranes. In the past the macula adherens has also been called desmosome. In addition to all these junctions the lateral cell membranes have an oblique and tortuous course with respect to the anterior-posterior axis of the cornea and show rather complex interdigitations. The interdigitations continue along the lateral cell membranes almost to the anterior chamber, where a marginal fold is frequently seen.

The anterior cell membrane is in contact with Descemet's membrane. Many small areas of increased density are seen along this membrane. These densities are produced by opened pinocytotic vesicles facing the membrane. The interior of such vesicles has an increased density, and when they become continuous with the cell membrane this density becomes part of the membrane.

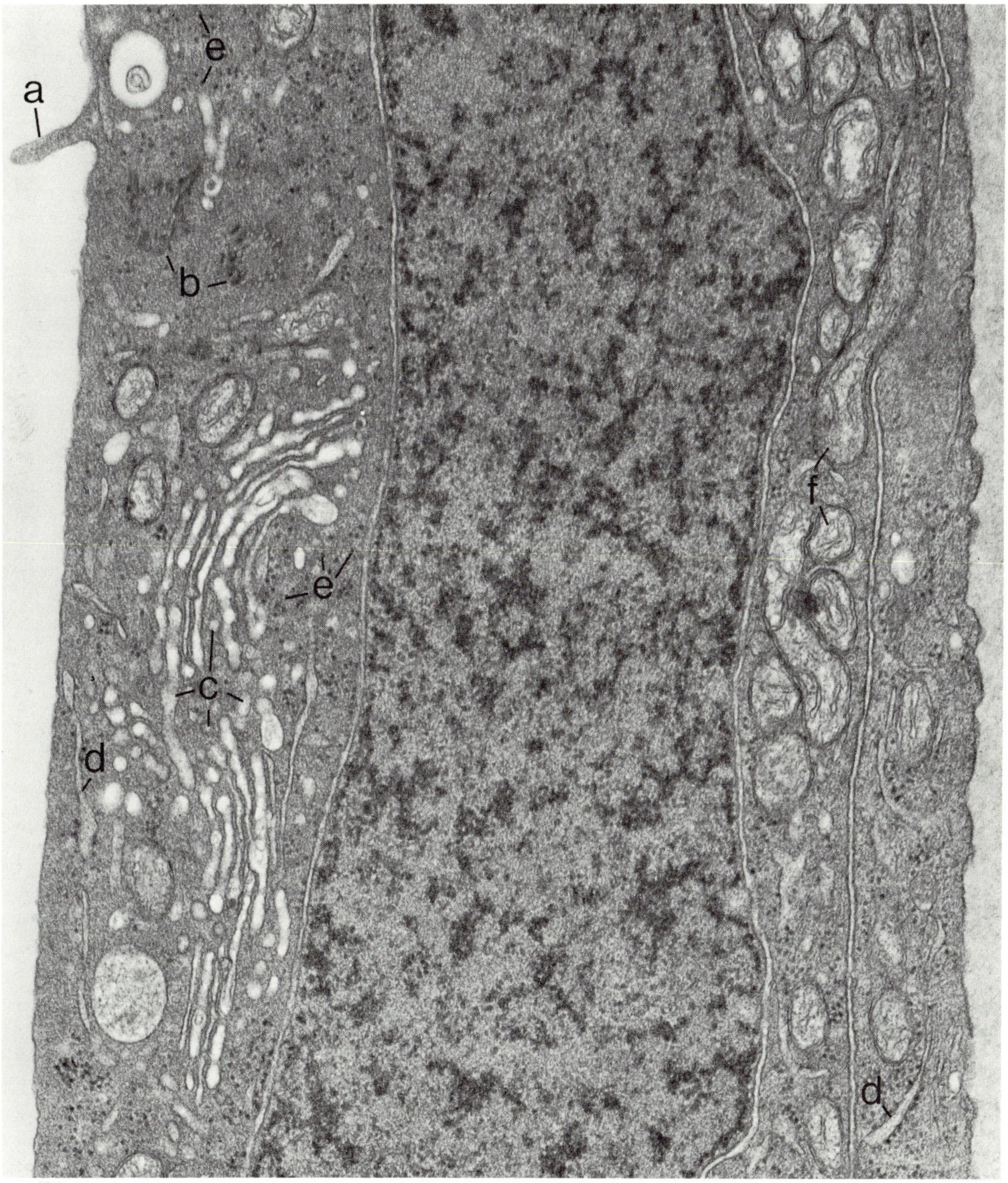

Figure 3-38. Endothelium. A microvillus protrudes into the anterior chamber at (a), and two centrioles (b) are in the posterior cytoplasm near the nucleus. A prominent Golgi complex is seen at (c) and cisternae of rough-surfaced endoplasmic reticulum (d) are scattered throughout the cytoplasm. There are numerous free ribosomes (e) and many closely packed mitochondria (f). (× 34,100.)

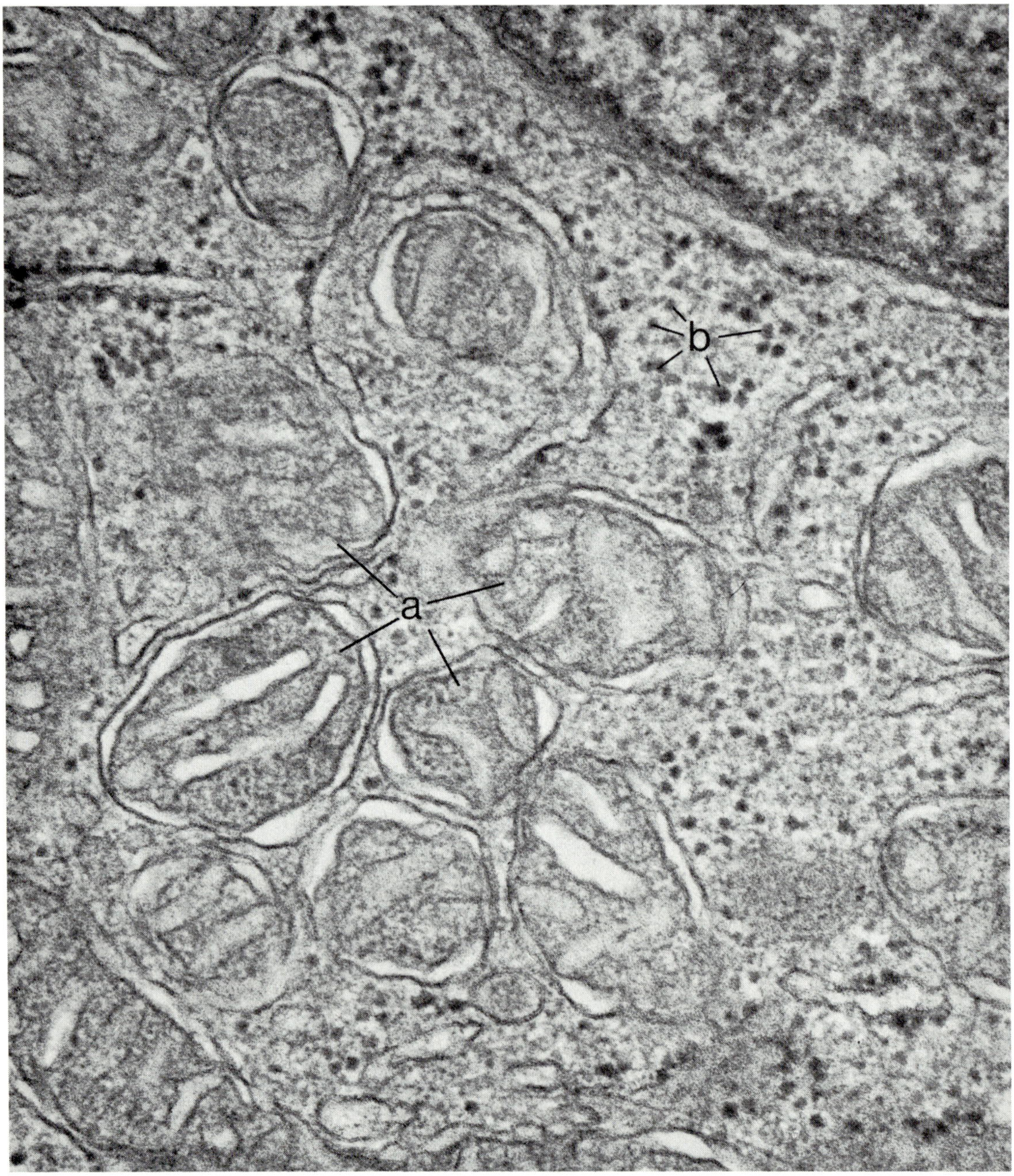

Figure 3-39. Endothelium. The cytoplasm of the endothelium is characterized by the large number of closely packed mitochondria with longitudinally disposed cristae (a) and by numerous free ribosomes (b). A portion of the nucleus with its dispersed chromatin (heterochromatin) is seen at the upper right. (× 84,000.)

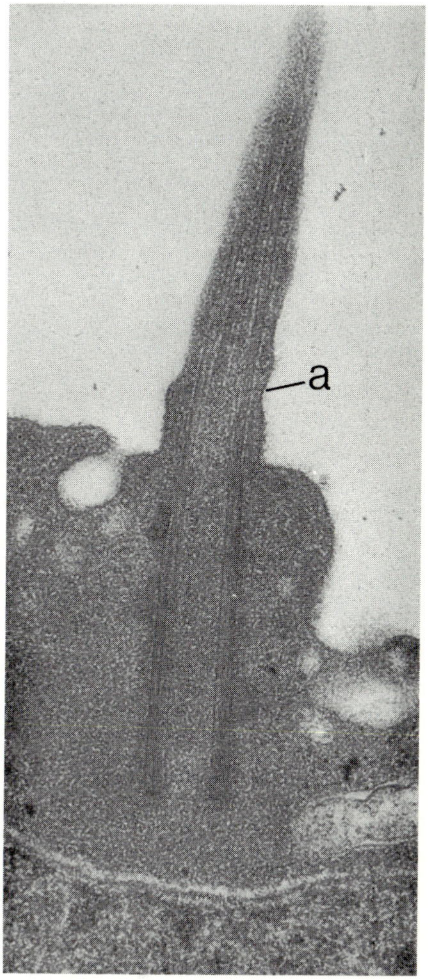

Figure 3-40. Endothelium. Occasional corneal endothelial cells have a cilium (a) which protrudes into the anterior chamber. Similar cilia are also present in cells on the anterior surface of the iris and on the endothelial cells covering the trabecular sheets. (× 62,500.)

Pinocytotic vesicles are also found along the inner surfaces of the posterior and lateral cell membranes. It is known that these vesicles are formed by the surface invaginations of the cell membrane and that they contain substances which will be used for the cells and the adjacent corneal stroma. The vesicles detach themselves from the cell membrane, traverse the cytoplasm, and release their contents either into the spaces between the endothelial cells anterior to the zonula occludens or in the region of Descemet's membrane. Their function has been studied by the use of labeled isotopes and radiopaque substances (Maurice, 1953; Kaye et al., 1961, 1962; Iwamoto and Smelser, 1965). For example, after injection into the anterior chamber, Thorotrast is removed from the aqueous humor into the endothelial cytoplasm by pinocytosis, and the pinocytotic vesicles have been observed to transfer the Thorotrast into the intercellular space anterior to the zonula occludens. The Thorotrast is later found to be concentrated at the inner surface of Descemet's membrane. Cold inhibits this removal, suggesting that its movement is a metabolic function involving active transport. Particles 58 A. in size can be transferred across the endothelium in this way. Water, however, does not pass from the anterior chamber to the corneal stroma by this method (Maurice, 1951).

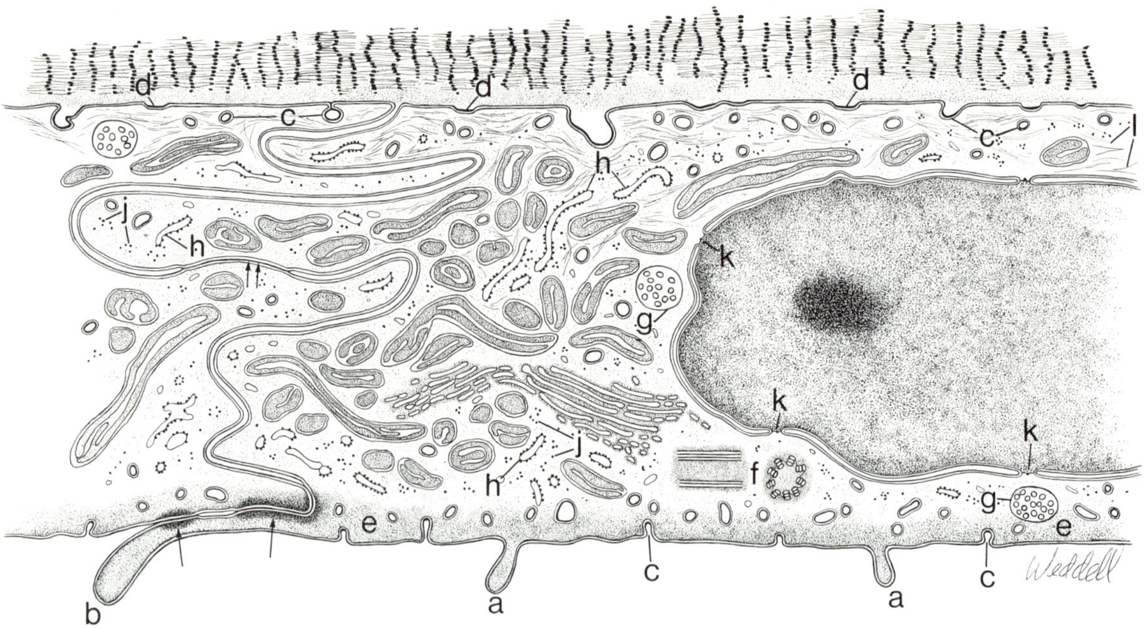

Figure 3-41. Summary drawing showing portions of two endothelial cells. The posterior surface of the cells shows short, club-like microvilli (a) and there is a marginal fold (b) at the cell junctions which protrudes into the anterior chamber. Pinocytotic vesicles (c) open into the anterior chamber and at the cell surface which faces Descemet's membrane. The membrane leaflet which lines the interior of the vesicles is more dense than the leaflet which faces the cytoplasm (d). On the lateral side a 200 A. wide space separates contiguous endothelial cells. The posterior intercellular space is closed by a zonula occludens (arrows). Because of the zonula occludens particulate matter must first pass through the endothelial cytoplasm to circumvent the tight junction. A macula occludens (double arrows) is frequently seen elsewhere along the lateral cell membrane. Maculae adherentes are rarely seen. The organelle-free terminal web (e) is seen in the cytoplasm adjacent to the anterior chamber. A pair of centrioles (f) and a prominent Golgi apparatus are usually found posterior to the nucleus. Multivesicular bodies (g), cisternae of the rough-surfaced endoplasmic reticulum (h), and free ribosomes (j) are indicated. The nuclear envelope with several nuclear pores (k) appears on the right. Thin cytoplasmic filaments are found mainly in the anterior cytoplasm (l). The mitochondria are a common feature of epithelial engaged in the active transport of water; they provide the high energy phosphates required by membrane-associated pumps which carry on such activities. Such a pump, however, has not been adequately characterized for the corneal endothelium.

The endothelial cell cytoplasm is rich in organelles. Near the posterior cell membrane is a terminal web, measuring about 0.2 μm. in thickness, composed of a thin meshwork of fine filaments that increases the density of the cytoplasm perceptibly (Iwamoto and Smelser, 1965). In other tissues where the terminal web is found it is usually associated with tight junctions. The corneal endothelium seems to have this same arrangement, since the web, at its lateral edges, lies in juxtaposition to the zonula occludens.

The number of mitochondria in these cells is striking, being more numerous than in any other cell of the eye, excepting the ellipsoids of the retinal receptor cells. They are long and their cristae are oriented longitudinally. The mitochondria are distributed throughout the cytoplasm, but they are most numerous around the nucleus and are scarce in the region of the terminal web. Both rough and smooth-surfaced endoplasmic reticulum are present, and free ribosomes occur throughout the cytoplasm. There is an extremely well developed Golgi apparatus in the usual perinuclear position, facing the posterior chamber. An interesting finding in some of these cells is a pair of centrioles in the posterior cytoplasm, with a cilium projecting into the anterior chamber. This finding of cilia suggests a common origin for these cells with those of the corneoscleral trabecular sheets and the cells on the anterior surface of the iris. The endothelial cytoplasm also contains vesicles in some areas; some are associated with the Golgi apparatus.

It is not uncommon to see pigment granules in the cytoplasm of the corneal endothelial cells. The granules apparently have been phagocytosed from the aqueous humor, and they appear to be melanin which has been released from the uveal cells. Lysosomes are occasionally seen in the cytoplasm, as are multivesicular bodies which are probably related to the lysosomes as residual structures following intracellular enzymatic digestion.

REFERENCES

Abraham, A.: Microscopic innervation of the cornea with reference to the neural connections of the fibrocytes. Acta Biol. Hung. *6*:31, 1955.

Adler, F. H.: Physiology of the Eye. 4th ed. St. Louis, The C. V. Mosby Co., 1965.

Bairati, A., and Grignolo, A.: Preliminary investigations of the submicroscopic structure of Descemet's membrane with the electron microscope. Boll. Soc. Ital. Biol. Sper. *30*:16, 1954.

Baud, C. A., and Balavoine, C.: The intimate structure of Descemet's membrane and its pathological derivatives. Ophthalmologica *126*:290, 1953.

Blümcke, S., and Morgenroth, K., Jr.: The stereo ultrastructure of the external and internal surface of the cornea. J. Ultrastruct. Res. *18*:502, 1967.

Blümcke, S., Rode, J., and Kudszus, G.: Feinstruckuselllе Veränderungen des Corneaepithels in der Gewebekultur. I. Die Lipoidschicht an der Epithelflöche. Z. Zellforsch. *82*:589, 1967.

Busacca, A.: The basal membrane of the corneal epithelium. Bull. Soc. Franç. Ophtal. *62*:133, 1949.

Calmettes, L., Deodati, F., Flanel, H., and Bec, P.: Étude histologique et histochemique de l'épithélium anterieur de la cornée et de ses basalés. Arch. Ophthal. (Paris) *16*:481, 1956.

Davson, H.: Some considerations on the salt content of fresh and old ox corneae. Brit. J. Ophthal. *33*:175, 1949.

Dohlman, C. H., and Balazs, E.: Chemical studies on Descemet's membrane in bovine cornea. Arch. Biochem. *56*:446, 1955.

Ehlers, N.: The pre-corneal film. Biomicroscopical, histological, and chemical investigations. Acta Ophthal. *43* (Suppl. 81), 136 pp., 1965.

Feeney, M. L., and Garron, L. K.: Descemet's membrane in the human peripheral cornea: A study by light and electron microscopy. *In* Smelser, G. K. (ed.): The Structure of the Eye. New York, Academic Press, Inc., 1961.

Garzino, A.: Le fibre collagene nella cornea normale e nei processi di cicatrizzazione corneale. Rass. Ital. Ottal. *24*:118, 1955.

Goldman, J. N., and Benedek, G. B.: The relationship between morphology and transparency in the nonswelling corneal stroma of the shark. Invest. Ophthal. *6*:574, 1968.

Grignolo, A.: Studies on the submicroscopical structure of the ocular tissues. Boll. Ocul. *33*:513, 1954.

Hanna, C., Bicknell, D. S., and O'Brien, J. E.: Cell turnover in the adult human eye. Arch. Ophthal. (Chicago) *65*:695, 1961.

Hanna, C., and O'Brien, J. E.: Cell production and migration in the epithelial layers of the cornea. A.M.A. Arch. Ophthal. *65*:536, 1960.

Henkind, P.: Migration of limbal melanocytes into the corneal epithelium of the guinea pigs. Exp. Eye Res. *4*:42, 1965.

Hogan, M. J., and Zimmerman, L. E.: Opthalmic Pathology—An Atlas and Textbook. 2nd ed. Philadelphia, W. B. Saunders Company, 1962.

Irvine, A. R., and Irvine, A. R., Jr.: Variations in normal human corneal endothelium; preliminary report of pathologic human corneal endothelium. Amer. J. Ophthal. *36*:1279, 1953.

Ishida, T.: A study of corneal tissue by electron microscopy. Acta. Soc. Ophthal. Jap. *62*:1324; 2220, 1958.

Iwamoto, T., and Smelser, G. K.: Electron microscopy of the human corneal endothelium with reference to transport mechanisms. Invest. Ophthal. *4*:270, 1965.

Jakus, M. A.: Studies on the cornea. II. The fine structure of Descemet's membrane. J. Biophys. Biochem. Cytol. (Suppl.) 2:241, 1956.

Jakus, M. A.: The fine structure of the human cornea. *In* Smelser, G. K. (ed.): The Structure of the Eye. New York, Academic Press, Inc., 1961.

Kaye, G. I., and Pappas, G. D.: Studies on the cornea. I. The fine structure of the rabbit cornea and the uptake and transport of colloidal particles by the cornea *in vivo*. J. Cell Biol. *21*:457, 1962.

Kaye, G. I., Pappas, G., and Donn, A.: An electron microscope study of the rabbit corneal endothelium in relation to its uptake and transport of colloidal particles. Anat. Rec. *139*:244, 1961.

Kaye, G. I., Pappas, G. D., Donn, A., and Mallett, N.: Studies on the cornea. II. The uptake and transport of colloidal particles by the living rabbit cornea *in vivo*. J. Cell Biol., *12*:481, 1962.

Kayes, J., and Holmberg, A.: The fine structure of Bowman's layer and the basement membrane of the corneal epithelium. Amer. J. Ophthal. *50*:1013, 1960.

Kinoshita, J. H.: Some aspects of the carbohydrate metabolism of the cornea. Invest. Ophthal. *1*:178, 1962.

Kinoshita, J. H., and Masurat, T.: Aerobic pathways of glucose metabolism in bovine corneal epithelium. Amer. J. Ophthal. *48*:47, 1959.

Kinoshita, J. H., Masurat, T., and Helfant, M.: Pathways of glucose metabolism in corneal epithelium. Science *122*:72, 1955.

Kohler, A., and Tobgy, A. F.: Mikroskopishe Untersuchungen einiger Augenmedien mit ultravioletten und mit polarisiertem Licht. Graefes Arch. Ophthal. *99*:263, 1929.

Kokott, W.: Das Spaltlinienbild der Sklera. Klin. Mbl. Augen. *92*:117, 1934.

Kokott, W.: Uber mechanischfunktionelle Strukturen des Auges. Arch. Ophthal. *138*:424, 1938.

Langham, M. E., and Taylor, I. S.: Factors affecting the hydration of the cornea in the excised eye and the living animal. Brit. J. Ophthal. *40*:321, 1956.

LaTessa, A. J., Teng, C. C., and Katzin, H. M.: The histochemistry of the basement membrane of the cornea. Amer. J. Ophthal. *38*:171 (Aug.), 1954.

Laurent, T. C., and Anseth, A.: Studies on corneal polysaccharides. II. Characterization. Exp. Eye Res. *1*:99, 1961.

Loewenstein, A.: Glass membranes in the eye; Bowman's membrane, Descemet's membrane, and lens capsule. Amer. J. Ophthal. *23*:1229, 1940.

Martola, E. L., and Baum, J. L.: Central and peripheral corneal thickness. Arch. Ophthal. (Chicago) *79*:28, 1968.

Maurice, D. M.: The permeability of sodium ions of the living rabbit's cornea. J. Physiol. *122*:367, 1951.

Maurice, D. M.: Preliminary notes. Intercellular spacing of the corneal endothelium. Biochim. et Biophys. Acta *11*:311, 1953.

Maurice, D. M.: The structure and transparency of the cornea. J. Physiol. *136*:263, 1957.

Maurice, D. M.: Cornea and sclera. *In* Davson, H. (ed.): Physiology of the Eye. 2nd ed. Boston, Little, Brown and Co., 1969, pp. 6, 14, 15.

Maurice, D. M.: Transparency of the Human Cornea by J. W. Smith. Letter to the editor. Vision Res. *10*:107, 1970.

Maurice, D. M., and Riley, M. V.: The Biochemistry of the cornea. *In* Graymore, C. N. (ed.): The Biochemistry of the Eye. New York, Academic Press, Inc., 1968.

Mawas, J.: The innervation of the human cornea. Bull Soc. Ophthal. France *2*:162, 1951.

McTigue, J. W.: The human cornea: A light and electron microscopic study of the normal cornea and its alterations in various dystrophies. Trans. Amer. Ophthal. Soc. *65*:591, 1967.

Mishima, S.: Some physiological aspects of the precorneal tear film. Arch. Ophthal. (Chicago) *73*:233, 1965.

Otorí, T.: Electrolyte content of the rabbit corneal stroma. Exp. Eye Res. *6*:356, 1967.

Payrau, P., Pouliquen, Y., Faure, J. P., and Offret, G.: La Transparence de la Cornée. Les Mechanismes de ses Altérations. Paris, Masson et Cie., 1967.

Pedler, C.: The fine structure of the corneal epithelium. Exp. Eye Res. *1*:286, 1962.

Peschell, D.: Die strukturlosen Augenmembranen im Ultramikroskop. v. Graefes Arch. Ophthal. *60*:557, 1905.

Polack, F. M.: Morphology of the cornea. I. Study with silver stains. Amer. J. Ophthal. *51*:179, 1961.

Ramachandran, G. N.: Chemistry of Collagen. New York, Academic Press, Inc., 1967, Vol. 1, Chapter 1, pp. 1-75.

Redslob, E.: Le Développement de la cornée. Arch. d'Anatomi, Histologie et Embryologie *19*:137, 1935.

Schwarz, W.: Electron microscopical studies of the fibrillogenesis in the human cornea. *In* Smelser, G. K. (ed.): The Structure of the Eye. New York, Academic Press, Inc., 1961.

Schwarz, W., and Keyserlingk, D. G.: Über die Feinstrukter der Menschlichen Cornea, mit Desonderer Ber Berüksichtigung des Problems der Transperenz. Z. Zellforsch *73*:540, 1966.

Smelser, G. K., Polack, F. M., and Ozanics, V.: Persistence of donor collagen in corneal transplants. Exp. Eye Res. *4*:349, 1965.

Smith, J. W.: The transparency of the human cornea. Vision Res. *9*:393, 1969.

Teng, C. C., and Katzin, H. M.: The basement membrane of corneal epithelium. A preliminary report. Amer. J. Ophthal. *36*:895, 1953.

Toussaint, D.: A study of the corneal nerves using various histological techniques. Bull. Soc. Belg. Ophtal. *120*:589, 1958.

Virchow, H.: Graefe-Saemisch Handbuch der gesammten Augenheilkunde. Vol. 1, 2nd ed. Leipzig, Engelmann, 1910.

Weimar, V.: Healing processes in the cornea. *In* Duke-Elder, W. S., and Perkins, E. S. (eds.): The Transparency of the Cornea. Oxford, Blackwell Scientific Pub., 1960.

Whitear, M.: An electron microscope study of the cornea in mice, with special reference to the innervation. J. Anat. *94*:387, 1960.

Wislocki, G. B.: The anterior segment of the eye of the Rhesus monkey investigated by histochemical means. Amer. J. Anat. *91*:233, 1952.

Wolf, J.: Pit-like islets of corneal endothelium. Docum. Ophthal. *25*:195, 1969.

Wolter, J. R.: Innervation of the corneal endothelium of the eye of the rabbit. A.M.A. Arch. Ophthal. *58*:246, 1957.

Zander, E., and Weddell, G.: Observations on the innervation of the cornea. J. Anat. *85*:68, 1951.

Chapter Four

THE LIMBUS

The limbus is not a separate structural entity. In the past, some limbal components have been described with the cornea, and the aqueous humor outflow pathways have been included in the anatomy of the anterior chamber angle or even with the aqueous humor itself. However, the limbal components are so important for the maintenance of the intraocular pressure and they provide such a valuable landmark for surgical procedures that this area merits a separate chapter. During recent years so much new information has accumulated on the physiology of the aqueous outflow and the morphology of the limbus that it seems desirable to attempt a separate description.

The limbal transition zone is composed of elements of both the cornea and the sclera. The contribution of each tissue to the structure of the limbus varies in its superficial compared to its deep portion, as well as in the various sectors around the limbal circumference.

The pathologist considers the anterior limit of the limbus to be formed by a plane joining the peripheral termination of Bowman's layer and Descemet's membrane and the posterior limit to be formed by another plane constructed perpendicular to the surface of the eye about 1.5 mm. posterior to the first plane, passing through the scleral spur (Fig. 4-1). These limits are useful for the description of pathologic specimens, so that surrounding tissue changes can be related to the limbus.

Figure 4-1. Drawing of a meridional section of the limbal area. The histologic limit of the corneolimbal junction is outlined by the dotted plane commencing at the termination of Bowman's layer and curving posteriorly toward Schlemm's canal, then extending forward to end at Descemet's membrane. Another definition of the limbus is that used by the pathologist; the anterior limit (corneolimbal junction) is formed by a plane joining the ends of Bowman's layer and Descemet's membrane; the posterior limit by a plane constructed 1.5 mm. posterior to the corneolimbal junction at a right angle to the scleral surface in the superior and inferior limbus, and 2 mm. in the horizontal meridian. The limbus has the following gross anatomic parts: Conjunctival epithelium (a), conjunctival stroma (b), Tenon's capsule and episclera (c), and the limbal or corneoscleral stroma at (d). The longitudinal portion of the ciliary muscle is indicated at (e) and circular and radial bundles of the muscle at (f). The microscopic subdivisions of the limbus are seen in Figure 4-9.

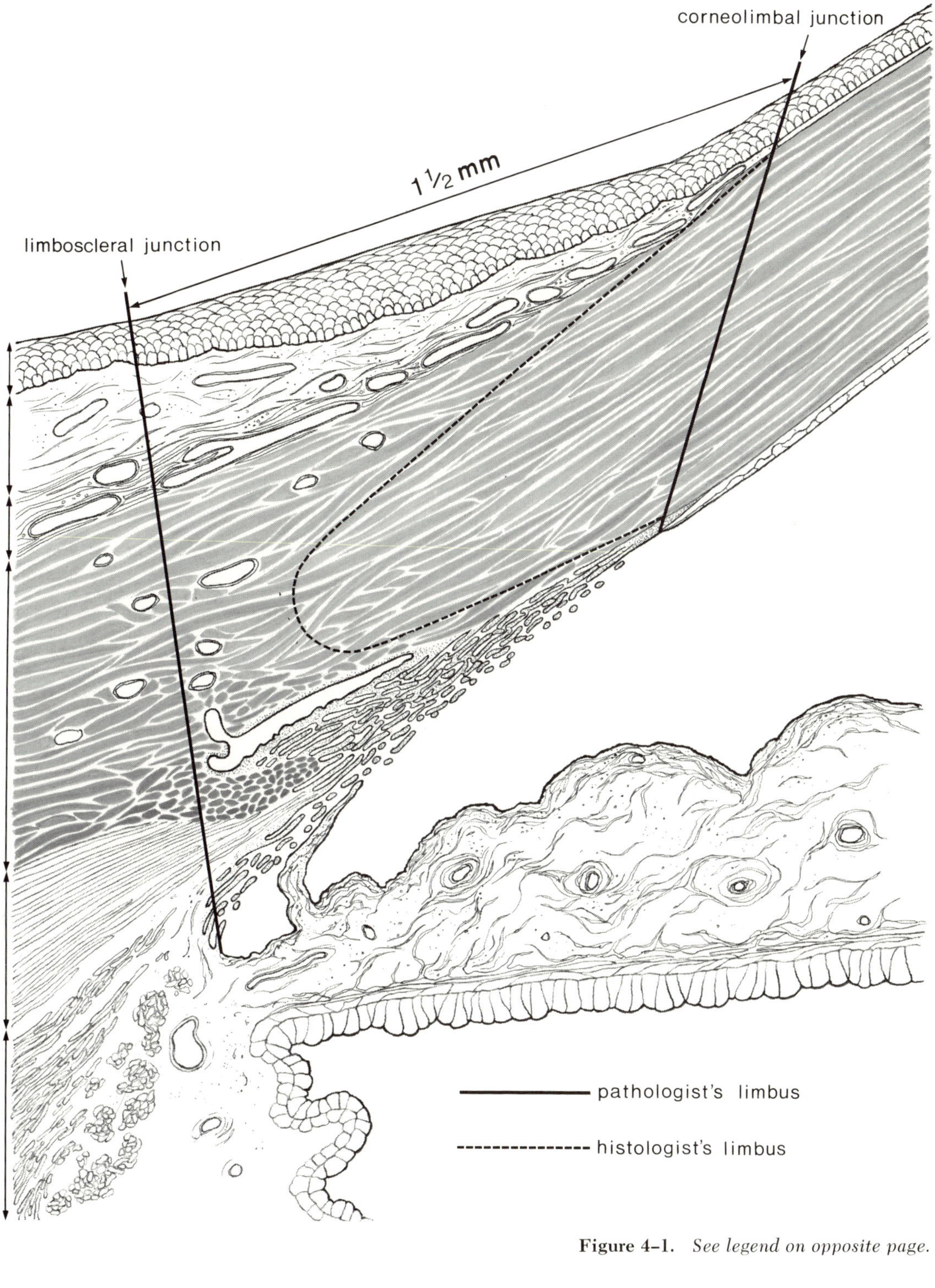

Figure 4-1. *See legend on opposite page.*

It is not easy to demonstrate the junction of the cornea with the sclera in ordinary histologic sections because the transition from opaque sclera to clear cornea is gradual. The junction, however, commences at the end of Bowman's layer and extends posteriorly into the stroma in a concave arc (Fig. 4-1). The deepest posterior extension of the corneoscleral junction is adjacent to the midpart of the canal of Schlemm. From here the junction curves forward external to Schlemm's canal; it ends close to Descemet's membrane in the anterior part of the trabecular meshwork. This histologic arrangement of the corneoscleral junction places the corneoscleral trabecular meshwork and Schlemm's canal within the sclera, and part of the venous system draining the canal within the cornea.

PHYSIOLOGY

The limbus has two important functions: to provide nourishment for the peripheral cornea and to provide a pathway for removal of aqueous humor.

Both the limbal and the peripheral conjunctival capillaries contribute to the nutrition of the peripheral cornea. Substances diffuse from these capillaries and can be detected in the peripheral cornea of experimental animals. Most of them diffuse at a very slow rate in the corneal stroma, however, and finally leave the cornea through the epithelium and the endothelium. Maurice (1960) found the rate of flow of water across the peripheral cornea from these vessels to be very slow. The fact that extensive incisions can be made around the peripheral cornea without interfering significantly with the corneal nutrition and transparency indicates that only a small part of the peripheral cornea is nourished by this route.

Most of the aqueous humor leaves the eye via limbal structures which, from an anatomic standpoint, are specially developed for this purpose. Many aspects of the exact mechanism for the removal of aqueous humor are unclear, but much information is available which demonstrates that the limbus is the *principal site* for aqueous drainage in the eyes of man and primates (Kinsey et al., 1942; Seidel, 1921). Other possible sites for the removal of aqueous humor have been investigated both in man and in other vertebrates; these include the *iris* and the *ciliary body* region.

The role of the iris in the removal of aqueous humor appears to be insignificant because the evidence is that there is little or no bulk flow out of the eye in the iris vessels. The iris, however, plays an important role in changing the composition of the aqueous humor because of diffusion across its surface.

There is good evidence to suggest that part of the aqueous humor leaves the eye in the ciliary body region by the uveoscleral route, the amount being removed varying among different species (Bill, 1965, 1966; Bill and Hellsing, 1965; Bill and Walinder, 1966; Bill and Bárány, 1966). These authors traced the course of ^{131}I-labeled albumin after injection into the anterior chamber of animals and found a *bulk flow* of aqueous humor into adjacent tissues. This radioactive substance could be followed into the ciliary body, the choroid and the suprachoroidal tissues, where it probably was removed by the vessels of these tissues. The flow was found not to be dependent on the level of the intraocular pressure, and the flow varied in different species. For example, in the cynomologus monkey, 35 per cent of aqueous humor was found to be removed by the uveal route; in the vervet monkey the amount removed by the uvea was 23 per cent; in the cat and rabbit only about 3 per cent of the aqueous humor was removed in this manner. The outflow of aqueous humor via this route has not been assessed completely in man, but it may be significant. François and co-workers (1965, 1967) demonstrated such a pathway in enucleated human eyes by microradiography after placing Thorotrast into the anterior chamber. Fine (1964) employed an electron opaque tracer, ferritin, in human and primate eyes, injecting it at physiologic pressures and at a steady state prior to enucleation of the eye. The tracer could be found in the ciliary body, suprachoroidal region and scleral vessels. It seems likely that a small but significant amount of aqueous humor is removed from the eye of man by the uveal route, and the removal appears to be independent of the intraocular pressure. The *principal route* by which aqueous humor leaves the eye in man seems to be quite well established, but the *mechanism* by which it traverses this system of channels is not entirely clear.

The aqueous humor leaving the peripheral anterior chamber moves through the trabecular meshwork and into Schlemm's canal. The uveal part of the meshwork is coarse, with wide spaces, and it offers no hindrance to the passage of the fluid. The openings in the corneoscleral meshwork are of a size which would not be expected to offer significant obstruction to outflow. The intertrabecular spaces are thought to become narrower in the deep meshwork, and there is much more intricate bridging of the spaces by endothelial cells, so that if there is any selective process in the flow of aqueous humor it would be expected to occur in this region. Finally, as the wall of the canal of Schlemm is approached, its wall is interposed between the deepest trabecular spaces and the lumen of the canal, possibly providing another area regulating the flow of aqueous humor. The fineness and complexity of the anatomic arrangement makes it difficult to determine the mechanism by which the aqueous humor crosses the deep meshwork and canal wall to enter the lumen of the canal of Schlemm.

Giant vacuoles have been found in the cytoplasm of some endothelial cells along the inner wall of the canal of Schlemm; it has been suggested that they are important for the removal of aqueous humor. Some observers have traced connections of the vacuoles into the nearest intertrabecular space, and others have found openings from the vacuoles into the lumen of the canal of Schlemm. This suggested that the vacuoles might act intermittently to provide a direct pathway for aqueous humor from the deepest intertrabecular space into the lumen of the canal of Schlemm. More recent studies, employing newer fixation techniques and embedding materials, have not shown these vacuoles connecting into the deepest intertrabecular spaces.

The existence of small canaliculi (internal collector channels; Sonderman's canals) arising from Schlemm's canal and extending into the trabecular meshwork suggested that aqueous humor might bypass the deep trabecular meshwork and enter the canal directly through the canaliculi. Most anatomic studies have shown these canaliculi to extend into the meshwork only a short distance, and physiologic studies seem to indicate that they do not play an important part in removal of aqueous humor.

Perfusion with chromium phosphate and bacteria in rabbit and human eyes (Huggert, 1955) showed that particles 1.2 μm. in size passed through the trabecular meshwork easily in human eyes, and that the maximum size which could traverse the meshwork was betweeen 1.5 and 4.4 μm. Karg and associates (1959) perfused enucleated human eyes with latex spheres. They found that spheres with a diameter of 1.2 μm. passed through easily, that there was some hindrance to passage of spheres with diameters 3.0 μm., while spheres 5.6 μm. in size did not appear in the episcleral veins at all. Utilizing microradiography and radiopaque substances injected into the anterior chamber of freshly enucleated human eyes and in vivo in monkey eyes, François and co-workers (1955) concluded that aqueous humor passes directly from the anterior chamber into Schlemm's canal through openings larger than 1.5 μm. and smaller than 2.25 μm. in diameter.

All these studies show that aqueous humor flows into the canal of Schlemm through openings, then into the external venous branches from the canal and into the episcleral veins. Berggren (1963) found that larger molecules of starch in solutions passed through the filtration meshwork of rabbits more easily than small molecules of glucose, xylose and mannitol in solution. This suggested to him that the movement of substances across the meshwork and venous system could be compared with "gel filtration," a phenomenon shown by a column filled with particles of cross-linked dextran, which allows larger molecules to pass more rapidly than smaller ones. He suggested that the comparable gel in the eye is hyaluronic acid. This mucopolysaccharide is thought to be present in the intertrabecular spaces, and Bárány (1955) has shown experimentally that if a chicken eye is perfused with hyaluronidase there is a significant increase in the facility of outflow. However, the facility returns to normal after about six hours.

From the evidence presented, it seems likely that the aqueous humor passes through the outflow channels by a process similar to filtration. The rate of flow, as determined by calculation from tonography in the human eye, is about 2 μl. per minute.

The outflow channels for aqueous humor include all the structures of the trabecular meshwork, the canal of Schlemm and the collecting veins. The sum total of the resistance to flow of aqueous humor offered by these structures is the reciprocal of the facility of outflow of aqueous humor from the eye. Measurement of this facility is important in the study of the intraocular pressure in normal and glaucomatous eyes. There is some variation in the facility, but it has a mean value of 0.28 ± 0.05 μl. per minute per mm. Hg intraocular pressure; any value below 0.18 is suspect (Becker and Shaffer, 1961). The movement of fluid occurs as a result of a pressure gradient between the mean intraocular pressure (16 ± 2.8 mm. Hg, Schiotz; 15.4 ± 2.5 mm., applanation) (Becker and Shaffer, 1961) and the episcleral venous pressure (9.0 ± 1.4) (Podos et al., 1968).

The ciliary muscle may play a part in the change of facility of outflow because of its attachment to the scleral spur and to the trabecular meshwork. Movement of the spur and the trabecular meshwork under the influence of accommodation or miotics tends to "fan out" the trabecular sheets, diminishing the compact arrangement of the deeper lamellae and reducing the resistance to flow. Flocks and Zweng (1957) studied the effects of pilocarpine on the trabecular meshwork in the primate and demonstrated widening of the intertrabecular spaces in the pilocarpinized eye.

The work of Ascher (1942, 1953) provided the groundwork for important studies on the flow of aqueous humor into the episcleral veins. He described venous channels in the limbal region of the eye which contained clear aqueous humor (the aqueous veins of Ascher). Other veins of this type were also described, either containing diluted blood or exhibiting lamination, one side of the lumen being occupied by blood and the other by clear aqueous humor. The laminated veins are formed by the confluence of a venous channel with an aqueous vein. Ascher showed that if pressure is made with a glass rod on a laminated vein it might fill either with pure aqueous humor or with blood, depending on the relative pressures in the afferent vessels to the laminated vein. Goldmann (1946, 1949) injected fluorescein intravenously and found that the episcleral veins fluoresced earlier than the aqueous veins, providing additional evidence that the fluid in the aqueous veins is derived from aqueous humor. Goldmann also found that if fluorescein were injected into the aqueous humor prior to enucleation of a human eye the aqueous veins fluoresced immediately.

There appears to be no important connection between the system of vessels removing aqueous humor from the canal of Schlemm and the venous system removing aqueous humor through the uveoscleral route in the human eye. Jocson and Grant (1965) studied these systems after silicone rubber injections into the arterial as well as the venous systems of the limbal region and were unable to demonstrate anastomoses. The studies of Ascher (1942, 1953), Theobald (1934), Ashton (1951), and Jocson and Grant (1965) provide clear evidence that the fluid in those veins which leave the canal of Schlemm is aqueous humor and that these veins are the main pathway for movement of aqueous humor from the canal of Schlemm to the episcleral veins.

EMBRYOLOGY

The cornea begins to develop by the sixth week (12 mm. stage) of embryonic life, with the formation of a simple epithelium and endothelium. The corneal stroma appears by the end of the seventh week (24 mm.) and contains collagen. Scleral condensation does not commence in the paraxial mesoderm until about the end of the sixth week (18 mm. stage) when it is seen in the region anterior to the equator. By the seventh week (24 mm. stage) the condensation has passed anterior to the rectus muscle insertions and is extending toward the limbus; this area shows definite condensation by the tenth week (49 mm. stage). The scleral spur can be recognized at this time, and the fibrils of the mesoderm in the internal corneosclera are arranged in parallel bundles in this region as the precursors of the corneoscleral meshwork. By the twelfth week (65 mm. stage) Schlemm's canal is present on the venous side of the recently developed vascular channels in the associated mesoderm. The angle of the anterior chamber also begins to form at this time as a result of the forward growth of the neuroectoderm, which will become the epithelial layers of the iris.

During the period between the third and the fifth month of early fetal life, growth and differentiation of the eye leads to a series of events in the limbal region. First, the orientation of the deep cells of the mesodermal tissue in the anterior chamber angle region is parallel to the surface of the eye. Growth and forward extension of the tissues leads to a separation of the corneoscleral meshwork from the surface of the developing iris. Second, there is progressive migration of the canal of Schlemm in an anterior direction as the anterior chamber angle widens and deepens. Development is slow after this period, and organization of the mesodermal tissue to form the trabecular meshwork does not occur in the chamber angle until the seventh to eighth month of fetal life.

The ciliary muscle differentiates from its anlage between the third (65 mm. stage) and the fifth month, at which time the meridional part of the muscle is seen to be attached to the scleral spur. The tendinous fibers of the meridional part of this muscle are partially continuous with the posterior part of the corneoscleral meshwork.

The conjunctiva and its stroma are derived from the surface ectoderm and the associated mesoderm, appearing soon after formation of the optic vesicle in the first month. By the sixth week (16 mm. stage) the rudimentary lid folds are present and are covered by the surface ectoderm, which is continuous with the corneal epithelium. The lid folds grow toward each other, fuse at about the ninth week (31 to 35 mm. stage) and remain closed horizontally until the fifth or sixth month of fetal life (110 to 200 mm.). During this time the limbal conjunctiva reaches its definitive development.

Many variations have been reported in the formation of the canal of Schlemm. Most common is the complete absence of the canal, especially in some infants with other anomalies and congenital glaucoma. The trabecular sheets also have shown considerable variation in their development, particularly in the uveal portion, where there may be thick, heavily pigmented, rope-like bands crossing the angle recess to join with the remainder of the meshwork. These rope-like bands resemble those seen in some mammals which have spaces of Fontana and pectinate fibers. In congenital glaucoma there may be a thin membrane covering the trabecular sheets (Barkan's membrane), possibly the result of persistence of embryonic mesodermal tissue over the meshwork. Many observers have denied the existence of this membrane.

Another type of faulty development has been emphasized by Maumenee (1958), who found incomplete cleavage of the iris from the trabecular meshwork, producing the effect of a forward insertion of iris into the meshwork. He showed that goniotomy could be done to separate the iris from trabecular tissue, facilitating the exit of aqueous humor through the meshwork and into Schlemm's canal.

GROSS ANATOMY

When the living eye is examined with a loupe or slit-lamp microscope the anterior limit of the limbus appears at the site where the opaque sclera joins the transparent cornea. The sclera extends farther forward in the superior and inferior half of the eye than in the medial and lateral region, resulting in the elliptical shape of the outer corneoscleral junction (Fig. 3–1). The external surface of the limbus is covered by the conjunctiva, which ends at the periphery of Bowman's layer.

The conjunctival vessels are seen with the slit lamp as fine arcades that extend into the clear cornea for about 0.5 mm. beyond the limbal edge. The palisades of Vogt of the peripheral cornea and limbal conjunctiva commence in the epithelium of the cornea and extend into the limbus as spoke-like radiations arranged at right angles to the peripheral cornea. The palisades, which measure 0.5 mm. in width by 2 to 4 mm. long, are more prominent in the inferior conjunctiva and frequently are heavily pigmented in darker races. These palisades are formed by the epithelial rete pegs and the conjunctival stromal papillae. The latter first appear in the conjunctival epithelium at the corneal edge and contain blood vessels, lymphatics and nerves.

In the anterior limbus a loose, vascular connective tissue lies between the limbal conjunctiva and Tenon's capsule. Tenon's capsule lies beneath this connective tissue as far forward as its insertion into the episclera near the peripheral cornea. The arterial, venous, capillary and lymphatic systems are quite visible in the transparent tissues of this region. Veins containing clear aqueous humor can often be seen emerging from the deep tissues around the limbus to join the episcleral veins.

The corneoscleral relations of the limbus can be defined more clearly in enucleated eyes after removal of the conjunctiva and other surface tissues. The anterior limit of the limbus at the edge of Bowman's layer is known as the *corneolimbal junction* and constitutes an important surgical landmark. The posterior limit is located by measurement; a circular line 1.5 mm. from the corneolimbal junction in the horizontal meridian and 2 mm. from it in the vertical meridian and running parallel to it around the circumference of the eye is known as the *limboscleral junction.*

The limbus, then, is composed of a narrow, circular strip of tissue which extends circumferentially around the eye in the corneoscleral region. Its depth is almost 1.0 mm. and its shape is roughly that of two ellipses whose ends lie at the horizontal meridian; the widest portion is superiorly and inferiorly. The gray color of the surface of the limbus is due both to the transition from opaque sclera to transparent cornea and to underlying filtration meshwork and vessels in this area. Hence, this area is known as the *gray zone.* The flat curve of the sclera meets the steeper one of the cornea in the limbus, producing a surface indentation or depression which is known as the *external scleral sulcus.*

On the internal side the limbus is bathed by aqueous humor over its entire surface. The corneoscleral tissues are hollowed out on the internal surface to form the *internal scleral sulcus.* Within the sulcus are the corneoscleral meshwork and Schlemm's canal, which completely fill the cavity of the sulcus, with Schlemm's canal lying in the posterolateral part of the sulcus.

The posterior margin of the limbus lies in the sclera so that its deep edge is close to the scleral spur, in the vicinity of the insertion of the meridional portion of the ciliary muscle and the anterior chamber angle recess.

BLOOD VESSELS (Figs. 4-2 to 4-6)

Conjunctival Arterial Vessels and Lymphatics. Most of the arterial channels are arterioles which terminate in a complex subconjunctival capillary network (Fig. 4–2). The superficial marginal plexus of the limbus is derived from the branches of the anterior ciliary arteries. It encircles the cornea and provides branches which supply the peripheral cornea. These small branches pass forward in the papillae of the palisades of Vogt, giving off two sets of vessels (Fig. 4–3): (1) *terminal* ones which form the peripheral corneal arcades and then become venous, and (2) *recurrent* ones which form some of the peripheral corneal arcades and run posteriorly to supply 3 to 6 mm. of the perilimbal conjunctiva; they then anastomose with the recurrent conjuncti-

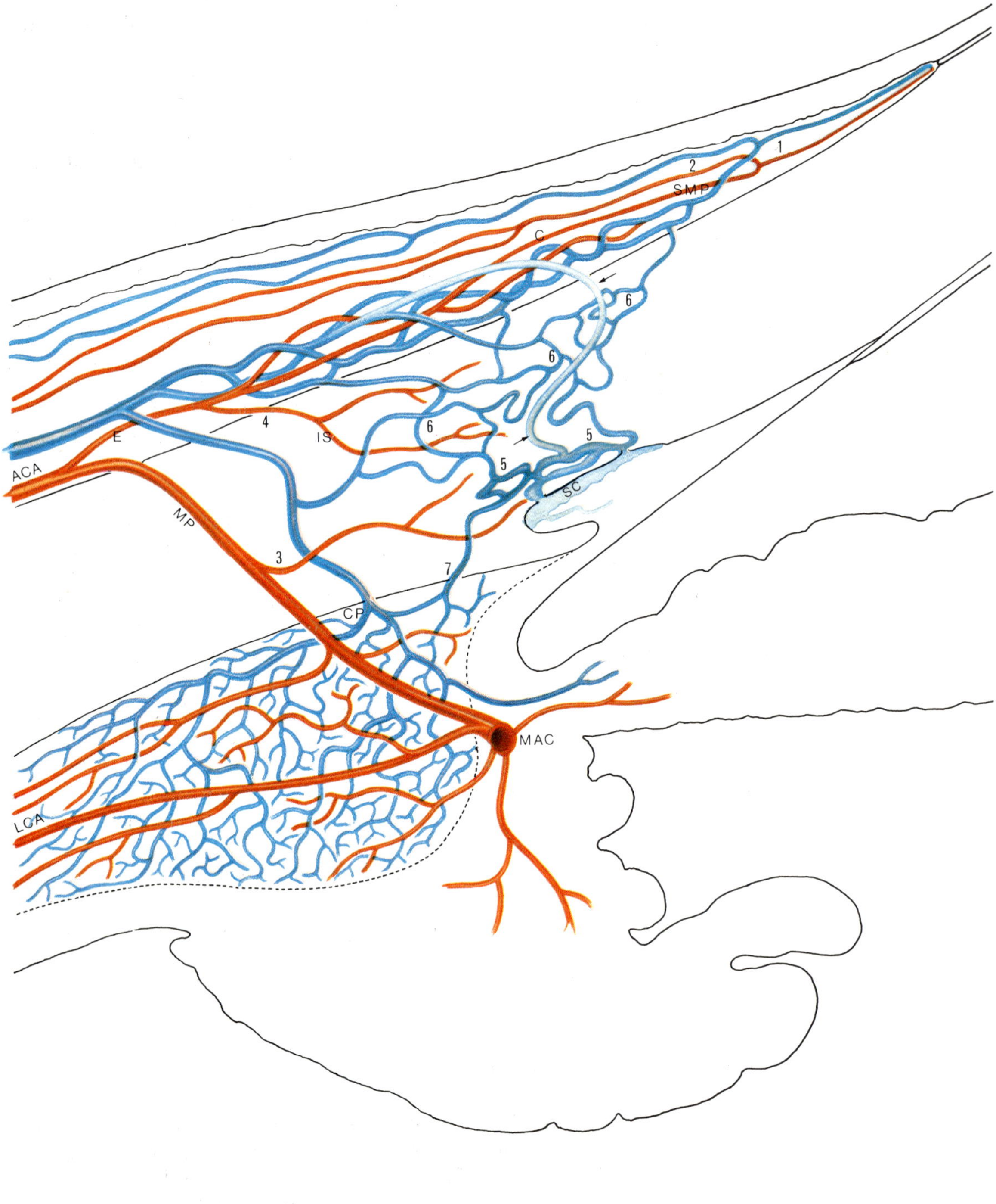

Figure 4-2. Drawing of a meridional section of the eye to show the blood supply of the limbal area.

Red indicates arterial channels. An anterior ciliary artery (ACA) divides to form an episcleral (E) and a major perforating (MP) branch. The episcleral branches produce episcleral, conjunctival (C) and intrascleral (IS) nutrient vessels. The conjunctival vessels form the superficial marginal plexus of the cornea (SMP). Two sets of vessels arise from the superficial marginal plexus: one (1) extends forward to form the peripheral corneal arcades; the other forms recurrent vessels (2) which run posteriorly to supply 3 to 6 mm. of the perilimbal conjunctiva. The latter eventually anastomose with the recurrent conjunctival vessels from the fornices. The

val vessels from the fornices. The arterial channels have much the same microscopic structure as they do elsewhere.

The conjunctival *capillaries* mainly are of the nonfenestrated continuous type that occurs in skeletal muscle and iris (Fig. 4–6). The endothelium has a relatively uniform thickness and a well defined basement membrane, but some capillaries show areas where the endothelium is thin and fenestrated. The lateral endothelial cell membranes show extensive interdigitations, and a zonula occludens is found near the capillary lumen. Pericytes are sparse; these cells are surrounded by a basement membrane which is continuous with that of the adjacent endothelial cells.

Episcleral Arterial Vessels. Most of these vessels arise from the branches of the anterior ciliary arteries. They supply all the subconjunctival tissues and anastomose with the more superficial conjunctival vessels. Their tributary veins carry blood to the ophthalmic veins. The capillaries of the episclera have a structure similar to those in the conjunctiva.

Scleral Arterial Channels. The scleral arterial channels arise directly from the main trunks of the anterior ciliary arteries and form their branches as they traverse the sclera to join the major circle of the iris. The scleral branches do not anastomose with Schlemm's canal, but they lie close to it or are even embedded in its wall (Theobald, 1934; Ashton, 1951).

Venous System. The venous return from the conjunctival capillaries flows posteriorly into the episcleral vessels, and the small veins at the level of Tenon's capsule and the episclera also drain into the episcleral vessels. The limbal stroma has two venous nets (Fig. 4–2 *B*): (1) the *deep scleral* plexus, which lies close to the canal of Schlemm, and (2) the *intrascleral* plexus, which forms a vast interconnecting network in the limbal sclera and receives blood both from the deep scleral plexus and from the highly developed ciliary plexus. Many venous channels pass from the venous plexus in and around the ciliary body into the deep scleral plexus. For this reason the veins of these scleral plexuses become engorged in anterior uveal inflammations (ciliary flush). These two plexuses drain posteriorly into the episcleral veins. Some venous (external collector) branches from the canal of Schlemm merge immediately with the deep scleral plexus, while others pass through the sclera to its surface without anastomosing as the aqueous veins of Ascher. All the scleral veins have much the same structure as the capillaries except that they are of larger caliber.

Lymphatics (Figs. 4–4 and 4–5). The conjunctival lymphatics comprise three groups (Busacca, 1952): (1) a peripheral system which lies either subepithelially or deep in the conjunctiva and is associated with the terminal arcades of the limbal arterial system; (2) radial lymphatics, extending through the palisades of Vogt deep to the blood vessels; and (3) branches from the radial lymphatics that become deep in the subconjunctival region, forming an

Text continued on page 126

Figure 4–2. *Continued.*
major perforating artery passes through the sclera to join the major arterial circle (MAC) of the iris. At (3) a branch from the major perforating artery passes forward to form the intrascleral arterial channels of the limbus. This region often is supplied by a vessel which arises directly from the anterior ciliary artery as an episcleral vessel, such as the one indicated at (4).

Venous channels are blue. The major venous drainage from the limbus is into the episcleral veins, which then unite with the ophthalmic veins. The deep scleral venous plexus (5) is close to Schlemm's canal (SC). An aqueous vein (arrows) arises from the deep scleral plexus and joins the episcleral veins. The intrascleral venous plexus (6) forms an extensive network in the limbal stroma. An important part of the drainage from the ciliary plexus (CP) is into the deep and intrascleral venous plexuses. One of these channels is seen at (7).

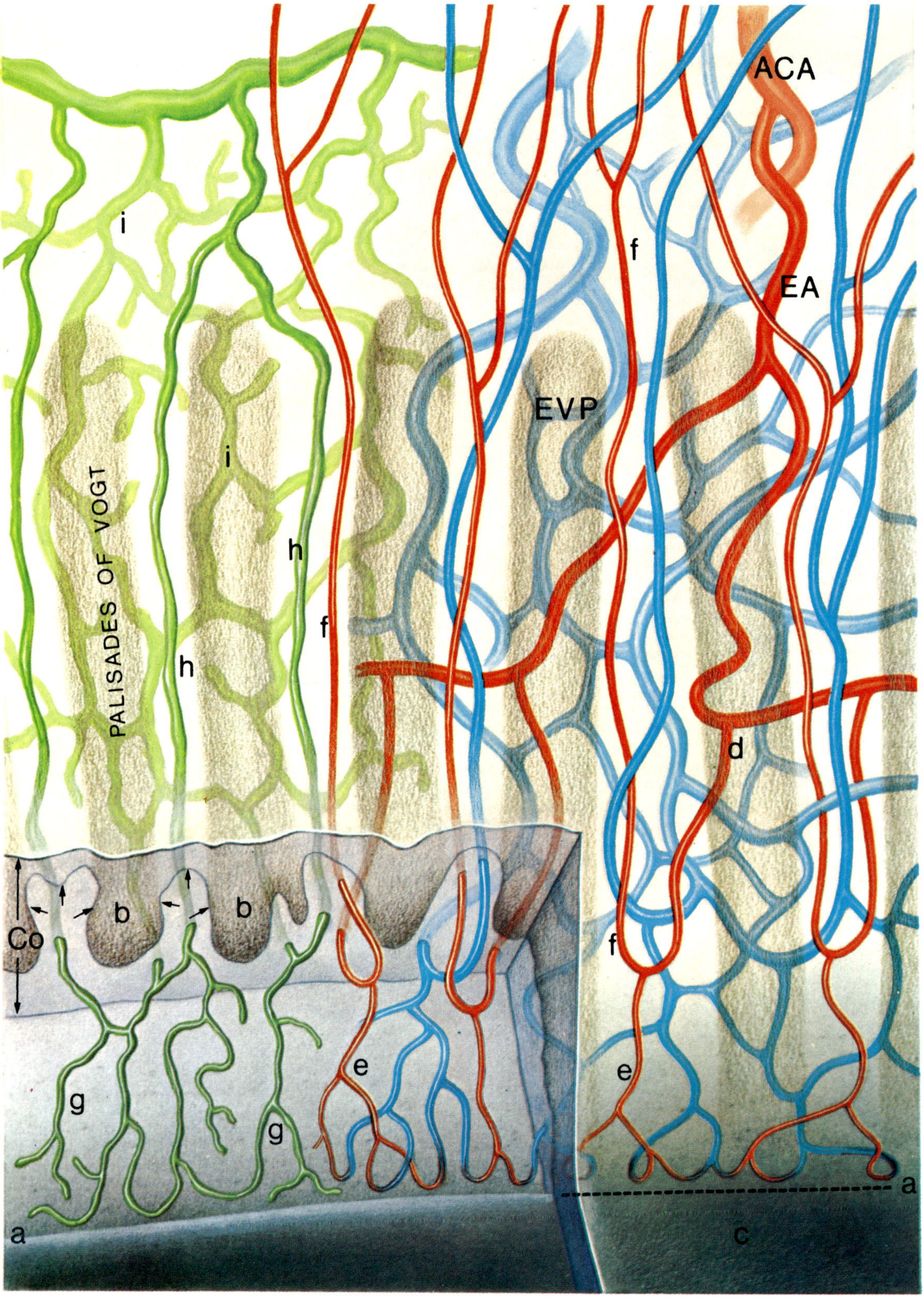

Figure 4–3. *See legend on opposite page.*

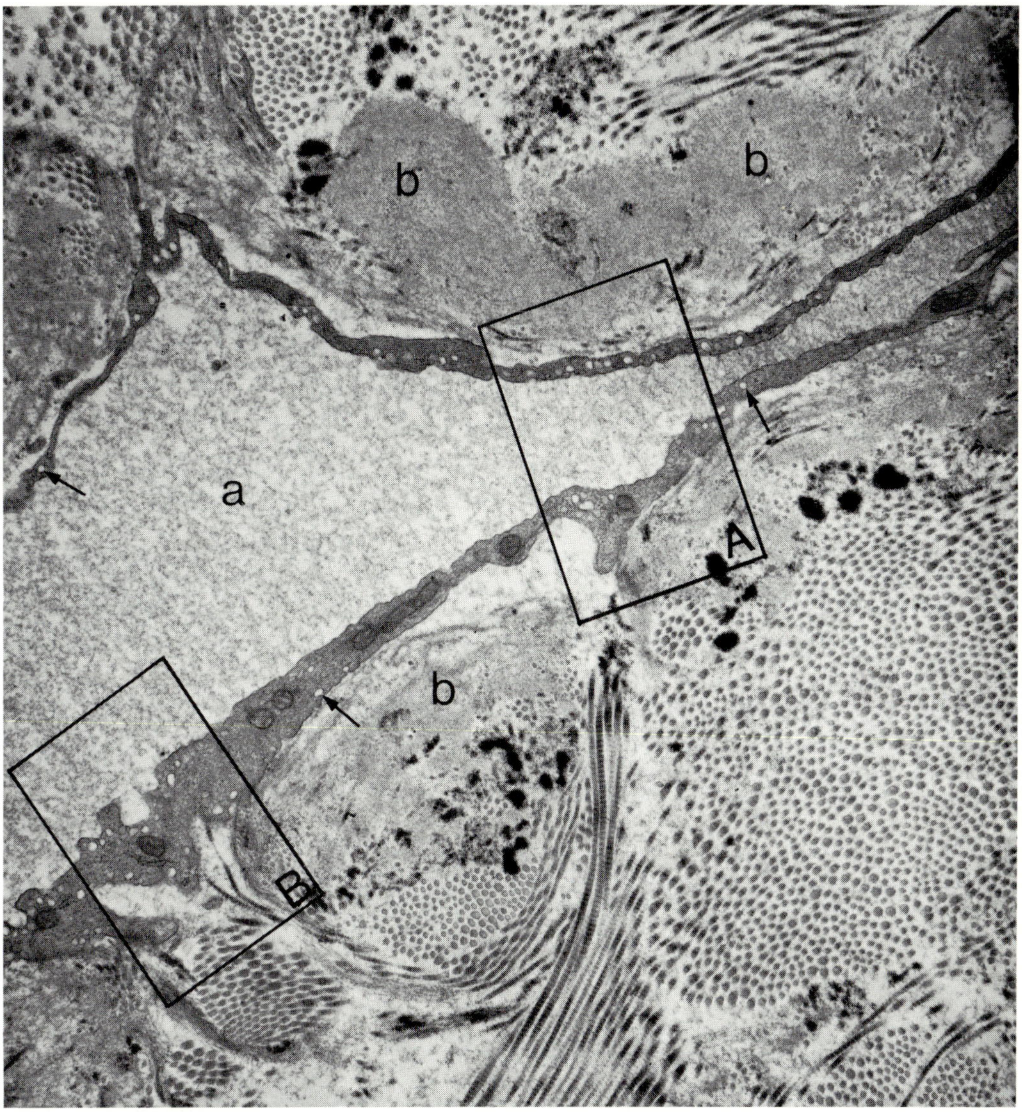

Figure 4-4. Lymphatic vessel. The lumen (a) is filled with precipitated plasma and the endothelial wall is thin. There is no endothelial basement membrane and the wall contains no pericytes or other adventitial cells. Several pinocytotic vesicles are seen (arrows) in the endothelial cytoplasm. A finely granular material (b) is aggregated along the surface of the lymphatic wall, and some bundles of collagen fibrils also lie close to the endothelium. Areas blocked and labeled A and B are shown at higher magnification in Figure 4-5 *A* and *B*, respectively. (× 10,000.)

Figure 4-3. A drawing of the peripheral corneal vascular arcades and the palisades of Vogt. Bowman's layer terminates (a) at the periphery of the cornea (c). A cross-section of the conjunctiva (Co) shows the palisades of Vogt. The palisades are formed by stromal papillae (arrows) and the epithelial rete pegs (b). An anterior ciliary artery (ACA) is seen at the upper right corner; it forms the episcleral arteries (EA). The superficial marginal arterial plexus of the limbus is at (d). Two sets of vessels originate from this plexus: (1) *terminal* (e), forming the peripheral corneal arcades near the termination of Bowman's layer; and (2) *recurrent* (f), which also form part of the peripheral arcades; these run posteriorly through the palisades to supply the perilimbal conjunctiva. The recurrent vessels anastomose with conjunctival vessels from the fornices. The episcleral venous plexus (EVP) is deep to the palisades of Vogt.

The lymphatics are colored green; two groups of lymphatics, superficial and deep, extend through the palisades of Vogt. The peripheral lymphatic system is indicated at (g), and a superficial radial group is shown at (h). The deep radial lymphatics form a network at (i).

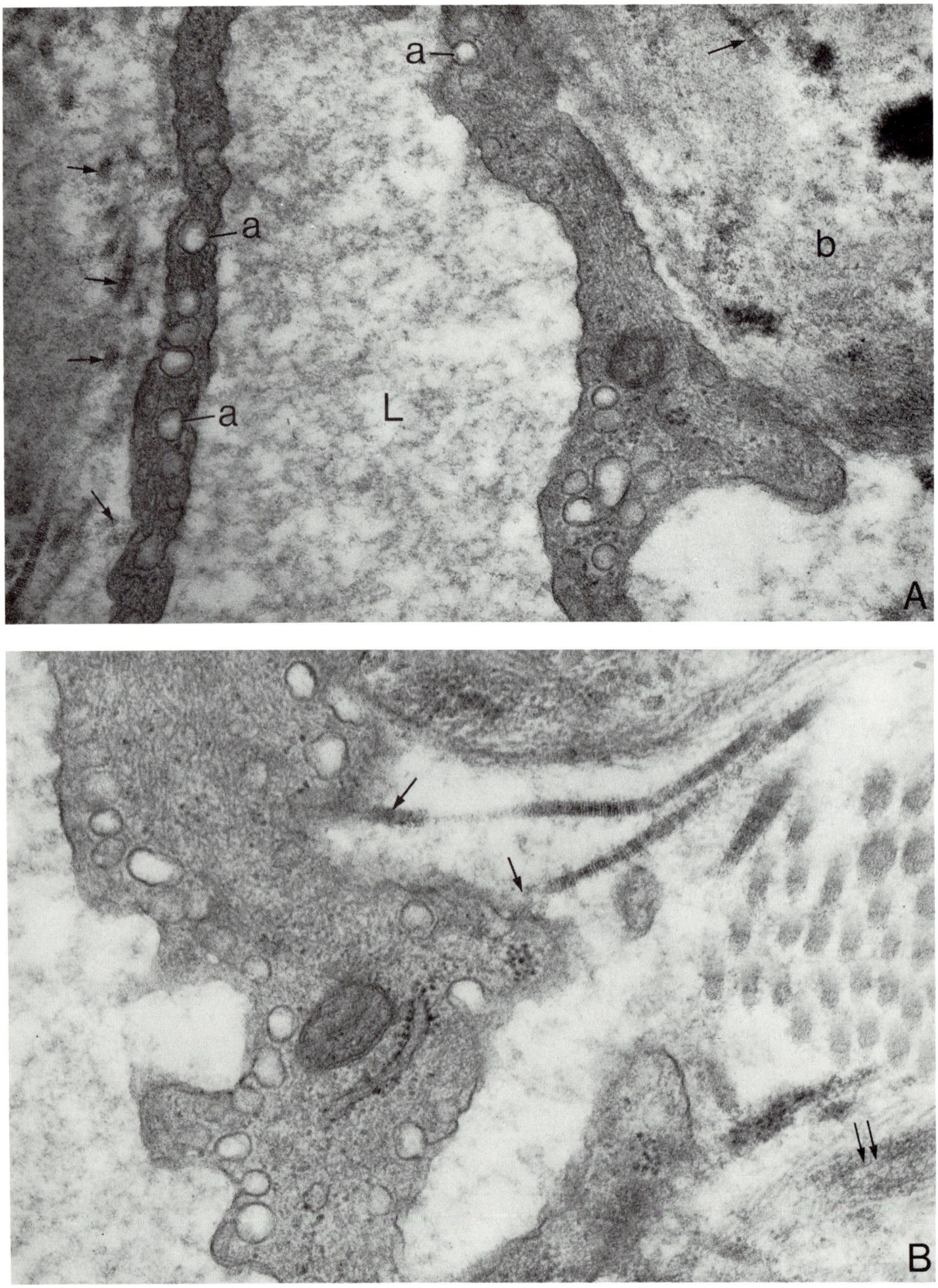

Figure 4–5. *See legend on opposite page.*

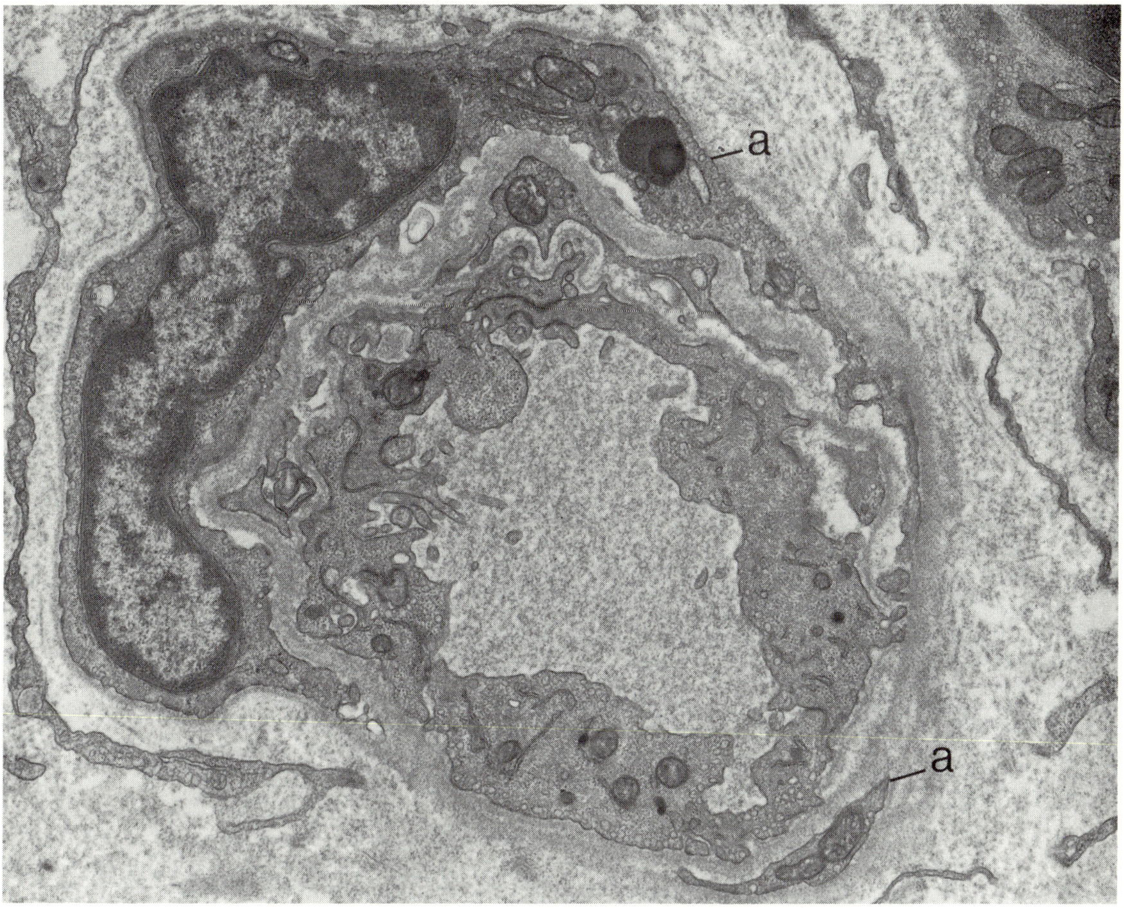

Figure 4–6. Capillary in the terminal arcade. A subepithelial vessel (a) is similar to that shown in Figure 4–13. These capillaries most often do not have fenestration of the endothelium in their walls, but occasional endothelial cells may show a few fenestrations. Pericytes are found (a) along the capillary wall. (× 13,000.)

Figure 4–5. Lymphatic vessel wall. *A*, Detail of an area enclosed in Figure 4-4. Pinocytotic vesicles are seen at (a) facing the lumen (L) of this vessel. A basement membrane comparable to that possessed by arterial capillaries is not evident. Masses of a finely granular and fibrillar material (b) resembling basement membrane material appear here and there along the wall. Mature collagen fibrils (arrows) are present in this material, some of them being close to the endothelial cells. (× 50,000.)

B, Detail of an area enclosed in Figure 4–4. Two collagen fibrils (arrows) approach and appear to merge with the endothelium. According to some observers, collagen disposed in this manner acts as support for the lymphatic wall. The fibrillar nature of the material described in Figure 4-4 is shown here (double arrows); note that these fibrils also approach the endothelium. (× 45,000.)

irregular net that drains either temporally or nasally. A large superior and inferior lymphatic trunk is formed about 7 to 8 mm. from the limbus and parallel to it. Nasal and temporal trunks are formed from these two vessels, the nasal trunk draining into the submaxillary and the temporal into the preauricular lymph nodes.

These lymphatics differ from arterial capillaries in many respects. The caliber of the lymphatic channels often is larger and its endothelial lining is much thinner. There is an absence of the basement membrane of the arterial capillaries and no pericytes are found on their walls, even in the large lymphatic trunks. An intercellular space measuring approximately 200 A. separates the endothelial cells and there are no tight or other specialized junctions.

Nerves

The fifth nerve distribution to the cornea and limbus via the long posterior ciliary nerves has been discussed (Fig. 3–2). Branches from the intrascleral and conjunctival nerves form several nets in the limbus: (1) conjunctival, (2) episcleral, and (3) stromal. The conjunctival and episcleral nerves supply the epithelial and subepithelial tissues of the limbal pericorneal region. Limbal stromal branches are both myelinated and unmyelinated, with endings around blood vessels and in the connective tissue. Other unmyelinated branches from the ciliary nerves supply the trabecular meshwork and the region of Schlemm's canal. Most of these branches appear to be sensory nerves.

MICROSCOPIC ANATOMY

The structure of the limbus will be discussed as follows (Fig. 4-7):

1. Conjunctiva
   a. Epithelium
   b. Stroma
2. Tenon's capsule
3. Episclera
4. Limbal or corneoscleral stroma
5. Aqueous outflow apparatus

Figure 4–7. Drawing of the limbus to illustrate the structures discussed in the section "Microscopic Anatomy." The limbal conjunctiva (A) is formed by an epithelium (1) and a loose connective tissue stroma (2). Tenon's capsule (B) forms a thin, somewhat ill-defined connective tissue layer over the episclera (C). The limbal stroma occupies the area (D) and is composed of the scleral and corneal tissues which merge in this region.

The conjunctival stromal vessels are seen at (a); they form the peripheral corneal arcades, (b) which extend anteriorly to the termination of Bowman's layer (arrow). The episcleral vessels (c) are cut in different planes. Vessels forming the intrascleral (d) and deep scleral plexus (e) are shown within the limbal stroma. The scleral spur with its coarse and dense collagen fibers is shown at (f). The anterior part of the longitudinal portion of the ciliary muscle (g) merges with the scleral spur and the trabecular meshwork. The lumen of Schlemm's canal (h) and the loose tissues of its wall are clearly seen. The sheets of the trabecular meshwork (i) are internal to the cords of the uveal meshwork (j). An iris process (k) is seen to arise from the iris surface and join the trabecular meshwork at the level of the anterior portion of the scleral spur. Descemet's membrane terminates (double arrows) within the anterior portion of the triangle, outlining the aqueous outflow system.

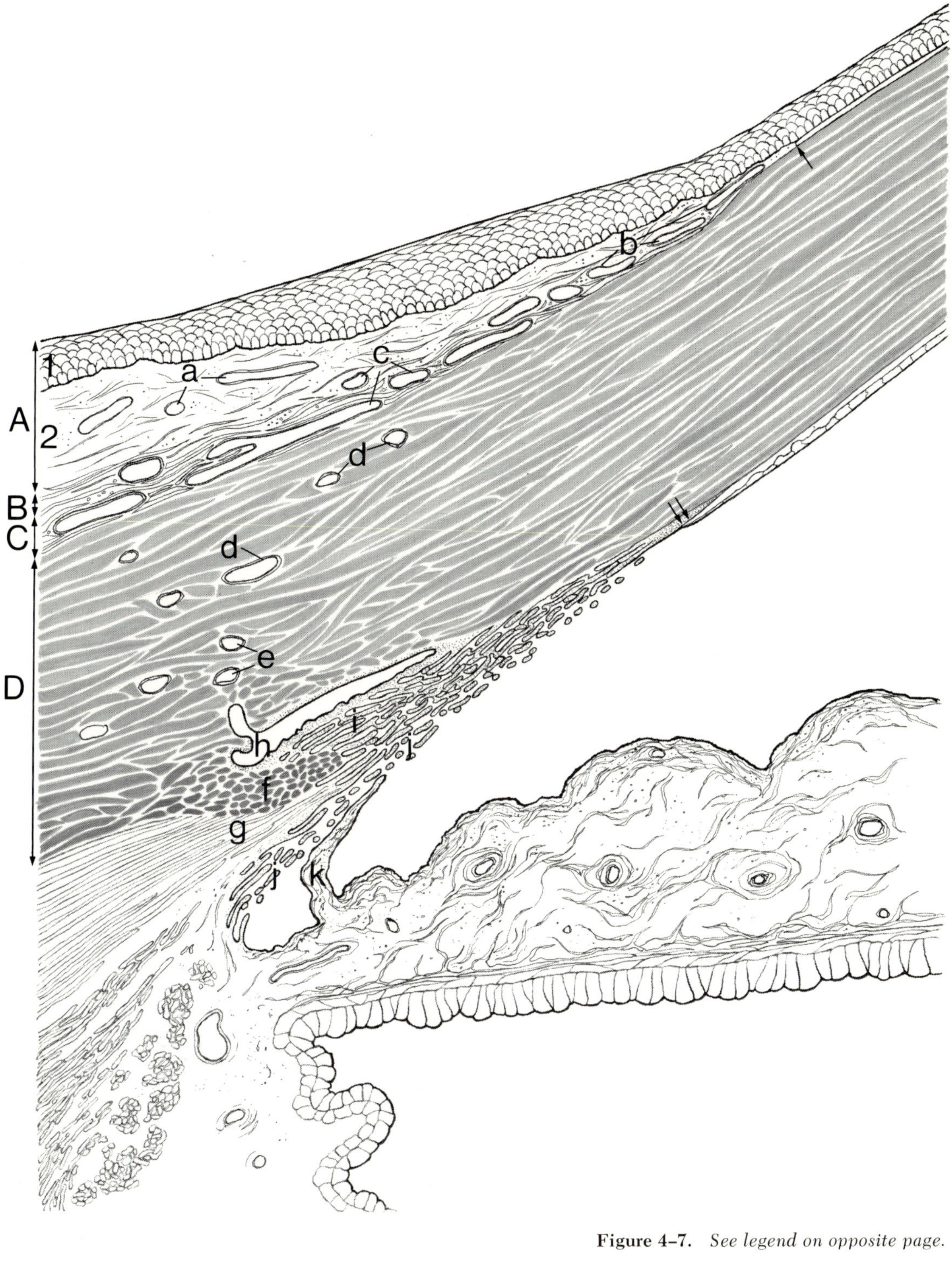

Figure 4–7. *See legend on opposite page.*

CONJUNCTIVA

Epithelium (Figs. 4-8 to 4-11). At the corneal edge the number of layers of epithelium in the limbal conjunctiva increases to 10 or 15, the increase occurring mainly in the wing cells. Goblet cells are not present in the limbal epithelium, but some are found at its periphery. The general appearance and organization of the epithelium is similar to that of the cornea. The superficial cells contain some glycogen, but their surfaces are not so smooth as those of the cornea. The conjunctival stroma is somewhat folded and the basal cells follow the folds. The cells in the basal layer are like those of the cornea but are smaller and more closely packed. Their basement membrane, however, has the same thickness and structure as that of the cornea. Melanin granules are frequently seen in the cytoplasm of the basal and wing cells; the pigment is produced by melanocytes of the basal layer and is transferred to the epithelial cells. The amount of pigment is smaller in blue eyes than in heavily pigmented ones.

The ultrastructure of the limbal epithelial cells is only slightly different from the corneal epithelium. The conjunctival cells have larger mitochondria and their cytoplasmic tonofilaments form dense bundles, some of which are closely associated with desmosomes. The cell membranes, intercellular spaces, junctional complexes and interdigitations are like those of the cornea. Like the cornea, the cytoplasm of the wing and surface cells shows many vesicles with the same relation to the Golgi apparatus (p. 75); these vesicles become less prominent in the posterior limbus. The surfaces of the superficial cells show the same type of microplicae and size of microvilli as are seen in the corneal epithelium.

Lymphocytes and melanocytes are found in the basal and suprabasal layers of the limbal conjunctival epithelium. The melanocytes are located at or close to the epithelial basement membrane but do not form specialized attachments to the adjacent epithelial cells. Dendritic processes extend from their cell bodies into the wing cell layers. The melanocyte cytoplasm is less dense than that of the basal epithelial cells because of its paucity of filaments. Mature pigment granules are found in the cytoplasm near the nucleus as well as in the dendritic processes. A Golgi complex is located in the apical

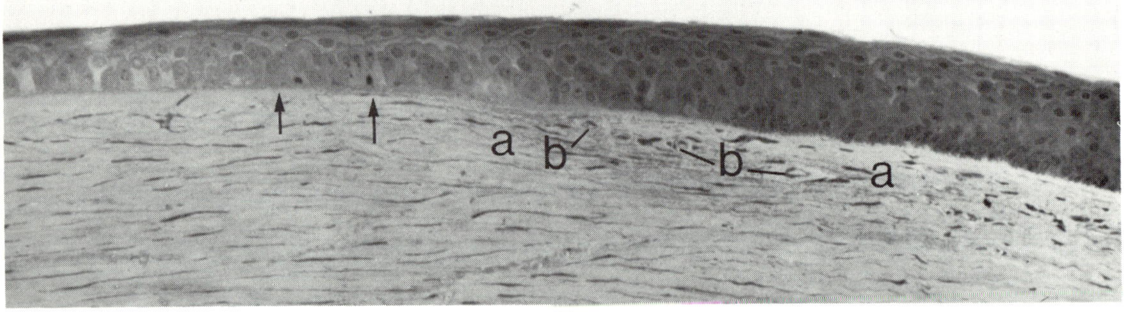

Figure 4–8. Corneolimbal transition, light micrograph. The corneal epithelium is at the left; it gradually thickens as it becomes the limbal epithelium. Bowman's layer tapers until it finally disappears (arrows) in the conjunctival stroma. The conjunctival stroma (a) is denser in this region than further posteriorly. A few vessels of the peripheral corneal arcades (b) are seen in cross-section. (× 190.)

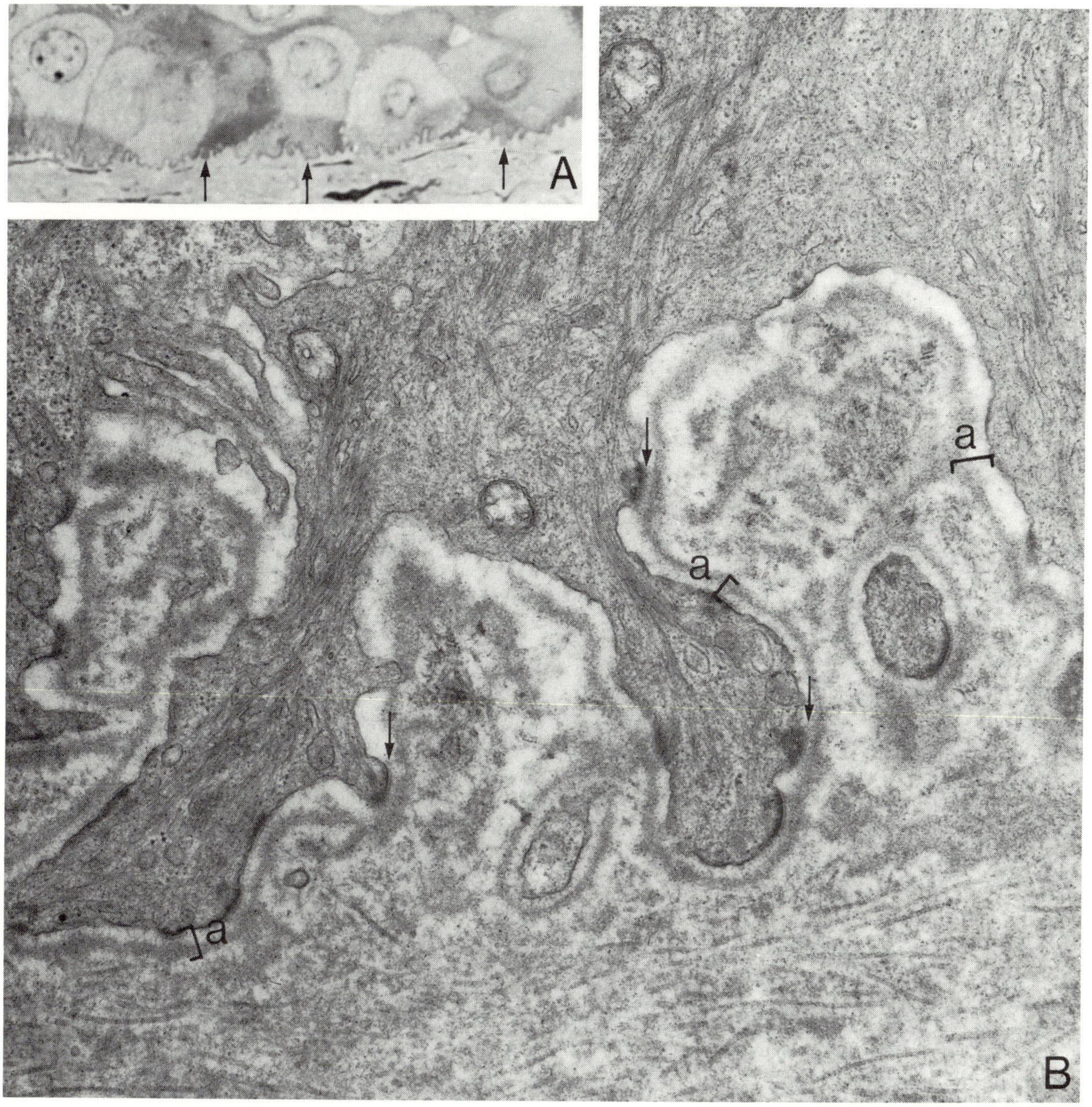

Figure 4-9. Basal epithelium at the limbus. *A*, Light micrograph showing the serrated basal portion of the epithelium at the limbus (arrows) (× 960.) *B*, Electron micrograph illustrating cytoplasmic extensions that form the serrated base of the conjunctival epithelial cell. The basement membrane (a) is composed of an electron-dense granular lamina measuring approximately 0.1 μm. in thickness and an electron-lucent space measuring 0.1 μm. in width. The total thickness of the basement membrane measures approximately 0.2 μm. Extremely fine fibrils (arrows) cross this electron-lucent space and connect the half-desmosomes with the basement membrane. (× 27,500.)

cytoplasm, and many mitochondria are present near the nucleus and in the processes. Smooth and rough-surfaced endoplasmic reticulum is dispersed in the cytoplasm, and some pinocytotic vesicles are seen near the cell membrane. Sugiura and Matsuda (1968) described Langerhans' cells in the suprabasal portion of the epithelium. These cells also have dendritic processes but do not contain pigment; they are negative when stained for dopa and melanin but can be demonstrated with gold chloride stains. The relation

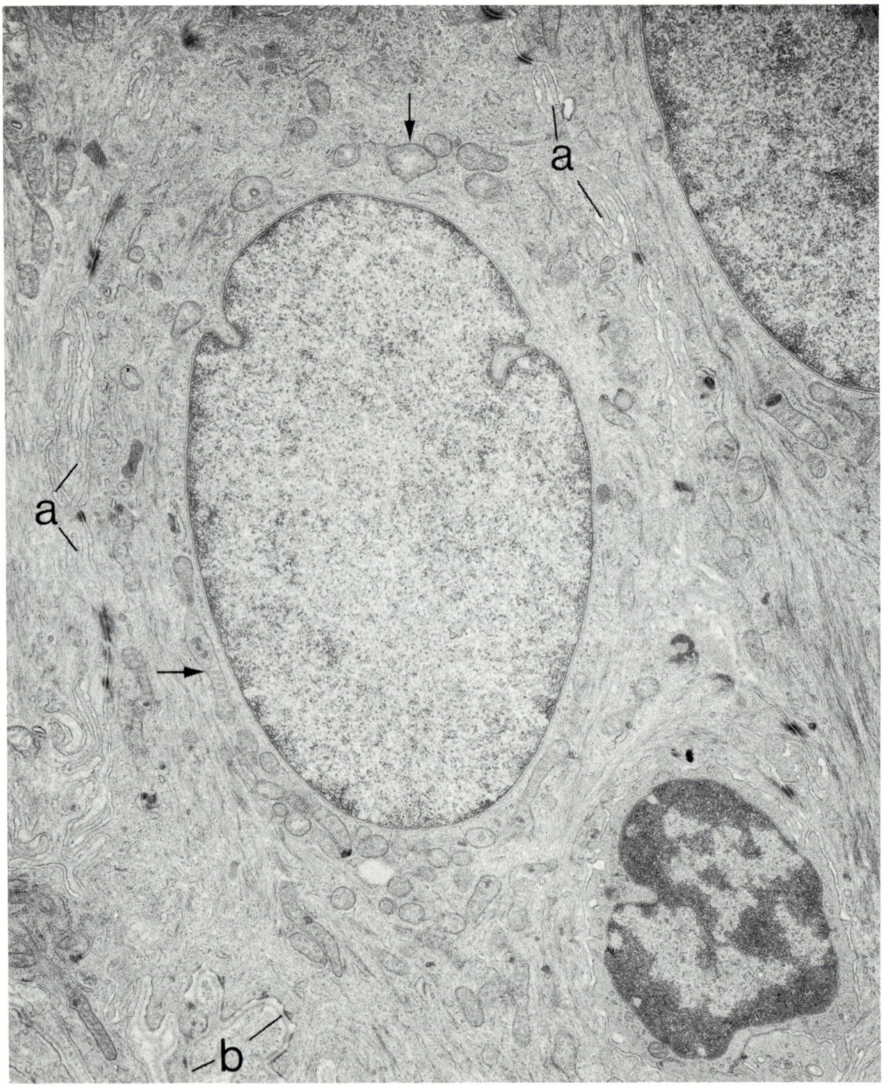

Figure 4–10. Basal epithelial cell at the limbus. The limbal basal epithelial cells have a greater number and size of mitochondria than the corneal epithelial cells (arrows). Interdigitating infoldings (a) are commonly seen in the basal epithelial cells of the limbus. The basement membrane is shown at (b). (× 10,000.)

of these cells to melanocytes is not known. Some observers believe them to be worn-out melanocytes, whereas others consider them to be specialized cells of unknown function because they can be demonstrated in the skin of embryos. Some cytoplasmic organelles have a distinctive feature in Langerhans' cells. They measure 2 μm. in length in their immature stages and have a tennis racket-like shape. The "handle" portion of the racket first forms as a bud from a cisterna of the Golgi apparatus, with the cisterna becoming the "racket" portion. In the mature granule the handle appears as a cross-striated organelle with the striations spaced about 90 A. apart. A striated linear lamella lies midway between the limiting membrane of the granule.

Conjunctival Stroma (Figs. 4-12 to 4-14). The epithelium and conjunctival stroma form rete pegs and papillae at the periphery of the cornea.

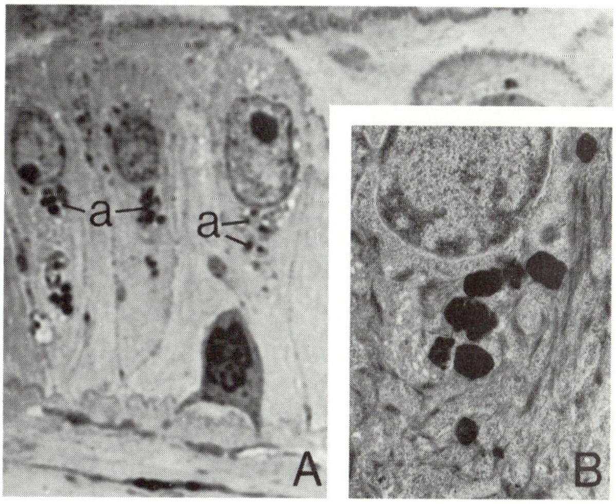

Figure 4-11. *A*, Basal epithelial cells at the limbus. Pigment granules (a) are observed in the limbal epithelium of individuals from darker races. (× 800.) *B*, Electron micrographs of pigment granules (arrows) in the limbal epithelium. (× 9000.)

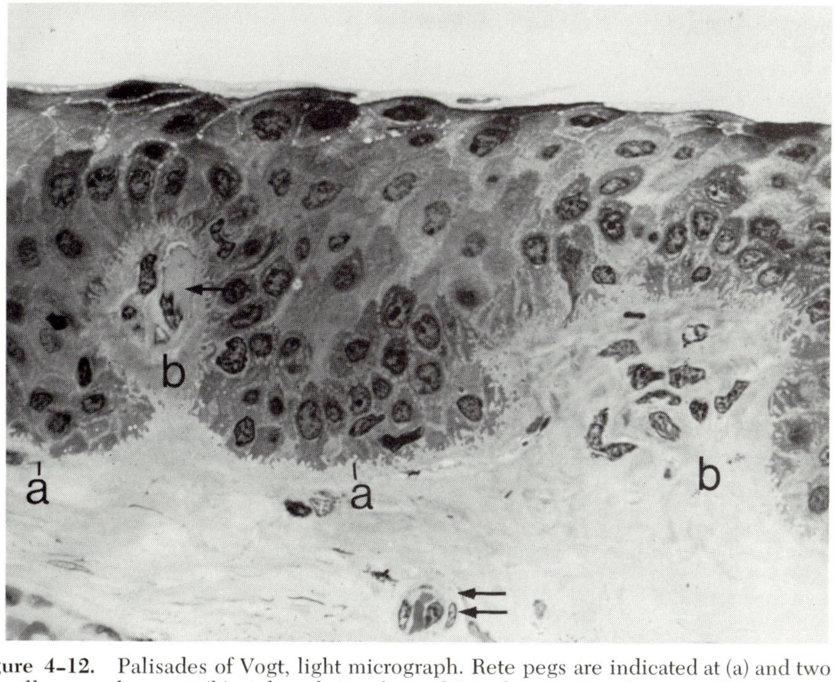

Figure 4-12. Palisades of Vogt, light micrograph. Rete pegs are indicated at (a) and two dermal papillae are shown at (b). A lymphatic channel (single arrow) and some cells are seen within a papilla. A vascular channel, probably belonging to the terminal arcades, is shown (double arrows). (× 600.)

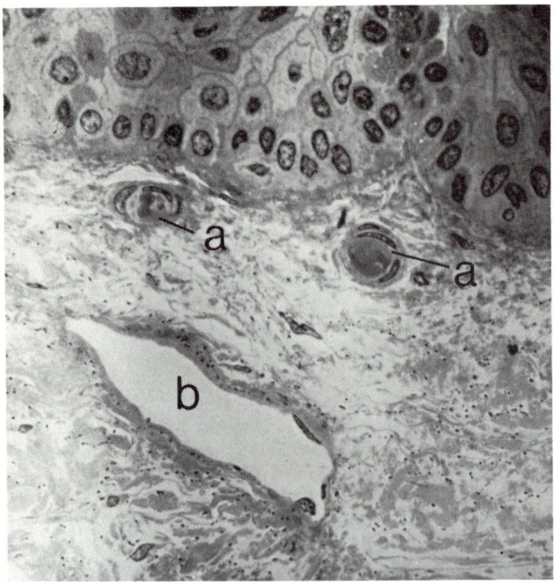

Figure 4-13. Light micrograph of a palisade of Vogt. Three vessels are shown in a peripheral corneal arcade. Two small arterioles are seen at (a). A large lymphatic channel is seen at (b). The lymphatic luminae usually contain no cells except for an occasional leukocyte. The lymphatic channel has a thin wall which can easily be differentiated from that of the arterial channels. (× 560.)

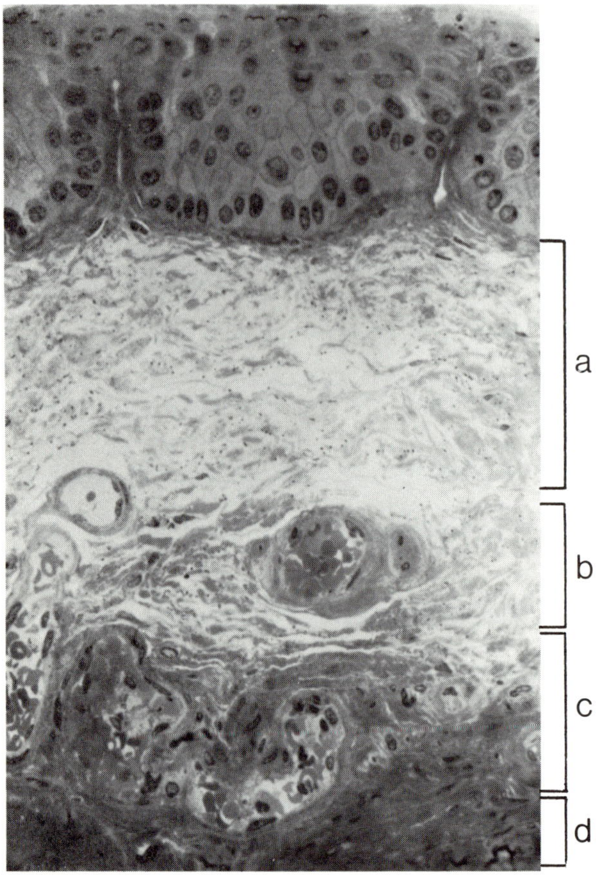

Figure 4-14. Light micrograph of the conjunctival stroma at the limbus. The epithelium is seen at the top. The loose connective tissue of the conjunctival stroma is shown at (a), while the denser connective tissue of Tenon's capsule (b), the episclera (c) and the sclera (d) are beneath it. (× 300.)

The papillae are oriented like the spokes of a wheel, radiating outward from the corneal edge into the conjunctiva to form the palisades of Vogt. The small vessels and nerves which run the length of the papillae are located along their lateral edges, while the lymphatics are central and deeper. The nerves are unmyelinated and branch considerably upon entering the conjunctival stroma and the basal epithelial layer, whose sensory nerve supply they provide.

The connective tissue of the conjunctival stroma has a varying degree of compactness and is arranged in two layers: a more dense portion near the end of Bowman's layer and in the vicinity of the epithelium; and an intermediate portion which is very loosely arranged beneath the first layer. The conjunctival stroma is composed almost entirely of loosely arranged bundles of coarse collagenous tissue containing numerous fibroblasts. The bundles of collagen are generally oriented parallel to the surface of the eye, but they intermingle in a random fashion at various levels.

Fibroblasts, melanocytes, macrophages, mast cells, lymphocytes, plasma cells and occasional polymorphonuclear and eosinophilic leukocytes are found in the loose connective tissue of the conjunctiva.

Fibroblasts. The fibroblast is the principal cell seen in this area. The organelle composition of these fibroblasts is the same as described for the corneal fibroblast. The conjunctival fibroblasts are not so compressed between collagen lamellae and tend to be round and shorter than the corneal fibroblasts.

Macrophages. Macrophages are commonly seen in the conjunctival stroma. They are large cells with an irregular contour and frequently show villous protrusions of cytoplasm from the surface. The abundant cytoplasm contains many vesicles that vary considerably in size and shape. Some of these vesicles are lysosomes that may contain pigment granules, lipids and other substances which are being digested by the lysosomal enzymes.

Mast Cells. Mast cells are common in the conjunctiva. They have been studied extensively because of their possible relation to allergic reactions. Their ultrastructure in the conjunctiva was described by Iwamoto and Smelser (1965). These cells are round or oval and, at times, elongated. They usually show cytoplasmic projections from their surfaces. The cytoplasm contains many organelles, including mitochondria, a Golgi apparatus, rough-surfaced endoplasmic reticulum, free ribosomes and many filaments. The characteristic feature of the cytoplasm is the mast cell granule, which is present in large numbers and is the probable site for storage of histamine, serotonin and heparin. The granules measure about 0.5 to 0.6 μm. in diameter and are surrounded by a single limiting membrane. The structure of the granules can be resolved into three main components: (1) finely particulate, (2) round, and (3) rod-shaped. A fourth component may consist of fine particles arranged in a lamellar pattern. Their structural variation may be a function of the direction in which they are cut, so that it is probable that the round granules are cross-sections of the rod-shaped ones. The rod-shaped granules have a diameter of about 0.1 μm. and often exhibit concentric rings which are arranged as lamellae or scrolls (Figs. 6–16 through 6–18).

Polymorphonuclear Leukocytes, Eosinophils and Lymphocytes. All these, especially the lymphocytes, are seen extravascularly in the limbal tissues. The polymorphonuclear leukocyte (Fig. 4-15) has an abundant cytoplasm and the lobed nucleus characteristic of these cells as well as the cytoplasmic granules which are their distinguishing feature. The granules

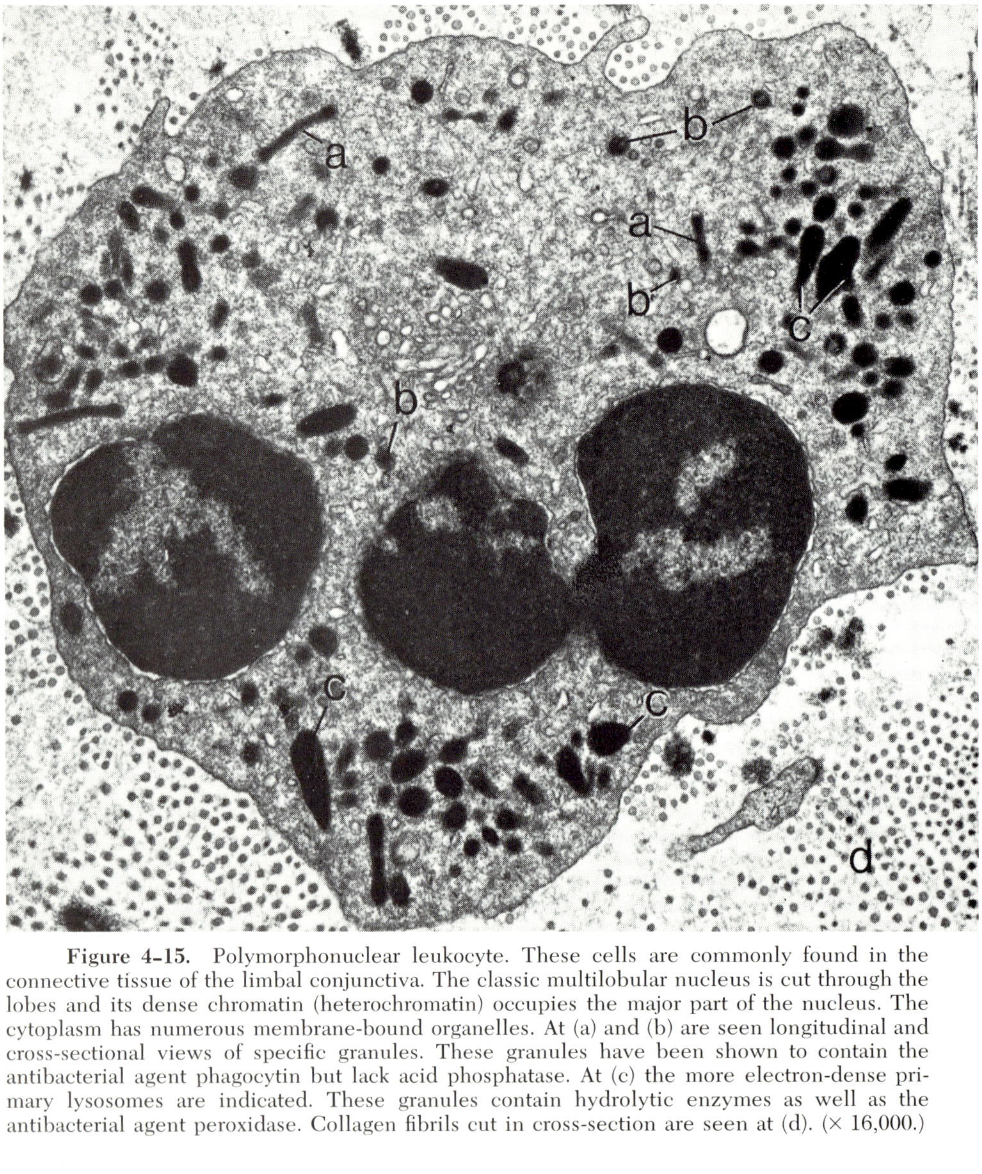

Figure 4-15. Polymorphonuclear leukocyte. These cells are commonly found in the connective tissue of the limbal conjunctiva. The classic multilobular nucleus is cut through the lobes and its dense chromatin (heterochromatin) occupies the major part of the nucleus. The cytoplasm has numerous membrane-bound organelles. At (a) and (b) are seen longitudinal and cross-sectional views of specific granules. These granules have been shown to contain the antibacterial agent phagocytin but lack acid phosphatase. At (c) the more electron-dense primary lysosomes are indicated. These granules contain hydrolytic enzymes as well as the antibacterial agent peroxidase. Collagen fibrils cut in cross-section are seen at (d). (× 16,000.)

vary in density, are surrounded by a single membrane and have a larger ovoid or smaller bacillary shape. These membrane-bound structures contain packets of hydrolytic enzymes which can digest proteins, lipids, nucleic acids and other substances. The granules also have been shown to contain the antimicrobial agent phagocytin.

The morphology of the eosinophils is striking; the cytoplasm of these cells contains granules which differ from those of the polymorphonuclear leukocyte. They are large and are surrounded by a single membrane. Their shape is either round or oval and their matrix has two zones, a light, granular outer one, and a more electron-dense sharply demarcated crystalloid core. These granules also contain numerous hydrolytic enzymes but have a very high concentration of the enzyme peroxidase, which occurs in the crystalloid portion of the granule.

Plasma Cells. Plasma cells can be recognized easily because of their abundant cytoplasm, an eccentric nucleus with its chromatin arranged like the face of a clock, and the cytoplasmic perinuclear halo. With the aid of the electron microscope the peripheral nuclear chromatin is found to be more dense and clumped while the central chromatin is less dense. The less dense appearance of the perinuclear halo is found to be the result of the presence of the Golgi apparatus, centrioles and mitochondria in this area. The distinctive feature of the plasma cell is the extensive development of rough-surfaced endoplasmic reticulum in its cytoplasm. The cisternae of this endoplasmic reticulum are filled with a granular material. Antibody protein is manufactured by the ribosomes and stored in the lumina of this very convoluted endoplasmic reticulum.

TENON'S CAPSULE

Tenon's capsule is a dense, collagenous layer which lies between the episclera and the loose conjunctival stroma (Fig. 4-7). It extends forward from the rectus muscle insertions over the surface of the episclera as a more condensed fascia-like layer and becomes thinner anteriorly. It finally terminates in the limbal episclera a short distance from the cornea. Tenon's capsule is thicker in the eyes of children, but it thins and atrophies with increasing age. It is composed almost entirely of compactly arranged collagen and a few fibroblasts. The collagen bundles are oriented parallel to the scleral surface.

EPISCLERA

The episcleral tissue is a thin, dense connective tissue layer that is part of the superficial sclera, but it differs from the sclera in its looser texture (Fig. 4-7). Both the episclera and Tenon's capsule can be distinguished from the loose conjunctival tissue by their greater compactness and the orientation of their collagen. The episcleral collagen bundles are circumferentially arranged and contain relatively few cells. The collagen fibrils of the episclera are larger than those of the conjunctival stroma but are smaller in cross-sectional diameter than those of the midsclera.

THE LIMBAL OR CORNEOSCLERAL STROMA (Fig. 4-7)

The regular arrangement of the corneal lamellae and cells is gradually lost in the dense connective tissue framework of the limbus, and the interweaving of larger collagen bundles becomes increasingly apparent. Anteriorly the collagen bundles are arranged like those of the cornea, while posteriorly they are more like those of the sclera. In the superficial limbal stroma the collagen bundles are oriented meridionally toward the rectus muscles, while near the scleral spur they are completely circular. The corneal collagen in the limbus is less eosinophilic than that of the sclera. Collagen fibrils of the corneal size persist for a considerable distance in the limbus posterior to the end of Bowman's layer and Descemet's membrane. Instead of a regular lamellar arrangement, however, these collagen bundles branch more often and form extensive intercommunications. The fibrils are not so uniformly spaced as they are in the cornea and there is less ground substance. Posteriorly the fibrils assume dimensions more like those in the sclera, their diameter being between 700 and 1000 A. The fibroblasts of the limbal stroma are like those of the cornea and sclera. Only occasional macrophages and leukocytes are seen here.

Most of the vessels encountered in the limbal stroma are the veins of the deep and intrascleral plexuses. Small arterial channels are found throughout the stroma and a net of small arteries appears in the region of Schlemm's canal, but those vessels do not communicate directly with the lumen of the canal.

Myelinated and unmyelinated nerves are seen throughout the limbal stroma, most of them being branches of the ciliary nerves which are destined for the cornea.

Aqueous Outflow Apparatus (Figs. 4-16 and 4-17)

The limbus contains structures which are specially developed for the removal of aqueous humor. The elements involved in removal of the aqueous humor are mostly found in the internal scleral sulcus. The outflow apparatus is composed of tissue derived from the cornea, sclera, iris, and ciliary body and will be described as follows:

1. Schlemm's canal and collector channels
   a. Schlemm's canal
   b. External collector channels
   c. Internal collector channels
2. Trabecular meshwork
   a. Corneoscleral meshwork
   b. Uveal meshwork
   c. Pectinate fibers or iris processes
3. Scleral spur
4. Deep corneolimbus
5. Innervation

Figure 4-16. Drawing of the aqueous outflow apparatus and adjacent tissues. Schlemm's canal (a) is divided into two portions. An internal collector channel (Sondermann) (b) opens into the posterior part of the canal. The sheets of the corneoscleral meshwork (c) extend from the corneolimbus (e) anteriorly to the scleral spur (d). The rope-like components of the uveal meshwork (f) occupy the inner portion of the trabecular meshwork; they arise in the ciliary body (CB) near the angle recess and end just posterior to the termination of Descemet's membrane (g). An iris process (h) extends from the root of the iris to merge with the uveal meshwork at about the level of the anterior part of the scleral spur. The longitudinal ciliary muscle (i) is attached to the scleral spur but has a portion which joins the corneoscleral meshwork (arrows). Descemet's membrane terminates within the deep corneolimbus. The corneal endothelium becomes continuous with the trabecular endothelium at (j). A broad transition zone (double-headed arrows) begins near the termination of Descemet's membrane and ends where the uveal meshwork joins the deep corneolimbus.

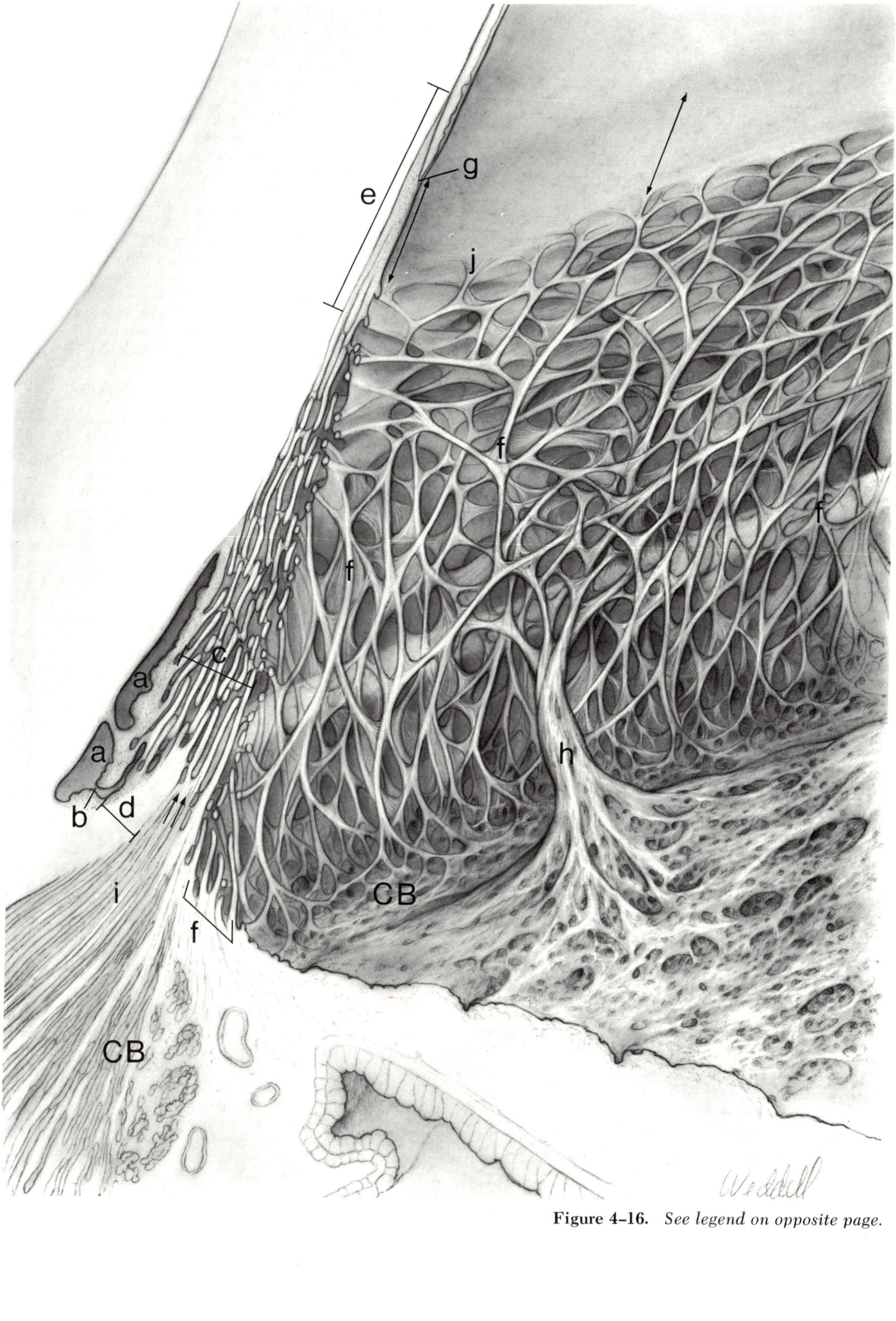

Figure 4–16. *See legend on opposite page.*

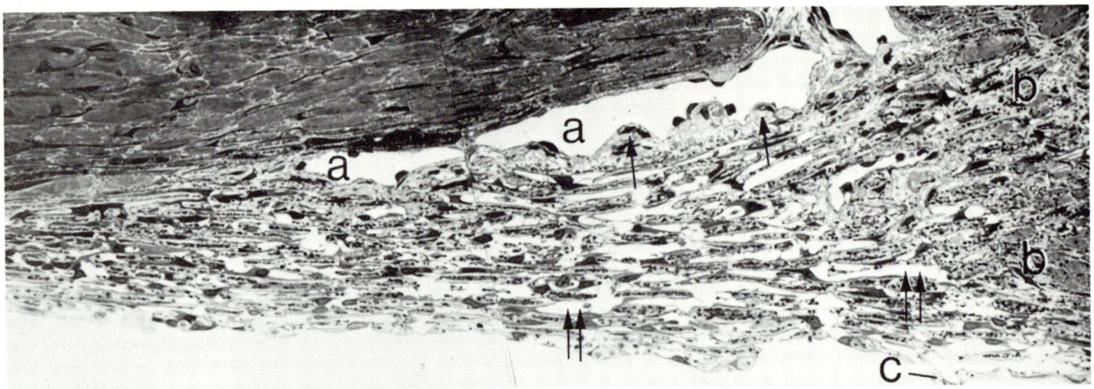

Figure 4-17. Light micrograph of the aqueous outflow apparatus. Schlemm's canal (a) is split into two portions. The external wall of the canal is relatively smooth in comparison with the inner wall. The inner canal wall is identified by single arrows. The scleral spur (b) with its denser collagenous tissue is seen posteriorly. The empty intertrabecular spaces (double arrows) are formed by the sheets of the corneoscleral meshwork. The thin cords of the uveal meshwork are adjacent to the anterior chamber; one cord (c) is shown. (× 310.)

Schlemm's Canal and the Collector Channels

Schlemm's Canal (Figs. 4-18 to 4-29). This circular venous channel lies in the outer portion of the internal scleral sulcus. The external wall of the canal is located quite close to the limbal stroma but is separated from it by the thin layers of connective tissue that form the canal wall. The internal wall of the canal of Schlemm is adjacent to the deepest part of the corneoscleral meshwork. The deep sclera is close to the posterior boundary of Schlemm's canal, and on its anterior side are the sheets of the corneoscleral meshwork.

The ring formed by the canal measures 36 mm. in circumference (McEwen, 1965), and it has a flattened elliptical cross-section. Its meridional width varies between 350 and 500 μm. in adults, being somewhat smaller in children, and the lumen frequently becomes very narrow or even splits into branches which enclose islands of tissue. Salzmann (1912) likened this configuration to that of a river that is subdivided by islands along its course. The surface of the canal is varicose, the varicosities having cross-sectional shapes from round to oval, or even triangular (Ashton, 1951). When the shape is triangular, the base is posterior and measures 50 μm. in width, while the anterior apex narrows to 5 or 10 μm.

A thin connective tissue wall surrounds the endothelial lining of Schlemm's canal. On the external side the wall is 5 to 10 μm. in thickness and can be differentiated easily from the adjacent limbal stroma by its cellularity and large deposits of finely fibrillar material. The greater part of this layer is composed of fibroblasts having numerous arrays of rough-surfaced endoplasmic reticulum, a well developed Golgi apparatus and many mitochondria. It is likely that the fine granular material present near these fibroblasts is synthesized by the cells. If this material is tropocollagen, it will undergo further polymerization to form the mature collagen fibrils. The collagen fibrils in the external adventitia resemble those of the corneal stroma, measuring approximately 300 A. in cross-sectional diameter. The fibrils are irregularly dispersed in an abundant matrix composed of a slightly osmiophilic, amorphous ground substance.

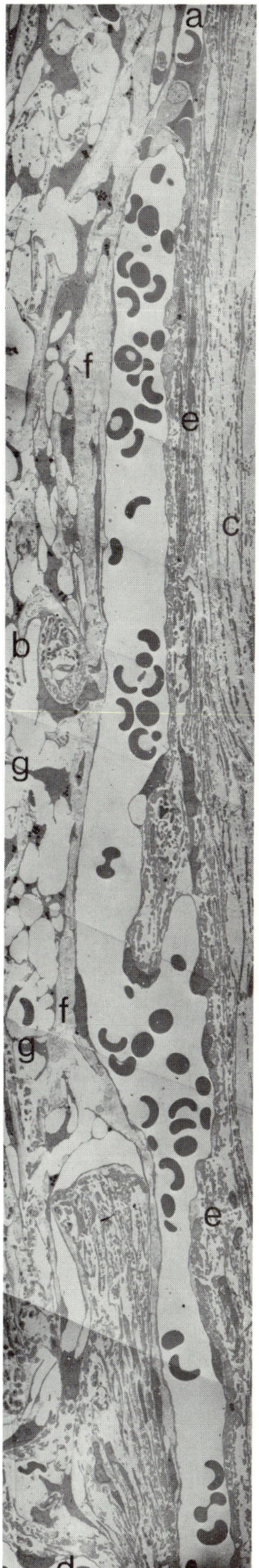

Figure 4-18. Composite electron micrograph of Schlemm's canal. The anterior canal is near (a), the inner side is at (b) and the limbal stroma is at (c). The canal has a length of 500 μm. and an average width of 40 μm. Numerous red blood cells occupy the lumen of the canal, probably as a result of backflow into the canal at surgery. An internal collector channel (d) or canal of Sondermann is seen at the bottom of the photograph near the posterior canal. The external wall of the canal is at (e) and the internal wall is at (f). In this photograph the inner wall of the canal shows no giant vacuoles in the endothelium. The bridging of the intertrabecular spaces by endothelial cells and subdivisions of the trabecular sheets is evident at (g). (× 760.)

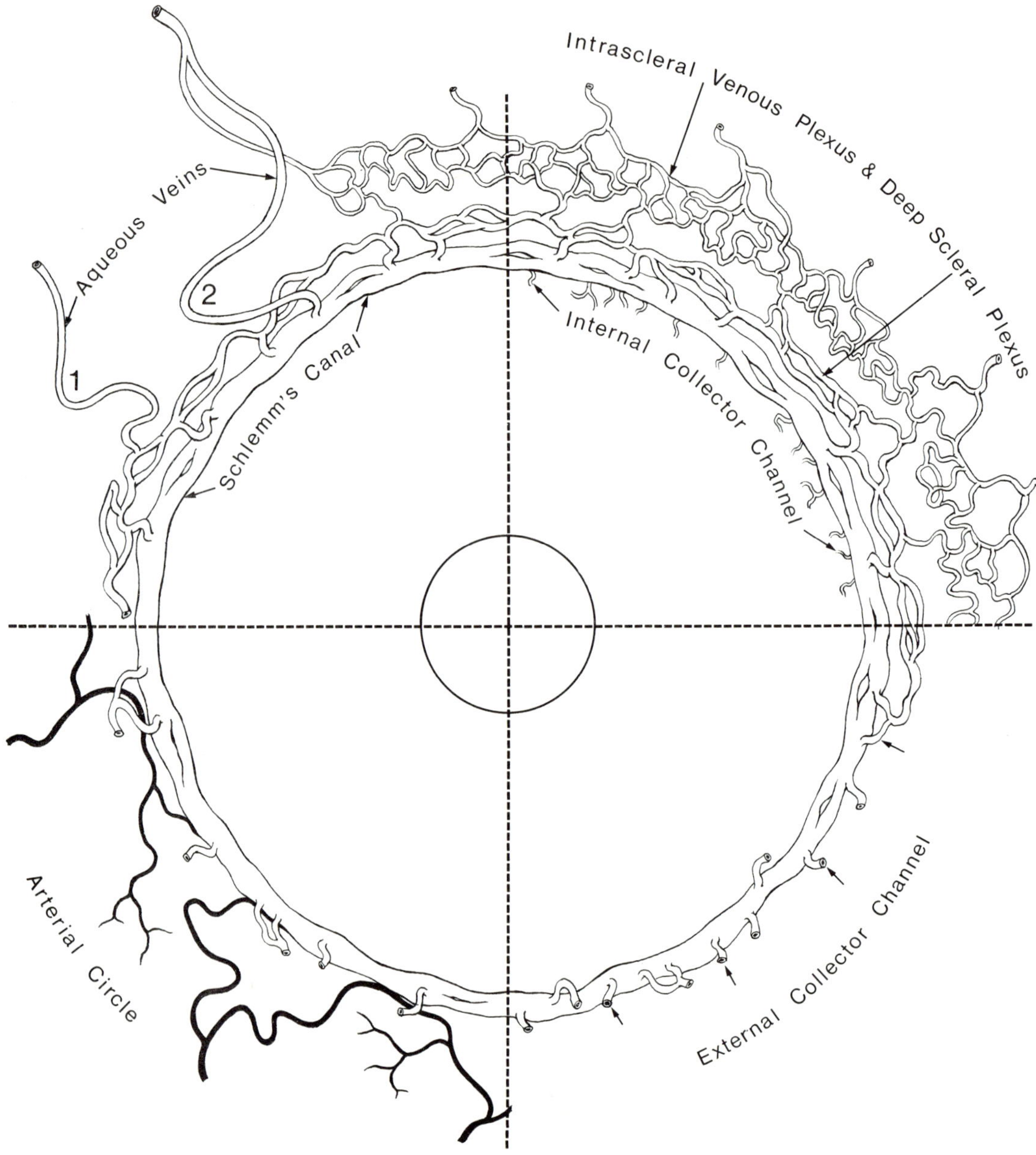

Figure 4-19. Schematic drawing showing the circular course and related vessels of the canal of Schlemm. The canal divides into two or more portions intermittently. The drawing is divided into four portions by the dotted lines. The internal collector channels of Sondermann are labeled in the upper right sector as they extend into the trabecular meshwork. The external collector channels are seen in the upper and lower right sectors, arising from the canal and uniting with the deep intrascleral plexus or extending directly to the episcleral veins. The deep and intrascleral venous plexuses are external to the canal.

In the upper left sector an aqueous vein (1) arises from the deep scleral plexus and another (2) arises from Schlemm's canal and runs directly to the episcleral venous plexus. External collector veins are seen to arise from the canal and join the deep scleral plexus.

In the lower left sector the arteries of the deep sclera are seen to be in close relation to the canal of Schlemm.

Polymorphonuclear leukocytes, macrophages and mast cells are seen occasionally in this narrow cellular connective tissue layer. It is surrounded by a transition zone measuring 20 to 30 μm. in thickness and composed of 8 to 10 lamellae of collagenous tissue. These collagenous lamellae run in all directions and are separated from each other by long fibroblasts. The collagen fibrils of the lamellae gradually increase in cross-sectional diameter from 300 A. to 800 to 1000 A. in diameter so that they come to resemble scleral collagen.

The cell wall internal to Schlemm's canal continues posteriorly around the wall of the canal and joins the external wall. This internal wall has been studied for many years by light microscopists, who noted the presence of many cells and a complete absence of trabecular spaces in the zone adjacent to the canal. It has been called the pore tissue by Flocks (1956), the cribriform area by Rohen (1961, 1963, 1964), and the juxtacanalicular connective tissue by Fine (1966). If a title has to be applied, juxtacanalicular tissue is most satisfactory, but we prefer to consider it as the inner wall of Schlemm's canal.

The structure and thickness of this canal wall vary in different sections along its sinuous outline. Many areas are seen in the wall where the ground substance has been extracted during the processing of the tissue, causing further changes in its character. Extracted areas of this type have been mistaken in the past for trabecular spaces, introducing an additional error in estimation of the actual thickness of the canal wall. In general, this layer measures between 10 to 20 μm. in thickness between the "basement membrane" of the endothelium and the nearest intertrabecular space. In well fixed specimens a complete endothelial layer is generally demonstrable at the junction of the outermost trabecular space with the canal wall.

The relationship between the trabecular spaces, the cell wall and the canal of Schlemm is as follows: (1) a layer of endothelium lines the outermost trabecular space; (2) next to this is found connective tissue of the canal wall which is composed of the same cells, collagen, tropocollagen and amorphous ground substance as we have described in the external canal wall; and (3) the endothelium of Schlemm's canal and its basement membrane. However, even in well fixed specimens there may be a few areas where the first and second components are lacking, and in such regions only the endothelium of the inner canal wall and its basement membrane separate the canal of Schlemm from the nearest intertrabecular space.

The lumen of Schlemm's canal is lined by an endothelium which has a rather smooth luminal surface everywhere except for its sinuous inner side. Most of the endothelial cells are small, having an average diameter of 10 μm. and a thickness of 0.2 μm. (Holmberg, 1965). Those along the inner wall, however, have a diameter of 20 to 50 μm. An endothelial basement membrane has been described, especially at the inner wall of the canal (Garron et al., 1958). This membrane is quite different from basement membranes found in other tissues, such as those of the corneal epithelium and of capillary endothelium. It is poorly defined, inconstant, frequently interrupted and of variable thickness; it is often separated from the endothelium by an irregular space. The lateral walls of the endothelial cells are joined by tight junctions, mainly zonulae occludentes, near their luminal surfaces. The points of membrane fusion are unusually small, measuring between 100 and 200 A., and occasionally the intercellular space is not closed by a tight junction.

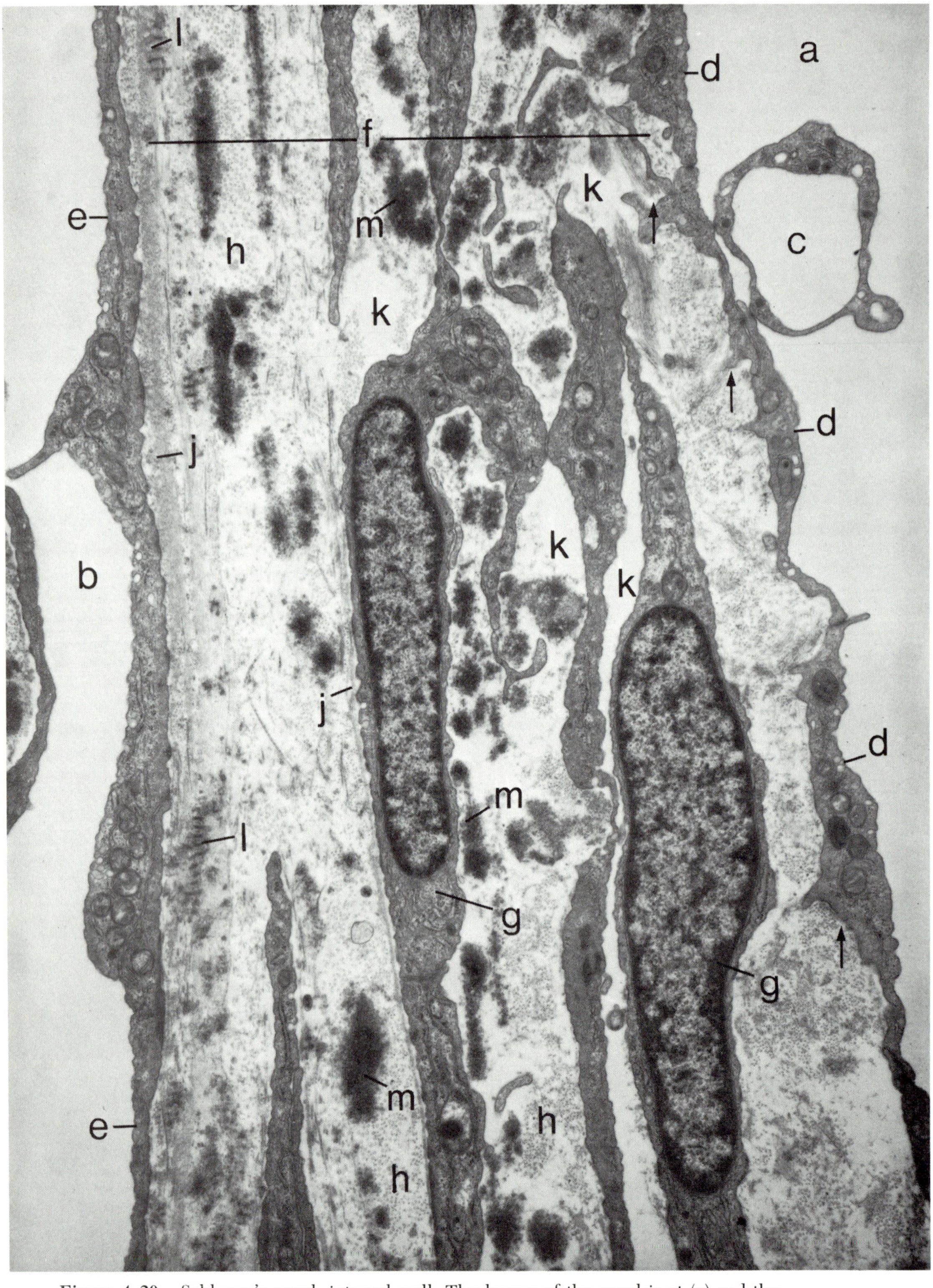

Figure 4-20. Schlemm's canal, internal wall. The lumen of the canal is at (a) and the nearest trabecular space is at (b). One endothelial cell lining the canal contains a giant vacuole (c) which measures 2.5 μm. in diameter and protrudes into the lumen of the canal. Four endothelial cells (d) line the inner canal wall. The trabecular space (b) is lined by portions of

The cytoplasm of these endothelial cells is mainly characterized by its content of filaments and free ribosomes. The mitochondria are very small, and the Golgi apparatus and profiles of rough-surfaced endoplasmic reticulum are seen only occasionally. Numerous pinocytotic vesicles, similar in size and distribution to those seen in the endothelium of capillaries, are found along the cell membranes of this endothelium.

Many of the cells along the internal canal wall possess cytoplasmic vesicles or vacuoles of extraordinary dimensions and of specific distribution. These have come to be known as giant vacuoles and are found only in the cells of the inner wall of Schlemm's canal. The vacuoles are outlined by a single membrane, with the largest vacuole measuring up to 14 μm. in length by 5 μm. in width. Holmberg (1965) made serial sections of 10 μm. portions of canal wall and found an average of 0.5 vacuoles per 10 μm. The range for six eyes was from 0.3 to 0.9 vacuoles for 10 μm. These giant vacuoles have been the subject of numerous studies, but their role and importance in aqueous humor transport into the lumen of Schlemm's canal is not entirely clear. In some early studies the vacuoles were shown to have an opening into the lumen of Schlemm's canal measuring about 0.3 to 2.0 μm. in diameter. A number of investigators (Speakman, 1960; Rohen, 1961; Holmberg, 1959, 1965) have also seen openings from these vacuoles into the nearest trabecular spaces. It has been suggested that the vacuoles might provide a direct pathway for the movement of aqueous humor from the innermost trabecular space into the canal of Schlemm (Garron et al., 1958; Garron and Feeney, 1959; Holmberg, 1959, 1965; Leeson and Speakman, 1961; Spelsberg and Chapman, 1962; Iwamoto, 1967a; Kayes, 1967; Vegge, 1963, 1967; and Tripathi [Rhesus], 1968).

The presence of the canal wall as a practically continuous layer between the endothelial lining of the canal and the nearest trabecular space makes it difficult to believe that the vacuoles can provide a constant pathway for the flow of aqueous humor. The vacuoles may actually open into the connective tissue, but in recent studies they have not been observed to open into the nearest trabecular space. Feeney and Wissig (1966), using an electron-opaque tracer (ferritin), showed that the vacuoles are not constantly open. When tracer material was perfused into the anterior chamber it accumulated in high concentration within some vacuoles, while it was entirely absent in others. It seemed to these investigators that the vacuoles must

---

Figure 4–20. *Continued.*
two endothelial cells (e). One cell branch almost crosses the intertrabecular space to join the endothelial cell of a trabecular sheet. The cells lining the spaces of the trabecular meshwork are thicker and more extensive than those lining Schlemm's canal.

The inner wall of the canal (f) includes all the tissue between the endothelium (d) of the canal and the endothelium (e) of the nearest trabecular space (b). The canal wall contains numerous fibroblasts (g) and thin collagen fibrils (h). The collagen fibrils measure 300 A. in diameter and most often are seen in cross-section when the sections are meridional. Adjacent to the canal some collagen fibrils are in close contact with its endothelium (arrows). This arrangement is similar to that found in lymphatic channels. The endothelial cells lack a basement membrane in this portion of the canal for 20 μm. At (j) a fibroblast appears to have what has been described as a "basement membrane." The abundant ground substance of the canal wall has been extracted during preparation of the tissues, leaving numerous empty spaces (k) which were formerly misinterpreted as trabecular spaces. Wide-spacing fibers (l) are found near the trabecular space, and dense clumps of very fine filaments (m), possibly tropocollagen, are scattered throughout the wall. (× 12,400.)

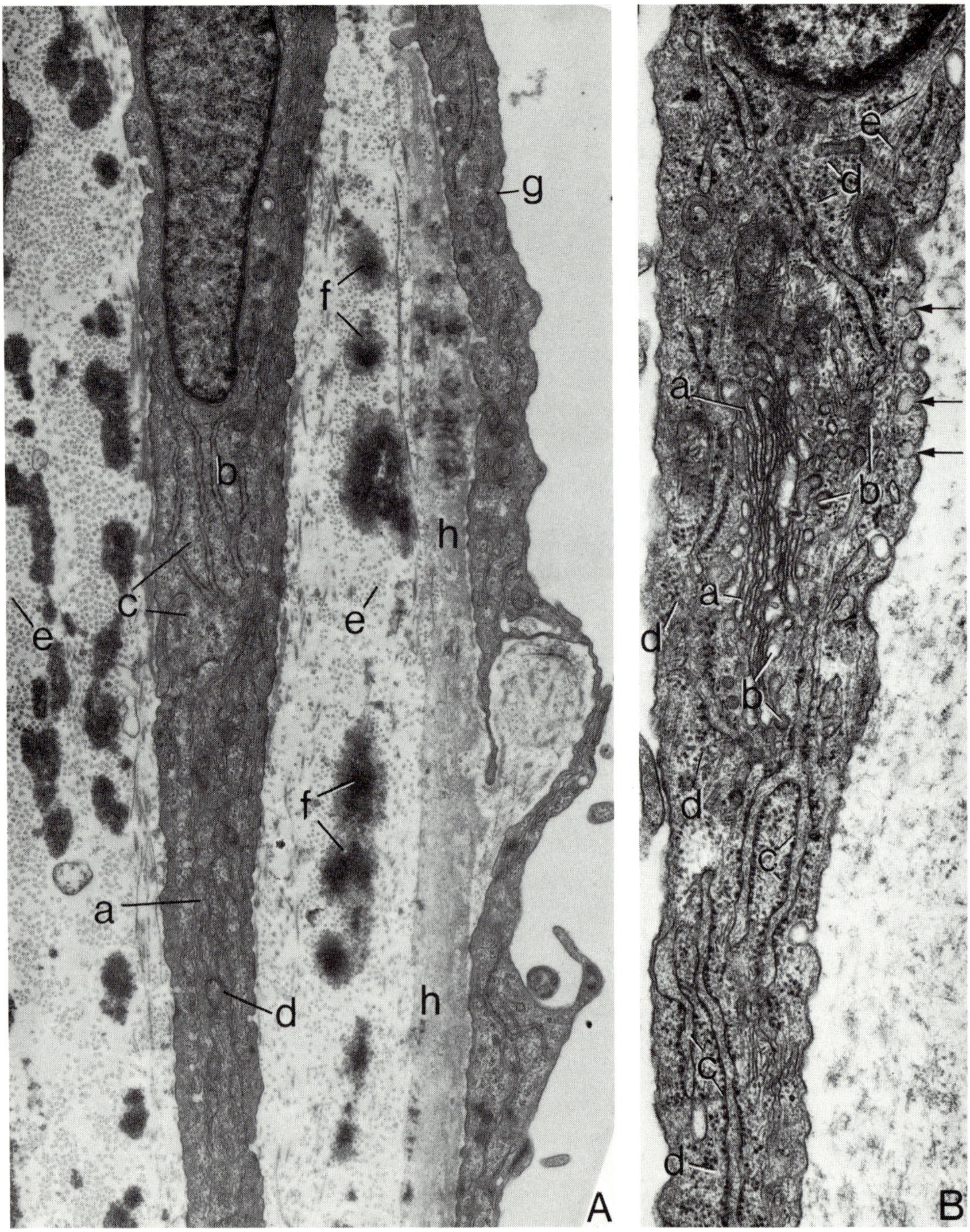

Figure 4-21. The inner wall of Schlemm's canal. *A*, The fibroblasts (a) resemble those of the cornea in their thickness and length. Long interconnecting cisternae of the rough-surfaced endoplasmic reticulum (b) and free ribosomes (c) are indicated. The mitochondria are small (d) and relatively sparse, and the nuclear chromatin is dispersed. The collagen fibrils (e) seen here measure less than 300 A. in diameter and are cut mostly in cross-section. Some of these fibrils are associated with masses of an electron-dense material (f). The endothelium of a trabecular space (g) is seen on the right. There is a layer of fibrillar material which varies in thickness adjacent to the endothelium, but it does not clearly represent a basement membrane. It contains clumps of wide-spacing fibers. (× 13,000.)

open and close intermittently, emptying their contents into the canal. The main function of the vacuoles would appear to to be in the active transport of large molecules such as proteins across the endothelium in order to circumvent the barrier presented to these molecules by closure of the intercellular space by the zonulae occludentes. The smaller pinocytotic vesicles also found in the endothelium of Schlemm's canal probably work in conjunction with the large vacuoles in the active transport of substances.

It is not clear whether a barrier to aqueous outflow is presented by the endothelium of the trabecular space nearest the juxtacanalicular tissue. Since this endothelium is not always continuous, aqueous humor may freely enter the connective tissue of the canal wall and then be incorporated into those vacuoles which are open. Finally, it should be emphasized that the greatest volume of aqueous humor diffuses passively through the wall of Schlemm's canal and that active transport may be needed only for large macromolecules and electrolytes.

The External Collector Channels (Fig. 4-28). Twenty-five to 35 veins emerge from the external wall of the canal of Schlemm and either join the deep scleral plexus directly or pass to the surface of the eye as aqueous veins. They are the principal route for the flow of aqueous humor from the canal of Schlemm into the episcleral veins. The channels are unevenly distributed around the circumference of the canal, being more numerous nasally than temporally, and are often connected to it in groups (Theobald, 1934). Theobald showed in serial sections of human eyes that these channels connect with each other and with the deep scleral plexus of veins, but not with arterial channels. Ashton (1951), using neoprene injections, verified the existence of these channels in human eyes and verified their origin from the canal of Schlemm. In addition to those veins which arise from the canal of Schlemm and pass directly to the episcleral plexus, he found others that joined the deep scleral plexus of veins; from this plexus, collector channels then joined the episcleral vessels. Ashton also confirmed the absence of arterial connections to these veins even though the arteries were located close to, or even embedded in, the wall of Schlemm's canal. His preparations also showed the presence of veins connecting the ciliary venous plexus with the deep scleral plexus.

When studied with the electron microscope, the external collector vessels are seen to be lined by an endothelium similar to that along the outer wall of Schlemm's canal. The connective tissue of the wall of Schlemm's canal continues outward along the external collector channels as a very simple layer which may show an occasional muscle cell. The adventitia disappears from the walls of those vessels which join the deep scleral plexus.

Internal Collector Channels (Fig. 4-29). Sondermann (1933) was the first to indicate that endothelial-lined canaliculi might connect the anterior

---

Figure 4–21. *Continued.*

B, Area similar to *A* to show the details of another fibroblast. The Golgi complex with its flattened cisternae (a) and associated vesicles (b) is prominent in the cytoplasm. Branching cisternae of rough-surfaced endoplasmic reticulum (c) also are prominent. Several vesicles are also observed, with an opened end toward the extracellular region (arrows). Free ribosomes (d) and cytoplasmic filaments (e) are indicated. (× 31,000.)

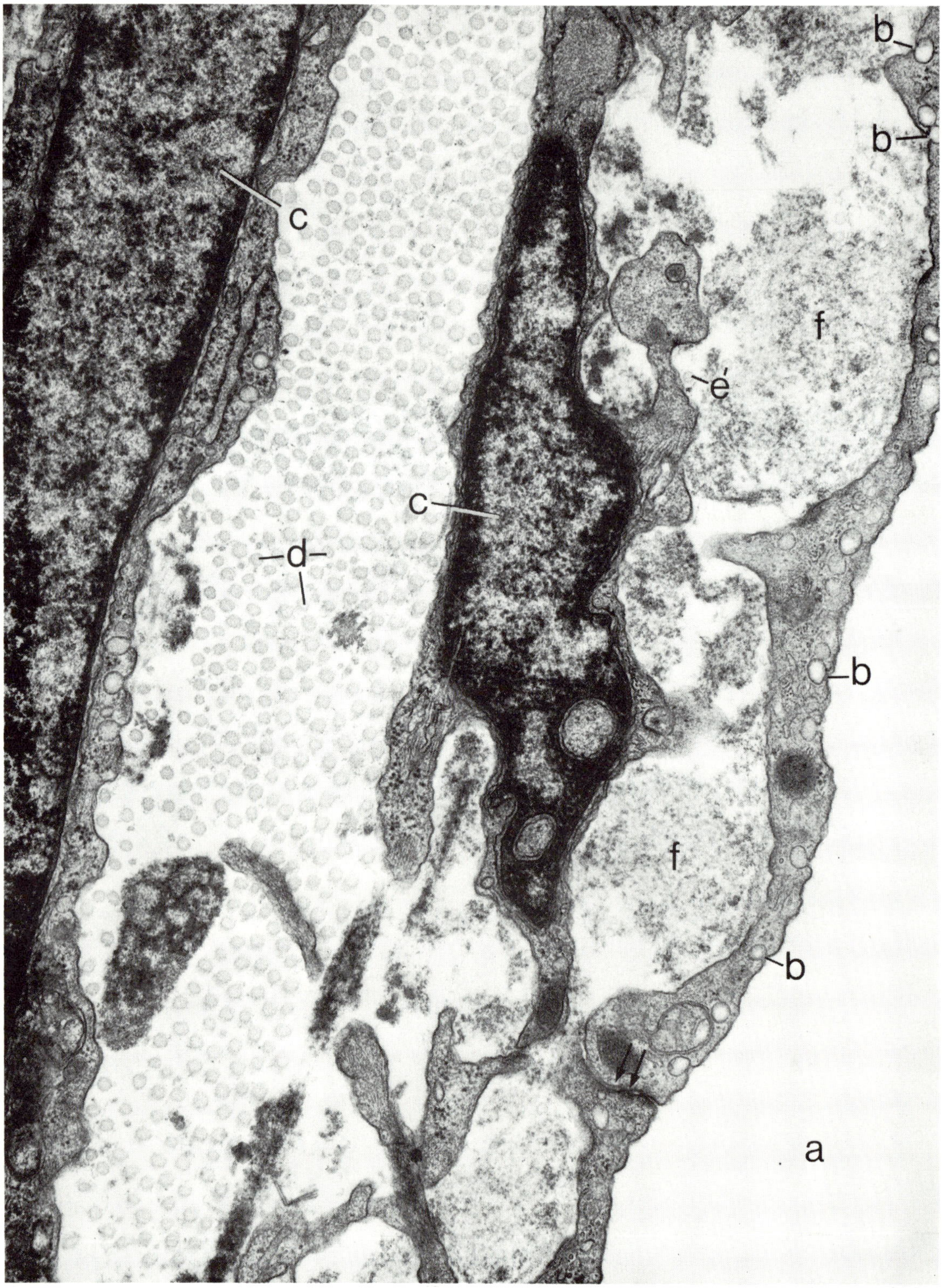

Figure 4–22. *See legend on opposite page.*

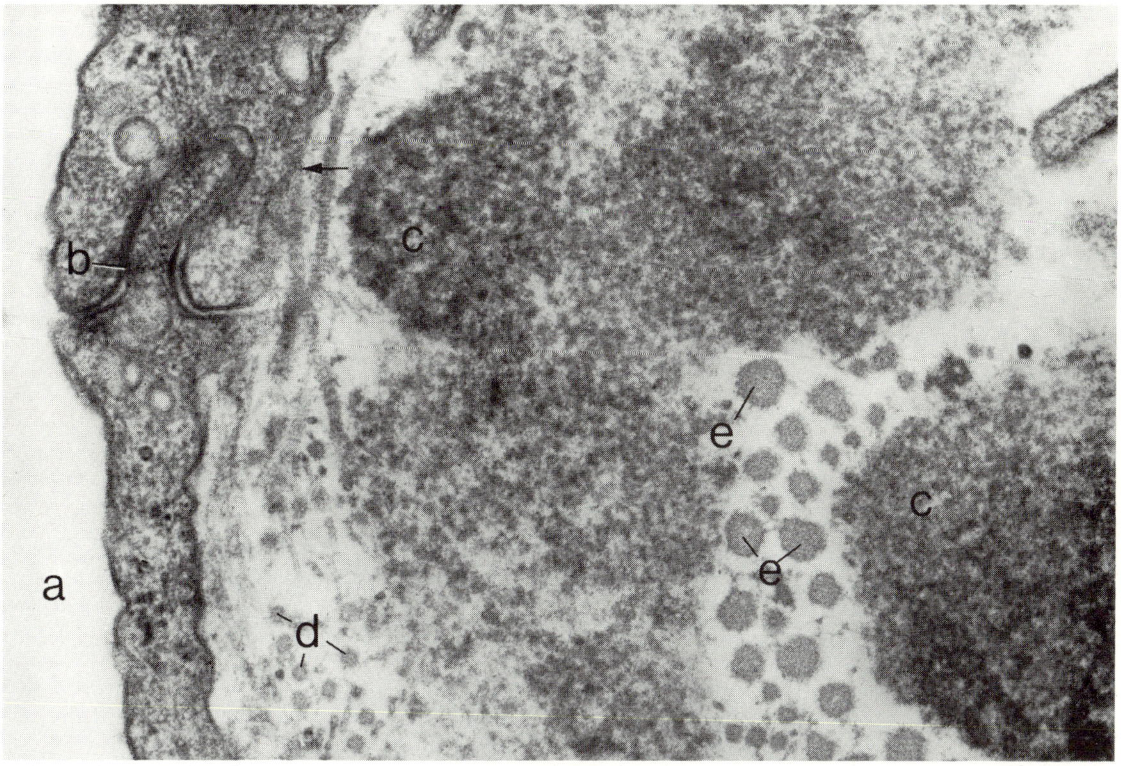

Figure 4-23. Schlemm's canal, external wall. The lumen of Schlemm's canal is at (a), while the junction of two endothelial cells is seen at (b). The granular, particulate nature of the material (c) is quite evident. Mature collagen fibrils are seen in cross-section (d,e), measuring 1000 A. and 2000 A., respectively. A collagen fibril (arrow) is in contact with the endothelium, a relationship often seen in lymphatics. (× 67,500.)

chamber to Schlemm's canal. Such channels were also described by Theobald (1934); Thomassen and Bakken (1951); François and associates (1955); Ashton (1956); Unger and Rohen (1959) and Iwamoto (1967 a, b). Other observers have denied their existence, including Fortin (1942); Flocks (1956); Garron and Feeney (1959); Feeney and Wissig (1966); and Vegge (1967). Sondermann demonstrated at least five internal collector channels per external collector channel through serial sections and reconstructions of this region in a number of human eyes. Theobald observed that these channels are easy to overlook unless serial sections are made, since they are not evenly distributed around the eye.

Routine histologic sections of human eyes often show small endothelial-

Text continued on page 153

Figure 4-22. Schlemm's canal, external wall. The lumen of the canal is at (a). Pinocytotic vesicles (b) lie adjacent to both the outer and inner endothelial cell membrane. Two tight junctions or areas of membrane fusion are identified between two endothelial cells (arrows). The nuclei of two adjacent fibroblasts are shown at (c). Most of the mature collagen fibrils (d) are found a short distance from the canal wall; the cross-sectional diameter of the largest of these fibrils is approximately 600 A. A few collagen fibrils (e) appear within the fine particulate material (f) adjacent to the canal wall. This granular particulate material appears to be the ground substance of the canal wall. It is probably produced by both the fibroblasts and endothelial cells. (× 31,000.)

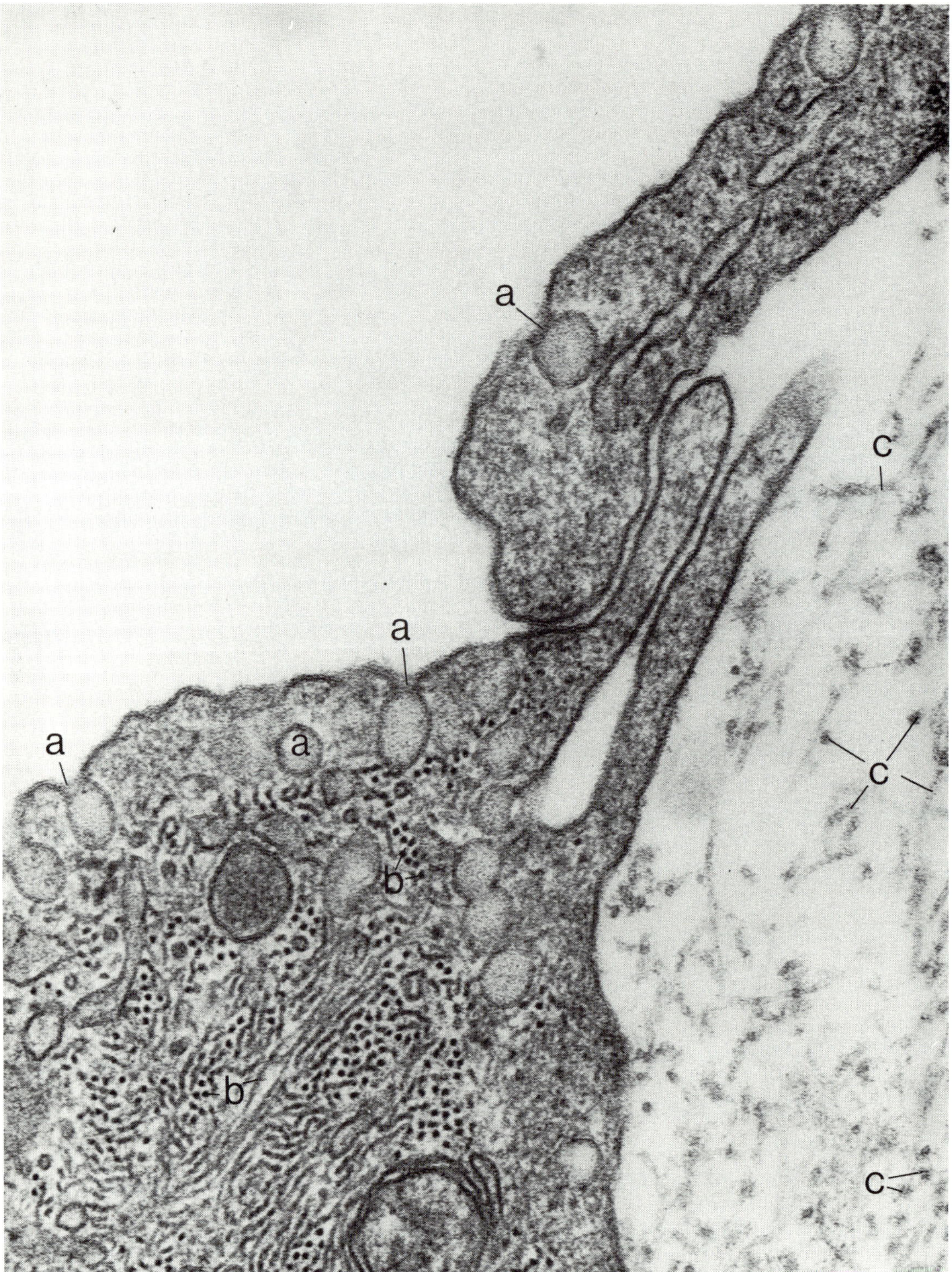

Figure 4-24. Schlemm's canal, internal endothelium at the junction of two cells. There are numerous pincoytotic vesicles (a) which are filled with a finely granular material. These cells contain a large number of cytoplasmic fibrils (b). The intercellular space measures 200 A. except for a small area of contact. Small collagen fibrils (c) measuring approximately 200 A. are seen in longitudinal and cross-section. (× 88,000.)

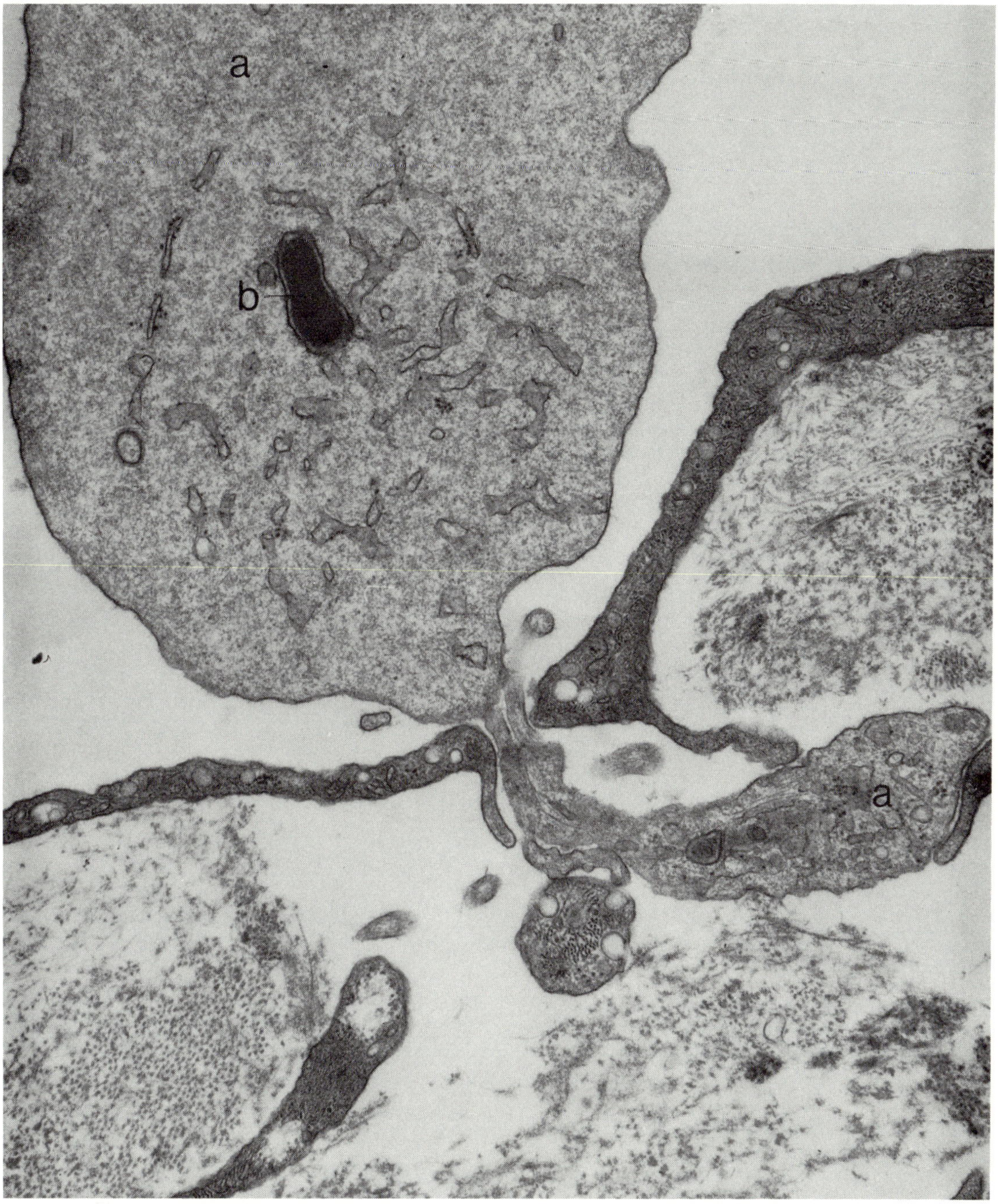

Figure 4-25. Schlemm's canal, inner wall. Red blood cells and other cells are seen occasionally "in transit" between contiguous endothelial cells. A leukocyte (a) containing a bacterium (b) is mostly within the lumen of Schlemm's canal, but a small portion is in the canal wall. (× 32,000.)

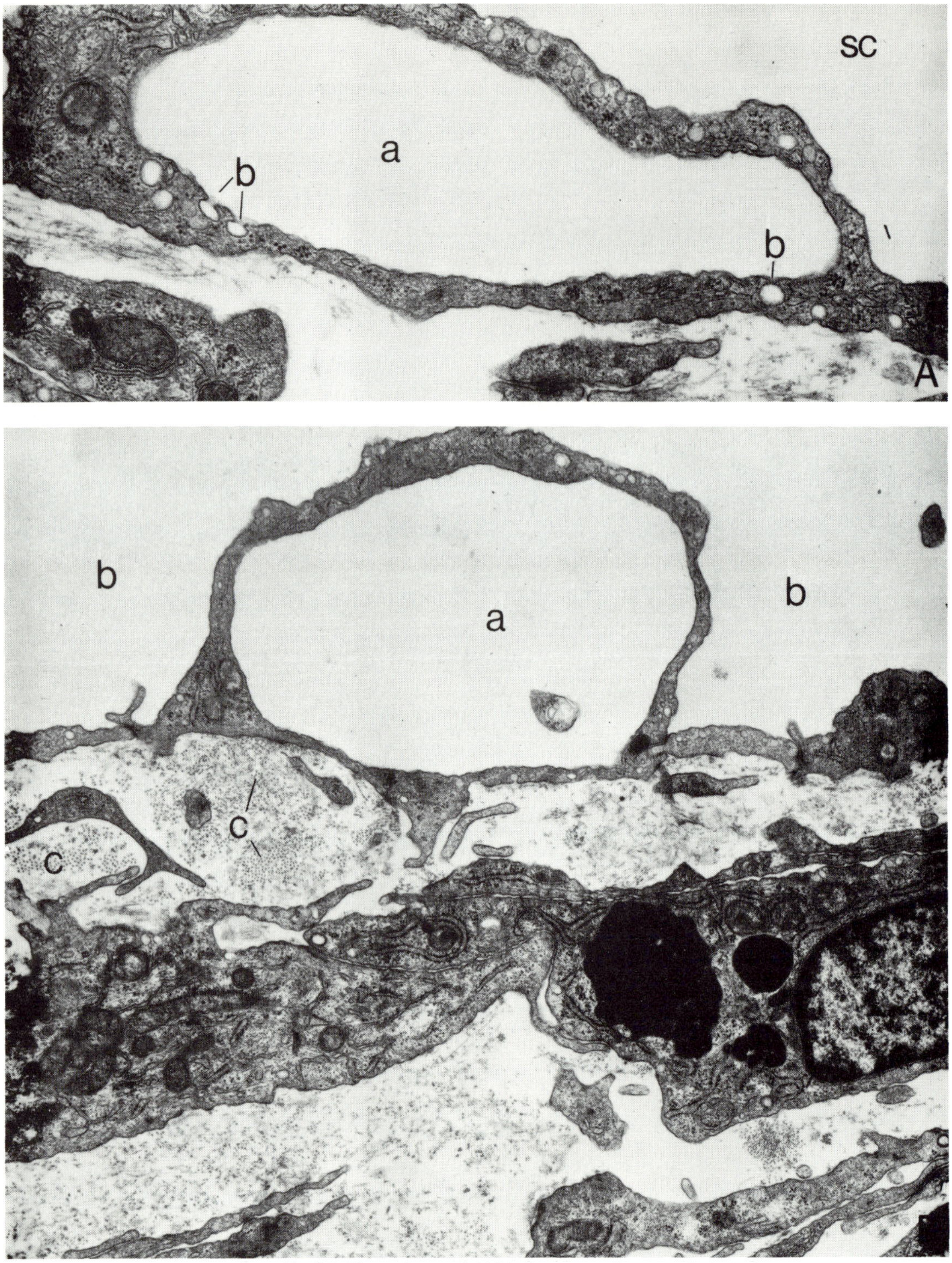

Figure 4-26. *A*, Inner wall of Schlemm's canal (SC) showing a large endothelial vacuole. Large vacuoles are found only in the inner wall of the canal. The giant vacuole (a) or vesicle measures 5 μm. by 1.5 μm; its endothelial lining has several pinocytotic vesicles (b) opening into the lumen. (× 25,000.)

B, Inner wall of Schlemm's canal. A giant vacuole (a) protrudes into the lumen of the canal (b). This vacuole measures 3 by 5 μm. The internal canal wall has a number of fine collagen fibrils (c) measuring around 200 A. in diameter. Some fibroblasts are seen at the bottom of the figure. (× 14,000.)

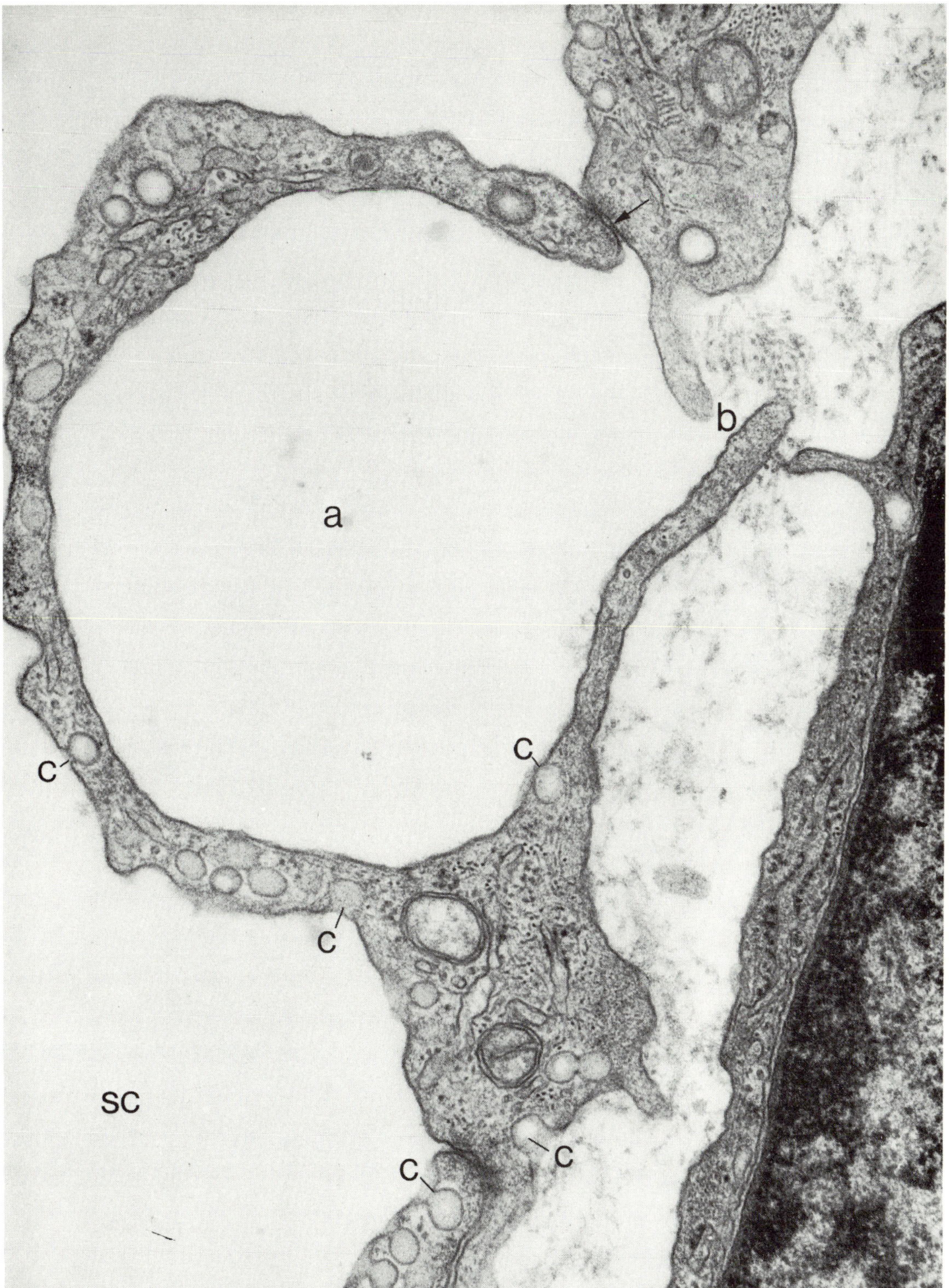

Figure 4-27. Inner wall of Schlemm's canal (SC). A giant vacuole (a) has an opening (b) which provides a clear passageway into the canal wall. Pinocytotic vesicles (c) are abundant. The arrow points to a tight junction between two endothelial cells. Pictures such as this suggest that some "vacuoles" may be formed by large marginal folds. When such large folds appear, however, they rarely extend freely into the canal lumen. (× 46,500.)

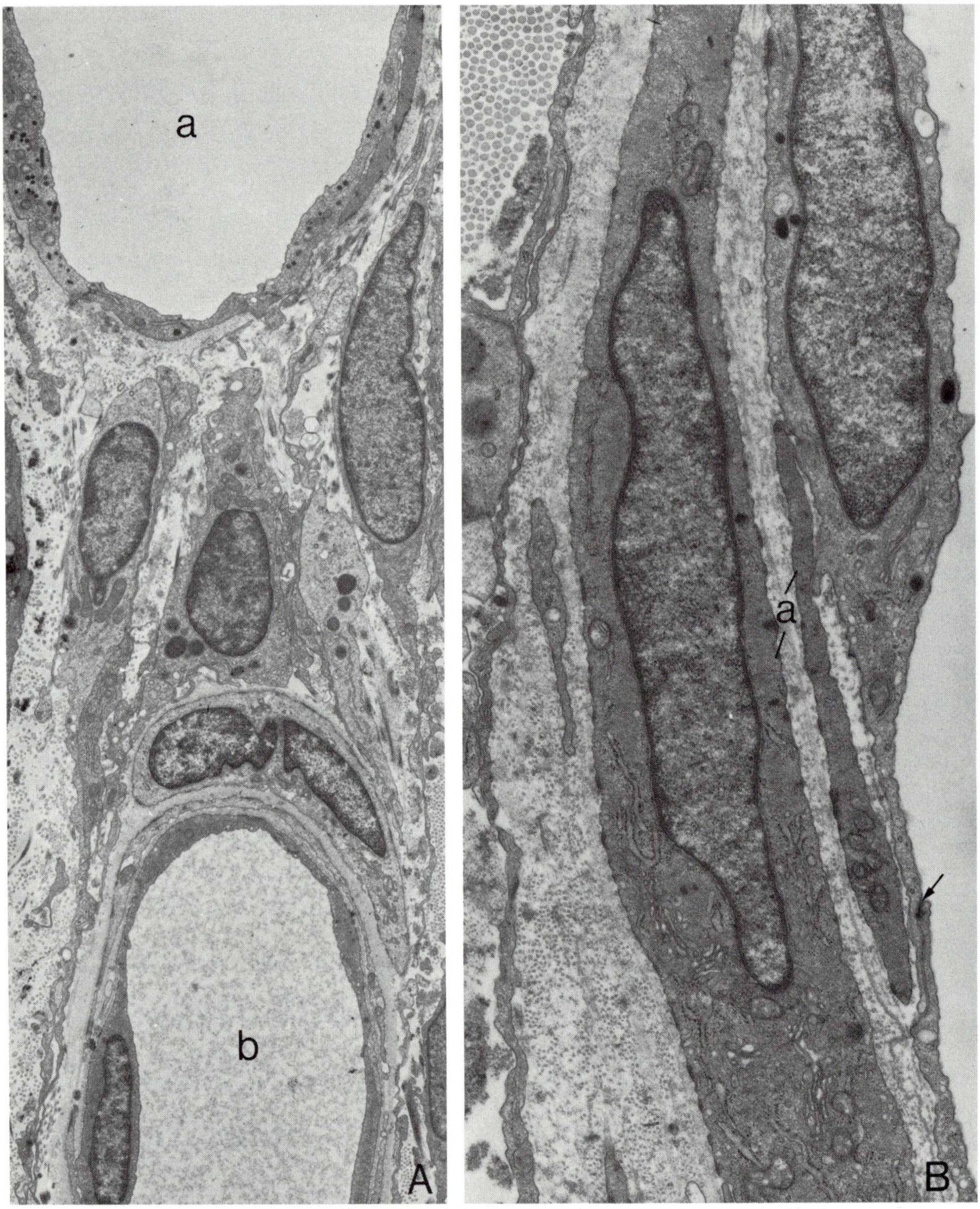

Figure 4-28. External collector channels and the deep scleral venous plexus. The external collector channels may join the deep scleral venous plexus or extend directly to the surface of the eye, where they join the episcleral venous plexus.

A, An aqueous vein (a) can be differentiated from a deep scleral vein (b) by the absence of plasma in its lumen. The wall of the aqueous vein is thinner and less developed. (× 6200.)

B, Higher magnification view of the wall of an aqueous vein. The endothelial cells are like those in other vessels and they are joined to each other by a zonula occludens (arrow). Occasional smooth muscle cells (a) may be seen in the wall of the aqueous vein. (× 13,000.)

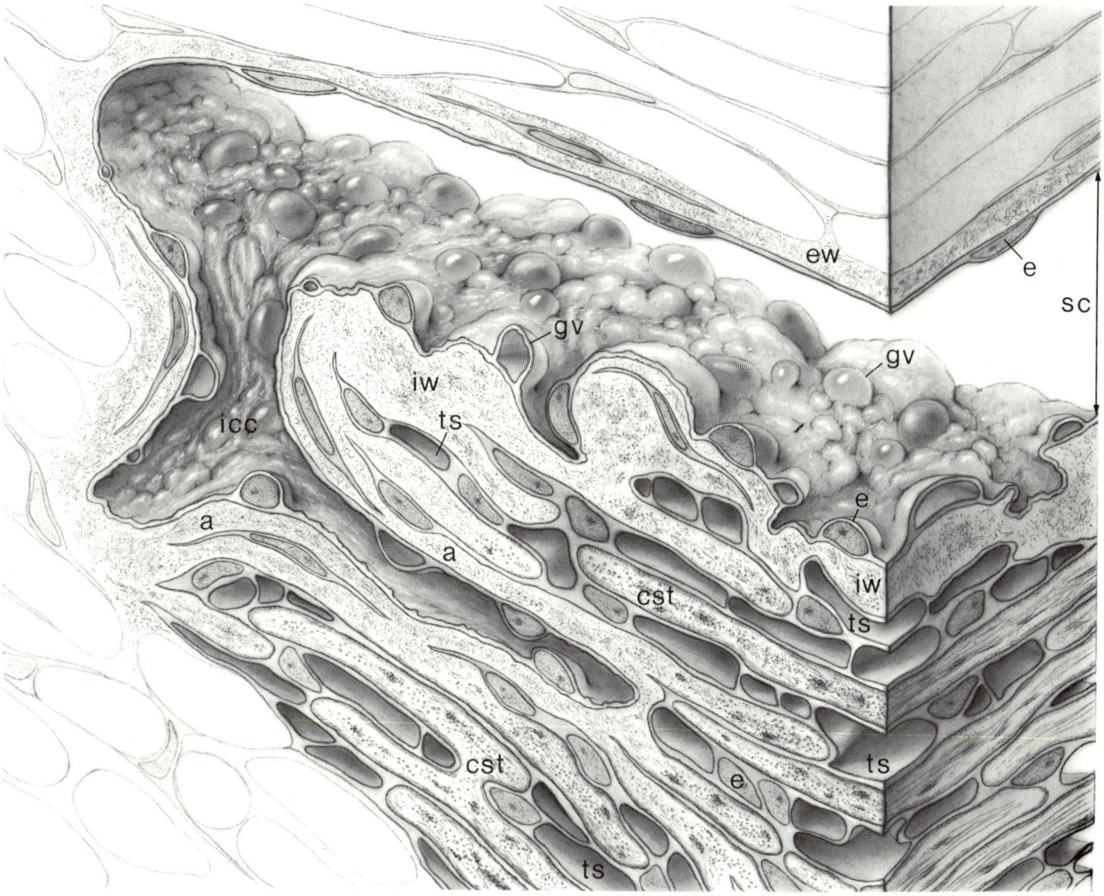

Figure 4–29. Drawing of the canal of Schlemm, an internal collector channel and adjacent tissues. The lumen of the canal (SC) is lined by endothelium (e). The endothelium of the inner wall is quite irregular, with many folds and outpouchings. Giant vacuoles (gv) are seen in the endothelial cells along the inner wall. The external wall of the canal (ew) is shown. The internal wall (iw) lies between the endothelium and the nearest trabecular space (ts). An internal collector channel (icc) arises near the posterior canal wall and extends into the trabecular meshwork, where it is lost. Like Schlemm's canal, it also is surrounded by a wall (a) which separates its lumen from the adjacent trabecular spaces. The corneoscleral trabecular sheets (cst) branch frequently, and their endothelial cells often form bridges between adjacent sheets.

lined channels arising near the posterior part of Schlemm's canal and curving forward into the trabecular meshwork. Some of these channels can be traced for a fairly long distance into the meshwork, but they almost always terminate in the inner trabecular meshwork. They have not been shown to traverse the entire corneoscleral meshwork into the anterior chamber.

Iwamoto (1967a, b) employed light and electron microscopy to study these collectors and did find endothelial-lined channels that opened into Schlemm's canal from the deep intertrabecular spaces in both human adult and infant eyes. He followed some of these channels a considerable distance toward the anterior chamber; he failed, however, to demonstrate that they are uninterrupted channels from Schlemm's canal to the anterior chamber.

We have studied these channels carefully in a number of eyes. The internal collector channels most often commence near the posterior part of Schlemm's canal as right-angle branches which are lined by endothelium and surrounded by adventitia. Shortly after emerging from the canal they turn to become parallel with it. The width of the collector channel at its opening into Schlemm's canal may be as large as 12 to 15 μm. The diameter diminishes rapidly and soon is the caliber of the intertrabecular spaces. The internal collector channels are tortuous and branch frequently. We have been unable to establish a clear direct connection of the lumen of the collector with an intertrabecular space. We feel that the internal collectors are simply diverticulae of Schlemm's canal that serve to increase the total surface area of the inner wall. They are always surrounded by a wall which separates their endothelium from the nearest trabecular space. Those opposed to the theory of the existence of through-and-through channels from the anterior chamber to the canal of Schlemm argue that the size and number of Sondermann's canals are too great to be consistent with known facts about the bulk flow of aqueous humor.

Trabecular Meshwork (Fig. 4–16).

The trabecular meshwork occupies most of the internal scleral sulcus. It has a somewhat triangular shape, its apex being near the end of Descemet's membrane and its base at the scleral spur. The anterior meshwork contains three to five layers and the posterior meshwork 15 to 20 layers. The larger number of posterior sheets is due to formation of new sheets from the wall of the internal scleral sulcus, and also from branching of pre-existing sheets as they extend posteriorly.

Virchow (1910) was the first to divide the trabecular meshwork into scleral or corneoscleral and uveal portions. The former comprises the bulk of the meshwork, the latter forming only a thin, loose network on the inner surface of the corneoscleral meshwork.

Corneoscleral Meshwork (Figs. 4–30 to 4–37). The corneoscleral meshwork extends from the region of the end of Descemet's membrane and deep cornea to the sclera, scleral spur and ciliary body. Most of the meshwork inserts into the sclera. Two to three sheets of the corneoscleral

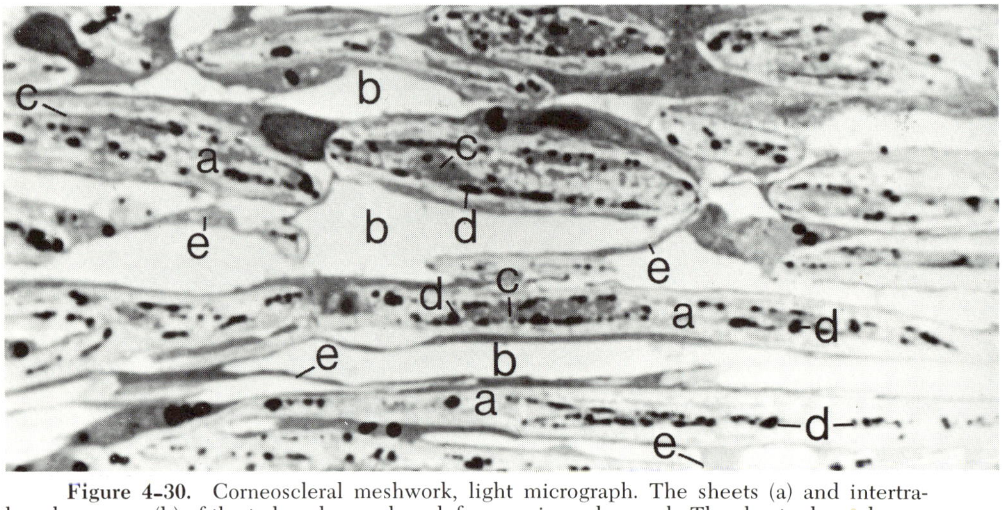

Figure 4–30. Corneoscleral meshwork, light micrograph. The sheets (a) and intertrabecular spaces (b) of the trabecular meshwork form an irregular mesh. The sheets show clumps and strands of pale material (c) and prominent clumps of dense material (d). The corneoscleral trabecular sheets vary in size, thickness and shape. Each sheet is surrounded by a continuous endothelium, and the sheets branch and merge with other sheets, causing the intertrabecular spaces to vary considerably in size and shape. Endothelial cells also branch and cross the intertrabecular spaces (e). (× 688.)

meshwork pass internal to the scleral spur to join the ciliary body stroma and the meridional portion of the ciliary muscle. The meshwork is thicker posteriorly near the scleral spur, where it measures 120 to 150 μm.

The corneoscleral meshwork is composed of a large number of flattened perforated sheets which branch and interlace with each other. The branches may lie in a single plane or connect to more superficial or deeper sheets. The general arrangement of the collagen in the sheets is circular and parallel to the circumference of the limbus. Meridional sections, therefore, show the collagen to be cut in cross-section, while tilted frontal sections show the collagen to be cut longitudinally. Routine histologic sections show the trabecular sheets in the corneoscleral portion of the meshwork to measure about 5 μm. in thickness. The intertrabecular spaces probably are slightly collapsed in routine histologic preparations, where they measure about 0.5 μm. in width (Huggert, 1955; Ashton, 1956). Openings which connect adjacent intertrabecular spaces exist in the trabecular sheets. These openings are not superimposed on each other in successive sheets. The sizes of the openings vary considerably; Ashton (1956) observed them to measure between 12 and 20 μm. in diameter. The corneoscleral trabecular sheets, therefore, form a circular, three-dimensional grid within which are the intertrabecular spaces. The grid contains apertures which allow aqueous to pass from the anterior chamber through the meshwork toward Schlemm's canal. Conventional studies have shown that these apertures are irregular in size and shape and that they become progressively smaller as Schlemm's canal is approached. No apertures are found in the inner wall of Schlemm's canal.

When viewed with the light microscope, each trabecular sheet has been considered historically to have four components (Salzmann, 1912): (1) a central core of connective tissue, with fibrils circularly oriented; (2) a dense layer of elastic tissue, which surrounds the core; (3) a glass membrane, believed to be derived from Descemet's membrane, lying external to the two inner layers; and (4) an endothelium covering the sheets and forming the lining of the intertrabecular spaces.

This concept of the structure of the sheets persisted until the tissues of this region could be studied with the electron microscope. Garron and Feeney (1959) first studied the fine structure of the corneoscleral and uveal meshwork. They found the center of each corneoscleral sheet to be composed of numerous circularly oriented collagen fibrils of standard size and 640 A. banding. They found no "dense layer of elastic tissue" external to this collagen. In its place they found a sheath of banded material with a periodicity of around 1000 A. Instead of a glass membrane derived from Descemet's membrane, a light-density matrix of ground substance was found in the region of the basement membrane of the endothelium. Ten years have elapsed since these early studies were performed, and many improvements have been made in fixation and embedding techniques. This original electron microscopic description of the trabecular sheets, however, is still partially correct.

By electron microscopy the thickness of the trabecular sheets varies considerably, their dimensions being between 6 and 12 μm. They are separated from each other by intertrabecular spaces measuring between 6 and 12 μm. in width. The endothelial cells covering these sheets may be as long as 40 μm.; they are mostly oriented meridionally. The cells are very thin, measuring an average of 4 to 5 μm. in thickness, except near the nuclear region, where they may measure 12 μm. Elaborate infoldings of adjacent cells occur along the lateral cell walls, but specialized junctions are rarely

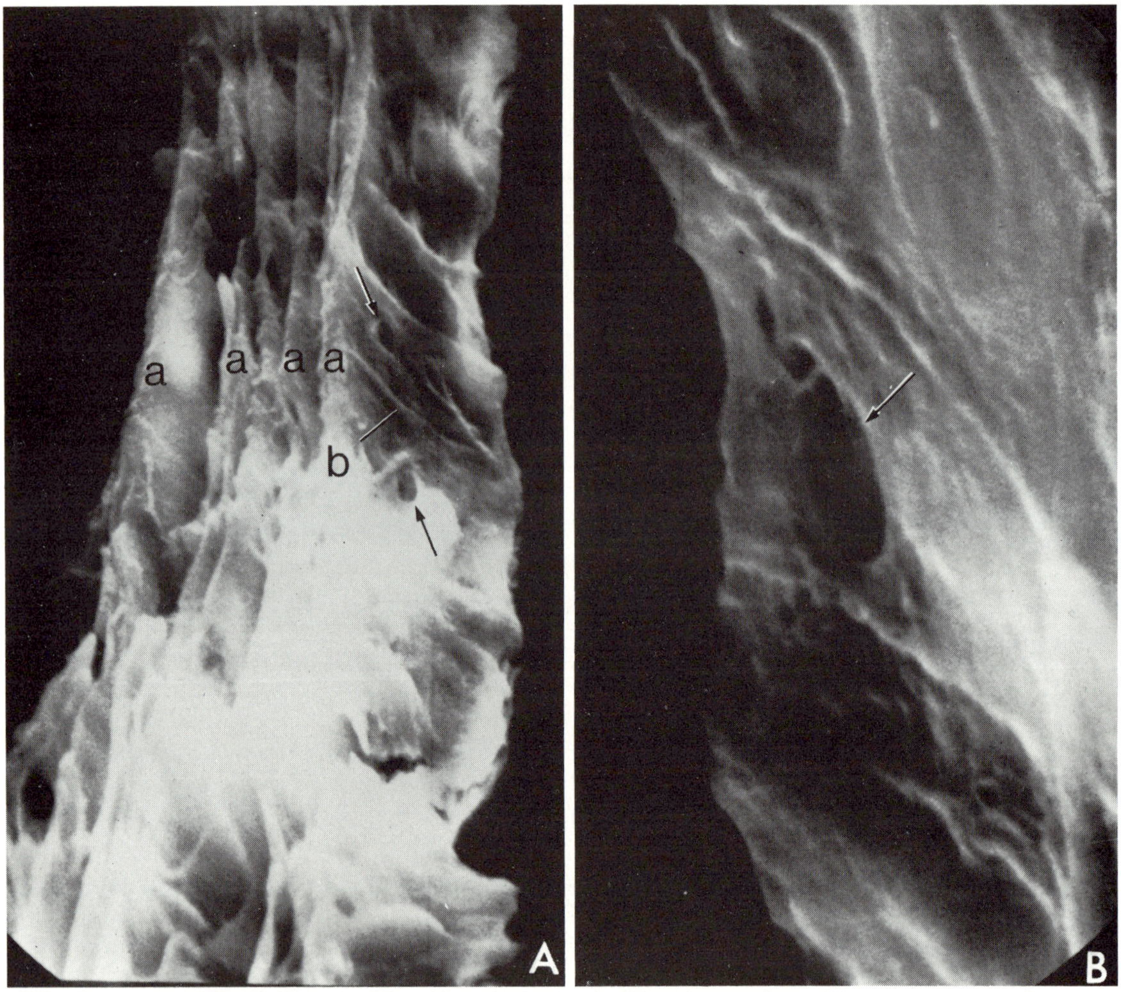

Figure 4–31. *A*, A 30 μm. cross-section of the corneoscleral trabecular sheets, viewed obliquely. A number of layers of sheets are seen (a). Openings through the sheets from one level to the next are seen (arrows). The contiguous border of two cells is seen at (b). (× 1000.)

B, The hole (*A*) is seen at higher power. It has depth and resembles a tunnel. Its diameter is 8 μm. (× 3000.) (Spencer, W. H., Alvarado, J., and Hayes, T. L.: Invest. Ophthal. 7:651, 1968.)

C, Corneoscleral meshwork, electron micrograph. The photograph shows two sheets (a) of the corneoscleral meshwork, each measuring between 3 and 4 μm. in width and separated from each other by an intertrabecular space (b). Single arrows indicate the intercellular space between contiguous endothelial cells. The cells are quite thin in this region, measuring 0.5 to 1.0 μm. in thickness. The collagen fibrils (c) are mostly cut in cross-section and are quite small, measuring around 200 A. in diameter. The sheet on the left shows isolated patches of a particulate, very electron-dense material (d); this same material is found in the midportion and runs almost the whole length of the sheet on the right (d). The fine collagen fibrils are intimately associated with these areas of marked electron density. A finely granular material of variable width is observed near the endothelial cells; in the past this material has been called a basement membrane. Fine collagen fibrils (double arrows) are observed within this material. Wide-spacing collagen (e) is observed in the sheet on the right. (× 13,000.)

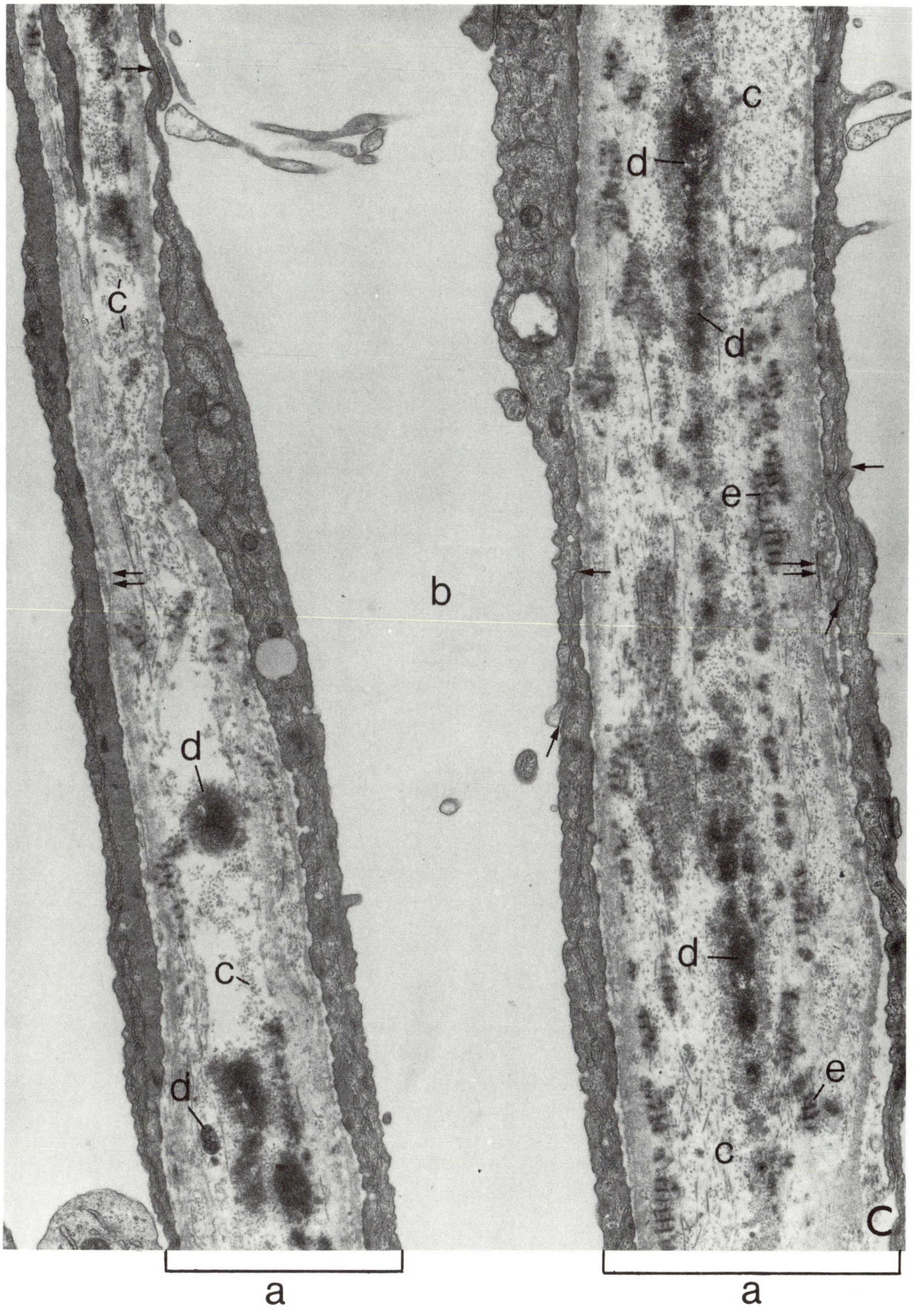

Figure 4–31, *C. See legend on opposite page.*

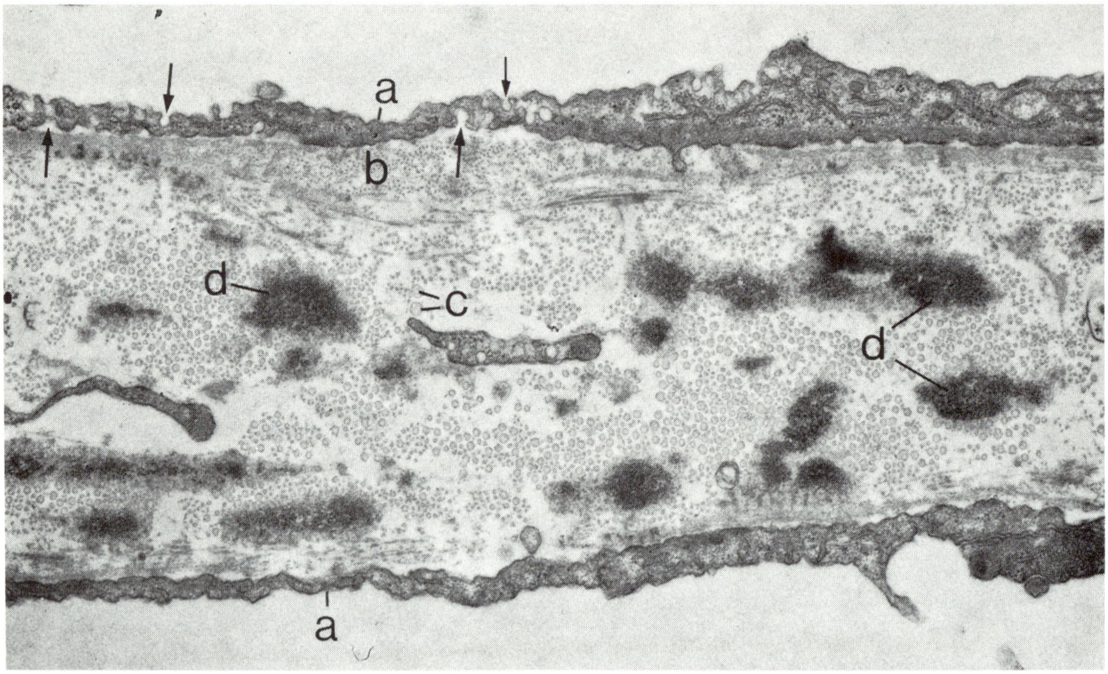

Figure 4-32. Corneoscleral sheet, meridional section. The thin endothelial lining (a) of the trabecular sheets may measure as little as 0.1 μm. in thickness in some areas. The cytoplasm often contains numerous pinocytotic vesicles (arrows) which face either the trabecular space or the interior of the sheet. The collagen fibrils are distributed throughout the entire width of the sheet, and there is no continuous "basement membrane" under the endothelial cells. This sheet contains collagen fibrils of various sizes, unlike those in the sheets previously shown. At (b) there are fibrils which measure between 100 and 200 A. in diameter, while at (c) there are two fibrils measuring approximately 800 A. in diameter. Meridional sections of this type show the collagen fibrils to be cut in cross-section, indicating a circular disposition of the collagen fibrils parallel to the limbus. The electron-dense clumps of fibrils (d) which are scattered through the sheet correspond to the dense clumps seen in Figure 4-31. They are not elastic tissue, but appear to be tropocollagen fibrils. The presence of the finer collagen fibrils in the endothelial region suggests they are being produced by these cells. (× 15,000.)

seen. The intercellular space occasionally is seen to become narrow at the site of a macula adherens. The cytoplasm of these cells is filled with many free ribosomes and a great number of filaments measuring 80 to 100 A. in thickness. Pinocytotic vesicles are numerous, and they open both toward the intertrabecular space and the connective tissue of the sheets. The mitochondria are small and scanty except in the perinuclear cytoplasm, where many more are seen. Many profiles of cisternae of the rough-surfaced endoplasmic reticulum and the Golgi apparatus are commonly found in the perinuclear region. The perinuclear cytoplasm also contains many filaments and free ribosomes. The nucleus generally bulges toward the connective tissue of the sheets and contains a moderate amount of dense chromatin or heterochromatin.

The endothelial cells of the trabecular sheets are richly endowed with the cytoplasmic organelles responsible for protein synthesis and secretion, and it seems likely that they are involved in the synthesis of the collagen, fibrils and matrix of the sheets. Unfortunately there is no direct information on this subject or on the rate of turnover for collagen in this tissue. The presence of large deposits of tropocollagen fibrils, however, may be indicative of a rather rapid rate of turnover. If the endothelium is indeed involved

Text continued on page 164

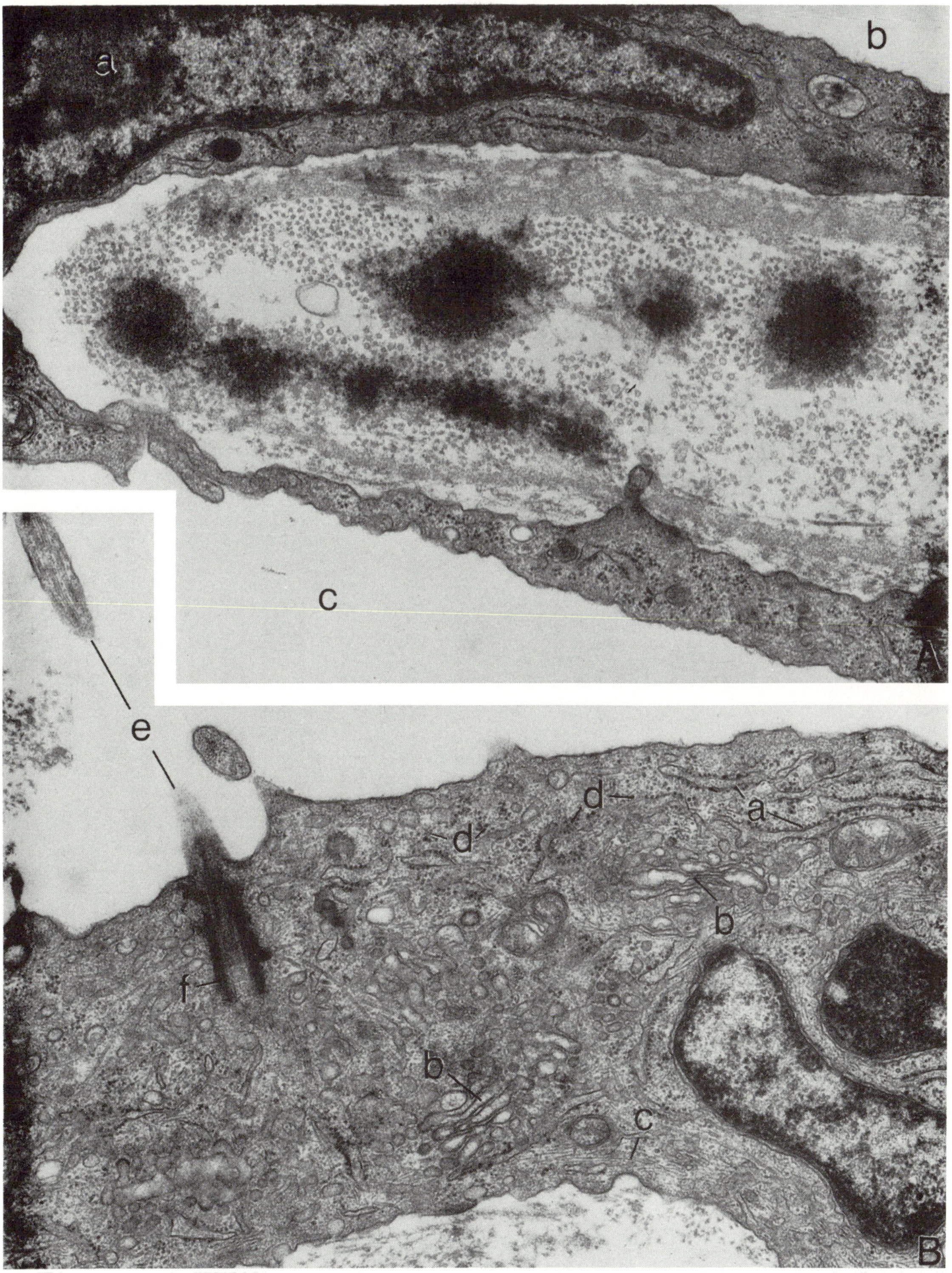

Figure 4-33. Corneoscleral sheet, meridional section. *A*, The endothelial nucleus frequently occupies a position on the edge of the trabecular sheet; it has a prominent nucleolus (a) and dispersed chromatin. This endothelial cell covers both sides (b, c) of the trabecular sheet. (× 26,000.)

B, The cytoplasm of the trabecular endothelium is more abundant in the nuclear region. Cisternae of rough-surfaced endoplasmic reticulum (a) are seen, as well as a Golgi complex (b), filaments (c) and free ribosomes (d). A cilium (e) is seen to protrude into the trabecular space; its basal body is at (f). (× 28,000.)

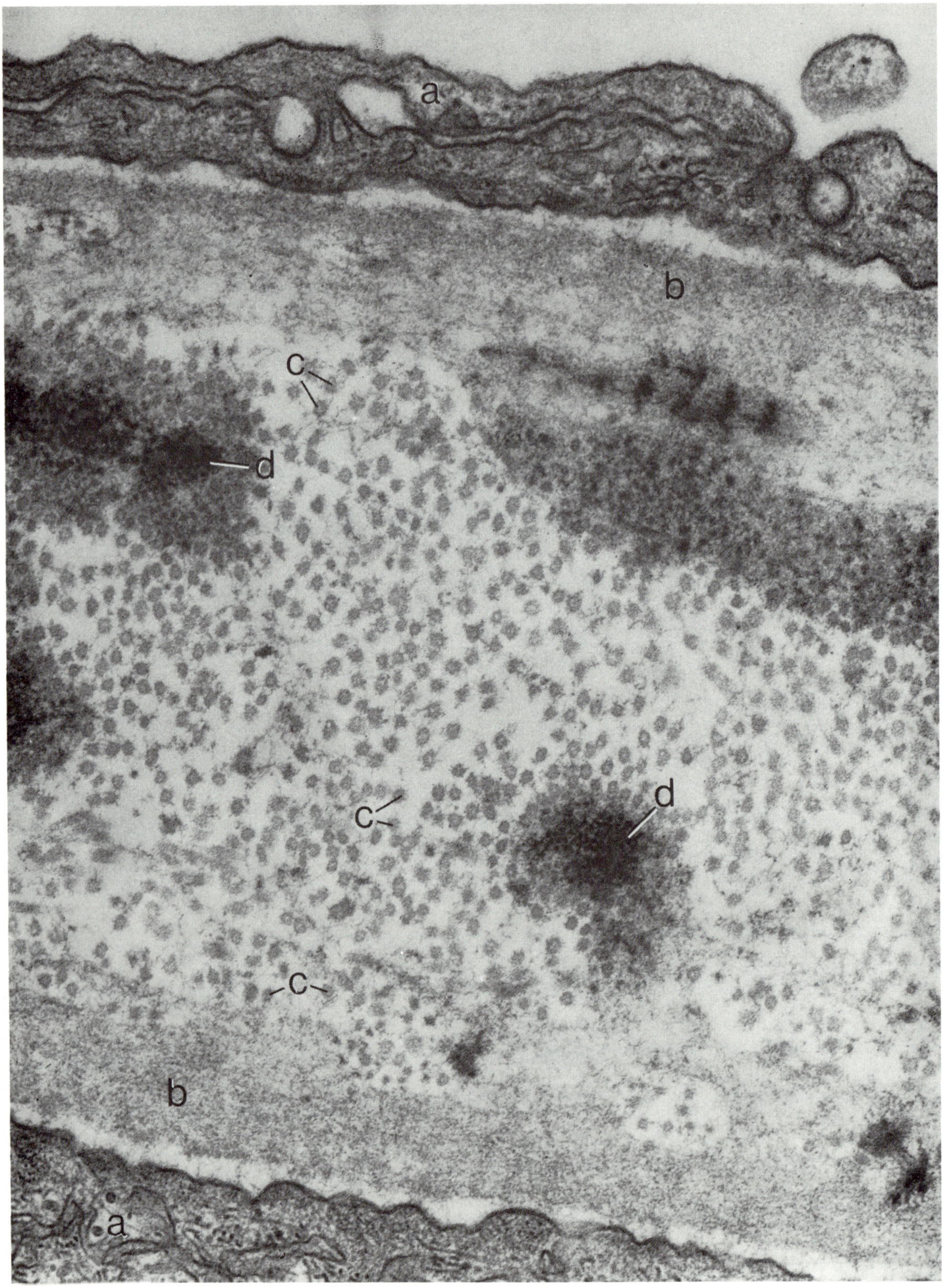

Figure 4–34. Corneoscleral sheet, meridional section. Higher magnification to show the composition of the sheet. The endothelium is at (a), and the fine granular material (b) adjacent to the endothelium is seen to be part of the ground substance and not a basement membrane. It contains some filaments which join the endothelial cell membrane. Collagen fibrils (c) are dispersed throughout the sheet. The collagen fibrils are approximately 300 A. in diameter. There are clumps of finer and denser fibrils with an electron-dense core at (d). (× 56,000.)

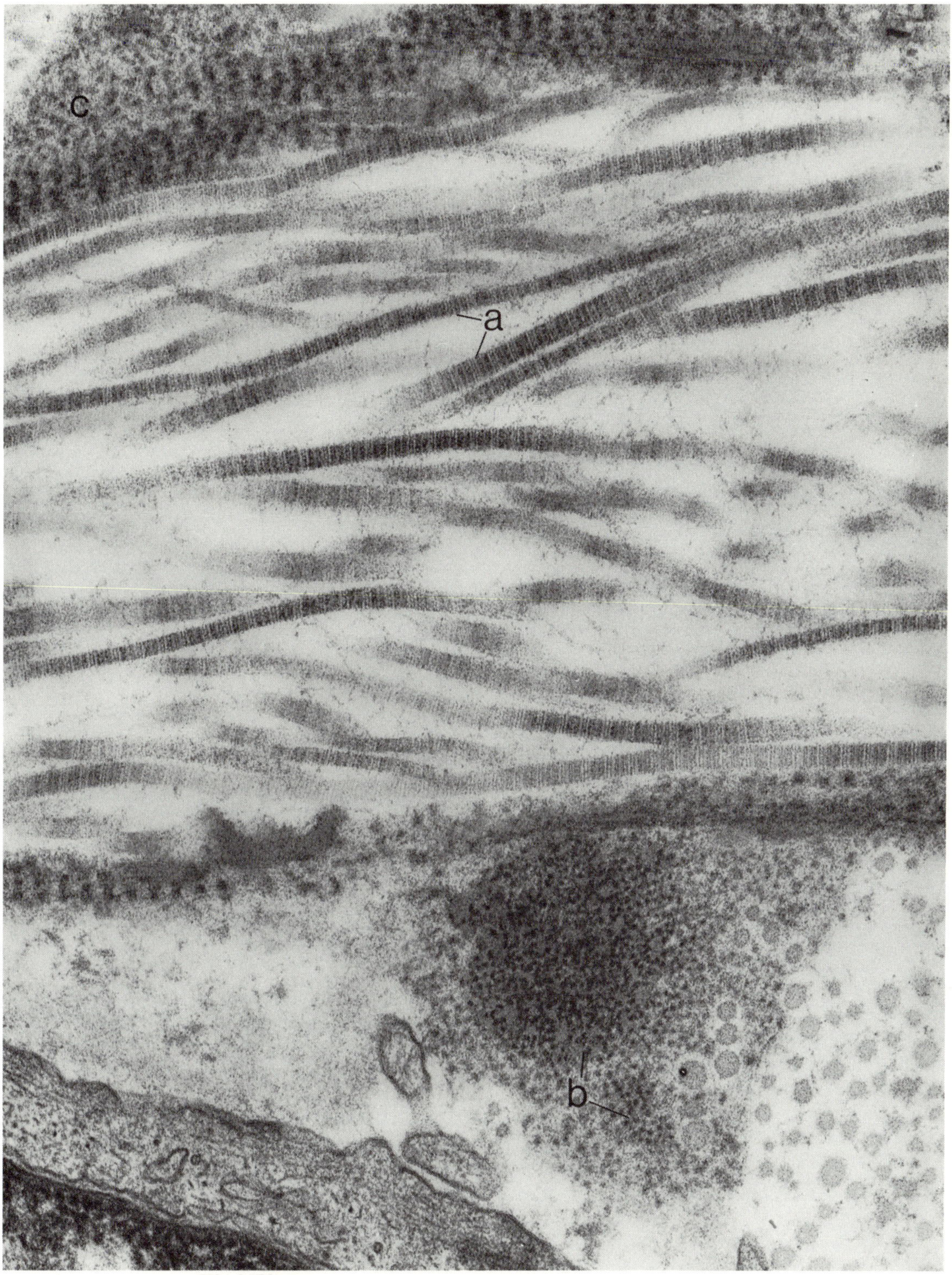

Figure 4–35. Corneoscleral sheet. The collagen fibrils (a) show the usual periodic striations, which repeat every 600 A. At (b) is a more osmiophilic structure composed of tiny, dense particles. These are associated with mature collagen fibrils. At (c), above, a mass of collagen is cut longitudinally; it has a striated appearance. (× 19,600.)

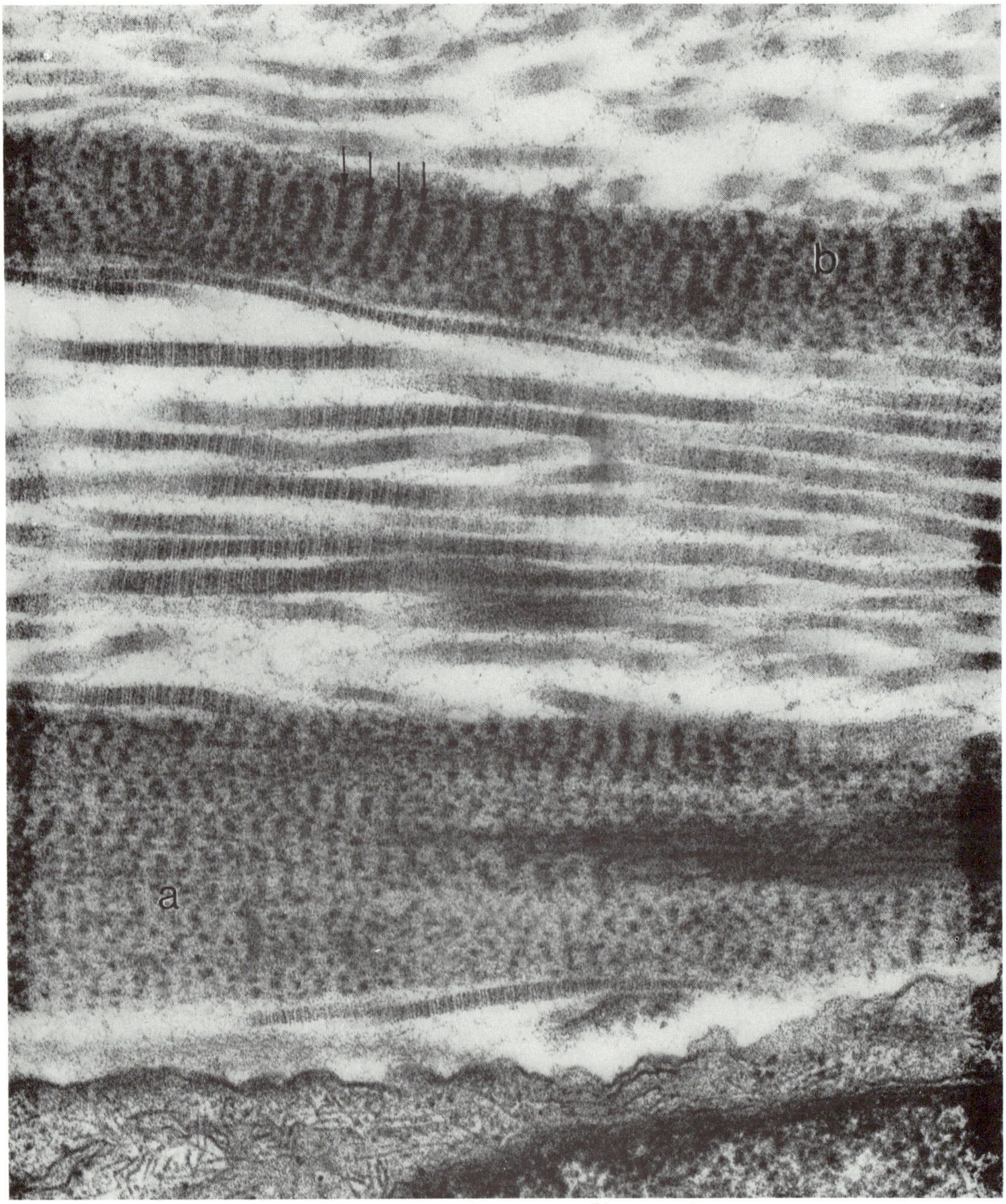

Figure 4–36. Corneoscleral sheet. Two large masses of collagen are cut longitudinally (a, b). They are composed of fibrils with the usual 600 A. repeating striations. The upper mass shows coarse striations which also repeat every 600 A. (arrows). These masses stain strongly with basic dyes and they have been mistaken for elastic fibers. (× 19,500.)

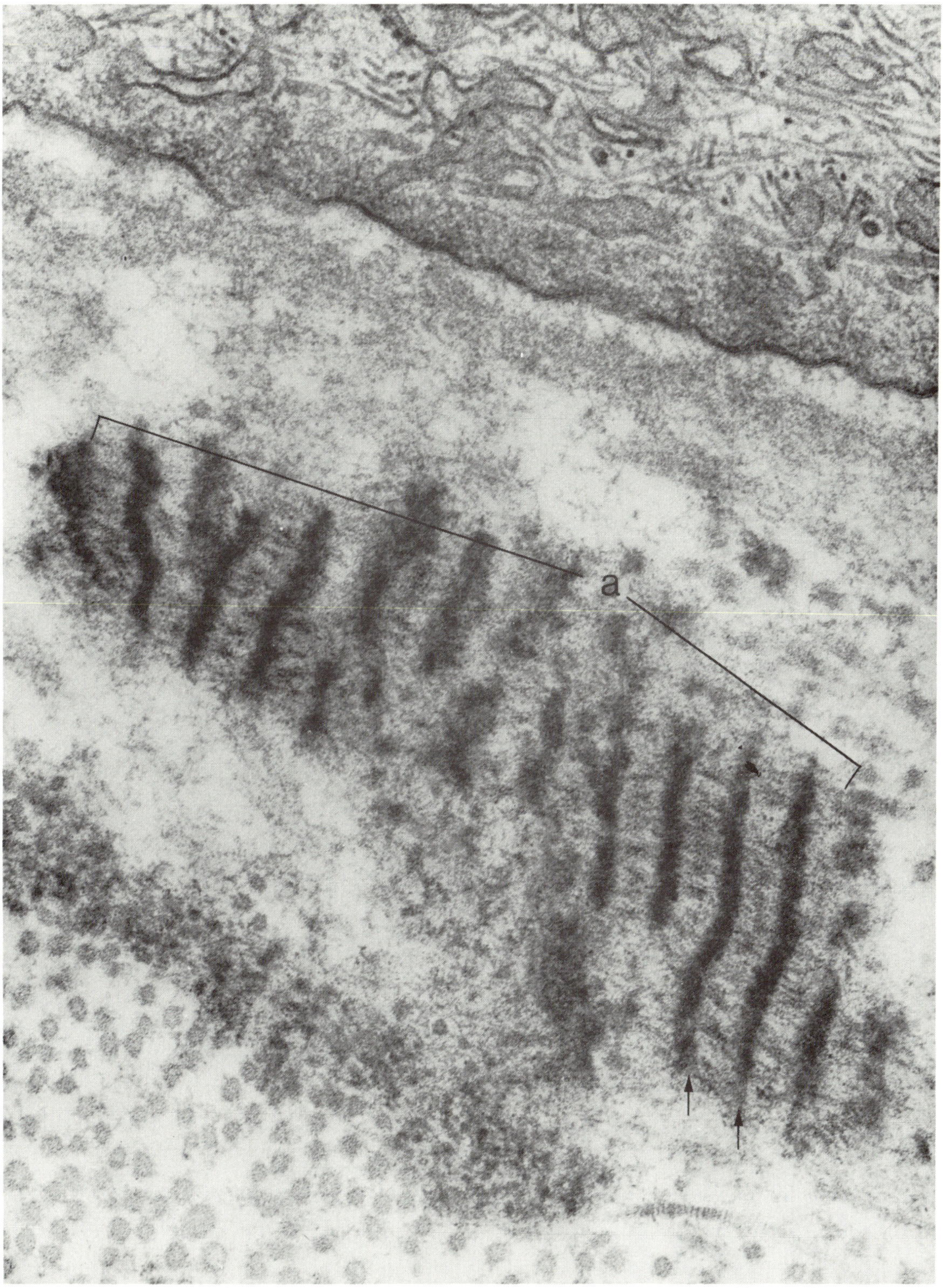

Figure 4–37. Corneoscleral sheet. A clump of wide-spacing collagen is shown at (a). Its coarse striations are separated from each other by a distance of 1200 A. (arrows). The heavy collagen masses which are shown in Figures 4-35 and 4-36 are found in both young and old eyes; wide-spacing clumps of this type, however, appear as an aging phenomenon. In very old eyes they occupy a larger portion of the interior of the corneoscleral sheets. (× 84,000.)

in fibrillogenesis, it is possible that the so-called basement membrane represents deposits of collagen precursors recently secreted by the endothelium. The endothelium would seem to carry out a dual function in this tissue: (1) it serves as a lining for the trabecular spaces, and (2) it probably synthesizes the matrix and fibrils of the trabecular sheets.

The interior of the trabecular sheets is typically devoid of cells, except for nerves and an occasional macrophage or other wandering cell. Beneath the endothelial envelope the sheets contain (1) collagen fibrils, (2) tropocollagen aggregates, (3) wide-spacing collagen deposits and (4) a layer of a finely granular material traditionally called a basement membrane but not organized as a true basement membrane.

The *collagen fibrils* are dispersed through the ground substance of the trabecular sheet. These fibrils vary widely in diameter between 100 and 400 A. The smallest of the fibrils are considered to be tropocollagen fibrils which have become aggregated lengthwise and transversely to produce the mature collagen fibril with a diameter of around 400 A. The smaller fibrils predominate near the periphery of the sheets, close to the granular material lying under the endothelium. The larger fibrils predominate in the center or core of the trabecular sheet.

The *tropocollagen fibrils* form bundles that measure as much as 0.4 μm. in cross-section. These bundles are composed of minute fibrils which are oriented in the same direction as the mature collagen fibrils. These tropocollagen aggregates are very osmiophilic; they are especially abundant in the trabecular sheets of young eyes. Rhodin (1967) pointed out that such small fibrils are commonly found in rapidly growing connective tissues and especially during development. We find these fibrils in all the connective tissues of the eye, but they are especially abundant in the trabecular meshwork and the sclera. The fibrils stand out clearly when the tissues are examined with the light microscope, under which they resemble elastic fibers. They do stain with elastic tissue stains, but are not sensitive to elastase.

With increasing age the trabecular sheets have large deposits of *wide-spacing collagen*, but we have not been able to find such deposits in young eyes (first decade). The wide-spacing collagen deposits are also osmiophilic; by light microscopy they cannot be differentiated from the aggregates of tropocollagen. The wide-spacing collagen and the tropocollagen fibrils were originally described as a layer around the central collagen core, but they really have no special orientation around the central collagen. They are, however, frequently found around the central portion of the sheet where 400 A. diameter collagen fibrils are located. A layer of very finely *fibrillar material* of varying thickness is interposed between the endothelium and the collagen fibrils. This fibrillar layer is separated from the endothelium by a less dense area of variable thickness. The fibrillar layer is not continuous, however, but it increases to several times the thickness of the endothelium. In the region of Descemet's membrane the fibrillar material often contacts the cell membrane, but it is not a continuation of Descemet's membrane onto the trabecular sheets. It is not a typical basement membrane because it is discontinuous and varies in its relation to the endothelial cells. The best that can be said is that it is a basement membrane-like material and that it is probably ground substance.

Intertrabecular Spaces. Light microscopic studies have indicated that a mucopolysaccharide may occupy these spaces. This observation has not been confirmed by studies with the electron microscope, and no additional information is available on this point. The spaces communicate with each other, and Holmberg (1965) showed in serial section studies that the communicating orifices measure 50 to 60 μm. in diameter. He also found a decrease in the size of these channels to 1 or 2 μm. in the deep meshwork. Spencer and co-workers (1968) studied these communicating orifices with the scanning electron microscope, using sectioned, paraffin-embedded specimens as well as fixed, air-dried specimens. Contrary to the classic conceptions, these investigators were unable to show a decrease in the size of the holes connecting the intertrabecular spaces from the innermost portion to the outer part of the meshwork.

Uveal Meshwork (Figs. 4–38 to 4–40). There have been some differences of opinion about the presence and attachments of the uveal meshwork. Rohen (1963) and Holmberg (1965) believe that the uveal cords do not extend anteriorly to the region of Schwalbe's ring and that they are rudimentary in the human eye. Salzmann (1912), Burian and associates (1955), Flocks (1956) and Ashton (1956), on the other hand, believe that the uveal bands do attach anteriorly at Schwalbe's ring. Spencer and associates (1968), using the scanning microscope, found the uveal meshwork to attach near Schwalbe's ring at the zone of transition between the corneal and trabecular endothelium. The uveal portion of the trabecular meshwork arises in the ciliary body, and the cords of this meshwork pass forward medial to the scleral spur and attach anteriorly near Schwalbe's ring. The meshwork is never more than two or three layers thick.

In children the posterior portion of the uveal meshwork is prominent, but it becomes less so with increasing age. The anterior portion of the uveal meshwork is especially difficult to demonstrate in the eyes of very old persons, but we have been able to identify the cords in the region of Schwalbe's ring in such eyes. Posteriorly most of the uveal bands merge with the ciliary body, but occasionally one joins the iris root. The uveal cords branch frequently as they extend forward from the ciliary body, and the branches form narrow or wide angles. They either unite with branches from other cords or merge with the underlying corneoscleral meshwork and enclose meshes measuring 30 to 40 μm. The cords have a diameter of 4 to 6 μm. in the midportion of the meshwork and are slightly larger posteriorly.

Microscopically the difference in the structure of the uveal cords and corneoscleral trabecular sheets is seen clearly in cross-section. The uveal meshwork is cord-like, in contrast to the flattened sheets of the corneoscleral trabecular meshwork. The electron microscope shows the cords of the uveal meshwork to be covered by an endothelium similar to that of the corneoscleral sheets. The endothelial cytoplasm frequently shows pigment granules which are enclosed by a thin membrane. These pigment granules are more common in older individuals and in the inferior portion of the meshwork.

The endothelium encloses a connective tissue matrix containing the same fibrils and components that are found in the corneoscleral sheets. Unlike the circularly oriented collagen fibrils of the corneoscleral sheets, the disposition of the collagen fibrils in the uveal cords is parallel to their long axes.

Iris Processes or Pectinate Fibers (Figs. 4–41 and 4–42). These are large processes which arise from the iris and bridge the angle of the anterior

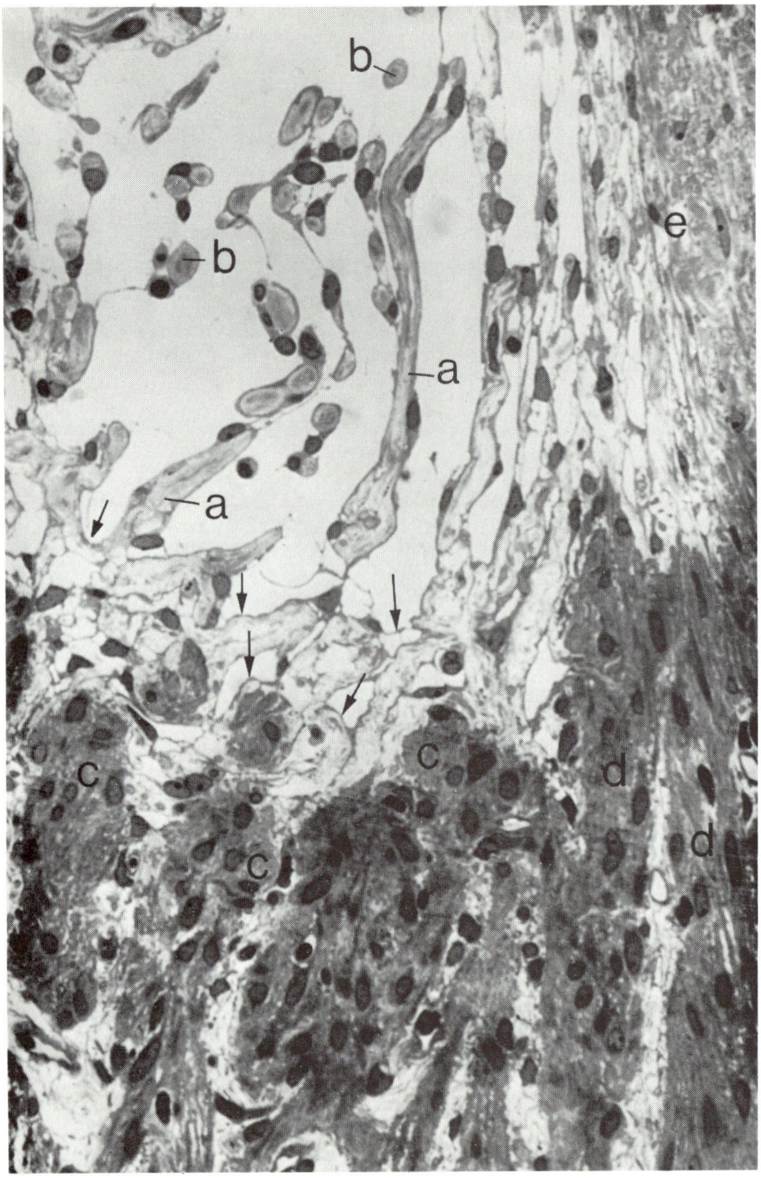

Figure 4-38. Uveal meshwork, light micrograph. The uveal meshwork is better developed in young eyes than in those of older individuals. This is the anterior chamber angle of a child. Some uveal cords are cut longitudinally (a) and others are seen in cross-section (b). Endothelium (arrows) covers all the structures in the angle. The radial part of the ciliary muscle (c) lies in proximity to the chamber angle. The longitudinal portion of the ciliary muscle (d) has a close relation to the corneoscleral meshwork (e). (× 400.)

chamber. Most often they insert at the scleral spur region, but at times they extend forward as far as the midportion of the trabecular meshwork. In congenitally anomalous eyes, iris processes may extend to the region of Schwalbe's ring. Most eyes, however, possess only a few iris processes; there usually are fewer than 100 of them around the entire circumference of the anterior chamber angle.

The iris processes have the same morphology as the anterior iris stroma from which they arise. They are covered by fibrocytic cells identical

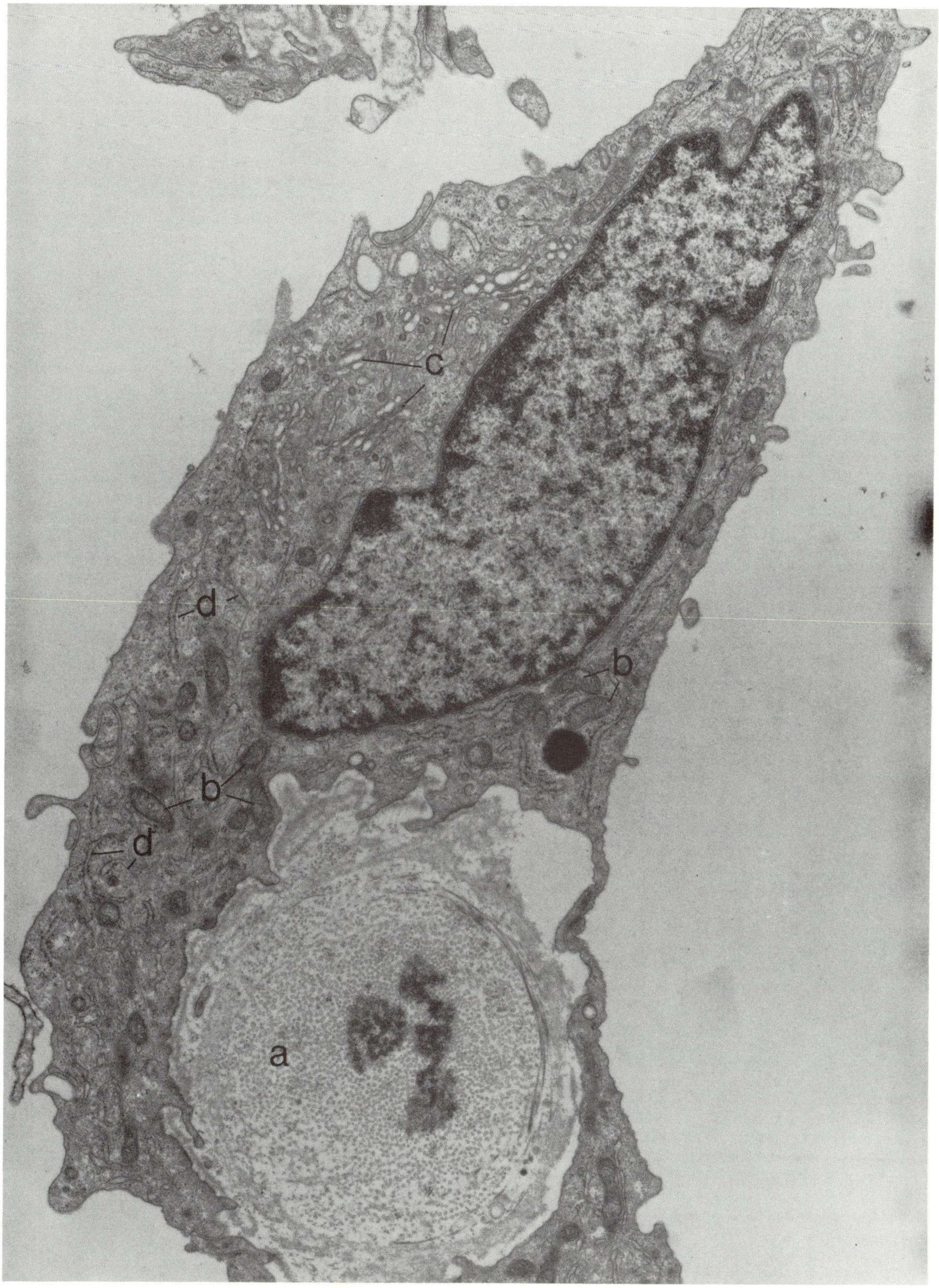

Figure 4–39. Uveal cord, cross-section. The round collagen fibrils of the interior of the cord (a) are cut in cross-section. For the most part the collagen fibrils of the cords are oriented parallel to its long axis. Endothelial cells surround the cords, and their cytoplasm away from the nuclear region is rather thin and may measure 1 μm. or less in thickness. The cytoplasm in the nuclear region has a number of mitochondria (b), a well developed Golgi complex (c), cisternae of rough-surfaced endoplasmic reticulum (d), free ribosomes and filaments. (× 13,000.)

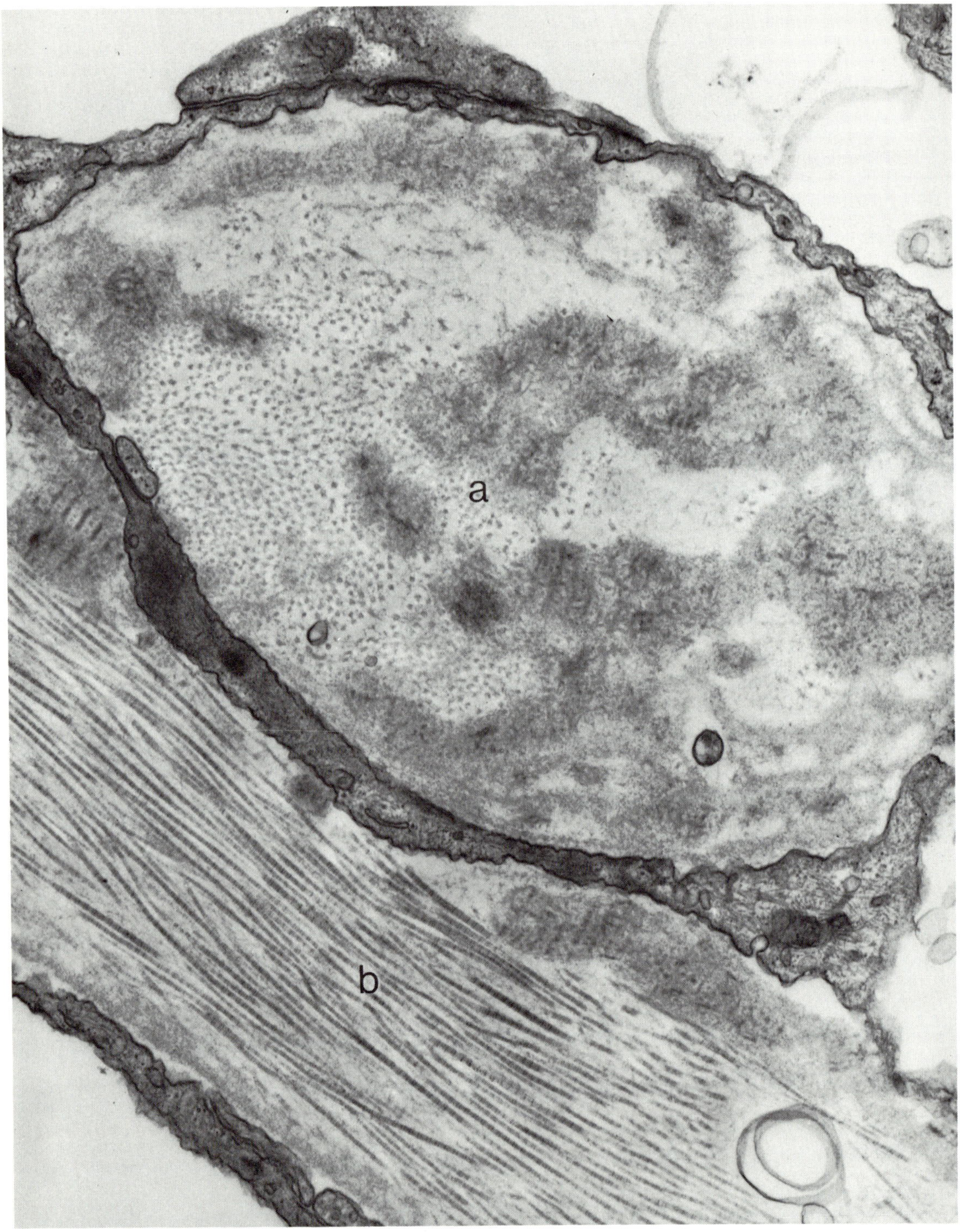

Figure 4-40. Uveal meshwork, electron micrograph. The section passes through two uveal cords which are joined but are oriented at right angles to each other. The upper cord (a) is cut in cross-section so that its collagen fibrils are seen in cross-section; the lower cord (b) is sectioned longitudinally, and its collagen also is sectioned in a longitudinal plane. Wide-spacing collagen forms clumps in the cord. (× 26,000.)

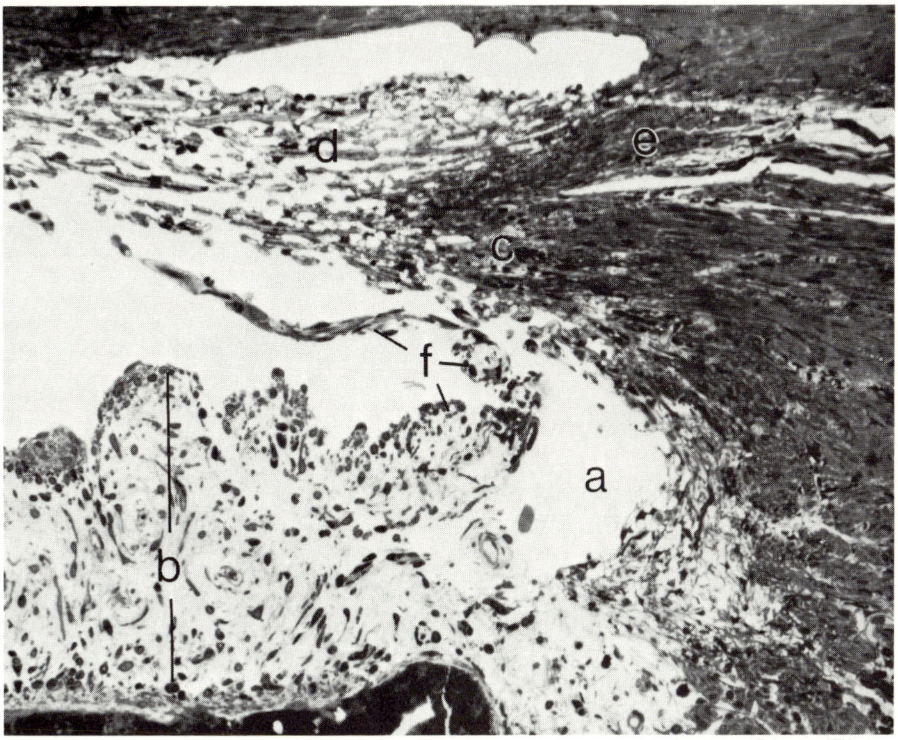

Figure 4-41. Iris process, light micrograph. The anterior chamber angle is seen at (a). A portion of the iris (b), ciliary muscle (c), trabecular meshwork (d) and scleral spur (e) are included. An iris process (f) arises from the anterior iris stroma and crosses the anterior chamber to join the trabecular meshwork. Ordinarily this process would insert near the scleral spur. (× 260.)

to and continuous with those of the anterior iris surface (p. 209). Melanocytes and fibroblasts are found in their interior. The iris processes measure as much as 100 μm. in diameter near their origin in the iris but become narrower at the scleral spur or trabecular meshwork. Near the trabecular meshwork, as they merge with it, the fibers develop the morphology of the uveal cords, losing their melanocytes and fibroblasts.

Finally, it is worthwhile to indicate the reasons for the dual terminology used in describing these structures. The term pectinate fibers has been adopted by some observers to indicate an anatomic relationship between these structures and the pectinate ligament found in some ungulates; to others the term only suggests a similar morphology between these fibers and the pectinate ligament. The use of the term iris process is simpler since it indicates only the relationship of these fibers to the adjacent tissues and avoids the connotations of pectinate fibers.

Scleral Spur (Figs. 4–43 to 4–45).

The scleral spur is the posterior site of insertion of a good part of the corneoscleral meshwork, and it provides the anterior insertion for most of the longitudinal part of the ciliary muscle. The collagen of the spur is oriented in the same circular direction as that of the corneoscleral sheets, and it is continuous with their collagen. Most of the collagen fibrils of the spur resemble those of the trabecular meshwork, measuring around 340 A. in diameter, but there are also many smaller fibrils. The collagen fibrils increase in size in the

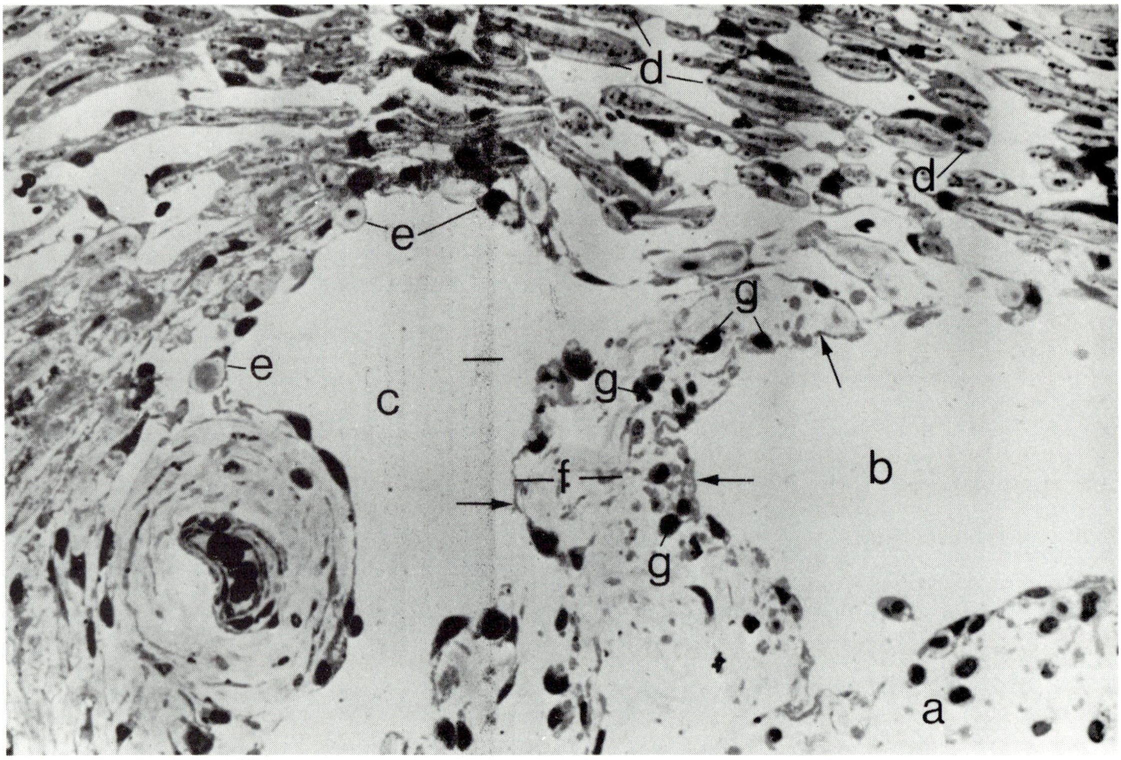

Figure 4-42. Iris process, light micrograph. Iris tissues (a), anterior chamber (b) and anterior chamber angle (c), corneoscleral sheets (d) and uveal meshwork (e) are indicated. An iris process (f) crosses the anterior chamber from the iris to join the trabecular meshwork. The surface of the process is covered by thin cells (arrows) like those covering the uveal meshwork. Numerous fibroblasts and pigmented cells (g) are seen within the iris process. (× 400.)

external portion of the spur, where they become around 800 A. in diameter. In young persons the scleral spur has numerous aggregates or clumps of circularly oriented, electron-dense tropocollagen fibrils measuring 100 A. in diameter. In adult eyes these tropocollagen aggregates form masses of wide-spacing collagen fibers. Early histologists reported the presence of elastic tissue in the scleral spur; it is likely that the basophilic, electron-dense tropocollagen aggregates and wide-spacing collagen correspond to this elastic tissue. These are not elastic fibers, however. The corneoscleral trabecular sheets lose their endothelial cells rather abruptly at the spur, and their collagen enters into the framework of the spur.

At the insertion of the longitudinal part of the ciliary muscle into the scleral spur the muscle cells do not pass through the spur to the trabecular sheets and there is no distinct tendinous structure at the muscle termination. The inner portion of the longitudinal part of the ciliary muscle bypasses the scleral spur and terminates in the posterior corneoscleral sheets. The muscle cells, however, do not extend anteriorly beyond the spur, but the connective tissue of this part of the muscle does extend forward to merge with the sheets. Unger (1959) and Rohen (1963), and Unger and Jankovsky (1966) have studied the relation of the ciliary muscle to the corneoscleral trabecular meshwork and the scleral spur. They found tendinous extensions of the longitudinal portion of the ciliary muscle through the spur into the posterior part of the corneoscleral trabecular sheets. After entering the posterior mesh-

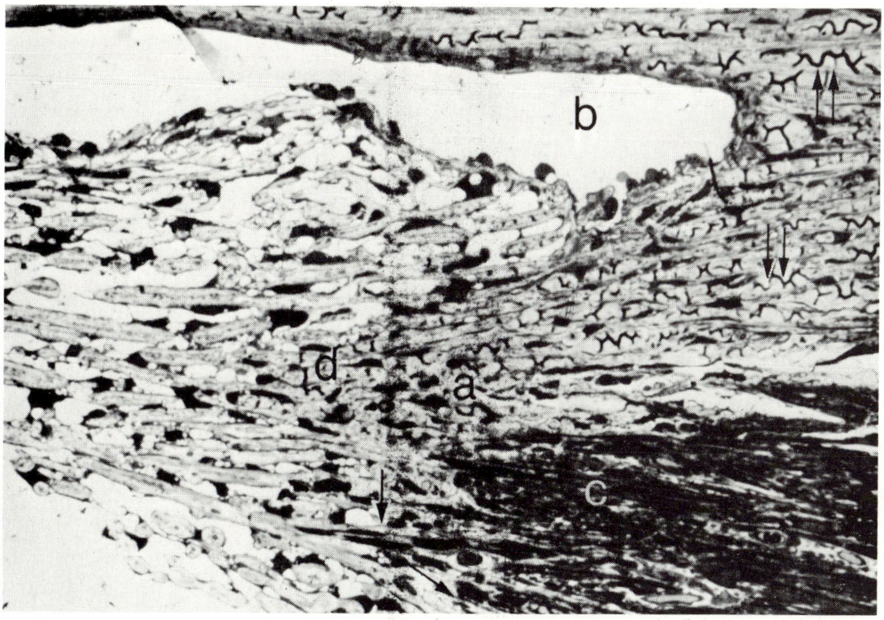

Figure 4–43. Scleral spur, light micrograph. The spur (a) lies between the posterior portion of Schlemm's canal (b) and the insertion of the longitudinal ciliary muscle (c). The sheets of the corneoscleral meshwork insert into the scleral spur at (d). The ciliary muscle inserts largely on the spur, but some cells are continuous with the corneoscleral sheets (arrows). The spur is composed of a very dense collagen which is difficult to demonstrate because sections of this tissue are difficult to stretch. The double arrows point out artefactual wrinkles in the spur and sclera. (× 400.)

work these tendon-like extensions were found to fan out and become oriented in the same direction as collagen fibers of the trabecular sheets. We have not been able to demonstrate this extension in light or electron microscopic sections, however.

Deep Corneolimbus (Figs. 4–46 to 4–48).

The deep corneolimbus contains the anteriormost portion of the trabecular meshwork, the termination of Descemet's membrane and Schwalbe's ring. It commences where the collagenous corneal lamellae, which are oriented in many directions, gradually change to become circularly oriented trabecular collagen. This zone is roughly triangular in shape, with its apex at the cornea external to the end of Descemet's membrane and its base where the first intertrabecular spaces appear. The external border is formed at the junction of dense corneal collagen and the looser trabecular connective tissue. The internal border of the deep corneolimbus is formed mostly by the anterior chamber, except for the tip of the triangle, which runs anterior and external to the termination of Descemet's membrane for as much as 100 μm. The deep corneolimbus varies a good deal in size in various eyes and different regions; it may measure from 150 to 200 μm. in length.

In this anterior triangle of the deep corneolimbus the endothelium lining the intertrabecular spaces continues forward in layers, preserving the arrangement of the sheets. In young eyes this region has a greater proportion of tropocollagen aggregates than the corneoscleral sheets, and the endothelial cells of this region seem to have more rough-surfaced endoplasmic reticulum and a better developed Golgi apparatus. With aging, sheets of wide-spacing collagen are found within the tropocollagen aggregates.

Text continued on page 178

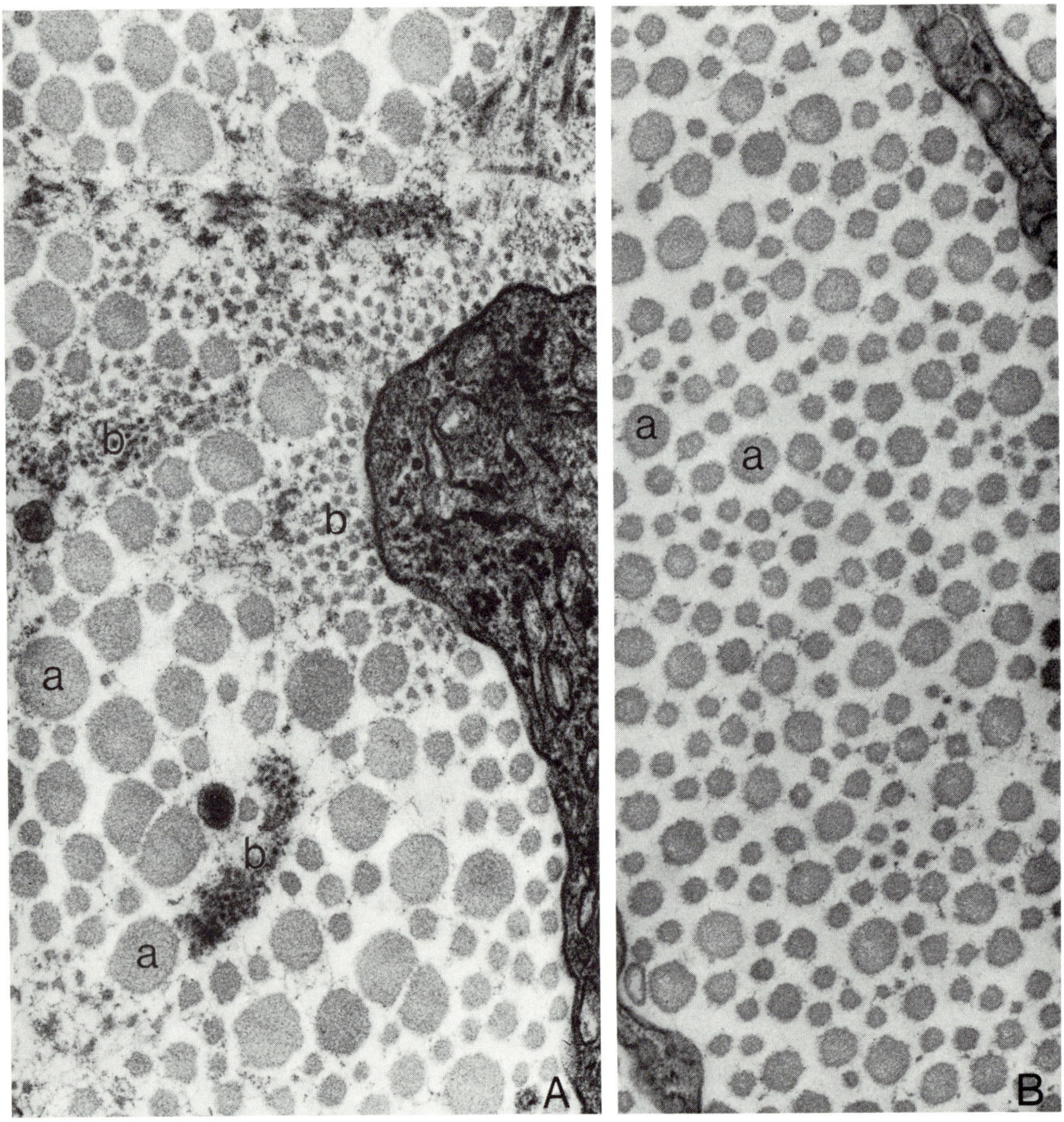

Figure 4-44. Collagen of the scleral spur. The collagen of the scleral spur, like that of the trabecular meshwork, is oriented circularly and parallel to the limbus. Its cross-sectional diameter varies considerably; very large fibrils are found posteriorly in the scleral region, and much smaller fibrils are found anteriorly near the trabecular meshwork.

A, Posterior scleral spur. The largest collagen fibrils (a) have a diameter of about 2000 A. Clumps of smaller, denser fibrils (b) measuring around 200 A. are seen in the vicinity of a fibroblast. These clusters of fine fibrils formerly were believed to be elastic tissue, but they probably are tropocollagen. (× 50,000.)

B, Scleral spur, midportion. The largest fibrils seen in this area are generally smaller than those in the posterior portion. The largest fibrils (a) have a diameter of about 1000 A. and the smallest are 500 to 700 A. The fibrils in the anterior part of the scleral spur near the trabecular meshwork measure between 300 and 600 A. (× 50,000.)

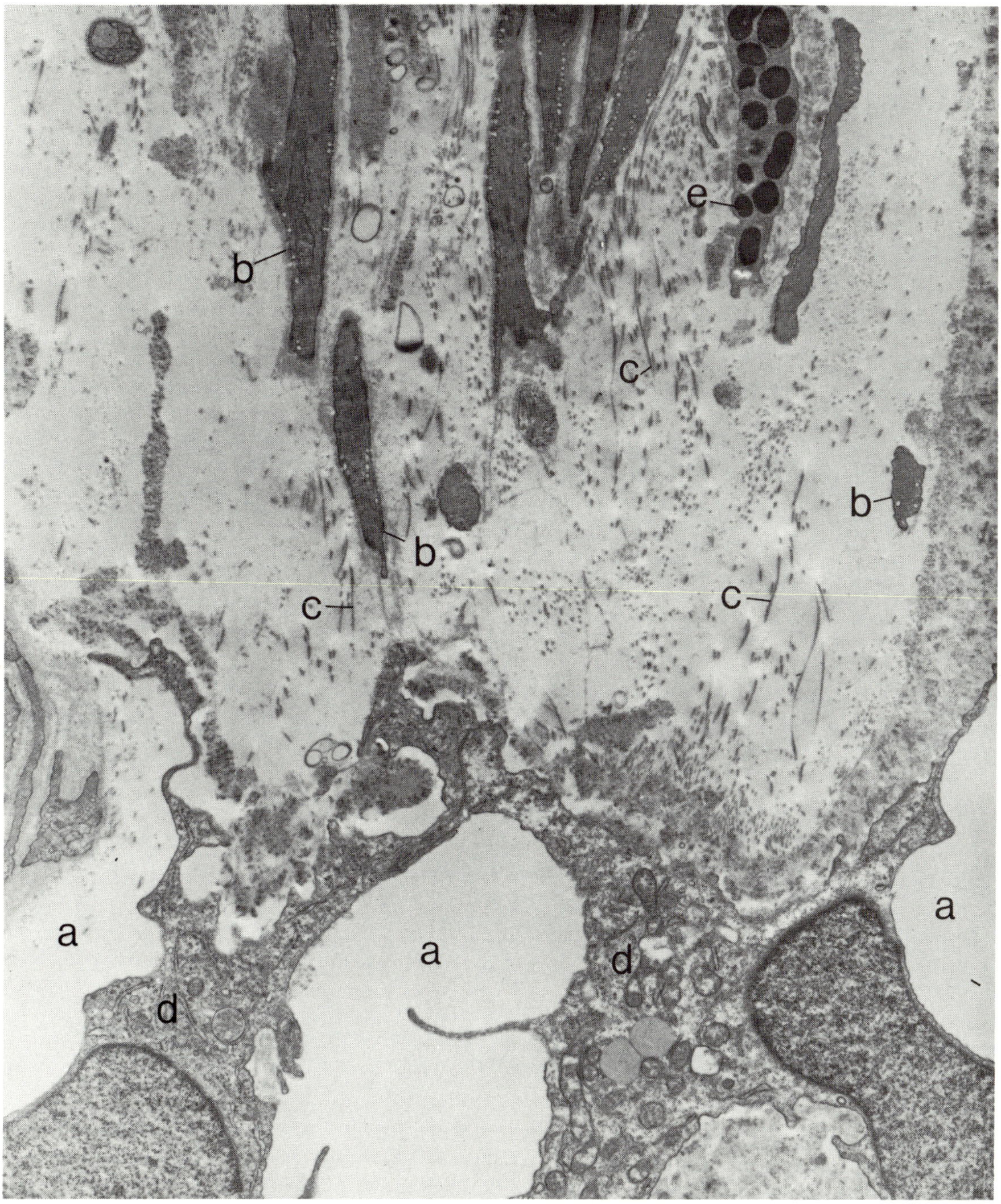

Figure 4-45. Ciliary muscle insertion. The major portion of this muscle inserts into the collagen of the scleral spur, but some muscle tendon fibrils continue into the corneoscleral sheets. Trabecular spaces are seen at (a) and ciliary muscle cells are seen at (b). The muscle cells have bypassed the scleral spur and terminate close to the trabecular sheets. The collagen fibrils (c) associated with the muscle are oriented longitudinally and are sparse. The trabecular endothelial cells (d) cover the terminations of the intertrabecular spaces, and some of their processes end in the ciliary body stroma. Part of a melanocyte is seen at (e). (× 10,000.)

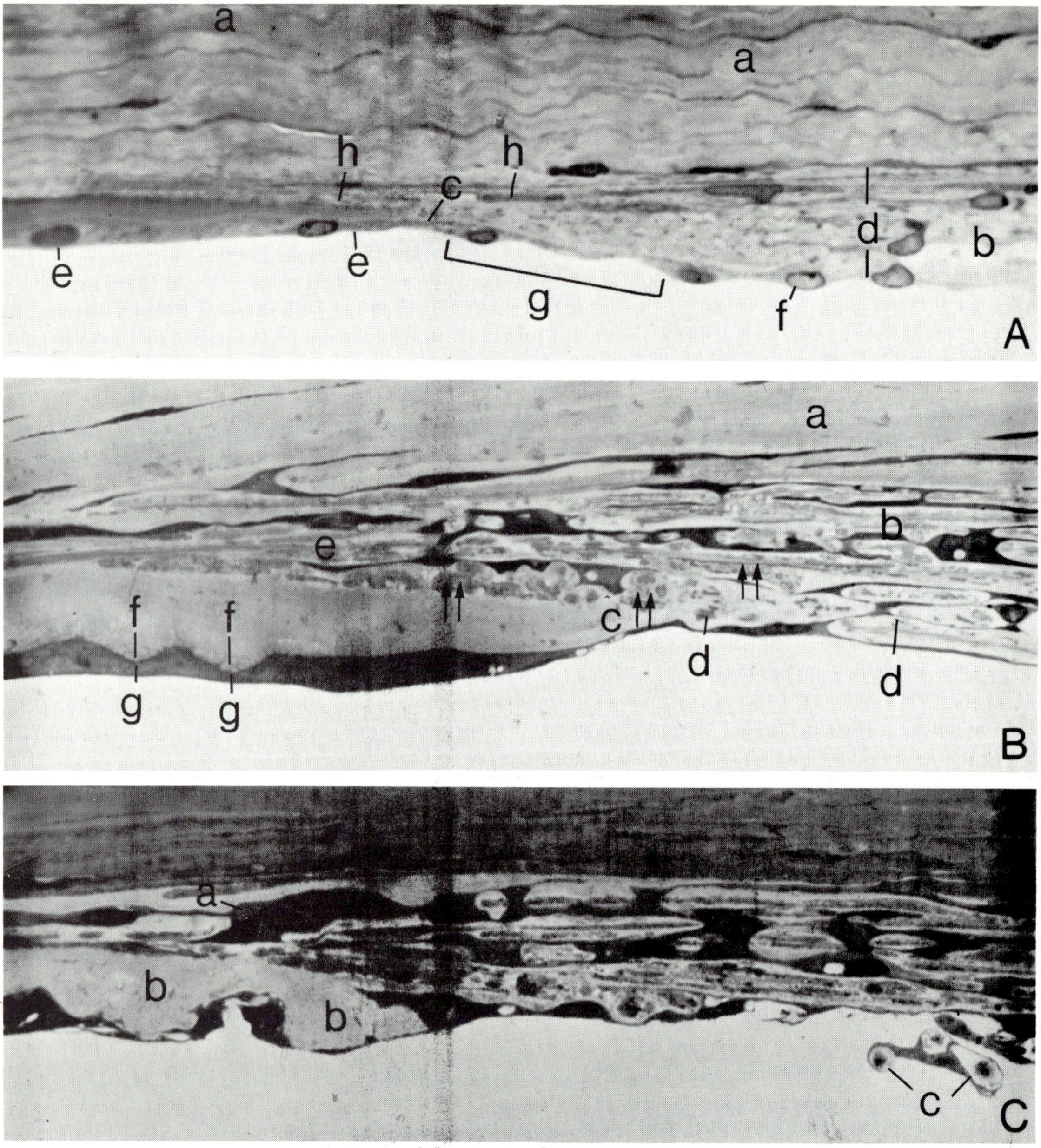

Figure 4-46. Deep corneolimbus, light micrographs. *A*, This photograph shows the transition zone between the cornea and the trabecular meshwork in the eye of a young individual. The corneal stroma is seen at (a), the trabecular meshwork at (b), the end of Descemet's membrane at (c) and Schwalbe's ring at (d). The corneal endothelium (e) gradually becomes thinner as the limbus is approached, and it is continuous with the trabecular endothelium at (f). The "flat zone" of endothelial transition is seen at (g). The extension of some trabecular sheets anteriorly behind Descemet's membrane is seen at (h). (× 700.)

B, Transition zone in an older individual. The corneal stroma is at (a), the trabecular endothelium at (b), the end of Descemet's membrane at (c), Schwalbe's ring at (d) and the anterior extension of the trabecular sheets behind Descemet's membrane at (e); Hassall-Henle warts showing fine "fissures" are seen at (f). The corneal endothelium (g) is atrophic over the warts and also becomes quite attenuated over Schwalbe's ring. Deposits of wide-spacing collagen are found in Descemet's membrane and in the collagen external to the membrane (double arrows) in the eyes of adults. The corneal stroma does not show this change. (× 800.)

C, This figure is similar to *B*. It shows more clearly the extension of the endothelial cells and collagen of the corneoscleral meshwork anteriorly behind Descemet's membrane in the deep corneolimbus (a). The Hassall-Henle warts (b) are also more pronounced in this specimen than in the previous one. The endothelial cells over these warts show severe thinning and degenerative changes. Several branches of a uveal band are seen at (c). (× 700.)

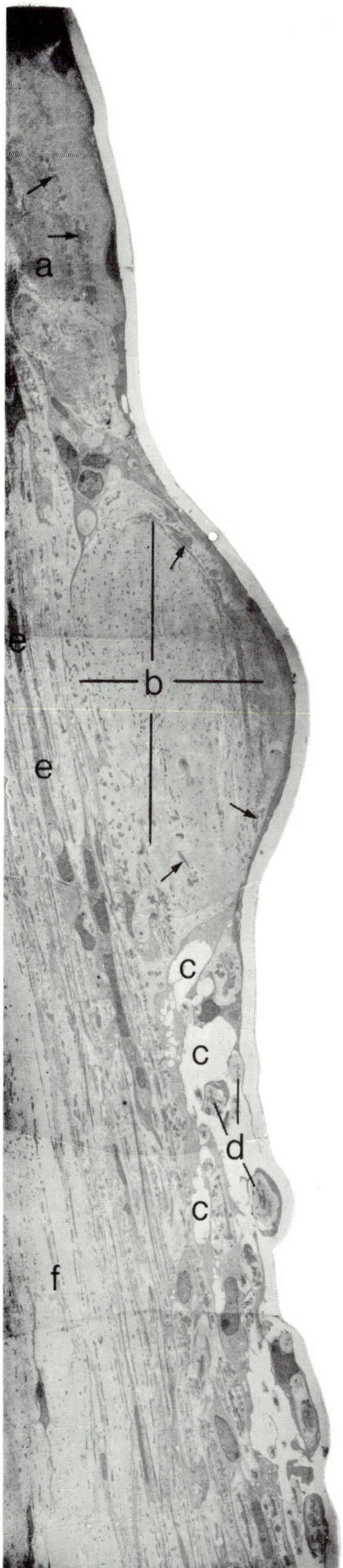

Figure 4–47. Montage of the deep corneolimbus to show a hypertrophied Schwalbe's ring and other structures; electron micrograph. The end of Descemet's membrane is seen at (a), the hypertrophied Schwalbe's ring at (b), the first trabecular sheets and intertrabecular spaces at (c), cross-sections of uveal bands at (d), the anterior extension of trabecular sheets behind Schwalbe's ring and Descemet's membrane at (e) and the limbal stroma at (f). This type of Schwalbe's ring is found in about 15 per cent of eyes. The collagen in Schwalbe's ring is oriented concentric to the limbus, but it frequently is interrupted. Dense, dark-staining clumps of wide-spacing collagen are seen in the ring and in Descemet's membrane (arrows). (× 800.)

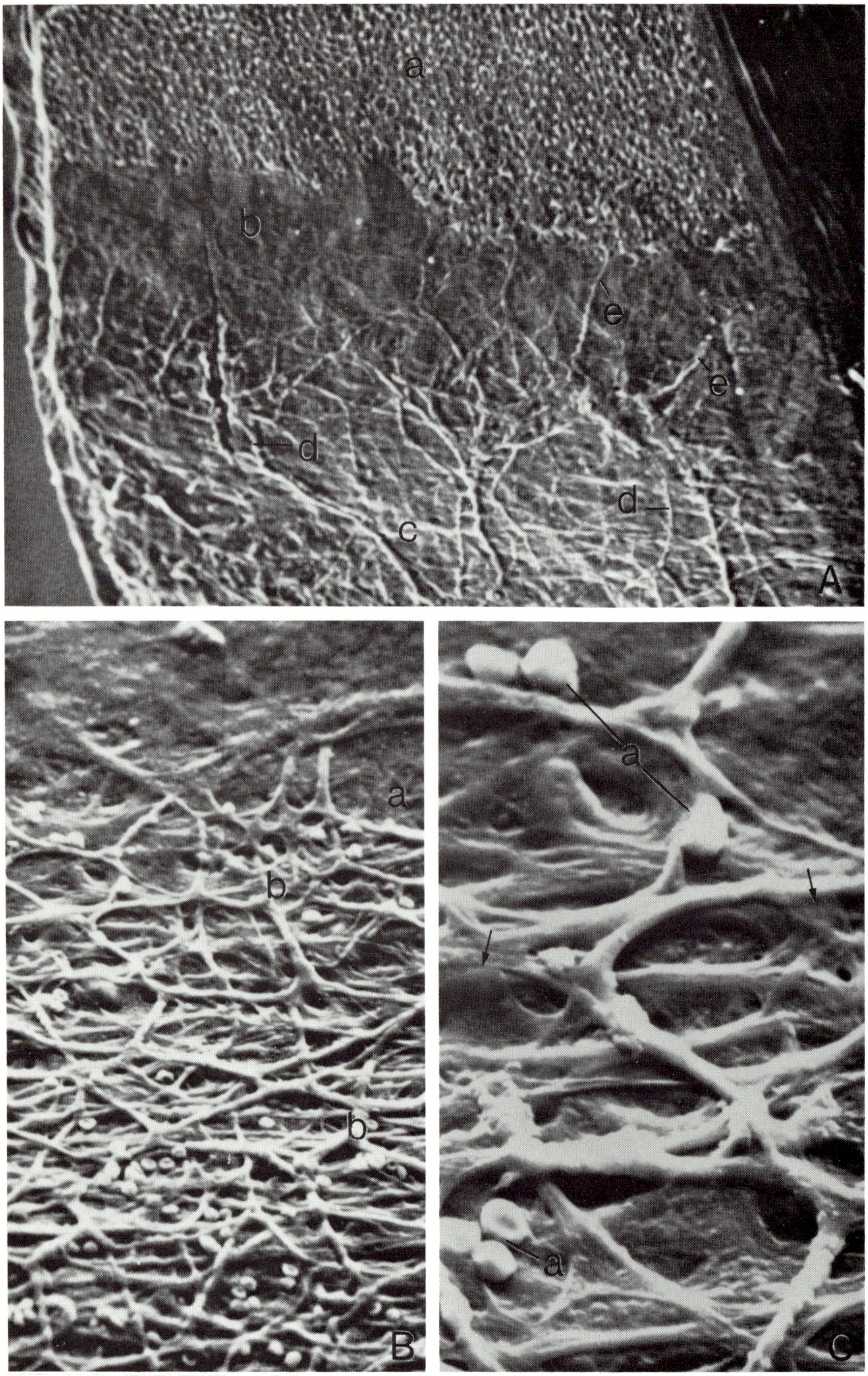

Figure 4–48. *See legend on opposite page.*

Figure 4–48. *A*, Limbal transition zone in a 13 year old girl showing the corneal endothelium (a), the smooth endothelial transition zone (b) and the trabecular zone (c). Most of the cords of the uveal meshwork terminate in the anterior trabecular region (d), but occasional ones extend forward into the smooth zone (e). (× 270.)

B, Deep corneolimbal region in the eye of a 90 year old man. The posterior edge of the smooth endothelial zone is at (a). The cords of the uveal meshwork interconnect with those of the trabecular sheets in a random fashion and cover the underlying corneoscleral trabecular sheets (b). The meshwork spaces are quite large. (× 300.)

C, Enlargement of the trabecular meshwork at the posterior edge of the smooth zone shown in *B*. The uveal cords are 3 to 4 μm. in diameter, and they are covered by an endothelium which frequently extends externally to cover adjacent cords (arrows). Some red blood cells (a) lie on the trabecular sheets. (× 1400.)

D, Three-dimensional drawing of the deep corneolimbus to show the transition zone between the peripheral cornea and the trabecular meshwork. Near the corneal periphery the endothelium is regular and polygonal, but over Hassall-Henle warts (1) it is thin, irregular and atrophic. The warts are represented as lighter areas on the flat surface view. At the end of Descemet's membrane (heavy arrow) the endothelial cells are larger but still somewhat polygonal. Posterior to Descemet's ending is a transition area, the "flat zone," measuring 100 μm. wide, where the endothelium is large and irregularly polygonal.

The cords of the uveal meshwork first appear at the posterior end of the flat zone. They are covered by endothelial cells which are about 60 μm. in diameter and have poorly defined borders.

The anterior extension of the corneoscleral trabecular meshwork forms a wedge-shaped tissue (2) external to and 100 μm. anterior to the end of Descemet's membrane. The trabecular endothelial cells are closely packed here. The collagen between them is oriented circularly and is embedded in an abundant mucopolysaccharide matrix. External to the wedge is some corneal lamellar tissue containing fibroblasts (3). The region of Schwalbe's ring is at (4). The most anterior trabecular spaces are seen at (5). The endothelium (6) lining these spaces is continuous anterior to the trabecular insertion at the wedge. (Spencer, W. H., Alvarado, J., and Hayes, T. L.: Invest. Ophthal. 7:651, 1968.)

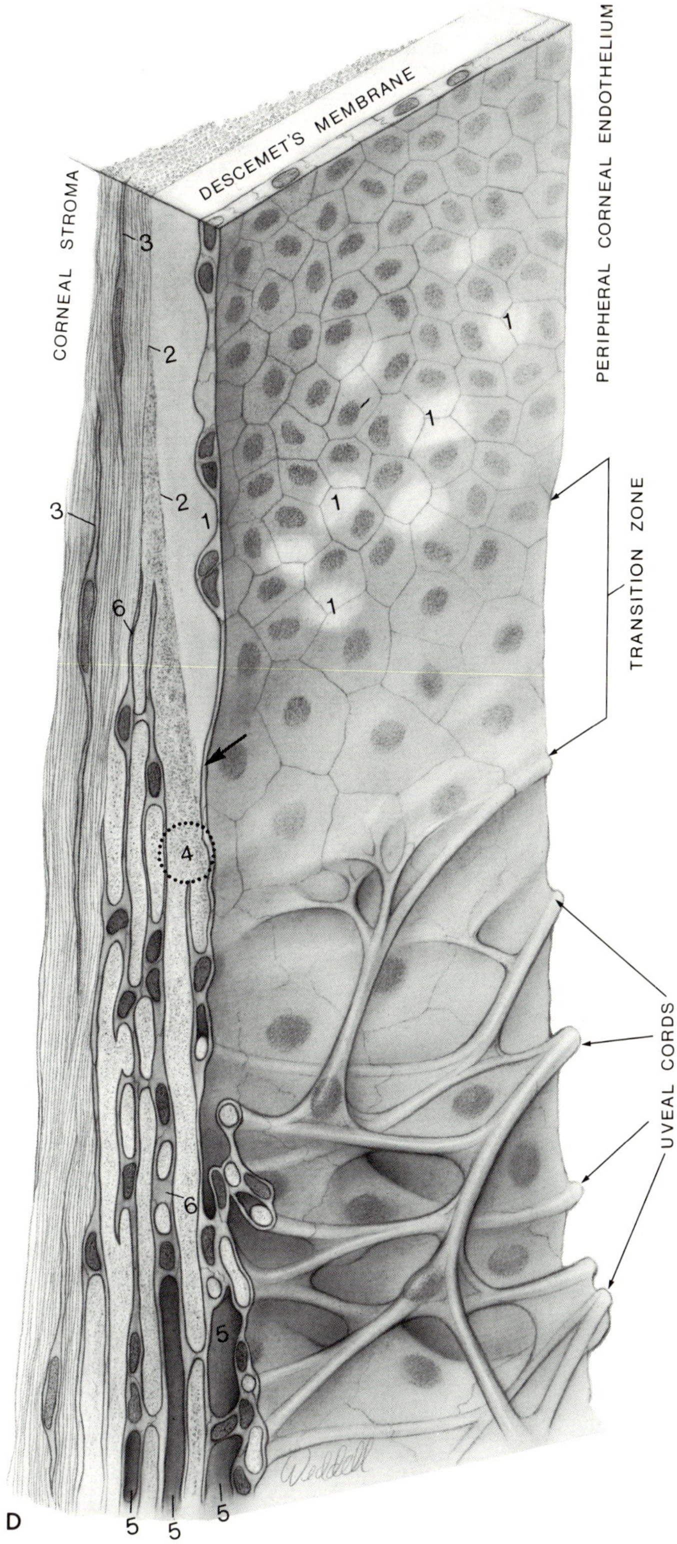

D

Anterior to the deep corneolimbus on the internal side, the Hassall-Henle warts appear, especially in persons over 20 years of age. The endothelium becomes attenuated over these warts, and Descemet's membrane becomes correspondingly thickened. Wolf (1968) studied this area with replicas of the inner portion of the deep corneolimbus. He showed that the endothelium overlying the warts spreads out to form a relatively flat and smooth zone which extends posteriorly for a short distance as the end of Descemet's is approached. The cells of this zone have clear outlines and still show the hexagonal shape that is typical of the corneal endothelium, but they are slightly larger. The uveal cords and innermost corneoscleral sheets are attached at the posterior border of this smooth zone. Near this insertion Wolf identified the large spaces formed by the uveal cords, as well as small openings in the corneoscleral sheets. Spencer and co-workers (1968) confirmed all these findings with the scanning electron microscope. They also showed that Schwalbe's ring when present occupies the posterior border of the smooth zone and that this ring does not extend continuously along the circumference of the deep corneolimbus.

Salzmann (1912) found the ring of Schwalbe to be located just external to the termination of Descemet's membrane; this ring was distinguished from adjacent tissue because of the circular disposition of its collagen. Some textbooks show a prominent area of thickening or elevation at the site of Schwalbe's ring, usually posterior to the termination of Descemet's membrane. Allen and associates (1955) and Burian and co-workers (1955) made a histologic study of this region in 600 human eyes. They found a prominent ring of Schwalbe in 72, or 15 per cent, of all these eyes. This observation correlated well with the findings obtained by gonioscopic observation of large numbers of eyes. These authors also found this prominent ring to be frequently associated with a severe hypoplasia of the anterior stromal layer of the iris, correctopia, polycoria and even glaucoma. They believed that a prominent ring results from the overgrowth of tissue in this region, rather than from a failure to absorb pre-existing tissue.

Since Schwalbe's ring is difficult to demonstrate in most eyes, the finding of a prominent Schwalbe's ring in histologic sections is indicative of some type of developmental abnormality of the deep corneolimbus and is characterized by its protrusion into the anterior chamber. The term Schwalbe's ring (or, incorrectly, line) is used in gonioscopy to describe the anteriormost portion of the trabecular meshwork at the end of the internal scleral sulcus, but we feel that the term corneolimbal junction is preferable.

Nerves (Figs. 4–49 and 4–50).

Nerves have been demonstrated in the trabecular meshwork of animals and humans with the light and electron microscopes by Vrabec (1954, 1961); Holland and associates (1956, 1957); Kurus (1958); Wolter (1959); Feeney (1962); Lamers (1962); and Valu (1963). There has been considerable speculation on the function of these nerves. Holland and associates (1956, 1957) believed them to have sensory, sympathetic and parasympathetic functions in the rabbit eye. Lamers (1962) believed that all these nerves are sensory. Some observers have reported special end-organs, and others have found only fine filamentous nerve endings.

In the human eye the nerves to this region arise from the supraciliary and ciliary plexuses near the scleral spur. From here axons extend forward and externally, branching as they enter the meshwork; they finally end as free

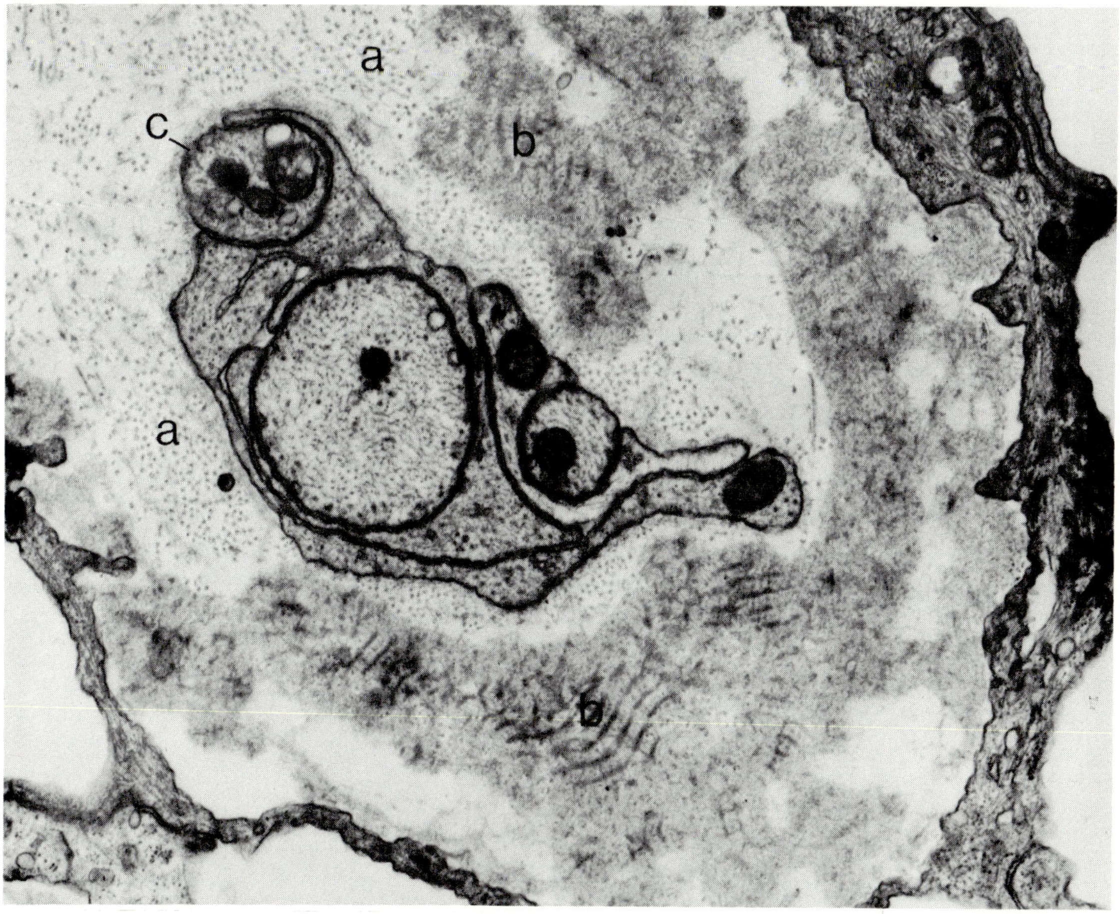

Figure 4-49. Nerves in the trabecular meshwork. A trabecular sheet containing collagen fibrils (a) and clumps of wide-spacing collagen (b) also shows several nerve axons (c) surrounded by a Schwann cell. These nerves are usually seen more easily in the posterior portion of the trabecular meshwork than in the anterior portion. (× 23,000.)

filaments without a constant relation to the endothelial cells of the meshwork. Generally the filaments have a plexiform pattern, and occasional filaments have a swelling at their endings. All parts of the meshwork have nerve fibers, but they are especially numerous in the region of the scleral spur. Feeney (1962) found both myelinated and unmyelinated nerves in the human trabecular meshwork, the former being located only in the region of the scleral spur. Unmyelinated nerve fibers were found in all parts of the trabecular meshwork with the exception of the uveal bands, the meshwork near Descemet's membrane and the outer 7 μm. of the corneoscleral meshwork adjacent to the lumen of Schlemm's canal. The nerves were found to penetrate the trabecular bands through the collagenous core of the trabecular sheets and were wrapped by Schwann cells. Occasional nerves were seen to cross the intertrabecular spaces. Feeney also found that the nerve endings often closely resembled axonal endings. Axons containing numerous mito-

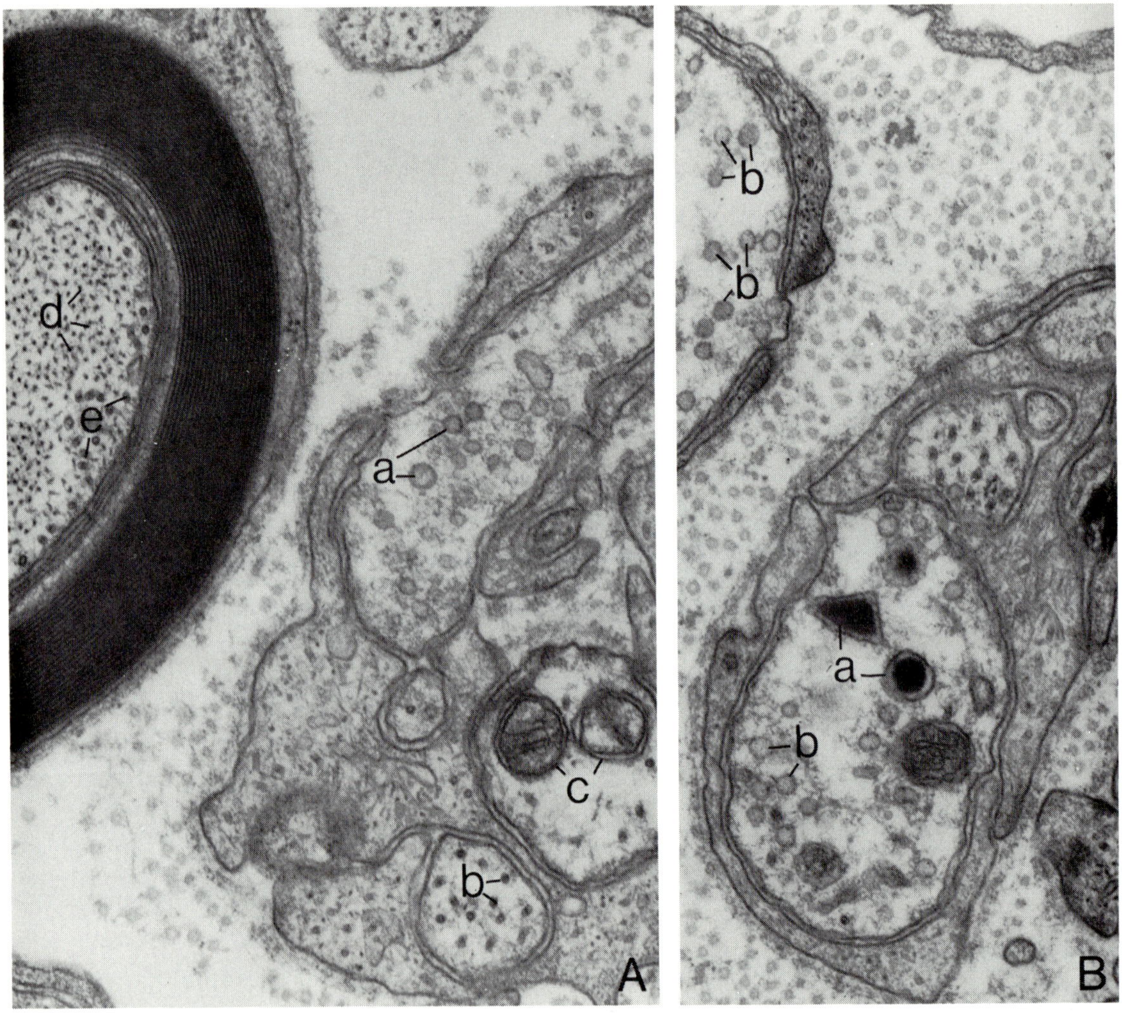

Figure 4-50. Nerves in the posterior trabecular meshwork. *A*, A Schwann cell surrounding several axons is seen on the right side. Synaptic vesicles (a), neurotubules (b) and small mitochondria (c) are indicated. A myelinated axon is seen on the left side. Neurofilaments (d) and neurotubules (e) are found in the axon. Myelinated axons are uncommon; when present, they are usually found only in the posterior of the meshwork. (× 37,500.)

B, Two types of vesicles are observed within these axons: (1) large vesicles containing an electron-dense limiting membrane and a dark homogeneous material in their core (a); and (2) more numerous small vesicles (b). (× 37,500.)

chondria and vesicles of the type associated with synaptic endings were found to be enveloped by endothelial cell cytoplasm. This study provided clear evidence that the majority of nerves observed in the meshwork terminate here.

REFERENCES

Allen, L., Burian, H., and Braley, A.: The anterior border ring of Schwalbe and the pectinate ligament. Arch. Ophthal. 53:799, 1955.

Ascher, K. W.: Aqueous veins: A preliminary note. Amer. J. Ophthal. 25:31, 1942.

Ascher, K. W.: Aqueous veins: Their status eleven years after their detection. Arch. Ophthal. 49:438, 1953.

Ashton, N.: Anatomical study of Schlemm's canal and aqueous veins by means of neoprene casts. Part I. Aqueous veins. Brit. J. Ophthal. 35:291, 1951.

Ashton, N., Brini, A., and Smith, R.: Anatomical studies of trabecular meshwork of normal human eye. Brit. J. Ophthal. *40*:257, 1956.

Bárány, E. H.: Physiologic and pharmacologic factors in influencing the resistance to aqueous outflow. First Josiah Macy Conference on Glaucoma, 1955, pp. 123–213.

Becker, B., and Shaffer, R. N.: Diagnosis and Therapy of the Glaucomas. St. Louis, The C. V. Mosby Co., 1961, pp. 59, 76.

Berggren, L.: Passage out of the eye of substances of low and high molecular weight. Invest. Ophthal. *2*:305, 1963.

Bill, A.: The protein exchange in the eye. Structure of the eye. VIIIth International Congress of Anatomists, Wiesbaden, Germany, 1965.

Bill, A.: Formation and drainage of aqueous humor in cats. Exp. Eye Res. *5*:185, 1966.

Bill, A., and Bárány, E. H.: Gross facility, facility of conventional routes, and pseudofacility of aqueous humor outflow in the cynomolgus monkey. The reduction in aqueous humor formation rate caused by moderate increments in intraocular pressure. Arch. Ophthal. (Chicago) *75*:665, 1966.

Bill, A., and Hellsing, K.: Production and drainage of aqueous humor in the cynomolgus monkey (Macaca irus). Invest. Ophthal. *4*:920, 1965.

Bill, A., and Walinder, P. E.: The effects of pilocarpine on the dynamics of aqueous humor in a primate (Macaca irus). Invest. Ophthal. *5*:170, 1966.

Burian, H., Braley, A., and Allen, L.: External and gonioscopic visibility of the ring of Schwalbe and the trabecular zone. Trans. Amer. Ophthal. Soc. *52*:389, 1955.

Busacca, A.: Biomicroscopy and Histology of the Eye. Vol. I. Zurich, S. Karger, 1952.

Feeney, M. L.: Ultrastructure of the nerves in the human trabecular region. Invest. Ophthal. *1*:462, 1962.

Feeney, M. L., and Wissig, S.: Outflow studies using an electron dense tracer. Trans. Amer. Acad. Ophthal. Otolaryng. *70*:791, 1966.

Fine, B. S.: Observations in the drainage angle in man and rhesus monkey: A concept of the pathogenesis of chronic simple glaucoma; a light and electron microscopic study. Invest. Ophthal. *3*:609, 1964.

Fine, B. S.: Structure of the trabecular meshwork and the canal of Schlemm. Trans. Amer. Acad. Ophthal. Otolaryng. *70*:777, 1966.

Flocks, M.: The anatomy of the trabecular meshwork as seen in tangential section. Arch. Ophthal. *56*:708, 1956.

Flocks, M., and Zweng, H. C.: Studies on the mode of action of pilocarpine on aqueous outflow. Amer. J. Ophthal. *44*:380, 1957.

Fortin, P.: Existence of a true ocular organ of filtration: The pectinate fiber. Ophthal. Ibero-Am. *4*:251, 1942.

François, J., Neetens, A., and Collette, J. M.: Microradiographic study of the inner wall of Schlemm's canal. Amer. J. Ophthal. *40*:491, 1955.

François, J., Neetens, A., Leroux, G., and Collette, J. M.: A propos des voies postérieures d'écoulement de l'humeur aqueuse. Bull. Soc. Belg. Ophtal. *141*:641, 1965.

François, J., Neetens, A., Leroux, G., et al.: Concerning the posterior routes for the drainage of aqueous humor. Ophthalmologica (Basel) *153*:215, 1967.

Garron, L. K., and Feeney, M. L.: Electron microscopic studies of the human eye. II. Study of the trabeculae by light and electron microscopy. Arch. Ophthal. *62*:966, 1959.

Garron, L. K., Feeney, M. L., Hogan, M. J., and McEwen, W. K.: Electron microscopic studies of the human eye. I. Preliminary investigations of the trabeculae. Amer. J. Ophthal. *46*:27, 1958.

Goldmann, H.: Outflow of aqueous humor in man. Ophthalmologica *111*:146, 1946.

Goldmann, H.: Do the aqueous veins contain aqueous fluid? Ophthalmologica *117*:240, 1949.

Holland, M., Sallmann, L. V., and Collins, E.: A study of the innervation of the chamber angle. Amer. J. Ophthal. *42*:148, 1956.

Holland, M., Sallmann, L. V., and Collins, E.: Study of the innervation of the chamber angle. II. The origin of the trabecular axons revealed by degeneration experiments. Amer. J. Ophthal. *44*:206, 1957.

Holmberg, A. S.: The fine structure of the inner wall of Schlemm's canal. Arch. Ophthal. *62*:956, 1959.

Holmberg, A. S.: Schlemm's canal and the trabecular meshwork. An electron microscopic study of the normal structure in man and monkey (cerecopithecus ethiops). Docum. Ophthal. (Den Haag) *19*:339, 1965.

Huggert, A.: Pore size in the filtration angle of the eye. Acta Ophthal. (Kbh.) *33*:271, 1955.

Iwamoto, T.: Light and electron microscopy of Sondermann's channels of the human trabecular meshwork. Graefe's Arch. Ophthal. *172*:197, 1967a.

Iwamoto, T.: Further observation on Sondermann's channels of the human trabecular meshwork. Graefe's Arch. Ophthal. *172*:213, 1967b.

Iwamoto, T., and Smelser, G. K.: Electron microscopic studies of the mast cells and blood and lymphatic capillaries of the human corneal limbus. Invest. Ophthal. *4*:815, 1965.

Jocson, V. L., and Grant, W. M.: Interconnections of blood vessels and aqueous vessels in human eyes. Arch. Ophthal. *73*:707, 1965.

Karg, S. J., Garron, L. K., Feeney, M. L., and McEwen, W. K.: Perfusion of human eyes with latex microspheres. Arch. Ophthal. *61*:68, 1959.

Kayes, J.: Pore structure of the inner wall of Schlemm's canal. Invest. Ophthal. *6*:381, 1967.

Kinsey, V. E., Grant, M., and Cogan, D. G.: Water movement and eye. Arch. Ophthal. *27*:242, 1942.

Kurus, E.: Versuch einer morphologischen Analyse der Funktion and Dysfunktion der intraocularen Drukregulierung. Klin. Mbl. Augen. *132*:201, 1958.

Lamers, W.: The innervation of the corneoscleral trabecula. Ophthalmologica *144*:455, 1962.

Leeson, T. S., and Speakman, J. S.: The fine structure of extracellular material in the pectinate ligament (trabecular meshwork) of the human iris. Acta Anat. *46*:363, 1961.

McEwen, W. K.: Application of Poiseuille's law to aqueous outflow. Arch. Ophthal. *4*:815, 1965.

Maumenee, A. E.: The pathogenesis of congenital glaucoma: A new theory. Trans. Amer. Ophthal. Soc. *56*:507, 1958.

Maurice, D. M.: The movement of fluorescein and water in the cornea. Amer. J. Ophthal. *49*:1011, 1960.

Podos, S. M., Minas, T. F., and Macri, F. J.: A new instrument to measure episcleral venous pressure. Comparison of normal eyes and eyes with primary open-angle glaucoma. Arch. Ophthal. *80*:209, 1968.

Rhodin, J. A.: *In* Wagner, B. M., and Smith, D. E., (eds.): The Connective Tissue. Baltimore, The Williams & Wilkins Co., 1967.

Rohen, J. W.: The histologic structure of the chamber angle in primates. Amer. J. Ophthal. *52*:529, 1961.

Rohen, J. W.: Experimental studies on the trabecular meshwork in primates. Arch. Ophthal. *69*:335, 1963.

Rohen, J. W.: Das Auge und seine Hilfsorgene. *In* Möllendorff, (ed.): Handbuch der mikroskopischen Anatomie den Menschen. Berlin, Erganz zu Bd. III/2, 1964.

Salzmann, M.: The Anatomy and Histology of the Human Eyeball. Translated by E. V. L. Brown. Chicago, University of Chicago Press, 1912.

Seidel, E.: Further experimental studies on the origin and pathways of intraocular fluids. XI. Information on the mechanics of glaucoma. Graefe's Arch. Ophthal. *106*:176, 1921.

Sondermann, R.: The formation, morphology and function of Schlemm's canal. Acta Ophthal. (Kbh) *11*:280, 1933.

Speakman, J. S.: Drainage channels in the trabecular wall of Schlemm's canal. Brit. J. Ophthal. *44*:513, 1960.

Spelsberg, W. W., and Chapman, G. B.: Fine structure of human trabeculae. Arch. Ophthal. *67*:773, 1962.

Spencer, W. H., Alvarado, J., and Hayes, T. L.: Scanning electron microscopy of human ocular tissues: The trabecular meshwork. Invest. Ophthal. *7*:651, 1968.

Sugiura, S., and Matsuda, H.: Ultrastructure of Langhans' cells in human corneal limbus. Trans. Soc. Ophthal. Jap. *72*:2435, 1968.

Theobald, G. D.: Schlemm's canal. Its anastomosis and anatomic relations. Trans. Amer. Ophthal. Soc. *32*:574, 1934.

Thomassen, T. L., and Bakken, K.: Anatomical investigations into the exit channels of aqueous humor. A preliminary report. Acta Ophthal. (Kbh) *29*:257, 1951.

Tripathi, R. C.: Ultrastructure of Schlemm's canal in relation to aqueous outflow. Exp. Eye Res. *7*:335, 1968.

Unger, H. H.: Anatomy of the angle of the anterior chamber. Klin. Mbl. Augen. *135*:161, 1959.

Unger, H. H., and Jankovsky, F.: Tendons and supporting elements in the corneoscleral trabecula. Graefe's Arch. Ophthal. *170*:355, 1966.

Unger, H. H., and Rohen, J. W.: Studies on the histology of the inner wall of Schlemm's canal. Amer. J. Ophthal. *48*:204, 1959.

Valu, L.: Innervation of the uveal trabecular system. Amer. J. Ophthal. *56*:677, 1963.

Vegge, T.: Ultrastructure of normal human trabecular endothelium. Acta Ophthal. (Kbh) *41*:193, 1963.

Vegge, T.: The fine structure of the trabecular cribriform and the inner wall of Schlemm's canal in the normal human eye. Z. Zellforsch. *77*:267, 1967.

Virchow, H.: Graefe-Saemisch Handbuch der gesammten Augenheilkunde. 2nd ed. Leipzig, Engelmann, 1910.

Vrabec, F.: Innervation of the trabecular system of the iris angle. Ophthalmologica (Basel) *128*:359, 1954.

Vrabec, F.: The topography of encapsulated terminal sensory corpuscles of the anterior chamber angle of the eye. *In* Smelser, G. K., (ed.): The Structure of the Eye. New York, Academic Press, Inc., 1961.

Wolf, J.: Inner surface of regions in the anterior chamber taking part in the regulation of the intraocular tension, including the demonstration of the covering viscous substance. Doc. Ophthal. Advances in Ophthal. *25*:113, 1968.

Wolter, J. R.: The trabecular endothelium. Arch. Ophthal. *61*:928, 1959.

Chapter Five

THE SCLERA

The sclera forms the principal part of the outer coat of the eye. It is almost entirely collagenous, relatively avascular and roughly spherical in shape. Except for a turnover of collagen and cells, the sclera has a rather inactive metabolism. The viscoelastic properties of the sclera are of interest in the study of the distensibility of the eye and its relation to the intraocular pressure.

PHYSIOLOGY

The sclera and cornea comprise the outer coat of the eye, and one of their functions is to provide constant protection for the intraocular tissues. Ninety-four per cent of the area of the outer coat of the eye is composed of sclera; therefore, the characteristics of the outer coat will be described in terms of the sclera.

The intraocular pressure stabilizes the tissues in the outer coat of the eye in the same way as inflation of a collapsed pigskin makes a resilient football. This pressure and its complex interwoven collagenous structure make the sclera a tough layer that stabilizes the positions of the structures concerned with normal vision.

The intraocular pressure always creates a certain degree of tension or stretch on the scleral collagen. However, the amount that the sclera stretches when the intraocular pressure increases is not directly proportional to the change in pressure, because it has been found that the *rigidity* of the sclera increases with increasing stretch of its collagen bundles. A small amount of fluid injected into an eye at a pressure of 40 mm. Hg will cause a greater increase in pressure (a greater increase in tension in the coat) than when the same volume of fluid is injected into an eye at 15 mm. Hg.

The ratio of change of *pressure* to a change of *volume* in the eye is called the *immediate ocular rigidity*. In addition to this relation of pressure to volume is the relation of *pressure* to *time*. When fluid is injected into an eye, the pressure immediately rises (immediate ocular rigidity) and then begins to fall. Originally it was believed that the fall in intraocular pressure was due to removal of fluid from the eye via the outflow channels. It was found, however, that even if the outflow channels were blocked, there was some decrease in pressure soon after the initial rise. This decrease in pressure has been shown to result from a relaxation of the tension in the sclera itself for a short period of time after an initial stretch. This relation is now known to be caused by a decrease in the ocular rigidity for a time after the increase in pressure and is known as *time-dependent ocular rigidity*. The sclera is capable of limited distension and contraction to accommodate to minor variations in ocular volume. The total extensibility of excised strips of sclera, as well as extensibility within physiologic ranges, were studied by Gloster and co-workers (1957), who found that the scleral elasticity allows for rapid stretching in response to application of a measured force, and that the initial lengthening is followed by slow stretching due to a viscous component. The sclera was thus shown to be a viscoelastic tissue. These viscoelastic properties of the sclera also have been studied by St. Helen and McEwen (1961), who confirmed the observations of Gloster and associates that there is a quantitative time-dependent relationship between stress and strain in scleral segments. St. Helen and McEwen found that the scleral fibers elongate rapidly and briefly after the initial application of pressure. This rapid phase is followed immediately by a period of slower relaxation, both phases of which are dependent on its viscoelastic properties. These scleral changes, which are the basis for time-dependent ocular rigidity, occur a few seconds to 10 to 20 minutes after a change in pressure. When the eye has returned to its initial pressure, it shows no permanent change in ocular rigidity.

When a Schiötz or other indentation tonometer is placed on the eye, the fluid which formerly occupied the volume of indentation is not displaced from the eye but finds room within it as a result of the distension of the sclera, thereby raising the intraocular pressure. The calculation of pressure from a Schiötz reading involves the immediate ocular rigidity of an eye. Variations in ocular rigidity can be caused by different-sized eyes. For instance, if the diameter of two eyes differs by 2 mm., the smaller eye would give a Schiötz pressure reading of 19 mm. Hg, compared to a reading of 15 mm. Hg for the larger eye. Therefore, it is important to determine the ocular rigidity of eyes which may be considered to be larger (myopic) or smaller (hyperopic) than normal when using Schiötz tonometry alone.

The gradual distensibility of the eye in cases of infantile glaucoma, and possibly myopia, appears to result from an actual stretching of the scleral coat beyond its elastic limit. Since the sclera of the enucleated human eye suffers no permanent change when pressures of many hundreds of mm. of Hg are applied acutely, the permanent scleral stretching which occurs in glaucomatous and myopic eyes subjected to much less pressure must be caused by another mechanism.

There has been much speculation about the opaqueness of the sclera, and the reason for its opaqueness as compared to the cornea has been studied intensely (see p. 57).

There is less water in the sclera than the 72 to 82 per cent found in the cornea. Most studies suggest that the sclera is around 65 per cent water, although Krause (1932) found it to contain 72.24 per cent, and Pénzes and Pataky (1964) found 75.5 per cent. Recent studies by electron microscopy have shown very little elastic tissue in the sclera, revealing that collagen is the principal component. The collagen amounts to about 75 per cent of the dry weight of the sclera and, in addition to the collagen protein, contains about 10 per cent of other proteins and 1 per cent of mucopolysaccharide. The mucopolysaccharide content of the sclera is about one fourth that of the cornea. The irregular arrangement of the scleral collagen and the low mucopolysaccharide content create part of the lack of scleral clarity. The hydration of the sclera is important for its clarity, for if the water content is reduced below 40 per cent or increased above 80 per cent, the sclera becomes almost as transparent as the cornea. Maurice (1969) believes that the alteration of transparency occurs because of a change in the hydration of the ground substance so that it has the same index of refraction as the scleral collagen. The sclera swells to a maximum increase of 15 per cent of its original weight when placed in physiologic saline, compared to a maximum increase of 100 per cent for the cornea. The scleral swelling pressure is 20 to 30 gm./cm.^{2} compared to 75 to 85 gm./cm.^{2} for the cornea.

The sclera becomes somewhat thicker during early life, especially in the anterior portion. Its rigidity also increases, particularly in older age groups, possibly because of the increased amount of collagen, reduction in the amount of ground substance and deposition of calcium salts. The turnover of scleral collagen is not known, but it is probably similar to the corneal collagen and that of other connective tissues. Vannas and Teir (1960) found the sclera to stain less intensely with age, especially with lead acetate, mercury bichloride and the Mallory stain. The diminution in staining was especially marked in the region of Schlemm's canal. They also found a zonal concentration of mucopolysaccharide in the anterior sclera with increasing age. Friedenwald (1937) found that the sclera is thinner, denser and less hydrated in older age groups. The slight yellow color observed in the sclera of older individuals is believed to be the result of an increased amount of fat. The sclera of older persons may show focal areas of calcification; it is not unusual to find crystals scattered throughout the posterior sclera in the eyes of very old persons. Focal senile translucency of the sclera appears anterior to the insertion of the medial and lateral rectus muscles of some older persons; this is due to a deposition of calcium among the scleral fibers, rendering them more transparent.

EMBRYOLOGY

The sclera develops from that part of the associated mesoderm which surrounds the optic vesicle. It first appears as a condensation in the mesoderm external to the primitive choroid. Before the 18 mm. stage the mesoderm external to the cup is undifferentiated, but by the 20 mm. stage the mesodermal cells rearrange around the cup so that their long axes are parallel to its surface. The scleral condensation then appears near the anterior cup at the future site of attachment of the extraocular muscles. This condensation extends forward to the level of the anterior chamber. By the 35 mm. stage scleral condensation of the mesoderm is evident around the posterior pole of the eye. Near the end of embryonic life the condensation has approached the choroid. The entire sclera becomes more defined as a result of condensation of the collagen during the fourth month; by the fifth month it forms a complete layer around the cup. After the fifth month the sclera increases in thickness and becomes even more dense, so that its inner surface is quite distinct from the outer choroid.

GROSS ANATOMY

Anteriorly the sclera terminates at the limbus. Posteriorly it ends at the optic nerve, but some scleral collagen continues across the optic nerve canal as the scleral portion of the lamina cribrosa. At the optic nerve ending, the outer third of the sclera is continuous with the dural sheath of the optic nerve (Fig. 5-1). On its external side the scleral surface is in close contact with Tenon's capsule, with fine collagenous bands joining these two layers (Fig. 5-2 *A* and *B*). At the optic nerve Tenon's capsule joins that portion of the sclera which is reflected as the dural sheath. Anteriorly the episclera is in contact with the loose subconjunctival tissues, and the rectus muscle tendons insert into the superficial scleral collagen, producing an increase in thickness of the anterior sclera. On its internal surface the sclera is adjacent to the choroid and the ciliary body. The suprachoroidal tissues lie close to, and to a certain extent blend with, the internal collagen or lamina fusca of the sclera. Some bundles of smooth muscle from the ciliary muscle insert into

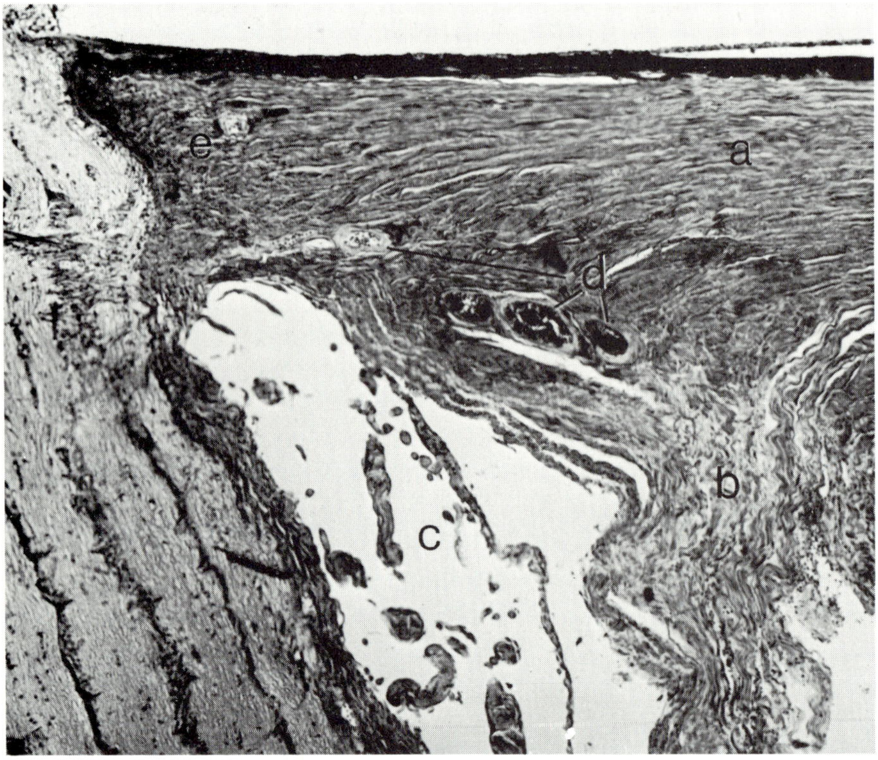

Figure 5-1. Light micrograph of the posterior sclera and optic nerve. The inner two thirds of the sclera (a) joins the optic nerve. The outer one third (b) bends posteriorly to join the dura mater. The subdural and subarachnoid spaces are at (c). Short posterior ciliary vessels (d) extend in other sections to the circle of Zinn (e). (× 110.)

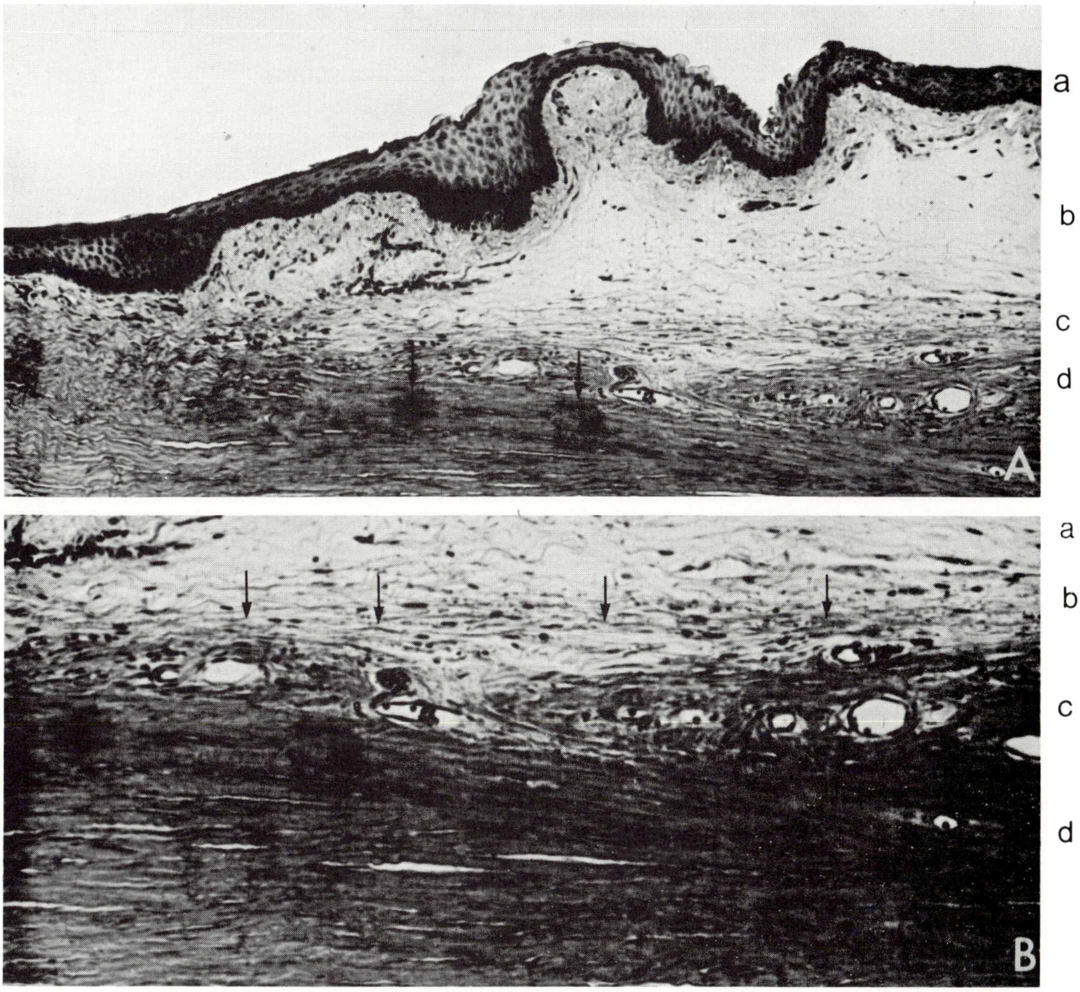

Figure 5–2. *A*, Light micrograph of the anterior scleral region. The conjunctiva (a) is external to the loose subconjunctival tissue (b). Tenon's capsule (c) covers the vascular episclera (d). The sclera contains calcium deposits (arrows), a common finding in older eyes. (× 130.)

B, Higher magnification view of *A*. The conjunctiva (a), Tenon's capsule (b), episclera (c) and sclera (d) are shown. The scleral calcium is more evident at this magnification. Tenon's capsule becomes more attenuated (arrows) as it reaches the limbus, where it blends with the episclera. (× 190.)

the inner sclera anteriorly, as do most of the supraciliary lamellae. The scleral spur is found at the deep limbal border of the anterior sclera (p. 112). The spur is an important anatomic structure because of its relation to the ciliary muscle insertion, the anterior chamber angle and the corneoscleral trabecular sheets.

The sclera covers four fifths of the surface of the globe and forms a segment of a sphere approximately 22 mm. in diameter. The anterior sclera near the limbus measures 0.8 mm. in thickness; behind the insertions of the rectus muscles it has a thickness of just 0.3 mm. Anterior to the tendon of insertion of the rectus muscles, it is 0.6 mm. in thickness; at the equator it varies between 0.4 and 0.6 mm.; and near the optic nerve it is about 1.0 mm. thick.

Two potential openings exist in the sclera, one anteriorly for the cornea, and one posteriorly for the optic nerve. The anterior one has been discussed previously (p. 60). The posterior opening is the optic nerve canal, which has the shape of a truncated cone, with an internal opening 1.5 to 2.0 mm. in width and an external one 3.0 to 3.5 mm. in width. The sclera forms the principal wall of the optic nerve canal, with the remaining part formed by the choroid. Bundles of scleral collagen extend across the canal and form a meshwork known as the lamina cribrosa through which axons of the optic nerve pass.

A number of channels or emissaria exist in the sclera for the passage of arteries, veins and nerves into or out of the eye. These can be divided into anterior and posterior groups. Most of the anterior channels are found in the limbus and consist of venous branches of the deep and intrascleral plexuses that join the episcleral venous plexus and small vessels from the anterior ciliary arteries, which supply the limbal and peripheral corneal tissues (p. 121). The principal channels that traverse the anterior sclera are the main trunks of the anterior ciliary arteries (Fig. 5-3). There are two anterior ciliary arteries in the sheaths of each rectus muscle except the lateral rectus, which has only one. Near the insertion of the muscle tendon into the sclera these arteries leave the muscles and penetrate the sclera to join the major circle of the iris. Their channels through the sclera frequently can be recognized on the scleral surface by a small cuff of uveal pigment.

The posterior emissaria are more important and comprise three groups: the vortex veins, the long posterior ciliary arteries and nerves, and the short posterior ciliary arteries and nerves. We have seen that, based on oph-

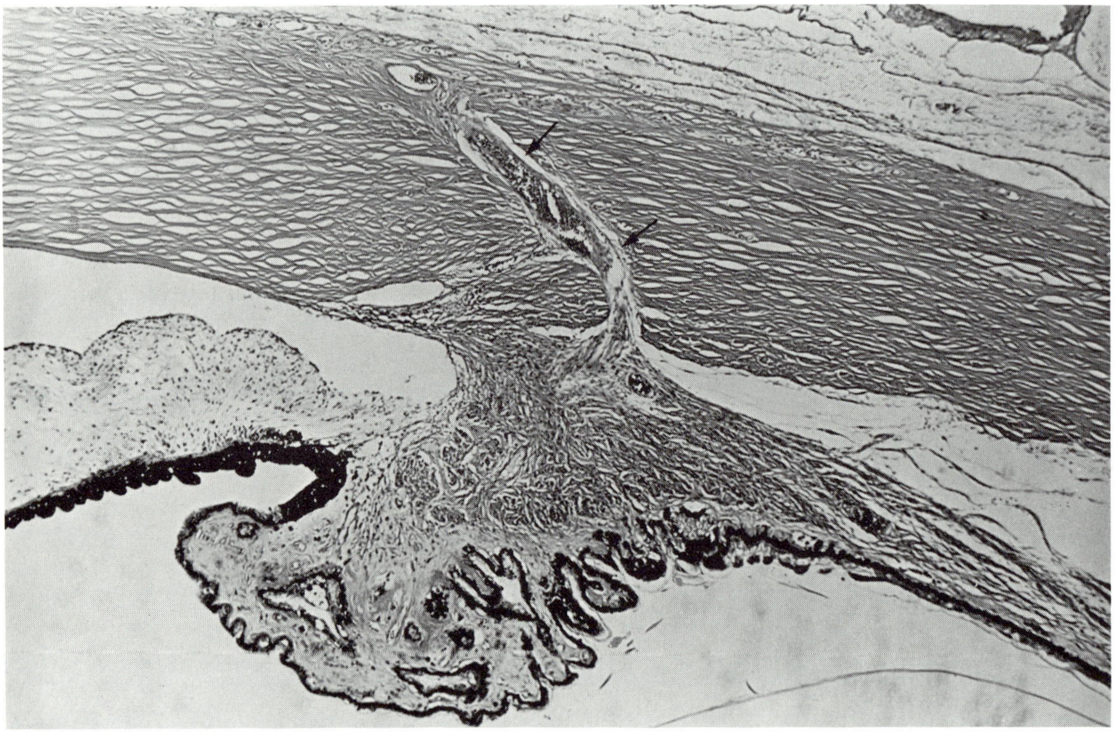

Figure 5-3. Light micrograph of the anterior sclera to show an anterior ciliary artery traversing the sclera into the ciliary body (arrows). (× 50.)

thalmoscopy, the average eye has six to seven vortex veins (see p. 52). There are, however, four main vortex veins. Their locations and approximate distances in millimeters from the limbus to their external and internal orifices are as follows (Salzmann, 1912):

	External Orifice (mm.)	*Internal Orifice (mm.)*
Superoexternal	22	18
Superointernal	20	16
Inferoexternal	19	15
Inferointernal	18	14.5

It can be seen that the four channels are about 4 mm. long and that their direction through the sclera is oblique. The superoexternal vortex is 8 mm. and the superointernal 7.0 mm. posterior to the equator. The inferoexternal vortex is only 5.5 mm. from the equator, while the distance to the inferointernal one is 6.0 mm.

Two long posterior ciliary arteries and nerves pierce the sclera along the horizontal meridian of the eye (Fig. 5–4, and p. 50). One artery and nerve are nasal, and the other artery and nerve are temporal to the optic nerve. Additional long ciliary nerves may be present superiorly and inferiorly, mainly the latter, but are usually smaller. The entrance of the long ciliary arteries and nerves into the sclera is about 3 to 4 mm. from the dural sheath of the optic nerve. They pass through the sclera in long oblique channels surrounded by a loose connective tissue. The nerve and artery are separated from each other by a small amount of pigmented tissue. The length of the long ciliary emissaria is about 3 to 5 mm., depending on the obliquity of their courses. After passing through the sclera, the nerves and arteries lie in the suprachoroidal space and run forward to the ciliary body.

Approximately 20 short ciliary arteries and 20 short ciliary nerves pass through the sclera, surrounding the optic nerve at a right angle to its surface (Fig. 5–5 *A* and *B*, and p. 50). They provide the principal blood and nerve

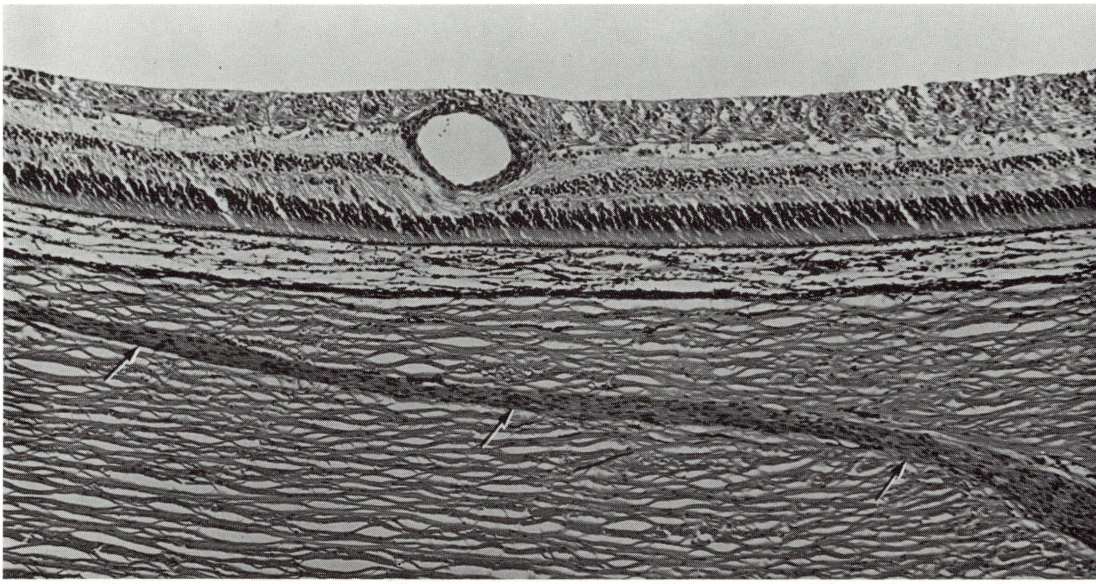

Figure 5–4. Light micrograph of a long posterior ciliary nerve (arrows) traversing the sclera toward the choroid. (× 85.)

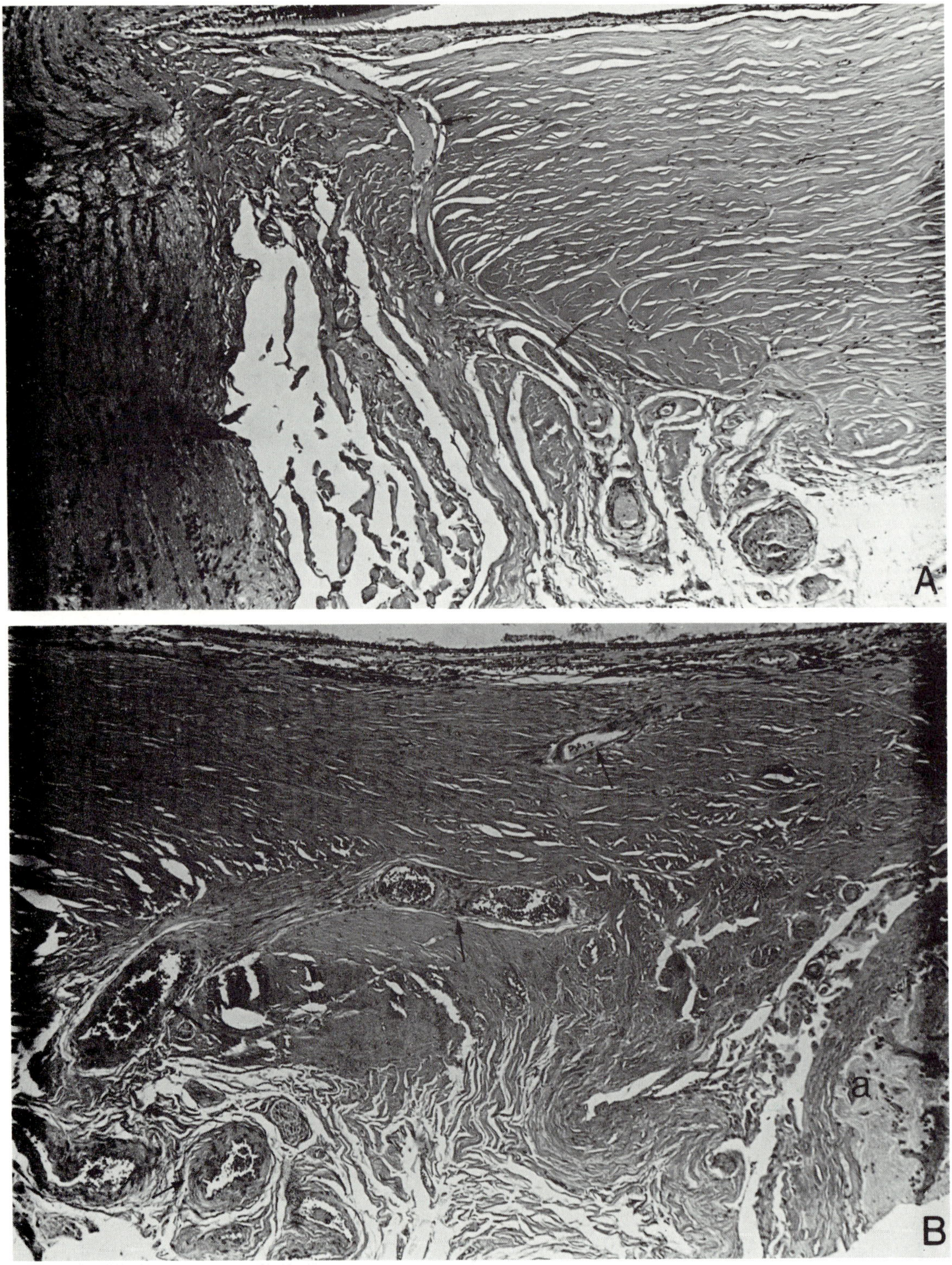

Figure 5-5. *A*, Light micrograph of a short posterior ciliary artery (arrows) passing through the sclera to the choroid. (× 85.)

B, Another view of a short posterior ciliary artery (arrows). The optic nerve is at (a). (× 85.)

supply to the posterior sclera and to the choroid. The arteries also send branches to the circle of Zinn, which is located in the sclera at the edge of the optic nerve and furnishes some of the blood supply to the optic disc.

The choroid is anchored firmly to the sclera at the sites where the vortex veins pass from the choroid through the sclera to the orbit. For this reason, if the choroid becomes detached from the sclera after cataract removal or other intraocular surgical procedure, the detachment usually occurs between two of the vortex veins.

An additional anterior emissarium is found in some eyes, the intrascleral nerve loop of Axenfeld (Fig. 5-6). This nerve loop appears in the anterior sclera, either in the region of the channels of the anterior ciliary arteries or between the rectus muscle insertions. Clinically the nerve loop is smooth and dome-shaped, measuring 1 to 2 mm. in size. At times the loops appear cystic, and an attempt is made to remove them. Axenfeld's nerve loops occur on branches from the long posterior ciliary nerves which ramify in the ciliary body. Occasionally one of these branches loops out through the sclera in the anterior suprachoroidal region and then returns to the ciliary body. Stevenson (1963) found a nerve loop of Axenfeld in 12 per cent of 2000 human eyes examined. One per cent of all patients had these nerve loops in both eyes, and in 10 eyes there was more than one loop. Almost all loops were associated with blood vessels, and all were pigmented. Most of the loops were located in the upper half of the sclera, and in 12 patients the nerve protrusions produced clinical symptoms.

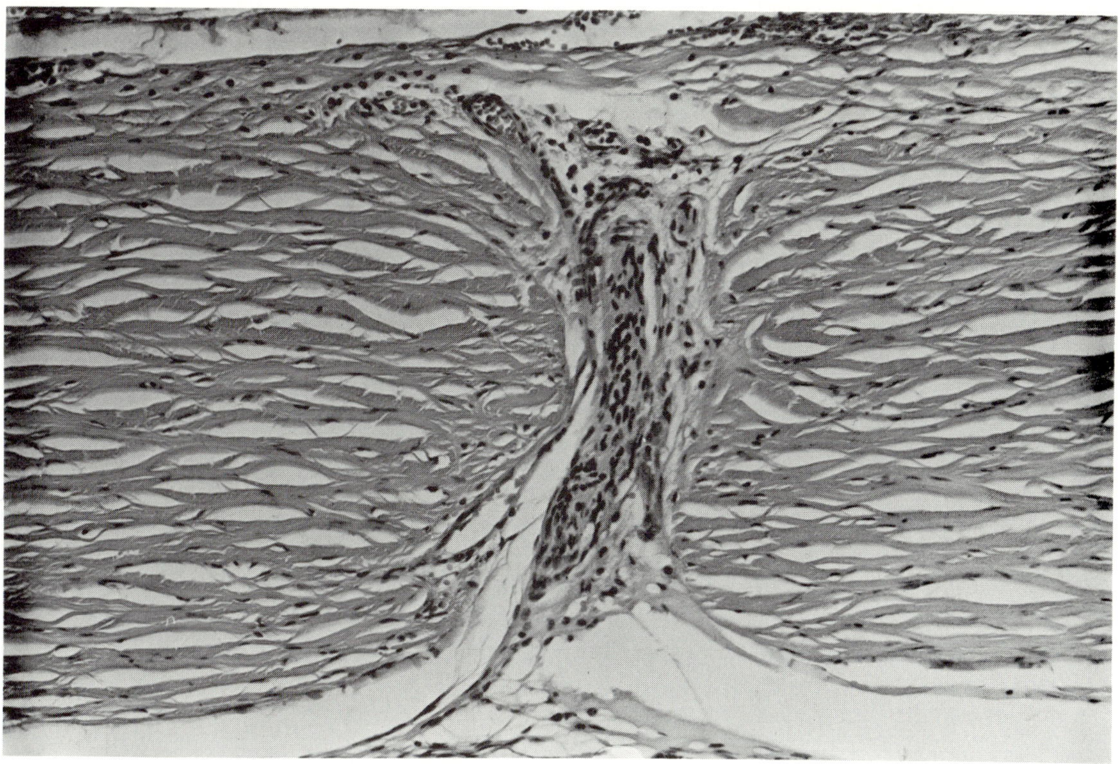

Figure 5–6. Light micrograph of the anterior sclera and a nerve loop of Axenfeld. The episclera is at the top. (× 170.)

Blood Supply

The sclera is relatively avascular, with the principal blood supply coming from the anterior and posterior ciliary arteries. Small branches from these spread out in the episclera to form a coarse network, which sends smaller branches to the scleral stroma. The internal sclera receives some nourishment from the choroidal vessels.

Branches from the anterior ciliary arteries go to the episcleral tissue anterior to the rectus muscle insertions to form an episcleral vascular layer, which extends forward to the limbus. Other branches supply the deep sclera and the region of Schlemm's canal. At the equator there are very few episcleral or scleral vessels. Posteriorly the branches of the short posterior ciliary vessels form a rich plexus known as the circle of Zinn in the sclera around the optic nerve. Small branches from the circle supply the posterior sclera.

Nerves

The short posterior ciliary nerves pierce the sclera around the optic nerve. They send some branches to supply the scleral surface before entering the emissarium and others to the scleral stroma within the emissarium. The remainder of the sclera is supplied by branches from the long posterior ciliary nerves. The limbal region of the sclera contains many fine nerves derived from the long posterior ciliary nerves. Some of these are on their way to supply the cornea, some supply the trabecular meshwork, and still others end in the sclera itself. They are probably mainly of sensory origin. Ehinger (1964) has shown that the sclera contains no adrenergic fibers except where vessels penetrate the emissaria.

MICROSCOPIC ANATOMY

The sclera is composed of the following parts: (1) episclera, (2) scleral stroma, and (3) lamina fusca.

Episclera

The anterior episclera is a dense, vascular connective tissue which is really a part of the superficial scleral stroma (see p. 193). It merges with the scleral stroma and the overlying subconjunctival tissue and Tenon's capsule. Its collagenous bundles are finer and more irregular in their disposition and are slightly less compact than in the sclera. The increased thickness of the anterior episclera is the result of its incorporation of Tenon's capsule and the vascular tissues which surround the rectus muscles. It also contains pigmented melanocytes, some macrophages and a few lymphocytes.

The equatorial episclera posterior to the rectus muscle insertions is thinner than the anterior portion. It is loosely joined with Tenon's capsule by fine strands of collagen and is relatively avascular. The vessels it contains are derived mainly from the posterior ciliary arteries.

The episcleral collagen is like that of most connective tissues. There is some variation in the diameter of the collagen fibrils, but they are mostly smaller than those of the sclera and the bundles they form are more widely separated from each other. The ground substance of the episclera is more abundant than that of the sclera. The episcleral fibroblasts are not unusual; because of the looser structure of this tissue, they are not so thin and elongated as those of the cornea and sclera. Except for the main branches of the anterior ciliary arteries, the blood vessels are mostly capillaries, venules, small veins and arterioles. The walls of these vessels are constructed like those of similar vessels in other tissues, and the capillaries have an unfenestrated, continuous endothelium. Myelinated and unmyelinated nerves are found frequently, ending without specialization.

Scleral Stroma (Figs. 5-7 to 5-12)

The scleral stroma is composed entirely of bundles of collagen and fibroblasts, with a moderate amount of ground substance. The dimensions and course of the scleral collagen bundles are not completely understood, but they are different in the anterior equatorial and posterior portions, and in the superficial as compared to the deep portions. The collagen bundles of the sclera vary considerably in size and shape, depending on the degree to which they subdivide. They do branch extensively and intermingle in various planes. The bundles are basically composed of parallel collagen fibrils which vary in diameter and length, and they appear to be fusiform in shape.

Figure 5-7 shows the general arrangement of the scleral collagen in various portions of the eye. Anteriorly the superficial and deep collagen is oriented parallel to the limbus, especially in the deep portion and near the scleral spur. Within the limbus the intermediate and superficial collagen forms loops which have a posterior convexity. This orientation gradually becomes more meridional, especially in the region of the rectus muscle insertions. The collagen bundles that form the scleral spur are 30 to 50 μm. wide and up to 10 μm. thick (Salzmann, 1912). Elsewhere in the anterior sclera the bundles are less uniform, but Salzmann found many of them to be about 10 to 16 μm. in thickness and 100 to 140 μm. in width.

The peripapillary collagen also has a circular direction parallel to the circumference of the optic nerve, so that in meridional sections it appears cut in cross-section. This circular pattern persists beyond the entrance of the short posterior ciliary arteries and nerves for a distance of approximately 4 mm.

Posterior to the rectus muscle insertions the scleral collagen bundles are coarse and difficult to define because their branches have such an irregular course. In the equatorial sclera the bundles are more circular and form long loops with a posterior convexity. Meridional sections of this area show collagen bundles cut in cross- or very oblique sections. Around the equator the superficial collagen bundles form layers which intermingle in a single plane, like the cords in the net of a balloon, while in the deeper sclera the bundles have a more meridional course. The definitive length of the bundles in any part of the sclera could be elucidated only by serial section, but such a study would be impractical because of their large dimensions.

The scleral insertions of the rectus muscle tendons are characterized

Text continued on page 199

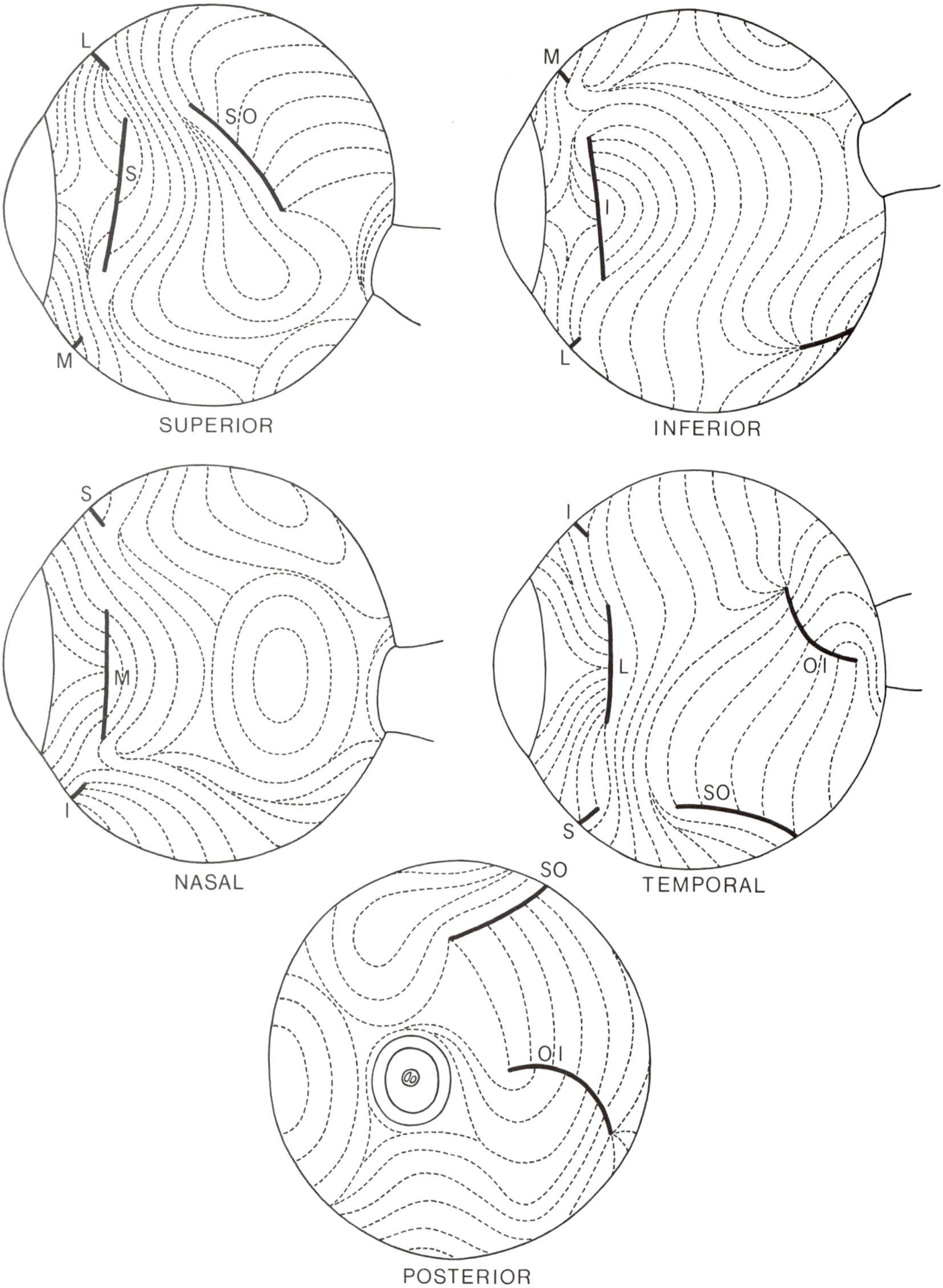

Figure 5–7. Orientation of the scleral collagen in different areas of the eye. For the most part, the collagen is circular, especially in the equatorial region. Anteriorly it is meridional in the limbal region nasally and temporally, and oblique in the vertical meridian. In the deep limbal region and scleral spur and around the optic nerve it is circular. (W. Kokott: Das Spaltlinienbild der Sklera. Klin. Mbl. Augen. 92:117, 1934.)

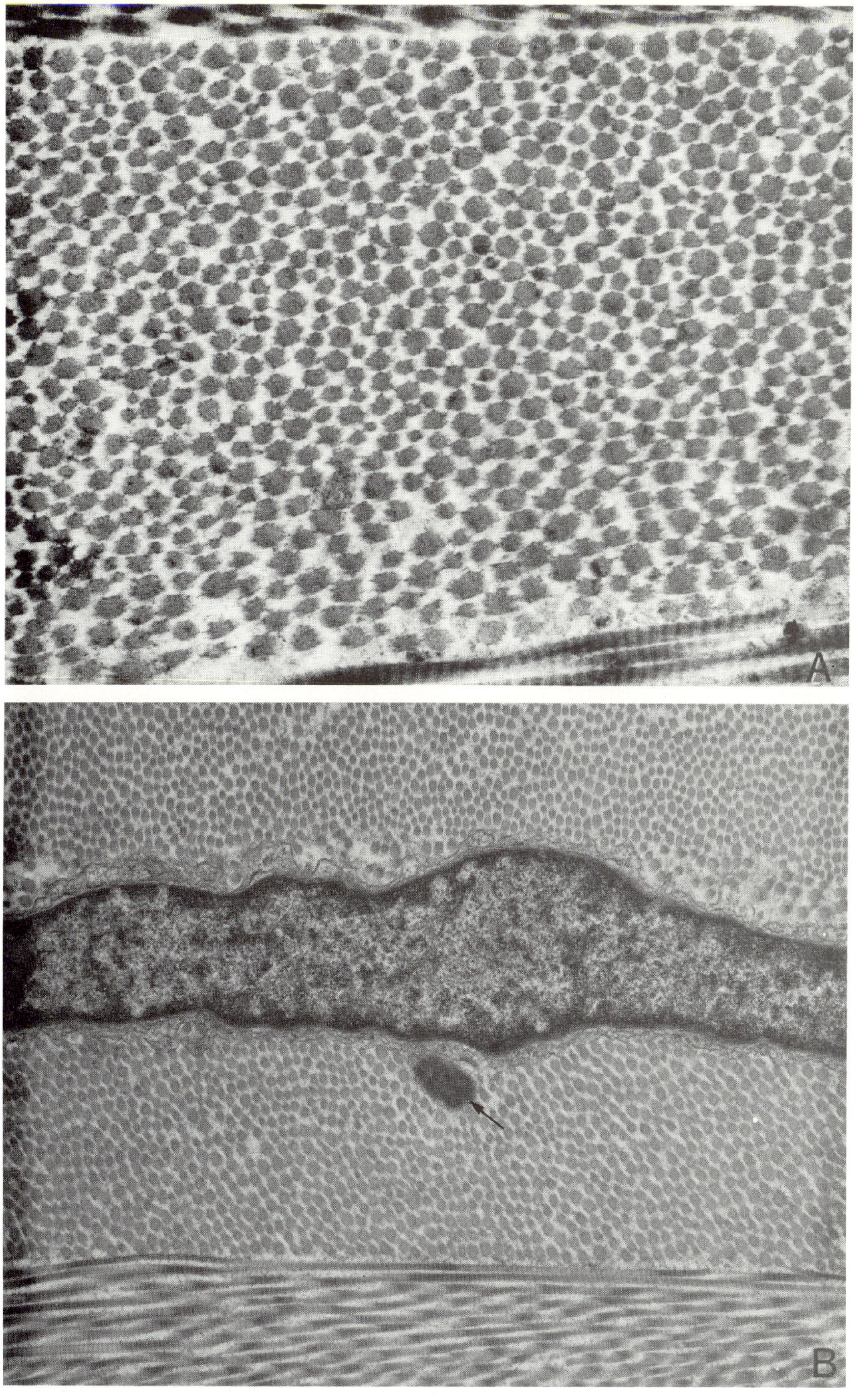

Figure 5–8. Scleral stroma. *A,* Outer scleral stroma; three bundles are shown to be sectioned longitudinally, in cross-section and obliquely. Because of the fusiform shape of the fibrils, the cross-sectional diameter is variable. (× 30,000.)

B, Inner scleral stroma, showing a fibroblast amidst the closely packed fibrils of a collagen bundle. These cells have an elongated nucleus surrounded by a scanty cytoplasm and long, thin processes. Note the presence of an electron-dense mass (arrow) adjacent to the fibroblast. Such masses are commonly found near these cells. Note the difference in size of the outer and inner collagen fibers. (× 12,000.)

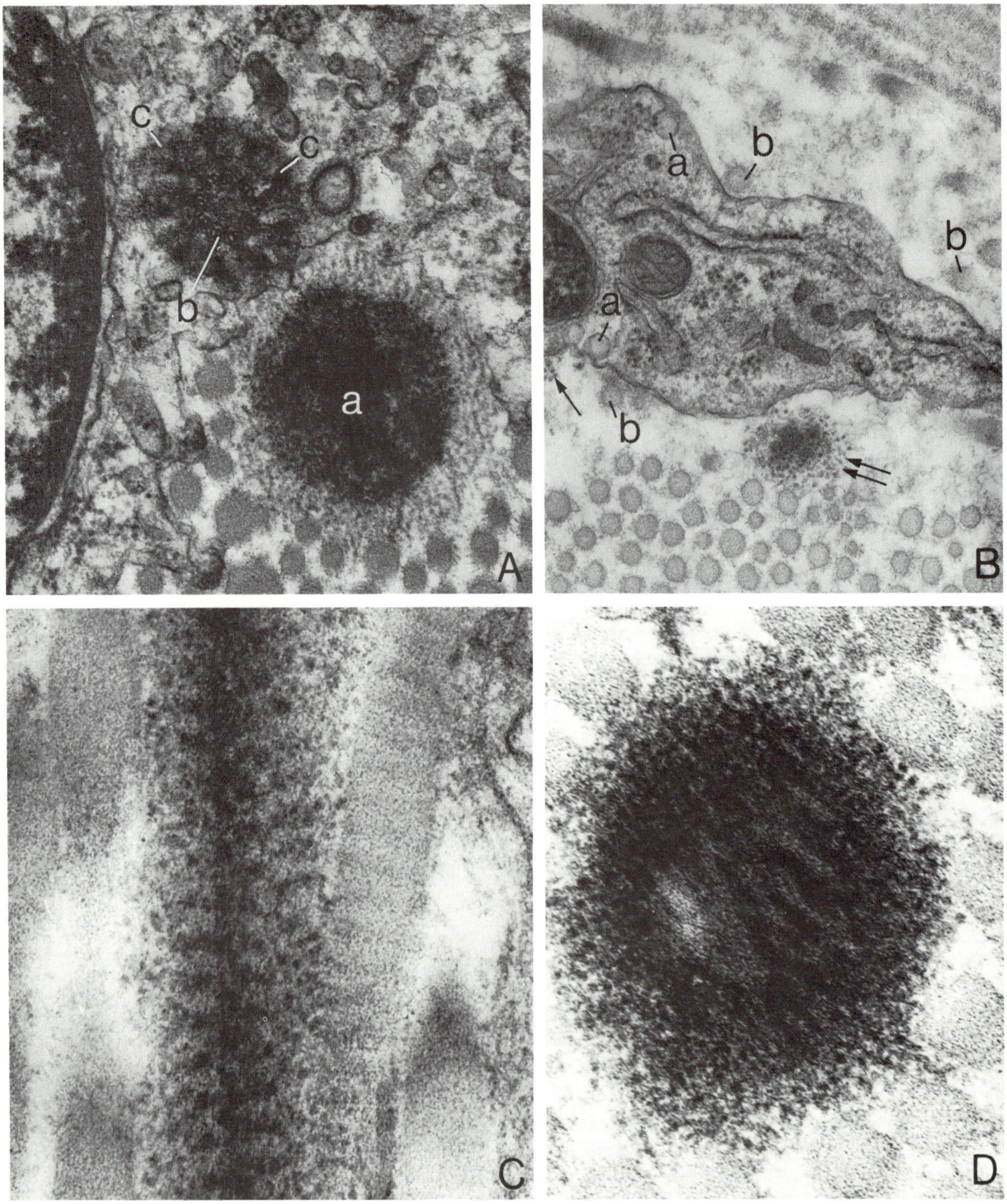

Figure 5–9. Collagenous electron-dense masses. This material stains strongly with basic dyes and it is often classified as elastin. It is not elastase-sensitive and is more abundant in very young eyes. *A*, At (a) an electron-dense mass appears in cross-section near the periphery of a fibroblast. A fibroblast contains a centriole with its nine triplets (b) and elaborate pericentriolar structures (c). (× 45,000.)

B, Scleral fibroblast showing some cisternae of the rough-surfaced endoplasmic reticulum, polyribosomes and pinocytotic vesicles (a). Five electron-dense collagen fibrils (single arrows) measuring around 150 A. in thickness are seen near its periphery in addition to some much larger "mature" collagen fibrils (b). An electron-dense mass (double arrows) is formed by aggregation of the smaller fibrils. (× 30,000.)

C, Longitudinal view of an electron-dense mass showing its striations. (× 90,000.)

D, Cross-section of an electron-dense collagenous mass. The individual fibrils can be discerned at the periphery. (× 90,000.)

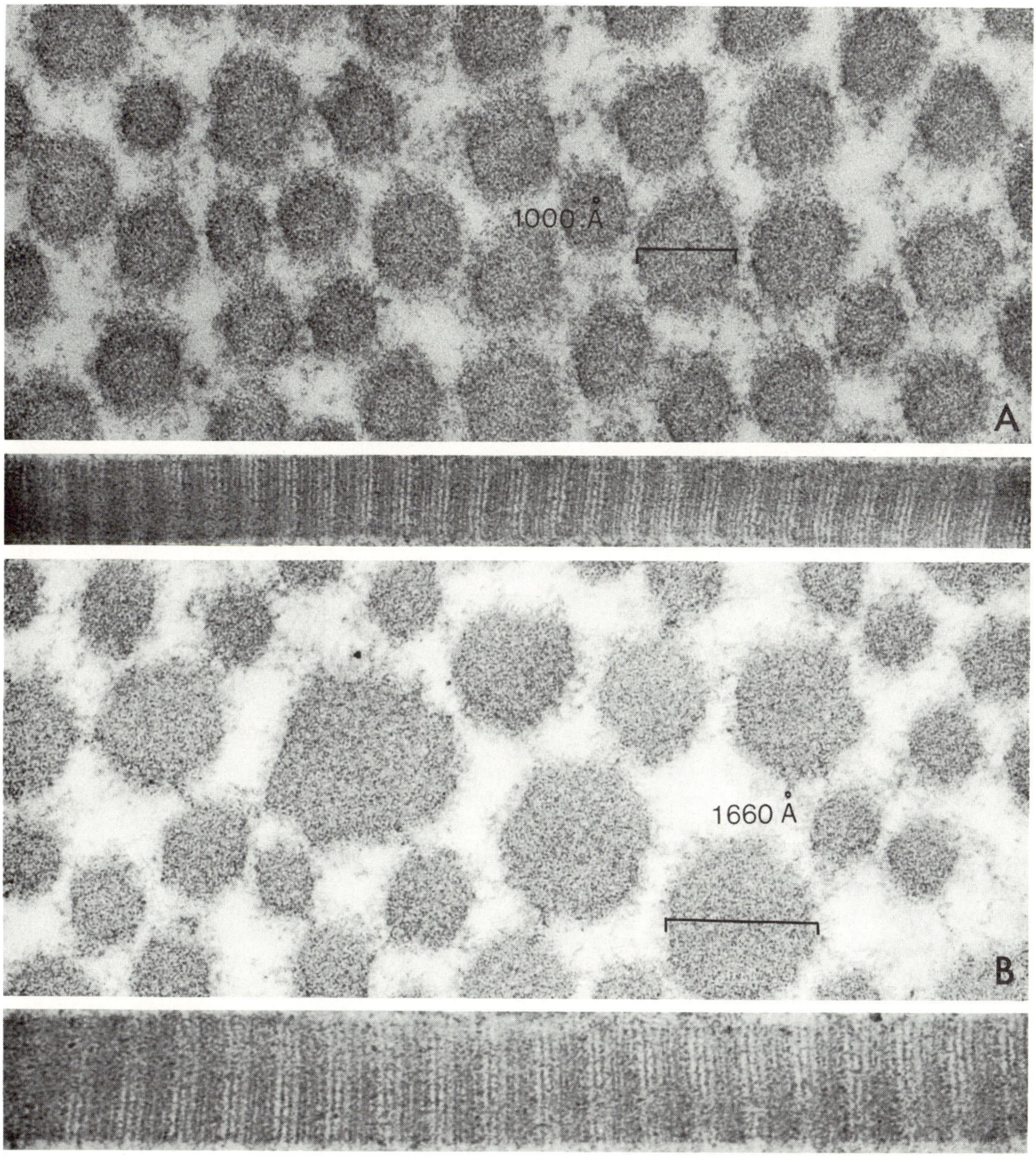

Figure 5–10. *A*, Inner scleral stromal collagen. The largest fibrils in this region measure 1000 A.

B, Outer scleral stromal collagen. The largest fibrils measure 1660 A. in diameter. The fibrils in the outer sclera are not only larger than those in the inner sclera but also show a greater variation in the size of the midsection, as well as in the tapering ends of the fibrils. (× 120,000.)

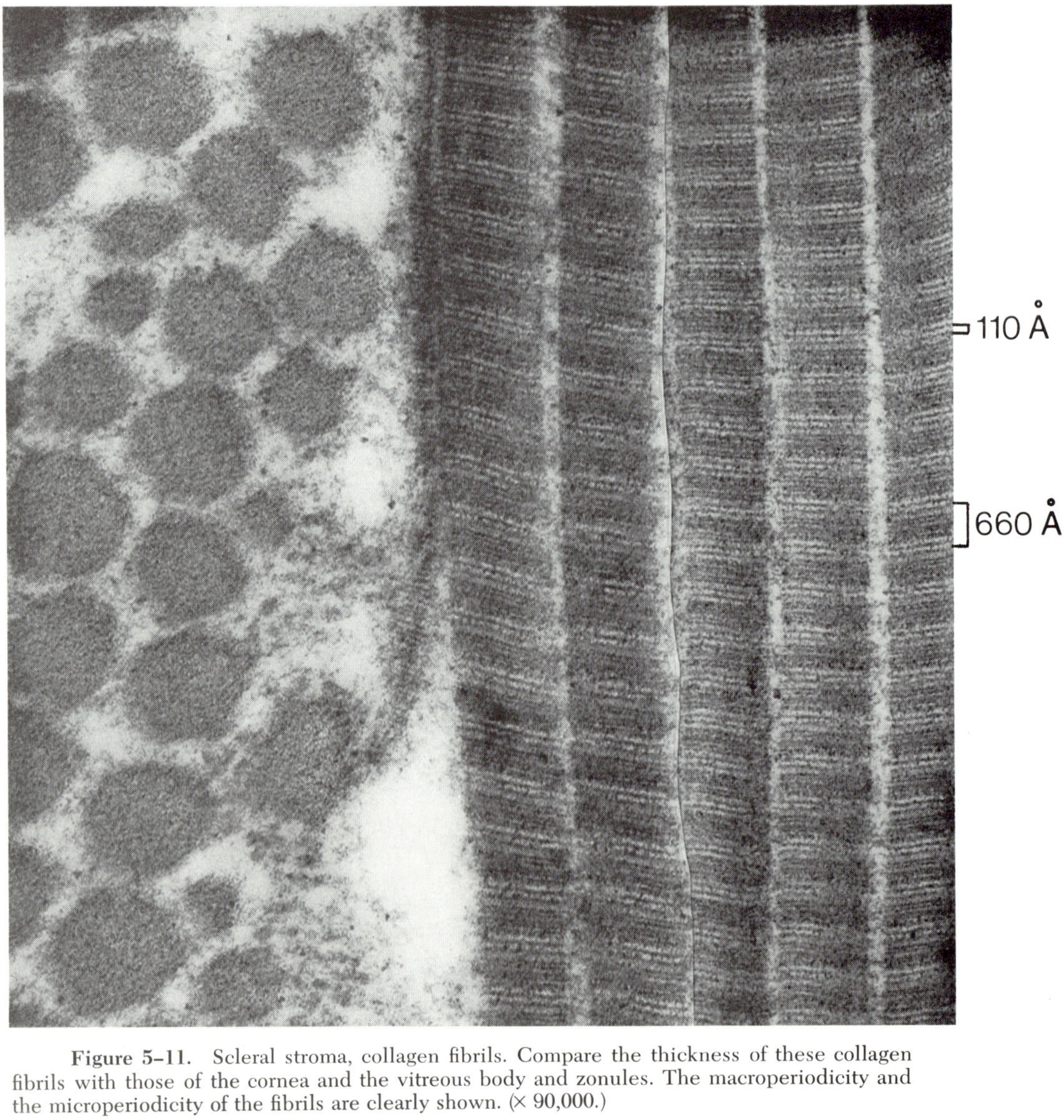

Figure 5–11. Scleral stroma, collagen fibrils. Compare the thickness of these collagen fibrils with those of the cornea and the vitreous body and zonules. The macroperiodicity and the microperiodicity of the fibrils are clearly shown. (× 90,000.)

by the merging of the well oriented meridional tendon collagen and the oblique and meridional collagen bundles of the sclera. The tendon collagen subdivides, spreads out and interweaves with that of the sclera, and from the insertion forward into the limbus the scleral bundles have the same meridional course. Around the emissaria the scleral collagen forms a thin zone which is oriented parallel to the course of the nerve or vessel.

The scleral collagen bundles are found to be composed of fibrils that are identical to those of tendon and skin when examined with the dark-field microscope (Grignolo, 1954). X-ray diffraction (Hertel, 1933) shows the scleral collagen to be like other collagen.

Using different methods, various authors have given the following dimensions for the fibrils (after Grignolo):

Author	*Species*	*Preparation*	*Diameter*	*Periodicity*
Schwarz	Man	Fixation with osmic acid; fragmentation with ultrasound	280–2800 A.	800 A.
Van den Hoff	Ox	Nonfixed and fixed material in osmium; mechanical fragmentation	350–1250 A.	570 A.
François et al.		Mechanical fragmentation	400–3300 A.	640 A. microperiodicity 210 A.

It has been believed that there is little or no coating on the collagen fibrils of the sclera, in contrast to those seen in the cornea. Schwarz (1953 *a*, *b*) found that fetal scleral collagen fibrils were coated with acid mucopolysaccharide but that the coating is diminished considerably when the sclera becomes opaque during fetal development. A comparison of high quality electron micrographs of the cornea and sclera, however, shows just as much or more ground substance in the sclera as in the cornea. The scleral collagen also differs from that of the cornea by its greater birefringence, by an absence of fixed spacing between the fibrils, and by considerable variation in the diameter of the scleral fibrils. Spitznas and co-workers (1970) have shown in human and rabbit eyes that the collagen fibrils of the superficial sclera are larger in diameter than those of the deeper sclera, the former having diameters around 1660 A., while the latter measure approximately 1000 A. in diameter.

The scleral cells are fibroblasts, but they are not numerous. They are very thin cells with small nuclei and long, branching processes. The processes of these cells come close to each other but do not have intimate contact.

Lamina Fusca (Fig. 5-12)

This layer is a modification of the inner scleral lamellae to form thin bundles which blend imperceptibly with the suprachoroidal and supraciliary lamellae. The innermost scleral collagen bundles become separated from each other, show broader branchings and form thin bundles which intermingle with the outer ciliary body and choroid. Because of the intermingling of fibers and bundles, the line of separation between the inner sclera and

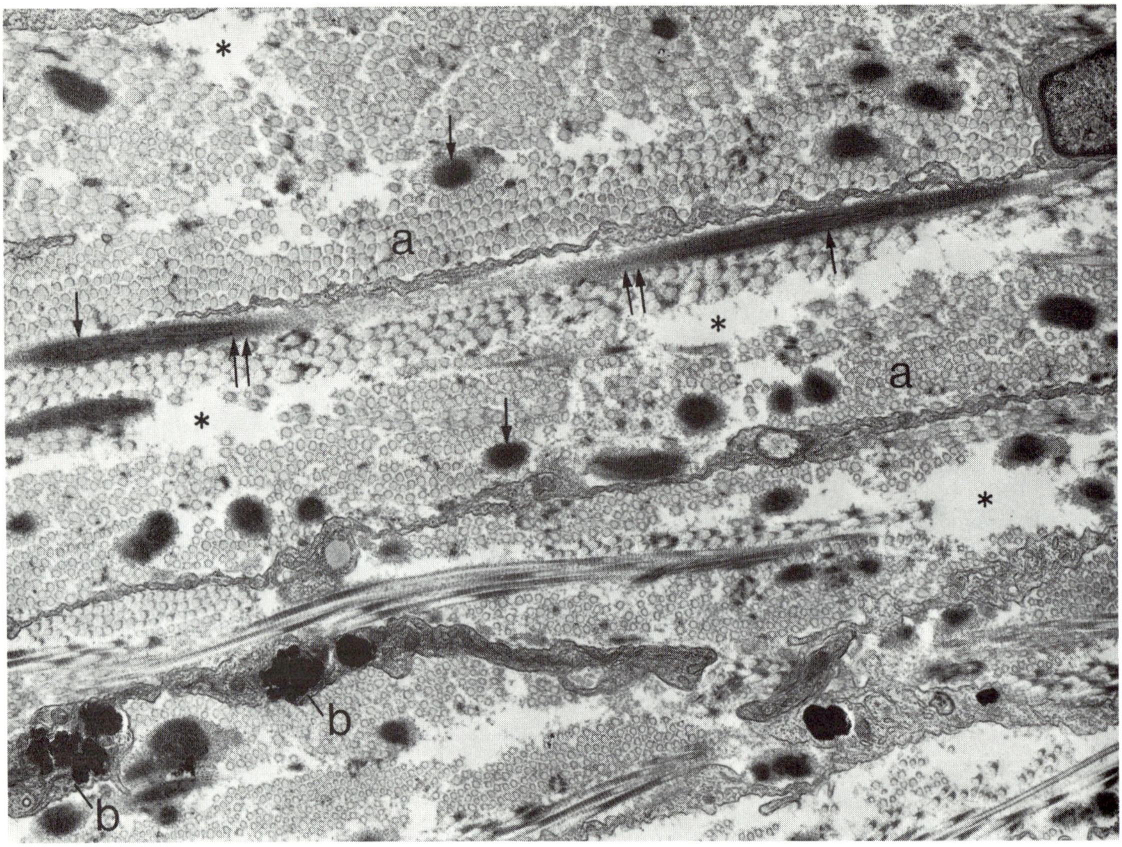

Figure 5-12. The lamina fusca of the sclera gradually blends with the choroid. It is rather cellular and its collagen is more loosely arranged than in the scleral stroma. In some fibril-free areas (asterisks) ground substance material probably has been extracted during preparation of the tissue. Numerous electron-dense masses are cut in longitudinal (double arrows) and cross-sections (arrows). Striations are clearly seen in those masses cut longitudinally. Several fibroblasts (a) and a melanocyte (b) are indicated. (× 15,000.)

outer choroid and ciliary body is not sharp. In this region there is a considerable increase in the amount of pigment because of the number of melanocytes and pigmented macrophages. These cells are found on the surface of and between the collagenous bundles. The ultrastructure of the lamina fusca will be considered in the chapter on the Choroid.

REFERENCES

Ehinger, B.: Distribution of adrenergic nerves to orbital structures. Acta Physiol. Scand. *62*:291, 1964.

Friedenwald, J.: Contribution to the theory and practice of tonometry. Amer. J. Ophthal. *20*:985, 1937.

Gloster, J., Perkins, E., and Pommier, M.: Extensibility of strips of sclera and cornea. Brit. J. Ophthal. *41*:103, 1957.

Grignolo, A.: Studies on the submicroscopical structure of the ocular tissues. Boll. Ocul. *33*:513, 1954.

Hertel, E.: The use and value of X-rays for the examination of structures in ophthalmology. Arch. Augen. *107*:259, 1933.

Krause, A.: The chemical constitution of the sclera. Arch. Ophthal. *7*:598, 1932.

Maurice, D.: The Cornea and Sclera. *In* Davson, H., (ed.): Physiology of the Eye. 2nd ed. Boston, Little, Brown and Company, 1969, p. 489.

Pénzes, T., and Pataky, G.: Determination of the calcium and water content of the sclera in calf and cattle eyes. Klin. Mbl. Augen. *144*:908, 1964.

St. Helen, R., and McEwen, W. K.: Rheology of the human sclera. I. Anelastic behavior. Amer. J. Ophthal. *52*:539, 1961.

Salzmann, M.: The Anatomy and Histology of the Human Eyeball. Translated by E. V. L. Brown. Chicago, University of Chicago Press, 1912.

Schwarz, W.: Electron microscopic studies of the structure of human scleral and cornea. Z. Zellforsch. *38*:26, 1953a.

Schwarz, W.: Electron microscopic studies of the differentiation of human corneal and scleral fibrils. Z. Zellforsch. *38*:78, 1953b.

Stevenson, T. C.: Intrascleral nerve loops: A clinical study of frequency and treatment. Amer. J. Ophthal. *55*:935, 1963.

Spitznas, M., Luciano, L., and Reale, E.: Fine structure of rabbit scleral collagen. Amer. J. Ophthal. *69*:414, 1970.

Spitznas, M.: Scleral Collagen. Amer. J. Ophthal. *71*(1):68, 1971.

Vannas, S., and Teir, H.: Observations on structure and age changes in the human sclera. Acta Ophthal. *38*:268, 1960.

Chapter Six

IRIS AND ANTERIOR CHAMBER

Iris

The iris is the most anterior portion of the uveal tract. It forms a delicate and movable diaphragm between the anterior and posterior chambers, corresponding in function to diaphragms in optical systems.

The reason for the varying color of the iris has excited speculation for hundreds of years, and much study has gone into the hereditary aspects of its pigmentation. It is known that the brown iris is inherited as a dominant and the blue as recessive. Variations in texture and pigmentation lead to gray or yellowish irises. Heterochromia of the iris is a condition in which one portion of an iris has a different color than other areas; heterochromia also may exist between the two irises. Freckles or nevus-like structures frequently are seen in the anterior iris. These areas of hyperpigmentation are produced by clusters of melanocytes within the most anterior layers of the iris stroma. In the white race the iris is usually blue at birth because of the paucity of pigment in the stromal melanocytes and because of the small number of melanocytes. The blue color results from the stromal absorption of the long wave lengths, allowing the shorter blue waves to return to the observer's eyes. Light which enters the eye traverses the lightly pigmented anterior border layer and iris stroma without hindrance and is reflected back out of the eye from the pigment epithelium. In black and brown races the iris stroma is always denser and contains some pigmented melanocytes; therefore, the iris has a slate gray or deep muddy blue appearance at birth in persons of these races.

Because of the forward convexity of the anterior lens surface, the pupillary plane of the iris is farther forward in the eye than the iris root, and thus the iris plane forms the sides of a truncated cone. The magnification produced by the cornea causes the iris to appear to be larger by one eighth and causes its anterior surface to be slightly convex when viewed from the front. The pupil is a round opening near the center of the iris; it is displaced slightly downward and nasally with respect to the center of the cornea.

PHYSIOLOGY

The sphincter and dilator muscles of the iris change the size of the pupil automatically, depending on the amount of light to which the eye is exposed and its position of gaze. The pupillary aperture regulates the amount of light entering the eye and is located on an optical axis behind the most optimally corrected portion of the cornea. For this reason, incoming light reaches the macular region without distortion in the normal eye. Constriction of the pupil is important because it improves the depth perception of the eye. The focal length of the eye is about 20 mm., and the pupil can change in size from 1.5 to 8.0 mm. The effective aperture, therefore, is between f 13 and f 2.5, a ratio of 30:1 in the amount of light admitted (Adler, 1965).

The sphincter muscle is like other smooth muscles. It is located in the pupillary stroma of the iris, is circular in shape and concentric with the pupil. Its action is to reduce the size of the pupil evenly and uniformly when stimulated. It is not certain whether there is a concomitant relaxation of the dilator muscle when constriction occurs. The sphincter has the unique feature of being able to shorten more on contraction than all other smooth muscles. When the pupil is reduced from a maximal dilatation of 8.0 mm. to a minimum of 1.5 mm., the muscle shortens by 87 per cent of its length, a remarkable change, compared to striated and other smooth muscles (Adler, 1965). This shortening probably is produced by the telescoping of the muscle fibrils on contraction, similar to that seen in striated muscle. The fusiform shape of the muscle cells and the apparent termination of the myofibrils on densities along the cell membrane probably facilitate the telescoping. There are intimate connections between the sphincter muscle cells, the adjacent stroma and the dilator muscle that enable the sphincter muscle to maintain its pupillary constrictor function even after a sector of the iris has been removed surgically.

The nerves which supply the sphincter muscle enter the eye via the long ciliary nerves. These motor nerves come from the ciliary ganglion, whose efferent branches are derived from the third cranial nerve. They form branches in the anterior choroid near the ora serrata. Ganglion cells, which are found along their course, may contain the synapses for terminals that eventually supply the sphincter. The sphincter muscle also has an abundant sympathetic innervation (Ehinger, 1966), the fibers being distributed directly to the muscle cells and to the connective tissue around the muscle bundles.

The dilator muscle of the iris is developed from and is an integral part of the anterior iris epithelium; each cell of this region has an epithelial and a muscular portion. The muscular portion has all the histologic and pharmacologic characteristics of smooth muscle and is innervated primarily by sympathetic nerve fibers that originate in the superior cervical ganglion. Postganglionic nerve fibers enter the adventitia of the carotid artery and its branches and follow these vessels into the middle cranial fossa. In the orbit they leave the ophthalmic artery and enter the long posterior ciliary nerves. Some fibers possibly pass through the ciliary ganglion and enter the eye via the short posterior ciliary nerves. All these nerves eventually reach the iris, where they contact the anterior epithelial cells and their muscular extensions. Ehinger (1966) has demonstrated both sympathetic and parasympathetic endings in and around the dilator muscle cells. The parasympathetic fibers probably are extensions of those to the sphincter muscle.

The sphincter and dilator muscles react pharmacologically to various substances in specific ways. The sphincter muscle constricts in response to cholinergic and parasympathomimetic drugs, whereas the dilator responds to adrenergic compounds. The cholinergic or parasympathomimetic substances probably act at the level of the motor end-plate in the same way as acetylcholine. Other substances act by competitive inhibition, binding cholinesterase so that acetylcholine can accumulate in large amounts. The drugs that stimulate the sphincter muscle to contract are called miotics; those most commonly used, such as pilocarpine and carbamylcholine, act on the motor end-plate. The anticholinesterase drugs most commonly used to produce miosis are physostigmine, Prostigmin and di-isopropyl fluorophosphate. Other drugs are parasympatholytic, acting as depressors on the motor end-plate; these include atropine, scopolamine and homatropine. They are competitive antagonists of acetylcholine for the muscarinic receptors of the sphincter muscle. Their action may be overcome by increasing the concentration of acetylcholine at the effector organ, such as by giving an anticholinesterase drug.

Sympathomimetic drugs are used to produce mydriasis; substances such as epinephrine and phenylephrine stimulate the motor end-plate of the dilator muscle. Antioxidase drugs such as cocaine are valuable for production of mydriasis under certain conditions. The tissues contain some oxidases which destroy sympathin; cocaine inhibits their action. Since the sphincter and dilator muscles contain both sympathetic and parasympathetic nerve fibers, it is not clear whether they act reciprocally.

EMBRYOLOGY

By the sixth week of pregnancy (12 to 17 mm. stage) the mesoderm at the edge of the optic cup and the neuroectodermal layers of the cup itself are the precursors of the iris. The mesoderm is destined to form the stroma of the iris and the pupillary membrane, while the neuroectoderm will form the sphincter and dilator muscles as well as the posterior and anterior iris epithelium. The initial ingrowth of mesoderm into the optic cup to form the corneal endothelium is associated with a fibrillar matrix which lies posterior to the endothelium and will participate in the formation of the iris. Vascular buds arise from the region of the annular vessel during the seventh week (17 to 24 mm. stage) and gradually extend toward the surface of the lens. At the same time some of the fibrils in the mesodermal matrix form a thin zone of condensation at the site of the future anterior tunica vasculosa lentis. There also is continuous extension of the mesodermal elements centrally over the lens. During the eighth and ninth weeks (24 to 40 mm. stage) there is rapid development of the vascular system of the iris and pupillary membrane with formation of vascular arcades. This results from anastomosis of the long posterior ciliary arteries with the annular vessel. The anterior chamber appears during this time as a result of the disappearance of the mesoderm behind the cornea. The developing anterior chamber is separated from the lens by a layer of vessels and mesoderm. By the ninth week (40 mm. stage) the pupillary membrane is well formed; the anterior chamber is shallower at this period than during the eighth week because of the rapid development of this membrane.

The neuroectodermal margin of the optic cup now begins to grow forward so that it lies anterior to the lens equator, and the early ciliary processes appear as radial folds in the two epithelial layers of the cup, the folding occurring just posterior to its margin. During the tenth week (40 to 49 mm. stage) the forward growth of the two neuroectodermal layers interrupts the connection of the pupillary membrane to the lateral part of the tunica vasculosa lentis. By the end of embryonic life (twelfth week; 59 to 70 mm. stage) the forward edge of the neuroectodermal layers has reached the level of the anterior chamber. These two layers will become the epithelial layers of the iris. They are fused except at their growing edge, where there is persistence of a small circular opening which is known as the *marginal sinus*. The posterior epithelium has gradually become pigmented by this time. During the fourth month (70 to 110 mm. stage) the sphincter muscle appears in the anterior layer of unpigmented cells of the marginal sinus. The muscle cells develop from the epithelium near its free margin, then become separated completely from it by iris stroma. During the fifth month the anterior layer of epithelium also begins to differentiate into the dilator muscle; its development is fairly complete by the sixth month (160 to 200 mm. stage). The dilator muscle does not reach the pupillary margin, however, but terminates behind the sphincter muscle in its midportion. At the end of the sixth month, the major circle of the iris becomes complete as a result of forward growth of the long posterior ciliary arteries to meet the annular vessel. The vascular arcades of the iris also have formed three to four tiers in the pupillary membrane. The stroma of the iris becomes thicker as a result of proliferation of the mesodermal cells. During the seventh month (200 to 240 mm. stage) the marginal sinus closes, and the pigmentation of both epithelial layers has become complete into the base of the iris. The central vascular arcade of the pupillary membrane atrophies during this month. The minor vascular circle of the iris is formed during the eighth month (240 to 280 mm. stage) in the most peripheral arcade of the pupillary membrane; by this time the other arcades have atrophied, resulting in formation of the collarette. The sphincter is complete and functioning at this time.

The two epithelial layers of the iris are derived from the optic vesicle, so that upon the formation of the optic cup the cells of these two layers face each other apex to apex. Since the optic vesicle is developed from the cavity of the forebrain that is lined by ciliated ependymal cells, it is not surprising that ciliated cells are found along the apical surfaces of the iris epithelial cells in adult eyes.

GROSS ANATOMY

The diameter of the iris is about 12 mm. and its peripheral circumference is about 37.5 mm. The thickest part of the iris is at the collarette, where it measures about 0.6 mm.; the collarette is about 1.5 mm. from the pupillary margin and divides the iris into two zones, a narrow pupillary zone and a wider ciliary zone (Fig. 6-1).

The *iris root* is attached to the anteromedial surface of the ciliary body; it is approximately 0.5 mm. thick at this attachment. The anterior iris is immersed in the aqueous humor, which enters the iris stroma through openings or crypts along its anterior surface. The central iris terminates at the rounded free pupillary margin. The posterior iris is in loose contact with the lens in its central third. The lateral two thirds is in contact with the aqueous humor of the posterior chamber. More peripherally the pars plicata of the ciliary body is close to the posterior surface of the iris.

ANTERIOR SURFACE (Fig. 6–1)

In the pupillary and collarette regions the anterior surface shows numerous thick branching bands or trabeculae, especially around the collarette. They are oriented roughly parallel to the length of the iris, and the depressions in the iris surface which they enclose are shallow and deep troughs with a triangular or diamond shape. Fuchs' *crypts* are found adjacent to the collarette on both its pupillary and ciliary sides; these crypts have rounded or irregular openings and are continuous with loose spaces in the iris stroma. At the pupillary margin the posterior epithelial layers extend forward around the pupil and its adjacent iris stroma to form *crenations* (physiologic ectropion of the iris). The crenations or ruffs are broader in the superior iris and are produced by the continuation around the pupillary margin of the radial folds present in the posterior iris surface. Clinically the sphincter muscle can be seen in the stroma of the pupillary zone in gray or blue eyes, especially if the iris is examined with the slit-lamp microscope. The muscle forms a circular band 0.75 mm. wide in the stroma near the pupillary margin. The margins of the muscle are remarkably uniform and its surface shows few irregularities.

The anterior surface of the *ciliary portion* of the iris shows long radial ridges which are produced by the underlying blood vessels and their surrounding connective tissue as they extend from the iris periphery toward the collarette. These ridges become less distinct near the collarette because the vessels become smaller and more circular in direction. At the collarette the arteries form an incomplete *minor circle of the iris*. Between the collarette and the iris root, the iris surface shows a number of circular contraction folds that are concentric with the iris periphery. Additional smaller rounded crypts, the peripheral or ciliary crypts, are found in the iris near its attachment to the ciliary body. The iris stroma joins the ciliary body between and peripheral to the crypts.

Figure 6–1. Composite drawing of the surfaces and layers of the iris. Beginning at the upper left and proceeding clockwise, the iris cross-section shows the pupillary (a) and ciliary portions (b), and the surface view shows a brown iris with its dense, matted anterior border layer. Circular contraction furrows are shown (arrows) in the ciliary portion of the iris. Fuchs' crypts (c) are seen at either side of the collarette in the pupillary and ciliary portion and peripherally near the iris root. The pigment ruff is seen at the pupillary edge (d). The blue iris surface shows a less dense anterior border layer and more prominent trabeculae. The iris vessels are shown beginning at the major arterial circle in the ciliary body (e). Radial branches of the arteries and veins extend toward the pupillary region. The arteries form the incomplete minor arterial circle (f), from which branches extend toward the pupil, forming capillary arcades. The sector below it demonstrates the circular arrangement of the sphincter muscle (g) and the radial processes of the dilator muscle (h). The posterior surface of the iris shows the radial contraction furrows (i) and the structural folds (j) of Schwalbe. Circular contraction folds are also present in the ciliary portion. The pars plicata of the ciliary body is at (k).

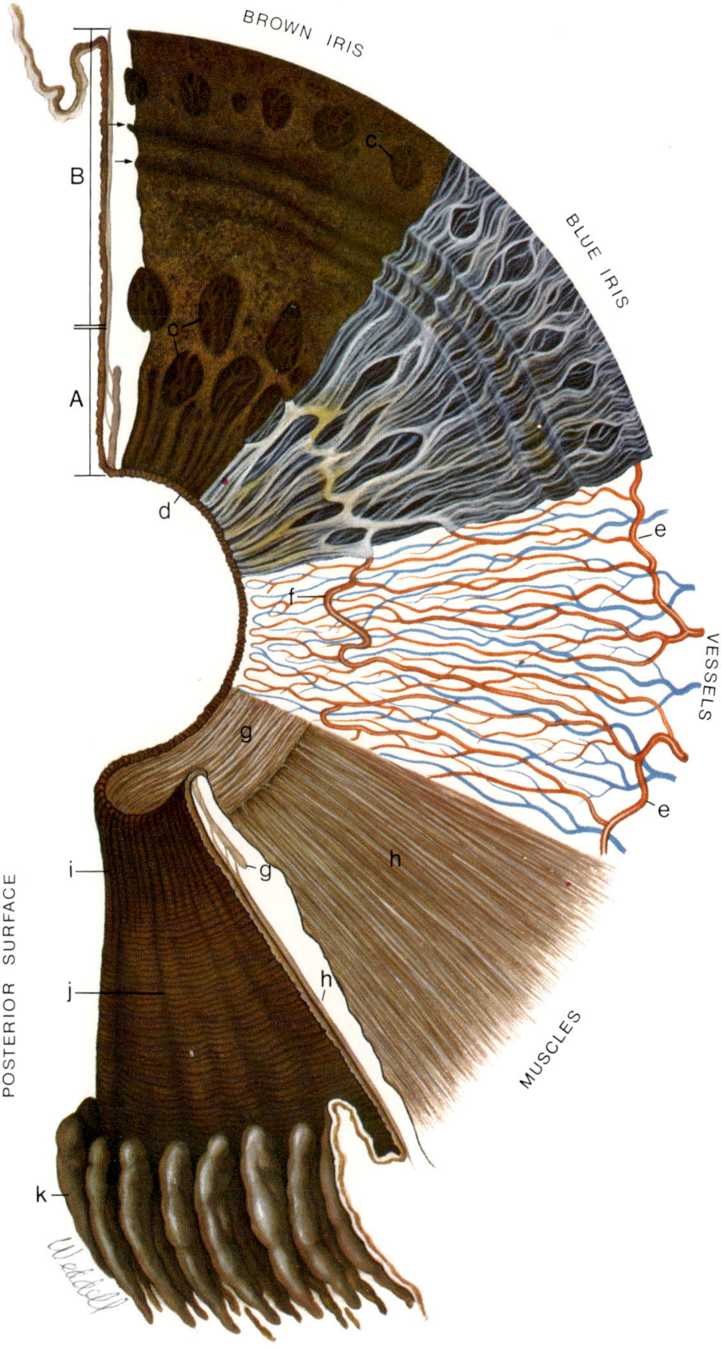

Figure 6–1. *See legend on opposite page.*

Posterior Surface (Fig. 6-1)

The posterior surface of the iris is black because of the pigmentation of the epithelial layers. The surface is quite smooth and contains several types of folds. The *radial contraction folds of Schwalbe* are in the pupillary portion. These radial folds extend outward from the pupil edge to the junction of the pupillary and ciliary parts of the iris. The *structural folds of Schwalbe* are arranged in a radial direction. These folds commence 1.5 mm. from the pupillary margin and their interspaces widen as the folds extend toward the peripheral iris; they then continue into the valleys between the ciliary processes. *Circular folds* are seen near the pupillary margin and result from variations in the thickness of the pigment epithelium. Circular contraction folds like those of the anterior surface also are found in the ciliary portion of the iris.

The central third of the iris is in loose contact with the anterior lens capsule, probably separated from it by a thin layer of aqueous humor. To a certain extent this contact creates a physiologic seclusion of the pupil. The flow of aqueous humor from posterior to anterior chamber, however, prevents constant contact between iris and lens capsule. The area of iris-lens contact may be more extensive in eyes with a shallow anterior chamber; under proper conditions (partial mydriasis) the physiologic seclusion may be effective in initiating the onset of angle closure glaucoma.

Blood Supply (Fig. 6-1)

The iris receives its arterial blood supply from the major arterial circle, which lies in the stroma of the ciliary body near the iris root (Fig. 8–3, p. 326). Branches from the major circle enter the periphery of the iris through its root. These branches occupy the anterior iris stroma as they extend toward the collarette. The branches of the these vessels supply the stroma and posterior iris. The main branches finally form an incomplete circular arterial ring at the collarette. The branches from the minor circle extend into the pupillary region to form capillary arcades; these then join venules behind the sphincter muscle. Branches from the minor circle also pass posteriorly between the bundles of the sphincter muscle to supply the muscle and the posterior iris. The iris venous channels roughly follow the arterial ones, the larger veins lying in the anterior stroma and the smaller ones near the dilator muscle. The collector trunks from these veins enter the ciliary body, where the blood then drains into the vortex system and the ciliary plexus.

Nerve Supply

The finer nerves to the sphincter and dilator muscles have been discussed in the section on physiology. The larger nerve trunks are myelinated or unmyelinated and enter the iris root from the ciliary body. They are principally sensory and vasomotor in function and are derived from the trigeminal nerve. The sensory nerves are diffusely distributed in the stroma and terminate as unmyelinated filaments without special endings. The sympathetic and parasympathetic nerves to the muscles enter the iris with the sensory nerves, then are distributed to the tissues surrounding the muscle cells.

MICROSCOPIC ANATOMY

The iris can be divided into the following parts: (1) anterior border layer, (2) stroma and sphincter muscle, (3) anterior epithelium and dilator muscle, and (4) posterior pigmented epithelium.

ANTERIOR BORDER LAYER (Figs. 6-2 to 6-9)

This layer is a modification of the stroma, differing from the stroma by its paucity of collagen and by the accumulation of cells, particularly melanocytes, which are oriented parallel to the iris surface. The anterior border layer varies in thickness, being thicker in brown than blue irises, and it may be absent or very thin near the openings of the iris crypts. The anterior border layer is thickest in the pupillary portion of the collarette and near the periphery of the ciliary region. Depending on its density and pigmentation, this layer has a great deal to do with the color of the iris. It is principally composed of melanocytes and fibroblasts whose processes branch frequently to form a dense meshwork. For many years it was believed that the anterior surface of the iris was covered by a layer of endothelium. Vrabec (1951, 1952) showed that an endothelium does exist over the anterior surface of the human iris at birth, but that it disappears after the first or second year of life when the cells are replaced by fibroblasts. Previous electron microscopic studies have also shown that there is no real endothelium on the anterior iris surface (Tousimis and Fine, 1959 a, b).

The density and arrangement of the meshwork of the anterior border layer varies from section to section and even within sections. In some areas it forms a thick layer, sufficient to cause an elevation of the iris surface, while in other areas it is only two to three cells thick. The thickness increases over the contraction furrows and the trabeculae. On its deep side the anterior border layer is fairly distinct from the adjacent stromal tissue of the iris. At the margins of the crypts the branching cell processes of this layer outline the openings into the crypts, but they may be absent in the edges of the crypts. Thin operculae have been described over the mouths of some crypts, but this observation has not been verified by recent light and electron microscopic studies. The anterior border layer becomes thicker and quite dense in the pupillary portion of the iris; at the pupillary margin the layer is firmly joined to the two epithelial cell layers of the pigment ruff. Localized accumulations of pigmented melanocytes frequently form freckle-like masses in the anterior border layer, especially in pigmented irises that are slightly elevated. Freckles may not be so distinct in blue irises because of their lesser pigmentation.

Nevus-like structures, probably derived from Schwann cells, also are observed in the anterior border layer. In eyes with congenital heterochromia of the iris there are more melanocytes in the pigmented areas of the anterior

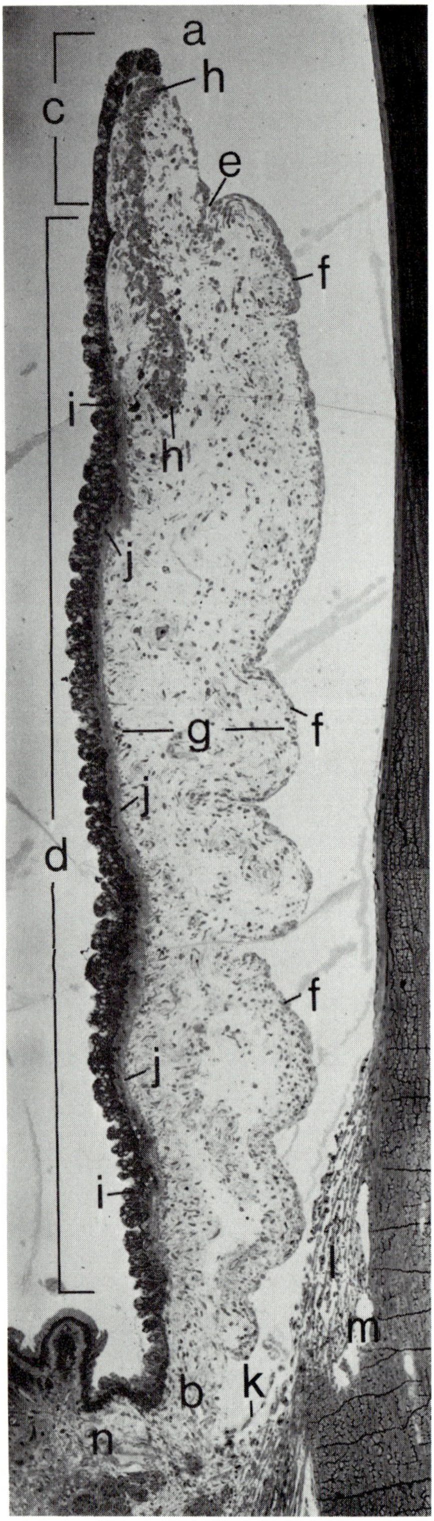

Figure 6–2. Iris and anterior chamber, light micrograph. The cornea, anterior chamber angle, trabecular meshwork, canal of Schlemm and part of the ciliary body are included. The anterior and posterior iris contraction furrows are accentuated by the slight dilatation of the pupil. The pupil and the pupillary ruff are at (a) and the iris root is at (b). The pupillary portion of the iris is at (c) and the ciliary portion at (d). The collarette (e) and minor arterial circle of the iris lie at the junction of these two portions. The cellular anterior border layer (f) is distinct from the very loosely arranged stromal tissue (g). The sphincter muscle lies in the stroma at (h). The posterior iris shows a posterior (i) and anterior (j) epithelium; the latter forms the dilator muscle. The anterior chamber angle shows part of a uveal band (k). The trabecular meshwork (l) and canal of Schlemm (m) lie external to the chamber angle. The ciliary body and its muscle are posterior to the iris (n). (× 60.)

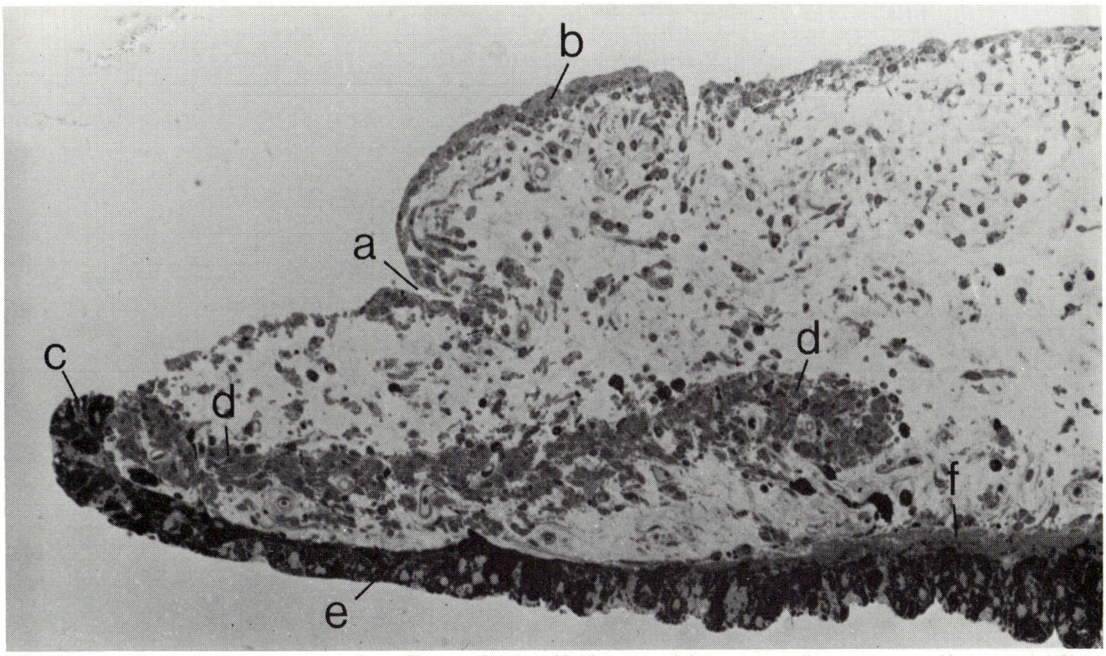

Figure 6–3. Pupillary portion of the iris. The pupil is slightly dilated so that the collarette is somewhat retracted into the stroma (a). The anterior border layer forms a distinct zone along the iris surface (b). The pigment ruff (c) is close to the termination of the sphincter muscle (d). The posterior epithelial layers are pigmented (e), and the dilator muscle ends behind the sphincter at (f). (× 450.)

border layer and fewer in the unpigmented areas. Capillaries are commonly seen in the anterior border layer and may be located very close to the surface of the iris. These vessels increase in number and size in iritis and diabetes, producing the condition known as neovascularization or rubeosis of the iris. Nerve filaments also approach this layer and terminate in the adjacent stroma.

The anterior border layer has been studied with the electron microscope by many investigators (Magari, 1957; Tousimis and Fine, 1959, a, b; Ueno, 1961; Iwamoto, 1961; Smelser and Ishikawa, 1966). The layer is composed of two types of cells, pigmented melanocytes and fibroblasts. The fibroblasts form a reasonably continuous single layer of cells over the surface of the iris from the base to the pupillary margin. These cells have branches which radiate out in many directions to form a thin layer on the iris surface. Wherever adjacent cells contact each other there is a narrow intercellular space of 200 A., but no intercellular junctions have been seen. Some of these fibroblasts show basal bodies in the cytoplasm with cilia projecting into the anterior chamber. At the periphery of the iris, the fibroblasts are continuous with those on the surface of the ciliary body and iris processes or pectinate fibers. At the pupillary margin they come into contact with the cells of the pigment epithelium but are not connected to them by special junctions. In the thickest parts of the anterior border layer pigmented cells are much more numerous than fibroblasts. The uveal melanocytes also are oriented parallel to the surface of the iris in the anterior border layer but are located beneath

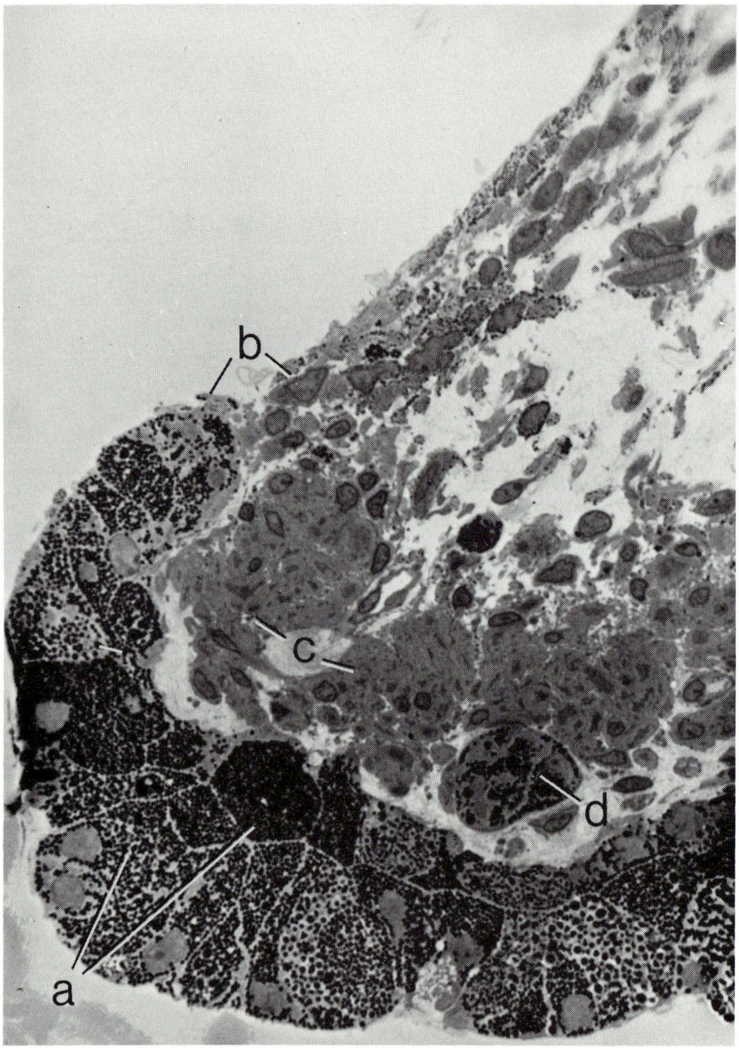

Figure 6–4. Pupillary margin of the iris to show the two pigment epithelial layers (a) and their continuity with the anterior border layer of the iris (b). The sphincter muscle of the iris (c) is slightly curved near the pupillary margin and is continuous with the anterior border layer by a thin layer of connective tissue. A clump cell measuring 90 μm. (d) is seen near the sphincter muscle. (× 680.)

the fibroblasts. Their many branching processes extend a great distance from the cell body and they frequently contact each other, as well as the processes of the fibroblasts, but no special junctions have been observed between any of the cells. The structure of these cells will be described in the iris stroma.

Iwamoto (1961) has subdivided the cells of the anterior border layer into several other varieties, based on their morphology, but all the cells we have observed are either fibroblasts or melanocytes. Around the margins of the crypts the fibroblasts continue to form a single layer over the surface of the iris, the melanocytes being disposed beneath them. The blood vessels of the anterior border layer are capillaries and venules, with the same structure as those found elsewhere in the iris.

Text continued on page 218

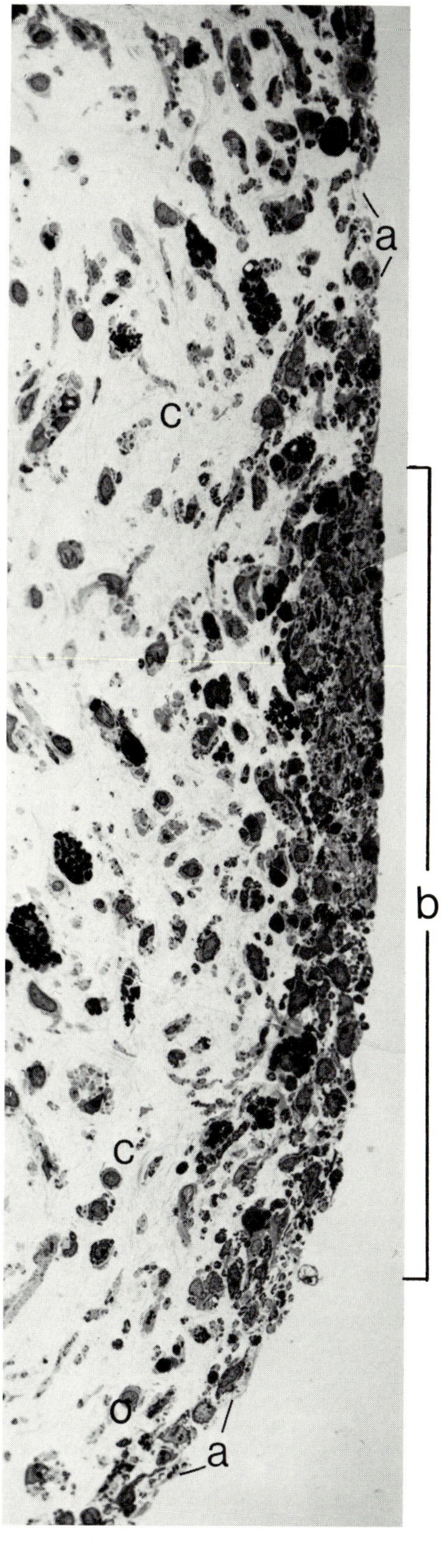

Figure 6–5. A pigmented iris showing the anterior border layer (a) and an iris freckle (b). In the area of the freckle the anterior border layer becomes more cellular. The iris stroma (c) beneath the freckle also is more cellular. (× 400.)

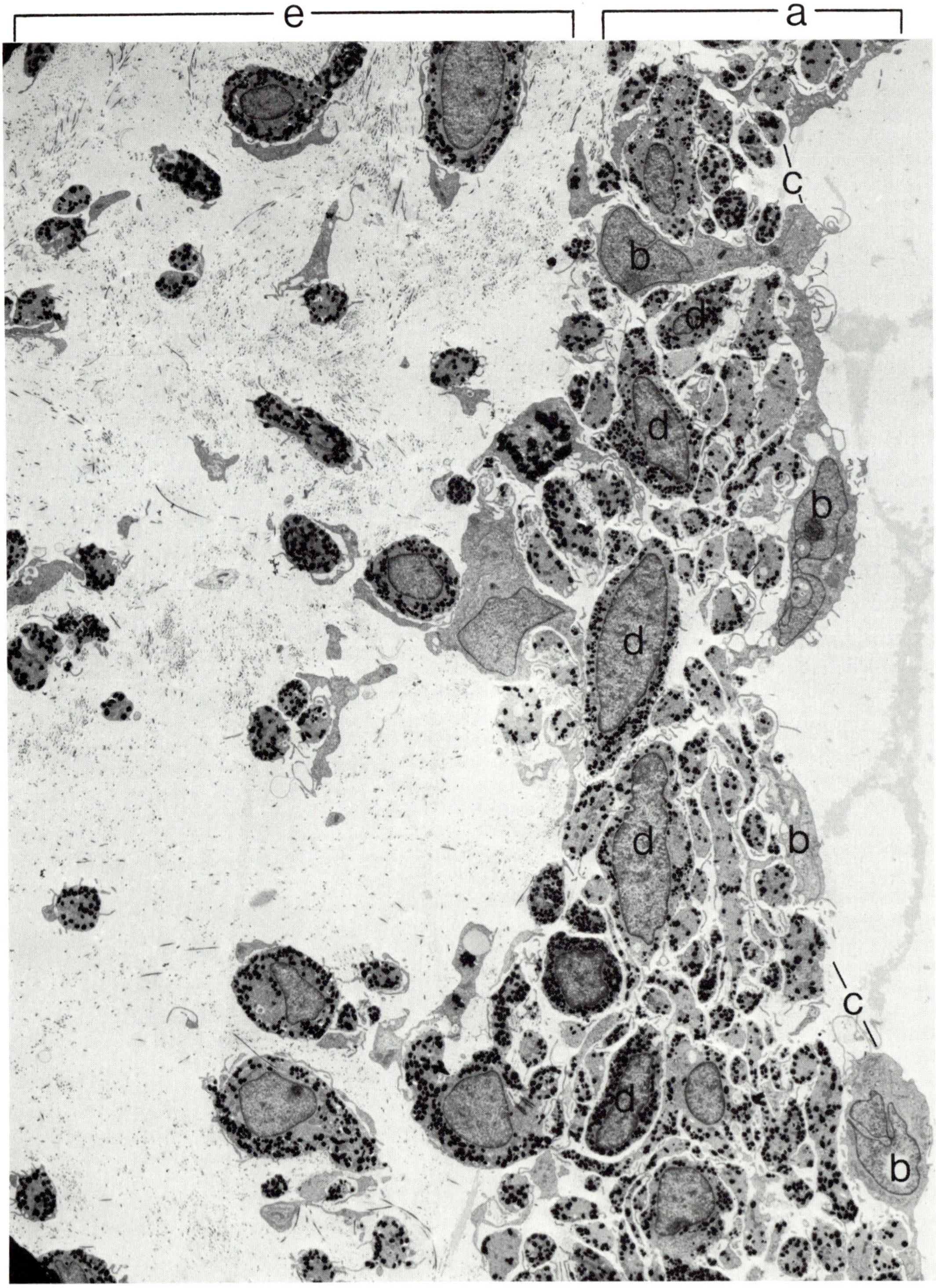

Figure 6-6. Anterior border layer, low-magnification electron micrograph. This layer (a) of the iris consists of an anteriormost layer of fibroblasts (b) which are interrupted here and there (c) by gaps. Melanocytes and their processes (d) also are found in this layer and adjacent stroma. The stroma (e) is distinguished from the anterior border layer by its lessened density and fewer cells. (× 2280.)

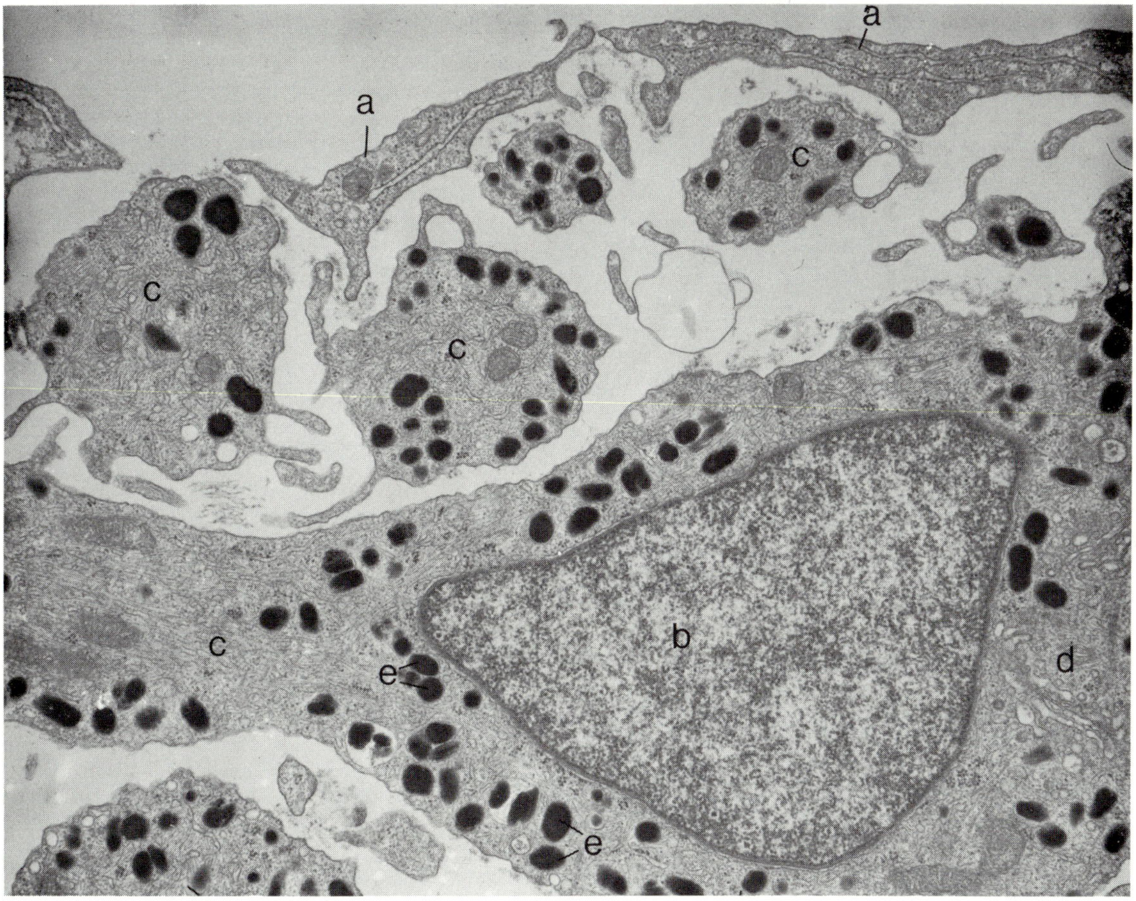

Figure 6–7. Anterior border layer, electron micrograph. The thin layer of fibroblasts on the anterior iris surface (a) is not continuous. Melanocytes (b) and their processes (c) form part of the anterior border layer. The Golgi apparatus (d) and melanin granules (e) are shown. (× 18,000.)

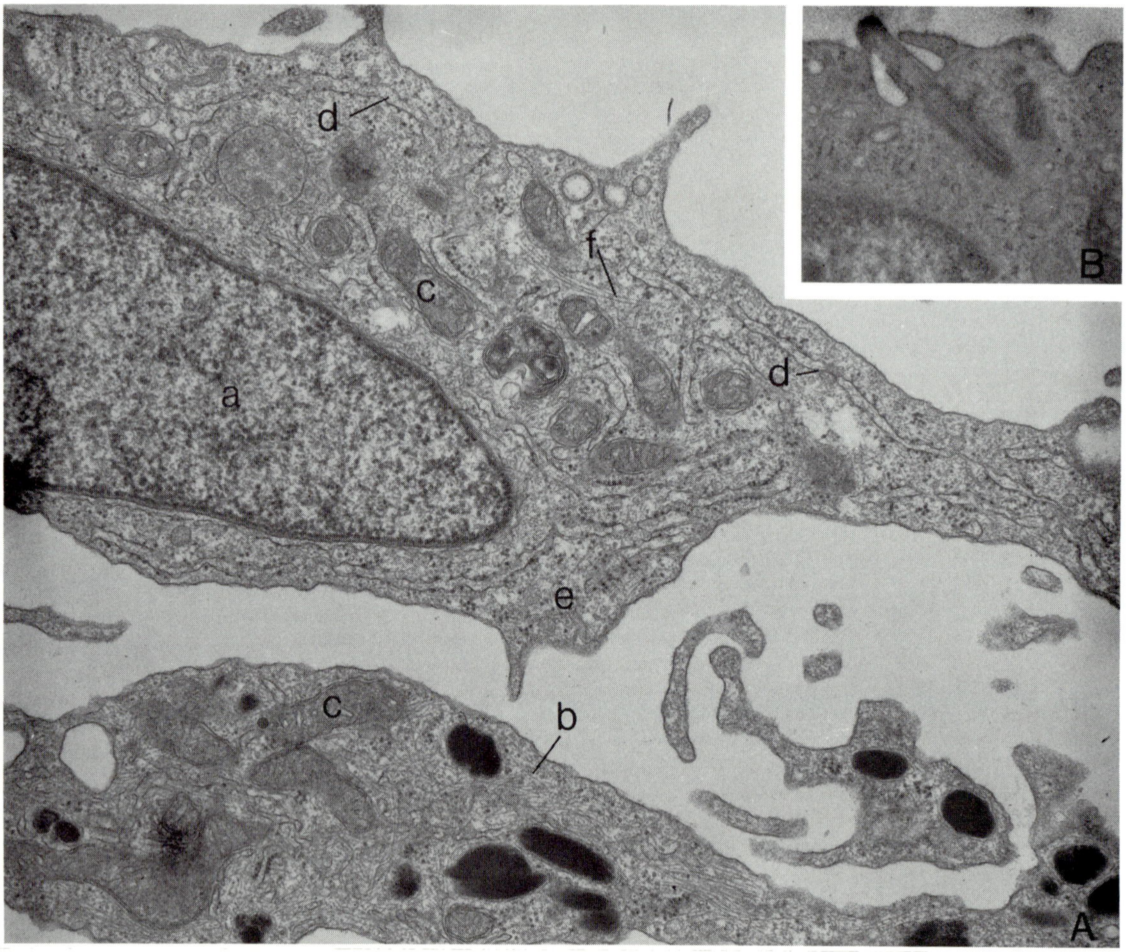

Figure 6–8. *A*, The nucleus of a fibroblast (a) on the anterior iris surface and a melanocyte (b) beneath it are indicated. The fibroblast contains abundant mitochondria (c), rough-surfaced endoplasmic reticulum (d), free ribosomes (e) and a moderate number of filaments which are arranged in bundles (f). The melanocyte cytoplasm is more filamentous and contains typical melanin granules. (× 30,000.)

B, A cilium projecting into the anterior chamber from a fibroblast on the anterior iris surface. (× 31,700.)

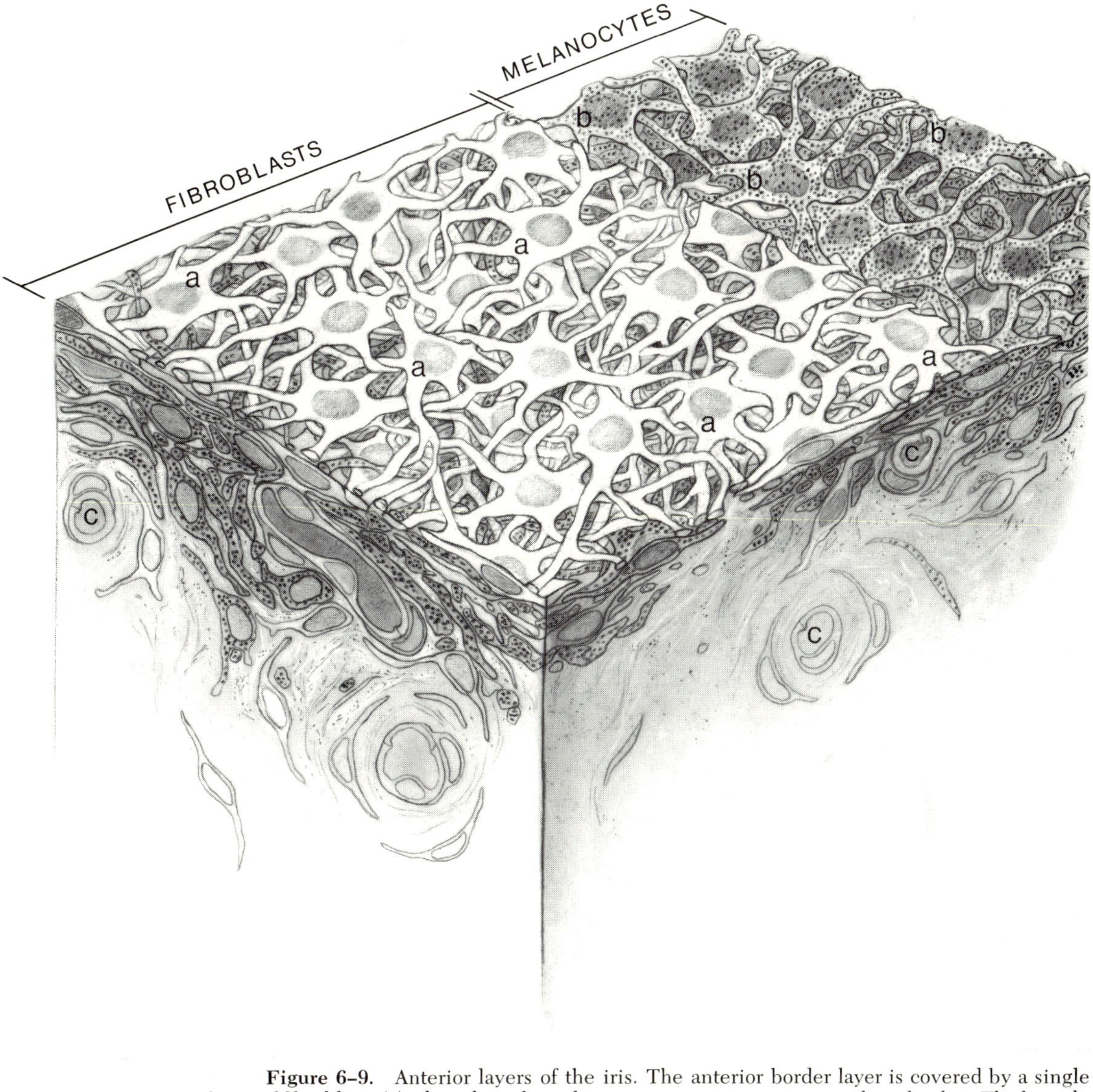

Figure 6–9. Anterior layers of the iris. The anterior border layer is covered by a single layer of fibroblasts (a) whose long, branching processes interconnect with each other. The branching processes of the fibroblasts form varying sized openings on the iris surface. Beneath the layer of fibroblasts is a fairly dense aggregation of melanocytes and a few fibroblasts. The superficial layer of fibroblasts has been removed at (b) to show these cells. The number of cells in the anterior border layer is greater than in the underlying stroma. The iris stroma contains a number of capillaries (c) which sometimes are quite close to the surface.

STROMA (Figs. 6-2 and 6-10 to 6-18)

The cells of the iris stroma are mostly fibroblasts and melanocytes, and the collagenous connective tissue framework is loosely arranged so that its open meshes contain a mucopolysaccharide ground substance and fluid; there is no elastic tissue. The sphincter muscle, blood vessels and nerves are located within this connective tissue framework. The framework is anchored to the anterior border layer and to the sphincter and dilator muscles, and it is continuous with the connective tissue of the ciliary body at the iris root. To a certain extent the iris stroma slides peripherally and centrally during dilation and constriction of the pupil, but for the most part it tends to fold or unfold rather than to slide. By light microscopy the collagen of the iris framework is extremely delicate; thus, intense staining is required to demonstrate it in the stroma. The collagen fibrils form small and large bundles which intersect at wide angles to form spaces of variable size. The collagen is more abundant and easier to demonstrate in the heavy sheaths around the blood vessels and nerves, in the iris trabeculae, and between the bundles of the sphincter muscle. Around the edge of the pupil the collagen bundles are oriented in a circular direction, whereas in the sphincter region they are more meridional.

Rohen (1961) found a precise pattern in the arrangement of the iris connective tissue fibers in birds and in many mammals. He observed that the collagen fibrils are organized in semicircular patterns, forming wide arches as they course toward the ciliary body from the pupillary region. Some of these arches are arranged clockwise, and others counterclockwise, forming a series of overlapping arcades. Rohen found a similar pattern in the human iris, except for the looser arrangement of the collagen and the presence of clefts and channels in the central stroma. This loose arrangement gives the impression that an empty space may exist between the anterior and posterior portions of the iris. An incomplete cleft can be seen in the stroma of some human irises, but there is probably no continuous cleft in the adult human eye. The human iris does contain tissue spaces, some of which are radial while others are meridional. If India ink is injected into the anterior chamber either intravitally or post mortem, it will pass deeply into the iris stroma. The ink enters the iris through gaps in the iris surface and Fuchs' crypts to pass into the adjacent connective tissue spaces. Injected killed cocci follow the same pattern of distribution in the stroma (Gregersen, 1960). Gregersen (1958) and Smelser and Ishikawa (1966), using substances of different molecular weight as well as bacteria and Thorotrast, showed that particles can enter the iris stroma rapidly both through the crypts and the other openings between the cells of the anterior border layer. These substances then diffuse into all the tissue spaces of the iris, around the endothelium of the blood vessels, and into the dilator muscle region. The iris appears to be freely permeable to fluids from the anterior chamber, as well as to particles measuring between 50 to 200 μm. in diameter. Dextran injected into the anterior chamber passes through the anterior border layer and eventually is distributed widely in the stroma, even in the spaces around the vascular endothelium (Gregersen, 1960).

By electron microscopy the collagen fibrils of the iris stroma are approximately 600 A. in width and have an axial periodicity of 500 to 600 A. (Tousimis and Fine, 1959). The iris stroma is in communication with the aqueous humor through many small openings in the anterior border layer.

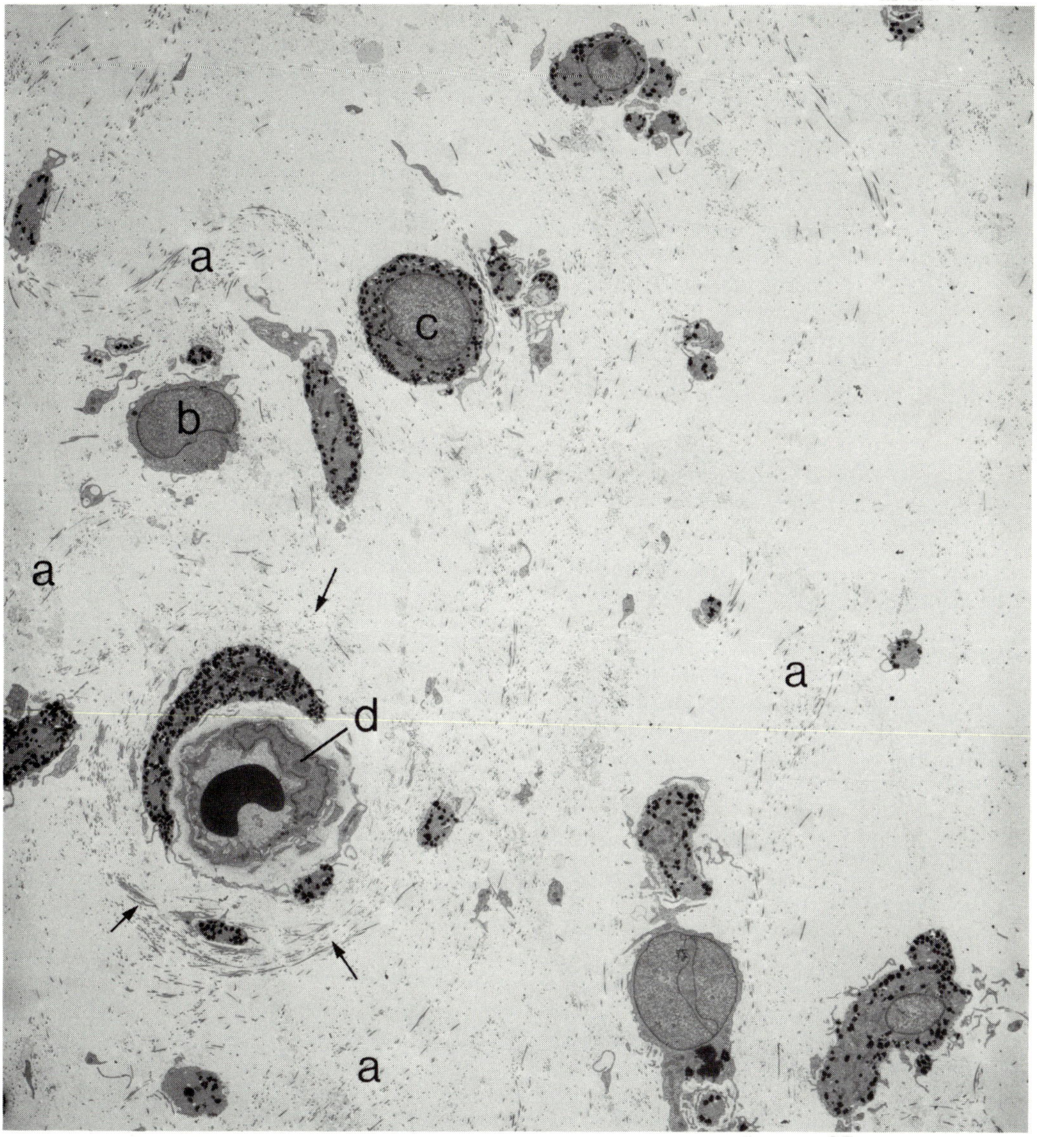

Figure 6–10. Iris stroma, electron micrograph. The loose iris connective tissue is composed of relatively few dispersed collagen fibrils (a) which increase in density in the adventitia of blood vessels (arrows). Fibroblasts (b), melanocytes (c), mast cells, nerves and blood vessels (d) are also found in the stroma. (× 2280.)

Since the collagen fibrils are so loosely arranged in the iris stroma, it is not surprising that particles 50 to 200 μm. in size can diffuse widely in the stroma after injection into the anterior chamber. Most of the ground substance of the iris stroma usually is extracted during preparation of tissues, so that sections show irregular, apparently empty spaces within the collagen fibrils and bundles. Occasionally a finely granular material is preserved, which may be the alcian blue-positive mucopolysaccharide, sensitive to hyaluronidase, that has been described by light microscopy (Zimmerman, 1957).

Iwamoto (1961) has described seven different types of unpigmented stromal cells in the iris. The cells we have identified in the iris are fibroblasts,

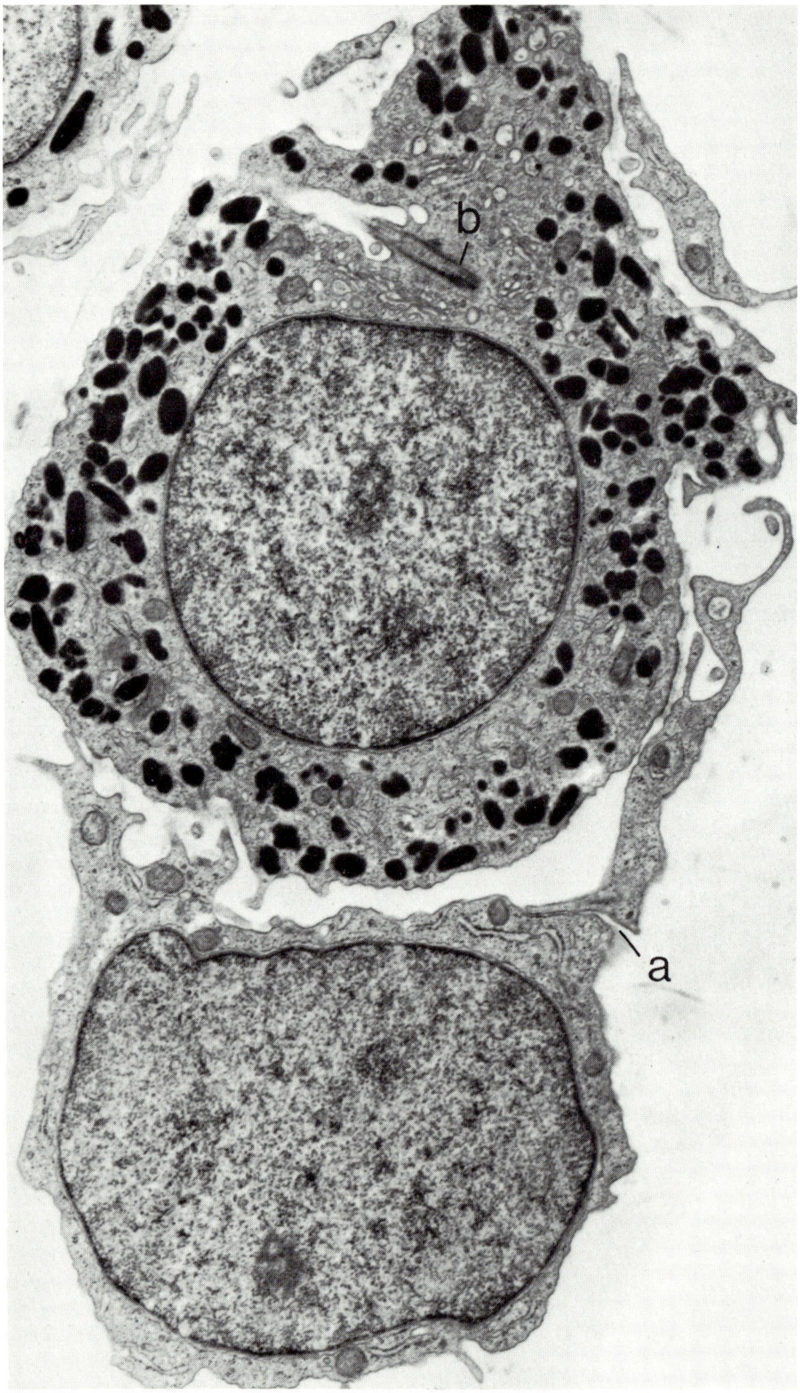

Figure 6–11. A melanocyte and a fibroblast in the iris stroma. The melanocytes of the stroma have a more abundant cytoplasm than those of the anterior border layer. The two cells shown here are separated from each other by a narrow intercellular space (a). A cilium projects into the iris stroma from the cytoplasm of the melanocyte (b). The melanocyte granules are completely melanized. (× 13,200.)

melanocytes, clump cells, mast cells, macrophages and lymphocytes. The principal cell of the iris stroma is the *fibroblast* (Figs. 6–11 and 6–12). Fibroblasts congregate around blood vessels, nerves and muscle tissue and are intimately associated with the support of these tissues. These cells are occasionally seen undergoing mitosis; they possess the usual organelle composition of the cells actively secreting large macromolecules. Cilia commonly are observed in the fibroblasts. The *melanocytes* have a small oval body, a prominent nucleus and nucleoli and heavy branching processes that measure up to 100 μm. in length. They often form plexuses with adjacent melanocytes and with the fibroblasts, and they are always arranged around the adventitia of a blood vessel. The cytoplasm has a moderate number of

Text continued on page 226

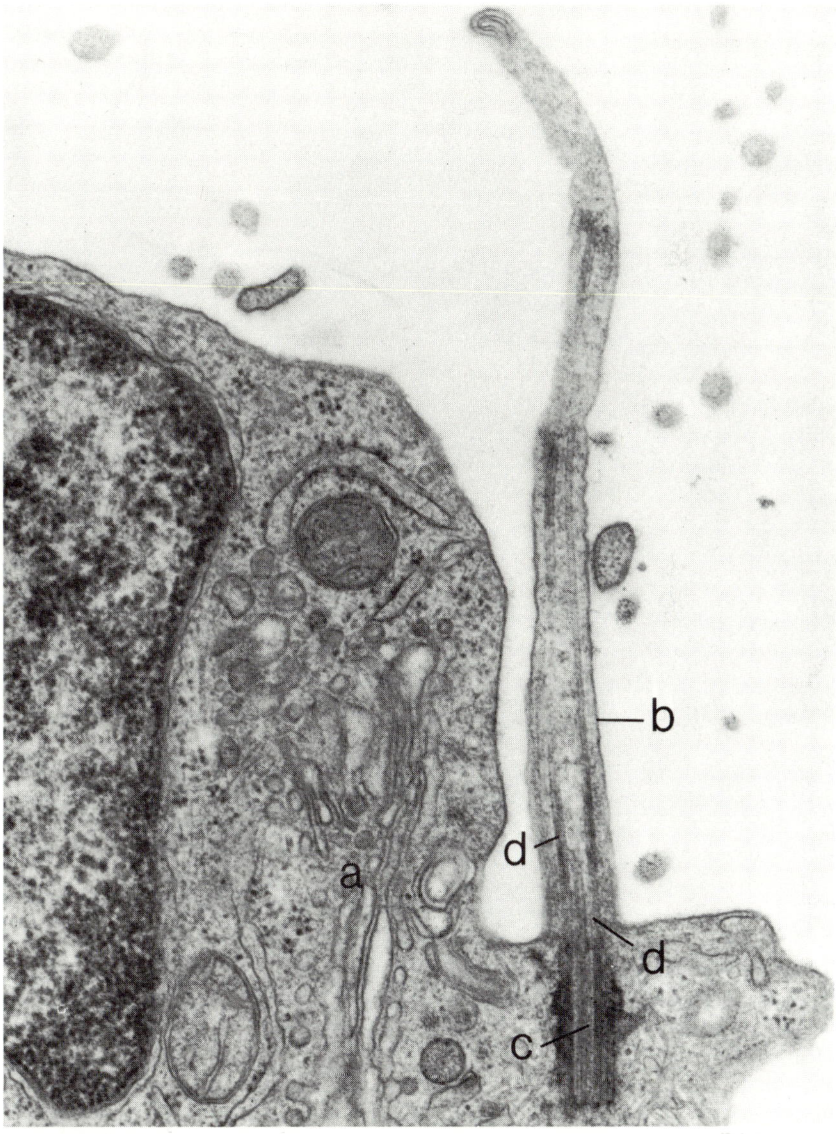

Figure 6–12. Iris stromal fibroblast. The Golgi apparatus is seen at (a) and a cilium (b) arises from the basal body (c) in the cytoplasm. The filaments from the basal body can be traced into the cilium (d). (× 32,000.)

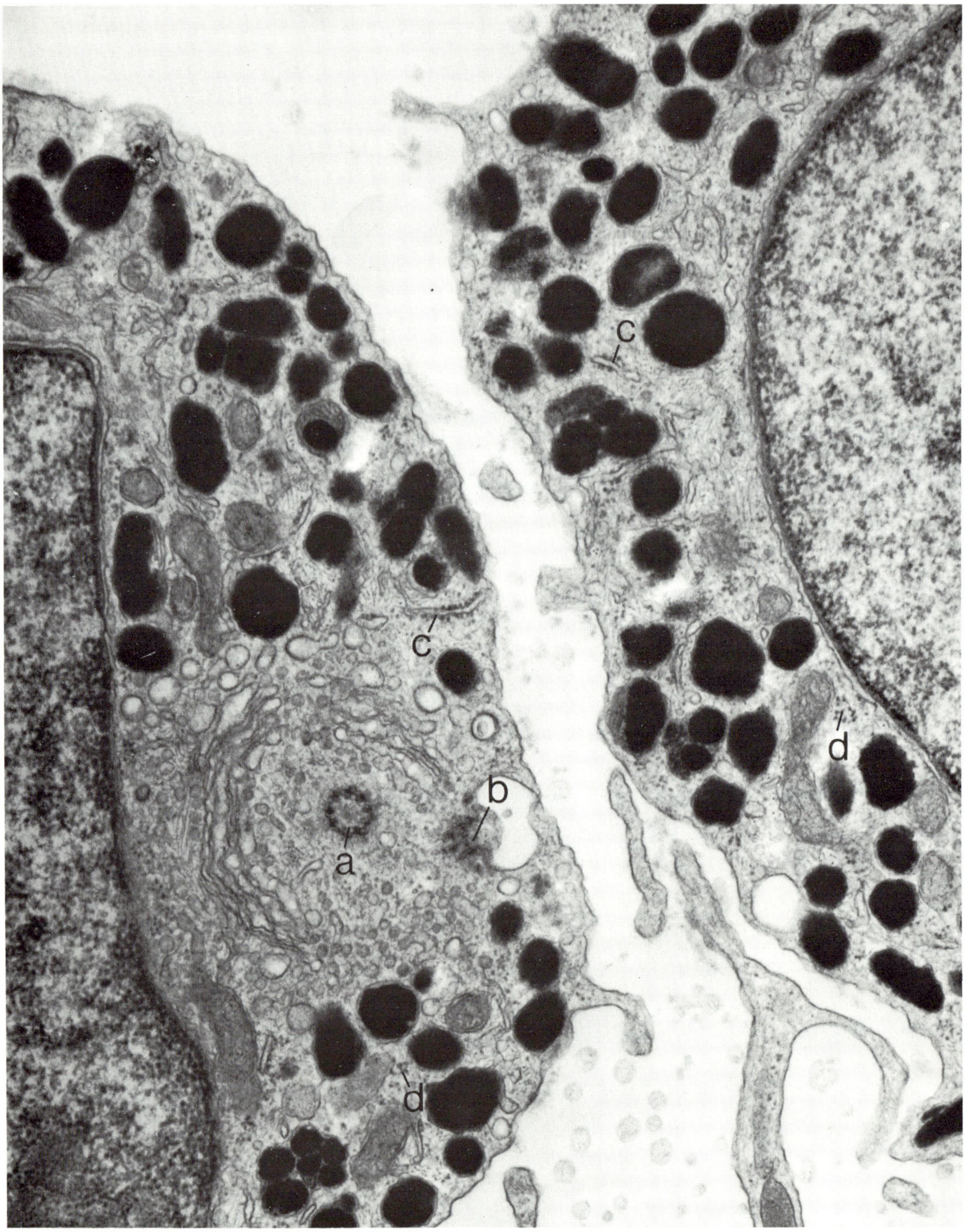

Figure 6–13. Iris stromal melanocytes. The melanin granules are enclosed by a membrane and are filled with melanoprotein. One cell has a well developed Golgi apparatus which surrounds a centriole (a). Part of a cilium is seen at (b). The cytoplasm is filamentous and contains rough-surfaced endoplasmic reticulum (c) and free ribosomes (d). (× 33,000.)

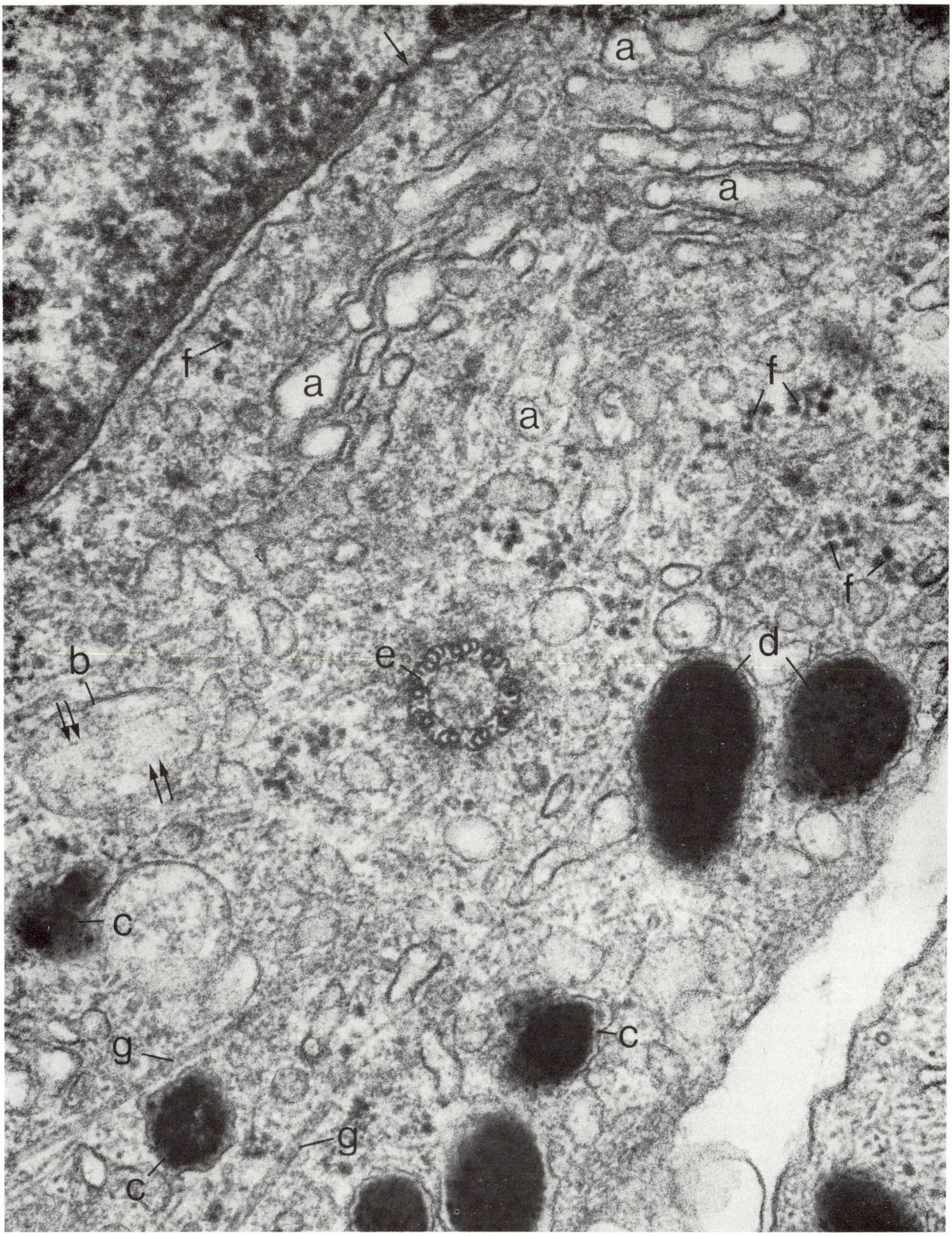

Figure 6–14. Iris stromal melanocyte. A portion of the nucleus is seen at the upper left and its nuclear envelope shows a pore (arrow) containing a diaphragm. The cisternae and vesicles of the Golgi complex (a) occupy a major portion of the cytoplasm. It is believed that the melanin granules are formed in the Golgi apparatus in large vesicles, which initially possess a protein skeleton. The amino acid units of melanin are polymerized on the filaments of this skeleton. The early vesicles are known as premelanosomes; one is shown at (b) with its striated protein skeleton (double arrows). Three partially melanized granules (c) and some fully melanized ones (d) are also seen. The membrane surrounding the granules is easily seen. The cytoplasm also shows a centriole (e), numerous free ribosomes forming close aggregates (f), microtubules (g) and microfilaments. (× 50,000.)

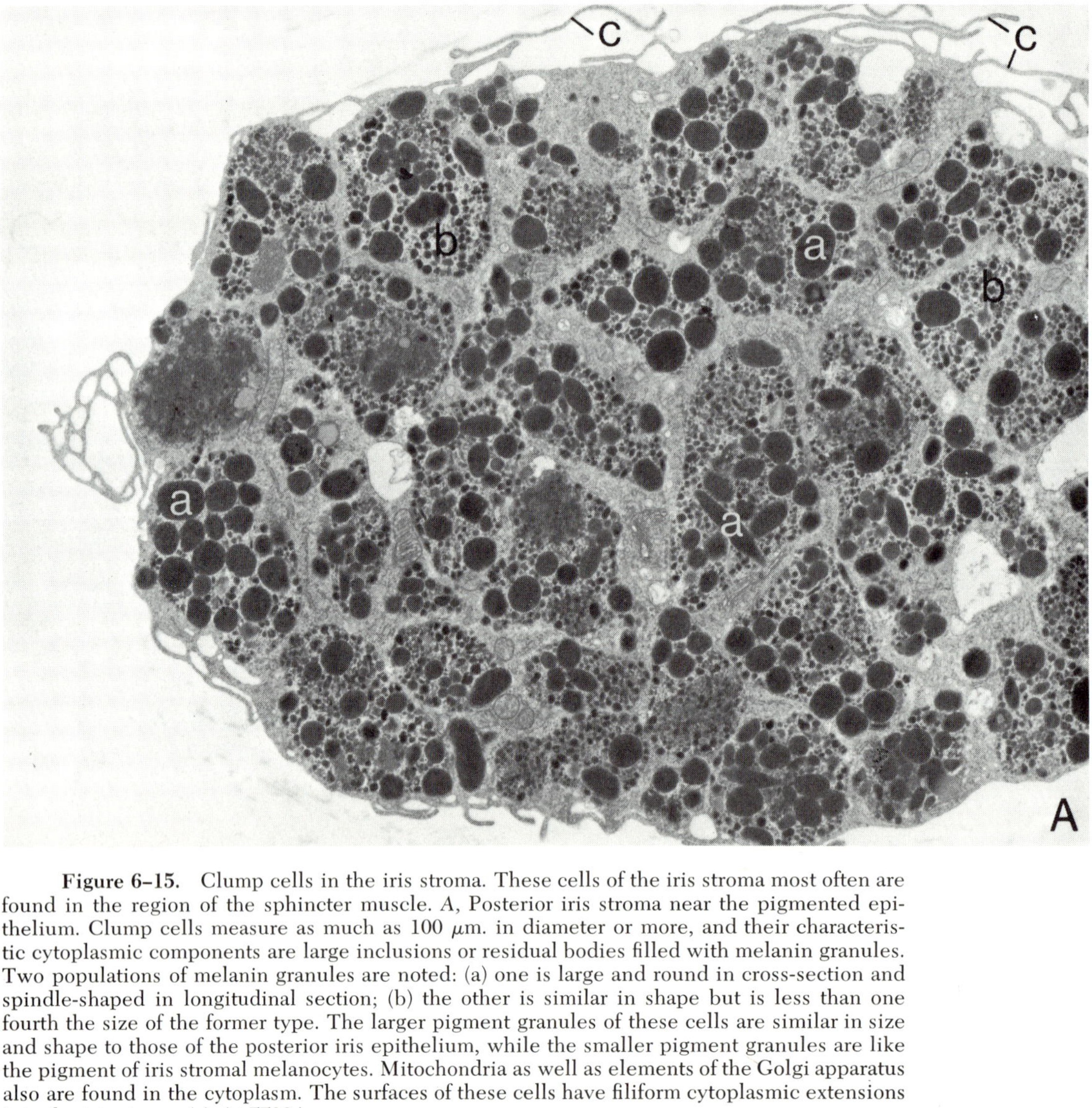

Figure 6–15. Clump cells in the iris stroma. These cells of the iris stroma most often are found in the region of the sphincter muscle. *A*, Posterior iris stroma near the pigmented epithelium. Clump cells measure as much as 100 μm. in diameter or more, and their characteristic cytoplasmic components are large inclusions or residual bodies filled with melanin granules. Two populations of melanin granules are noted: (a) one is large and round in cross-section and spindle-shaped in longitudinal section; (b) the other is similar in shape but is less than one fourth the size of the former type. The larger pigment granules of these cells are similar in size and shape to those of the posterior iris epithelium, while the smaller pigment granules are like the pigment of iris stromal melanocytes. Mitochondria as well as elements of the Golgi apparatus also are found in the cytoplasm. The surfaces of these cells have filiform cytoplasmic extensions into the iris stroma (c). (× 7700.)

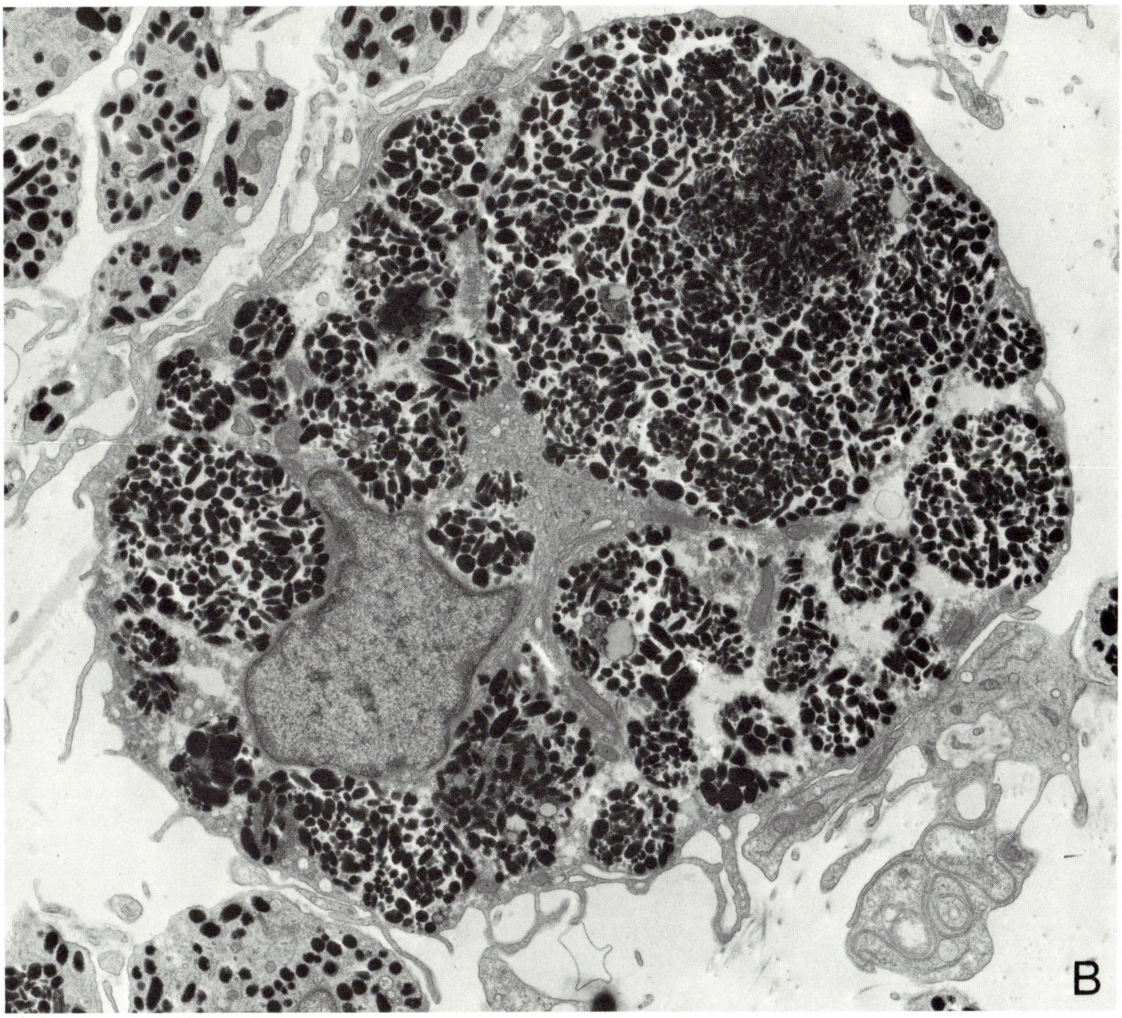

Figure 6–15. *Continued.*

B, Clump cell of the anterior stroma. The residual bodies of the clump cells of the anterior stroma are filled with small melanin granules like those in the stromal melanocytes. Note that the melanin granules of the melanocytes are identical to those in this clump cell. (× 10,500.)

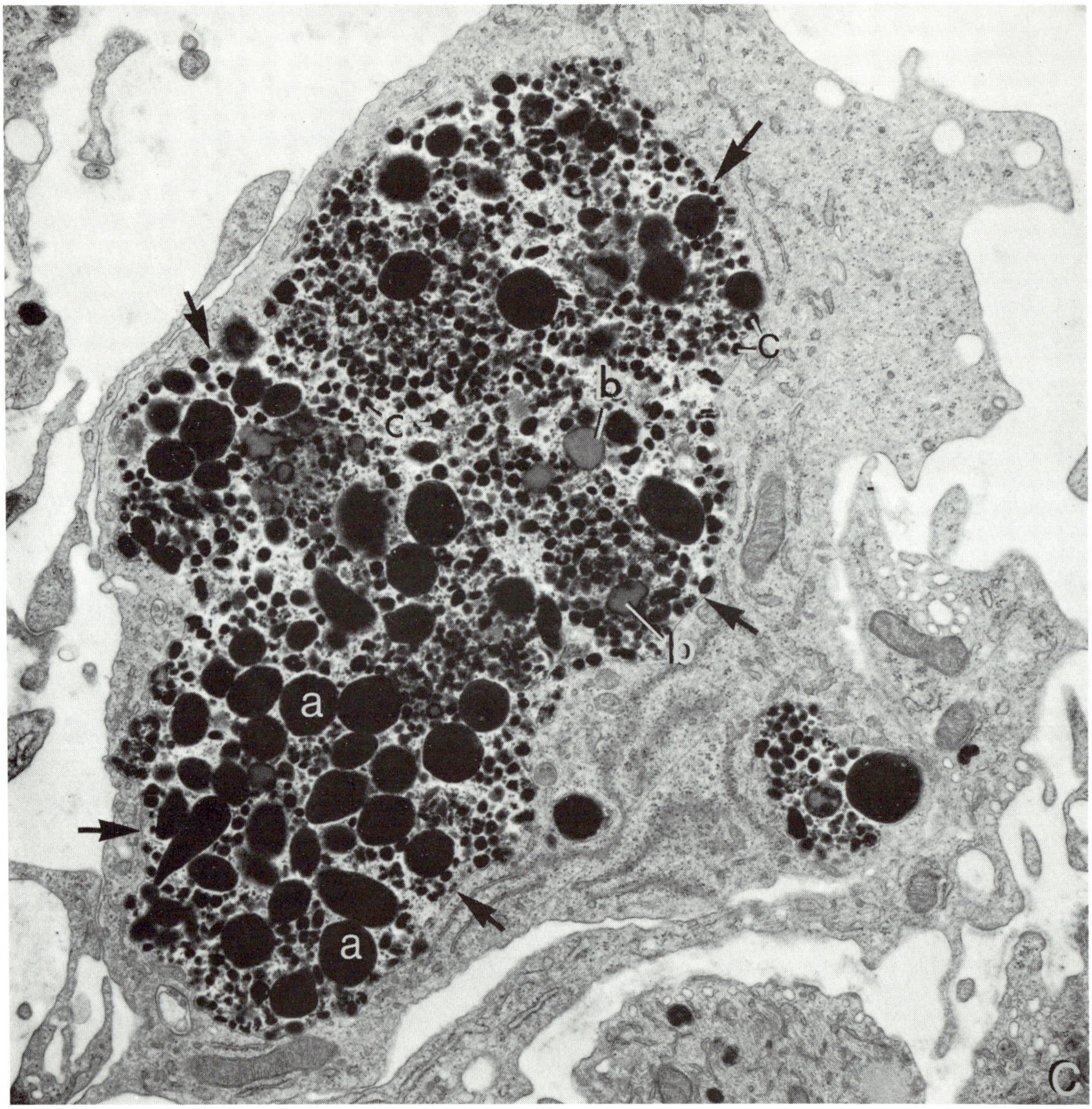

Figure 6–15. *Continued.*

C, Residual body in a clump cell to show its enveloping membrane (heavy arrows), large melanin granules (a), less dense lipid particles (b) and small pigment granules (c). The cytoplasm also contains cisternae of endoplasmic reticulum, free and attached ribosomes, mitochondria and filaments. (× 10,500.)

mitochondria, some vesicular profiles of both smooth- and rough-surfaced endoplasmic reticulum and free ribosomes. Melanin granules in various stages of development are seen in the cytoplasm, including premelanosomes, melanosomes and fully melanized granules. The granules are round to oval and measure up to 0.5 μm. in diameter. These granules are found in the cytoplasm and in the processes.

Clump cells commonly are found in the pupillary portion of the iris, especially around the sphincter muscle, but they also occur elsewhere. By light microscopy these cells appear as large round cells whose cytoplasm is filled with inclusion granules so large that they may obscure the nucleus.

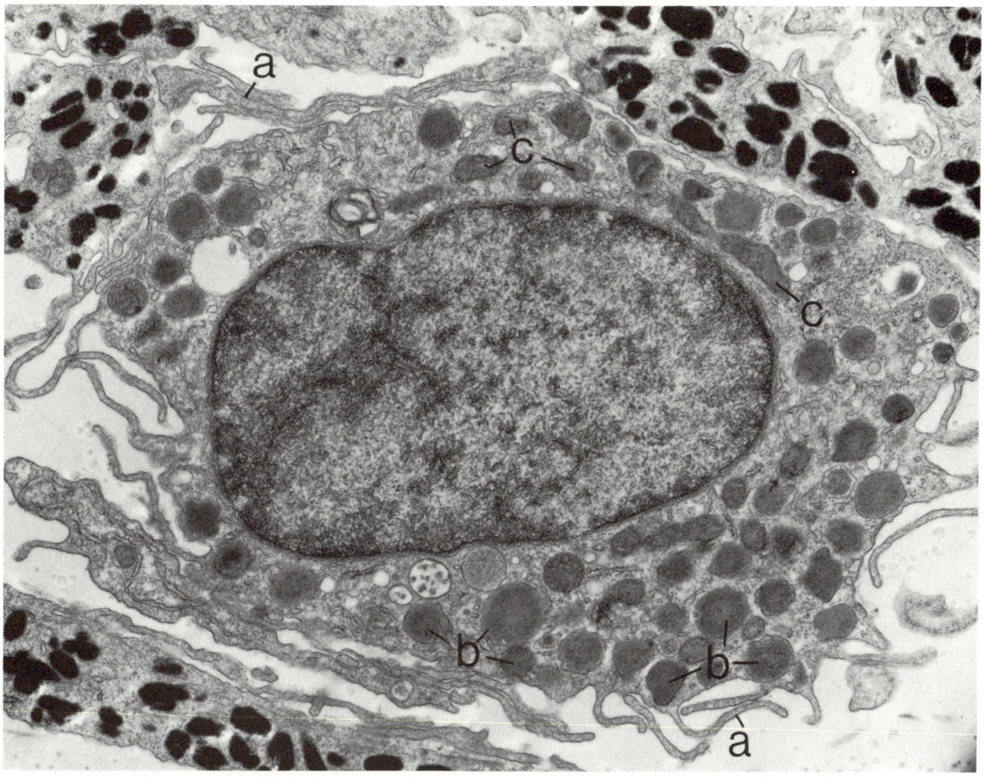

Figure 6–16. Iris mast cell, electron micrograph. The mast cells here are typically round, in contrast to the elongated mast cells of the limbus. There are long cytoplasmic processes (a) which extend from the cell surface into the iris stroma. Numerous typical mast cell granules are seen (b). The nucleus is centrally located, and the mitochondria (c) are similar in size to the granules. Several melanocytes are adjacent to this cell. (× 20,000.)

These cells may measure as much as 100 μm. in diameter, and their surfaces show villous processes measuring 1 or 2 μm. long and about 0.1 μm. wide (Tousimis and Fine, 1959; Iwamoto, 1961). The cytoplasmic granules observed by light microscopy are seen to be membrane-bound vesicles of varying size that can be up to 10 μm. in diameter when studied by electron microscopy. These vesicles contain mainly melanin granules and are considered to be residual bodies or secondary lysosomes. The clear and consistent appearance of these granules suggests they may not be susceptible to digestion by the lysosomal enzymes. Other substances found in these vesicles are lipid or lipoidal vesicles and a granular matrix. Clump cells are difficult to demonstrate in the irises of the young but are quite common in older eyes. Moreover, the type of melanin granule contained in the residual bodies varies according to the location of the clump cell. Those cells found in the posterior iris stroma contain a greater number of large melanin granules identical in size and shape to the pigment granules found in the neighboring epithelia, while those found in the anterior stroma have a greater number of small melanin granules similar to those found in melanocytes. Clump cells have traditionally been regarded as displaced neuroectodermal cells which exist in all irises, including blue irises. It is possible that these cells are altered macrophages which have ingested a large number of melanin granules.

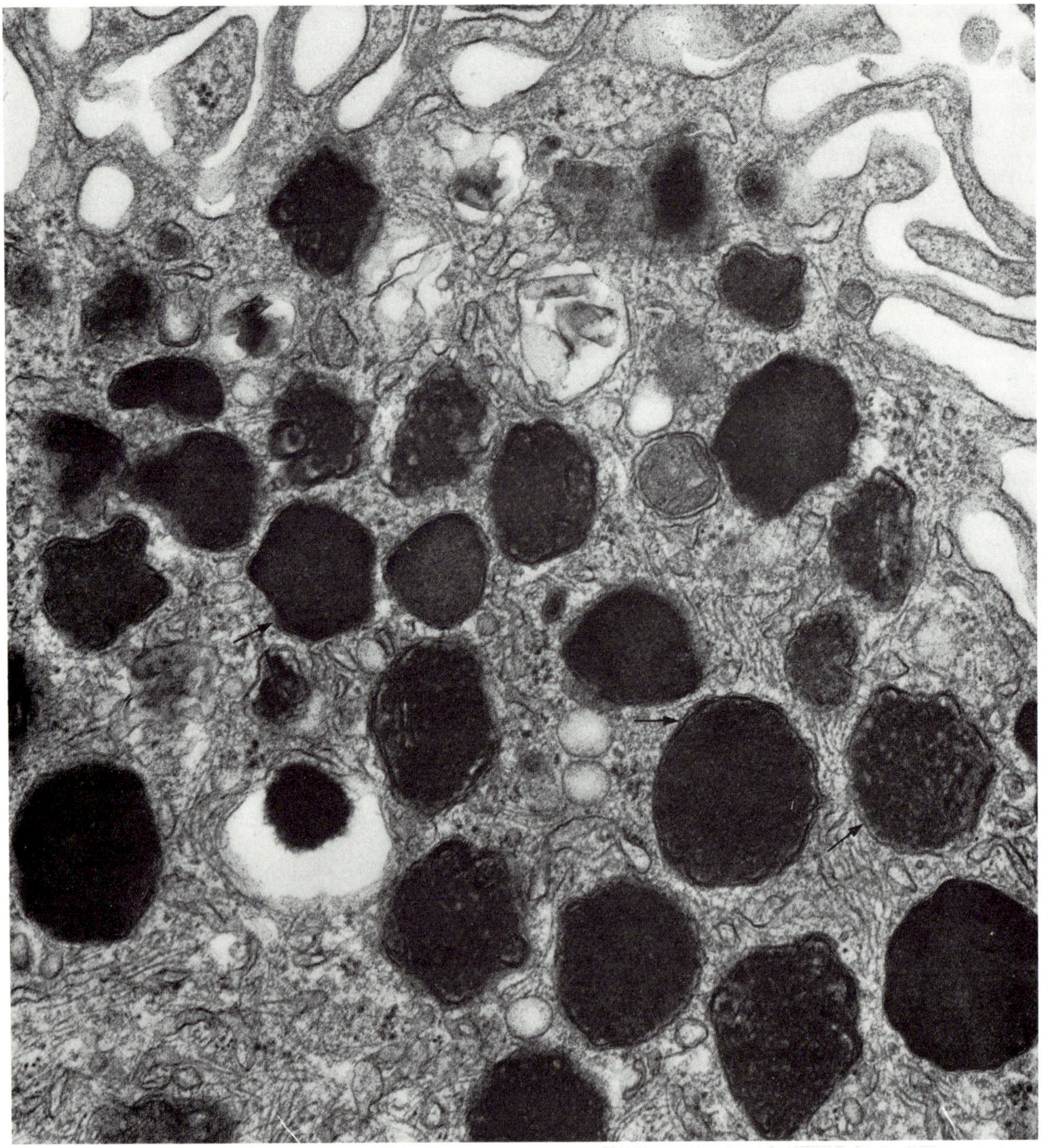

Figure 6–17. Mast cell depicted at higher magnification. Each mast cell granule has a surrounding membrane (arrows). The granules are filled with an electron-dense material which is believed to contain vasoactive substances and heparin. The cytoplasm also contains numerous filaments, unattached ribosomes, a few cisternae of the rough endoplasmic reticulum and a Golgi apparatus. (× 37,500.)

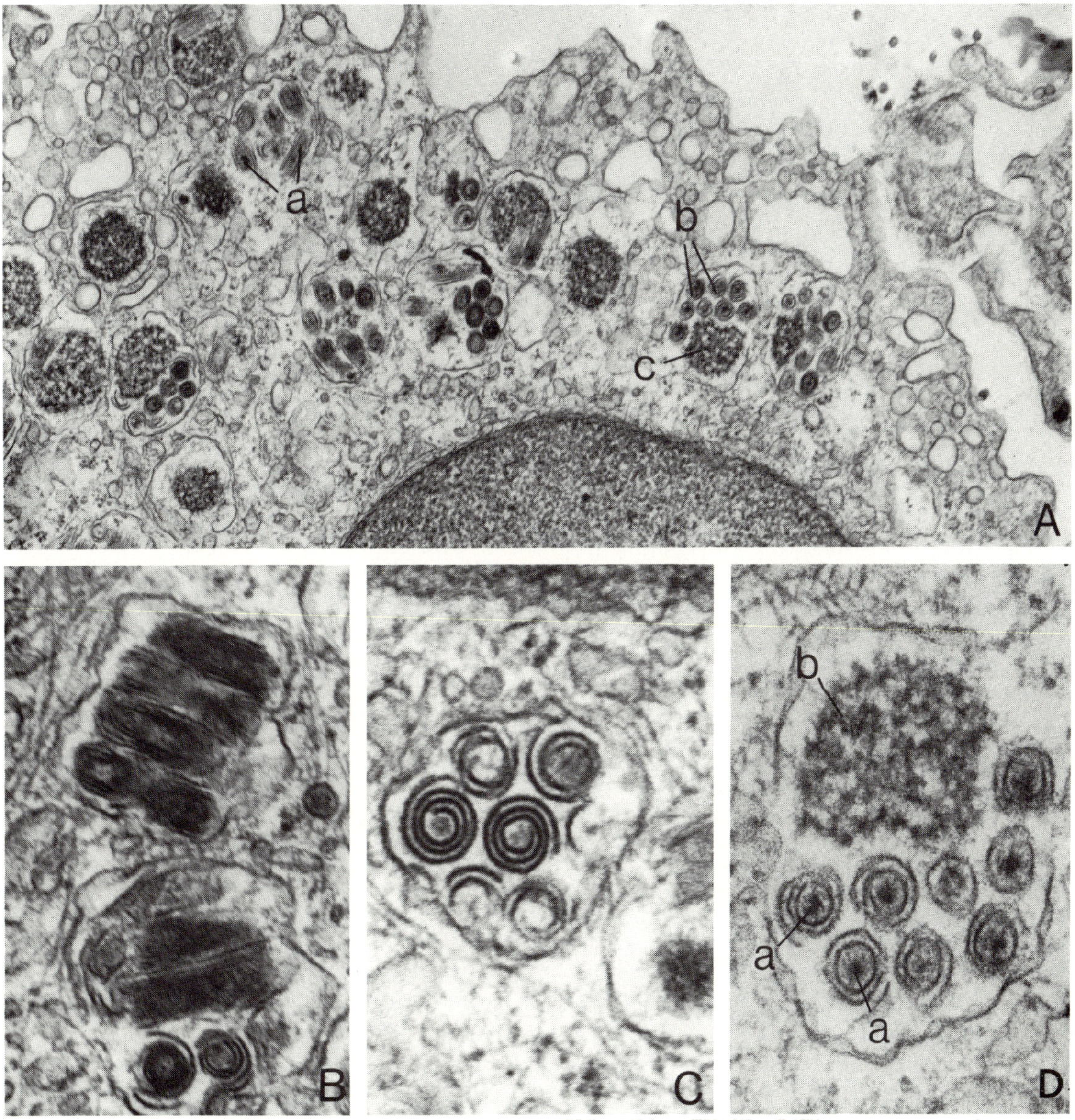

Figure 6–18. *A*, Iris stromal mast cell. This may be considered as a second type of iris mast cell, less commonly found in the iris than that seen in Figure 6–16. In the limbus this type of mast cell is more abundant than the one shown in Figure 6–16. This mast cell is distinguished by the fact that many of its granules contain cylindrical structures which are seen in longitudinal section (a) or in cross-section (b). A finely granular material is also contained (c) within the granules. (× 27,000.)

B, Higher magnification to show the cylindrical structures within the membrane of the mast cell granules. They are uniformly dense and of equal length. (× 60,000.)

C, View of the cross-sections of the cylindrical structures. Each cylinder is formed by a single lamellar membrane which is wound into a scroll. The core of the cylinder contains an electron-dense material. (× 90,000.)

D, Cylinders in mast cell granules seen in cross-section. The core material (a) and a mass of granular material (b) are found within the granules. (× 99,000.)

Indeed, the only difference between macrophages and clump cells of the iris is their size and shape. Macrophages are smaller and somewhat elongated and their residual bodies may contain substances other than melanin.

Mast cells frequently are found in the iris stroma. Unlike the elongated mast cells of the conjunctiva, those of the iris tend to be round, and their surfaces possess villous protrusions. Two morphologic types of mast cells are found, one having the structure of the conjunctival mast cell (p. 133), with the majority of the granules containing the characteristic rods with their scroll-like cross-sectional appearance. The other mast cell type has a larger proportion of its granules filled with an amorphous, electron-dense material. It is possible that these two types of mast cells merely represent different stages in the development of the granules or in the activity of the cells.

Sphincter Muscle (Figs. 6-1 to 6-4 and 6-19 to 6-24)

By light microscopy the sphincter muscle is identified in the pupillary portion of the stroma and appears as a ribbon-like band measuring 0.75 to 0.8 mm. in diameter and 0.1 to 0.17 mm. in thickness. At the pupillary margin the muscle edge is separated from the pigment epithelium by a narrow band of collagen. Posteriorly it is bound firmly to a dense layer of connective tissue which continues to the dilator muscle. The sphincter muscle cells are spindle-shaped and are oriented parallel to the pupillary margin. The bundles of muscle cells are closely packed and are separated by a thin but dense layer of collagen which runs from the stroma anterior to the muscle toward the dilator muscle. The collagen bands contain arterioles, capillaries and sensory and motor nerves.

By electron microscopy the sphincter muscle bundles are seen to be composed of smaller groupings of five to eight muscle cells. The muscle cell fibers are closely spaced and are in intimate contact with each other by means of tight junctions. In common with other smooth muscles, nerves do not enter into these tight groups of muscle cells but lie close to their periphery. Because of this arrangement of the nerves, it is believed that each muscle group functions simultaneously as a unit. Apparently only one cell of the group is innervated, and the tight intercellular junctions serve to spread the depolarizing current to the other muscle cells of the group. The

---

Figure 6–19. Pupillary portion of the iris. The dense, cellular anterior border layer (a) terminates at the pigment ruff (b) in the pupillary margin. The sphincter muscle is at (c). The arcades (d) from the minor circle extend toward the pupil and through the sphincter muscle. The sphincter muscle and the iris epithelium are close to each other at the pupillary margin. Capillaries, nerves, melanocytes and clump cells (e) are found within and around the muscle. The three to five layers of dilator muscle (f) gradually diminish in number until they terminate behind the midportion of the sphincter muscle (arrow), leaving low, cuboidal epithelial cells (g) to form the anterior epithelium to the pupillary margin. Spur-like extensions from the dilator muscle form Michel's spur (h) and Fuchs' spur (i), which extend anteriorly to blend with the sphincter muscle. The posterior epithelium (j) is formed by tall columnar cells with basally located nuclei. Its apical surface is contiguous with the apical surface of the anterior epithelium.

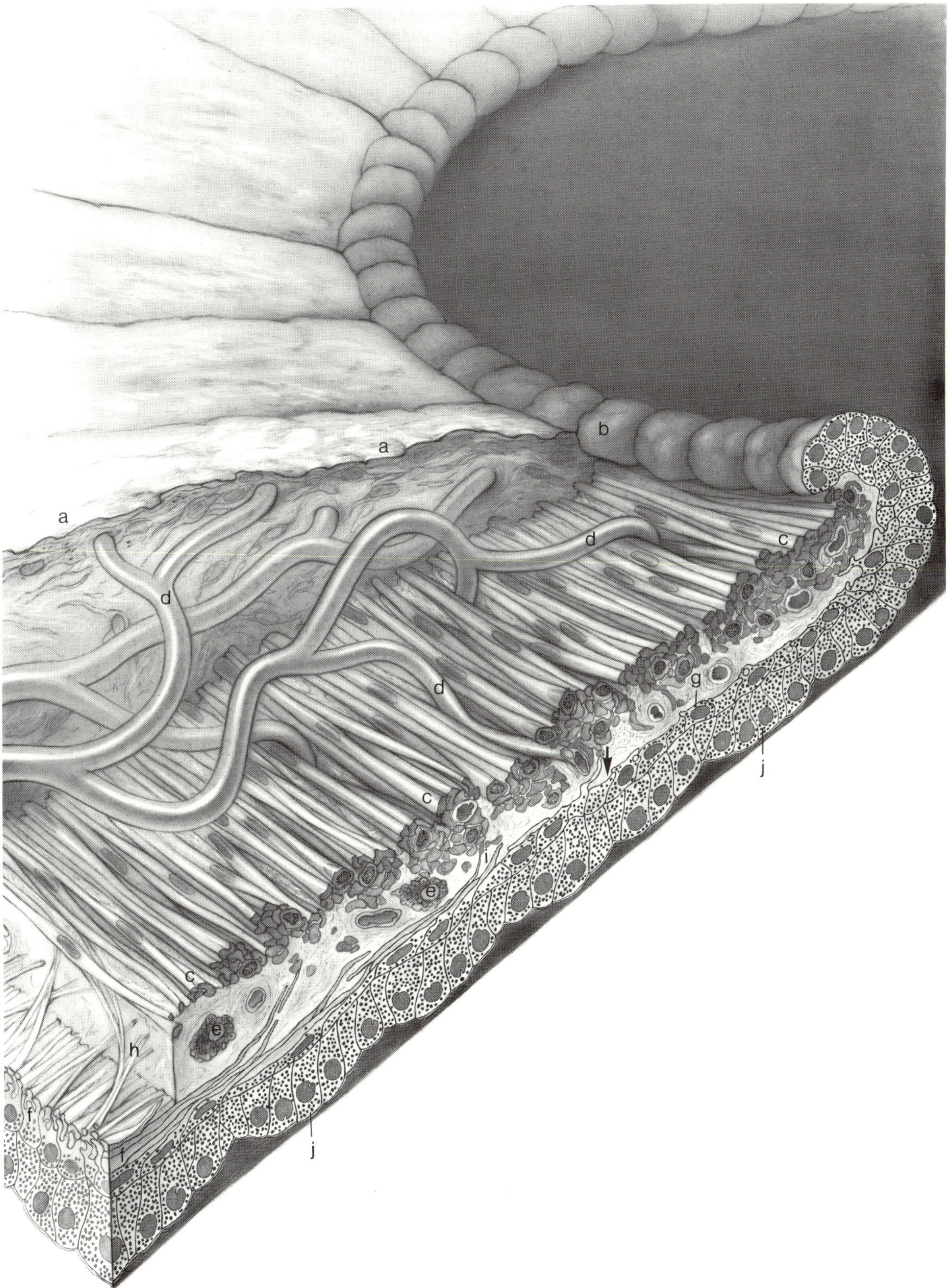

Figure 6–19. *See legend on opposite page.*

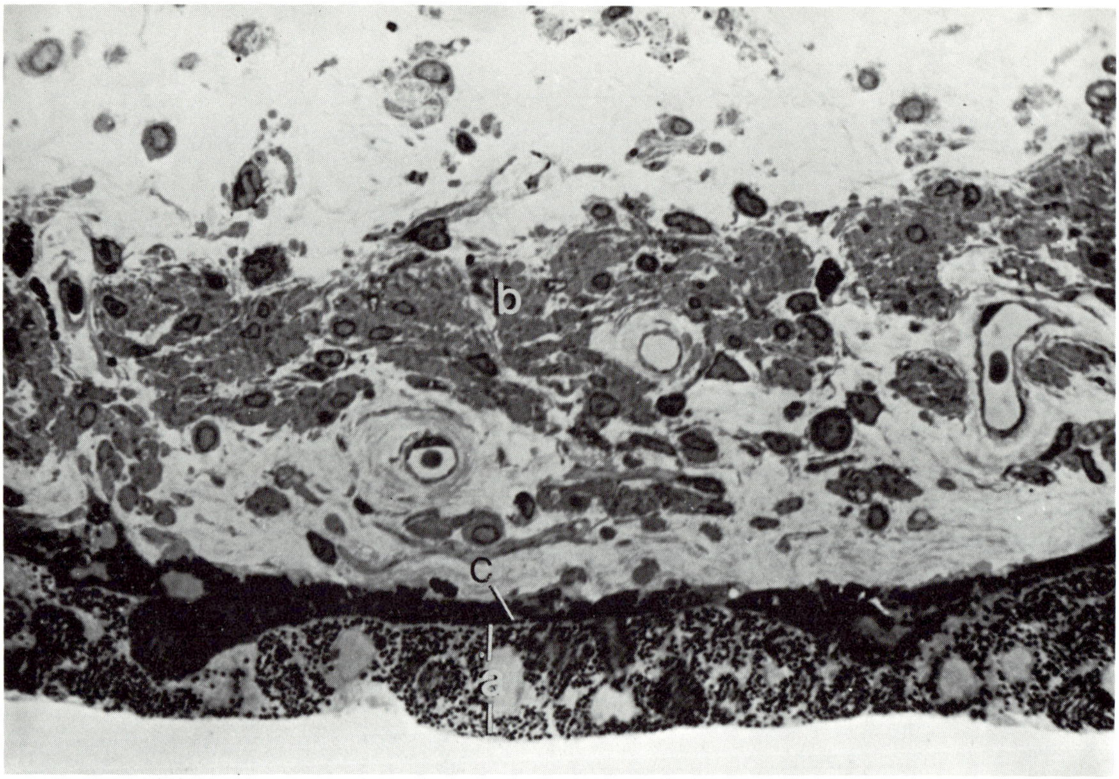

Figure 6–20. Posterior iris epithelium (a) and sphincter muscle (b) in the pupillary portion of the iris. The dilator muscle has terminated so that only two layers of pigmented epithelium (a and c) measuring 16 μm. in thickness are seen. (× 680.)

nucleus is centrally located somewhere around the midportion of these fusiform muscle cells. A number of cytoplasmic organelles are commonly found near the nucleus; these include a Golgi apparatus, small rod-shaped mitochondria, a few cisternae of the rough-surfaced endoplasmic reticulum and many unattached polyribosomes. The cytoplasm is filled with myofilaments of only one type. Scattered densities, similar to the Z-bands in striated muscle, are found among the filaments and may provide attachment areas for the myofilaments. Pinocytotic vesicles are found along the inner surface of the cell membrane.

A basement membrane similar to that found adjacent to other smooth muscle cells is also found in the sphincter muscle. This membrane comes in contact with the collagen fibrils separating the muscle groups. Melanocytes are numerous around and between the muscle cell bundles. Nerves are seen in the connective tissue separating the units of muscle cells. Upon approaching the smaller groupings of muscle cells the nerves form smaller bundles. Usually there is a small bundle of two to four nerve axons surrounded by a Schwann cell which approaches the muscle cells without coming closer to their surfaces than about 0.1 μm. Naked axons without a Schwann cell wrapping occasionally are seen to terminate in the sphincter muscle.

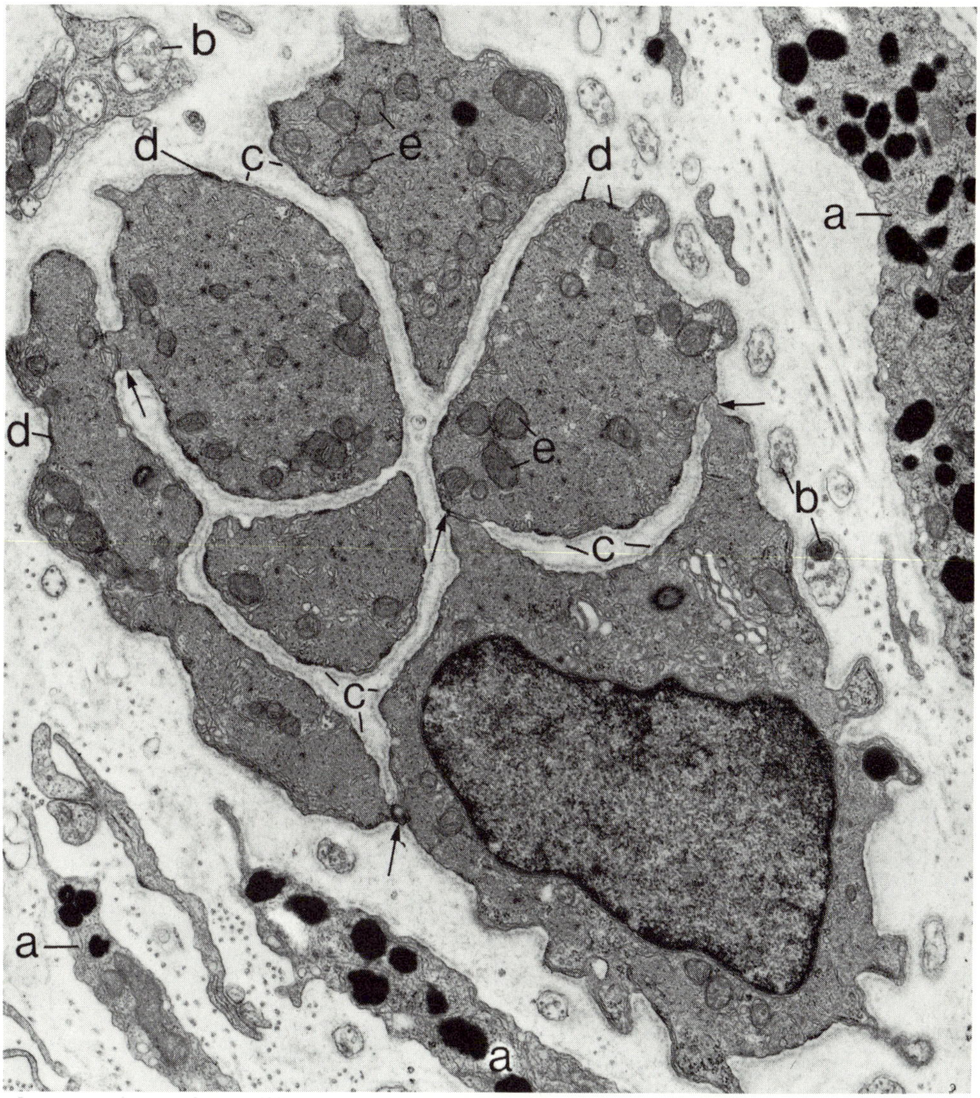

Figure 6–21. Sphincter muscle of the iris seen in meridional section. A bundle of six muscle cells is surrounded by collagen fibrils, processes of melanocytes (a) and several nerves (b). Four of the six muscle cells are seen to come into close contact with each other (arrows), and each muscle cell has a basement membrane (c). There are localized electron-dense patches along the cell membrane (d) and numerous mitochondria (e). One muscle cell is cut through the nuclear region where the cytoplasm is seen to contain a Golgi apparatus, a centriole and scattered ribosomes. (× 27,600.)

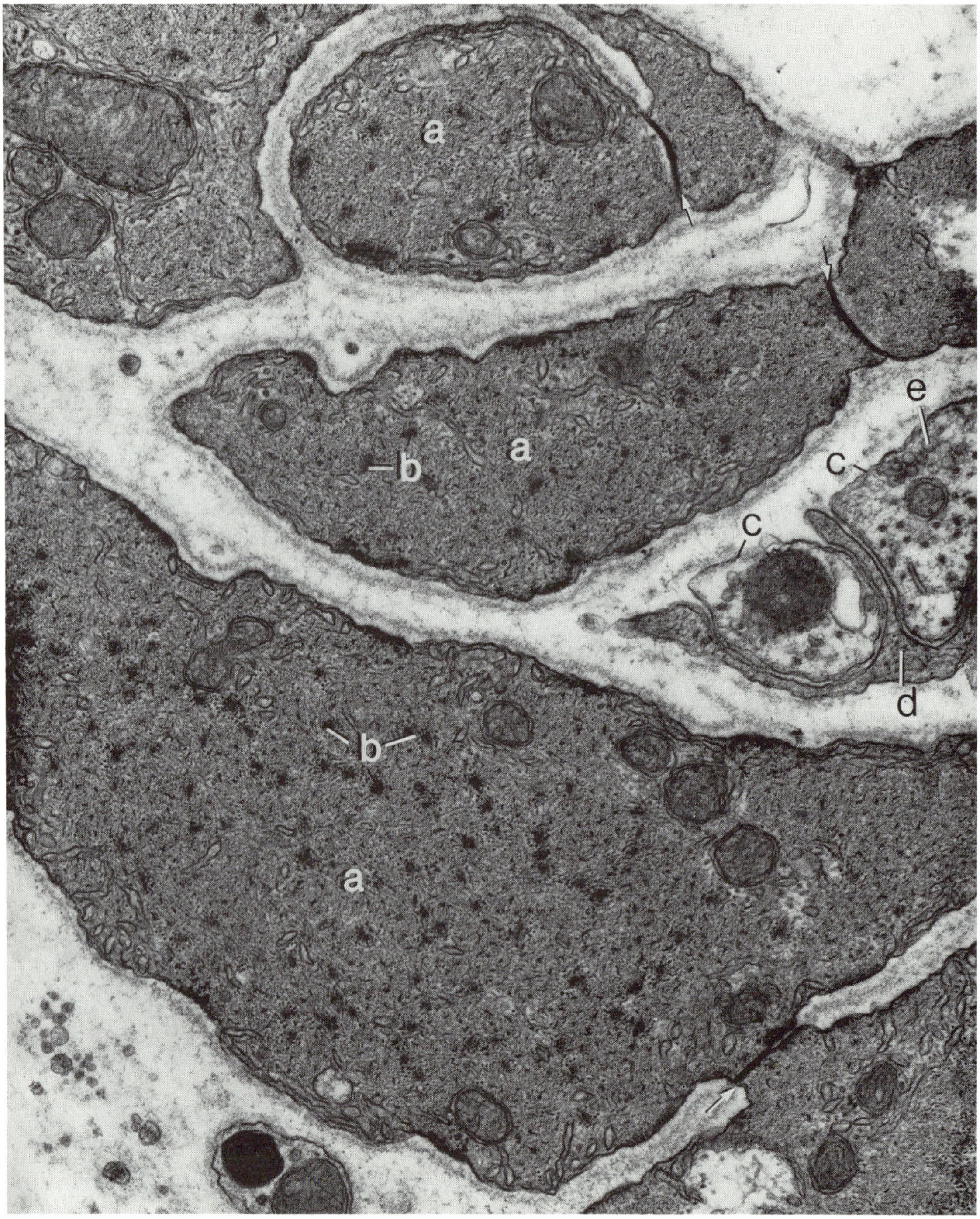

Figure 6–22. Sphincter muscle in meridional section. Groups of three to six muscle cells most often come into close contact with each other through tight junctions (arrows) or "gap" junctions. This arrangement is common to most smooth muscle cells. The muscle cell basement membranes are prominent and there is a finely granular ground substance. The cytoplasm of the cells is filled with fine myofilaments which are seen in cross-section (a). They form dense aggregations in the cytoplasm (b). Adjacent nerves (c) are seen to be partially enclosed by a Schwann cell (d) and they contain some vesicles (e) and neurotubules. (× 36,800.)

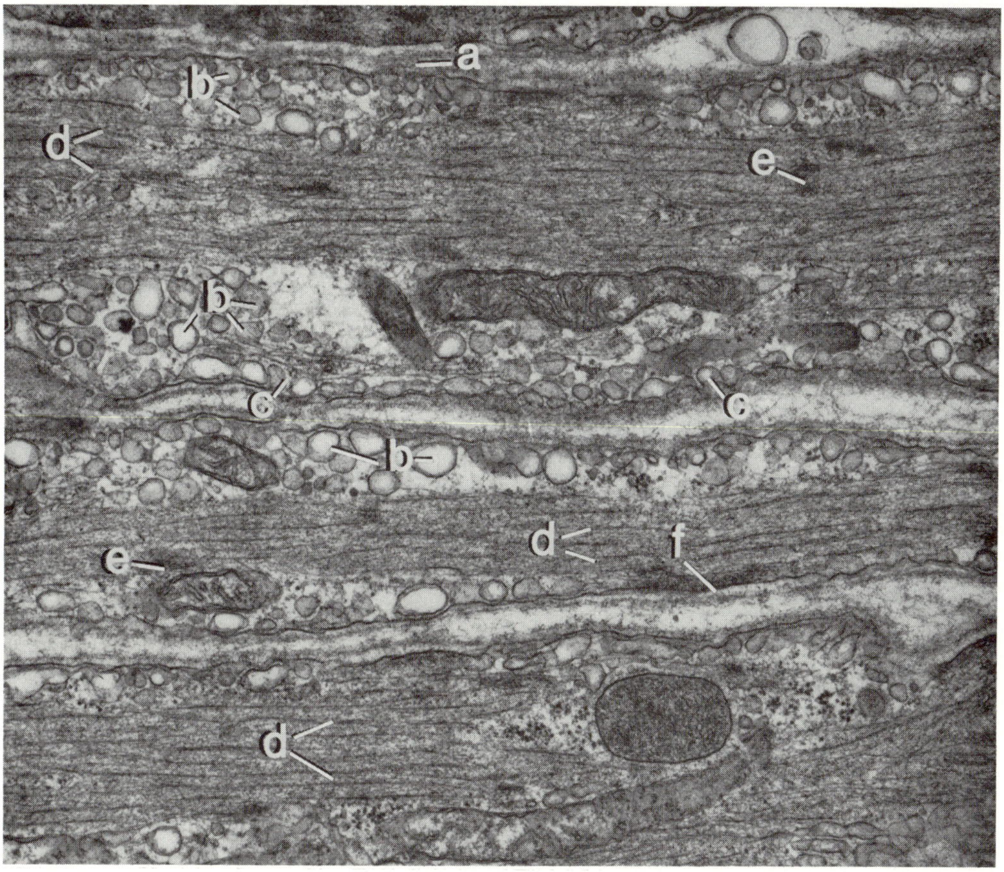

Figure 6–23. Iris sphincter muscle cut longitudinally. Several muscle cells are surrounded by basement membranes which fuse in areas of close apposition (a). The peripheral cytoplasm contains numerous pinocytotic vesicles (b), some of which seem to be open at the outside surface of the muscle cell (c). The myofibrils are quite distinct (d) and they are separated from each other by a fairly uniform space. A finely fibrillar material is found around the myofilaments, and there are areas of increased density (e) among the myofilaments as well as along the cell membrane (f). (× 25,000.)

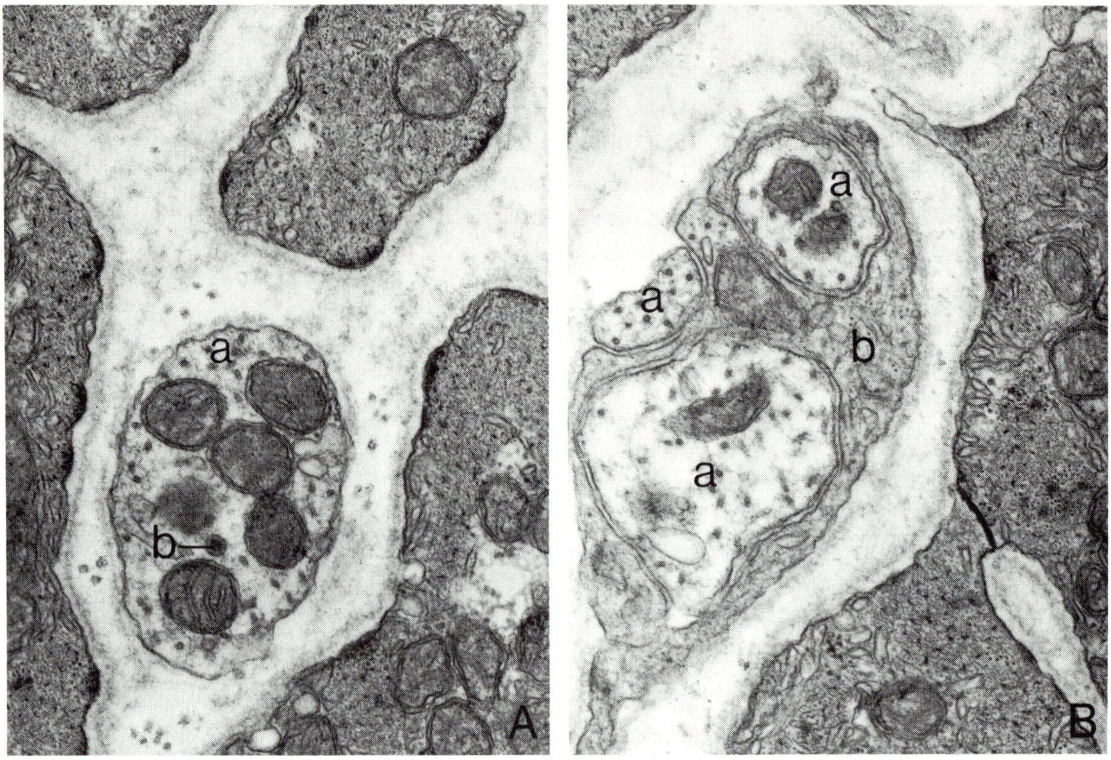

Figure 6–24. *A*, Iris sphincter muscle surrounding a single naked nerve axon. The nerves do not achieve close apposition with the muscle cell membrane, usually being separated from it by a space of about 0.1 or 0.2 μm. Several mitochondria, some neurotubules (a) and a synaptic vesicle (b) are shown in the nerve.

B, A nerve bundle (a) which possesses a Schwann sheath (b) lies adjacent to several muscle cells. (× 27,600.)

Blood Vessels (Figs. 6-1 and 6-25 to 6-33)

The blood vessels of the iris are believed to have a slight corkscrew shape so they can accommodate to the changes in the length of the iris during dilation and contraction. A striking finding in all the iris vessels is the presence of a thick, collagenous adventitia, the collagen being oriented circularly around the vessel. The thick adventitia is separated from the endothelium by a less dense space containing fewer fibrils and ground substance.

The *arteries* diminish in size rapidly near their entrance into the iris stroma from the major circle of the iris. These arteries possess some of the structural features of the major arterial circle, having one or two muscle layers and no internal elastic lamina. Upon entering the iris they become smaller and lose a layer of smooth muscle cells. The remaining muscle layer is oriented longitudinally. The adventitial collagen is oriented circularly around the muscle layer and is composed entirely of collagen, some fibro-

Text continued on page 240

Fig. 6–25

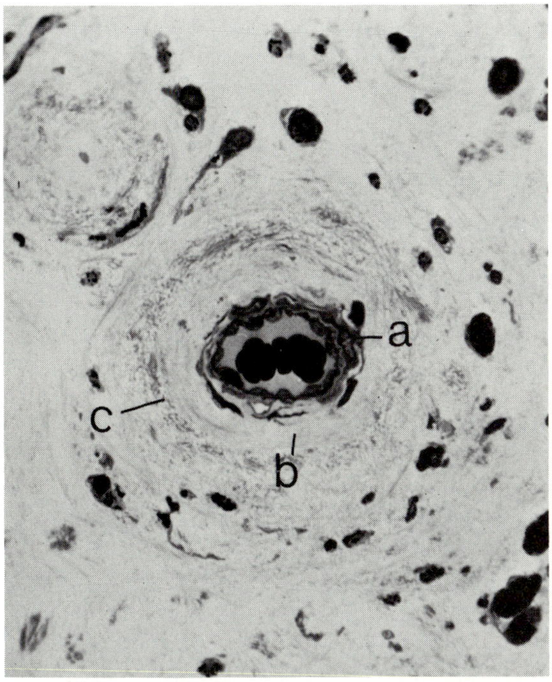

Fig. 6–26

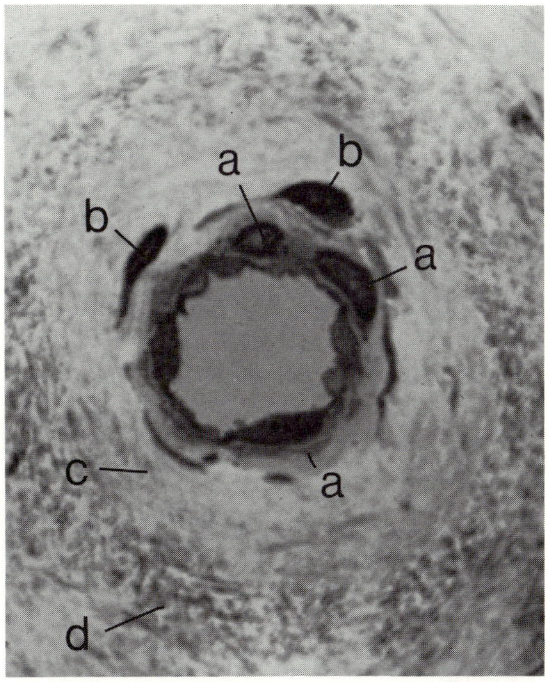

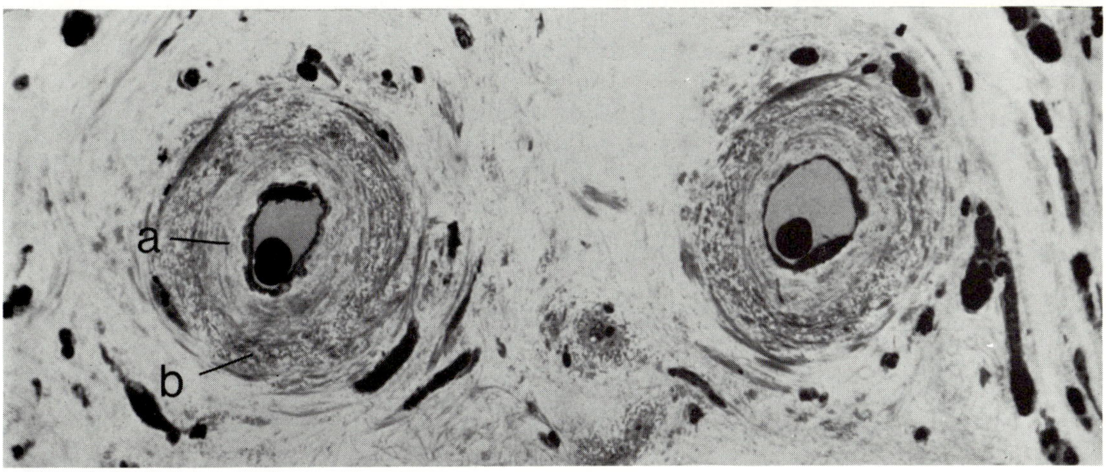

Fig. 6–27

Figure 6–25. Light micrograph of a small iris stromal artery, which has a muscular media (a) surrounded by a light collagenous zone (b) and a dense, coarse adventitia composed of circularly oriented collagen (c). The intima has no internal elastic lamina. Melanocytes and fibroblasts are found in the adjacent stroma. (× 640.)

Figure 6–26. A small iris stromal artery having a longitudinally oriented muscle coat (a). Several fibroblasts (b) lie external to the vessel. External to the muscle is a light collagenous zone (c) which, in turn, is surrounded by an outer, dense collagenous zone (d). This arrangement is typical of the iris vessels. (× 1220.)

Figure 6–27. Iris stromal artery and vein. The vessel on the left side is a small artery similar to that seen in Figure 6–25, and the other vessel is a small vein. The dense, coarse outer collagenous coat (b) of the vessels is quite distinct from the loose, randomly oriented iris stromal collagen. The inner less dense zone (a) is distinguished from the outer darker zone (b). The two vessels are similar except that the vein has no muscularis. (× 640.)

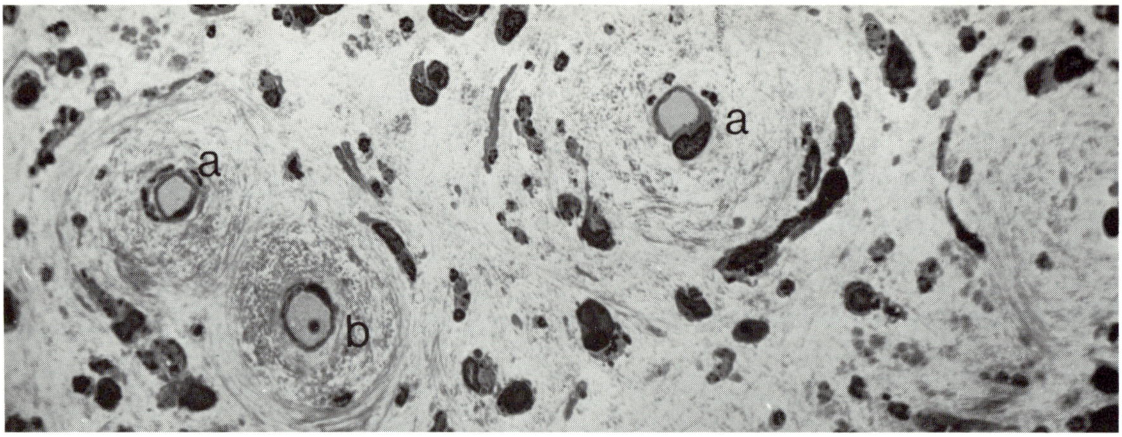

Figure 6–28. Light micrograph of some small iris vessels. These vessels measure between 7 and 10 μm. in diameter. Two appear to be capillaries (a) and one a venule (b). The lighter inner zone adjacent to the endothelium is less apparent in these small vessels. (× 640.)

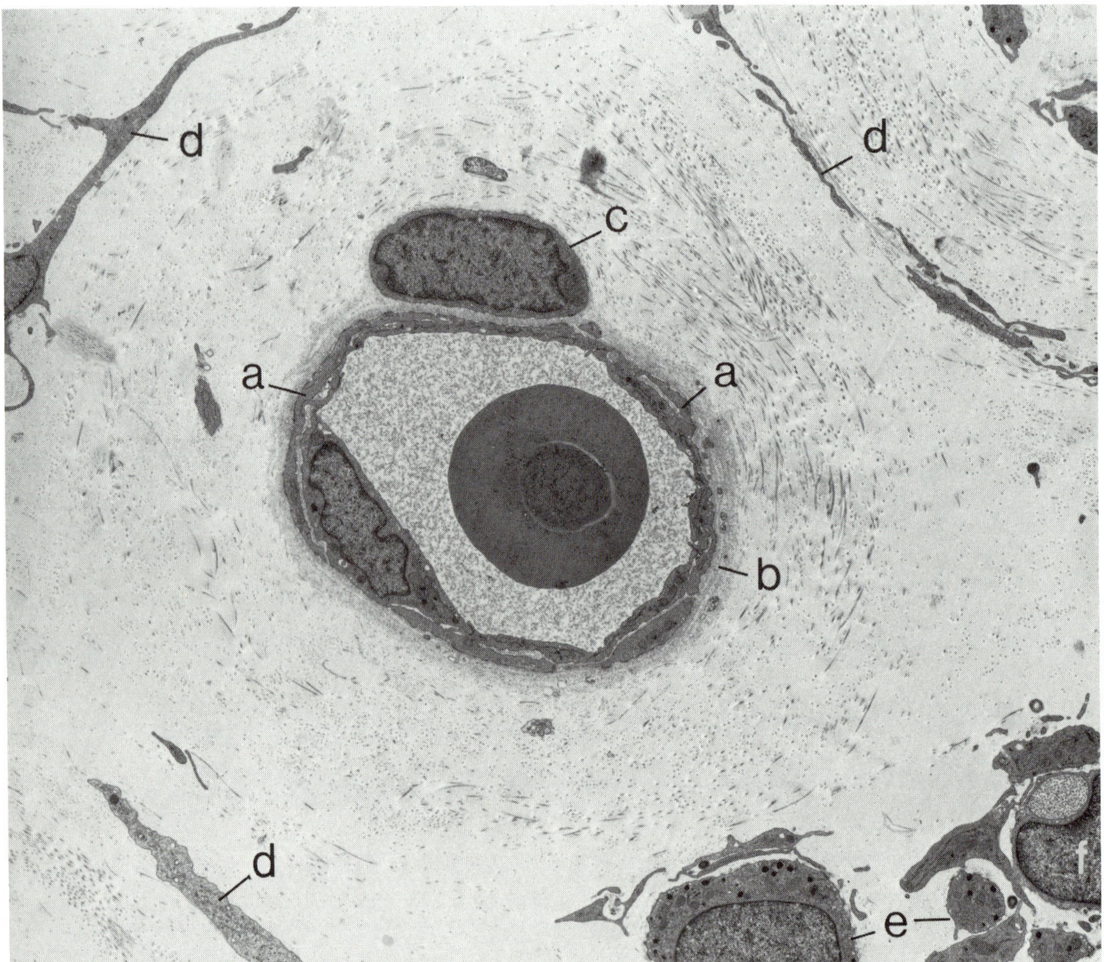

Figure 6–29. Electron micrograph of a medium-sized iris artery. A continuous layer of muscle (a) is close to the endothelium of this vessel. There is a thick laminated basement membrane (b) surrounding the endothelium. An adventitial cell (c) and numerous collagen fibrils occupy the perivascular zone. Long processes of fibroblasts (d) and melanocytes (e) as well as a Schwann cell (f) which encloses a nerve are also seen. (× 8500.)

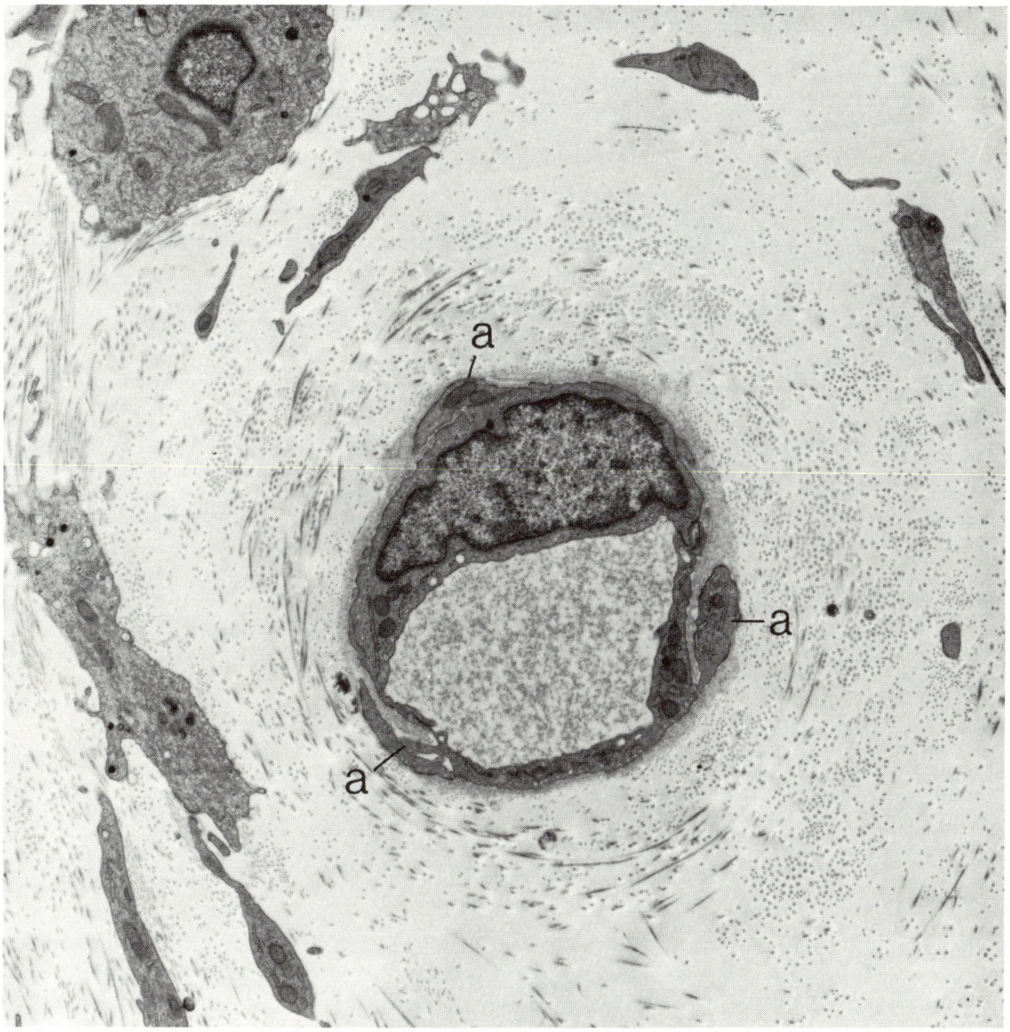

Figure 6–30. An iris stromal arteriole which shows a thick endothelial basement membrane and a semilongitudinally oriented muscularis (a). There is an abundant perivascular collagen coat. (× 8500.)

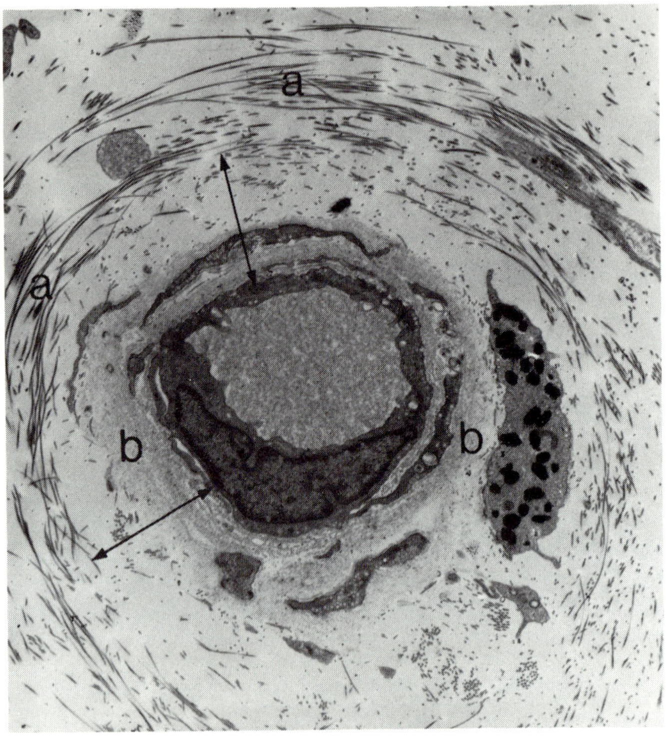

Figure 6–31. Iris arteriole. The thick endothelial basement membrane is seen at (b). A corona of circularly arranged collagen forms an adventitia (a) which is separated from the endothelium and its basement membrane by a zone containing very few collagen fibrils (arrows). This photograph can be compared with the light micrograph of the iris vessels in which the density of the perivascular collagen is more striking. (× 8600.)

blasts and melanocytes. The *veins* have thin walls, with an endothelium like that of the artery, and the media shows only scattered muscle cells.

Most of the vessels in the iris stroma are arterioles, venules and capillaries, the capillaries predominating in most areas. The *venules* have very thin walls, consisting of an endothelium which is surrounded by a thin layer of collagen. The *arterioles* have the characteristic interrupted muscular layer in the media, and a rather heavy adventitia of collagen fibers and fibroblasts. The *capillaries* are formed by a single layer of unfenestrated endothelium. The endothelial cells have a rather thick basement membrane. At the edge of this layer is a zone 7 μm. wide, containing sparse longitudinally oriented collagen fibers. A granular ground substance is enmeshed in this collagen. Outside all this is a thick layer of circularly oriented collagen measuring 10 μm. in thickness. Processes of fibroblasts and melanocytes are enmeshed in this collagen. This organization of the iris vessels has been described repeatedly by light microscopists, and it was postulated that the lighter intermediate zone outside the basement membrane of the endothelium is a perivascular space, allowing fluids to flow along the course of the vessel. Electron micrographs, however, do not show such a perivascular space. It is not apparent why the vessels are constructed in this way, except that such an arrangement may be necessary because of the movements of the iris.

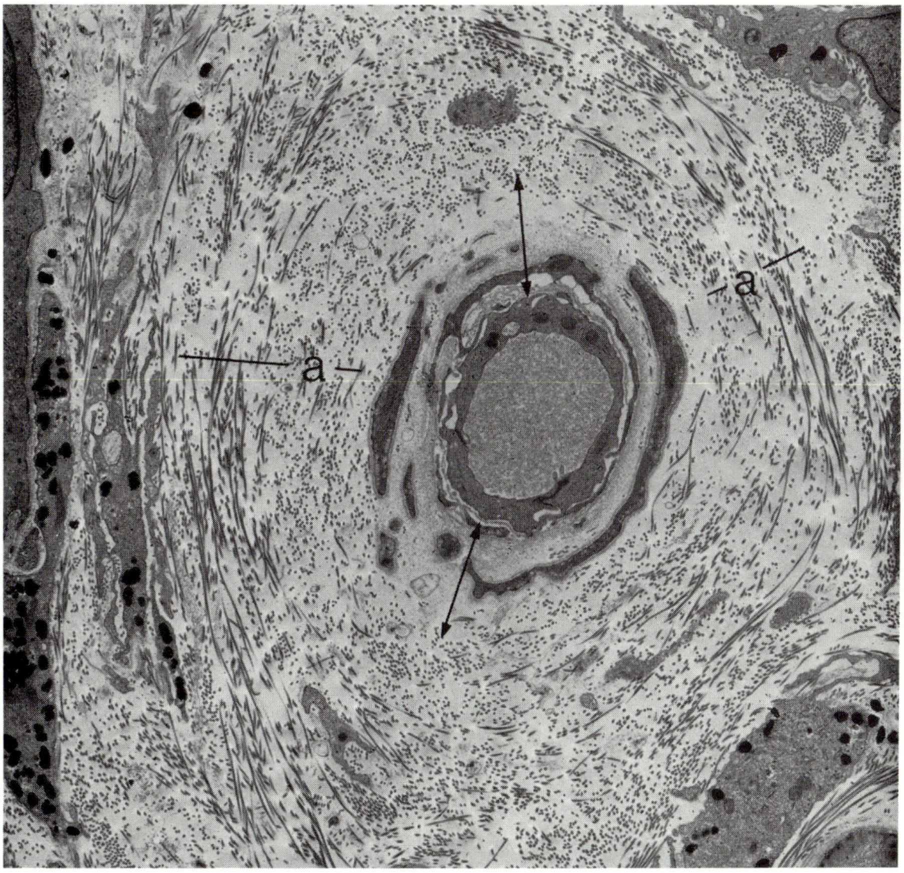

Figure 6–32. Small iris arteriole. The zone enclosed by arrows is the characteristic clear perivascular space which has been described by light microscopy. This clear zone contains a dense ground substance which is associated with the endothelial basement membrane, a few collagen fibrils and some cell processes. Outside this zone is the dense circular collagenous zone (a) which is so clearly seen with the light microscope. (× 2200.)

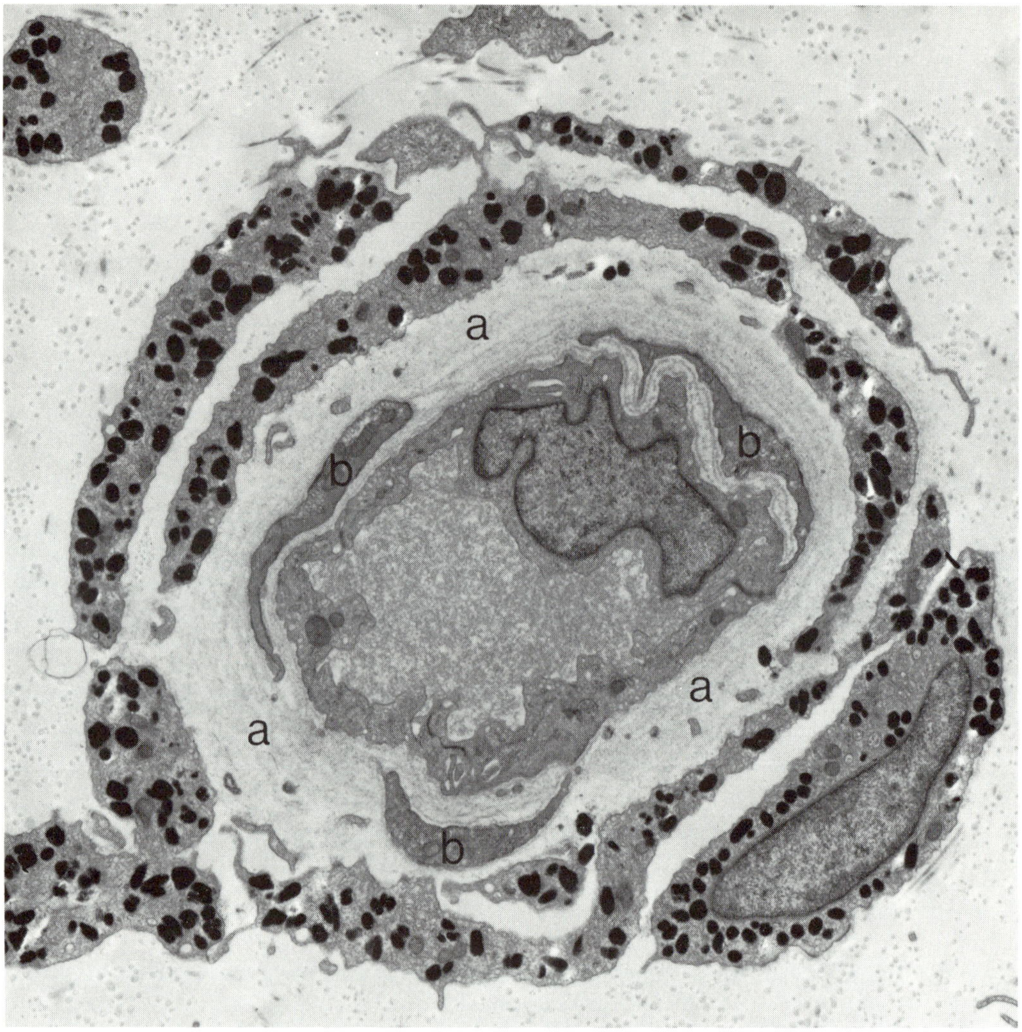

Figure 6–33. A small arteriole near the anterior border layer. Melanocyte processes are frequently seen around these vessels. The basement membrane is thick and laminated (a) and there are three muscle cells in the wall (b). Even the smallest iris vessels have occasional muscle cells in their walls. (× 9300.)

Nerves

Nerves can be seen occasionally in routine sections and are identified more easily with silver stains. They form fine plexuses along larger blood vessels, and filaments can be seen in the anterior border layer, in the stroma, and among the muscles, but not in the posterior pigmented epithelium. Nerves are found close to the anterior epithelial cell layer, however. Most of these nerves are unmyelinated, enclosed by Schwann cells.

Anterior Epithelium and Dilator Muscle Layer (Figs. 6–1 to 6–4, 6–20, 6–34 to 6–43 and 6–49)

This layer measures about 12.5 μm. thick; each cell is composed of an *epithelial apical portion* and a *muscular basal portion* which projects into the iris stroma. The muscular portion of these cells has a thickness of 4 μm.

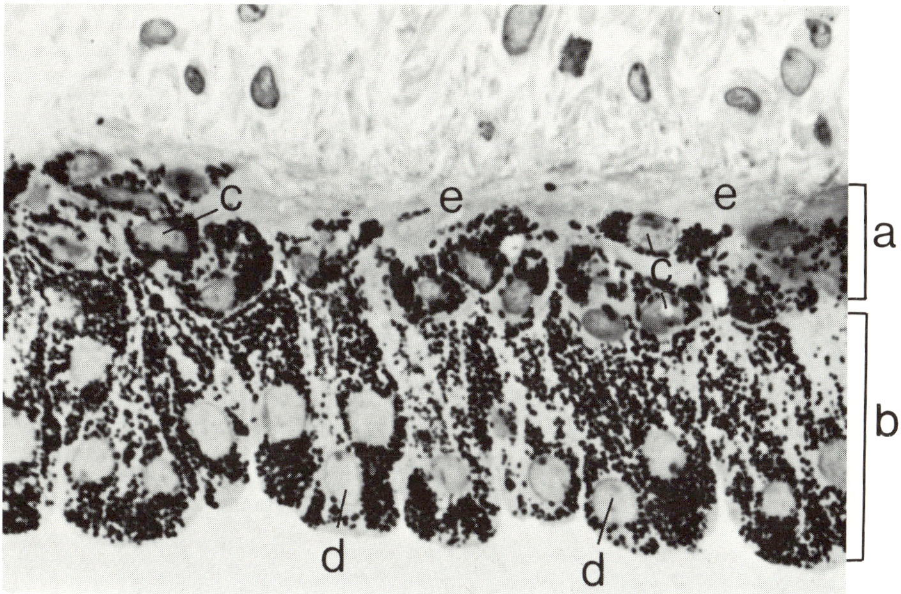

Figure 6–34. Light micrograph of the anterior (a) and posterior (b) iris epithelium. The nuclei of the anterior layer are at (c) and of the posterior layer at (d). The flattened muscular portion of the anterior layer is at (e). (× 500.)

Its anterior surface has a wavy outline, but the posterior border is indistinct because of the pigmentation of the cells. In meridional sections the muscular extensions of this anterior layer of epithelium are oriented in a radial direction from the iris root toward the pupil. Tangential sections of depigmented cells show the muscular processes to be spindle-shaped, measuring about 7 μm. wide and up to 60 μm. long. The nucleus is located in the epithelial portion of the cell; it is flattened and has a width of 4 to 6 μm. and a length of 14 μm. A great part of the pigment of these cells is found mainly in the epithelial portion, where the cytoplasm also contains the majority of the cell organelles. The muscular processes are filled with myofilaments, but the epithelial portion also contains some myofilaments.

The muscular portion of anterior epithelium disappears posterior to the midportion of the sphincter muscle (Fig. 6-2). Beyond this termination the cells become cuboidal in shape or are quite irregular (Fig. 6-20). Near its termination the dilator is sometimes seen to extend into the stroma behind the sphincter muscle or even unite with it, forming spur-like structures (Fig. 6-36). Peripherally the dilator muscle extends almost to the base of the iris, where the muscular portion disappears (Figs. 6-42 and 6-43). The epithelium then continues posteriorly onto the ciliary processes as a pigmented layer of cells.

By electron microscopy the *muscular portion* of the anterior epithelium consists of ribbon-like projections stemming from the apical portion. These processes are flattened in the plane of the iris, and they form three to five layers of dilator muscle. In common with other smooth muscles, these cells also possess a basement membrane. This membrane, as shown in Figure 6-49, disappears in the epithelial portion, where the intercellular space measures approximately 200 A. in width. Tight junctions similar to those described in the sphincter muscle are commonly found between the dilator

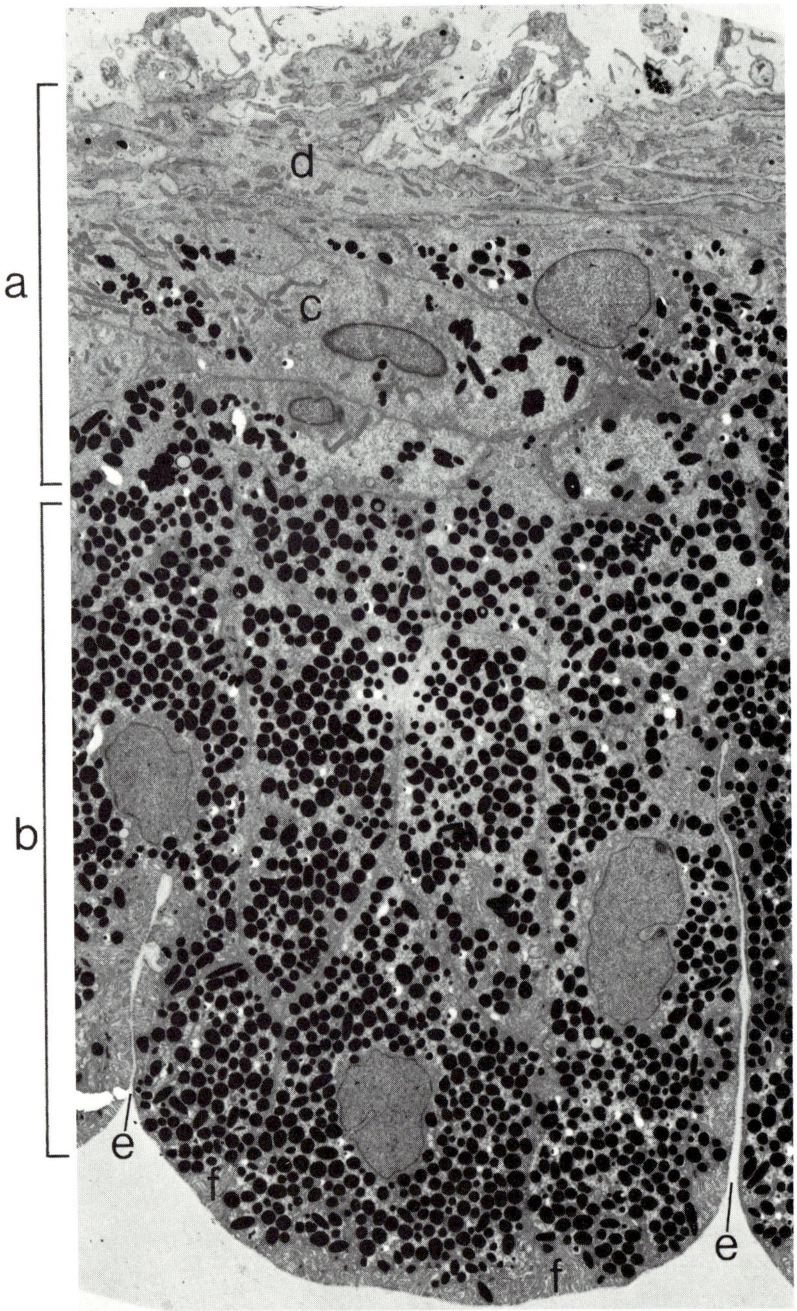

Figure 6–35. Low-power electron micrograph of the two layers of iris epithelium. The anterior epithelium and dilator muscle are shown at (a) and the posterior epithelium at (b). The epithelial portion of the anterior epithelium is at (c) and the muscular component at (d). Note the paucity of melanin granules in the anterior epithelium and their distribution in the apical portion near the nucleus. The posterior iris surface shows two deep furrows (e) and the basal epithelium shows extensive infolding (f). (× 2500.)

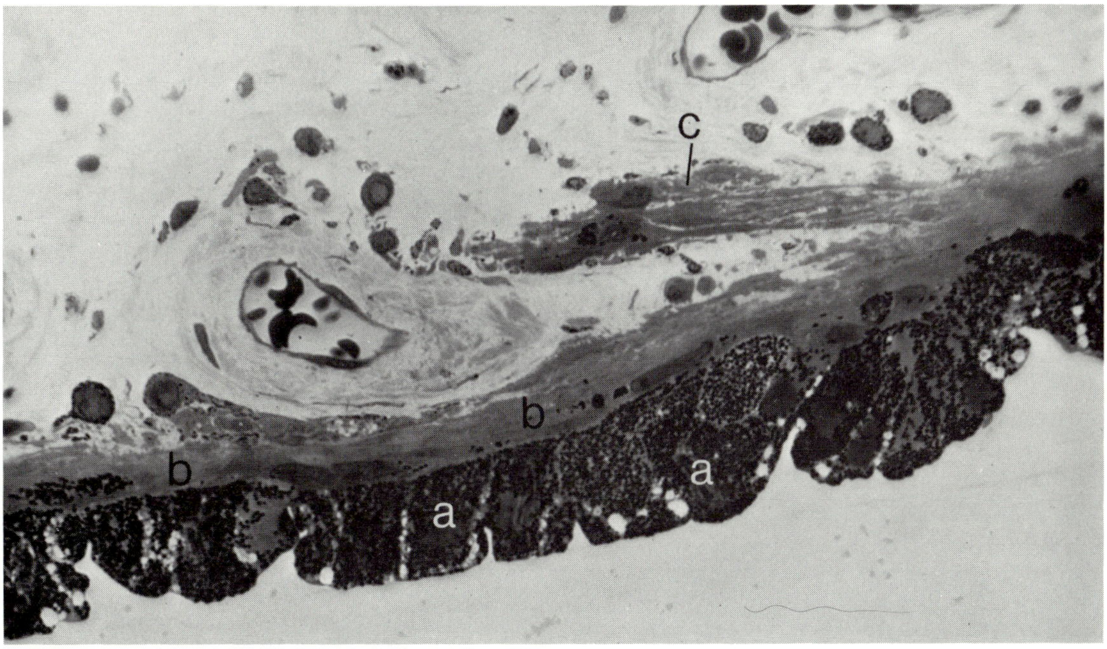

Figure 6–36. Posterior iris epithelium (a) and dilator muscle (b) in the pupillary region. A spur of dilator muscle tissue extends into the stroma toward the sphincter (c). (× 640.)

muscle fibers. These junctions may serve to electrically couple a number of fibers to function as a unit. The cytoplasm is filled with myofilaments measuring around 30 A. in diameter and a moderate number of mitochondria. Numerous densities are found throughout the cytoplasm; these are reminiscent of the Z-discs of skeletal muscle. These densities also are prominent along the cell membrane, producing thickenings that used to be called hemidesmosomes. Pinocytotic vesicles are not numerous, and pigment granules seldom are seen in this portion of the anterior epithelium.

Unmyelinated nerve fibers are seen near the muscle processes. These fibers often contain synaptic vesicles (Tousimis and Fine, 1959), but we have not been able to differentiate parasympathetic from sympathetic nerve endings in this area. The nerve endings come into very close contact with the muscle, being separated from the muscle cell membrane by a space measuring 200 A.

The apical portion of the anterior epithelium is the so-called *epithelial portion*. The apical cell surface joins that of the posterior epithelium, often being separated from it by spaces containing numerous microvilli which are formed by both the anterior and the posterior epithelium. Cilia frequently project into these spaces from the adjacent epithelium; they arise in the epithelial cell cytoplasm from a basal body. Elsewhere the two epithelial layers are separated by a space measuring about 200 A. Numerous desmosomes and tight junctions join the cells along their apical surfaces. The *lateral* cell membranes show moderate interdigitation. Tight junctions and desmosomes are found along these borders; the desmosomes disappear in the muscular portion, and only the tight junctions are found in that portion. The lateral intercellular space measures approximately 200 A. in width and, as previously mentioned, the basement membrane present in the muscular or basal portion is not found here. The majority of the cell organelles are

Text continued on page 251

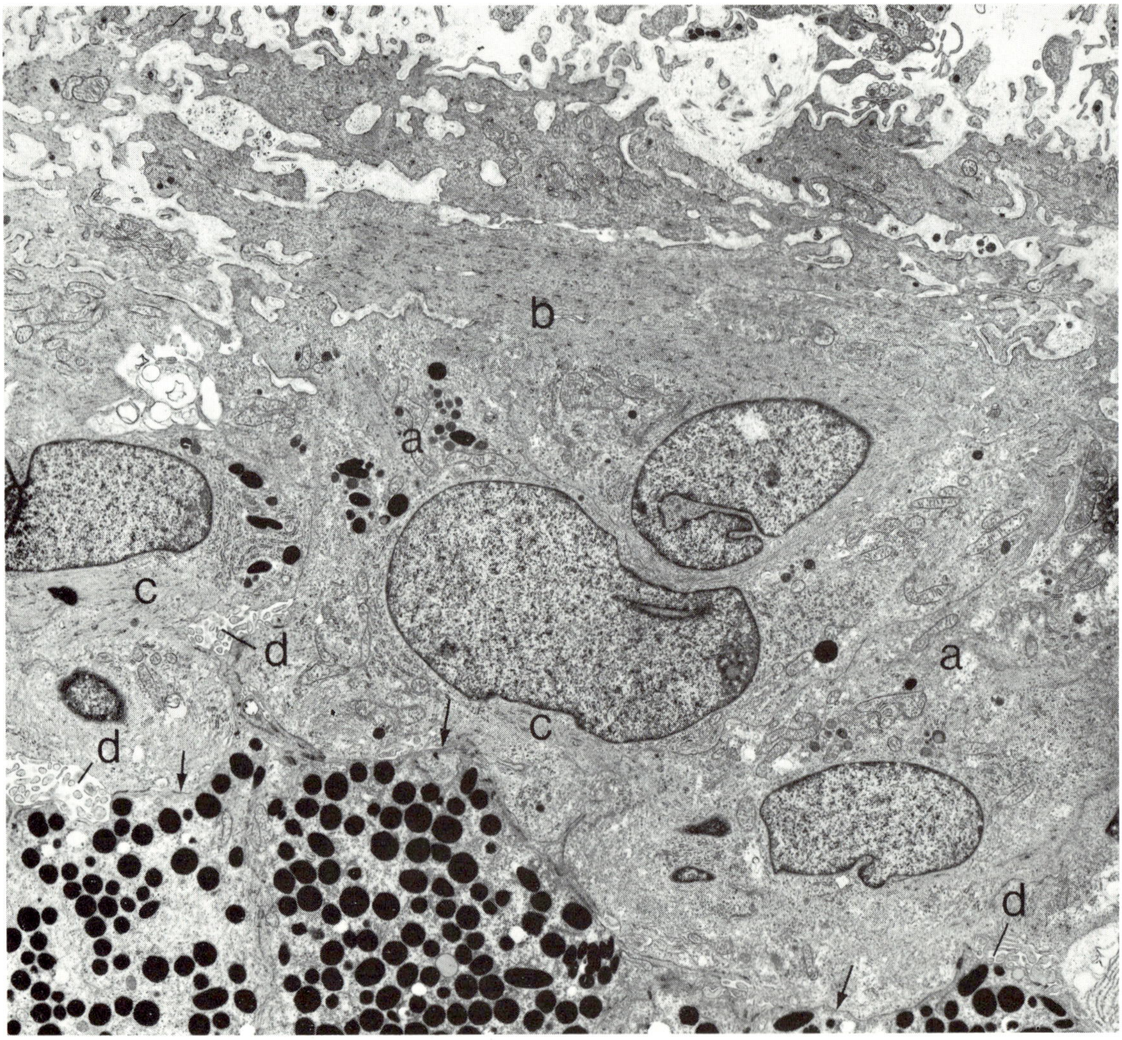

Figure 6–37. Anterior iris epithelium. The epithelial portion is at (a), and the muscular portion at (b). The majority of the cell organelles and melanin granules are found in the apical portion of the epithelium (a) around the nucleus. The myofilaments and the densities they form are best appreciated at (b), but they extend past the nucleus to the apex of the cell (c). The zone of contiguity between the apical portions of the two epithelial layers is seen at the bottom of the photograph (arrows). Both layers are joined tightly to each other by numerous intercellular junctions, but there are scattered intercellular separations (d). Villous cellular processes from both epithelial layers project into these spaces. (× 4000.)

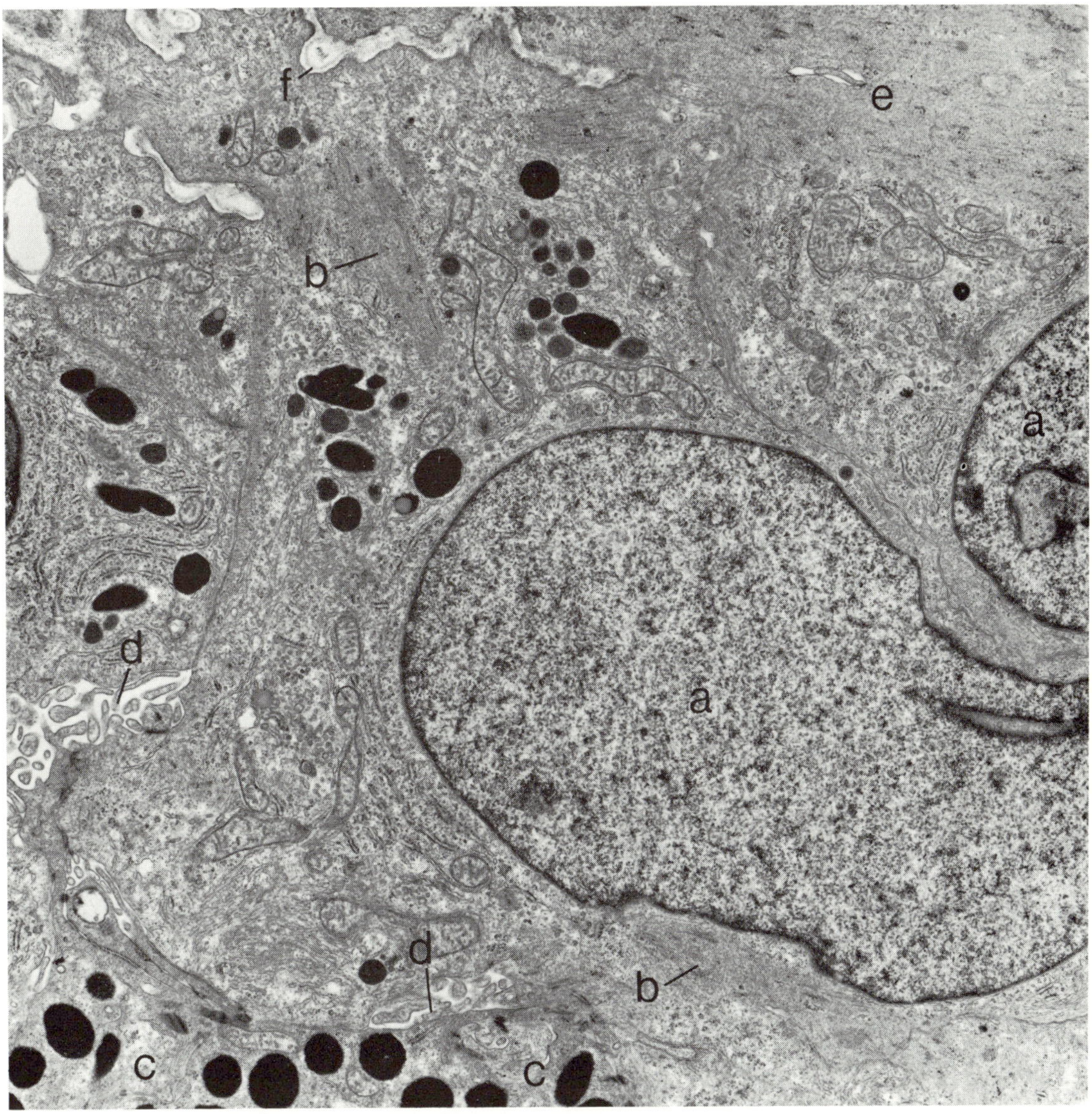

Figure 6–38. Anterior iris epithelium. The apical or epithelial portion of three cells with their nuclei (a), melanin granules, cell organelles and some clusters of myofilaments (b) are shown. These cells are in close contact with the posterior epithelium (c) by means of numerous desmosomes and tight junctions. Intercellular spaces containing villous processes are shown (d). The basal portion of the anterior epithelium sends tongue-like projections into the iris stroma. These cellular projections are filled with myofilaments (e) and form the dilator muscle. A basement membrane (f) surrounds the muscular portion of these cells. (× 8840.)

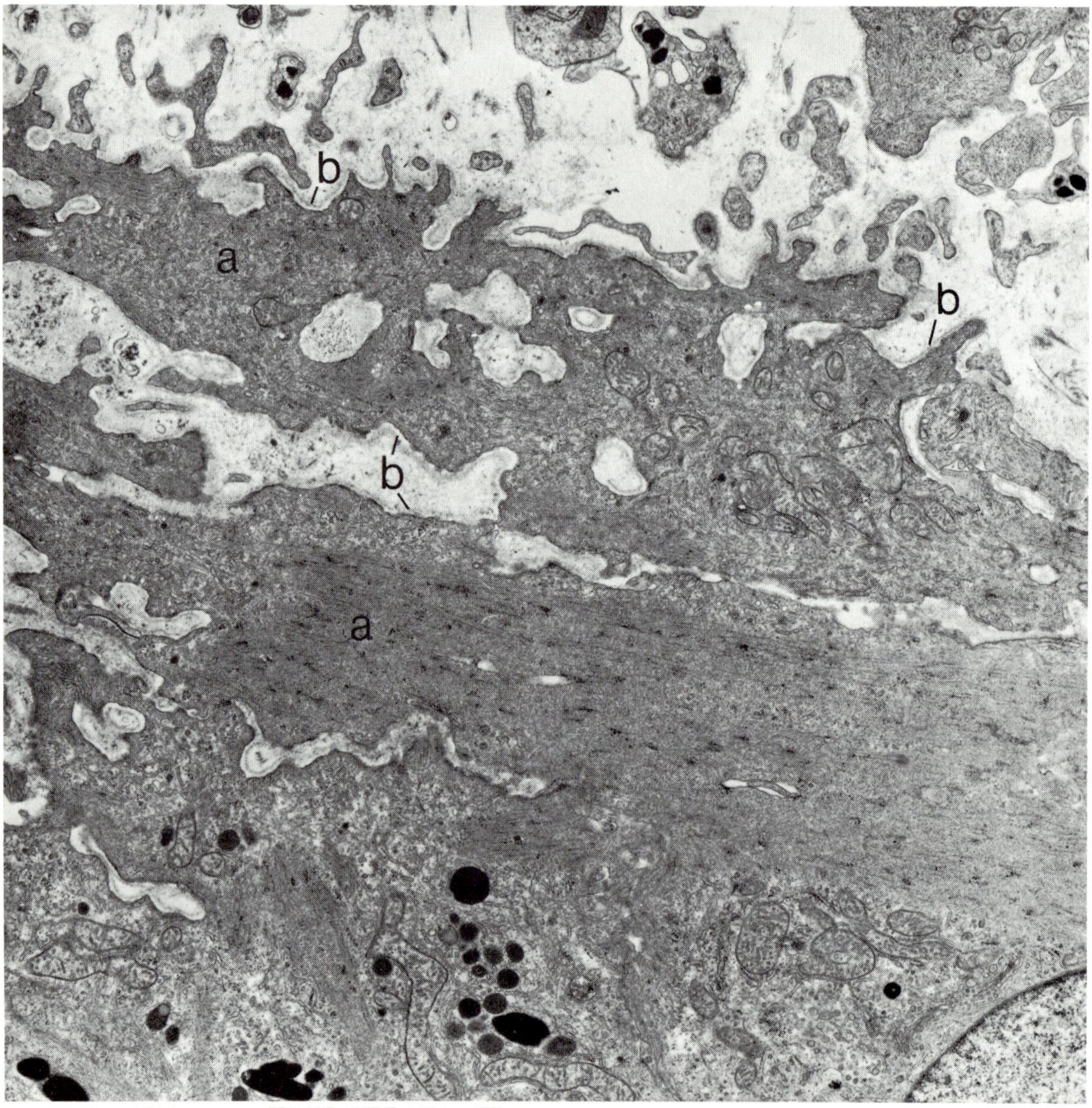

Figure 6–39. Anterior iris epithelium. A portion of the epithelial or apical portion of the anterior epithelium is seen at the bottom, while the tongue-like muscular projections are shown at (a). A basement membrane (b) surrounds the muscular portion. The muscle processes of the dilator muscle are oriented parallel to the iris plane and they overlap each other to form two to three layers. They branch in various directions, which makes it difficult to trace their extensions. The myofibrils are similar to those of the sphincter. (× 8840.)

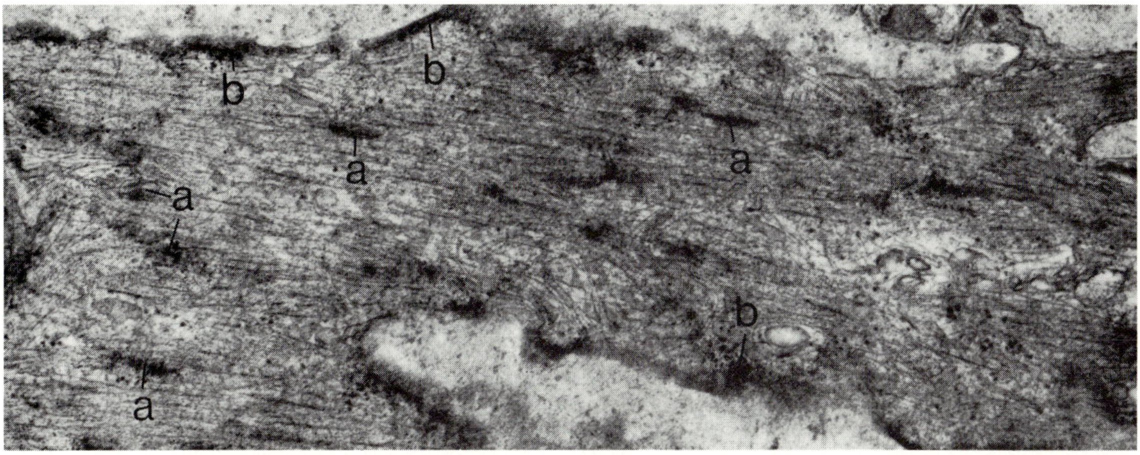

Figure 6–40. Anterior iris epithelium, to show the details of the myofilaments in the dilator muscle. The filaments appear to be of one type and they form areas (a) which are reminiscent of the Z-discs of skeletal muscle. The characteristic densities of the cell membrane of smooth muscle are also present (b). (× 27,600.)

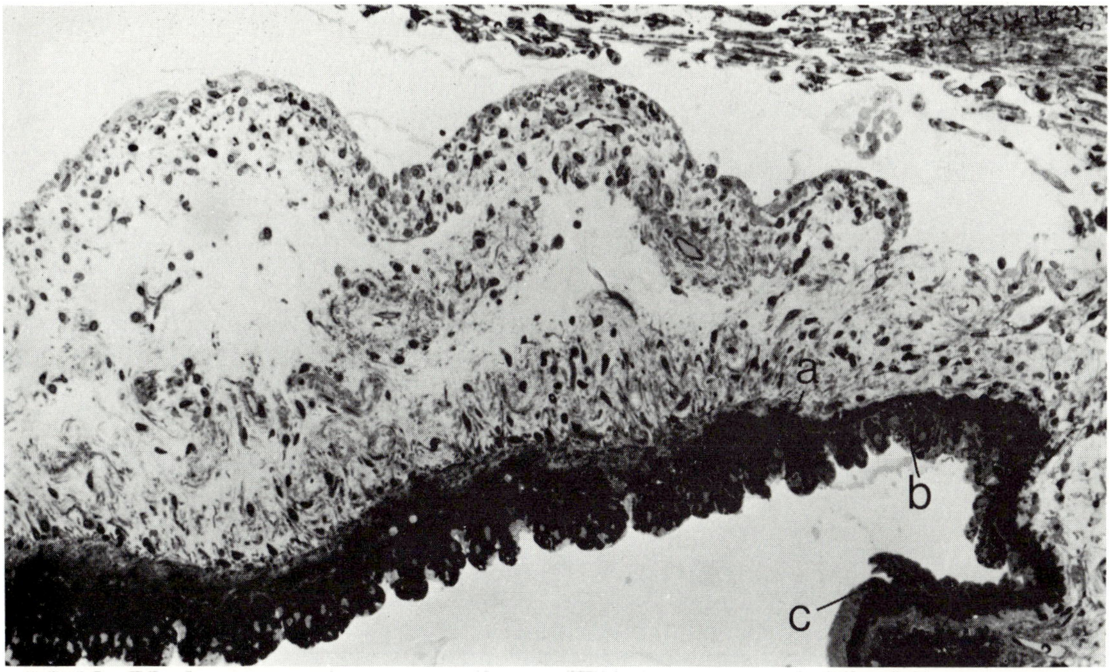

Figure 6–41. Periphery of the ciliary portion of the iris. The dilator muscle ends at (a). The posterior epithelium of the iris begins to lose its pigment at (b) and is completely unpigmented over the pars plicata at (c). (× 430.)

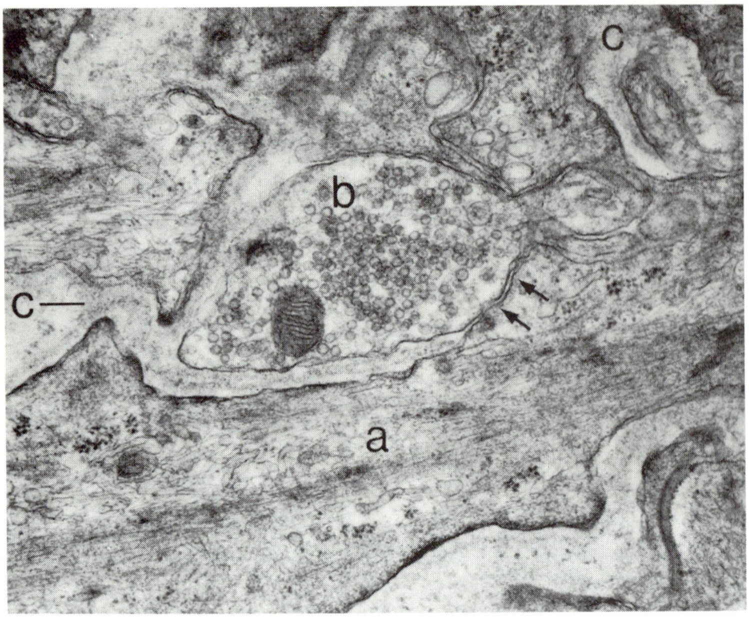

Figure 6–42. Dilator muscle fiber (a) innervated by a single axon (b) containing numerous synaptic vesicles and a mitochondrion. The nerve comes into close apposition with the muscle (arrows), being separated from it by a space measuring approximately 200 A.; the basement membrane (c) is excluded from this site. (× 21,000.)

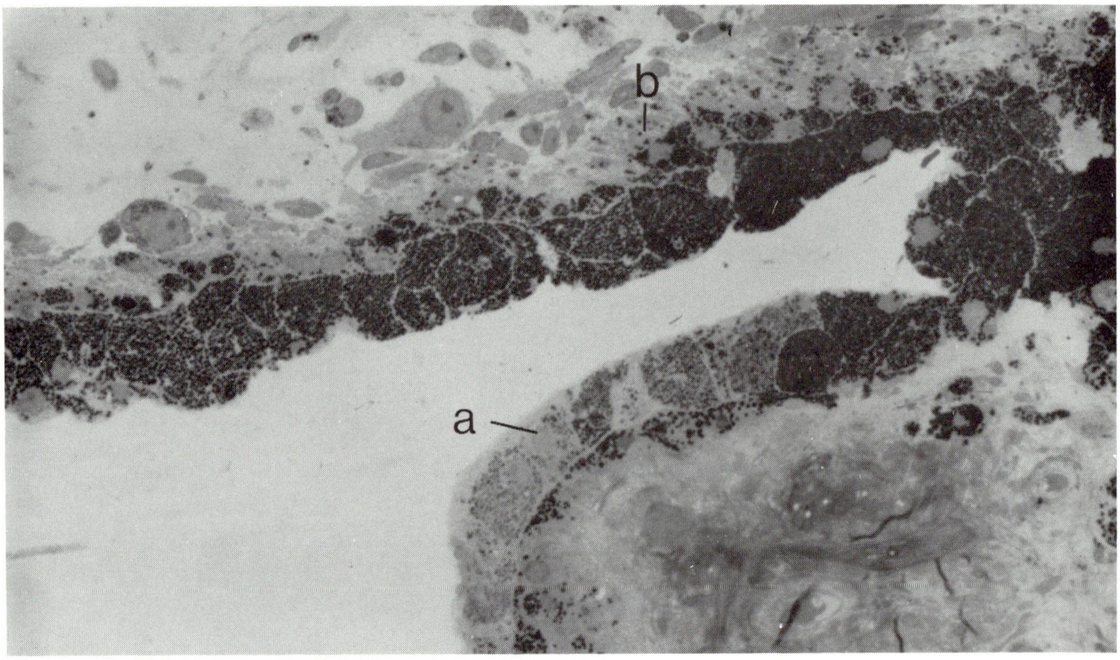

Figure 6–43. Peripheral iris and anterior pars plicata of the ciliary body. The transition of iris epithelium to that of the ciliary body is shown. The posterior epithelium loses most of its pigment at (a) and the dilator muscle begins to disappear at (b). (× 640.)

found in this portion. They consist of a moderate number of mitochondria, pigment granules, stacks of rough-surfaced endoplasmic reticulum and tubules of the smooth-surfaced endoplasmic reticulum. Clusters of unattached ribosomes also are abundant, usually located in the perinuclear region. The Golgi apparatus is poorly developed but one is usually seen. The nucleus also is found in this portion of the anterior epithelium. Myofilaments are seen here as well, bypassing the nucleus and cell organelles.

Posterior Pigment Epithelium (Figs. 6-1 to 6-4, 6-20, 6-36 and 6-42 to 6-49)

The cells of the posterior epithelial layer retain their purely epithelial character throughout life. The layer is so heavily pigmented that it is difficult to make out the details of the cytoplasm; the characteristics become

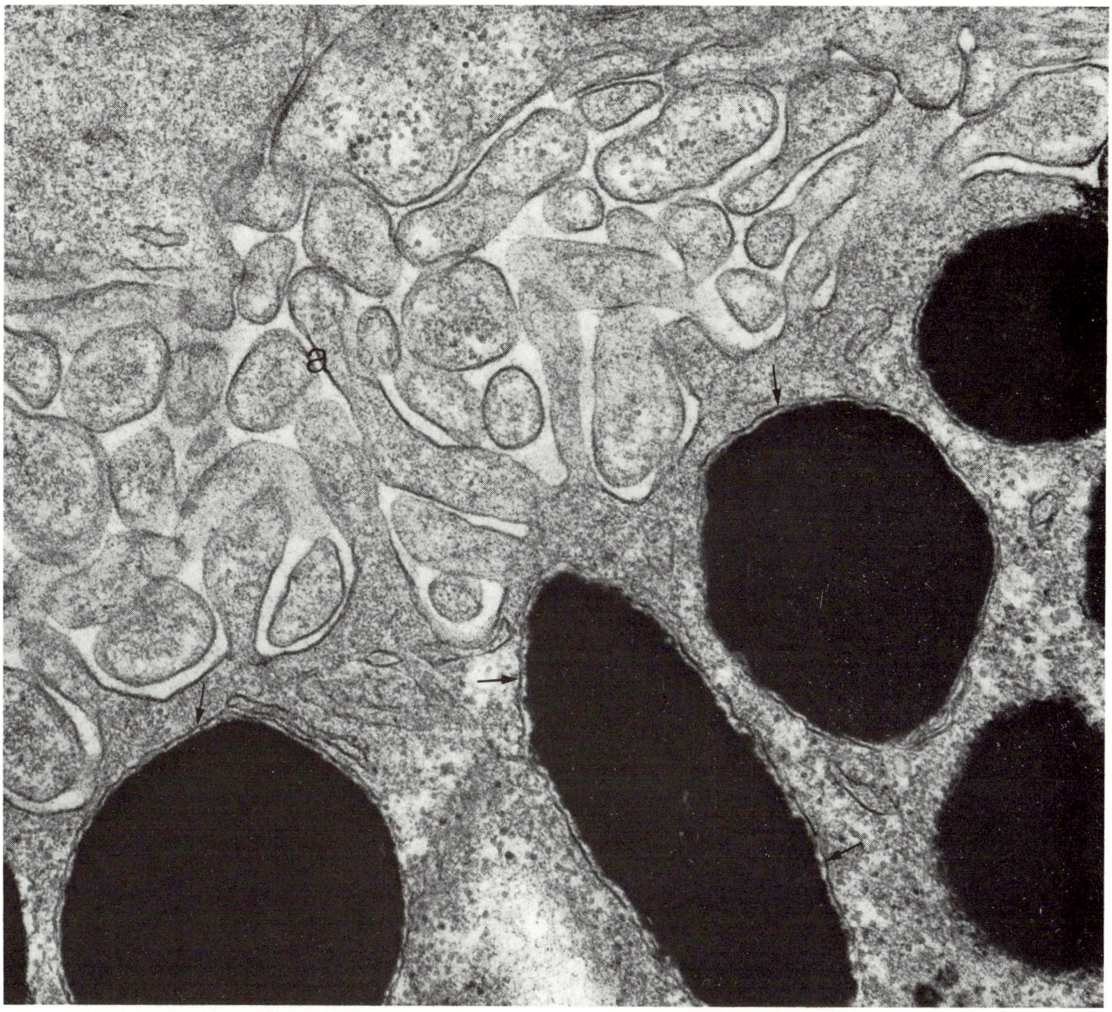

Figure 6–44. Posterior pigmented iris epithelium at its junction with the anterior epithelium. At (a) numerous obliquely sectioned microvilli from both epithelial layers fill a space found between the two epithelia. The membrane (arrows) encircling the melanin granules of the posterior epithelium is clearly shown. (× 45,000.)

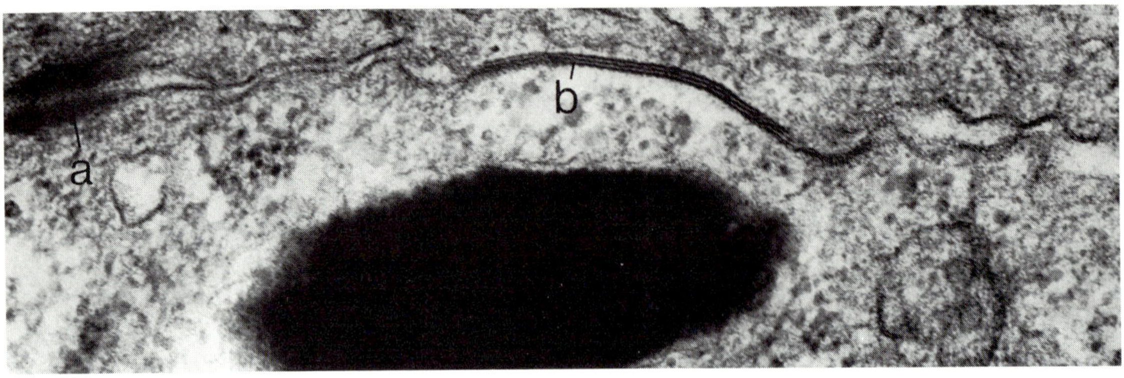

Figure 6–45. Junctions between the apical surface of the anterior and posterior epithelium. Desmosomes (a) are the most common type of junction in these epithelia, but numerous tight junctions (b) are also found. (× 75,000.)

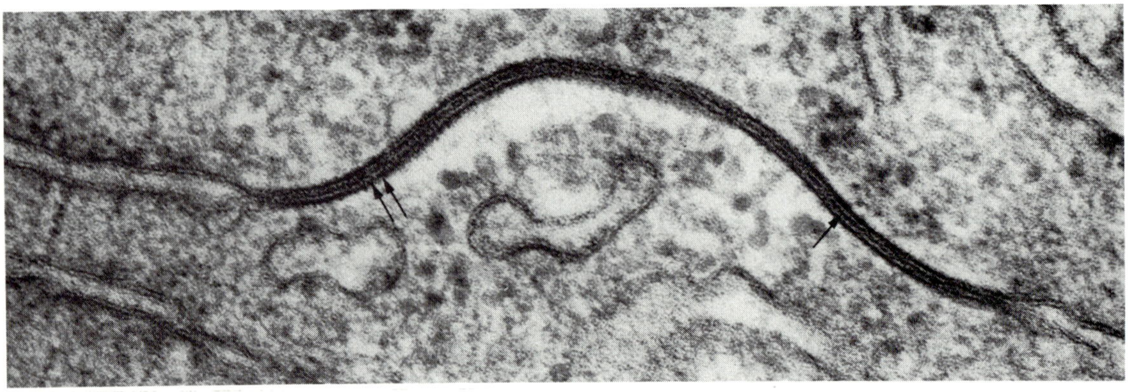

Figure 6–46. Junction between the apical surface of the iris epithelia, higher magnification. A tight junction similar to that shown in Figure 6–45 is shown here. Note areas of membrane fusion (single arrow) as well as areas of close apposition (double arrows) which could be classified as gap junctions. (× 90,000.)

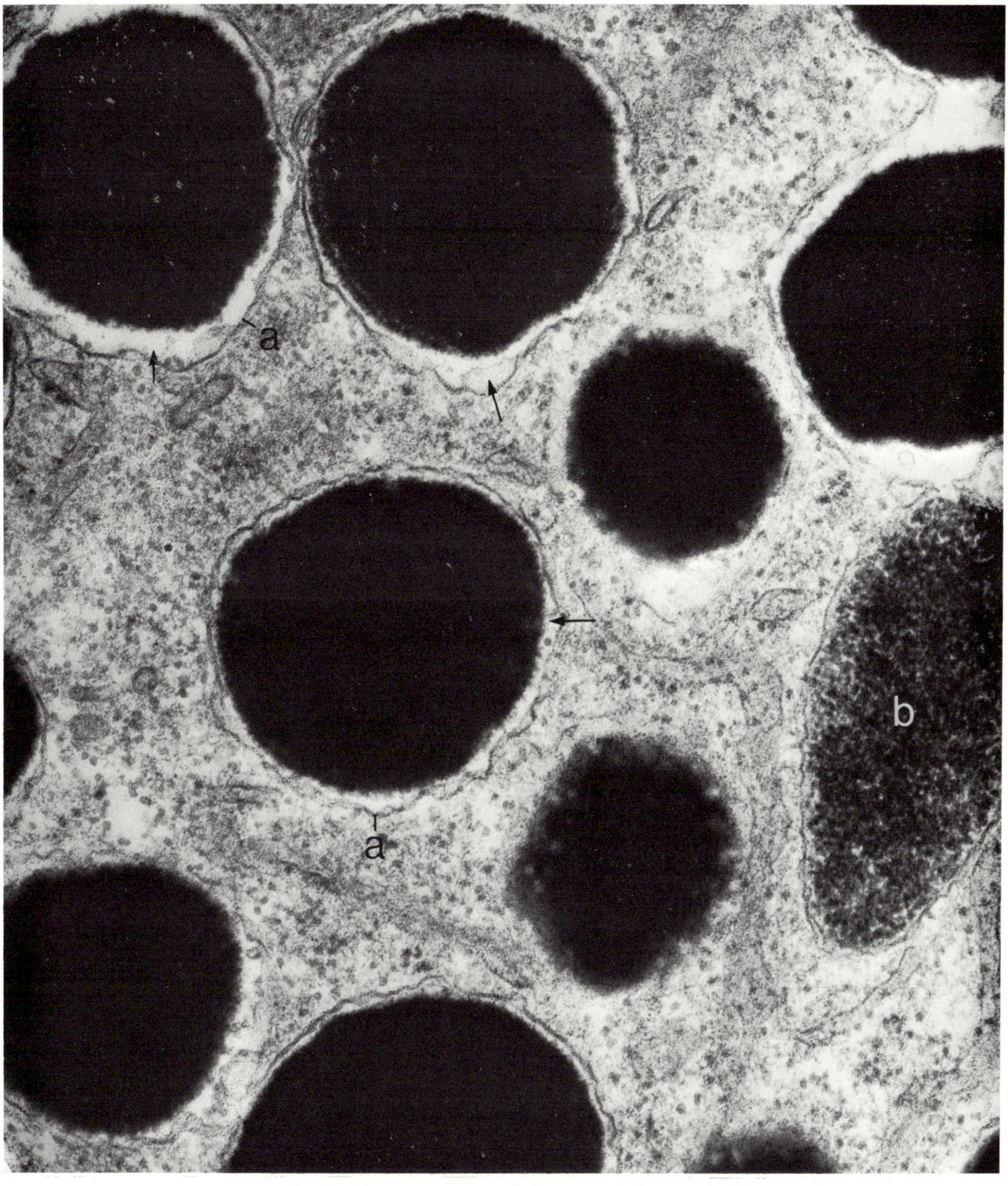

Figure 6–47. Posterior pigmented iris epithelium. The large melanin granules of the iris pigmented epithelium are round in cross-section, measuring 0.6 μm. and of spindle shape in longitudinal section, measuring 1.96 μm. in length. Note that these granules are membrane-bound (a) and that there is a narrow zone at the periphery of the granule (arrows) free of melanin. An incompletely melanized granule (b) is seen on the right. (× 62,500.)

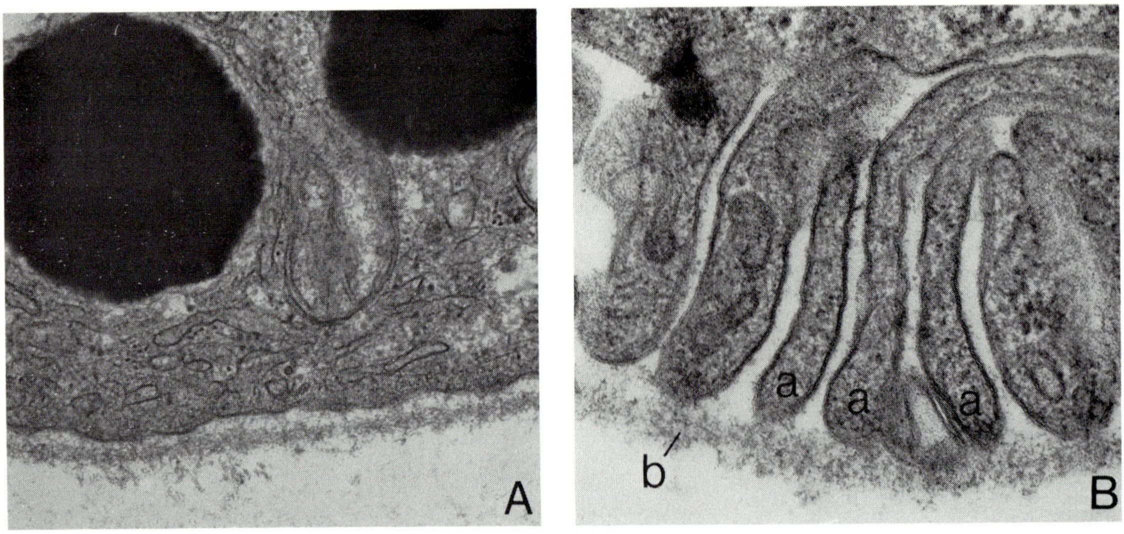

Figure 6–48. *A*, Iris posterior epithelium. The basal surface of the posterior epithelium faces the posterior chamber and the lens. A thin basement membrane is found on this surface. (× 45,000.)

B, Numerous infoldings (a) also occur on the basal surface of the posterior epithelium. Note that the basement membrane (b) continues along without entering the infoldings of the cell membrane. (× 60,000.)

evident only in depigmented specimens. The cells are somewhat rectangular, varying in shape only in the folds and contraction furrows, where they may become truncated or pyramidal. They have a height of 36 to 55 μm. and a breadth of 16 to 25 μm. (Salzmann, 1912). In the floors of the furrows the cells may be only 35 μm. in height, whereas they are taller elsewhere. The cytoplasm contains large numbers of round or cigar-shaped, brown-to-black pigment granules that are much larger than those of the stromal melanocytes (Feeney et al., 1965). In the pupillary region the cells become more pyramidal, but their pigmentation is unaltered. At the iris periphery this layer gradually becomes depigmented as it extends backward onto the ciliary body. A thin basement membrane is found adjacent to the posterior surface of the pigment epithelium in PAS-stained sections.

With the electron microscope (Figs. 6–44 and 6–48) the cell membrane at the base of the cell has a typical basement membrane. The basal cell membrane shows numerous infoldings which extend deep into the cell cytoplasm. The basement membrane, however, does not follow these infoldings. The lateral walls of the cells show some interdigitation but no infoldings; scattered maculae adherentes and occludentes are present along the lateral wall; otherwise, the cells are separated from each other by a space of 200 A. the apical cell wall is more undulating and these cells are frequently separated from the anterior epithelial cells by small spaces containing microvilli from the surfaces of the cells (Tousimis and Fine, 1959; Uneo, 1961; Tomita et al., 1961; Missotten, 1964).

The cytoplasm contains scattered large round and oval pigment granules, which are quite osmiophilic and measure 0.8 μm. in diameter by 2.5 μm. in length. The nucleus is smooth and rounded. The cytoplasm contains deposits of glycogen usually extracted during preparation of the tissues; mitochondria, stacks of rough-surfaced endoplasmic reticulum and a Golgi apparatus are commonly seen.

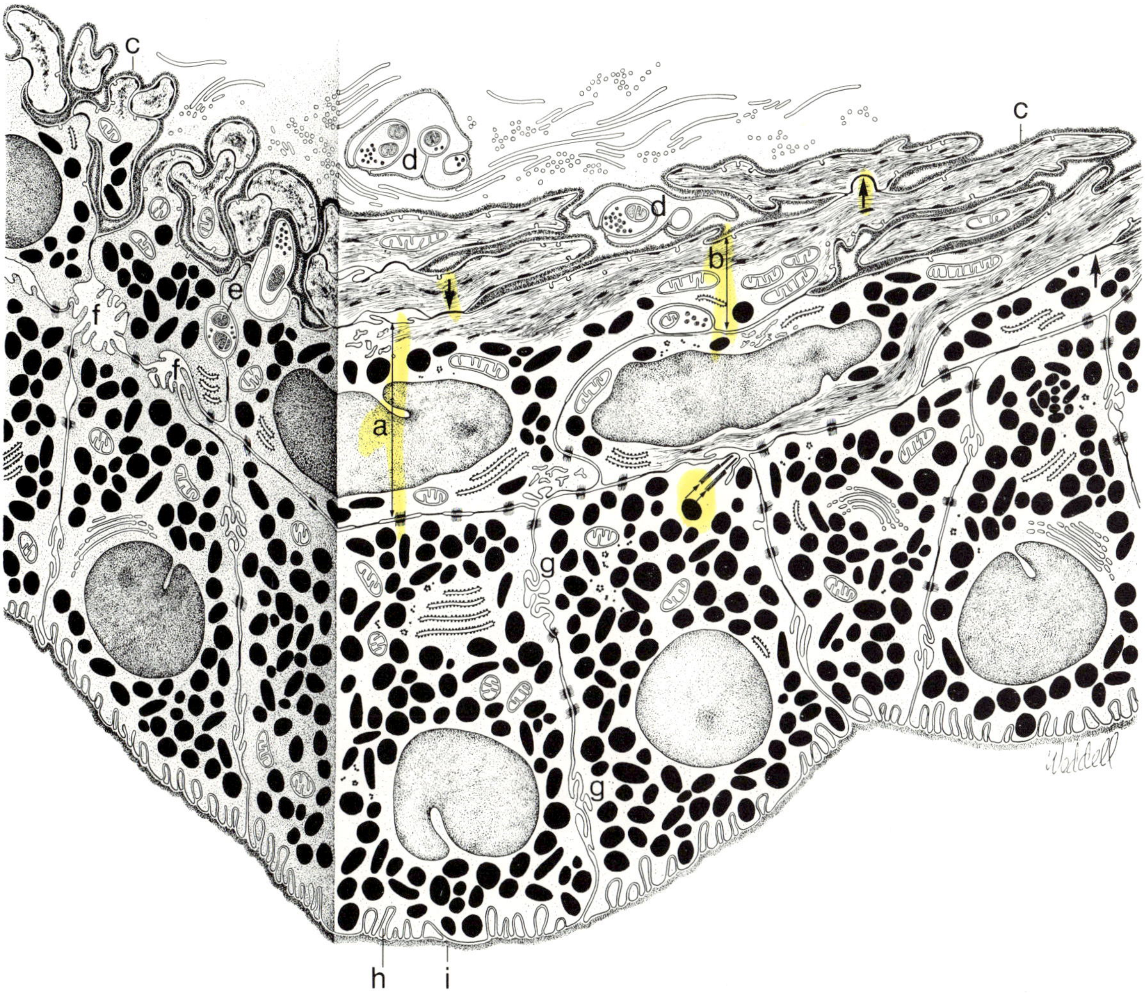

Figure 6-49. Posterior epithelial layers. The anterior iris epithelium has two morphologically distinct portions: an apical epithelial portion (a) and a basal muscular portion (b). The cytoplasm of the basal portion is filled with myofibrils and a moderate number of mitochondria. The tongue-like muscular processes overlap each other, creating three to five layers. Tight junctions (arrows) like those in the sphincter muscle are found between the dilator muscle cells. A basement membrane (c) surrounds the muscle processes. Unmyelinated nerves and their associated Schwann cells (d) as well as a few naked axons innervate the muscle. The axon at (e) is in close contact with the anterior epithelium, being separated from it by a space measuring 200 A. in width. The cytoplasm of the epithelial portions contains cell organelles, melanin granules, the nucleus and bundles of myofilaments. Most of the intercellular junctions present here are maculae occludentes and only a few desmosomes are present; desmosomes are not found in the muscular portion. The apical surface of the anterior epithelium is contiguous with that of the posterior epithelium. Desmosomes and tight junctions join the two layers, but there are some areas of separation (f) between the cells. The spaces so formed are filled with microvilli, and an occasional cilium is also found here (double arrows).

The posterior pigmented iris epithelium shows lateral interdigitations (g) and areas of infolding along its basal surface (h). A typical basement membrane is also found on the basal side (i). Numerous tight junctions and desmosomes occur along the lateral and apical walls. The cytoplasm of this epithelium has numerous melanin granules measuring around 0.8 μm. in cross-section and up to 2.5 μm. in length. Stacks of cisternae of the rough-surfaced endoplasmic reticulum, clustered unattached ribosomes, mitochondria and a Golgi apparatus are commonly observed.

Anterior Chamber

GROSS ANATOMY

The anterior chamber is bounded anteriorly by the corneal endothelium and posteriorly by the anterior surface of the iris and pupillary portion of the lens. Its periphery is bounded by the trabecular meshwork on the anterior side and by the ciliary body and periphery iris posteriorly. Endothelium lines the anterior chamber over the cornea and the trabecular meshwork, and a layer of fibroblasts and some melanocytes line it over the iris and ciliary body surfaces.

The anterior chamber is roughly ellipsoidal in shape, with the posterior surface of the ellipsoid flattened because of the shape of the iris. The plane of the iris root is about 4.2 mm. behind the vertex plane of the cornea, while the plane of the pupillary iris is about 3.6 mm. posterior to the corneal vertex, a difference of 0.6 mm. The distance from the corneal vertex to the peripheral iris plane is greater than that from the vertex to the central iris because of the forward displacement of the pupillary iris plane by the lens. In myopic eyes the difference between the two iris planes is smaller and the anterior chamber often is deeper. In some hypermetropic eyes the anterior ocular segment may be small in proportion to the size of the lens.

In emmetropic eyes the transverse diameter of the anterior chamber is approximately equal to that of the cornea, the chamber diameter varying between 11.3 and 12.4 mm. In the horizontal meridian the chamber angle is 1.0 mm. posterior to the peripheral cornea and in the vertical meridian it is 0.75 to 1.0 mm. posterior to the cornea (LaGrange, 1920). The anterior chamber is deepest centrally and narrower peripherally near the angle. A short distance from the angle, the chamber narrows slightly, then widens as it opens into the angle recess. This widening occurs because of a slight change in direction of the iris as it inserts into the ciliary body.

The depth of the anterior chamber and the width of the angle have been studied to determine their role in the causation of glaucoma. The refractive power of the cornea magnifies the iris and, therefore, makes the anterior chamber appear to be shallower than it actually is. Accurate measurements of the depth of the chamber can be made, however, with the slit lamp and special optical devices. The width of the angle of the anterior chamber is more difficult to measure because of the distortion induced by the corneal curvature and the need to observe the angle obliquely. Most observers have been content merely to estimate the width of the angle when it is viewed with the gonioscope.

Tornquist (1953) made a study of 45 sets of twins and concluded that the depth of the anterior chamber is genetically determined. Aizawa (1958) studied the anterior chamber depth in 451 emmetropic patients aged eight to 77 years and observed a wide distribution in depth, ranging from 2.6 and 4.4 mm., with an average of 3.54 $\pm$ 0.016 mm. The depth of the anterior chambers of two eyes in the same subject was quite similar. Aizawa also found a decrease in depth with increasing age. Calmettes and co-workers (1958) found that the anterior chamber decreases in depth with increasing age, whereas the radius of curvature and diameter of the cornea remain constant.

Stenström (1946) found the chamber depth to average 3.70 mm. in men and 3.65 mm. in women, while Calmettes and co-workers found a relation of 3.61 mm. in males to 3.41 mm. in females. Stenström was able to establish a correlation between the depth of the anterior chamber and the length of the eye, but he found no correlation between the radius of curvature of the cornea and the depth of the anterior chamber. Weekers and associates (1961a, b, 1963) showed a correlation between the diameter and the radius of curvature of the cornea, as well as between the diameter of the cornea and the depth of the anterior chamber, but no correlation was found between the radius of curvature and the depth of the anterior chamber. The following table from their studies gives the dimensions of the depth of the anterior chamber, the radius of curvature of the cornea and the diameter of the cornea in emmetropic subjects (0.050 to 1.0 diopters; n = number of cases; s = deviation; e = standard deviation from mean).

	Age, yrs.			
	Under 15	15–30	35–55	Over 55
Depth of the anterior chamber	3.61 n=27 s=0.21 e=0.040	3.60 n=40 s=0.25 e=0.039	3.27 n=40 s=0.34 e=0.054	3.18 n=40 s=0.34 e=0.054
Radius of curvature of the cornea	7.87 n=27 s=0.32 e=0.062	7.96 n=40 s=0.23 e=0.036	7.82 n=40 s=0.29 e=0.046	7.79 n=40 s=0.22 e=0.035
Diameter of the cornea millimeters	11.71 n=40 s=0.50 e=0.079	11.81 n=40 s=0.35 e=0.056	11.76 n=40 s=0.28 e=0.044	11.75 n=40 s=0.36 e=0.057

These same authors later made similar studies of 210 ametropic eyes and concluded that the anterior chamber was shallower in the hypermetropic and deeper in the myopic than in the emmetropic eye. They could demonstrate a mathematical relationship between the degree of ametropia and the depth of the anterior chamber in uncomplicated cases, but this did not hold in cases of complicated myopia or uni-ocular myopia.

EMBRYOLOGY

The anterior chamber first appears at the 18 mm. stage (end of the sixth week of embryonic life). At about the 12 mm. stage, a thin sheet of mesoderm growing in from the paraxial area separates the lens vesicle from the ectoderm. The posterior part of this mesoderm is destined to become the corneal endothelium. Posterior to this endothelium is some mesenchymal tissue that will later form the anterior chamber. Between the 12 and 18 mm. stages, a second wave of mesodermal ingrowth occurs between the surface ectoderm and the endothelium. This ingrowth forms the corneal stroma, as previously described (p. 59). At about the 18 mm. stage another wave of mesodermal cells extends into the cup from the lateral side near the lens, leaving a loose acellular matrix of fibrillar material between it and the corneal endothelium. This matrix liquefies behind the central cornea after the fifth month and leads to formation of the early anterior chamber.

The angle of the anterior chamber does not begin to differentiate until about the sixth month, or about two months after the appearance of the canal of Schlemm. The anterior chamber widens, causing separation of the corneosclera from the iris. During this time extensive changes occur in the relations of the various tissues in this area. The mesoderm internal to the canal of Schlemm fans out to form definitive trabecular sheets and spaces. The interrelationship of the canal of Schlemm, trabecular meshwork and scleral spur remains fairly constant, but all three change in position with respect to the chamber angle, which extends posteriorly. By the sixth month the angle is at the anterior trabecular meshwork; by the seventh month it is in the midtrabecular zone, with the canal and spur behind it; and at birth the angle is at the posterior part of the meshwork, with the spur and canal well in front of it.

AQUEOUS HUMOR

The anterior chamber is filled with aqueous humor that partially supports the cornea and is largely responsible for the intraocular pressure. It also provides nourishment for the avascular tissues of the eye, the lens and the cornea. The aqueous humor is produced by the pars plicata of the ciliary body, moves into the posterior chamber, circulates forward through the pupil to the anterior chamber, and leaves the eye mainly through the trabecular meshwork. Its rate of production and outflow is rather constant.

The aqueous humor contains the necessary ingredients for the metabolism of the lens and the cornea. It provides sugar and amino acids to assist in growth and replacement of tissue, transports oxygen to the tissues, and carries their waste products to the blood vessels of the iris and chamber angle. The aqueous humor does not carry sufficient oxygen, however, to meet all the metabolic needs of the cornea if the cornea is denied contact with air.

The aqueous humor is perfectly clear, and light which has traversed the cornea is transmitted through the aqueous humor to the lens aperture without interference. This fluid does have a lower index of refraction than the lens, however, and thus rays of light are refracted again at the aqueous-lens interface. The aqueous humor has a specific gravity of 1.0034 to 1.0036 and contains 1.0 gm. of solute per 100 ml., or about one tenth the amount of solids in the blood serum, chiefly because of its lower protein content.

The relative proportions of globulin and albumin in the aqueous humor are the same as in the blood serum, but the gamma globulin content is much lower. The protein content of human aqueous is between 0.019 and 0.034 gm. per 100 ml., compared to 7.0 per cent in the blood. The concentration of sugars seems to be lower in aqueous humor than in blood, probably because they are removed by the metabolism of the cornea and lens. The concentration of ascorbic acid is significantly higher in aqueous humor than in plasma, and in some animals, particularly the rabbit, it may be 10 to 15 times higher. The higher concentration of ascorbic acid in aqueous humor suggests active transport of this substance across the ciliary epithelium.

REFERENCES

Adler, F. H.: Physiology of the Eye: Clinical Application. 4th ed. St. Louis, The C. V. Mosby Co., 1965.

Aizawa, K.: The depth of the normal anterior chamber. Acta Soc. Ophthal. Jap. *62*:2283, 1958.

Calmettes, Deodati, Huron, and Bechac: Study of the depth of the anterior chamber; physiological variations. Arch. Ophtal. (Paris) *18*:513, 1958.

Ehinger, B.: Ocular and orbital vegetative nerves. Acta Physiol. Scand. 67(Suppl. 268):1, 1966.

Feeney, M. L., Grieshaber, J., and Hogan, M. J.: Studies on human ocular pigment. *In* Rohen, J. (ed.): The Structure of the Eye. II. Symposium. Stuttgart, F. K. Schattauer Verlag, 1965.

Gregersen, E.: The tissue spaces in the human iris and their communications with the anterior chamber by way of the iridic crypts. Acta Ophthal. *36*:819, 1958.

Gregersen, E.: Studies on the Spongy Structure of the Human Iris and Its Inhibition with the Aqueous Humor. Experimental and Histological Investigations. Copenhagen, Munksgaard, 1960, p. 102.

Iwamoto, T.: Electron microscopy of human iris stroma. Acta Soc. Ophthal. Jap. *65*:1296, 1961.

LaGrange, F.: Un moyen de rélévement de la tension oculaire. Ann. Occul. (Paris) *157*:447, 1920.

Magari, S.: The structure of the iris stroma and the question of an endothelium on its anterior surface. Graefes Arch. Ophthal. *159*:257, 1957.

Missotten, L.: L'ultrastructure des tissue oculaires. Bull. Soc. Belg. Ophthal. 136, Fascicle 1, p. 199, 1964.

Rohen, J.: Comparative and experimental studies on the iris of primates. Amer. J. Ophthal. *52*:384, 1961.

Salzmann, M.: The Anatomy and Histology of the Human Eyeball. Chicago, Deuticke, 1912.

Smelser, G. K., and Ishikawa, T.: Investigation of the porosity of the iris. Acta XIX Conc. Ofthal India *1*:612, 1966.

Stenström, S.: Untersuchungen über die Variation und Kovariation der optischen Elemente des menschlicken Auges. Acta Ophthal. *26*:1, 1946.

Tomita, I., Matsuo, T., and Kato, Y.: Electron microscopy of the pigment epithelial cells and dilator pupillae muscles in the human iris. Acta Soc. Opthal. Jap. *65*:1177, 1961.

Tornquist, R.: Shallow anterior chamber in acute glaucoma. Acta Ophthal. *31*(Suppl. 39):1, 1953.

Tousimis, A. J., and Fine, B. S.: Ultrastructure of the iris: The intercellular components. Amer. J. Ophthal. *48*:397, 1959 a.

Tousimis, A. J., and Fine, B. S.: Ultrastructure of the iris: The intracellular stromal components. A.M.A. Arch. Ophthal. *62*:974, 1959 b.

Ueno, K.: Some controversial points on the fine structure of the human iris. Negation of the existence of the continuous anterior endothelium and the fine structure of the dilator pupillae muscle and of the pigment epithelium. Kyushu J. Med. Sci. *12*:43, 1961.

Vrabec, F.: Investigations of the endothelium of the anterior surface of the human iris. Biol. Listy *31*:118, 1951.

Vrabec, F.: The anterior superficial endothelium of the human iris. Ophthalmologica *123*:20, 1952.

Weekers, R., Grieten, J., and Lavergne, G.: Study of the dimensions of the human anterior chamber. Ophthalmologica *142*:650, 1961a.

Weekers, R., and Grieten, J.: The measurement of the depth of the anterior chamber in clinical practice. Bull. Soc. Belg. Ophtal. *129*:361, 1961b.

Weekers, R., Grieten, J., and Lekeux, M.: Etude des dimension de la chambre antérieure de l'oeil humain. IV. L'intumescence cristallinienne et ses conséquences chirurgicales. Ophthalmologica (Basel) *146*:57, 1963.

Zimmerman, L. E.: Demonstration of the hyaluronidase-sensitive acid mucopolysaccharide in trabecula and iris in routine paraffin sections of adult eyes; a preliminary report. Amer. J. Ophthal. *44*:1, 1957.

Chapter Seven

CILIARY BODY AND POSTERIOR CHAMBER

Ciliary Body

The ciliary body has many functions that make it an important structure in the eye. The pars plicata of the ciliary body is responsible for the production of most of the aqueous humor, and it is probable that some of the vitreous mucopolysaccharide is secreted by the cells of the pars plana. The ciliary muscle occupies a large area of the ciliary body; its principal function is to facilitate accommodation of the lens. The vessels in the anterior ciliary body supply blood to the iris, limbal tissues, anterior choroid and the ciliary body. The nerve trunks that enter the ciliary body are distributed to almost all the anterior ocular structures.

The ciliary body is difficult to study in vivo because of its location in the eye. A small amount of its anterior surface can be seen indistinctly with the gonioscope, while the pars plana and ora serrata can be seen with the indirect ophthalmoscope and with the three-prism contact lens of Goldmann when the sclera is depressed.

PHYSIOLOGY

The ciliary body has three principal functions: (1) aqueous humor production and removal, (2) accommodation, and (3) restoration of vitreous mucopolysaccharide.

Aqueous Production and Removal

Most of the aqueous humor appears to be produced by the pars plicata of the ciliary body. The stroma in this part of the ciliary body contains many capillaries which lie close to the ciliary epithelium, and it is likely that both the capillaries and the epithelium are involved in the formation of aqueous humor.

The capillaries of the ciliary body are large and have a thin endothelium with many pores or fenestrations; these fenestrations facilitate the movement of substances into and out of the capillary lumen. These vessels, like those in the choroid, are very permeable, even to macromolecules such as myoglobin (Bill, 1968).

Diffusion of substances from the stroma through the ciliary epithelial cells probably occurs in much the same way as it does in the capillary endothelium. In addition to diffusion, there is secretion or active transport of many substances from the ciliary body stroma into the posterior chamber. Most of our knowledge about aqueous humor secretion is based on animal experiments, and it is possible that the results are not applicable to the human eye. Ascorbic acid, sodium and chloride ions, bicarbonate and free amino acids are present in higher concentrations in aqueous humor than in plasma.

Kinsey (1947) showed that there is an *ascorbic acid* carrier mechanism which exhibits the features of transport-maxima kinetics, like that present in the proximal kidney tubule for the transport of glucose. He found that increasing the concentration of ascorbic acid in the blood does not result in a proportional increment of ascorbate in aqueous humor. Rather, when a given concentration of ascorbic acid is reached, the sites in the ascorbate carrier mechanism are exhausted and the maximum rate of transport is reached. Thereafter, this plateau in the concentration of ascorbate in the aqueous remains unaltered even with increase in the concentration of ascorbate in the blood.

The increased concentration of *bicarbonate* in the aqueous humor is related to the presence of the enzyme carbonic anhydrase. This enzyme is found in many tissues involved in secretory processes, such as in the kidney and gastric mucosa, and it catalyzes the formation of carbonic acid from carbon dioxide and water. Inhibition of this enzyme in the ciliary body results in a marked decrease in the production of aqueous humor (Becker, 1959). There is also evidence for the presence of a Na^{+}-K^{+} activated ATPase in the inner or basal cell membrane of the unpigmented epithelium. *Sodium ions* are actively pumped into the posterior chamber, while water follows passively along the gradient established by this pump. Cole (1969) has presented experimental evidence indicating that *chloride ion* is also actively transported into the posterior chamber, but that the active chloride flux is considerably smaller than the active sodium flux. These ion pumps probably are responsible for the electrochemical potential across the ciliary epithelium. Kinsey (1947) found the "effective" electrochemical potential across the ciliary epithelium to be 2 to 4 mv., with the aqueous being positive and the stroma negative. Sugar and urea are in lower concentration in the aqueous humor than in the blood, but the lower concentration of sugar may result from its utilization by the lens and cornea.

If the intraocular pressure is lowered and the arterial pressure is maintained at a normal level, there is swelling of the ciliary processes, indicating that the ciliary epithelium offers resistance to the rapid passage of fluid into the posterior chamber. The precise anatomic site of this blood-aqueous barrier is not known. The lateral intercellular space between the cells of the pigmented and unpigmented epithelium measures around 200 A.

and does not appear to be obstructed by a zonula occludens; only a few maculae occludentes and adherentes are present. For this reason fluids move relatively freely along the lateral intercellular spaces. The apical intercellular space, on the other hand, is closed by many occluding junctions of the fascia and macula occludens type, but we are not sure about the presence of zonulae occludentes (Fig. 7-23 *A*, *B* and *C*). Because of the alignment of the cells of the two epithelial layers, it is probable that particles must traverse the apical intercellular space in order to reach the spaces between the unpigmented epithelial cells from those between the pigmented epithelium. At the cell apices of these two epithelial layers the occluding junctions could offer considerable obstruction to the passage of many substances. At any rate, the anatomic site of the blood-aqueous barrier probably exists at several levels for different substances. These sites may be the capillary endothelial cells, the basement membrane of the capillary endothelium, the pigmented epithelium and its basement membrane, and the junctional complexes between the apices of epithelial cells.

The ciliary muscle probably assists in the removal of aqueous humor because of its attachment to the scleral spur and because some of its longitudinal cells are connected directly to the corneoscleral meshwork (Fig. 4–16, p. 137). Through these insertions, the ciliary muscle can alter the size of the intertrabecular spaces of the meshwork. The action of pilocarpine in improving the facility of outflow in open angle glaucoma has been attributed to its action on the ciliary muscle and trabecular meshwork. Flocks and Zweng (1957) showed that, in the monkey, pilocarpine acts on the ciliary muscle and iris to cause the trabecular spaces to expand. Minor changes in the size of these spaces probably occur during accommodation, and for this reason the ciliary muscle may act as a pump to assist in the removal of aqueous humor. The accessory route for removal of aqueous humor through the ciliary body into the supraciliary and suprachoroidal region in various primates has been discussed (p. 114). The importance of this pathway has not been assessed in human eyes.

Accommodation

The second important function of the ciliary body is in the act of accommodation. The longitudinal part of the ciliary muscle is attached firmly to the scleral spur, to the stroma of the choroid and to the inner anterior sclera. The ciliary muscle is shortened meridionally during contraction; since the scleral spur is relatively unmovable, the muscle exerts its principal force on the choroid. During muscle relaxation the tension on the choroid is released, allowing this tissue to move posteriorly because of its inherent elasticity.

During accommodation the ciliary muscle overcomes the inherent choroidal tension so that the choroid is moved forward. As a result, the zonules are relaxed, allowing the normal elasticity of the lens capsule to increase its curvature and thus to increase the refractive power of the lens. The longitudinal, radial and circular cells of the ciliary muscle all seem to act jointly in regulating accommodation through their effects on the zonular fibers. The zonules are tightened or relaxed, depending on the movement of the ciliary muscle, the ciliary body and the choroidal stroma. The varying forces are transmitted to the zonules at their attachment into the inner limiting membrane of the unpigmented epithelial cells and into the capsule of the lens. It is possible that the occluding junction between the two epithelial layers at their apices is important in preventing separation of the two layers during accommodation.

RESTORATION OF VITREOUS MUCOPOLYSACCHARIDE

A final function of the ciliary body is believed to be the formation of mucopolysaccharide that is incorporated into the vitreous. Fine and Zimmerman (1963) demonstrated the presence of mucopolysaccharide in the cytoplasm and intercellular spaces of the epithelial cells of the pars plana; they suggested that these cells are actively engaged in synthesis of mucopolysaccharide.

EMBRYOLOGY

The ciliary body is derived from two tissues: (1) the associated mesoderm which forms the stroma, ciliary muscle, suprachoroidal lamellae and blood vessels; and (2) the neuroectoderm of the optic vesicle, which forms an outer pigmented and an inner unpigmented epithelium that line the ciliary body.

The ciliary body does not begin to form until early fetal life. Its first appearance is at the 50 mm. stage (third month), when folds appear in the outer neuroectodermal layer just behind the margin of the optic cup. The cells of the outer layer of the optic cup are pigmented almost to the cup margin. By the 65 mm. stage the folds involve the inner layer of epithelium. These folds will become the primitive ciliary processes, and they slowly increase in number and size. At the same time there is a change in the associated mesoderm which forms the stroma of the ciliary body and its processes. The primitive ciliary muscle also appears in this mesoderm during the third month.

After the 65 mm. stage the growing tip of the optic cup extends forward to form the iris, leaving the ciliary folds behind. These ciliary processes become more and more prominent and coincide with growth of the eye, also moving forward. Behind them a smooth area appears, the pars plana, which extends to the ora serrata. The pars plana develops very slowly and is barely discernible even at the fifth month. At the seventh month the ora serrata is still even with the midportion of the ciliary muscle. By the eighth month it is close to the posterior third of the muscle, and at the ninth month it is found at the posterior third of the muscle.

Each ciliary fold eventually develops into a ciliary process, the two epithelial layers covering the processes and the mesoderm forming a core containing small blood vessels. The inner surface of the inner epithelial layer shows no limitans interna and is irregular, with cone-shaped processes and filaments projecting from its surface. The surface becomes smooth over the summits of the processes in late fetal life, but it is always less differentiated in the cells of the ciliary valleys. The pars plicata changes little after the fourth month.

The ciliary muscle can be seen in the associated mesoderm at about the third month. It appears as an ill defined triangular area with its base directed anteriorly. The neuroepithelium is on its internal surface, and the early scleral condensation is lateral. The organization of the mesoderm into strands and fibers takes place between the third and fifth months, so that by the fifth month the meridional portion of the muscle is clearly visible, although its shape has been altered by growth of the eye and development of adjacent tissues. The muscle is still triangular, but the apex is now anterior at the scleral spur and the base is posterointernal. The radial and circular portions of the muscle do not become evident until after the sixth month and they are not completely developed at birth.

GROSS ANATOMY (Figs. 7–1 to 7–6)

In the living eye the ciliary body can be located by measurement. The anterior insertion is at the scleral spur, which is 1.5 mm. posterior to the corneolimbal junction. The posterior limit is at the ora serrata, 7.5 to 8.0 mm. from the limbus on the temporal side, 6.5 to 7.0 mm. on the nasal side, and 7.0 superiorly and inferiorly. The pars plana occupies the posterior 4.0 to 4.5 mm. of this area (see Fig. 2–2, p. 48).

Anteriorly the ciliary body forms part of the posterior surface of the anterior chamber angle. On the anterolateral side it is attached to the scleral spur and is joined by bands from the trabecular meshwork. The iris is attached to its anteromedial side. The ciliary body and iris, therefore, form the posterior surface of the anterior chamber angle; the ciliary body forms the angle through its connection to the trabecular meshwork and scleral spur (Fig. 7-5).

On the lateral side the ciliary body is connected to the sclera by the supraciliary lamellae. The supraciliary space, when present, lies between these two layers. Posteriorly on the lateral side are the long posterior ciliary arteries and nerves. Anterior to the rectus muscle insertions, the anterior ciliary arteries pierce the sclera and enter the outer ciliary body to form the major circle of the iris. A ciliary nerve branch (the nerve loop of Axenfeld) often passes through the sclera to the surface from the supraciliary space in the pars plana region, then loops back through the sclera into the supraciliary region (p. 191).

The posterior chamber is medial to the ciliary body in the region of the pars plicata, and the zonules and vitreous are medial to it in the pars plana region. The lens is close to the ciliary processes, being separated from them by an area containing the zonules and their surrounding vitreous matrix. The zonules arising from the posterior pars plana lie close to the ciliary epithelium through much of their course and are in intimate relation to each other in the valleys between the ciliary processes (Fig. 7-6).

Posteriorly the junction of the ciliary body with the choroid does not form a distinct boundary. The dentate processes of the retinal ora serrata terminate rather abruptly in the unpigmented ciliary epithelium at the posterior border of the ciliary body (Figs. 7-1 to 7-4).

The ciliary body is a circular structure, conforming on its outer aspect to the curvature of the sclera and presenting a somewhat triangular shape in cross-section (Fig. 7–1). The base of the triangle faces the anterior chamber

Text continued on page 269

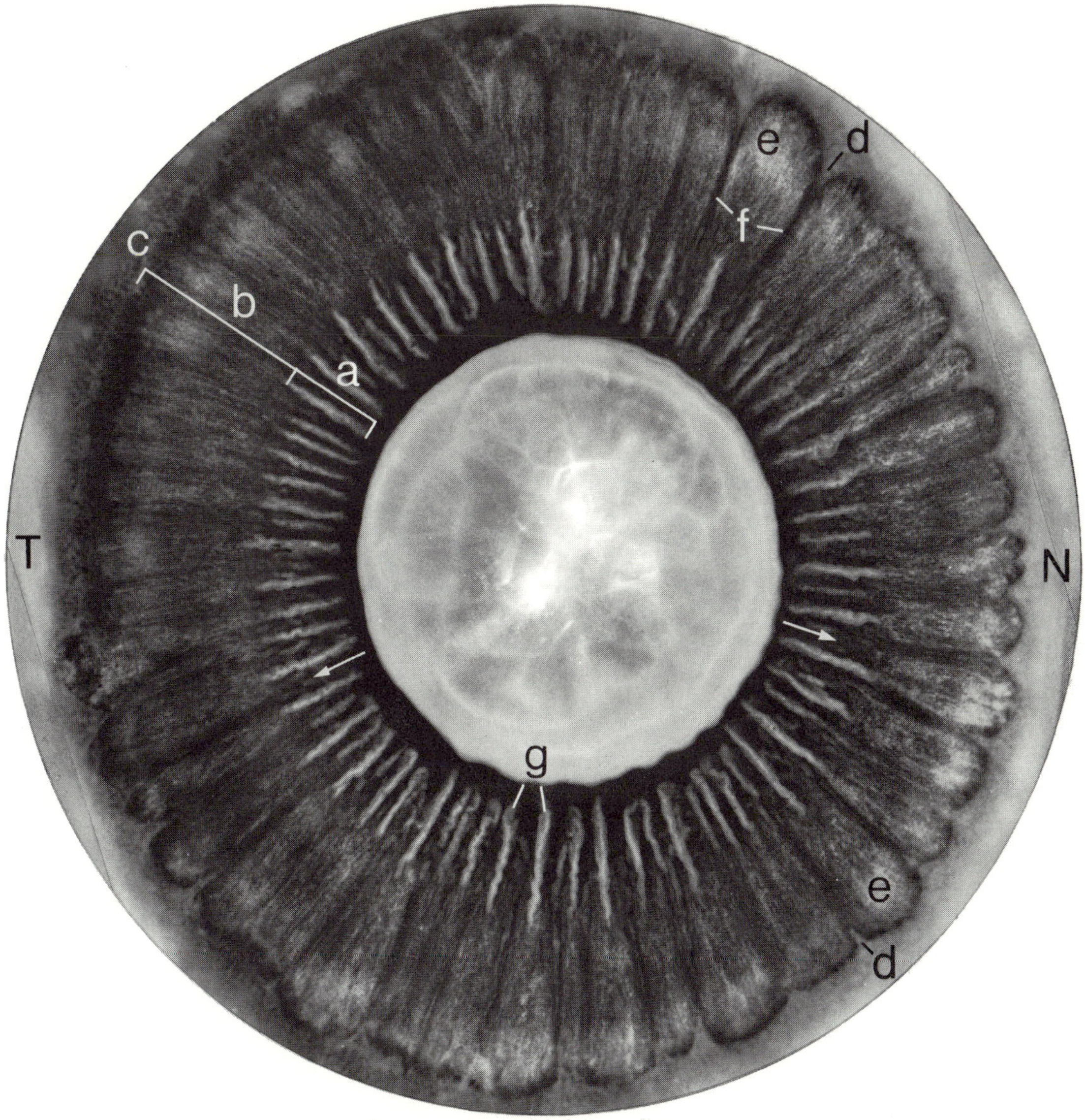

Figure 7-1. Light micrograph of the inner surface of the ciliary body and lens. The nasal side of the eye is at (N) and the temporal is at (T). The pars plicata (a), the pars plana (b) and the ora serrata (c) are indicated. The meridional length of the ciliary body is greater on the temporal side than on the nasal side. At the ora serrata the retina continues forward for a short distance, forming the dentate processes (d); the bays of the pars plana (e) are found between these processes. The bays and dentate processes are better defined on the nasal side than on the temporal side. Linear markings or striae (f) extend from the dentate processes across the pars plana into the valleys of the pars plicata (arrows). The valleys are flanked on either side by the ciliary processes (g), which number about 70. (Straatsma, B. R., Foos, R. Y., and Spencer, L. M.: The retina—topography and clinical correlations. *In* The New Orleans Academy of Ophthalmology: Symposium on Retina and Retinal Surgery. St. Louis, The C. V. Mosby Co., 1969.)

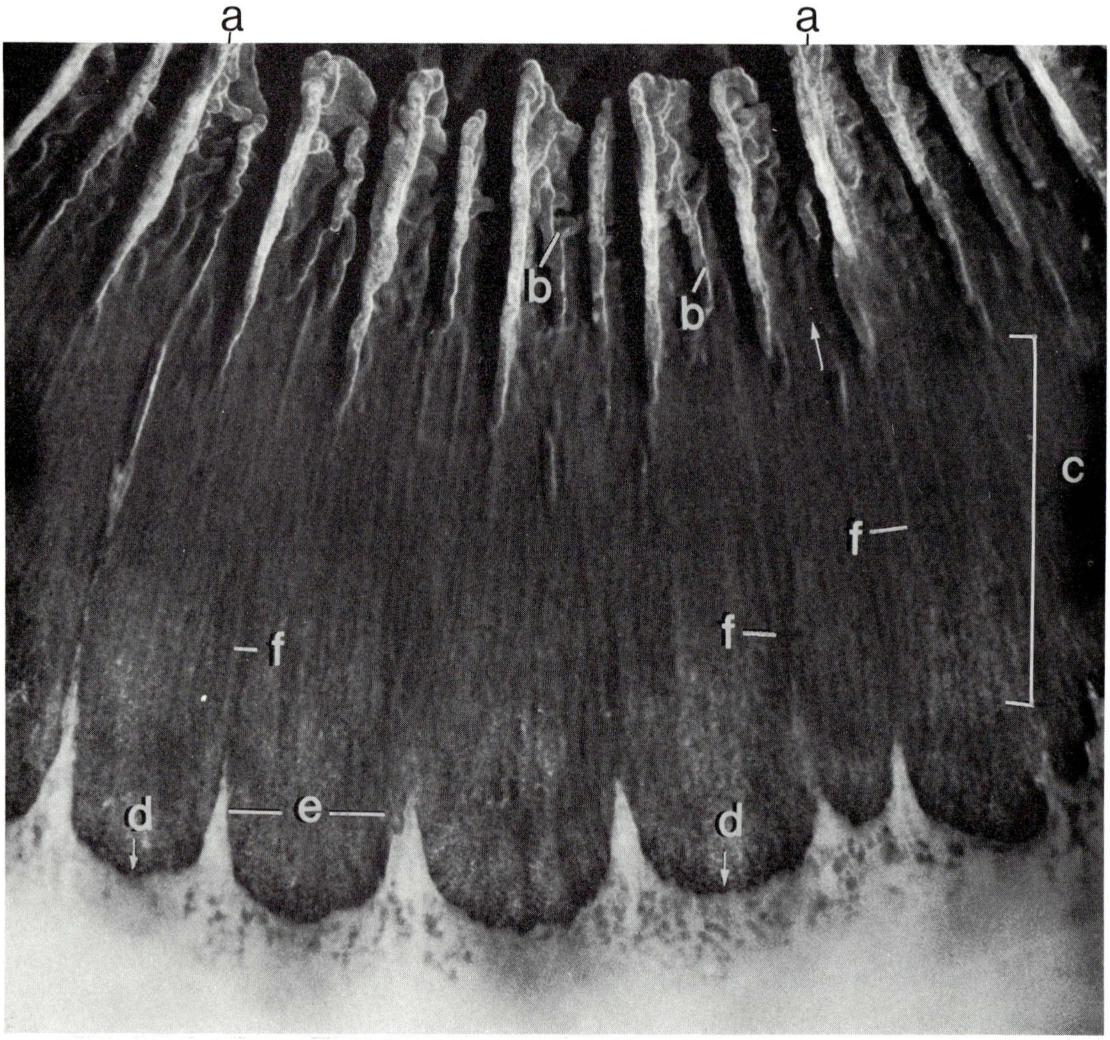

Figure 7–2. Higher magnification light micrograph of the ciliary body of a young person. The pars plicata is formed by the major ciliary processes (a) and smaller accesory or intermediate processes (b). The ciliary processes of the young eye are narrow and have smooth contours. The pars plana (c) ends posteriorly at the ora serrata where the scalloped bays (d) and dentate processes (e) are shown. Striae or linear markings (f) originate from the dentate processes and extend toward the valleys of the pars plicata (arrow). (Courtesy of Dr. R. Y. Foos from the Jules Stein Eye Institute, University of California, Los Angeles.)

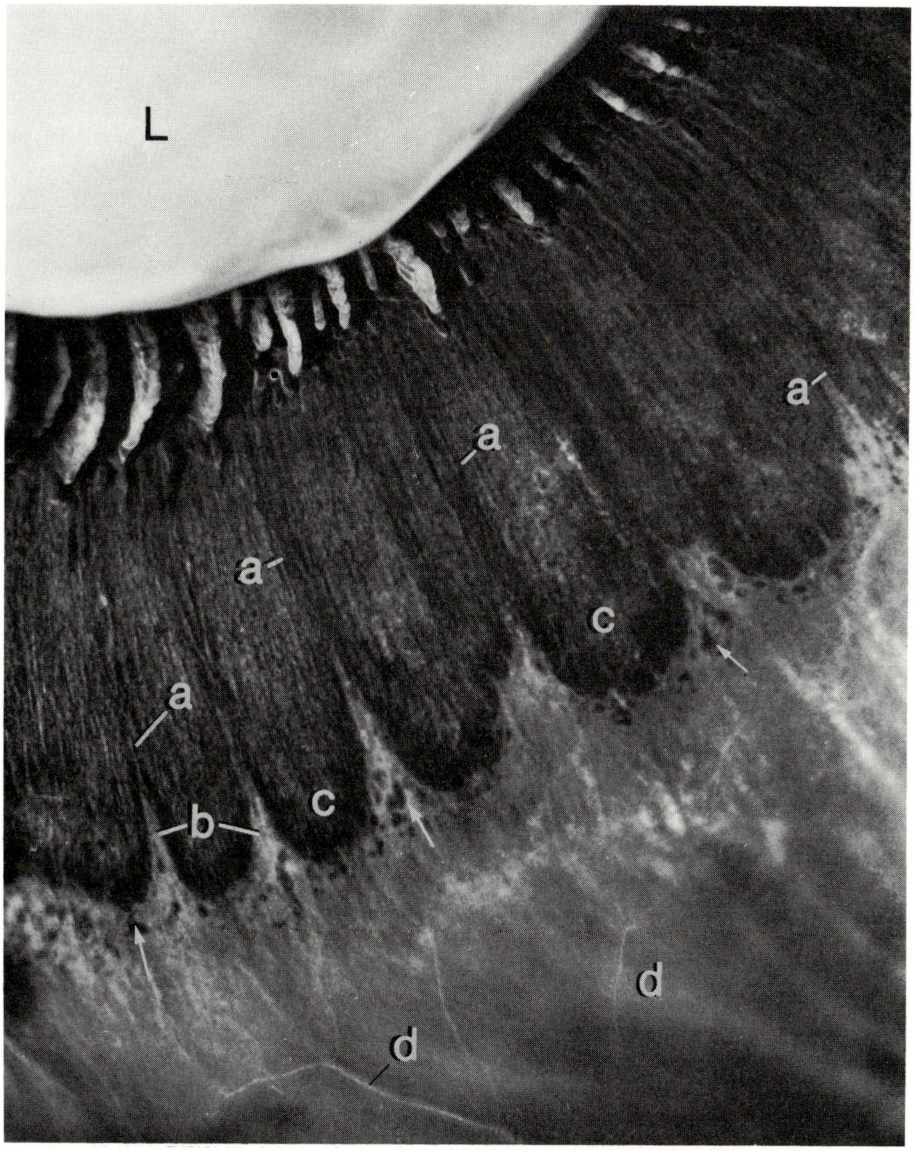

Figure 7-3. Detailed view of the ciliary body showing the lens (L) at the upper left and a partial view of the ciliary processes of the pars plicata. Linear markings (a) extend across the pars plana from the dentate processes (b) into the valleys of the pars plicata. The dentate processes are formed by the anterior extension of the peripheral retina. The scalloped bays (c) of the pars plana are clearly seen. Moderate cystoid degeneration (arrows) is shown in the peripheral retina; retinal vessels are seen at (d). (Courtesy of Dr. R. Y. Foos from the Jules Stein Eye Institute, University of California, Los Angeles.)

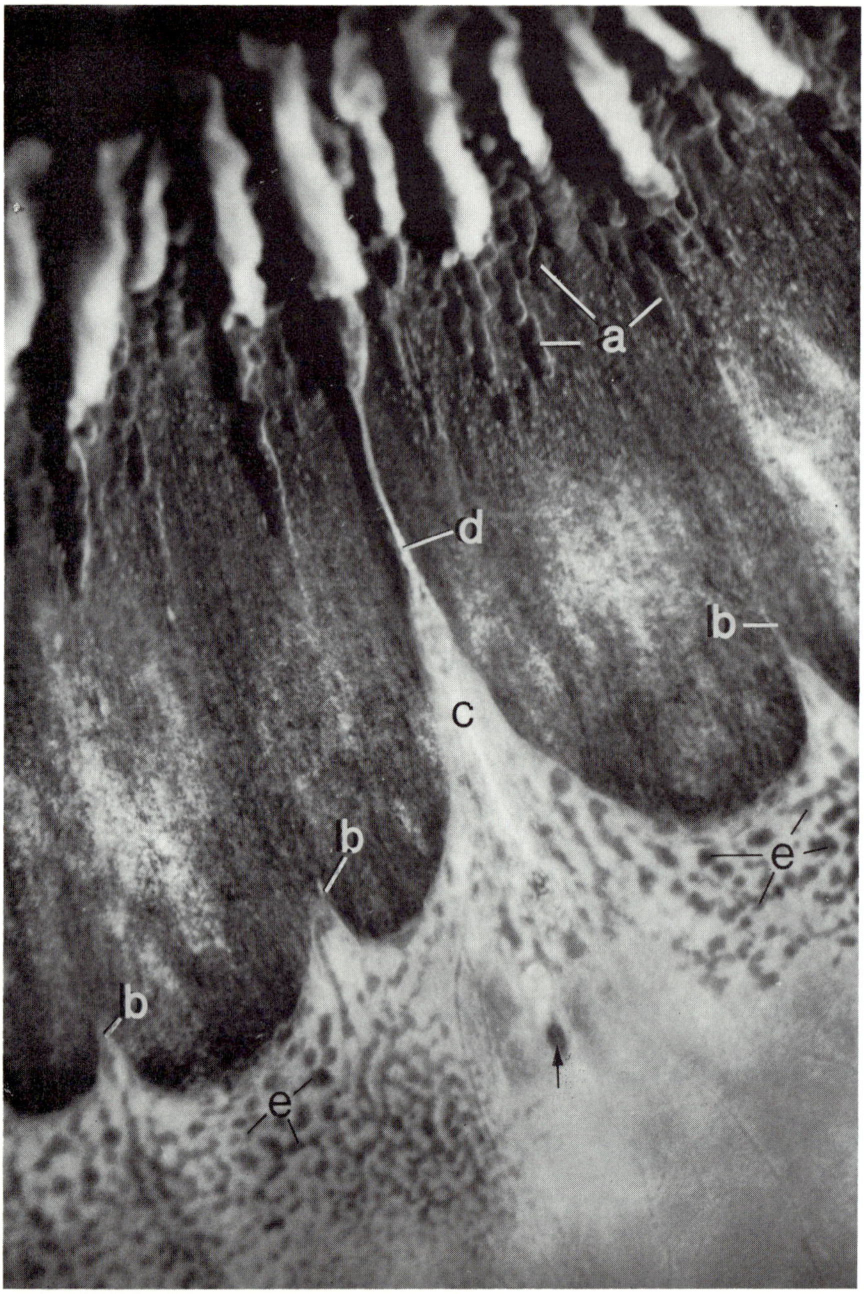

Figure 7–4. Ciliary body of an older person. The major ciliary processes are out of the focal plane, but the smaller accessory or intermediate processes (a) are clearly visible. Three typical dentate processes (b) are visible, and a less common dentate process (c) forms a meridional fold (d). The fold extends the length of the pars plana and merges with a major ciliary process. The peripheral retina shows typical cystoid degeneration (e) and a retinal hole (arrow). (Courtesy of Dr. R. Y. Foos from the Jules Stein Eye Institute, University of California, Los Angeles.)

and the apex is at the ora serrata (Fig. 7-6). The inner surface presents two zones, the corrugated pars plicata anteriorly and the smoother pars plana posteriorly (Figs. 7-1 and 7-5). The inner surface is free, whereas the outer surface is joined loosely to the sclera by long ribbon-like processes. The anteroposterior length of the ciliary body is shorter nasally, where it has a dimension of 4.5 to 5.2 mm.; its least length is in the upper nasal area. The ciliary body is longer temporally, where it measures 5.6 to 6.3 mm., the length being greatest inferiorly and temporally (Fig. 7-1).

The inner surface of the ciliary body is a dirty gray color, owing to the pigment in the outer layer of the ciliary epithelium. Epithelial cysts are often found along this surface, especially in the pars plana of older eyes. Cysts of a congenital type are also common in the anterior pars plicata portion.

The ciliary body commonly is subdivided into two portions, the pars plana (orbiculus ciliaris), and the pars plicata (corona ciliaris) (Figs. 7-1 to 7–6). The pars plana is about 3.5 to 4.0 mm. long and extends from the choroid-retinal termination to the posterior edge of the ciliary processes. At the posterior margin of the pars plana the retina terminates in the unpigmented epithelium of the ciliary body in a serrated fashion. The apices of the serrations are known as teeth or dentate processes, and the intervening scalloped zones are called bays (Fig. 7–3). The termination of the retina is more distinct at the apices of the teeth, and linear markings (striae) continue from the apices forward over the surface of the ciliary body into the valleys between the ciliary processes (Figs. 7–1 and 7–3). Spencer and co-workers (1969) described "meridional folds and complexes" also arising from the dentate processes but extending all the way to the ciliary processes (Fig. 7–4). They reported finding meridional complexes in 16 per cent of 400 autopsy cases studied and believe that approximately 20 per cent of normal eyes can be expected to contain one or more folds. The posterior zonules arise from the inner ciliary body about 1.5 mm. anterior to the termination of the retina, their zone of origin having a width of about 1.5 mm. From this origin the zonules extend anteriorly along the lateral edges of the striae into the valleys between the ciliary processes, where they are lost (Fig. 7-6). The base of the vitreous is also attached to the posterior ciliary epithelium, with its zone of attachment extending forward over the epithelium 1.5 to 2.0 mm. from the ora serrata. Posterior to this the vitreous base attaches to the inner retina.

The pars plicata has a meridional width of about 2 mm. It is so named because of the presence of about 70 to 80 prominent folds, the ciliary processes, which are oriented in a meridional direction and separated from each other by deep valleys. The processes are fairly symmetrical around the circumference of the ciliary body, but differ somewhat in their configuration and size, some being large and long, others small and short (Fig. 7-1). The processes measure around 2 mm. in length and 0.5 mm. in width. Their height is about 0.8 to 1.0 mm., but there are large variations in all dimensions. In the valleys between the processes are intermediate processes (Figs. 7-2 and 7-4).

A cross-section of the ciliary body reveals the differences in architecture between the pars plicata and the pars plana (Fig. 7-5). The former is much thicker; the latter tapers from anterior to posterior, where it meets the choroid and retina. The pars plicata is readily divisible into an outer muscular portion and an inner portion containing the stroma and processes. The

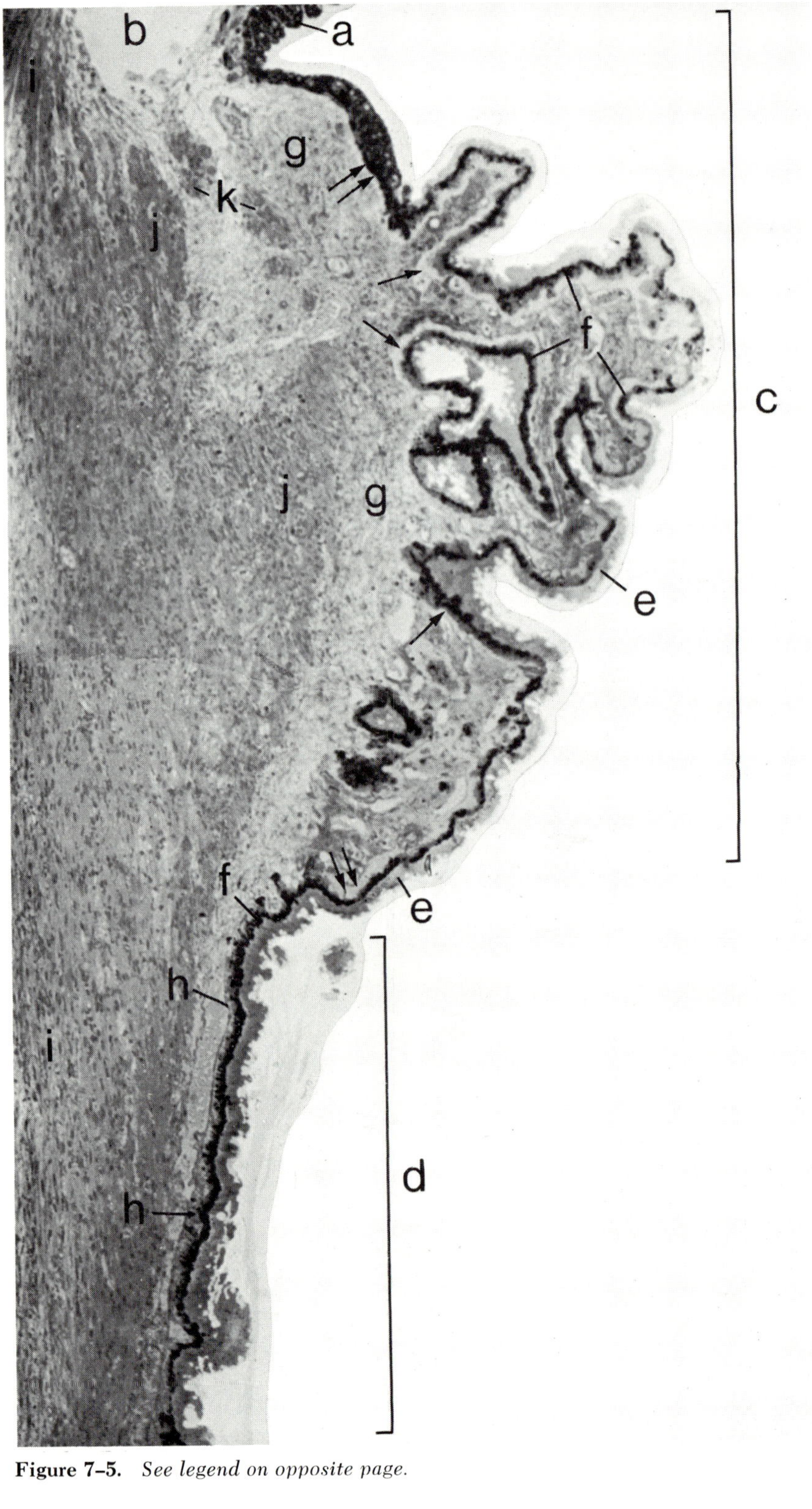

Figure 7–5. *See legend on opposite page.*

pars plana shows a thick muscular and much thinner stromal and epithelial portion. The ciliary processes lengthen and become taller with increasing age (Reese, 1934).

Blood Supply

The main arterial supply to the ciliary body is through the long posterior and the anterior ciliary arteries, which come together to form the major arterial circle of the iris just posterior to the anterior chamber angle recess. The principal route of venous drainage is posteriorly into the choroid and vortex system and, to a lesser extent, into the intrascleral venous plexus and episcleral veins in the limbal region (Fig. 8–3, p. 326). From the major arterial circle, branches pass to the anterior part of the ciliary processes, where they form a capillary bed underlying the epithelium. In this way an enormous diffusing surface is developed comprising an area of 6.7 cm.^{2} (Baurmann, 1930). Branches also go to the stroma and ciliary muscle, and others pass to the iris, anterior limbal region and anterior choroid. There are significantly fewer capillaries in the ciliary muscle than in the ciliary processes.

Nerves

The long posterior ciliary nerves first branch in the outer choroid near the ora serrata. A very rich plexus of myelinated and unmyelinated nerve fibers is formed, among which are many ganglion cells. Bryson and associates (1966) identified numerous ganglion cells in the human ciliary body by histochemical demonstration of the cholinesterase in their cytoplasm. Many of these resembled multipolar ganglion cells and were found along the inner border of the ciliary muscle, but some of them were found within the muscle itself (Fig. 7-15). Nerve branches pass into the ciliary body and iris from all these cells. These nerve fibers are from the oculomotor nerve and are of parasympathetic origin, destined for the ciliary and iris muscles. The fibers form a rich network among the bundles in the ciliary muscle. Fibers from the cervical sympathetic are also transmitted via the ciliary nerves from the carotid system and are distributed to the ciliary and iris muscles as well

---

Figure 7–5. Light micrograph of the meridional section of a ciliary body of a 50 year old man. The iris root (a) and the anterior chamber angle (b) are seen at the top. The pars plicata (c) and a portion of the pars plana (d) are included within brackets; they are lined by the unpigmented (e) and pigmented (f) epithelium. The stroma of the ciliary body may be divided into three parts: an innermost layer of a basement membrane-like material (single arrows) underlying the pigmented epithelium; a collagenous connective tissue (g); and the ciliary muscle. The basement membrane-like material is present mainly in the pars plicata, beginning near the root of the iris (double arrows) and terminating near the beginning of the pars plicata (double arrows). This material is not present in very young eyes, and its thickness increases with aging. The collagenous connective tissue contains numerous vessels which send capillaries toward the ciliary epithelium. The elastic lamina (h), which forms part of Bruch's membrane of the choroid, extends past the ora serrata into the pars plana. The ciliary muscle is formed by an external longitudinal portion (i), an internal radial portion (j) and an anterior circular portion (k). (× 52.)

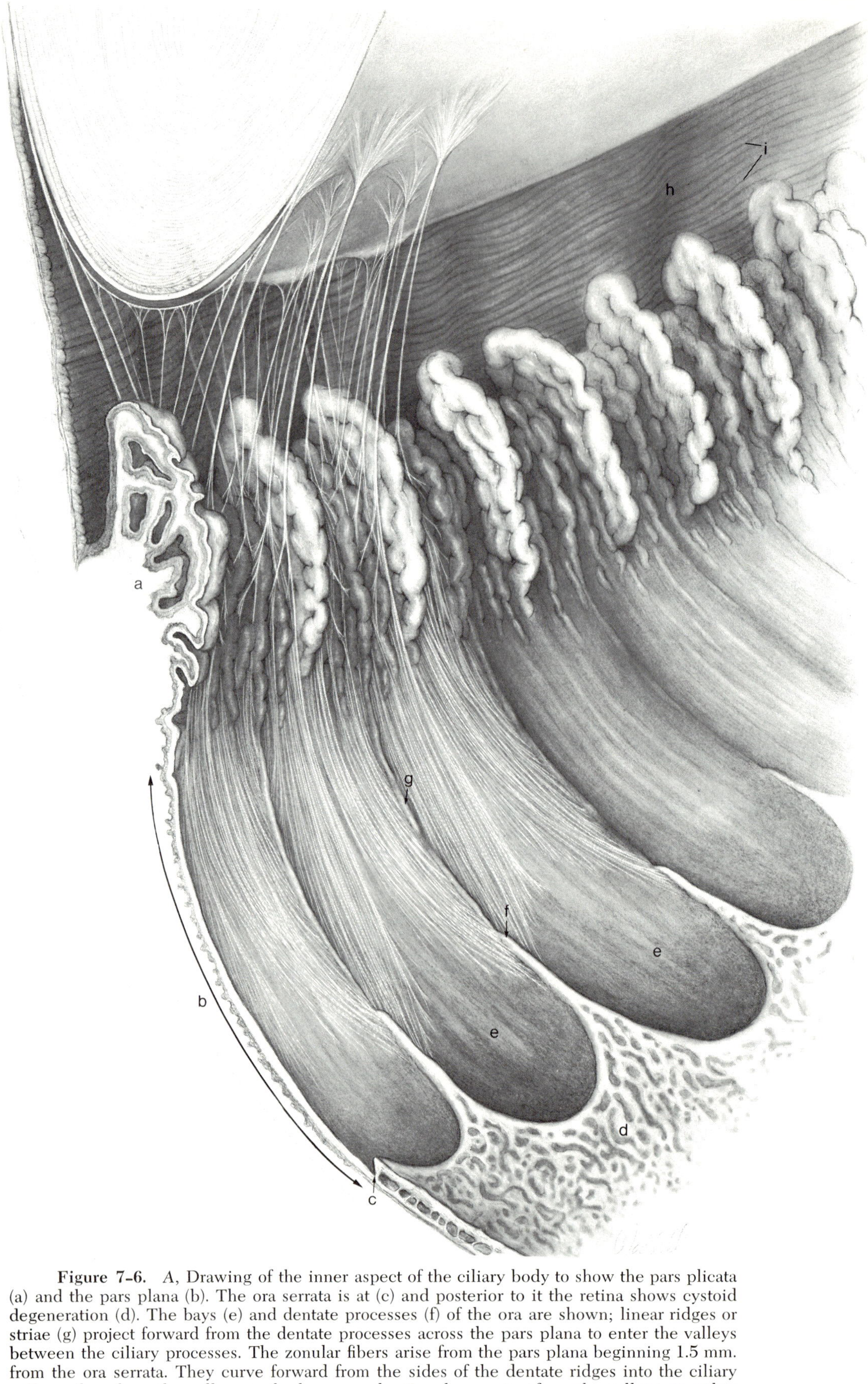

A

Figure 7-6. *A*, Drawing of the inner aspect of the ciliary body to show the pars plicata (a) and the pars plana (b). The ora serrata is at (c) and posterior to it the retina shows cystoid degeneration (d). The bays (e) and dentate processes (f) of the ora are shown; linear ridges or striae (g) project forward from the dentate processes across the pars plana to enter the valleys between the ciliary processes. The zonular fibers arise from the pars plana beginning 1.5 mm. from the ora serrata. They curve forward from the sides of the dentate ridges into the ciliary valleys, then from the valleys to the lens capsule. Zonules coming from the valleys on either

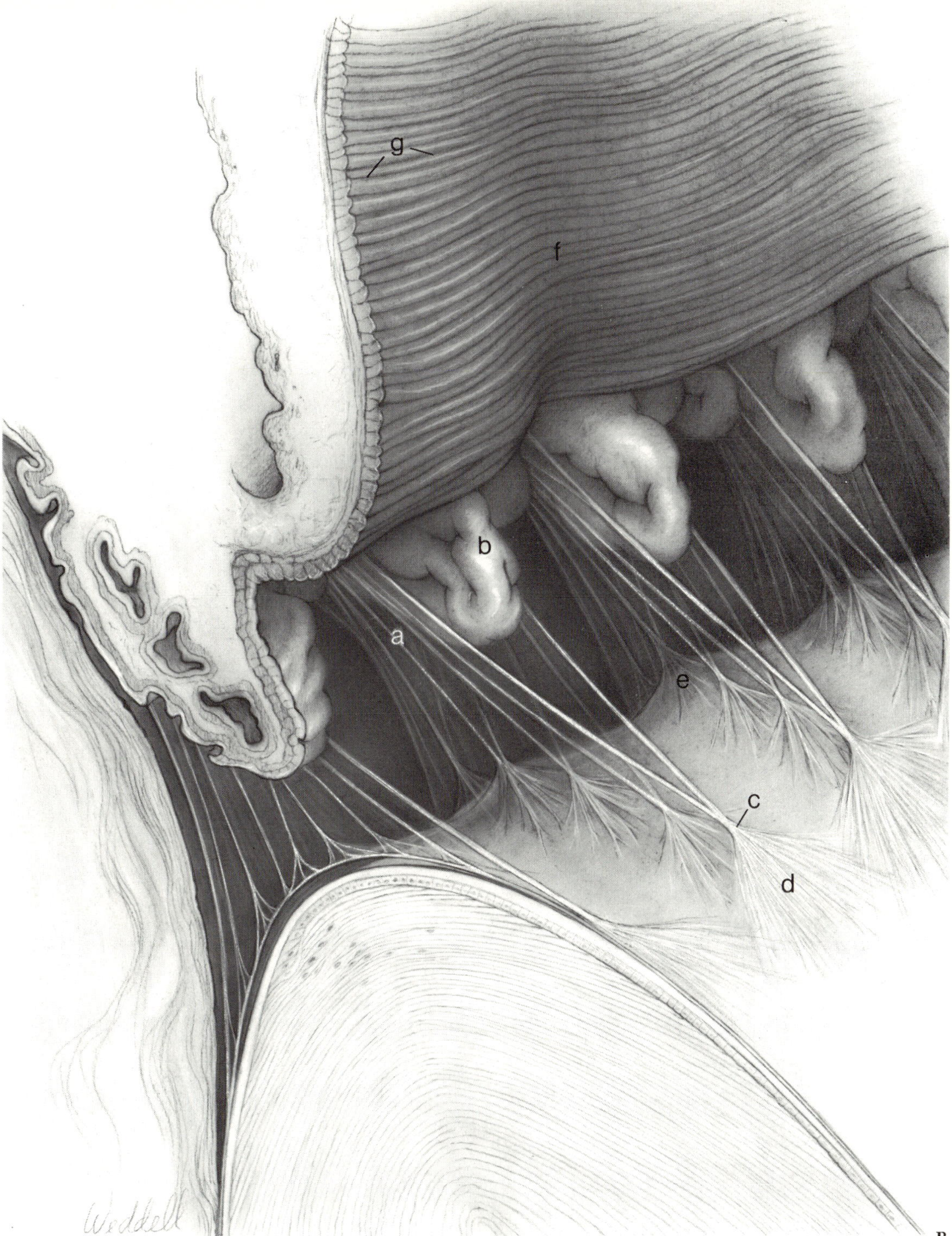

B

Figure 7–6. *Continued.*
side of a ciliary process have a common point of attachment on the lens. The zonules attach up to 1 mm. from the equator posteriorly, and up to 1.5 mm. from the equator anteriorly. At the equatorial border the attaching zonules give a crenated appearance to the lens. The ciliary processes vary in size and shape and often are separated from each other by lesser processes. The radial (h) and circular furrows (i) of the peripheral iris are shown.

B, Anterior view of the ciliary processes showing the zonules attaching to the lens. Zonules form columns (a) on either side of the ciliary processes (b), which meet on a single site (c) as they attach to the lens. These two columns form a triangle having its base on the ciliary body and its apex on the lens. The zonules form a tent-like structure (d) as they become attached to the lens capsule. The equatorial surface of the lens is crenated (e) by the attachment of the zonule. The iris is pulled upward, showing its posterior surface with the radial (f) folds and the circular furrows (g).

as to the blood vessels. Sensory nerve fibers from the ophthalmic division of the trigeminal nerve enter the ciliary body and terminate in all the anterior segment tissues.

MICROSCOPIC ANATOMY

For descriptive purposes the ciliary body can be divided into the following portions: (1) unpigmented ciliary epithelium, (2) pigmented ciliary epithelium, (3) stroma, and (4) ciliary muscle.

UNPIGMENTED CILIARY EPITHELIUM (Figs. 7–7 to 7–26)

The unpigmented ciliary epithelium forms the innermost layer of the ciliary body. It is a continuous layer from the base of the iris over the surface of the pars plicata and pars plana to its junction with the sensory retina at the ora serrata. It often contains some pigment anteriorly near the iris root (Fig. 7-7).

The unpigmented epithelium of the young eye is a single layer of fairly regular cells. Over the pars plicata the cells are low and cuboidal in shape, whereas over the pars plana they are tall and columnar. The cells are 12 to 15 μm. in width and 10 to 15 μm. in height over the crests of the ciliary processes, and their nuclei are rounded (Salzmann, 1912). The cells are flatter in the valleys between the processes and are quite irregular over the folds of the intermediate processes (Fig. 7-8). In the pars plana the cells may measure about 30 μm. in height by 6 to 9 μm. in width (Fig. 7-10). The nuclei are oval and lie near the pigment epithelium. The cells here may lie at odd angles to the inner surface of the ciliary body, depending on the attachments of adjacent structures such as the zonules and the base of the vitreous. Just anterior to the ora serrata the cells are more elongated, probably because of the traction produced by the vitreous (Fig. 7–14). In the anterior pars plana the cells are slightly flatter, but still are columnar.

The unpigmented epithelium is rather firmly united to the adjacent pigmented epithelium. The two separate from each other, however, when there is a fluid accumulation as a result of disease, such as a choroidal melanoma or an exudative process under the retina. The inner limiting membrane of the ciliary epithelium over the pars plicata and the pars plana in the young eye is thin and uniform in thickness.

With increasing age there is a significant alteration of the unpigmented ciliary epithelial cells and the inner limiting membrane over both the pars plicata and the pars plana. Over the crests of the ciliary processes the cells may show only moderate change, whereas in the valleys and along the side walls of the processes they develop a distinct irregularity of the basal (posterior chamber) cell surface (Fig. 7-11). Over the pars plana the cells become thinner and taller and have the appearance of being stretched, and their basal surfaces become extremely irregular and form thin, serrated or flame-shaped branching processes of varying length (Figs. 7-12 and 7-13). Particularly in the pars plana, the cells become less closely apposed. The intercellular space widens along the basal two thirds, and semiloculated spaces form that contain some granular material, probably mucopolysaccharide (Fine and Zimmerman, 1963).

The inner limiting membrane also changes with age, the alterations

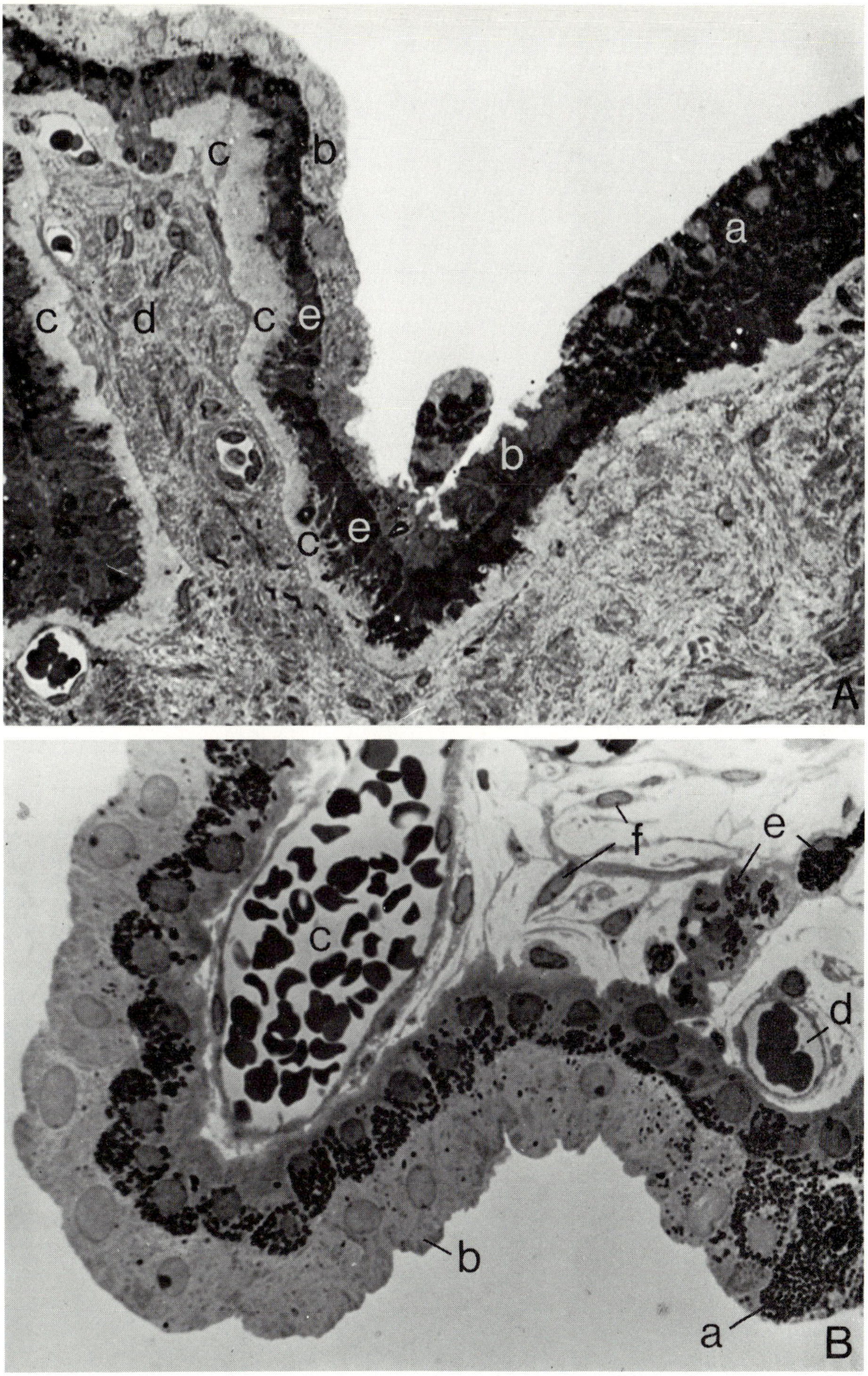

Figure 7-7. *A*, Ciliary body of an old person, light micrograph. The transition of the pigmented iris epithelium (a) into the unpigmented ciliary epithelium (b) is shown. Note the basement membrane-like strip (c) interposed between the dense collagenous connective tissue layers of this ciliary process (d) and the pigmented epithelium (e). (× 500.)

B, Ciliary body of a young person, light micrograph. The transition of the unpigmented ciliary body epithelium (b) into the pigmented iris epithelium. The epithelium shows increasing numbers of melanin granules until some of the cells become filled with pigment (a). A large vein (c) and a capillary (d) lie in the stroma close to the pigmented epithelium. Compare the stroma of the young eye with that shown in the preceding figure. Some melanocytes (e) and fibroblasts (f) are seen. (× 640.)

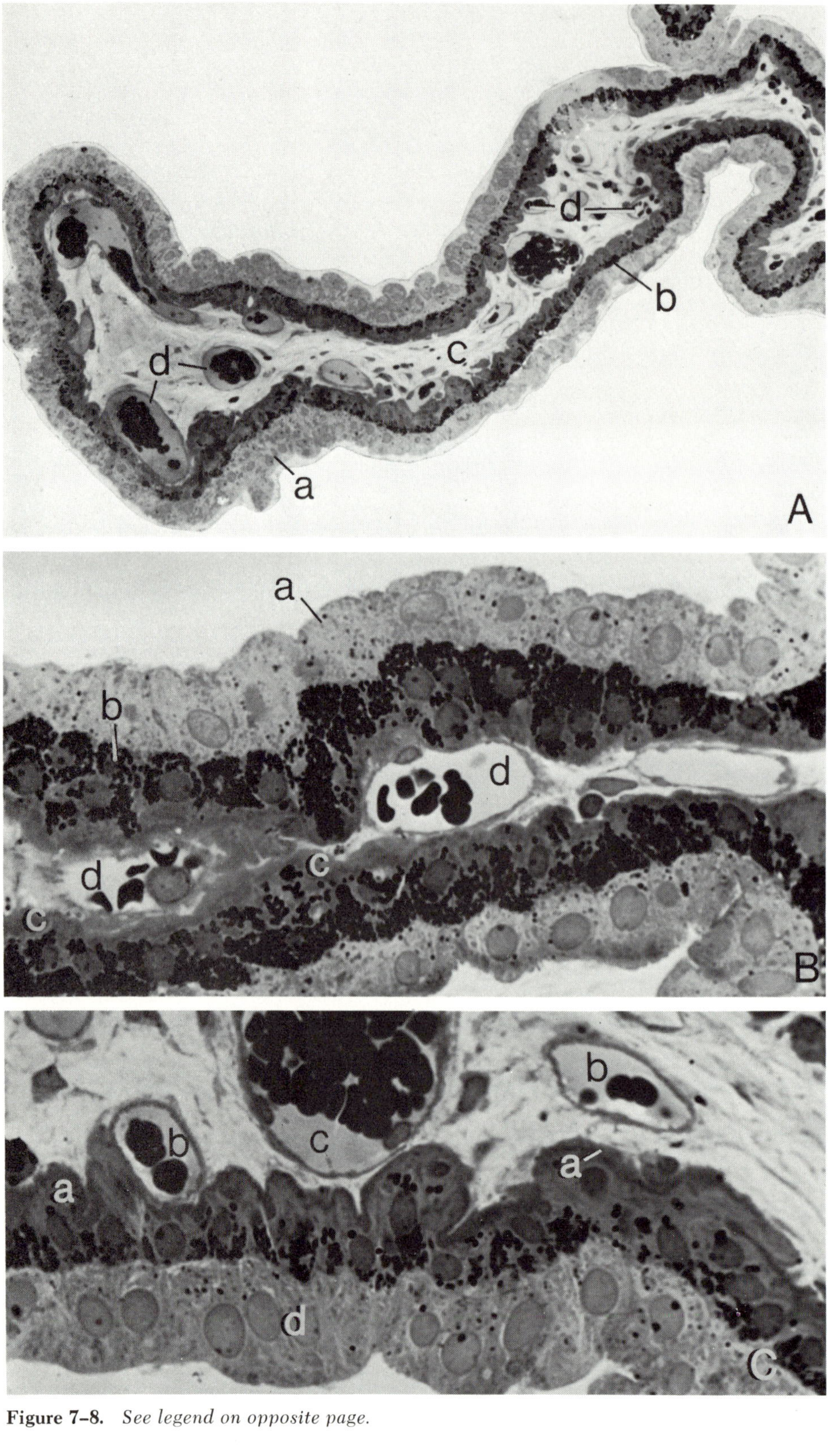

Figure 7–8. *See legend on opposite page.*

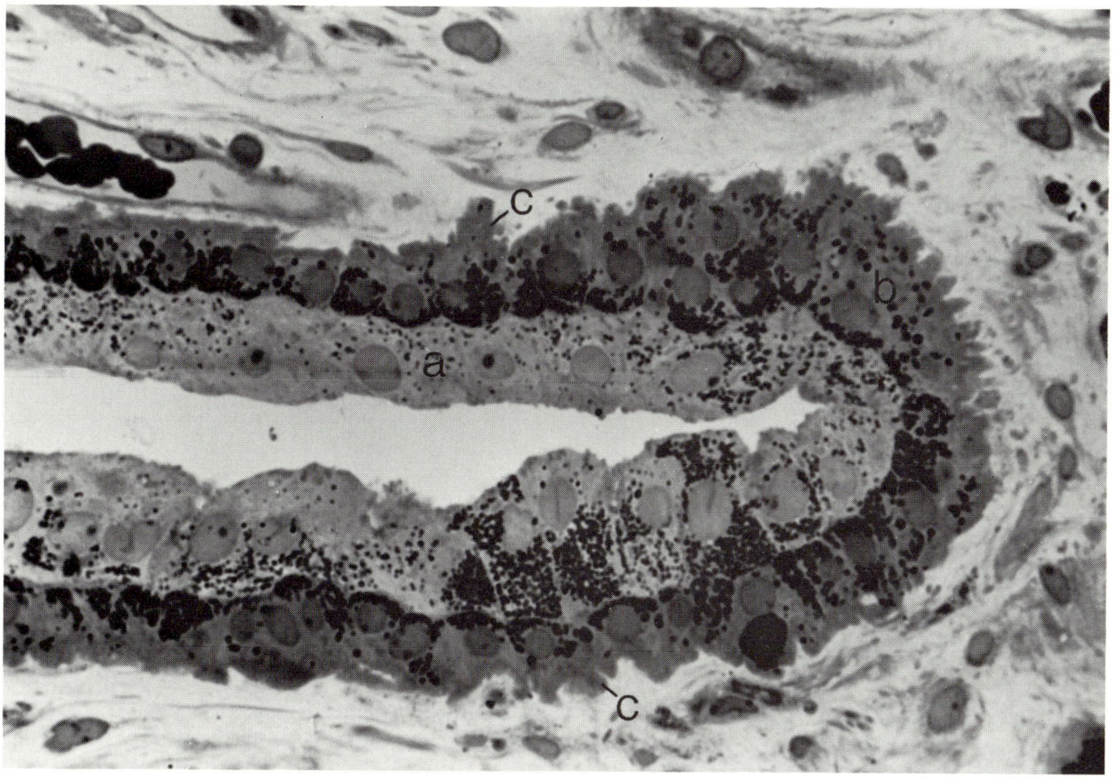

Figure 7-9. The eye of a young person, light micrograph. The pars plicata of the ciliary body near its junction with the iris is shown. The unpigmented epithelium (a) still contains some pigment here; the pigment in the pigmented epithelium (b) is located around the nucleus in the apical portion of the cell. The irregular outline of the basal surfaces of the pigmented epithelial cells is evident (c). Note the absence of a basement membrane-like material underlying the pigmented epithelium. (× 640.)

Figure 7-8. *A*, Ciliary process in a young eye, light micrograph. The unpigmented (a) and pigmented (b) ciliary epithelium cover the stroma (c) of the ciliary process. Longitudinal and cross-sections of small veins and capillaries are seen (d). Most of these vessels lie in close apposition to the pigmented epithelium. (× 200.)

B, Ciliary process in the eye of a young person, light micrograph. Note the smooth contours of the unpigmented epithelium (a). The pigmented epithelium contains considerable melanin (b), which often obscures the nuclei. The basement membrane is seen at (c), where it is sectioned obliquely. A capillary (d) containing red blood cells extends across the width of the stroma. (× 640.)

C, A ciliary process similar to that seen in *B*. The basement membrane (a) of the pigment epithelium is prominent because it is cut on the bias. Two capillaries (b) are closely related to the basement membrane. A vein occupies the central stroma of the process (c). The unpigmented epithelium is at (d). (× 640.)

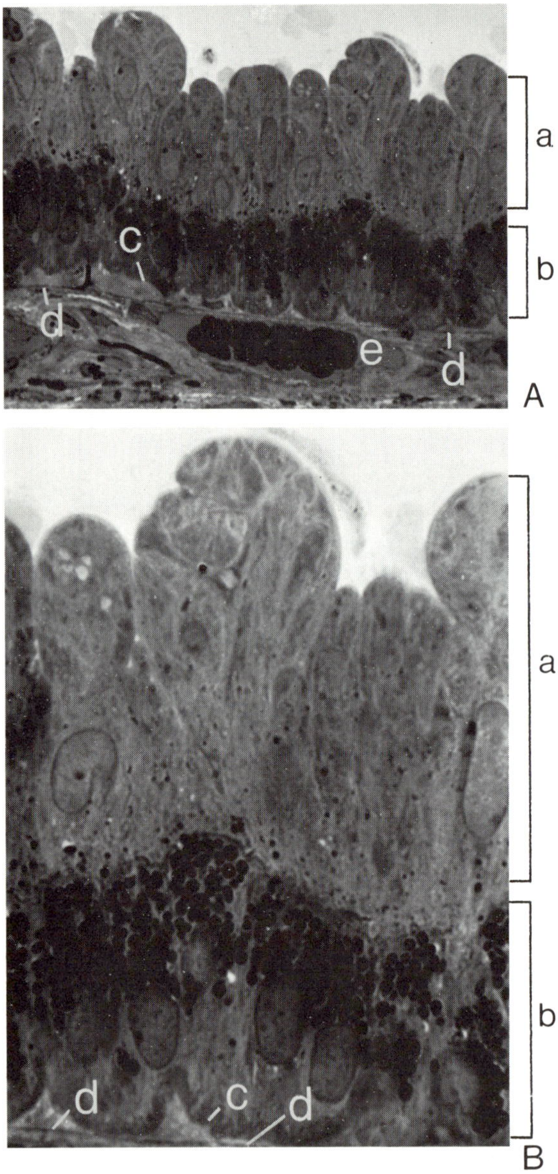

Figure 7–10. *A*, The eye of a young person, light micrograph. The epithelial layers and adjacent stroma of the pars plana of the ciliary body are shown. The unpigmented epithelial cells (a) are taller than those of the pars plicata, and no intercellular gaps are seen. (Compare this finding with that in older eyes.) The dense pigment in the pigmented epithelial cells (b) is aggregated toward the apex of the cell. The basement membrane (c) of the pigmented cells varies in thickness. The elastica of Bruch's membrane is seen as a thin, dark line at (d). The capillaries (e) are large and contain many red blood cells. (× 520.)

B, The eye of a young individual, higher magnification, light micrograph. The characteristics of the epithelial layers of the pars plana of the ciliary body are shown. The unpigmented cells (a) are quite tall, and the pigmented cells contain large pigment granules (b). The basement membrane of the pigmented cells is quite distinct (c). The elastic tissue of Bruch's membrane is at (d). (× 880.)

being easily seen with the light microscope. Over the pars plicata the membrane thickens somewhat above the crests of the ciliary processes and becomes much thicker in the ciliary valleys and along the sides of the processes. It fills the crevices between those cells, which are partially separated from each other, as well as the spaces formed by foldings of the epithelium. Over the pars plana the membrane also becomes greatly thickened along the inner surface and in the spaces between the cellular folds, but it does not become continuous with the intercellular material between these cells.

The zonules arise from the unpigmented epithelial cells in the posterior pars plana region and in the valleys between the ciliary processes. Various types of insertions of the zonules into the ciliary body have been

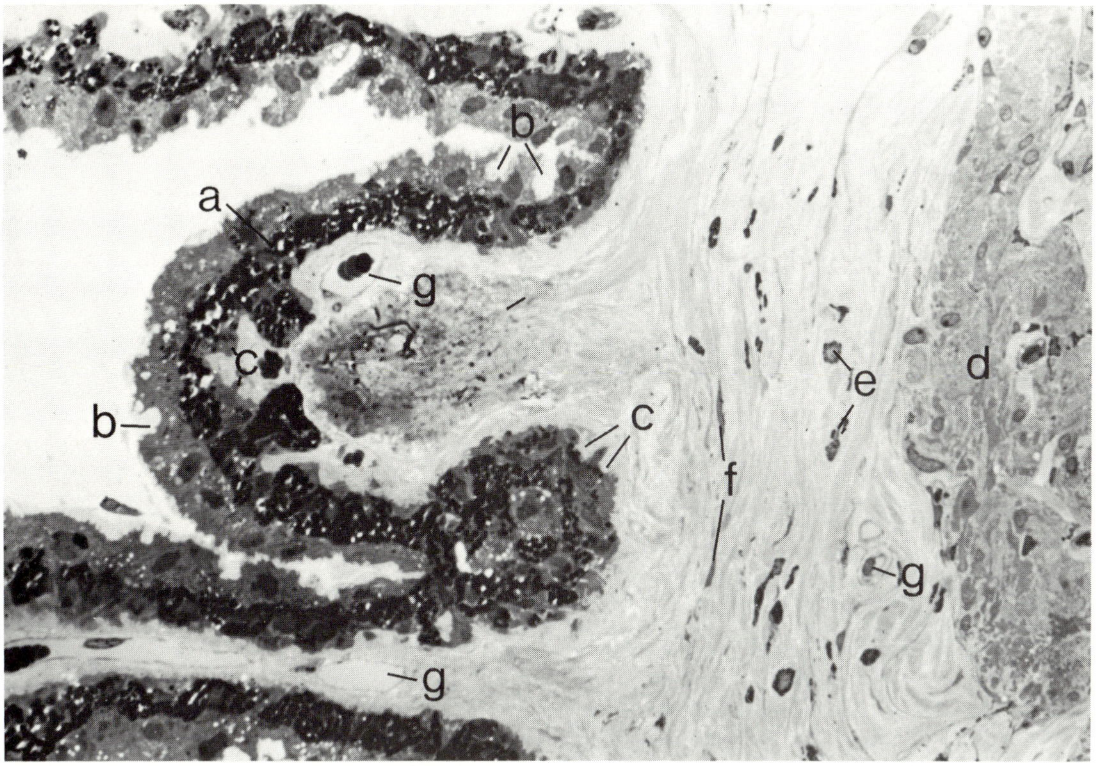

Figure 7–11. Epithelial layers and stroma of the pars plicata of a 42 year old patient, light micrograph. The epithelial layers are at (a). The unpigmented epithelium facing the posterior chamber has an irregular, serrated basal surface (b). The basal surface of the pigmented epithelium also is irregular where it faces the stroma (c). The ciliary muscle is shown at (d). Melanocytes (e), fibroblasts (f) and blood vessels (g) are found in the stroma. (× 560.)

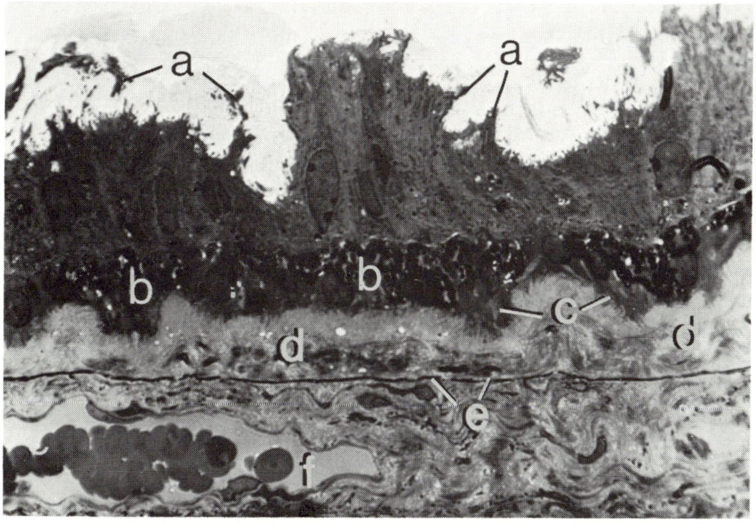

Figure 7–12. Posterior pars plana in an adult eye, light micrograph. The fraying of the basal surfaces of the unpigmented epithelium (a) is a phenomenon of aging. The pigmented epithelium (b) shows numerous protrusions into Bruch's membrane (c). A considerable amount of collagen (d) lies between the pigmented epithelium and elastic lamina (e) of Bruch's membrane. The capillary layer is at (f). (× 520.)

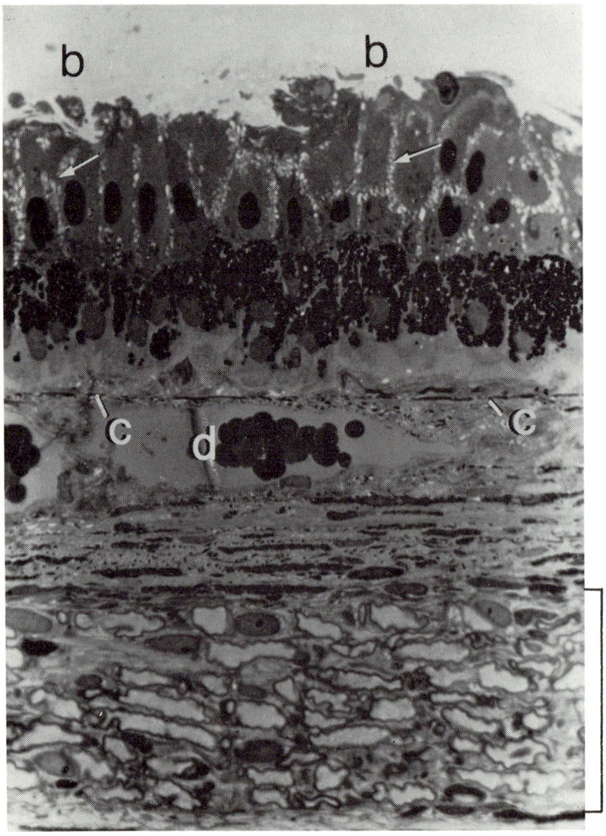

Figure 7–13. Pars plana of the ciliary body in an older eye. This light micrograph shows the long ciliary nerve (a) at the bottom. The unpigmented epithelium shows the basal fraying (b) and separation of the cells along their lateral surfaces (arrows). The elastic lamina of Bruch's membrane is at (c), and the capillaries are seen at (d). (× 480.)

described. When studied by light microscopy they most often seem to join the surfaces of the unpigmented epithelial cells and enter into the folds produced by these cells. Their course is parallel to the inner surface of the pars plana and at an angle to the surface in the valleys between the processes (Fig. 7-6).

In the young eye most of the unpigmented cells over the pars plicata show deep infoldings of the *basal cell membranes* when studied with the electron microscope (Fig. 7-20). The basement membrane, which is adjacent to the basal surface of these cells, continues as a regular layer without entering into the infoldings. Some 34 to 62 infoldings are seen in each epithelial cell in man (Holmberg, 1955). The infoldings are at right angles to the surface, are U-shaped and reach almost to the nuclear zone. Most of the infoldings occupy the peripheral zone of the basal cell surface, the central portion lacking them. The infoldings are better developed in the cells of the ciliary valleys. The *apical* cell membrane that faces the pigment epithelium is fairly straight (Figs. 7–22 and 7–23). Interdigitations along the *lateral* cell membrane in the human epithelium are found mainly in the basal or inner third of the cells, in contrast to rabbit eyes in which there are extensive interdigitations along the entire lateral side. The interdigitations of the lateral cell membranes and infoldings of the basal cell membranes are fewer in the pars plana. The lateral cell membranes exhibit junctions which are mostly desmosomal, located along the apical third of the cells (Figs. 7–17 and 7-22).

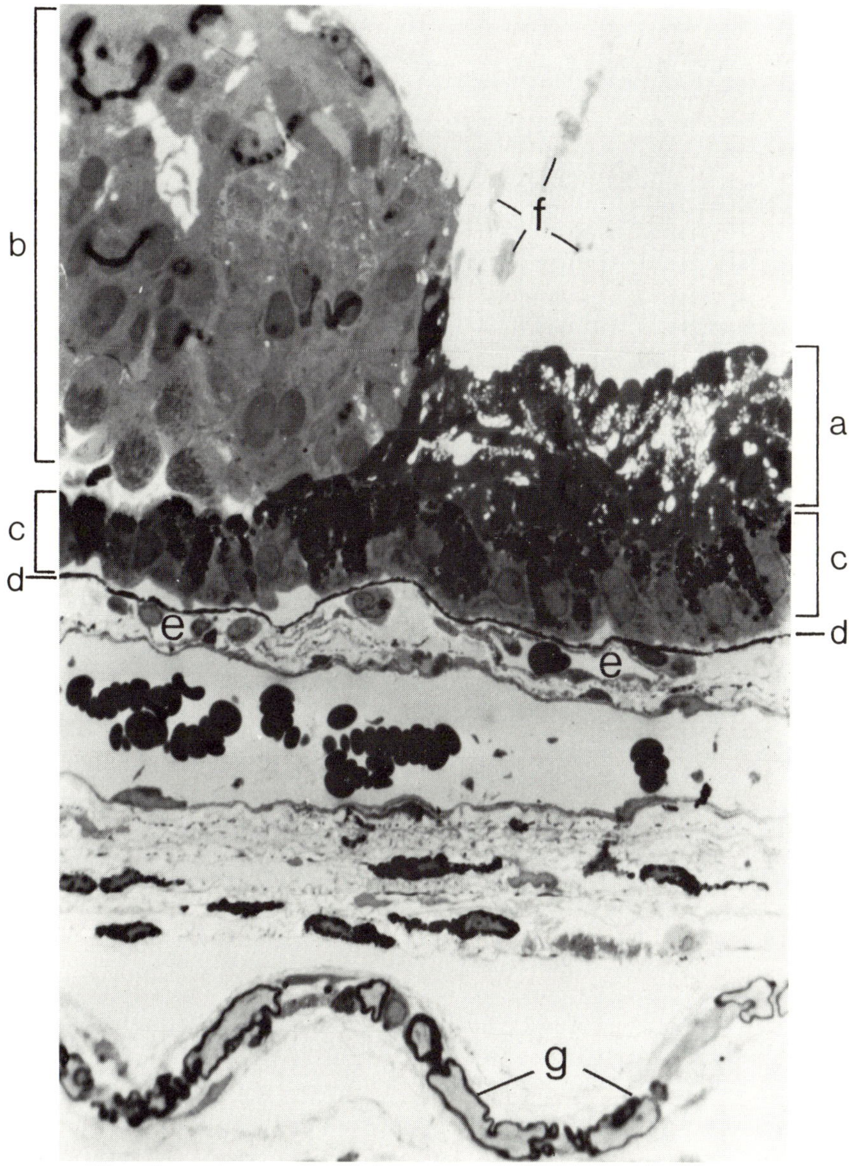

Figure 7–14. Ora serrata region in the eye of a middle-aged person, light micrograph. The ciliary epithelium is at (a) and the retina at (b). The pigmented epithelium of the ciliary body (c) is continuous with that of the retina. The elastic layer (d) of Bruch's membrane and the choriocapillaris (e) lie close to the pigmented epithelium. Vitreous collagen (f) joins the retina and ciliary body. A ciliary nerve is seen at (g). (× 560.)

As the eye ages the electron microscope shows that the spaces which form between the cells along their lateral sides are due to straightening and separation of the lateral interdigitations (Figs. 7-24 and 7-25). In the pars plana region the cells become separated from each other by a widened intercellular space which contains an electron-opaque material. The widening of the intercellular space is discontinuous, however, being interrupted by intercellular links at unbroken interdigitations. Fine and Zimmerman (1963) observed that the widened intercellular space contains a floccular

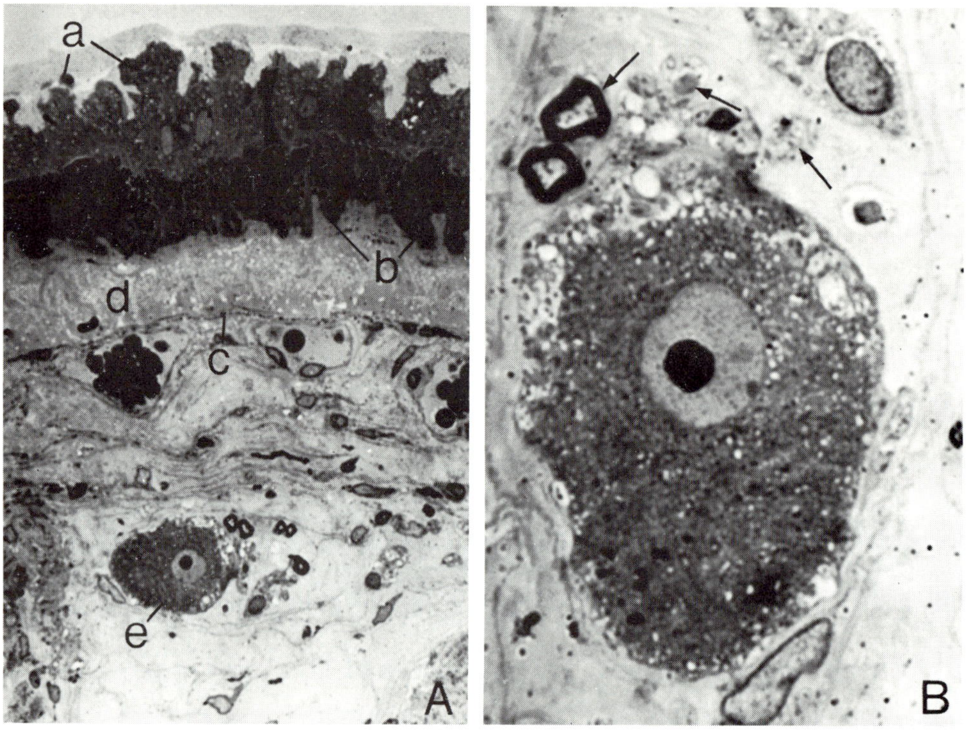

Figure 7-15. *A*, Pars plana of the ciliary body of a middle-aged person, light micrograph. Characteristic changes are seen in the serrated basal unpigmented epithelium (a). The basal surface of the pigment epithelium is folded (b). The elastic lamina (c) of Bruch's membrane is separated from the epithelial layers by a considerable amount of collagen (d). There is a ganglion cell in the stroma (e). (× 520.)

B, View of the ganglion cell in the stroma at higher magnification. A number of myelinated and unmyelinated nerves surround this cell (arrows). (× 800.)

substance and that the spaces containing this substance are continuous with the posterior chamber. Light and electron micrographs and histochemical studies convinced them that the intercellular substance is an acid mucopolysaccharide. A similar material also was demonstrated in the cytoplasm of the unpigmented epithelial cells of this region. Their study suggests that the acid mucopolysaccharide manufactured by these cells is secreted from cytoplasm to the intercellular space and then into the vitreous.

The unpigmented and pigmented epithelial cells face each other at their *apical* surfaces, with the cells joined by two types of junctions, adhering and occluding junctions (Figs. 7-16, 7-22 and 7-23). The occluding junctions are mostly maculae and fasciae occludentes, but it is difficult to be certain whether there are zonulae occludentes. The adhering junctions are mostly desmosomes and a few maculae adherentes.

In the young eye the inner limiting membrane of the unpigmented epithelium appears as an ordinary basement membrane with the electron microscope (Figs. 7-20 and 7-26). With increasing age this basement membrane becomes thicker, especially in the valleys between the ciliary processes, in the intercellular spaces near the base of the cells and within the areas produced by folding of the epithelium (Figs. 7-19, 7-25 and 7-43). The basement membrane has the same structure over the pars plicata as over the pars plana. Holmberg (1959a) found that in the human eye the membrane is

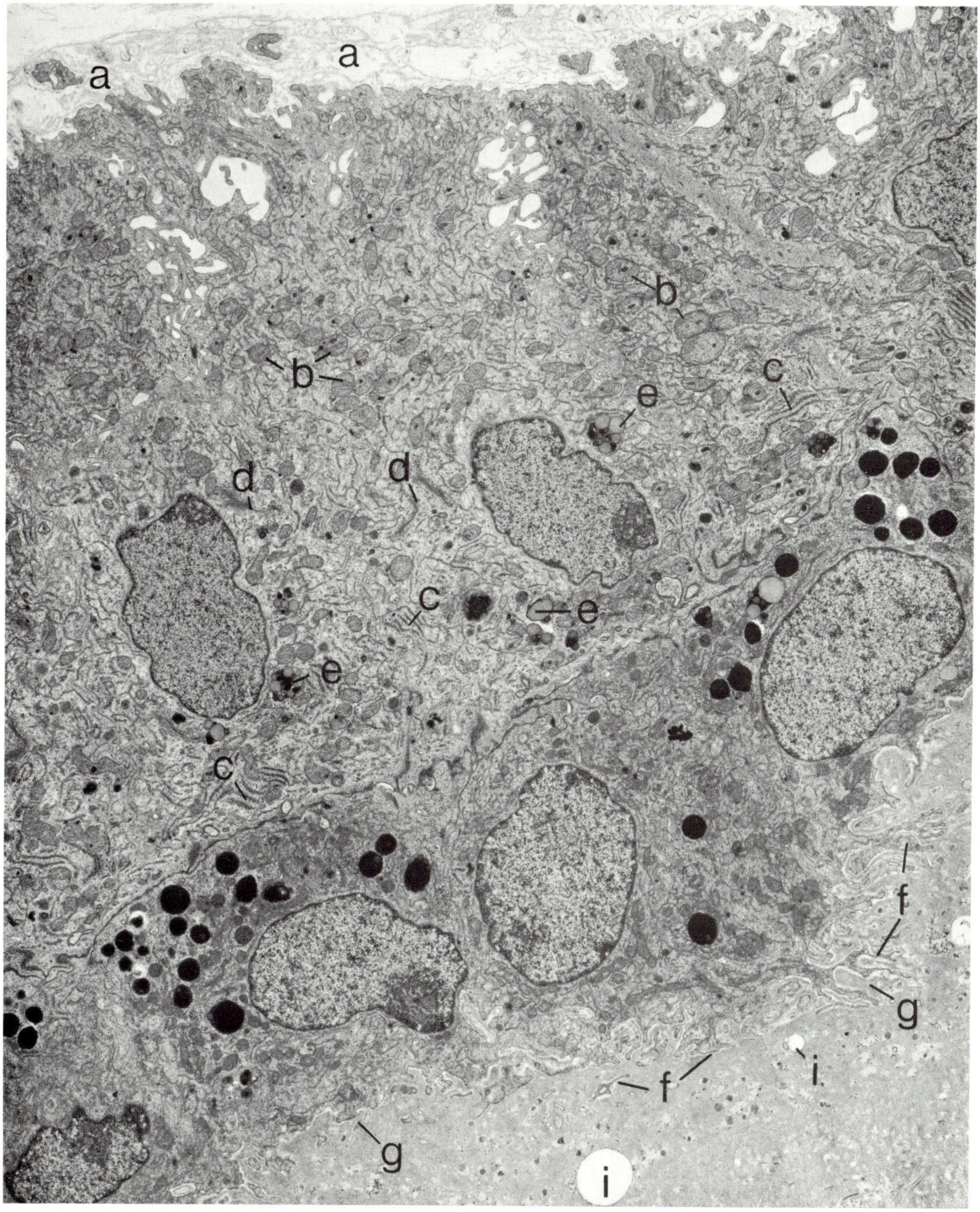

Figure 7–16. Pars plicata of the ciliary body showing the two epithelial layers in the eye of an older person. The unpigmented epithelial cells measure approximately 20 μm. high by 12 μm. wide. The cuboidal pigmented epithelial cells are approximately 10 μm. high. The thickened internal limiting membrane (a) is laminated and vesicular; such thickened membranes are a characteristic of older eyes. The cytoplasm of the unpigmented epithelium is characterized by its numerous mitochondria (b) and the cisternae of the rough-surfaced endoplasmic reticulum (c). A poorly developed Golgi apparatus (d) and several lysosomes and residual bodies (e) are shown. The pigmented epithelium contains many melanin granules, measuring about 1 μm. in diameter and located mainly in the apical portion. The basal surface is rather irregular, having many finger-like processes (f). The basement membrane of the pigmented epithelium (g) and a smooth granular material containing vesicles (i) and coarse granular particles are seen at the bottom of the figure. The appearance of the basement membrane is typical of older eyes and can be discerned with the light microscope. (× 5700.)

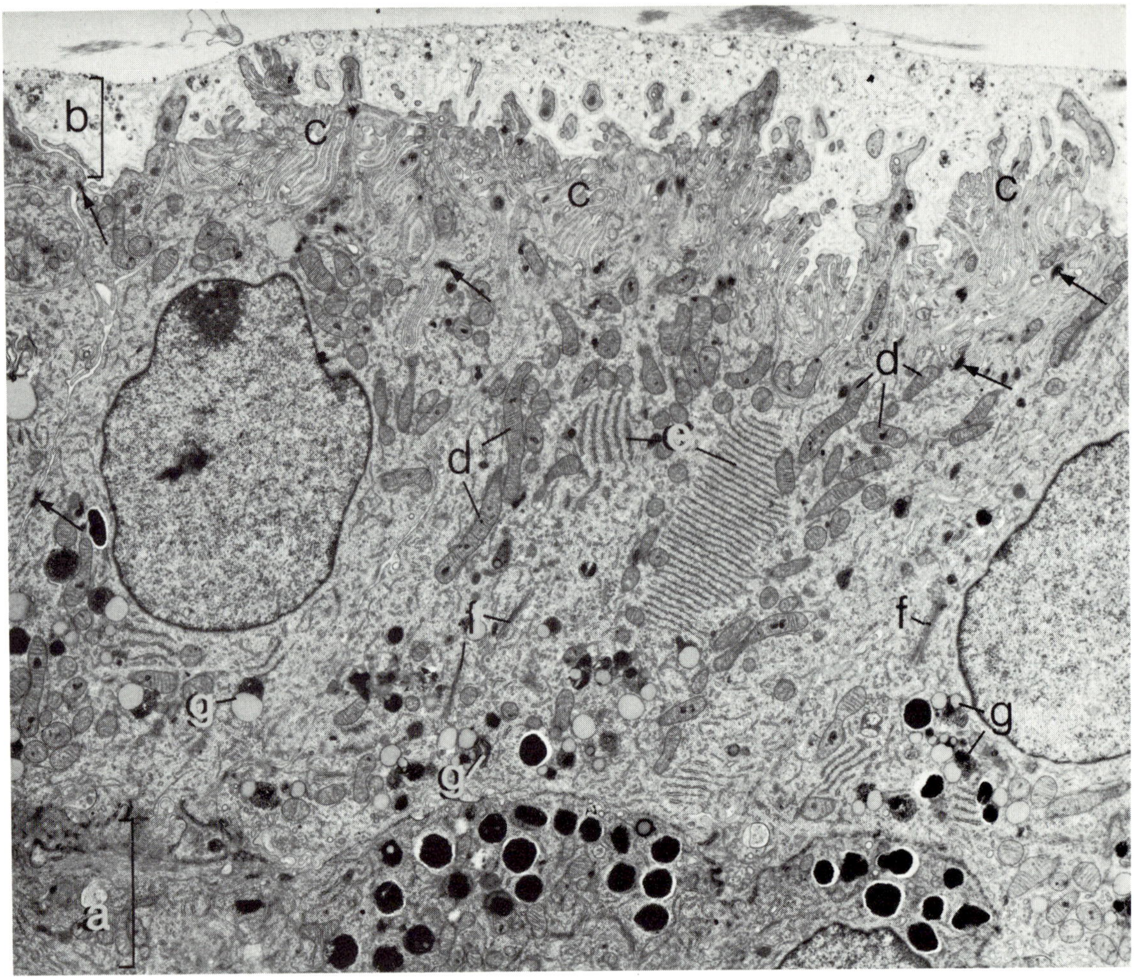

Figure 7-17. Unpigmented epithelium of the pars plicata of the eye of an older person. The full thickness of two unpigmented cells and the apical portion of the pigmented epithelium (a) are shown. At the top, the thickened, laminated internal limiting membrane (b) is seen. The basal surface contains numerous infoldings (c), while the lateral cell wall is rather straight, showing only a few interdigitations; a few desmosomes (arrows) are found in the lateral intercellular space. The apical surface is solidly bound to the pigmented epithelium by numerous occluding junctions and desmosomes. The cytoplasm contains many long mitochondria measuring 2 μm. or more (d), stacks of cisternae of the rough-surfaced endoplasmic reticulum (e), a poorly developed Golgi apparatus (f) and many lysosomes and residual bodies (g). (× 6250.)

reticular and stratified over the pars plicata. Fine and Zimmerman (1963) confirmed this finding in human eyes of patients aged 40 to 63 years. Missotten (1964) also found this alteration in the eyes of humans aged 30 and 50 years, but not in children of five and 10 years, and our observations confirm those of Missotten. We found that the basement membrane gradually becomes thicker as the result of formation of laminae of basement membrane-like material, and these layers form a reticular pattern. The laminae branch and interconnect in a complex manner, following the irregularities of the cell surface and filling out the spaces between the finger-like projections and folds between the cells. Over the crests of the ciliary processes the basement membrane is thinner and less reticular and it gradually

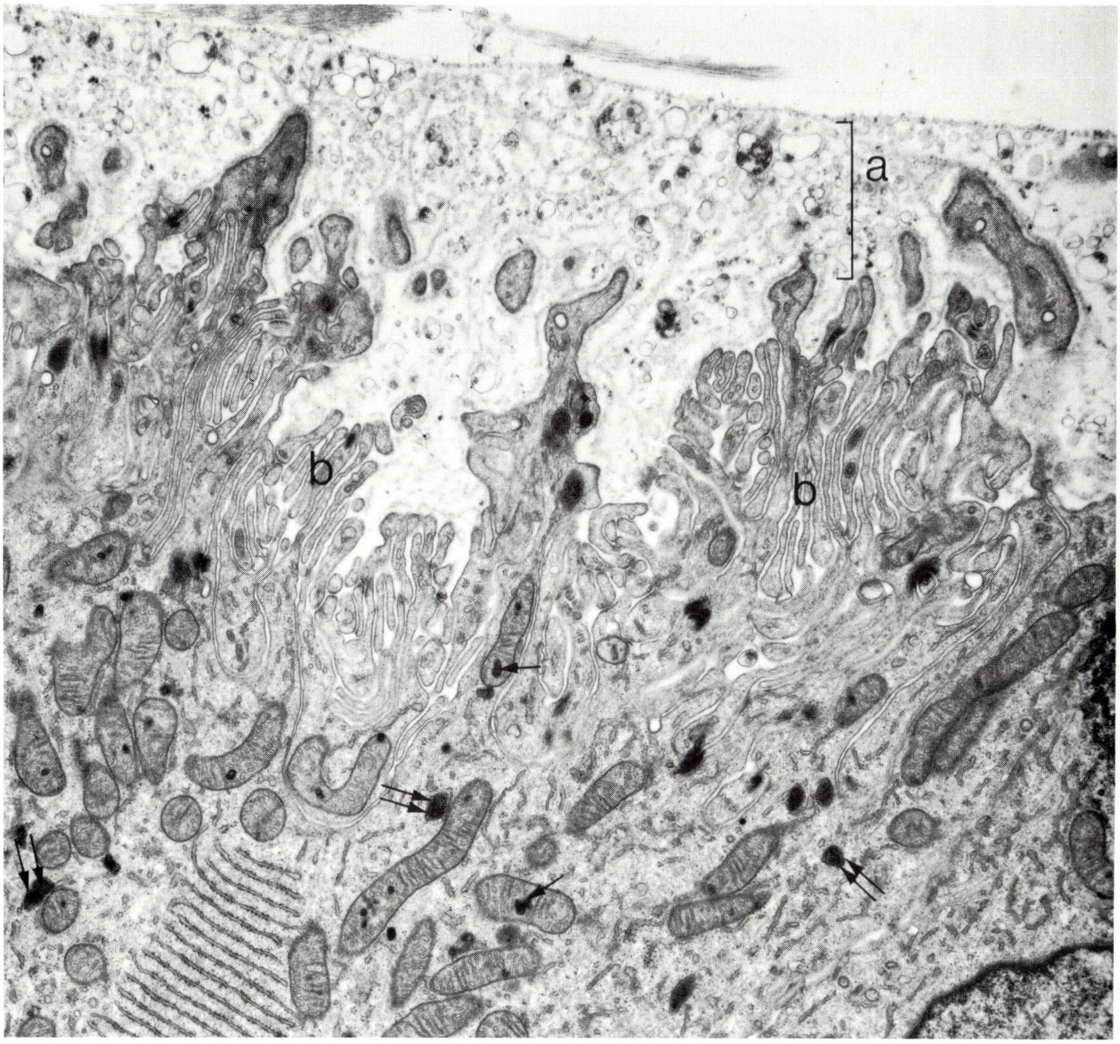

Figure 7–18. Higher magnification of Figure 7–17 showing the basal surface of the unpigmented epithelium. Note the vesicular structures contained within the thickened internal limiting membrane (a) and the infoldings (b) found in the inner portion of the lateral cell wall and the base of the cell. The mitochondria contain small, electron-dense bodies (arrows) in their interior; similar structures (double arrows) also are found in the cytoplasm. These structures are not present in the mitochondria or cytoplasm of the pigmented epithelium. (× 12,000.)

becomes thinner at the anterior part of the ciliary processes near the iris root, where it assumes the appearance of the usual basement membrane. The reticulated basement membrane measures as much as 2 μm. in the thickest areas and 0.5 μm. in its thinnest portions. Within the meshes of this reticular meshwork is a granular material, many deeply osmiophilic coarse and fine granules, and groups of membrane-bound vesicles like those seen in Bruch's membrane of the choroid as an aging phenomenon (Figs. 7-19, 7-25, 7-26 and 7-43). This reticulated inner limiting membrane was described many years ago by Salzmann (1912); some of his drawings were probably made from older human eyes. The basement membrane probably contains mucopolysaccharide, since it is PAS-positive. Its reticulated appearance in elec-

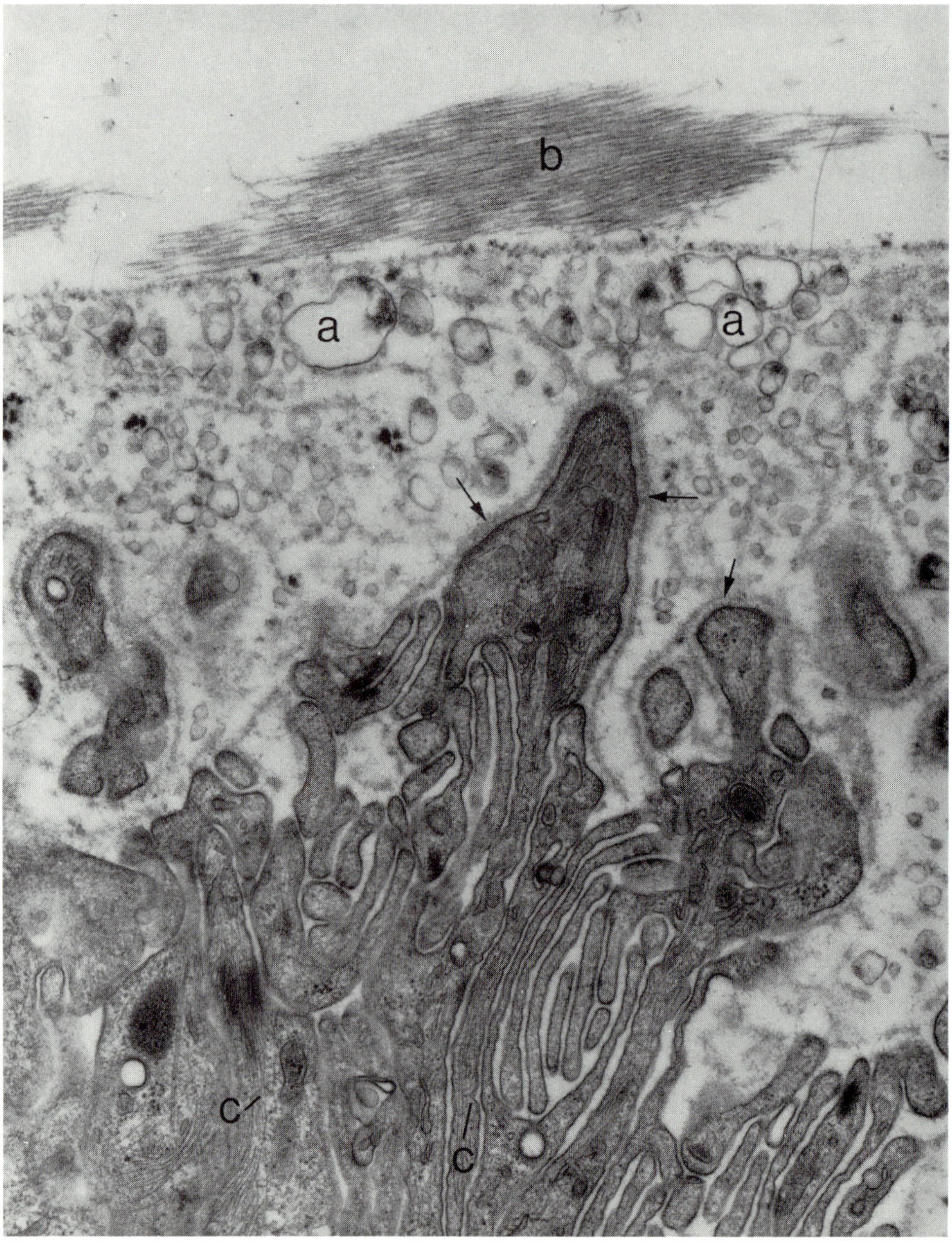

Figure 7–19. Higher magnification of the inner or basal surface of the unpigmented epithelium seen in Figure 7–18. The thickened internal limiting membrane measures as much as 2 μm. and contains membrane-bound vesicles (a). Note that the inner part of the membrane is fairly smooth and is seen to come in close contact with a zonule (b). The portion closest to the cell membrane (arrows) is identical to the internal limiting membrane in the young eye (see Figure 7–20). Numerous filaments are seen within the basal infoldings (c). (× 30,000.)

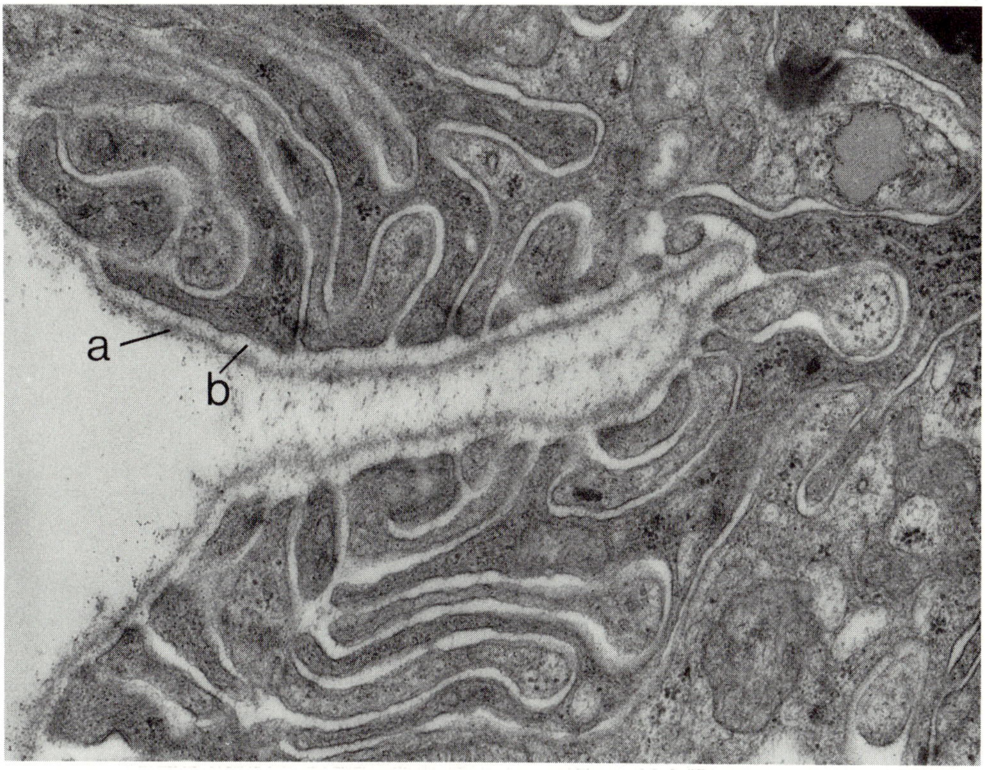

Figure 7-20. Unpigmented epithelium from the pars plicata of a young person. The internal limiting membrane is not thickened at this age and appears as a typical basement membrane. It is composed of an electron-dense band (a) measuring 300 A., separated from the cell membrane by an electron-lucent zone (b) measuring 500 A. in width. The basement membrane continues over the surface of the cell without entering the infoldings. (× 30,000.)

tron micrographs probably is caused by extraction of much of its mucoid during preparation of the specimens.

The cytoplasm of the unpigmented epithelium of the pars plicata is remarkable for its large number of moderate-sized mitochondria and its well developed rough-surfaced endoplasmic reticulum (Figs. 7-17 and 7-21). The mitochondria may measure 2 μm. in length and have small, round, lamellated osmiophilic inclusions in their matrix; similar structures are also found in the cytoplasm, but their nature and function are not clear (Figs. 7-18, 7-21 and 7-22). The rough-surfaced endoplasmic reticulum is frequently stacked in 10 to 20 parallel arrays located in the perinuclear region. Interconnecting single cisternae are spaced widely throughout the cytoplasm. The smooth-surfaced endoplasmic reticulum is not abundant, but cisternae of this reticulum are usually seen widely throughout the cytoplasm. The Golgi apparatus is present but poorly developed; its cisternal lumina are narrow and flattened. Many free, unattached ribosomes are found in the cytoplasm. A moderate number of cytoplasmic fibrils are present and microtubules occasionally are observed. Lysosomes and residual bodies are found most frequently in the apical part of the cell; lipid deposits and pigment granules also are present (Figs. 7-16, 7-17 and 7-22). The nuclear chromatin is mainly in the euchromatin or dispersed form, but a thin band of heterochromatin exists in the nuclear periphery (Figs. 7-16, 7-17 and 7-22).

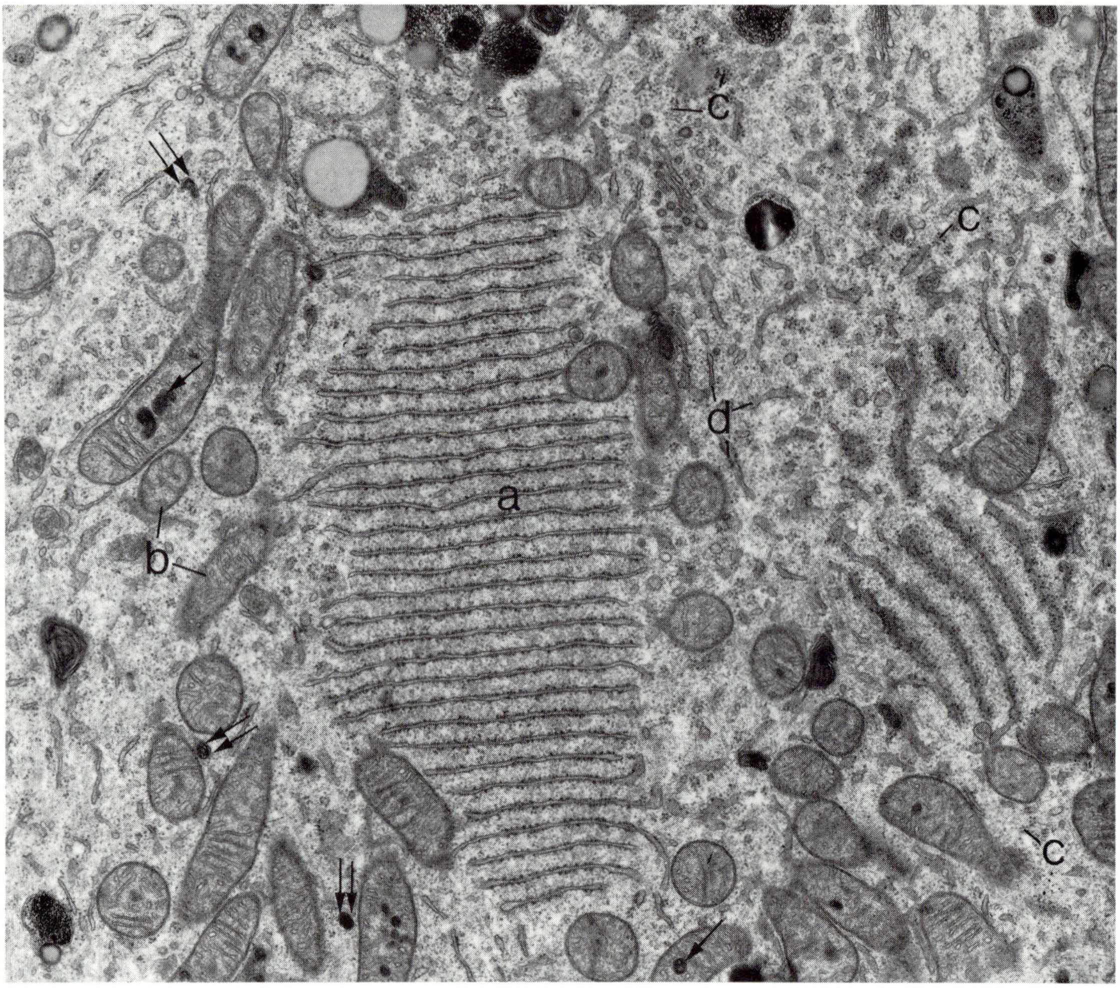

Figure 7–21. Detailed view of the cytoplasm of the unpigmented epithelium. A stack of cisternae of the rough-surfaced endoplasmic reticulum (a) is surrounded by many mitochondria (b). Some of the mitochondria have small, lamellated, electron-dense bodies (arrow) similar in appearance to others (double arrows) found in the cytoplasm. Aggregates of unattached ribosomes (c) are found throughout the cytoplasm, as well as many profiles of the smooth-surfaced endoplasmic reticulum (d). (× 20,000.)

The cytoplasm of the unpigmented epithelium of the para plana differs from that of the pars plicata in its higher content of smooth-surfaced endoplasmic reticulum and cytoplasmic fibrils. The latter are particularly abundant, giving the cytoplasm a dense and compact appearance (Figs. 7-25 and 7-26 *B*).

Aligned vesicles were found in the cytoplasm of the unpigmented epithelial cells in rabbit eyes by early observers. These vesicles were close to the lateral cellular interdigitations and measured 200 to 300 A. in diameter. Holmberg (1959a) investigated them in the rabbit ciliary epithelium and correlated their presence and increase in size and number with the reduction of aqueous humor production after administration of Diamox. He believed that these vesicles were involved in the production of aqueous humor and its release into the posterior chamber. Pappas and Smelser (1958) repeated this study but interpreted the aligned vesicles as resulting from an alteration of the interdigitating folds of the lateral cell surface. They believed that the reduced aqueous humor formation was secondary to a reduction in the area

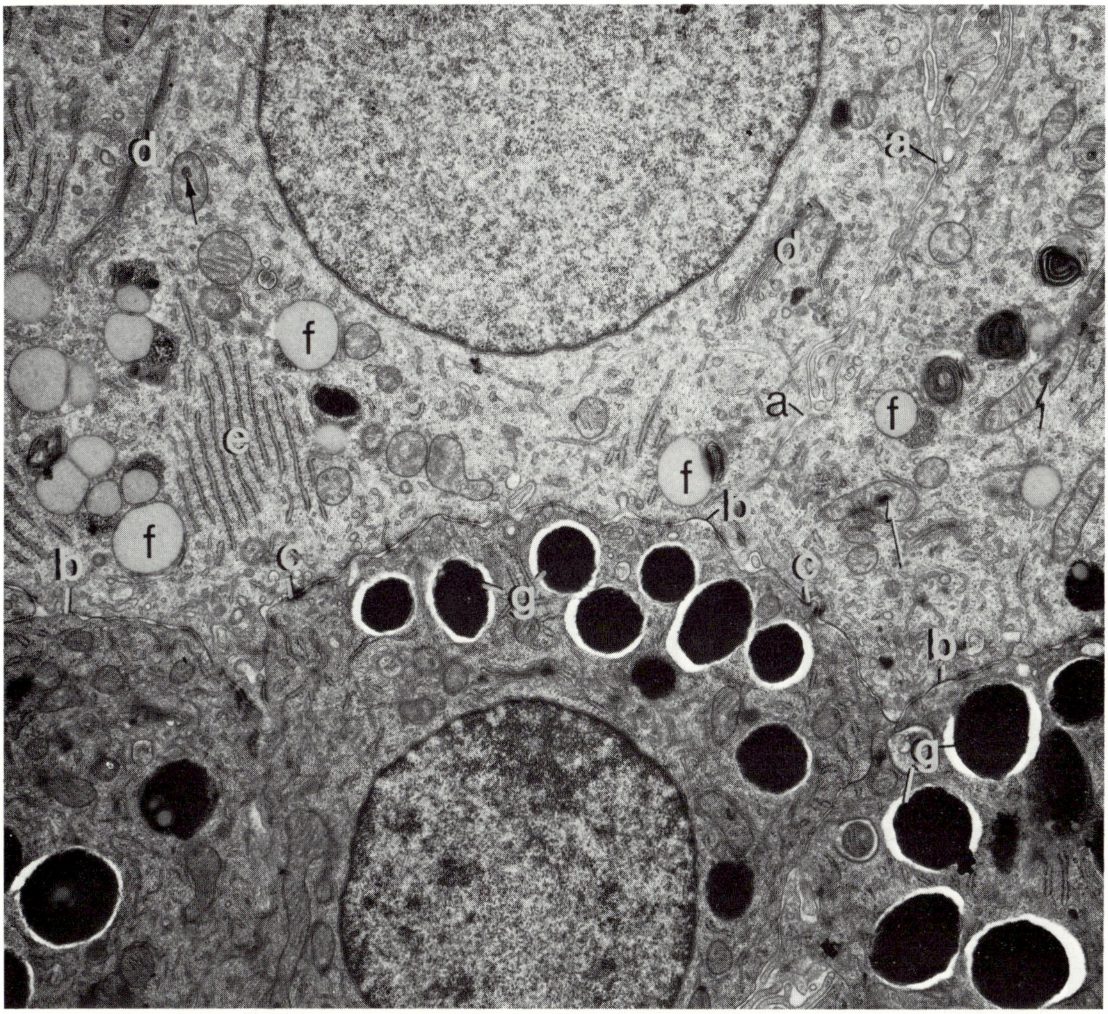

Figure 7–22. Apical portion of the unpigmented epithelium and the pigmented epithelium in the pars plicata. The lateral intercellular space (a) of the unpigmented epithelium has very few intercellular junctions, while the apical intercellular space is interrupted by many occluding junctions (b) and desmosomes (c). The cytoplasm of the unpigmented epithelium is lighter than that of the pigmented epithelium. Profiles of the cisternae of the Golgi apparatus (d) and of the rough-surfaced endoplasmic reticulum (e) are shown. Mitochondria containing electron-dense, lamellated bodies (arrows) are shown in the unpigmented epithelium; these structures are absent from the mitochrondria of the pigmented epithelium and other ocular tissues similarly fixed. Lipid droplets (f) commonly are found in the apical portion of the unpigmented epithelium. The pigmented epithelium contains numerous melanin granules (g) in its apical portion. (× 10,000.)

of the cell. Urayama and co-workers (1959) studied the epithelium after simple aqueous puncture and found a diminution in the number of interdigitations. After 24 hours these interdigitations returned to normal. Tormey (1964) studied this epithelium in rabbits. He produced a steady state of aqueous humor formation and intraocular pressure, then gave 20 mg. per kg. of Diamox. Fifteen minutes later the aqueous humor was removed and the eyes were fixed in osmium. He could find no difference between the ciliary epithelial cell cytoplasm of the test animals and that of the controls. He did not agree, therefore, with either Holmberg or Pappas and Smelser. Tormey showed that the aligned "rows of vesicles" described by the previous investigations were part of an unusual form of smooth-surfaced endoplasmic reticulum with many convolutions and interconnections. The sacs of endoplasmic

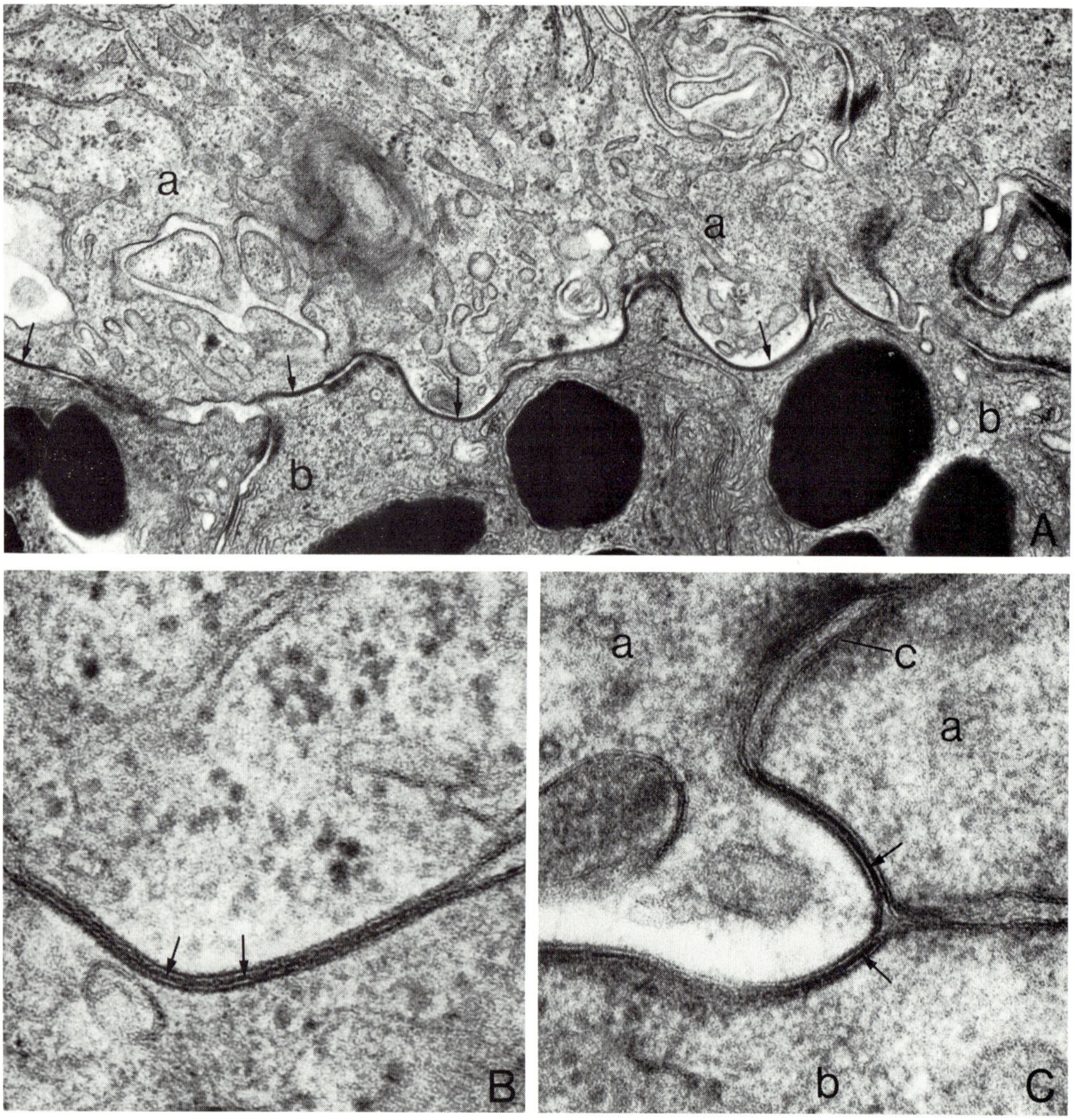

Figure 7–23. *A*, Apical intercellular space of the unpigmented (a) and pigmented (b) epithelium. The two layers of ciliary epithelium are solidly bound to each other by numerous occluding junctions; these junctions are mainly fasciae and maculae occludentes (arrows). (× 30,000.)

B, Higher magnification of a fascia occludens showing areas of membrane fusion (arrows). (× 120,000.)

C, Junctions between the unpigmented epithelium (a) and pigmented epithelium (b). Two occluding junctions (arrows) and part of a desmosome (c) are shown. (× 120,000.)

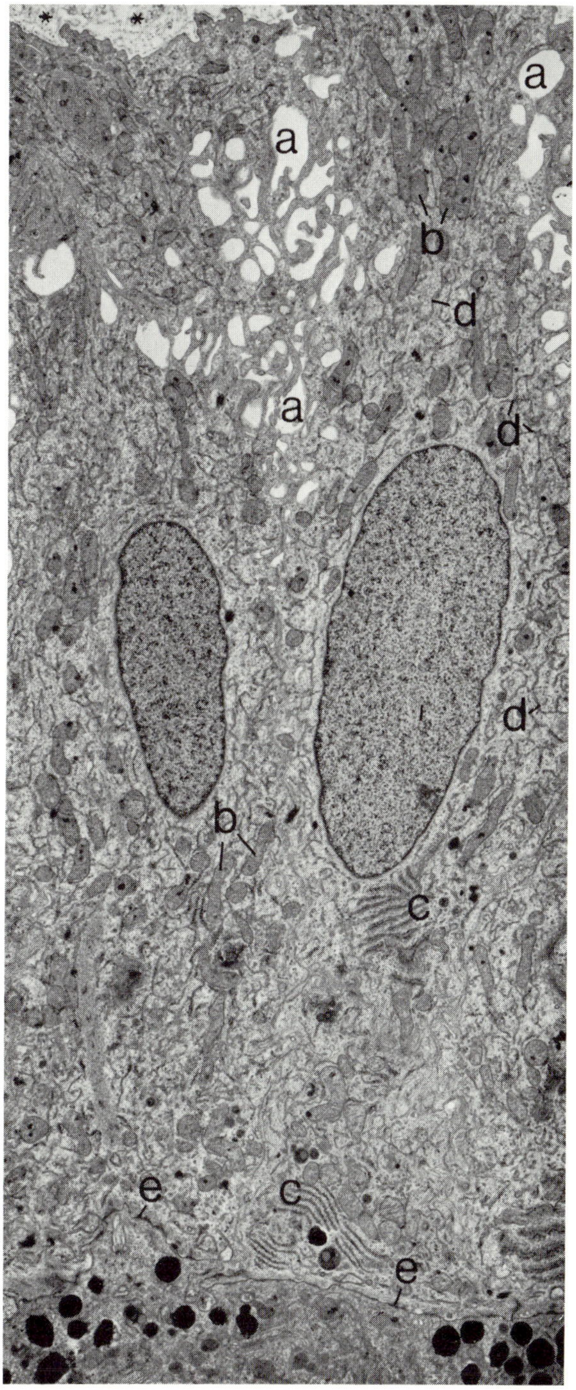

Figure 7–24. Unpigmented ciliary epithelium of the pars plana. These cells are tall and columnar, measuring 30 to 40 μm. in height. A small portion of the internal limiting membrane (*) is shown on the upper left. Wide intercellular gaps (a), a result of aging, appear on the inner third. The cytoplasm contains numerous mitochondria (b), arrays of cisternae of the rough-surfaced endoplasmic reticulum (c) and many tubules of the smooth-surfaced endoplasmic reticulum (d). The area of contiguity between the pigmented and unpigmented epithelium (e) is seen at the bottom. (× 5000.)

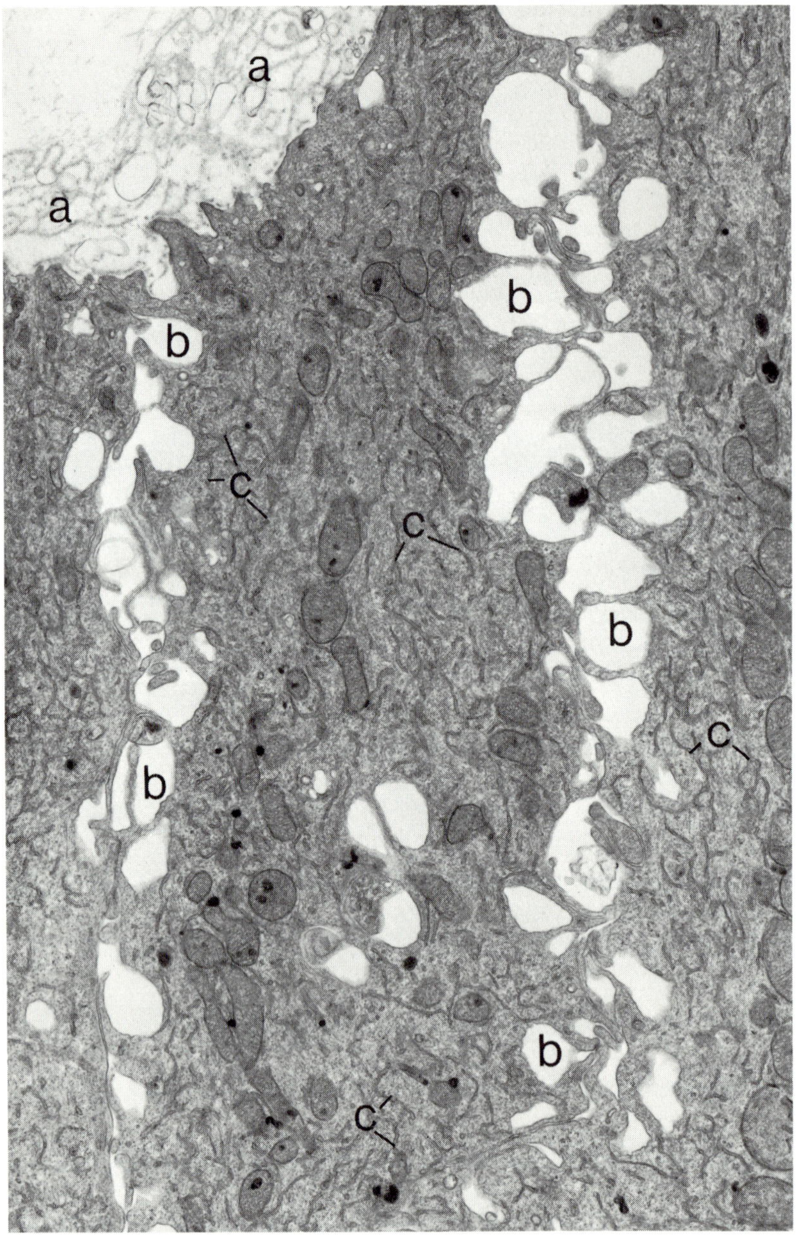

Figure 7–25. Unpigmented epithelium of the pars plana. Higher magnification of the inner third of the unpigmented epithelium showing the internal limiting membrane (a), with its laminated structure and the wide intercellular gaps (b) separating these cells in older eyes. The cytoplasm of the pigmented epithelium of the pars plana differs from that of the pars plicata by a greater filament content and a more developed, smooth-surfaced endoplasmic reticulum (c). Several mitochondria are also seen. (× 12,000.)

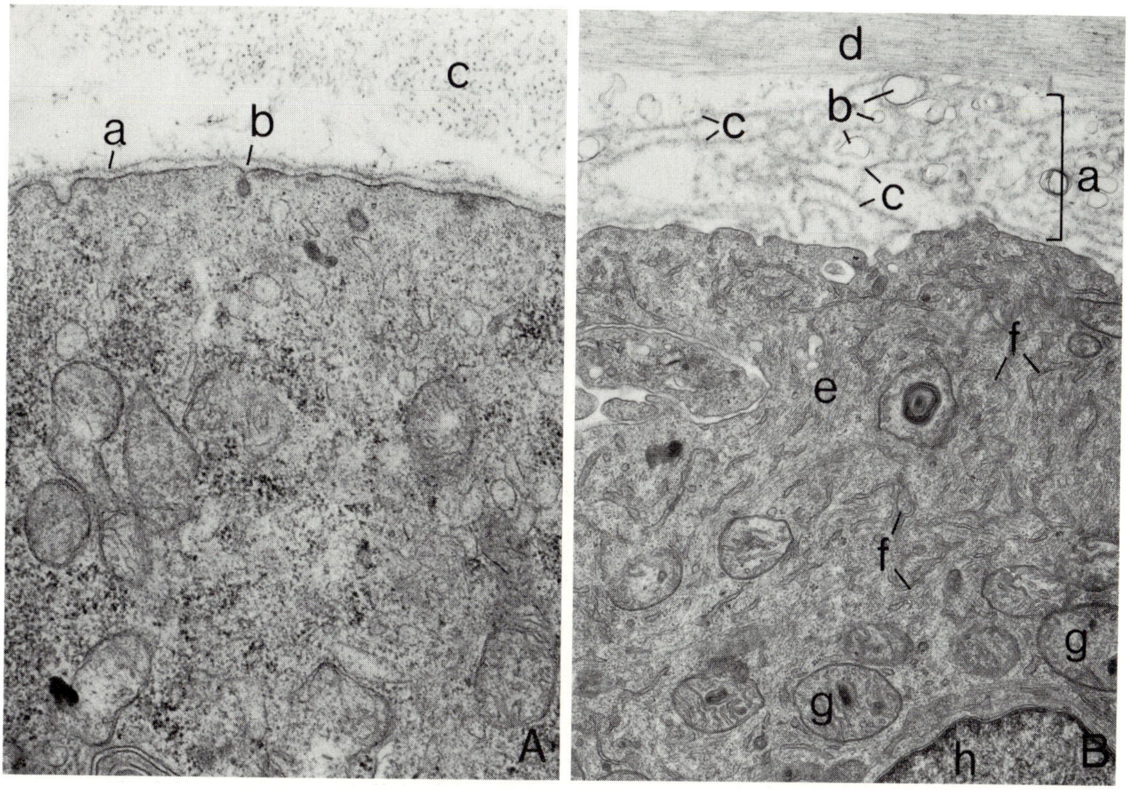

Figure 7–26. *A*, Unpigmented epithelium of a young eye. The internal limiting membrane of the young eye is a typical basement membrane composed of an electron-dense layer (a) 300 A. thick and an electron-lucent space (b) 500 A. thick. The collagen fibrils forming part of a zonule are seen at (c). (× 18,000.)

B, Unpigmented epithelium from an older eye. Note the multilayered, lamellated structure of the internal limiting membrane (a) of an older person. The membrane may be one or two microns thick and composed of numerous vesicles (b) and layers of an electron-dense lamina (c) identical in size and structure to those seen in the basement membrane of the young eye. A zonule is shown at (d). The cytoplasm of the unpigmented epithelium of the pars plana has numerous filaments (e) and cisternae of the smooth-surfaced endoplasmic reticulum (f). Mitochondria (g) and a portion of the nucleus (h) are shown. (× 13,000.)

reticulum were found to be arranged in sheets, so that a cross-section through the sheets produced the appearance of a row of vesicles. Missotten (1964) believed that the vesicles were an artifact, since the so-called vesicles were aligned similarly to the interdigitations of the lateral cell walls. He demonstrated occasional desmosomes in the membranes surrounding the so-called vesicles, signifying to him that they were related to the interlocking processes of adjacent cells. He found that the vesicles were absent in permanganate-fixed specimens and present in osmium-fixed material, therefore representing an artifact. Tormey (1965) subsequently studied serial sections of these cells and showed that the apparent vesicles really are the result of the interdigitating processes of adjacent cells. He further demonstrated that the so-called aligned vesicles are not seen in glutaraldehyde-fixed material but are present in osmium-fixed, and thus are artifactual. The most recent studies on human and primate eyes have shown that these aligned vesicles are not a normal component of the unpigmented epithelial cell.

Pigmented Epithelium (Figs. 7-5 to 7-14 and 7-27 to 7-29)

The pigmented epithelium is a single layer from the root of the iris to the ora serrata (Figs. 7-5 and 7-6). It is continuous with the dilator epithe-

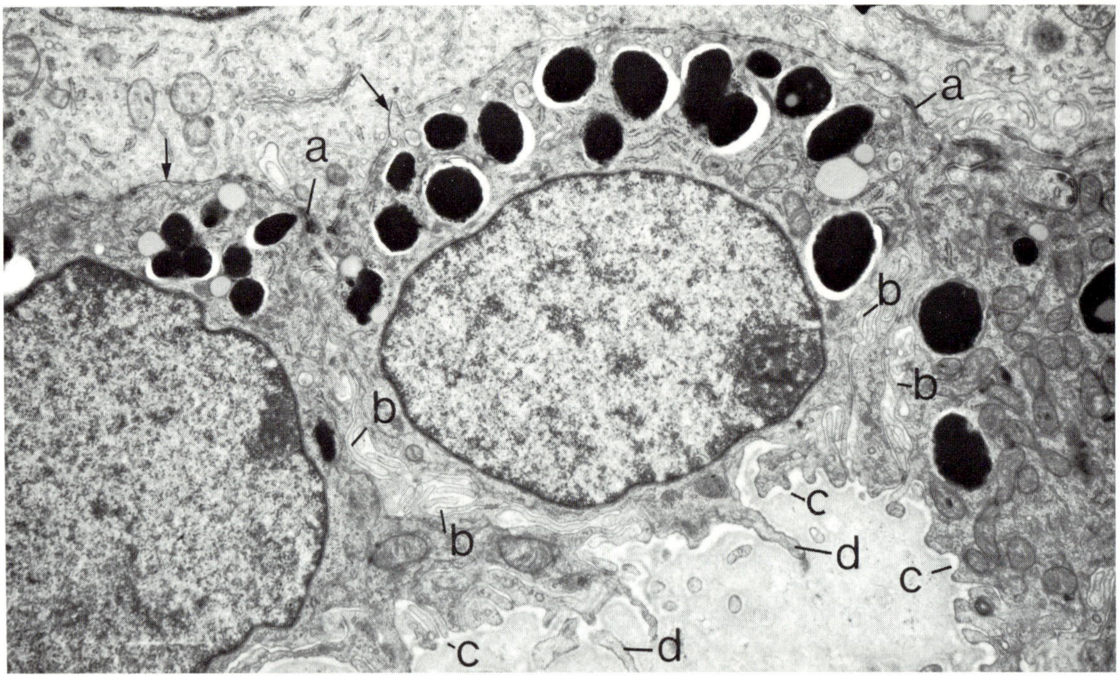

Figure 7–27. Pigmented epithelium from the pars plicata of an older person. Two cells of the pigmented epithelium measuring between 7 and 10 μm. in height are shown. They are joined to the unpigmented epithelium by many occluding junctions (arrows) and desmosomes (a). The lateral intercellular space has interdigitations (b) along its basal or outer third, but very few intercellular junctions are found here. The basal surface has a basement membrane (c) which has become considerably thickened and altered with aging. Cytoplasmic processes (d) project out from the basal surface. The cytoplasm of the pigmented epithelium is darker than that of the unpigmented epithelium and contains numerous melanin granules, located mainly in its apical portion. The white halo around the melanin granules represents a sectioning artifact. (× 11,000.)

lium of the iris anteriorly and with the pigmented epithelium of the retina posteriorly (Figs. 7–7 A and 7–14). This continuous epithelial portion represents the entire outer epithelium of the optic cup. It is a layer of neural ectoderm that has not differentiated into a specialized neurosensory tissue. This layer and the unpigmented epithelium, even though they develop specialized functions, retain some attributes of neural tissue in their ability to develop into benign and malignant neuroectodermal tumors.

By light microscopy the attachment of the pigmented to the unpigmented epithelium is rather smooth, without intervening tissue (Figs. 7–7 to 7–9). Over the pars plana the cells have smooth inner surfaces and measure 10 to 15 μm. in height by 10 μm. in width. Within the pars plicata their size and shape vary according to the tissue folds. Over the ciliary processes the cells are flattened, their height being 8 to 12 μm. and their width 8 μm.

On the external side the pigment epithelium is united with the ciliary body stroma by a basement membrane which is thin in young eyes and increases in thickness with age (Figs. 7–5, 7–8 and 7–29). In diabetic persons it also may show a considerable increase in thickness. This membrane is PAS-positive and is continuous posteriorly with Bruch's membrane of the choroid and anteriorly with the basement membranes of the dilator epithelium of the iris. At the lateral surfaces the cells are closely adherent to each other and at the base they are so firmly bound to the basement membrane

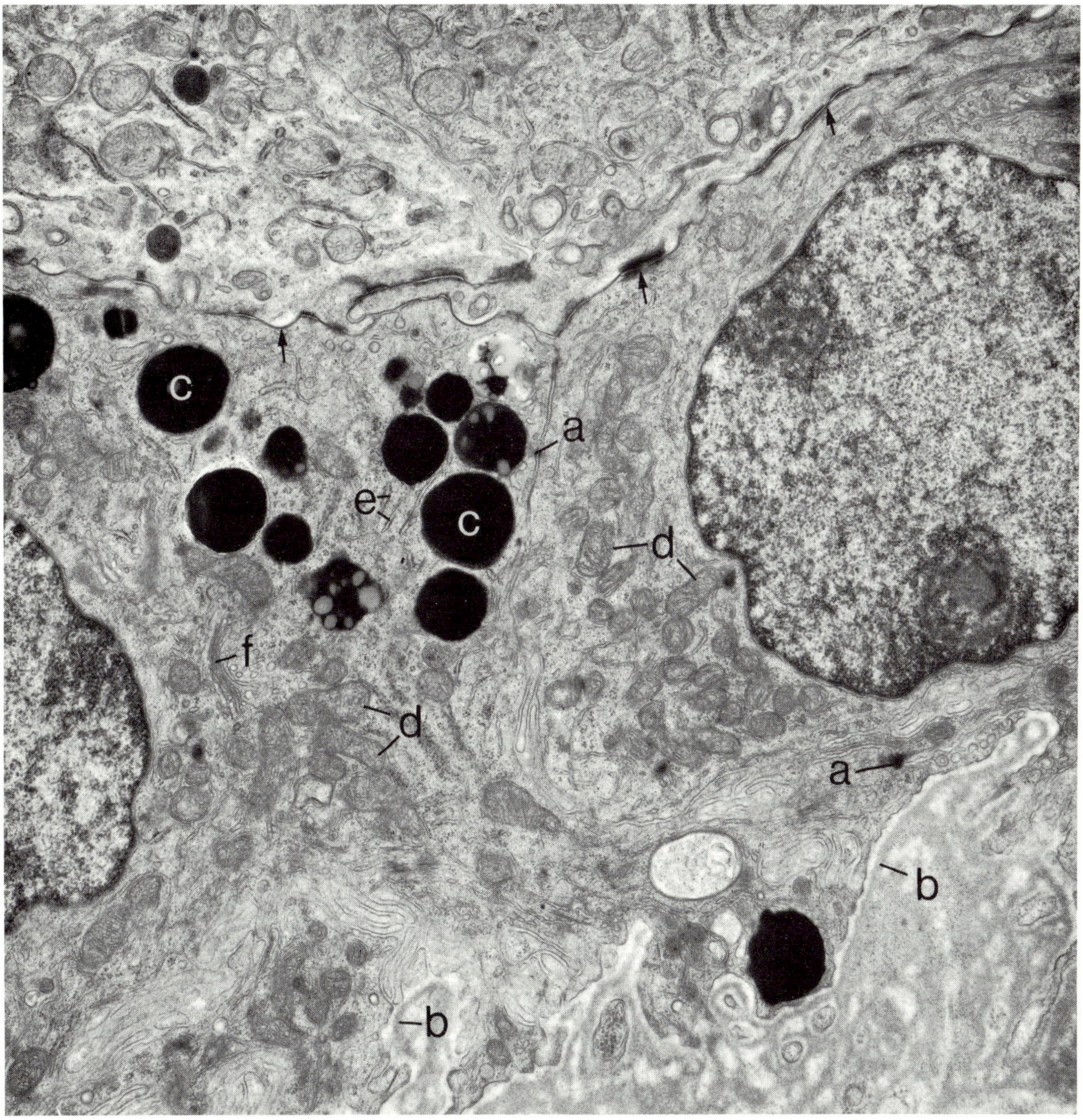

Figure 7–28. Pigmented epithelium of the pars plana. The apical intercellular space and the junctions with the unpigmented epithelium (arrows) appear at the top. The lateral intercellular space usually has only a few desmosomes (a). The basal surface and the basement membrane (b) appear at the bottom. The cytoplasm contains melanin granules (c) measuring 0.8 μm. to 1.0 μm. in diameter, a moderate number of mitochondria (d), rough-surfaced endoplasmic reticulum (e), a poorly developed Golgi apparatus (f) and numerous free ribosomes dispersed throughout the cytoplasm. (× 12,000.)

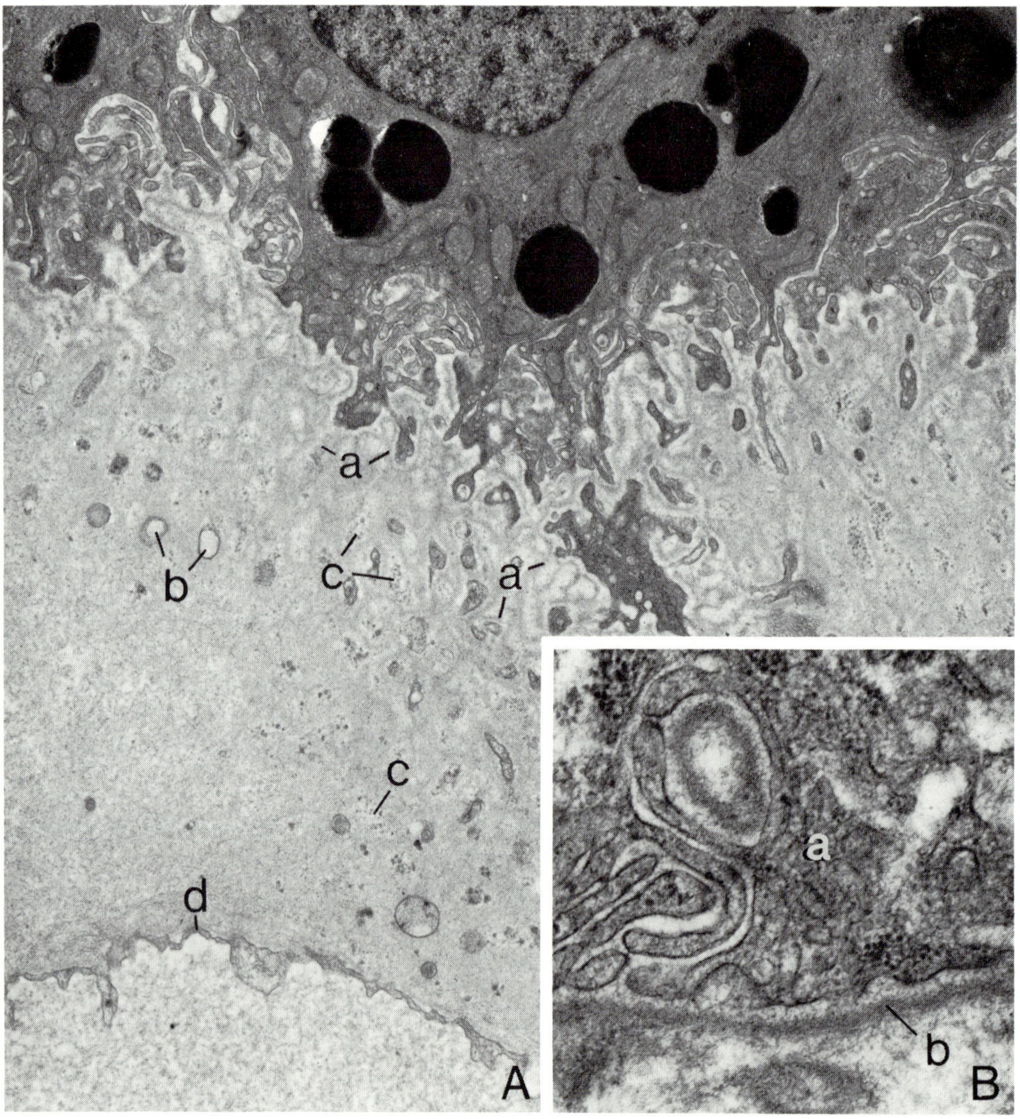

Figure 7–29. *A*, Pigmented epithelium and a capillary of the pars plicata. The basement membrane of the pigmented ciliary epithelium undergoes aging changes similar to those occurring in the internal limiting membrane of the unpigmented ciliary epithelium. The membrane (a) consists of several layers forming a network: vesicular structures (b), coarse electron-dense granules (c) and a finely granular material fill the zone separating the capillary endothelium (d) from the basement membrane. (× 7500.)

B, Basement membrane of the ciliary pigmented epithelium (a) in a young person. This membrane (b) resembles the internal limiting membrane of the unpigmented ciliary epithelium in the young. (× 12,000.)

and ciliary body stroma that attempts to remove them cause disruption of the cells. The pigment granules of these cells are like those of the iris and retinal epithelium. They are much larger than those of the stromal melanocytes, measuring 0.8 by 2.0 μm. in size, compared to 0.3 to 0.5 μm. in the melanocytes. Bleached preparations show the nuclei in cells over the pars plana to be somewhat oval, with their long axes at right angles to the height of the cell. More anteriorly the cells are rounded, with the nucleus arranged obliquely. Their cytoplasm is more dense than that of the unpigmented epithelial layer.

When viewed with the electron microscope, the basal side facing the ciliary body stroma (Fig. 7–29 *B*) has a basement membrane. This basement membrane is of the usual type and is uniform in thickness throughout the ciliary body. It follows the course of the cells but does not dip into infoldings. Anteriorly, in the region of the pars plicata, the membrane is separated by a narrow space from the capillaries (Fig. 7-29 *A*). Posteriorly, over the pars plana, it is related to the stromal collagen and blood vessels. The basal cell membrane shows only a few infoldings and no half-desmosomes. In the eyes of older individuals the basal cell membrane shows pronounced changes, characterized by irregularity of the surface, with long, finger-like processes projecting out through the basement membrane into a thick layer of amorphous tissue in the stroma of the ciliary body (Figs. 7-5 and 7-29 *A*). The cell membrane on the *apical* side is like that of the unpigmented epithelium, and there are numerous desmosomes and occluding junctions between these two layers of cells (Fig. 7-23). The *lateral* surfaces show interdigitations, but the infoldings are not so pronounced as in the unpigmented epithelium (Fig. 7–28). The cells along this wall are joined mainly by desmosomes and a few maculae occludens.

The cytoplasm of the pigment epithelium contains numerous round or oval pigment granules measuring 0.6 to 0.8 μm. in size. The granules are localized mainly in the apical portion, and all are completely melanized. Smooth and rough-surfaced endoplasmic reticulum is present, but is less abundant than in the unpigmented layer. The rough-surfaced endoplasmic reticulum is diffusely distributed and does not form so many parallel arrays as are found in the unpigmented epithelium. The mitochondria are smaller and less numerous in these cells. Ribosomes also are not so numerous. The Golgi apparatus is commonly found in the nuclear region of the apical part of the cell and is similarly developed as in the unpigmented epithelium. Characteristic of these cells and not of the unpigmented epithelium is the presence of grouped bundles of fine fibrils, which are like tonofilaments (Missotten, 1964).

STROMA (Figs. 7-30 to 7-42)

The following subdivisions of the ciliary body stroma will be described: (1) inner connective tissue layer and vessels, (2) Bruch's membrane, and (3) ciliary muscle.

Inner Connective Tissue Layer. This layer is composed of cells, collagen, vessels and nerves (Figs. 7-5 and 7-7 to 7-15). It is thick in the pars plicata, where it separates the epithelial layers from the ciliary muscle, and becomes thinner over the pars plana. The greatest thickness is over the apices of the ciliary processes, and the least is in the valleys between them.

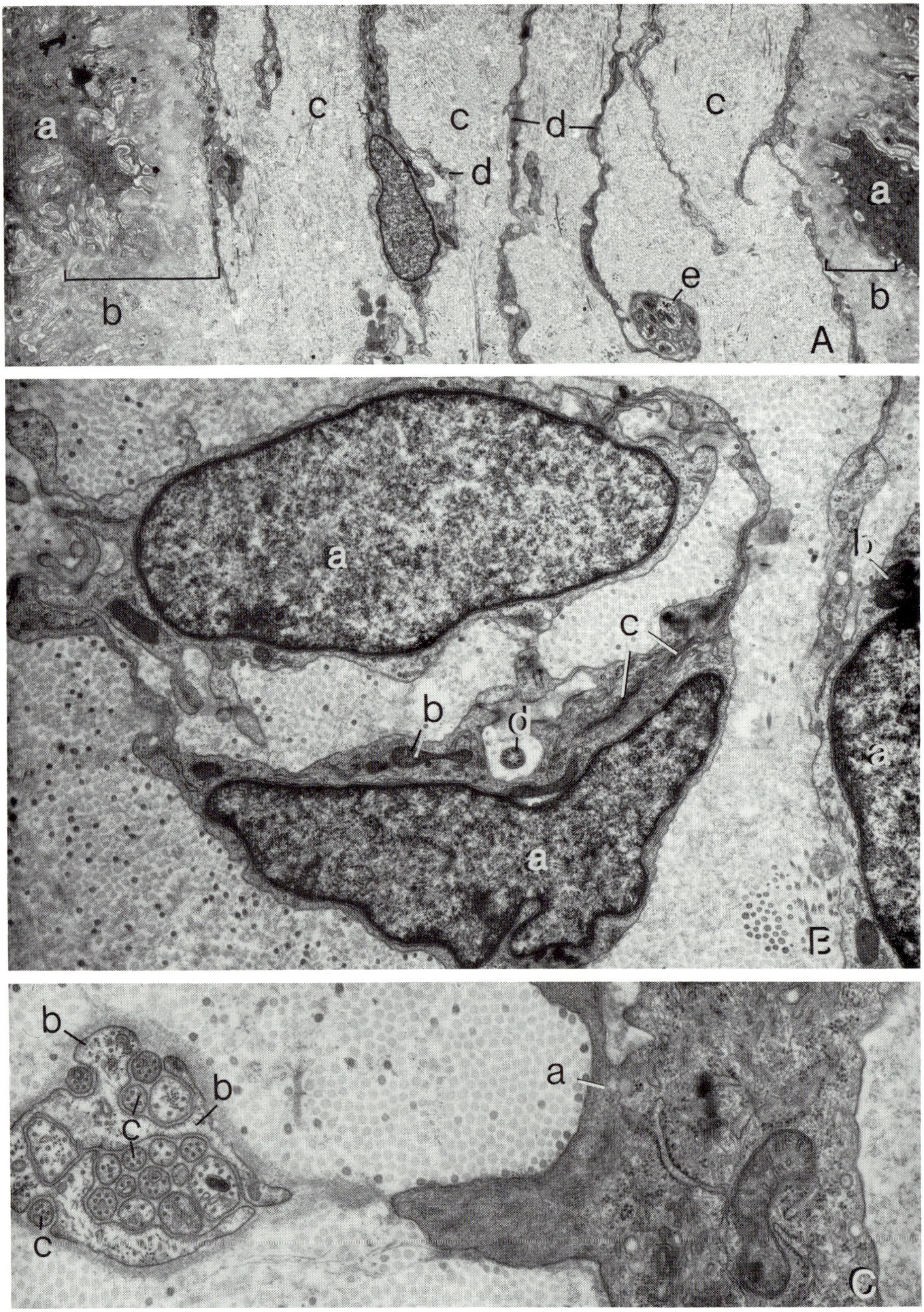

Figure 7–30. *See legend on opposite page.*

In the young eye the connective tissue is loosely arranged, whereas in older eyes the collagen becomes somewhat hyalinized. Except for the major arterial circle of the iris with its tributaries and branches, the vessels are mostly capillaries and veins. The smaller vessels lie close to the epithelium over the ciliary processes and valleys.

The inner connective tissue layer is continuous with that separating the bundles of ciliary muscle, and anteriorly it joins the connective tissue layer of the iris. Posteriorly it is continuous with the stroma of the choroid. Anteriorly, in the region of the root of the iris and the attachments of the trabecular meshwork, the connective tissue forms a thin, loose mantle between the ciliary muscle and anterior chamber (Fig. 7-5). The connective tissue is intimately related to the basement membrane of the pigment epithelial cells, and with aging an amorphous material is accumulated against the basement membrane, giving a thickened appearance to the latter (Figs. 7–5 and 7–8 A). The connective tissue in the muscular region is more compact than elsewhere. Its cellular components are fibroblasts, melanocytes, lymphocytes, a moderate number of mast cells and some macrophages. The collagen framework of this layer supports the epithelium and ciliary muscle and provides a passage for vessels and nerves to the ciliary processes, ciliary muscle and anterior eye structures.

The largest vessel in the connective tissue stroma of the ciliary body is the major arterial circle (Figs. 7-32 and 7-35). It is a typical small artery with two to three layers of smooth muscle cells in its media. The internal elastic lamina is very poorly developed; the endothelium and adjacent muscle cells have distinct basement membranes. The collagenous adventitia is loose and of medium thickness. Most of the capillaries are located close to the pigmented epithelium, and they often contact its basement membrane. The capillaries of the ciliary processes are large, like those in the choriocapillaris, and fenestrated. These capillaries measure between 15 and 30 μm. The capillaries in the ciliary muscle are smaller and less fenestrated. Taniguchi (1962) described fenestrae measuring 300 to 1000 A. in diameter. He found these fenestrations to be less numerous than in the choriocapillaris of the choroid. Occasionally pericytes are found outside the basement membrane of the endothelial cells. The capillaries merge into venules which are composed of an endothelium and endothelial basement membrane 300 to 400 A. thick.

Figure 7–30. *A*, Stroma of a ciliary process of the pars plicata. The basal portion of the pigmented epithelium is seen on either side (a), and associated with the thickened basement membrane is the finely granular, homogeneous material (b) seen in Figure 7–29 *A*. The stromal collagen (c) is tightly packed and oriented in several directions. Long, thin fibroblasts (d) and nerves (e) also are shown. (× 3200.)

B, Fibroblasts of the ciliary body, stroma of the pars plicata. The nuclei (a) of three fibroblasts and the scanty perinuclear cytoplasm are shown. Mitochondria (b), Golgi apparatus (c) and the cross-section of a cilium (d) are indicated. (× 13,500.)

C, Ciliary body stroma containing a fibroblast (a) and a nerve bundle. The cytoplasm of the fibroblast has many free ribosomes and some rough-surfaced endoplasmic reticulum. A Schwann cell (b) surrounds a number of axons; the microtubules (c) of the axons are clearly visible. (× 11,000.)

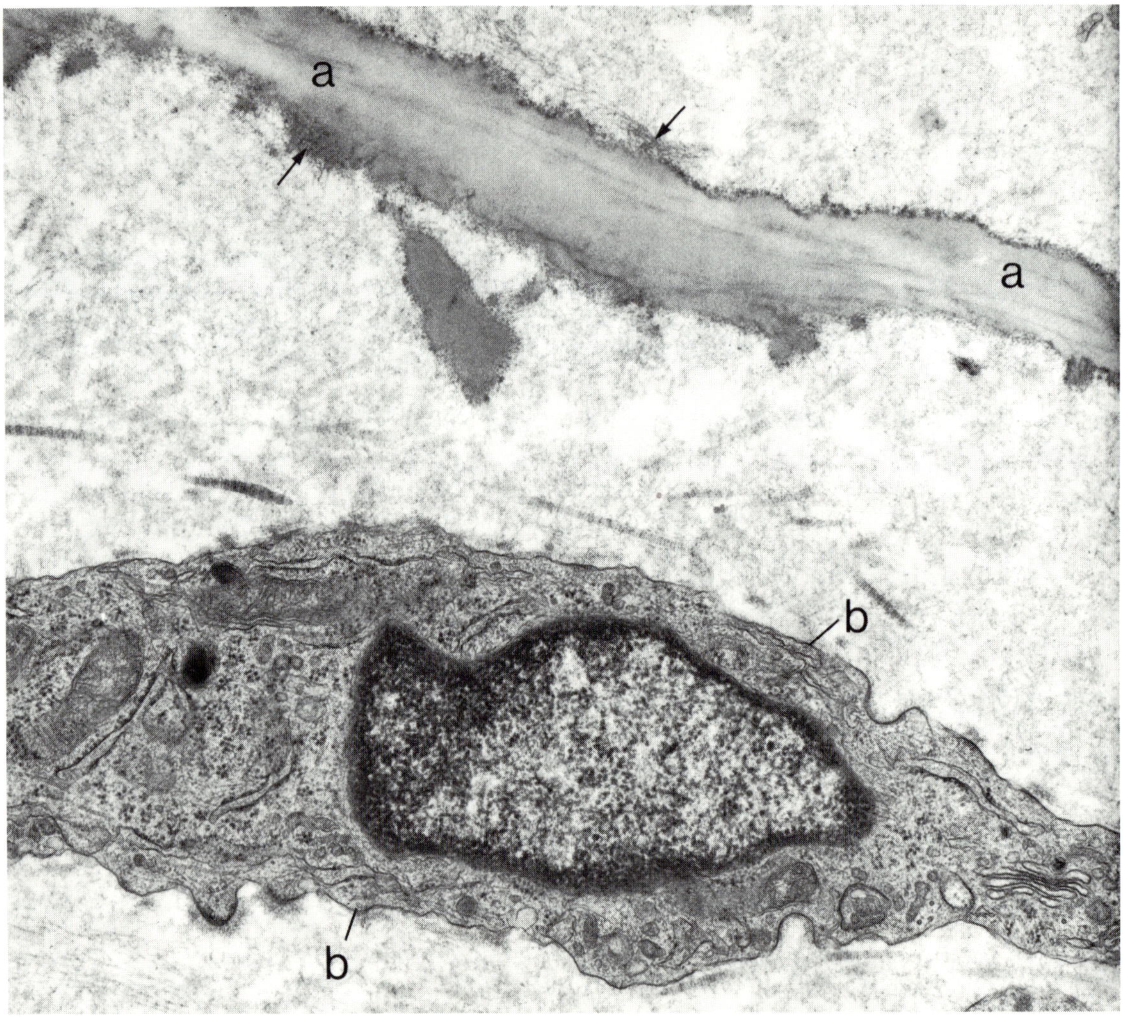

Figure 7–31. Ciliary body, stroma of the pars plana. The elastic tissue of Bruch's membrane (a) is present throughout the pars plana stroma. Note the fine filaments (arrows) found in the cortex, enclosing a lighter homogeneous mass of elastin. A fibroblast (b) containing all the organelles involved in protein synthesis and secretion is seen at the bottom. (× 25,000.)

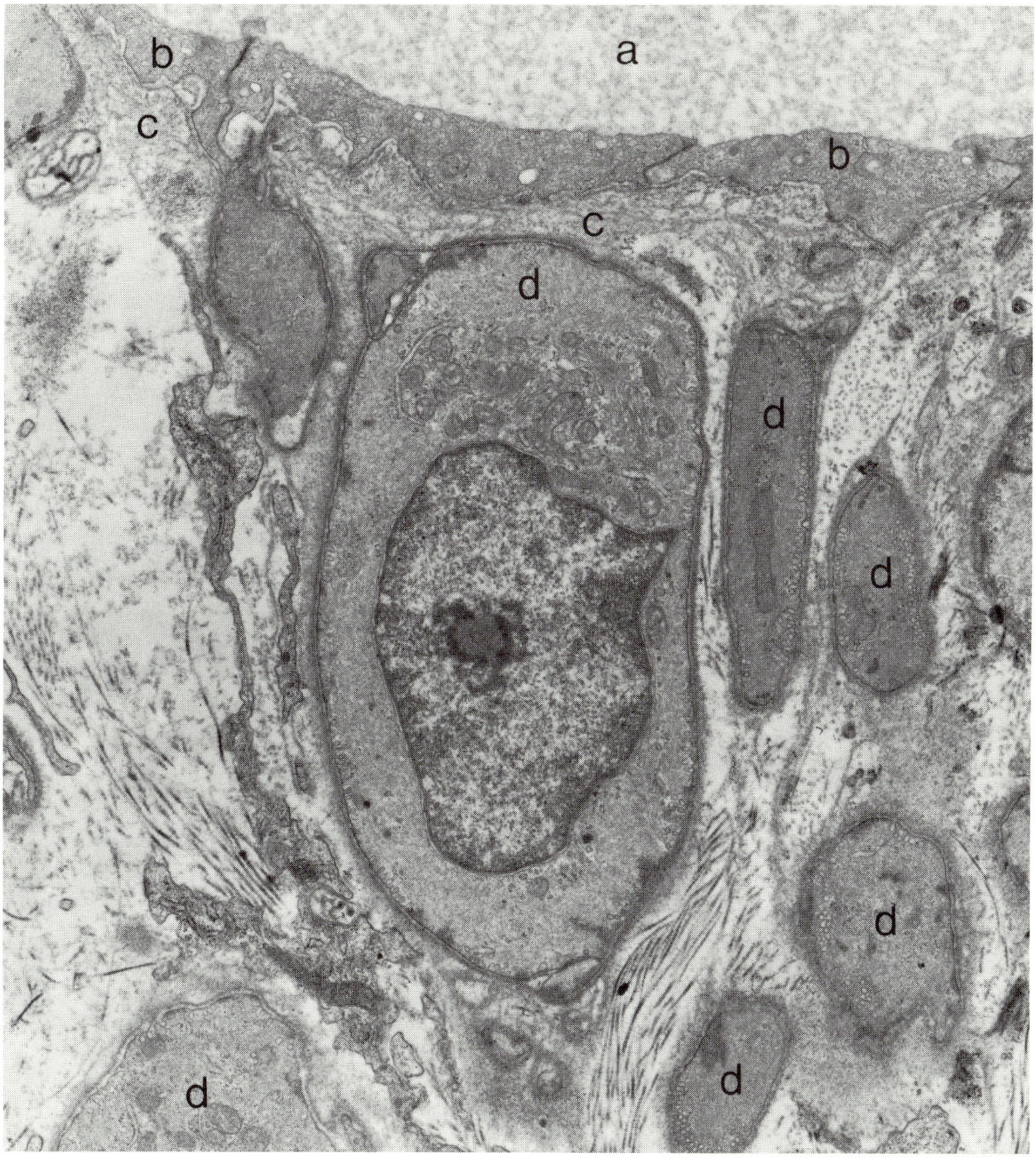

Figure 7–32. Wall of the major arterial circle in the anterior ciliary body stroma. The lumen is at (a), the endothelium at (b). The basement membrane of the endothelium (c) is thickened in some places. Note that there is no elastic tissue. The muscle cells (d) are cut in cross-section and are surrounded by their own basement membranes. Collagen fibrils separate the muscle cells. (× 11,480.)

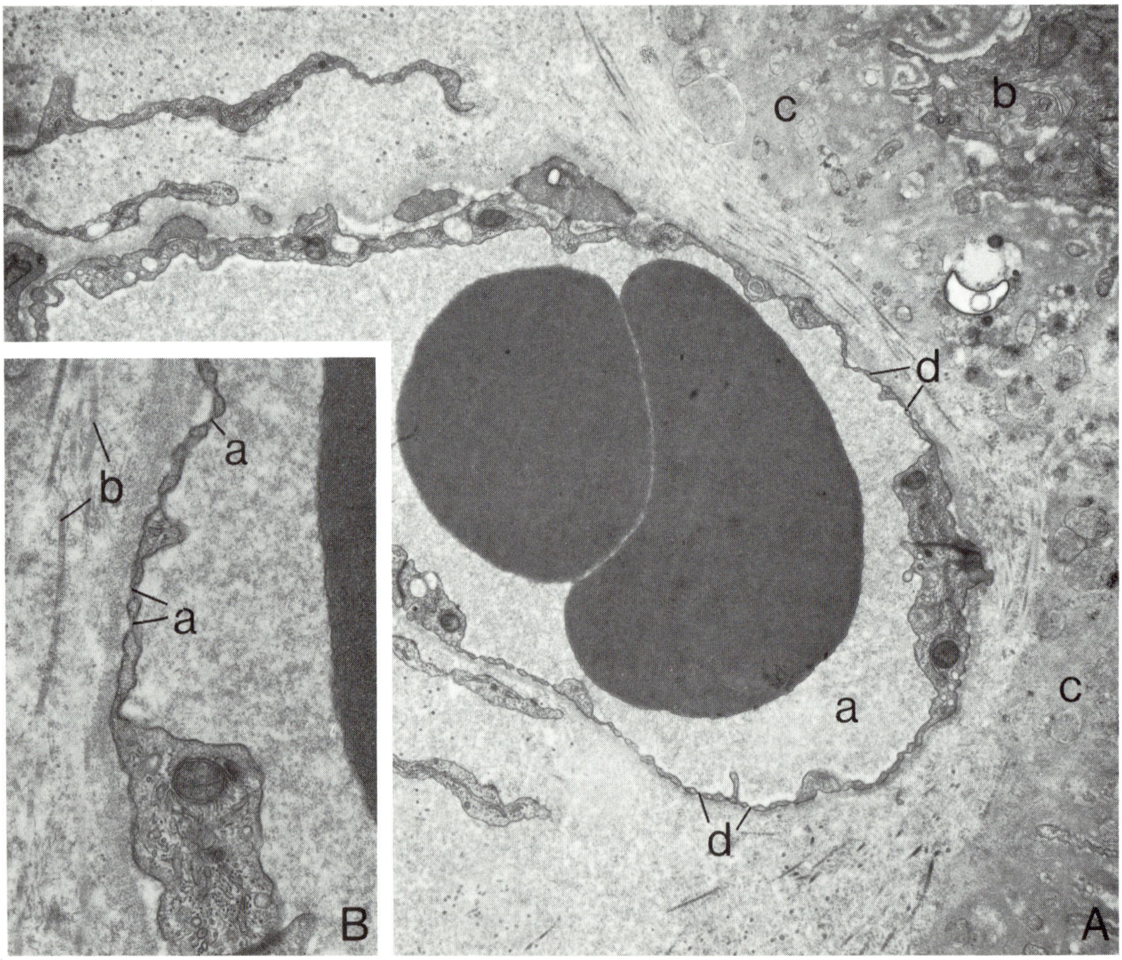

Figure 7–33. *A*, A capillary (a) adjacent to the pigmented epithelium of the ciliary body (b). The thickened basement membrane-like material of the pigment epithelium is at (c). The capillary wall is thin and has numerous fenestrations (d). (× 10,000.)

B, Higher magnification of the capillary wall. Note that a thin diaphragm (a) is present in the fenestrations of the endothelium. Collagen fibrils (b) are found between the capillary wall and the basement membrane of the pigmented epithelium. (× 30,000.)

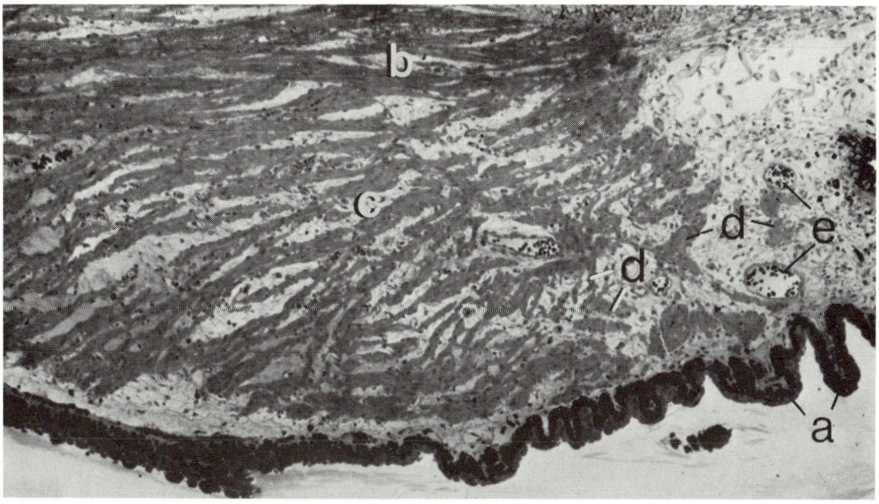

Figure 7–34. Low-magnification light micrograph of the ciliary body of a one and a half year old child. Ciliary processes of the pars plicata are seen at (a). The ciliary muscle in the eye of a child is not so compact as in the adult eye, and it is subdivided into distinct muscle bundles. Some vessels are seen coursing within the connective tissue separating the bundles of muscle. The longitudinal (b), radial (c) and circular (d) portions of the ciliary muscle are indicated. The major arterial circle of the iris and its components are seen at (e). (× 130.)

All the nerves found in the inner connective tissue layer are unmyelinated (Fig. 7–42). They are frequently observed in bundles containing 3 to 12 axons. Single nerve fibers are distributed to the vessels and to the stroma.

The *fibroblasts* found in this layer are like those described in the iris and limbus (Figs. 7-30 and 7-31). Mast cells are numerous and are identical to those of the iris.

Bruch's Membrane (Figs. 7-5, 7-6, 7-8 to 7-15 and 7-31). In the choroid Bruch's membrane is composed of the basement membrane of the pigment epithelium of the retina, some intermediate connective and elastic tissue, and the basement membrane of the choriocapillaris. Its principal components are collagen and elastic tissue. The so-called cuticular portion (basement membrane of the retinal pigment epithelium) of Bruch's membrane of the choroid continues forward as the basement membrane of the pigmented epithelium of the ciliary body. The elastic and collagenous portions of Bruch's membrane of the choroid become further separated from the basement membrane by layers of collagen and finally disappear in the stroma of the ciliary body near the posterior part of the pars plicata. The basic structure of this membrane will be described in the chapter on the choroid (p. 328).

Ciliary Muscle (Figs. 7–34 and 7–41) The ciliary muscle has always been considered to have three portions; meridional, radial and circular (Figs. 7–5, 7–34 and 7–35). This concept has been disputed, mainly by Rohen (1964), who thinks there is little justification for dividing the muscle into three parts. According to Rohen, the muscle cells form an orderly reticulum with a special architectural disposition (1952). Mollier (1938) originally described this reticular structure of the ciliary muscle; he described the muscle bundles enclosing meshes of varying size, which are more flat-

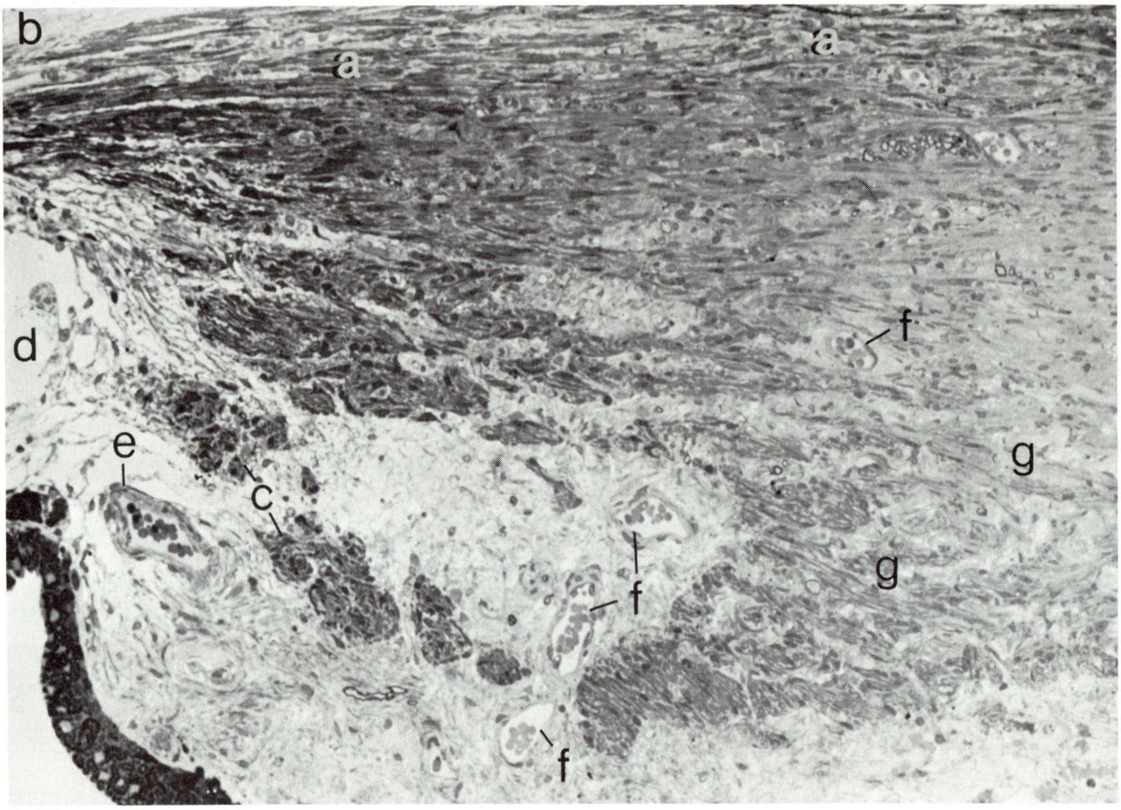

Figure 7–35. Ciliary muscle of an older person, meridional section. Compare the compact appearance of this ciliary muscle with that of a child shown in Figure 7–34. The longitudinal ciliary muscle (a) is shown near its attachment to the scleral spur (b). The circular muscle (c) is near the anterior chamber angle (d) and the major arterial circle of the iris (e). Some emissaries of this artery (f) are seen near the radial muscle (g). (× 200.)

Figure 7–36. Drawing of the ciliary body showing the ciliary muscle and its components. The cornea and sclera have been dissected away but the trabecular meshwork (a), Schlemm's canal (b) and two external collectors (c), as well as the scleral spur (d), have been left undisturbed.

The three components of the ciliary muscle are shown separately, viewed from the outside and sectioned meridionally. Section 1 shows the *longitudinal* ciliary muscle; in section 2 the longitudinal ciliary muscle has been dissected away to show the *radial* ciliary muscle; in section 3 only the innermost *circular* ciliary muscle is shown. According to Calasans (1953), the ciliary muscle originates in the ciliary tendon, which includes the scleral spur (d) and the adjacent connective tissue. The cells originate as paired V-shaped bundles. The *longitudinal* muscle forms long V-shaped trellises (e) which terminate in the epichoroidal stars (f). The arms of the V-shaped bundles formed by the *radial* muscle meet at wide angles (g) and terminate in the ciliary processes. The V-shaped bundles of the circular muscle originate at such distant points in the ciliary tendon that their arms meet at a very wide angle (h). The iridic portion is shown at (i) joining the circular muscle cells.

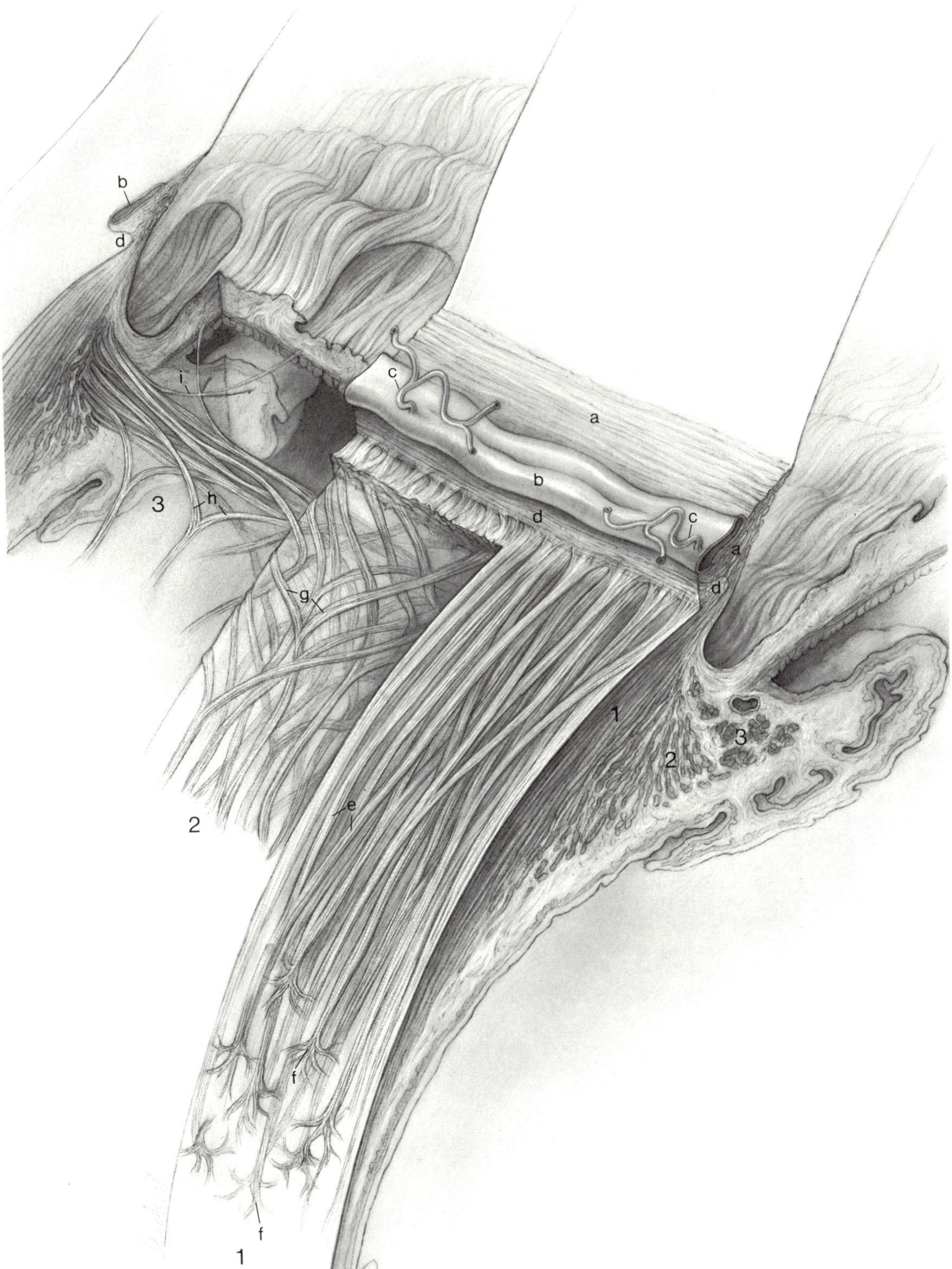

Figure 7–36. *See legend on opposite page.*

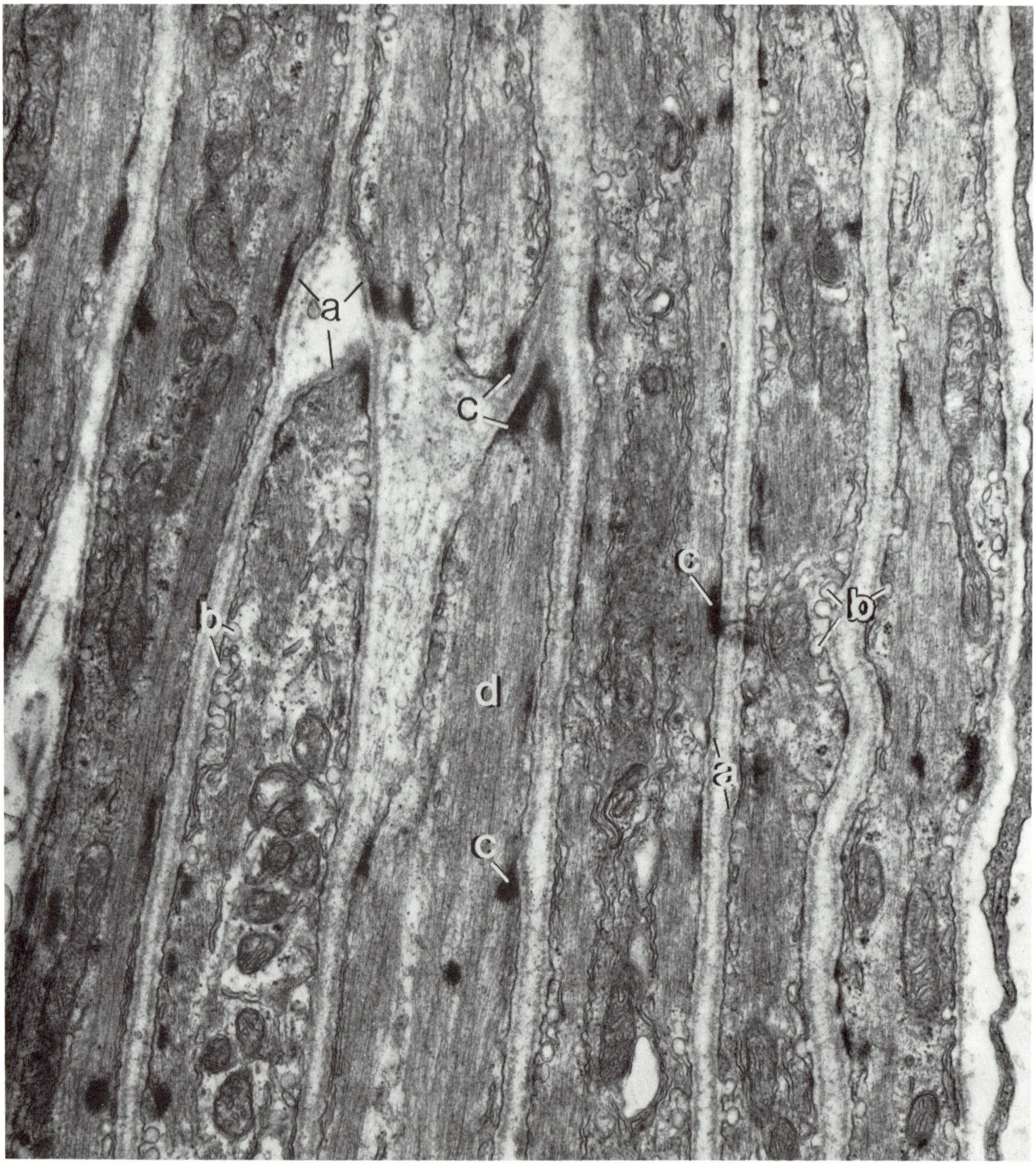

Figure 7-37. Longitudinal portion of the ciliary muscle. The muscle cells are surrounded by a basement membrane (a) and possess many pinocytotic vesicles (b) on their periphery. Desmosome-like thickenings (c) are scattered along the inner surface of the cell membrane; they probably fasten the myofilaments to the membrane. Myofilaments (d) fill the cytoplasm except where there are cell organelles. (× 24,000.)

tened in the meridional portion. Rohen believes that the whole muscle is interconnected, the muscle bundles forming a three-dimensional reticulum with considerable interweaving of the muscle cells from layer to layer (Fig. 7–36). Externally in the longitudinal or meridional portion, the muscle cell bundles cross at acute angles, creating a narrow meshwork. In the midportion (radial muscle), the muscle bundles cross at less acute angles to form a wider mesh; in the inner portion (circular portion), the muscle groups cross at very wide angles. The pattern of crossing of the muscle bundles at various levels differs because of the considerable interweaving from layer to layer. For example, in the meridional portion the bundles may at first cross at acute angles, then become more and more circular, or vice versa. Some muscle bundles may change from an external to a more internal position in the arcades of the meshwork. Rohen found the circular portion of the muscle to be connected by arcades to both the meridional and radial portions.

Calasans (1953) also studied the ciliary muscle and confirmed many of Rohen's observations. He also made new observations, some of which were not entirely confirmed by Rohen. According to Calasans, the entire ciliary muscle originates from the scleral spur region and inserts into the iris, the ciliary processes and the choroid. Calasans described the muscle as arising from the *ciliary tendon*, which includes the scleral spur and adjacent connective tissue. The muscle bundles of the longitudinal, radial and circular portions are oriented in the ciliary body in a certain pattern only because of their method of origin from the scleral spur and the direction of their muscle cells. He found meridional muscle bundles to form long V-shaped trellises whose bundles intersect at relatively narrow or wide angles. The most anterior of these bundles arise at such a wide angle from the spur region that they appear to have a circular direction.

The ciliary tendon gives rise to the many paired V-shaped bundles of the longitudinal muscle. The base of the V is at the scleral spur and its apex is in the choroid. The bundles of the longitudinal portion lie in the outer part of the ciliary body and they end in the so-called epichoroidal muscle stars in the anterior third of the choroid. This epichoroidal attachment of the muscle anchors it somewhat to the sclera and there is considerable interweaving of the V-shaped bundles with each other. Internal to the longitudinal muscle bundles is another group of bundles, the radial or oblique portion of the ciliary muscle. These interweaving and crossing cells also arise as paired V-shaped groups from the ciliary tendon. The origin of the arms of the V, however, is at a wider angle than is seen in the longitudinal portion and the bundles are arranged less compactly. All these V-shaped bundles insert by tendinous processes into the connective tissue of the anterior or posterior portion of the ciliary processes, depending on their origin from the scleral spur. The two arms of the V-shaped bands which form the circular muscle bundles, arise from very wide attachments to the ciliary tendon and insert into the connective tissue in the region of the anterior ends of the ciliary processes. Additional muscle bundles, the iridic portion, arise from the most internal region of the ciliary tendon as a pair of arms that also are united into a V. They form two thin, tendinous processes which insert into the iris near the termination of the dilator muscle (Calasans, 1953). By electron microscopy muscle cells can occasionally be seen to pursue a circular course in the iris root region, confirming the presence of the iridic portion of the muscle.

The connective tissue separating the muscle bundles is thin and

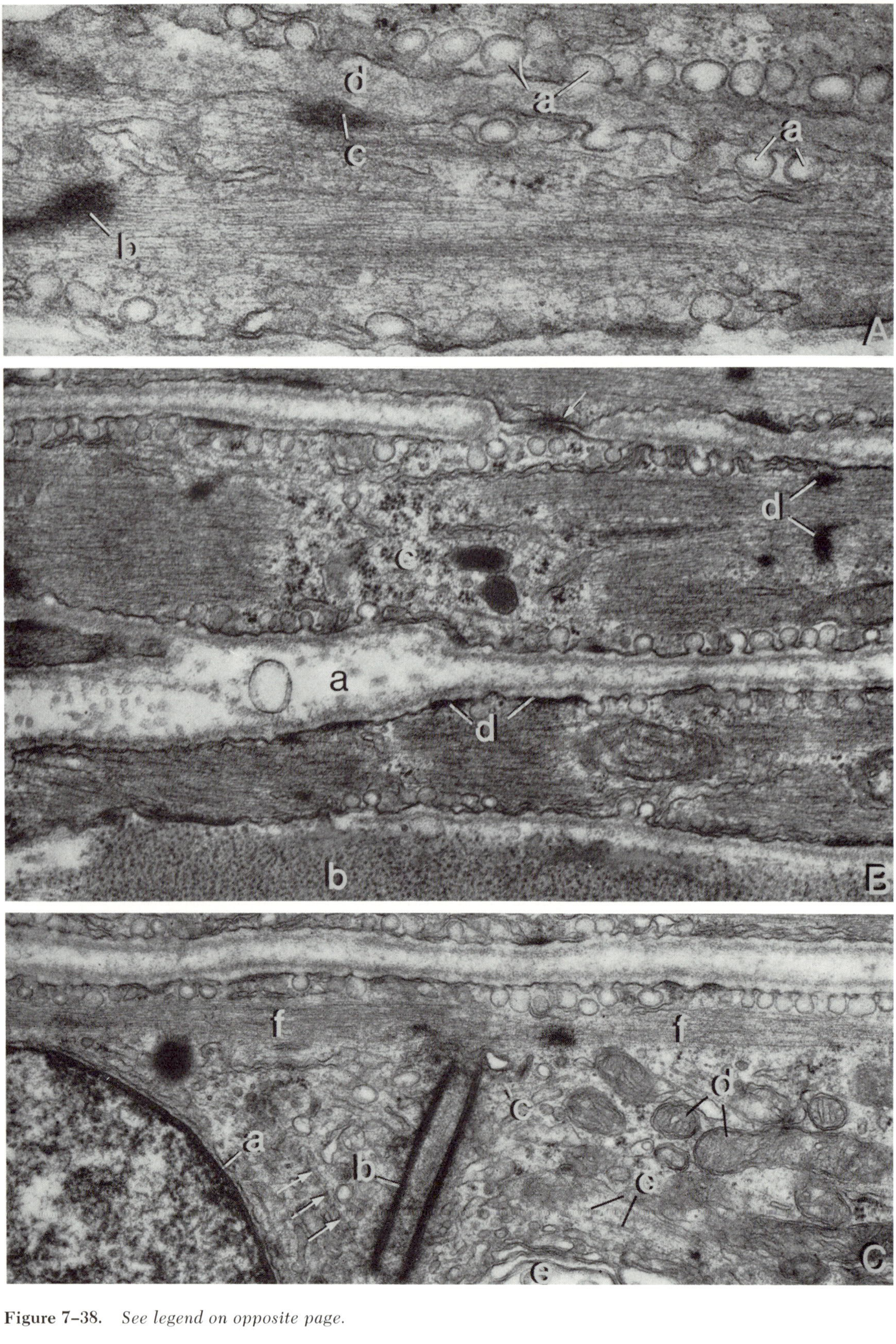

Figure 7–38. *See legend on opposite page.*

compact in the longitudinal portion and dense and thicker in the radial portion, so that it produces a greater separation of the muscle bundles. It is scanty in the circular portion of the muscle.

The anterior extension of the ciliary muscle and its relation to the trabecular meshwork has been studied by many histologists (Fig. 4–43, p. 171). According to Rones (1958) and Wolter (1953), part of the longitudinal portion of the muscle can be traced to the scleral spur, where the tendons pass through the spur into the posterior corneoscleral meshwork. Kupfer (1962) studied fetal eyes from five months to birth, as well as infant, child and adult eyes to determine the relationship of the meridional portion of the ciliary muscle to the corneoscleral trabecular meshwork. He found a continuity between the muscle and the meshwork and concluded that, except for the portion adjacent to Schlemm's canal, most of the meshwork represents a tendon of the meridional muscle that inserts into the cornea at Schwalbe's ring. Ultrastructural studies, however, do not confirm this opinion. Properly prepared sections do not show the extension of muscle tissue through the spur into the posterior meshwork and there are no real tendons. Slightly internal to the spur, muscle fibers are continuous with that portion of the corneoscleral meshwork which bypasses the scleral spur, but muscle cells do not extend forward in the meshwork beyond the level of the scleral spur (see Fig. 4–45, p. 173).

The principal electron microscopic study of the ciliary muscle is that of Ishikawa (1962), who investigated its structure and, to a certain extent, its nerve connections. The smooth muscle cells were found to be grouped in bundles surrounded by a thin sheath of fibroblasts and separated from each

---

Figure 7–38. *A*, Longitudinal portion of the ciliary muscle. Numerous pinocytotic vesicles (a) lie along the cell periphery; some open widely into the intercellular space, while others are closed. Myofilaments (b) are seen merging with an electron-dense structure in the cytoplasm; this arrangement is reminiscent of the Z-disc of skeletal muscle. These attachment bodies occur more frequently along the cell membrane (c), where they resemble the intracellular thickening seen at the site of desmosomes. In places where the muscle cells are closely apposed, their basement membranes are fused (d). (× 30,000.)

B, Longitudinal portion of the ciliary muscle. Mature collagen fibrils (a) and tropocollagen (b) separate the muscle fibers. The ciliary muscle cells, like those of the sphincter and dilator muscles of the iris, also come in contact with each other by means of intercellular junctions (arrows). Many clusters of unattached ribosomes (c) are observed in the cytoplasm, as well as electron-dense attachment bodies (d). (× 24,000.)

C, Longitudinal portion of the ciliary muscle, nuclear region. The nuclear envelope with its double membrane (a) encloses the centrally located nucleus. Near it is a complete longitudinal section of a centriole (b), which has a striated body (arrows) attached to one end and many microtubules (c) in its neighborhood. The perinuclear cytoplasm usually is occupied by a large number of mitochondria (d) and a Golgi apparatus (e) displacing the myofilaments (f) into the peripheral cytoplasm. Numerous pinocytotic vesicles are observed along the cell membranes. (× 30,000.)

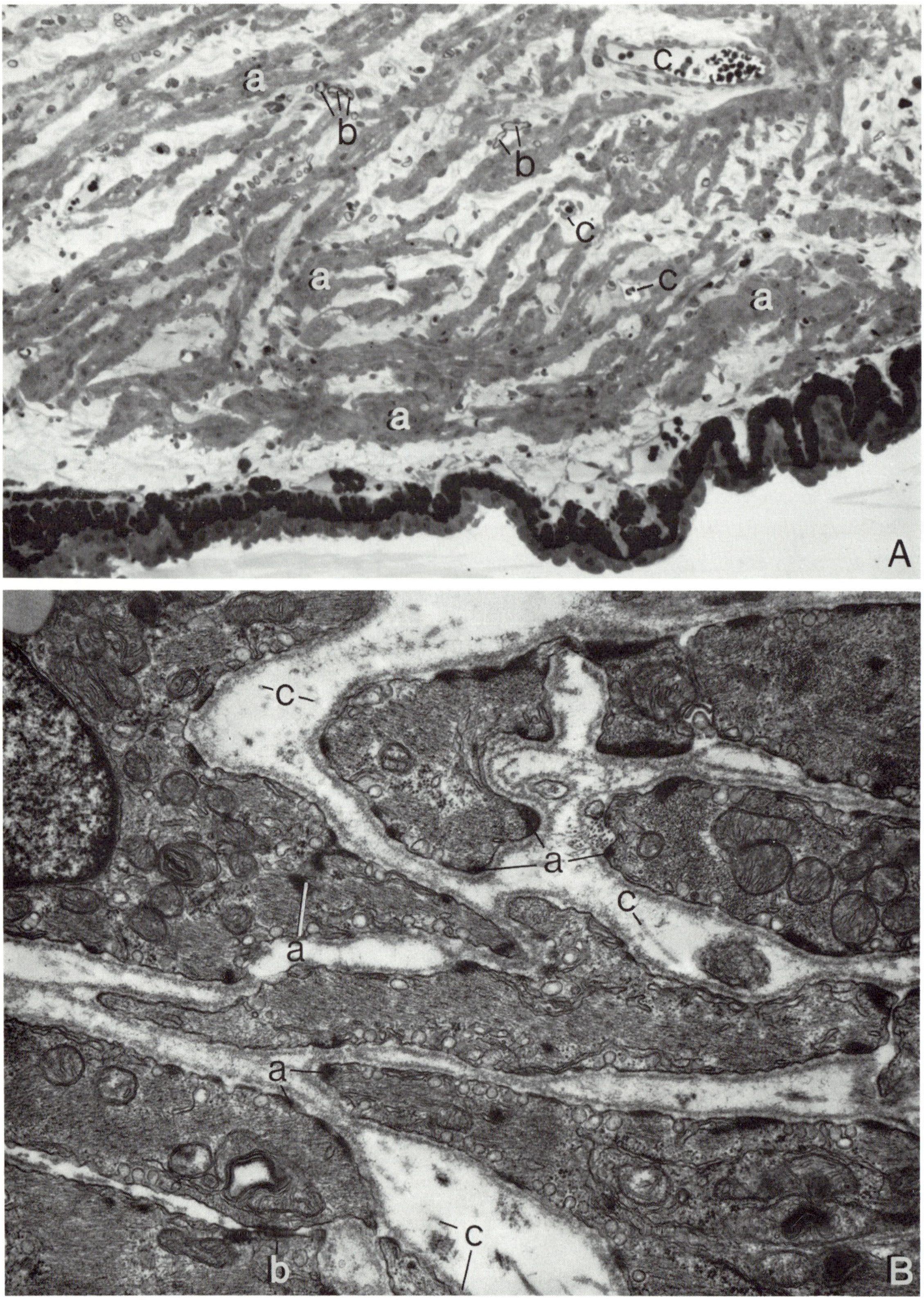

Figure 7–39. *See legend on opposite page.*

other by collagen, blood vessels and fibroblasts. In general, the structural differences between longitudinal and radial portions of the muscle seen by light microscopy are confirmed by electron microscopy (Figs. 7–34 to 7–41) The longitudinal muscle cells differ from radial cells in their smooth contours and great length. In common with most smooth muscle cells, the ciliary muscle cells all show a basement membrane that is separated from the cell membrane by about 300 A. Occasional muscle cells show interruptions of the basement membrane between two cells, and either a tight junction or a macula adherens is then formed between the adjacent membranes. Most cells show numerous pinocytotic vesicles along the inner surfaces of the cell membranes. In contrast to the smooth muscle cells of arteries and other tissues, the muscle cells here contain many mitochondria which may be closely related to the nucleus. The cells all contain longitudinally arranged myofilaments which are distributed throughout the cytoplasm. Dense osmiophilic bodies are found among the myofilaments and at the cell boundary; these probably are Z band-like attachments for the myofilaments. Ishikawa recognized three types of neuromuscular junctions (Fig. 7–42): (1) an indirect type of contact of the synaptic membrane with an intervening basement membrane which described the majority of the endings; (2) a more intimate contact of nerve and muscle without an intervening basement membrane, occurring rather infrequently and not having been seen in other smooth muscle; and (3) a rare ending in a depression in the muscle cell surface with a close attachment to the muscle cell membrane over a relatively large area. Many nerve fibers were observed throughout the ciliary muscle, both myelinated and unmyelinated.

The space between the muscle bundles in the ciliary body contains connective tissue, nerves and blood vessels. Occasionally vessels penetrate into the muscle bundles; these are of capillary dimension. The capillary walls are thicker than those in the ciliary processes and they usually have an unfenestrated continuous endothelium. The connective tissue is composed mainly of collagen and ground substance and shows occasional fibroblasts.

Supraciliaris

The supraciliary portion of the ciliary body is composed of pigmented ribbon-like layers of connective tissue which arise from the longitudinal portion of the ciliary muscle. They course outward from their origin at various angles to become continuous with the sclera. If the ciliary body is

---

Figure 7–39. *A*, Radial portion of the ciliary muscle, light micrograph, showing the bundles of radial muscle fibers (a), myelinated nerves (b) and vessels (c) coursing through the connective tissue. (× 120.)

B, Radial portion of the ciliary muscle. In a meridional section of the ciliary body, the fibers of the radial muscle appear to be sectioned obliquely. There are no structural differences in the different portions of the ciliary muscle. Attachment zones are shown along the cell membrane and in the cytoplasm (a). At (b) two muscle cells come closely together forming a macula adherens. Collagen fibrils (c) are found interspersed among the muscle fibers. (× 24,000.)

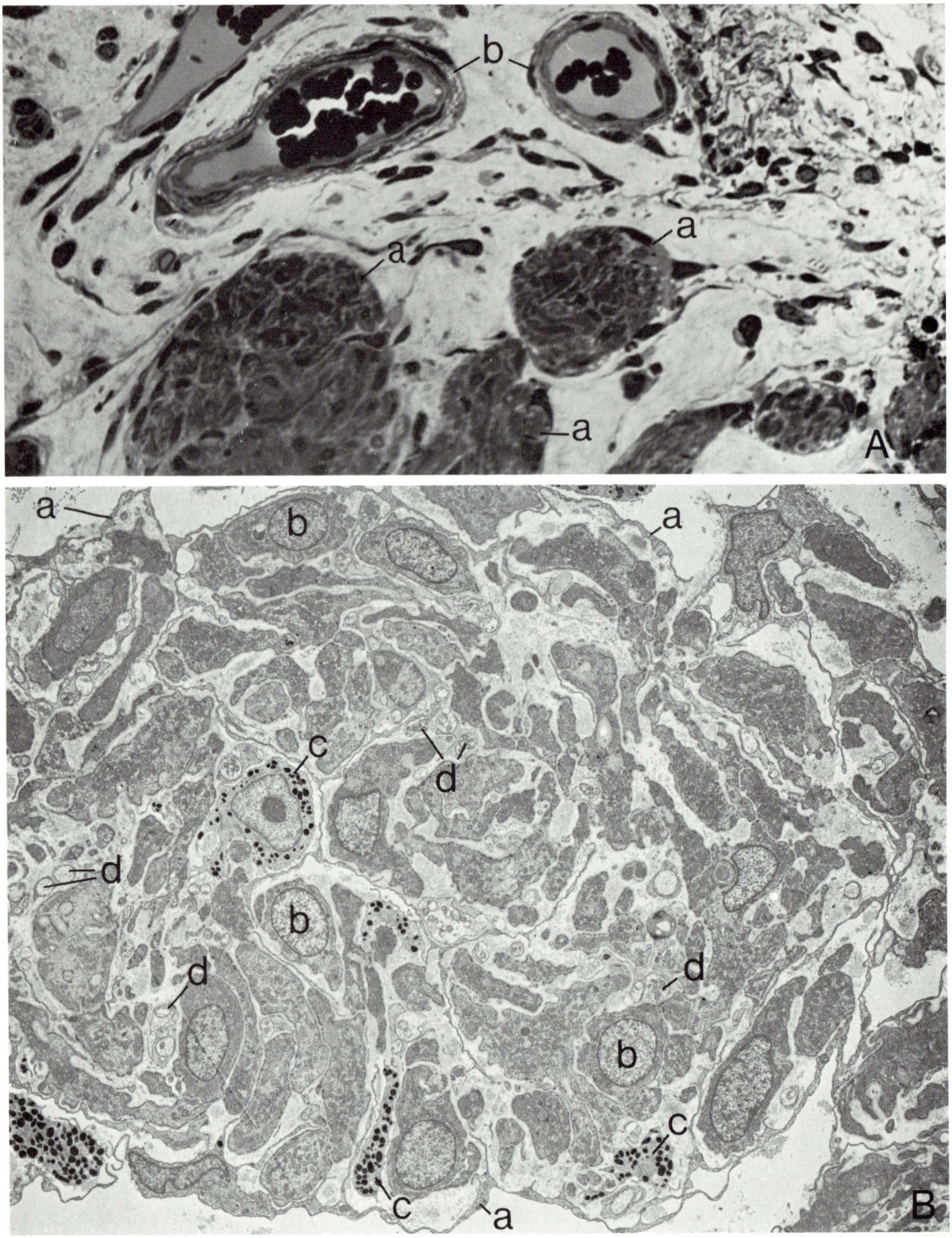

Figure 7–40. *A*, Circular portion of the ciliary muscle, meridional section. The circular portion occupies the anterior part of the ciliary body; this muscle (a) forms discrete bundles close to the angle recess of the anterior chamber. The major arterial circle (b) of the iris is usually found near this area. (× 500.)

B, Very low magnification electron micrograph to show a muscle bundle of the circular portion of the ciliary muscle. Long, thin fibroblasts (a) enclose a number of muscle fibers with their centrally located nuclei (b). Melanocytes (c) and many nerves (d) also are shown. (× 2580.)

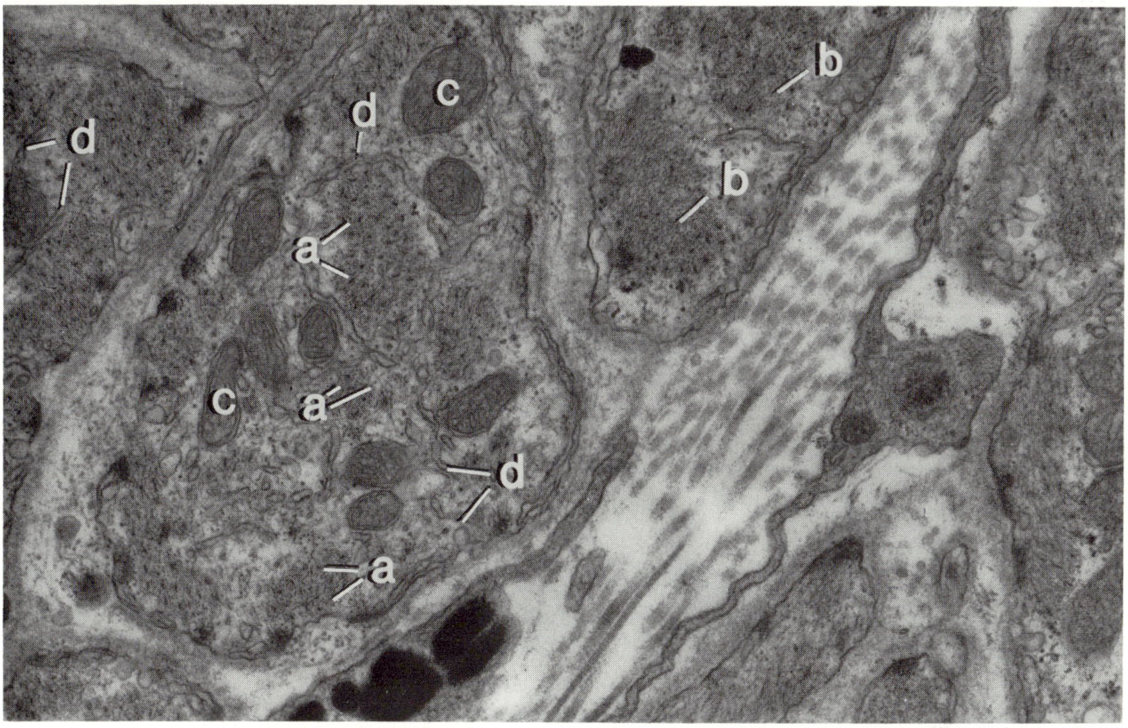

Figure 7–41. Circular portion of the ciliary muscle. This muscle appears cut in cross-section when the ciliary body is sectioned in a meridional plane. Two types of myofilaments are shown: thick (a) and thin (b). Mitochondria (c) and cisternae of the smooth-surfaced endoplasmic reticulum (d) separate the bundles of myofilaments. Numerous collagen fibrils are found among the muscle fibers. (× 30,000.)

separated from the sclera these ribbons remain attached to the ciliary body, leaving their tag ends on the sclera. If fluid accumulates in the supraciliary region, the layers become more distinct in microscopic sections. Ganglion cells are common in this area, especially in the region of the pars plana.

The bands of the supraciliary lamellae are composed of collagen of the usual type. Melanocytes and fibroblasts are enmeshed in this collagen, with no real endothelium covering their outer surfaces. At the juncture with the ciliary body, the collagen and cells are continuous with the connective tissue of the ciliary muscle. Under the sclera they blend with the collagen of the inner sclera.

Posterior Chamber

The posterior chamber of the human eye comprises a very small, irregular space whose dimensions cannot be defined exactly. Aqueous humor and other constituents enter it from the ciliary body, gradually flow toward the pupil, and enter the anterior chamber. Its size varies somewhat during accommodation, being narrow when the curvature of the lens is greater and wider in the nonaccommodated state.

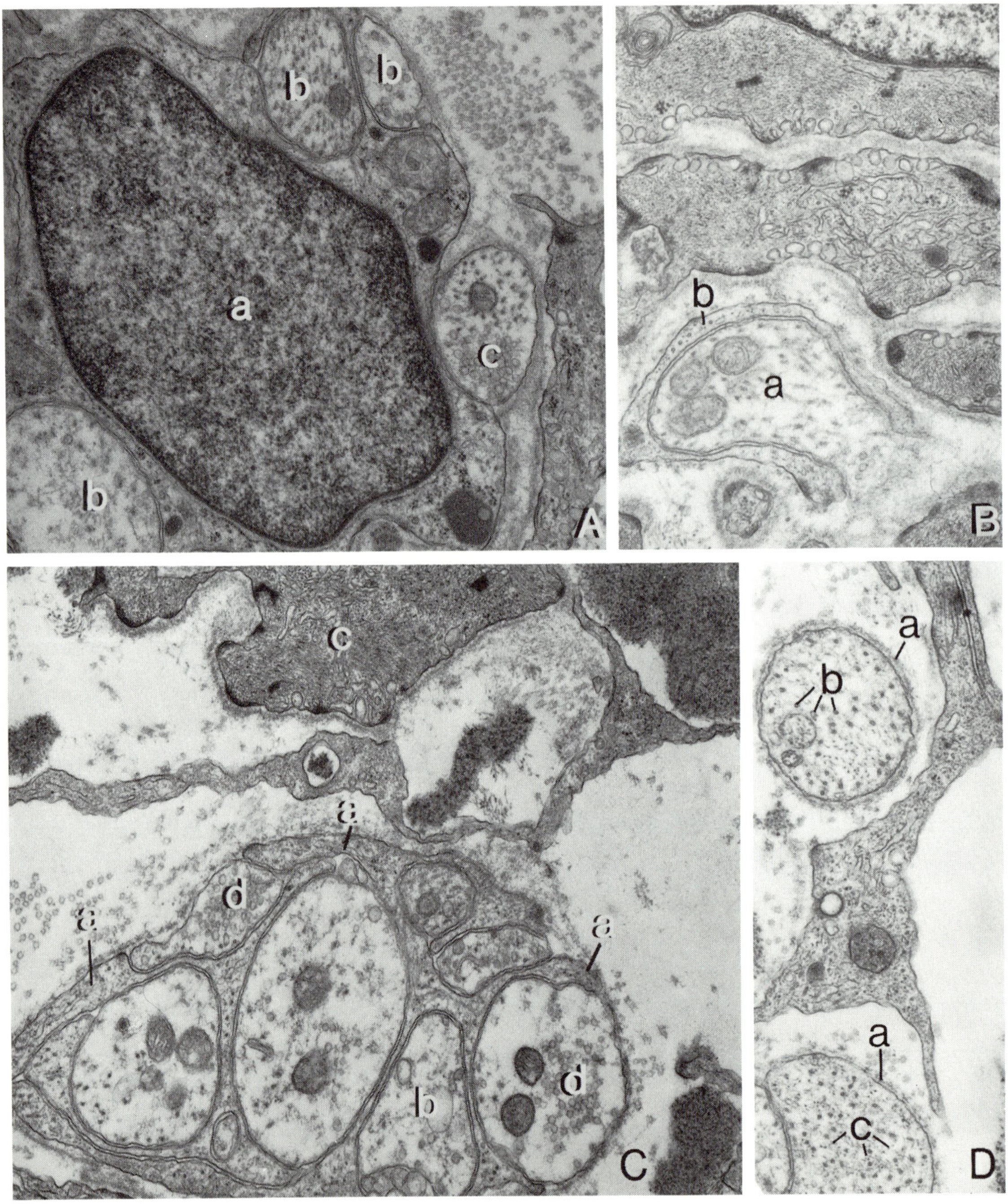

Figure 7–42. Nerves in the ciliary muscle. *A*, A Schwann cell (a) associated with four axons (b), one of which has many synaptic vesicles (c). (× 24,000.)

B, An unmyelinated axon (a) with its surrounding Schwann sheath (b) is seen separated from the muscle by the basement membrane and some collagen fibrils. (× 24,000.)

C, Schwann cell (a) surrounding seven axons (b) is seen in close proximity to a ciliary muscle cell (c). Note that the axons on the surface of the Schwann cell possess several synaptic vesicles (d). (× 24,000.)

D, Two naked axons (a) containing many microtubules (b) and neurofilaments (c) are shown within the connective tissue separating the ciliary muscle cells. (× 24,000.)

GROSS ANATOMY

The anterior boundary of the posterior chamber is formed by the pigment epithelium of the posterior iris, the anterolateral boundary is the iris and ciliary body junction, and the anteromedial boundary is the contact of the iris with the lens. The anteromedial dimension of the chamber varies in extent, depending on the amount of mydriasis or miosis. The medial portion, where the iris is in contact with the lens, is long and narrow if the iris is contracted, and more rounded if it is dilated. The area of contact between iris and lens may be considerable, and for the most part there is no real communication between posterior and anterior chambers. Physiologically, however, the constant secretion of aqueous humor into the posterior chamber separates the iris from the lens. The medial boundary is the equator of the lens and the lens zonules with their surrounding vitreous. The actual posterior border should be the surface of the vitreous. Because of differences of opinion about the relations of the zonules to the vitreous, some authors consider the posterior boundary to be the junction of the posterior zonulae with the anterior border layer of the vitreous. This junction is supposed to enclose the space of Petit.

The lateral border of the posterior chamber is the pars plicata of the ciliary body with its processes and valleys. The valleys between the processes form shallow recesses in the lateral chamber. If one considers the posterior chamber to comprise only that portion containing aqueous humor, the chamber lies anterior to the zonular attachments and includes only part of the anterior pars plicata. If the chamber is considered to contain the zonules and their surrounding investment material, it extends back to the face of the vitreous. It seems best not to argue too much about this point, since this serves no useful purpose. Rather, it is better to describe the zonules as part of the posterior chamber, because the fibers arise from the internal limiting membrane of the ciliary epithelial cells and extend forward through the chamber to the lens.

The posterior chamber customarily is divided into several zones:

1. The posterior chamber proper, which lies between the posterior iris and anterior face of the zonular-vitreous system. It contains aqueous humor which enters from the pars plicata.

2. The zonular portion, which lies between the anterior and posterior layers of the zonules. This area contains the aggregated collagenous fibrils that form the zonular fibers and their surrounding vitreous. The zonules pass through this area obliquely from the ciliary body to the anterior and posterior capsule, as well as directly across it from the valleys between the processes to the equatorial region. The final distribution of the zonular fibers will be discussed in the chapter on the lens (p. 638).

3. The retrozonular space, lying between the posterior zonules and the face of the vitreous and forming the slit-like canal of Petit.

MICROSCOPIC ANATOMY (Figs. 7–6 *A* and *B*, 7–43 and 7–44)

It is impossible to study the zonules and their surrounding mucoid material in routinely fixed specimens. If the tissues are fixed in glutaraldehyde containing CPC, better fixation is obtained and a better concept of the

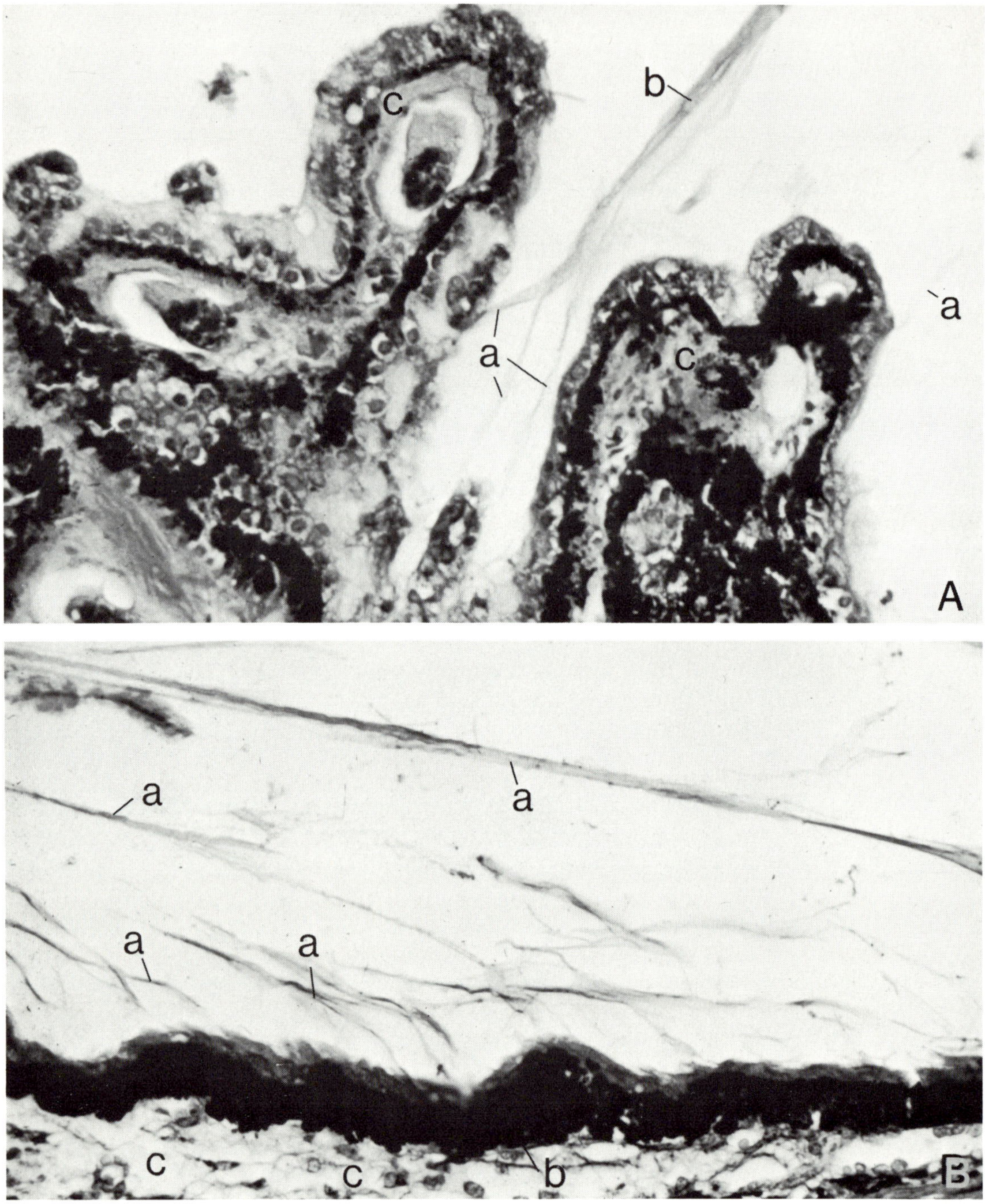

Figure 7–43. *A*, Pars plicata of the ciliary body, light micrograph. Formaldehyde-fixed, paraffin-embedded specimen. Three small zonules are seen at (a) originating from the walls of the ciliary processes to form a large zonule at (b). The stroma of the ciliary processes is at (c). (× 320.)

B, Pars plana of the ciliary body, light micrograph. Several zonules (a) are shown originating on the pars plana and extending toward the pars plicata. The pigmented epithelium (b) and the stroma (c) are shown. (× 320.)

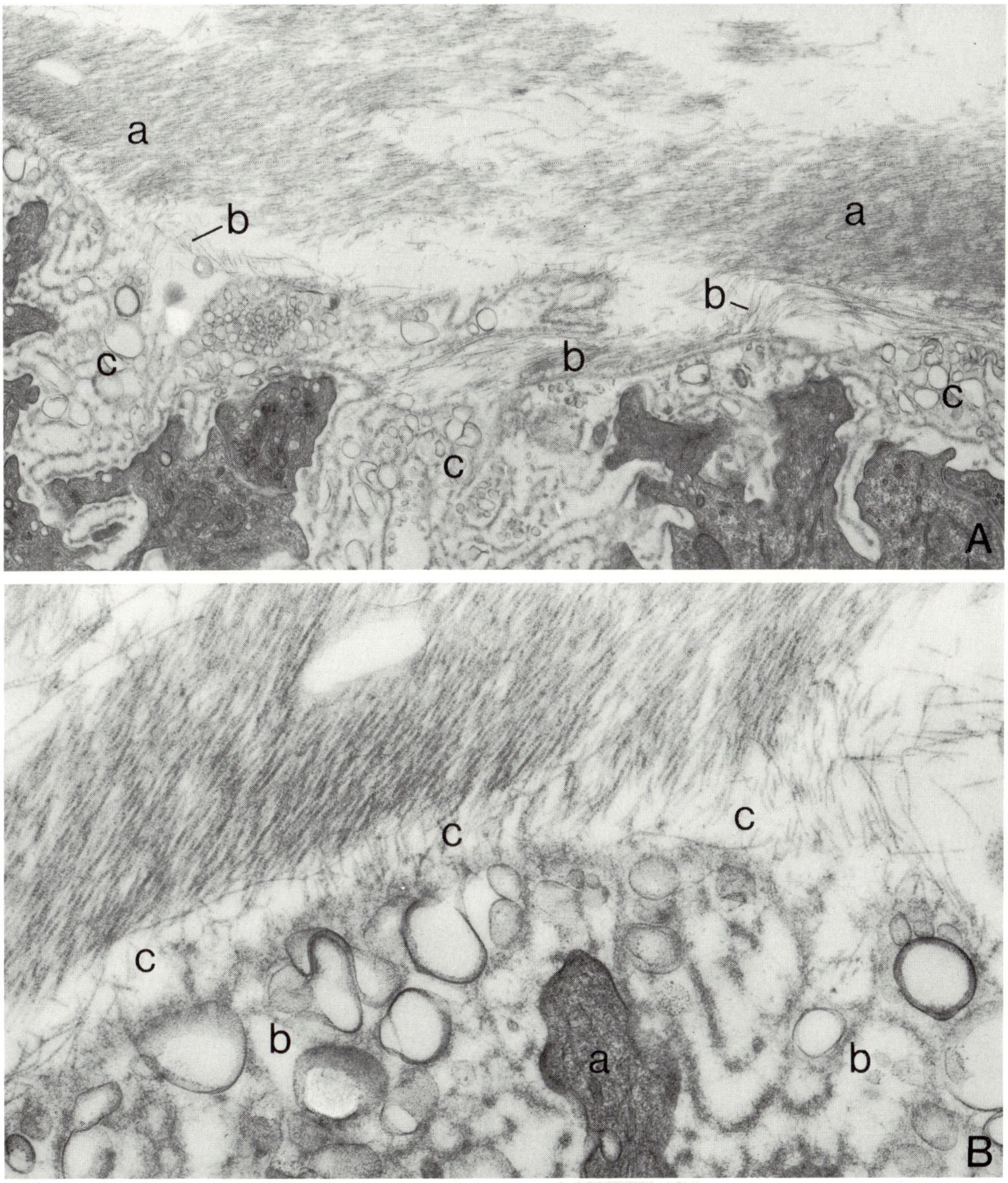

Figure 7–44. *A*, Low-power electron micrograph of the pars plana of the ciliary body. A zonule (a) is on the inner surface, sending fibrils (b) into the internal limiting membrane (c). The vesiculated, laminar internal limiting membrane is continuous into the folds of the epithelial cells. (× 6500.)

B, Zonular attachments at the inner surface of the ciliary epithelium. The unpigmented epithelium is at (a) and the internal limiting membrane is at (b). The zonular fiber sends numerous fibrils (c) to join the inner limiting membrane. The inner limiting membrane has vesicular structures within its lamellae. (× 35,000.)

structures can be obtained. Meridional sections are satisfactory for showing the attachments of the zonules to the lens, but these are not so valuable as sections that are tangential to the ciliary body or frontal sections. McCulloch (1954), in his classic thesis on the zonules, demonstrated the origin of the fibers from the posterior pars plana anterior to the spikes of the peripheral retina at the ora serrata and their extension forward between the valleys, where complex fusions and branchings occur, with the fibers arising from the deep sides of the ciliary processes.

Salzmann (1900) and Carlini (1912) postulated that the zonules arise from the internal limiting membrane of the ciliary epithelium. This was confirmed by Bruno (1936) and Garzino (1953) by phase-contrast microscopy, by Pappas and Smelser (1958) in the rabbit, and by Fine and Zimmerman (1963) in the human and primate by electron microscopy. The zonules are invested in a matrix which has the consistency of the vitreous. The zonule and vitreous matrix extend forward internal to the ciliary body into the spaces between the ciliary processes, then cross anteriorly to insert on the lens. The collagen fibers in this matrix form bundles which either merge or divide and subdivide. They finally form definitive bundles which attach to the lens capsule.

By electron microscopy the zonules are seen to arise at varying angles from the basement membrane of the unpigmented ciliary epithelium. In the posterior pars plana, where the membrane is thinner and more defined, the zonules are attached by a gradual blending with the basement membrane. The zonules enter into the folds along the inner surface of the epithelium to blend with the inner limiting membrane. Anteriorly, where the inner limiting membrane is thicker and more reticulated in the adult eye, the zonules blend with the reticular net and completely disappear so that no fibrils can be seen in the region of the cell membrane (Fig. 7–44).

Internal to the ciliary epithelium the zonules vary considerably in size and shape. Along their course they may widen or taper, possibly because of changes in their courses or branchings in another plane. Frequently there are fine bundles measuring 50 to 80 μm. in diameter, but more often they form larger aggregates measuring 130 to 150 μm. The individual fibrils appear to be collagenous, having a diameter of about 50 to 75 A. They have cross-banding, with a periodicity of about 80 to 100 A.

REFERENCES

Baurmann, M.: The vascular system of the ciliary process. Ber. Versamml. Dtsch. Ophthal. Ges. *48*:364, 1930.

Becker, B.: Carbonic anhydrase and the formation of aqueous humor. Amer. J. Ophthal. *47*:342, 1959.

Bill, A.: Capillary permeability to and extravascular dynamics of myoglobulin, albumin and gamma globulin in the uvea. Acta Physiol. Scand. *73*:204, 1968.

Bruno, G.: Sulla inserzione ciliare e sul probabile significato istologico dello fibre della zonula dello Zinn. Ann. Ottal. Clin. Ocul. *64*:400, 1936.

Bryson, J. M., Wolter, J. R., and O'Keefe, N. T.: Ganglion cells in the human ciliary body. Arch. Ophthal. *75*:57, 1966.

Carlini, V.: The structure and development of the zonula of Zinn. Graefes Arch. Ophthal. *82*:75, 1912.

Calasans, O. M.: The architecture of the ciliary muscle of man. Ann. Fac. Med. Univ. Sao Paolo *27*:3, 1953.

Cole, D. F.: Evidence for active transport of chloride in ciliary epithelium of the rabbit. Exp. Eye Res. *8*:5, 1969.

Fine, B. S., and Zimmerman, L. E.: Light and electron microscopic observations on the ciliary epithelium in man and Rhesus monkey. Invest. Ophthal. *2*:105, 1963.

Flocks, M., and Zweng, H. C.: Studies on the mode of action of pilocarpine on aqueous outflow. Amer. J. Ophthal. *44*:380, 1957.

Garzino, A.: A study of the zonular fibers of Zinn in fresh preparations, by phase contrast microscopy. Rass. Ital. Ottal. *22*:3, 1953.

Holmberg, A.: Studies of the ultrastructure of the non-pigmented epithelium in the ciliary body. Acta Ophthal. Scand. *33*:377, 1955.

Holmberg, A.: Differences in ultrastructure of normal human and rabbit ciliary epithelium. Arch. Ophthal. *62*:952, 1959a.

Holmberg, A.: The ultrastructure of the capillaries in the ciliary body. Arch. Ophthal. *62*:949, 1959b.

Ishikawa, T.: Fine structure of the human ciliary muscle. Invest. Ophthal. *1*:587, 1962.

Kinsey, V. E.: Transfer of ascorbic acid and related compounds across the blood-aqueous barrier. Amer. J. Ophthal. *30*:1262, 1947.

Kupfer, C.: Relationship of ciliary body meridional muscle and corneoscleral trabecular meshwork. Arch. Ophthal. *68*:818, 1962.

McCulloch, C. M.: The zonule of Zinn: Its origin, course, and insertion and its relation to neighboring structures. Trans. Amer. Ophthal. Soc. *52*:525, 1954.

Missotten, L.: Ultrastructure of the ocular tissues. Bull. Soc. Belg. Ophtal. *136*:3, 1964.

Mollier, G.: A quadruple stain for the demonstration of smooth and striated muscles and their relationship to the connective tissue. A. Wissensch. Mikr. *55*:472, 1938.

Pappas, G. D., and Smelser, G. K.: Studies on the ciliary epithelium and the normal aqueous humor formation in the rabbit. Amer. J. Ophthal. *46*:299, 1958.

Pappas, G. D., Smelser, G. K., and Brandt, P. W.: Studies on the ciliary epithelium and the zonule. II. Electron and flourescence microscope observations on the function of membrane elaboration. Arch. Ophthal. *62*:959, 1959.

Reese, A. B.: Ciliary processes; their relation to intraocular surgery. Amer. J. Ophthal. *17*:422, 1934.

Rohen, J.: Das Auge und seine Hilfsorgene. *In* W. V. Möllendorf (ed.): Handbuch der mikroskopischen Anatomie den Menschen. Erganz zu Bd. III/2. Berlin, 1964.

Rones, B.: A mechanistic element in trabecular function. Amer. J. Ophthal. *45*:189, 1958.

Salzmann, M.: Physiological optics and anomalies of refraction and accommodation. A. Augen. *3*:167, 1900.

Salzmann, M.: The Anatomy and Histology of the Human Eyeball. Chicago, Deuticke, 1912.

Spencer, L. M., Foos, R. Y., and Straatsma, B. R.: Meridional folds and meridional complexes of the peripheral retina. Trans. Amer. Acad. Ophthal. Otolaryng. *73*:204, 1969.

Taniguchi, Y.: Fine structure of blood vessels in the ciliary body. Jap. J. Ophthal. *6*:93, 1962.

Tormey, J. M.: Differences in membrane configuration between osmium tetroxide-fixed and glutaraldehyde-fixed ciliary epithelium. J. Cell Biol. *23*:658, 1964.

Tormey, J. M.: Artifactural localization of ferritin in the ciliary epithelium in vitro. J. Cell Biol. *25*:1, 1965.

Urayama, A., Kobayashi, M., Sato, S., and Mizuno, T.: Electron microscopic studies on the ciliary epithelium. Acta Soc. Ophthal. Jap. *63*:2664, 1959.

Wolter, J. R.: The innervation of the ciliary muscle of man. Ber. Dtsch. Ophthal. Ges. Heidelberg *58*:327, 1953.

Chapter Eight

CHOROID

The choroid is a long, thin, vascular, pigmented tissue which forms the posterior portion of the uveal tract. Because of its great vascularity, the choroid has some of the properties of erectile tissue. Its capillaries form a very unusual pattern, being arranged in a single layer restricted to the inner portion of the choroid; this arrangement enables the capillary layer to provide nutrition for the outer retina. The choroidal stroma contains a considerable number of pigmented melanocytes, which are distributed through all areas of the choroid, although they are more sparse in the innermost layers. The pigment in the melanocytes gives the choroid its characteristic dusky brown color. The choroidal vessels supply blood to and receive blood from the anterior portion of the eye. The nerves that supply the anterior part of the eye also pass through the choroid into the ciliary body. The choroid itself has an extensive nerve supply, and many ganglion cells can be found in the stroma and suprachoroidea.

PHYSIOLOGY

The principal functions of the choroid are to nourish the outer retina and to provide a pathway for the vessels that supply the anterior eye. The main arterial blood supply to the choroid is from three sources: the long posterior ciliary arteries, which send branches from the ora serrata region posteriorly to supply the choroid as far as the equator; the short posterior ciliary arteries that supply the choroid as far forward as the equator; and the anterior ciliary arteries, which send recurrent branches posteriorly to supply the choroid soon after they pierce the anterior sclera. The arteries of all three vessel systems rapidly extend internally to form the choriocapillaris. The main venous drainage of the choroid is outward through the vortex veins.

The choroid is unique in its capillary system, which lies in a single plane at the inner choroid. The normal intraocular pressure varies between 15 and 20 mm. Hg, so that both the arterial and venous pressures must be higher than this for normal circulation to occur. The systolic pressure in the ciliary arteries is about 65 to 70 mm. Hg, and the diastolic is around 50 mm.

Hg. The venous pressure probably is slightly above 20 mm. Hg. The difference between the pressure within the veins and venous capillaries and the pressure in the interstitial tissues is small; therefore, any change in orbital or intracranial pressure can produce venous stasis. Under ordinary conditions the amount of blood in the choroidal arteries and capillaries is adequate to maintain the retinal and anterior ocular nutrition.

The flow rates of blood through the choroid are high compared to other tissues and, as a result, the removal of O_2 from each milliliter of blood is low; in cats the O_2 content of choroidal venous blood is found to be only 3 per cent less than in arterial blood (Bill, 1970). It is possible that this high flow rate has some regulatory effect on the ocular temperature. The blood flow rate through the choroidal vessels is regulated by changes in caliber of the arterial vessels (Wudka and Leopold, 1951; Friedman and Oak, 1965).

The choroid has a rich nerve supply, probably for control of ocular blood flow. Alpha receptors are present for vasoconstriction, but sympathetic or parasympathetic fibers for vasodilation have not been demonstrated. In contrast to vessels in the brain, an increase or decrease in blood O_2 has no effect on the caliber of the uveal blood vessels. A change in systemic blood pressure, however, has an effect on uveal flow. In general, drugs which dilate the uveal blood vessels, such as acetylcholine, aminophylline, theophylline, amyl nitrate and papaverine produce an increase in blood flow only in doses that tend to produce a fall in arterial pressure. Retrobulbar administration of vasodilators produces vasodilation in the uveal blood vessels and a great increase in blood flow.

The permeability of the wall of the choriocapillaris to the various blood and tissue constituents is not known. Like other capillaries, they are probably readily permeable to lipid soluble substances such as O_2 and CO_2. Water and sodium enter and leave the capillary wall less easily. The capillary wall is permeable to many proteins that probably traverse the wall through the unusual number of pores in the endothelial cells. If ferritin is given intravenously to rabbits it can be demonstrated in the meshes of Bruch's membrane within a short period (Bernstein, 1965). It is probable that the fenestrations of the choriocapillary endothelium are important to facilitate the transfer of nutrients from the choroid to the retina.

The importance of the choroidal vascular system in the nourishment of the retina is borne out by experimental studies, and by the effects of disease on these vessels. If the choriocapillaris is lost in a fairly large area, as occurs in central areolar choroidal sclerosis, the overlying retina that is nourished by these vessels becomes atrophic. Embolic and thrombotic lesions of the human choroidal vessels are not ordinarily associated with retinal atrophy because of the extensive collateral blood supply. In the cat and dog, massive occlusion of the choroidal capillaries leads to retinal necrosis (Collier, 1967; Gray et al., 1964)

The choroid also plays a small part in the maintenance of intraocular pressure because of the blood contained in its vessels. The choroidal portion of the uveal tract has the largest sized and greatest number of vascular channels in the eye, and the amount of blood flowing through these channels at any one time has a certain effect on the intraocular pressure. The volume and flow of blood in these vessels in human eyes has not been completely assessed, however.

Another important function of the choroid is to provide a regular and smooth internal surface for support of the retina. The smoothness of Bruch's membrane is important for maintenance of exact relations between the retinal pigment epithelium and the outer segments of the adjacent rods and cones.

The exact function of the choroidal melanocytes has not been determined. They probably play a part in the absorption and reflection of whatever light passes the retinal pigment epithelium. To a certain extent, the melanocytes provide a dark background for the internal visual components of the retina.

EMBRYOLOGY

Prior to the 5.0 mm. embryonic stage (fourth week), the associated mesoderm surrounding the optic cup is undifferentiated. During the fourth week, endothelial cells differentiate in the mesoderm adjacent to the retinal pigment epithelium; these later differentiate into the choriocapillaris, which lies just outside the optic cup. Shortly after the fourth week, there is condensation of the mesoderm at the site of the future choroidal and scleral stroma. At the same time pigment appears in the outer layer of cells of the optic cup. By the 8 to 10 mm. stage (fifth week), the vascular net under the pigment epithelium has extended along the entire length of the cup, and this epithelium in the cup has become heavily pigmented. By the 12 to 17 mm. stage (sixth week), a well developed basement membrane lies external to the pigment epithelium. The collagenous portion of Bruch's membrane is present by this time, but the elastic portion of the membrane does not appear until the 70 mm. stage (twelfth week).

Rudimentary vortex veins appear in the upper and lower nasal and temporal quadrants of the eye during the sixth week. By the 25 to 30 mm. stage (eighth week), the choroidal capillary network is better developed and has become closely meshed. The short posterior ciliary arteries also appear in the mesodermal choroidal condensation. By the 50 to 60 mm. stage (eleventh week), these arteries have branched extensively throughout the choroid. Most of the choroidal vessel system develops after this stage (third and fourth months). Pigment first appears in the choroidal melanocytes between the 110 and 160 mm. stages (fifth month). The first pigment is seen in the cells of the outermost choroidal layers and it gradually becomes apparent in the innermost ones. The origin of these cells and their pigment has been the source of much controversy, but they are now believed to be derived from the neural crest during early embryonic life.

GROSS ANATOMY

External examination reveals that the choroid is light to dark brown in color, depending on the amount of pigment in the suprachoroidea and

---

Figure 8–1. Light micrographs of the retina, choroid and sclera. *A*, Compare the relative thickness of the choroid and retina in the macular region. The choroid measures 170 μm. in thickness here; its internal limit is the retinal pigment epithelium (a), and its external limit is the lamina fusca (b) of the sclera. (× 260.)

B, External retina and choroid in the macular region. The retinal photoreceptors (a) and pigment epithelium (b) lie internal to the choroid. Externally the suprachoroidea (c) is in contact with the lamina fusca (d) of the sclera. Two large veins (e) and arteries (f) lie in the choroid, while the choriocapillaris (g) is adjacent to the pigment epithelium. (× 200.)

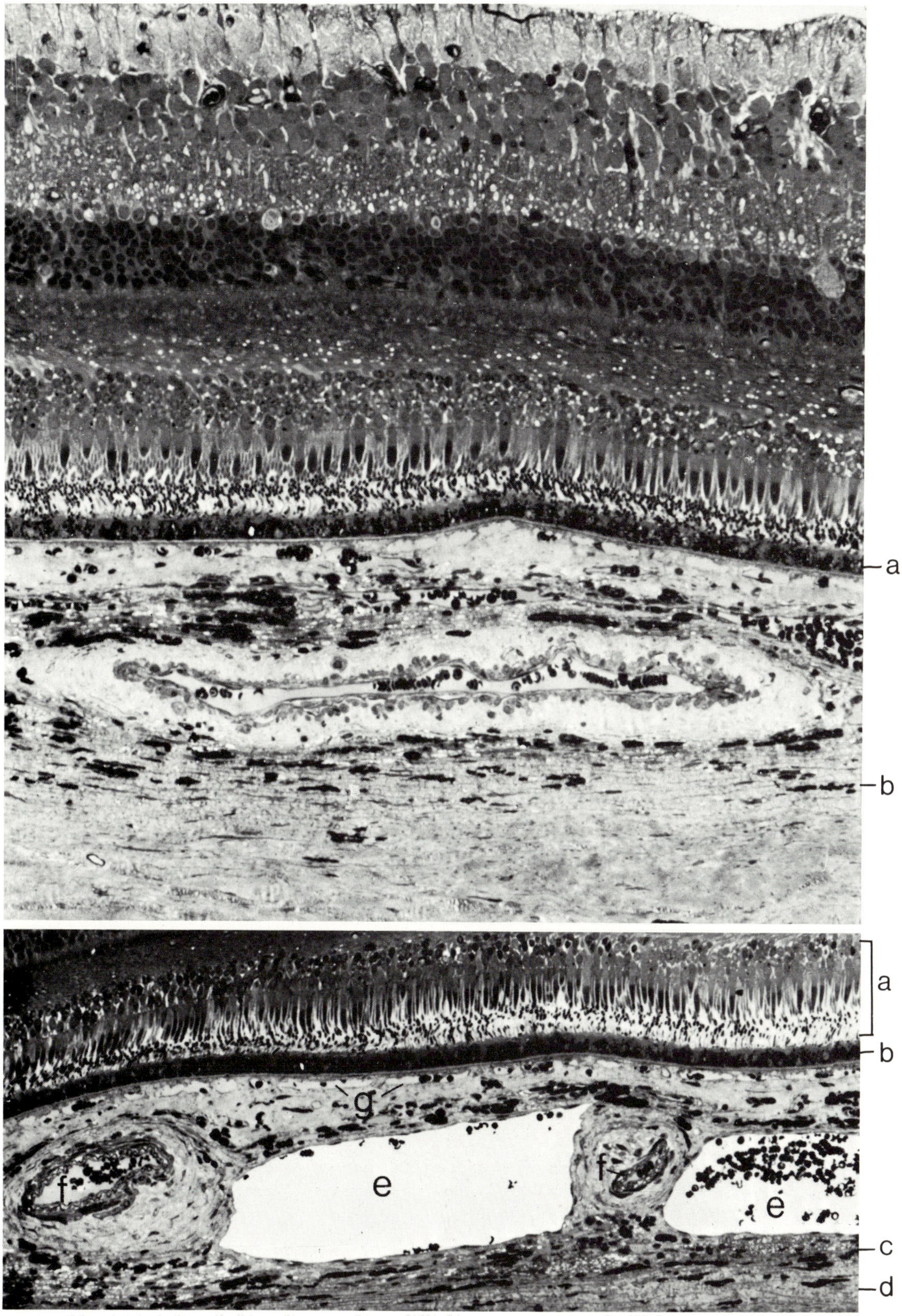

Figure 8–1. *See legend on opposite page.*

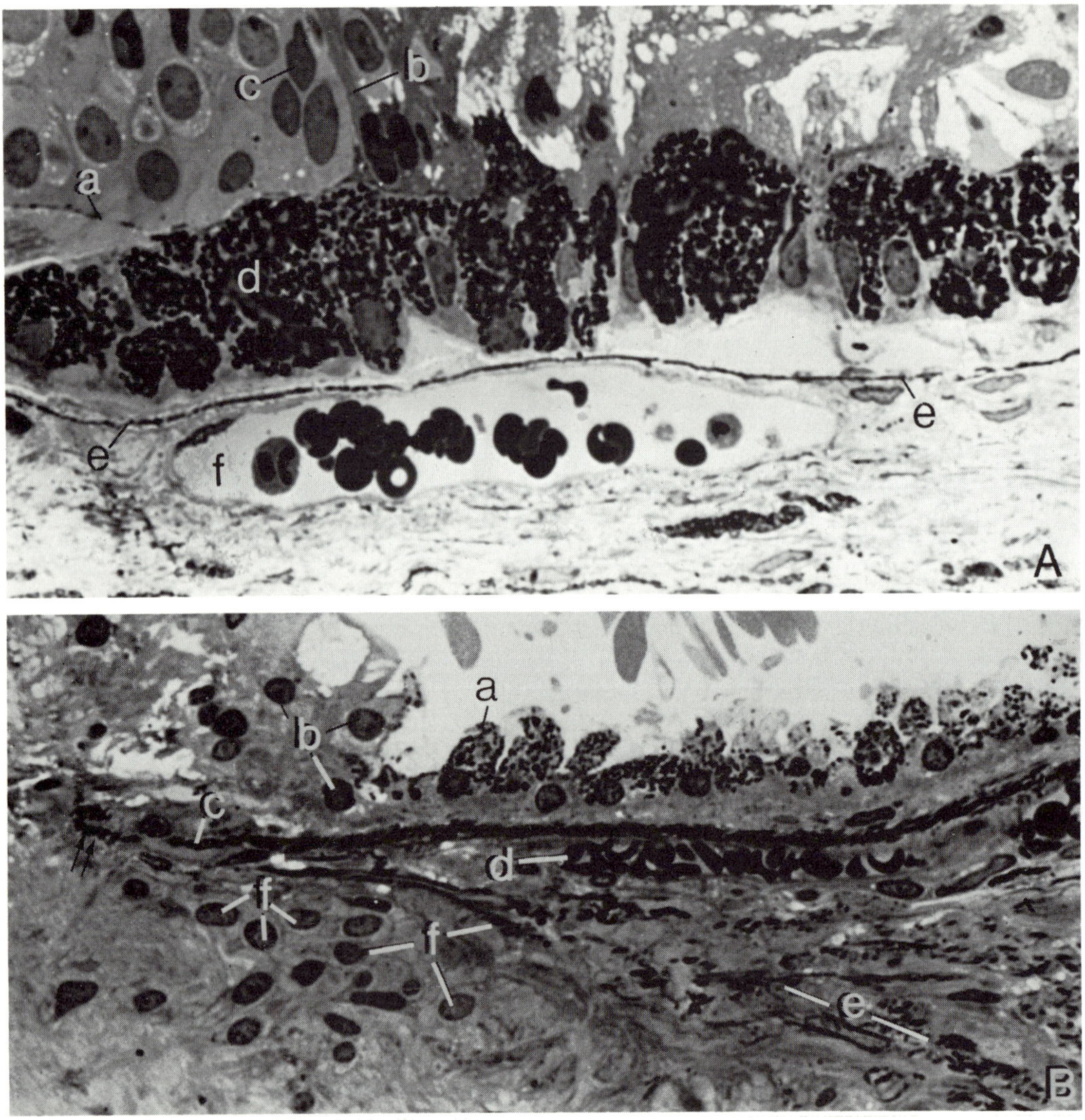

Figure 8–2. Light micrographs of the anterior and posterior choroid. *A*, Anteriorly the choroid is continuous with the pars plana of the ciliary body. The external limiting "membrane" (a) of the retina terminates as it merges with the pigment epithelium (arrows). The unpigmented epithelium (b) of the pars plana is contiguous with the sensory retina (c), while the retinal pigment epithelium becomes the pigmented epithelium of the ciliary body (d). Bruch's membrane extends forward into the pars plana; its elastic lamina is shown at (e) and the choriocapillaris is seen at (f). (× 640.)

B, The posterior termination of the choroid. The most posterior cell of the retina is the pigment epithelial cell shown at (a). Astrocytes form a layer between the posterior retina and optic disc nerve tissue (b). The internal portion of the choroid extends into the optic nerve more than the external, so that in this section the elastic layer of Bruch's membrane (c) is closest to the nerve. The rods of elastin in the posterior part of Bruch's membrane appear to be cut in cross-sections (arrows), indicating that they have become oriented circularly around the optic nerve. The choriocapillaris ends at (d). The choroid abuts on the edge of the nerve (e) and astrocytes lie between the posterior choroid and optic nerve surface (f). (× 500.)

stroma. Its numerous vessels give the choroid a spongy texture, and its very loose stroma fills the spaces between the blood vessels. The choroid is easily detached from the sensory retina and from the sclera, but it is firmly bound to the optic nerve, because its connective tissue is continuous with that of the nerve.

Internally the choroid is so closely attached to the retina that the retinal pigment epithelium adheres more to Bruch's membrane than to the retinal receptors (Fig. 8-1 *A* and *B*). If the sensory retina separates from the choroid, the disengagement occurs in the area of contact between the rods and cones and the pigment epithelium, rather than in the area between the epithelium and Bruch's membrane. This relationship exists throughout the entire retina, from the optic disc to the ora serrata.

Externally the pigmented suprachoroidal connective tissue lamellae are closely bound to those of the lamina fusca of the sclera. In diseased eyes the sclera and choroid often are separated by an accumulation of fluid or hemorrhage, but torn lamellae of one tissue may remain attached to the other. The long ciliary arteries and nerves lie in the suprachoroidal tissue along the horizontal meridian on either side of the eye as they pass forward to branch near the ora serrata region. The short ciliary nerves and arteries also occupy the suprachoroidal space briefly after piercing the sclera, but they quickly enter the choroidal stroma where they branch extensively.

The *anterior* termination of the choroid is at the ora serrata, where it is continuous with the ciliary body (Fig. 8–2 *A*; see Fig. 7–14). The transition from the choroid to ciliary body is gradual. Anteriorly on the external side the suprachoroidea is continuous with the supraciliary lamellae.

The *posterior* termination of the choroid is at the optic nerve, where the choroid forms part of the wall of the optic nerve canal (Fig. 8-2 *B*). (See Optic Nerve, p. 539.) The external layers of the choroid terminate first and the internal layers last, as is explained in the following section.

Blood Supply

The choroid is supplied by an extensive network of vessels, as shown in Figure 8-3. These vessels include two long posterior ciliary arteries, 15 to 20 short posterior ciliary arteries and the anterior ciliary arteries. The latter enter the eyeball anteriorly and send some branches to supply the anterior choroid. The posterior ciliary vessels have short arterioles that suddenly form the choriocapillaris, which is a most unusual network of closely meshed capillaries. Some branches from the short ciliary vessels pass medially through the sclera and choroid to form the circle of Zinn in the sclera at the edge of the optic disc (Fig. 8–3). This arterial circle is most important for the vascular supply of the optic nerve head.

The venous drainage of the choroid all occurs through the vortex system of veins. Direct and transmitted light through the exposed choroid reveals the choroidal vascular pattern. The vessels appear lighter, with dark space between them, because of the collagen in and around the vessels and the pigmentation of the intervening stroma. The vortex vessels create a striking picture, their afferent channels forming a true vortex as they radiate from all parts of the neighboring choroid toward the ampulla of the main vortex channel (Figs. 8-3, 8-4 and 8-36). The afferent veins to the vortex

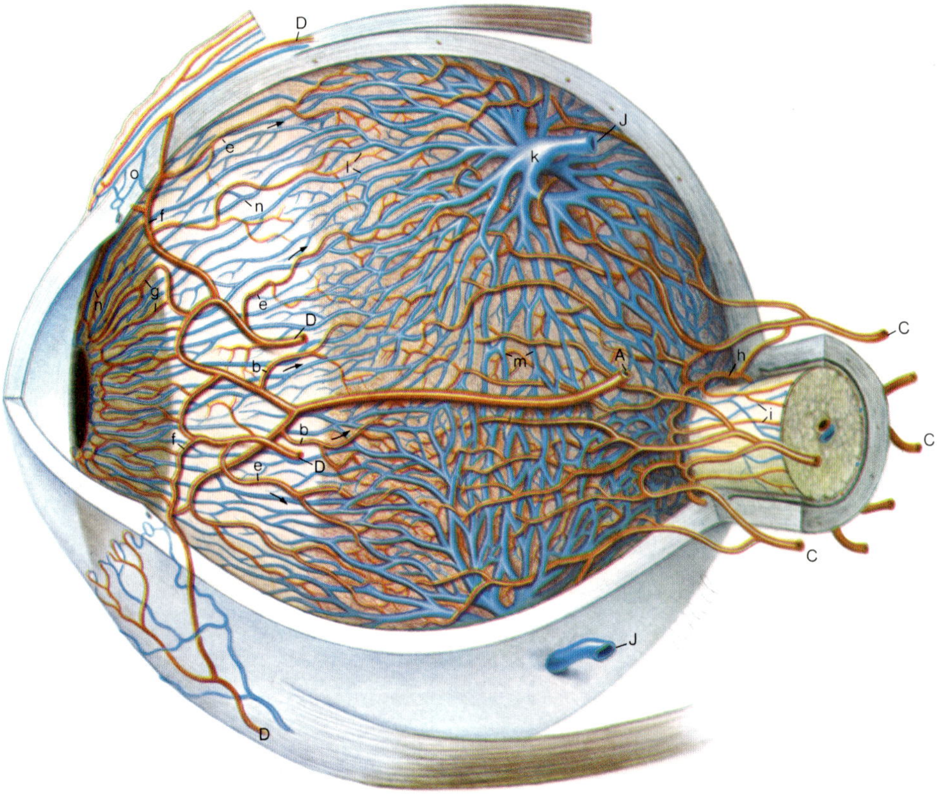

Figure 8–3. The uveal blood vessels. The blood supply of the eye is derived from the ophthalmic artery. Except for the central retinal artery that supplies the inner retina, almost the entire blood supply of the eye comes from the uveal vessels. There are two *long posterior ciliary arteries*, one entering the uvea nasally and one temporally along the horizontal meridian of the eye near the optic nerve (A). These two arteries give off three to five branches (b) at the ora serrata that pass directly back to form the anterior choriocapillaris. These capillaries nourish the retina from the equator forward. The *short posterior ciliary arteries* enter the choroid around the optic nerve (c). They divide rather rapidly to form the posterior choriocapillaris that nourishes the retina as far anteriorly as the equator (the choriocapillaris is not shown in this drawing). This system of capillaries is continuous with those derived from the long posterior ciliary arteries. The *anterior ciliary arteries* (D) pass forward with the rectus muscles, then pierce the sclera to enter the ciliary body. Before joining the major circle of the iris they give off eight to 12 branches (e) that pass back through the ciliary muscle to join the anterior choriocapillaris. The major circle of the iris (f) lies in the corona ciliaris and sends branches posteriorly into the ciliary body as well as forward into the iris (g). The circle of Zinn (h) is formed by pial branches (i) as well as branches from the short posterior ciliary arteries. The circle lies in the sclera and furnishes part of the blood supply to the optic nerve and disc. The vortex veins exit from the eye through the posterior sclera (J) after forming an ampulla (k) near the internal sclera. Venous branches that join the anterior and posterior part of the vortex system are meridionally oriented and are fairly straight (l), while those joining the vortices on their medial and lateral sides are oriented circularly about the eye (m). The venous return from the iris and ciliary body (n) is mainly posterior into the vortex system, but some veins cross the anterior sclera and limbus (o) to enter the episcleral system of veins.

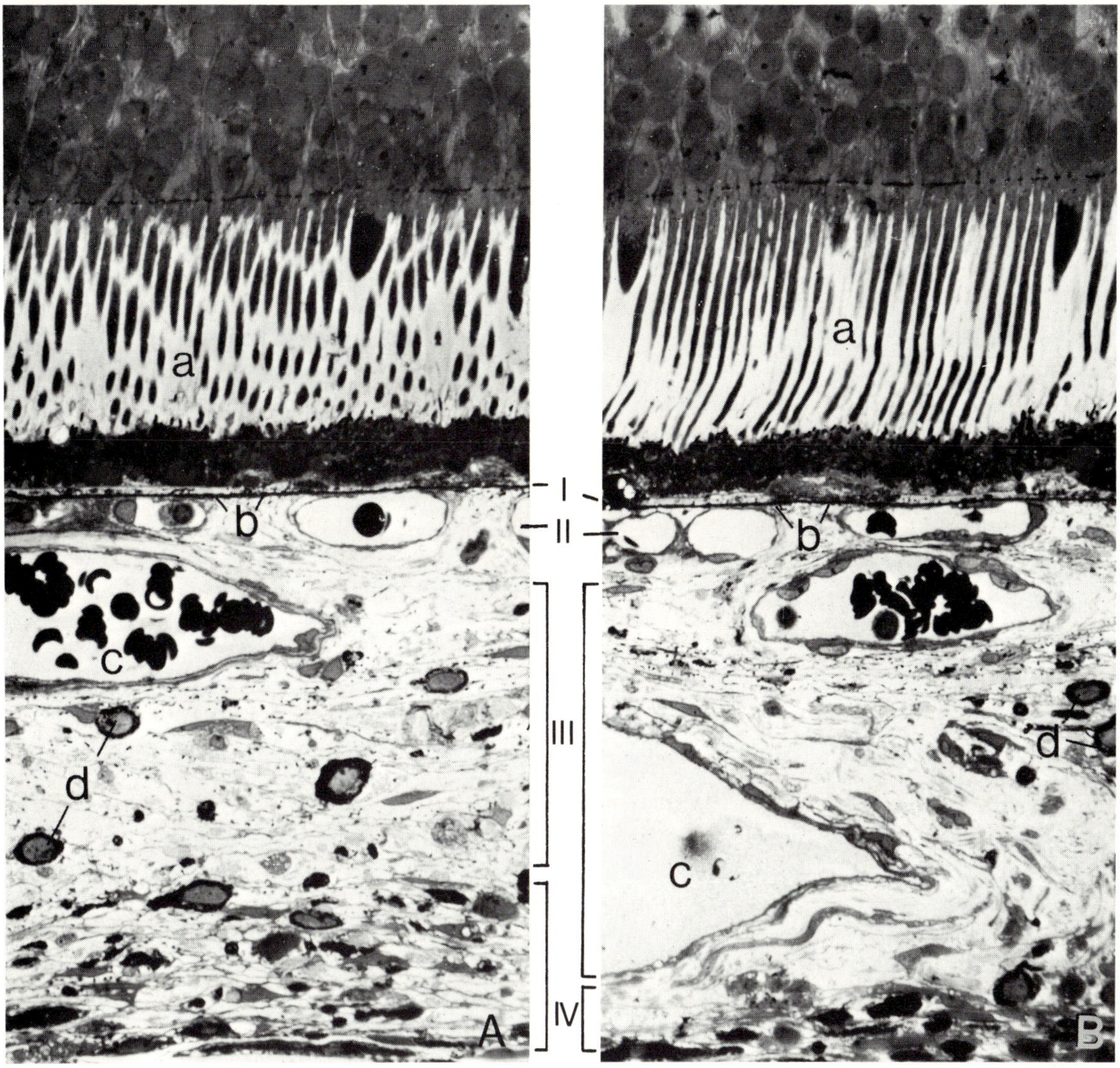

Figure 8–4. Light micrographs of the equatorial choroid and retina. The choroid here measures 130 μm. in thickness and is subdivided into the following portions: I, Bruch's membrane; II, choriocapillaris; III, stroma; IV, suprachoroidea. The outer processes of the photoreceptors merge with the retinal pigment epithelium at (a). The elastica of Bruch's membrane (b) is the thin dark line in I. Large veins are seen in the choroidal stroma (c), and melanocytes (d) are dispersed in the connective tissue. They become more numerous in IV. (× 430.)

system from the anterior part of the uvea pass straight back to the main vortex vein. Those from the lateral and equatorial regions and from the posterior eye are curved, the lateral branches curving toward the ampulla with their convexity directed backward. Near the inner sclera, where all these veins converge, the main vortex vein is dilated to form an ampulla that is about 1.5 to 2.0 mm. wide. The main vortex vein, which passes from the ampulla out through the sclera, is slightly narrower. The position and course of these veins have been discussed (pp. 52, 188). In the peripapillary region the choroidal vessels are more difficult to observe because of the density and thickness of the choroidal stroma and the increased amount of pigment. If most of the outer layers of the choroid are removed to expose the choriocapillaris, this vessel layer is seen to form a close-meshed net closely associated with Bruch's membrane.

MICROSCOPIC ANATOMY

Accurate measurements of the choroid's thickness are difficult to make because the vessels collapse from loss of blood in the vascular channels after death or enucleation. Salzmann (1912) found the thickness at the posterior pole of the choroid to be 0.22 mm., gradually decreasing to 0.10 to 0.15 mm. between the equator and periphery (Fig. 8-1).

The choroid is often subdivided into the suprachoroidea, large, medium and small vessel layers, the choriocapillaris and Bruch's membrane. The following divisions will be used because, as Salzmann (1912) pointed out, the vessel layers are rarely as regular as originally thought (Fig. 8-4 *A* and *B*):

I. Bruch's membrane
II. Choriocapillaris
III. Stroma
IV. Suprachoroidea

Bruch's Membrane

Early histologists called this layer the lamina vitrea, because of its resemblance to a glass membrane. Wolfrum (1908), however, noted that Bruch's membrane is composed of an inner thin basal membrane that is close to the retinal pigment epithelium, separated by a loose layer of collagen from an outer thick zone of elastic tissue (Fig. 8–5 *A*, *B* and *C*). Because of this collagen and elastic content, Wolfrum did not consider Bruch's membrane to be a true "glass membrane" like Descemet's membrane.

Bruch's membrane of the choroid extends from the margin of the optic disc to the ora serrata. It becomes modified beyond the ora serrata in the ciliary body (p. 303 and Figs. 7–5, 7–13). This layer is eosinophilic and PAS-positive. Mallory and other connective tissue stains show its collagen, and elastic tissue stains show that the membrane contains a well developed layer

---

Figure 8–5. Bruch's membrane. *A*, This remarkably accurate drawing of the structure of Bruch's membrane was made by Wolfrum in the early part of this century. He shows a fine collagenous zone between the pigment epithelium and the uninterrupted elastic layer of Bruch's membrane. This drawing correctly shows the elastic layer to be close to the wall of the choriocapillaris.

B, Light micrograph of Bruch's membrane fixed in formalin and embedded in paraffin. Bruch's membrane is at (a) and the choriocapillaris at (b). (× 800.)

C, Light micrograph of Bruch's membrane fixed with glutaraldehyde and osmium tetroxide and embedded in araldite. The pigment epithelium of the retina (a) is internal and the choriocapillaris (b) is external to Bruch's membrane. The elastic layer (c) divides Bruch's membrane into an inner collagenous zone (d) and a narrower outer collagenous zone (e). The basement membrane (f) of the retinal pigment epithelium is internal to the inner collagenous zone. The intercapillary zone (g) is continuous with the subcapillary collagen (h). (× 1600.)

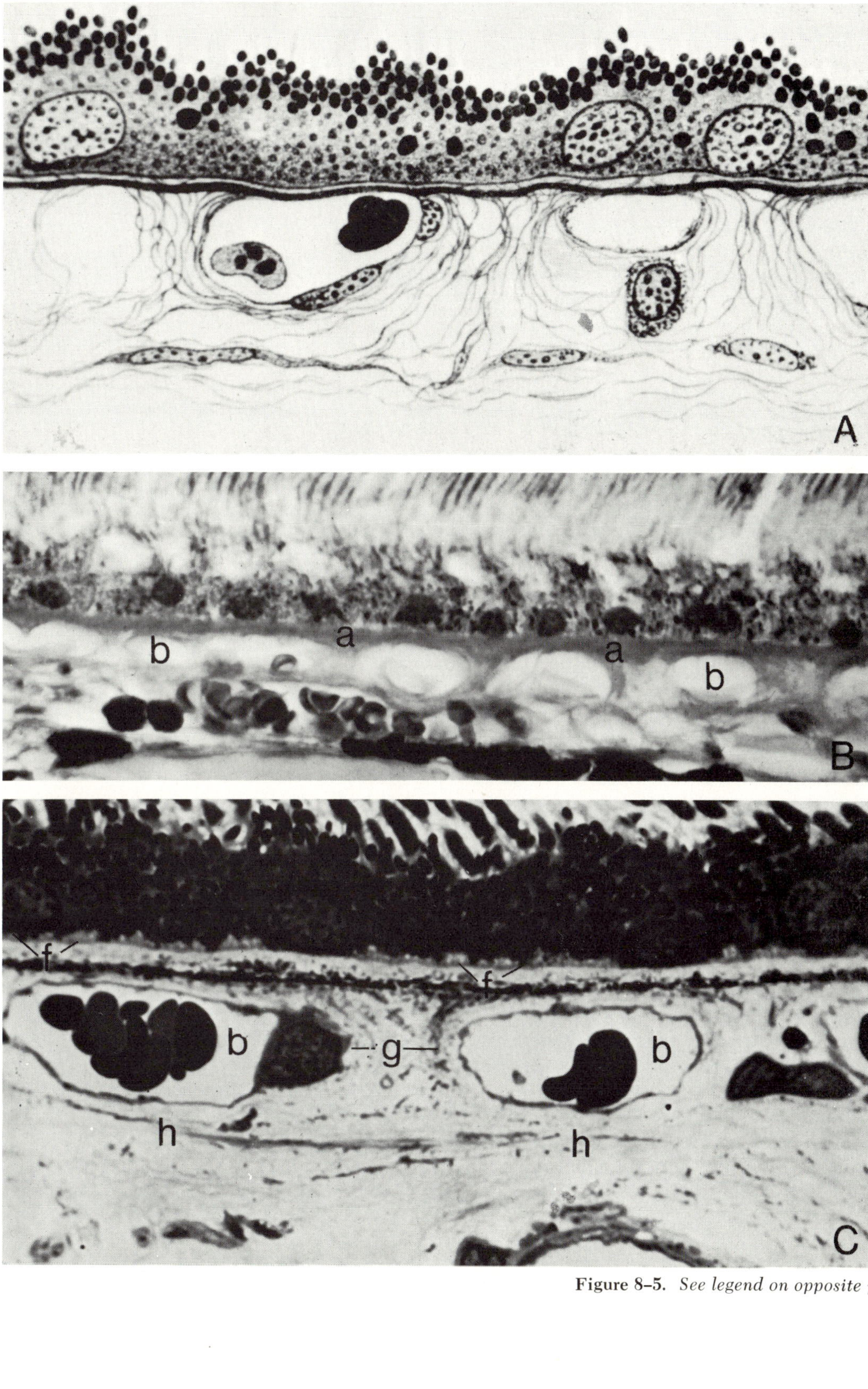

Figure 8–5. *See legend on opposite page.*

of elastic tissue. The membrane is about 2 μm. thick in the young eye, but thickens with increasing age. It is not uncommon for Bruch's membrane to show areas of basophilia in persons over age 50; this basophilia is more prominent in the peripapillary and macular regions. PAS staining also may become more intense with increasing age, because the membrane contains an increased amount of ground substance.

Examination with the light microscope reveals that Bruch's membrane is composed of the following portions: (1) a basement membrane of the pigment epithelium (cuticular layer); (2) a collagen layer; and (3) an elastic zone (elastic layer).

The collagen in the external part of Bruch's membrane is arranged differently internal to the capillaries than it is in the intercapillary zone (Fig. 8-5 *B* and *C*). In the capillary region some of the collagenous tissue adjacent to the internal wall of the capillaries is oriented toward the retina, traversing Bruch's membrane between the bundles of elastic fibers. In the intercapillary zone most of the collagen external to the elastic layer is oriented toward the intercapillary collagen. Wolter (1955) described the collagen in Bruch's membrane as having a brush-like arrangement, with the fine collagen fibers radiating from the capillary and intercapillary regions toward the pigment epithelium. This description is correct, but the number of radiating fibers diminishes in the intercapillary region. Fibroblasts and other cells are not seen in Bruch's membrane except in the extreme periphery, and we have identified no nerves in this tissue.

The layer previously designated as the cuticular layer is now known to be the basement membrane of the retinal pigment epithelium; it measures about 0.3 μm. thick. This layer is PAS-positive and can be recognized as a fine line which is closely apposed to the retinal pigment epithelial cells. Fehér and Valu (1967) studied meridional and tangential sections of Bruch's membrane in fixed as well as fresh choroidal tissue with the polarization microscope. The membrane was shown to be composed of collagen and elastic fibers woven together like a lattice, running parallel to each other or in arcades or brush-like patterns. Collagen fibers are seen to traverse the membrane in all directions when sections are stained with the Masson stain. In the peripheral choroid Bruch's membrane is modified by the presence of somewhat larger choroidal vessels in the choriocapillary layer. It becomes thinner over these vessels and its elastic layer is less continuous, but it is uniformly smooth internally where it abuts on the basement membrane of the retinal pigment epithelium. The elastic layer is approximately 0.8 μm. thick. It is separated from the basement membranes of the retinal pigment epithelium and endothelium of the choriocapillaris by a narrow space. This elastic portion of Bruch's membrane lies in a single plane throughout the choroid; in meridional sections it appears to be interrupted frequently by narrow spaces. Flat sections show the elastic layer to form a net-like meshwork along the whole inner choroid. The openings in the meshwork are triangular or irregularly polygonal and vary in size. The meshes of this elastic tissue framework are filled with loosely arranged collagen fibers which pass from the pericapillary and intercapillary connective tissue into the area between the elastic layer and the basement membrane of the retinal pigment epithelium.

The earliest electron microscopic studies of Bruch's membrane and its development in the human eye were those of Sumita (1961); Lerche (1963,

1965); Garron (1963); and Hogan (1961). Bruch's membrane has been studied with the electron microscope in a variety of animals with and without a tapetum; it has the same structure in all species, although it is thinner in small animals. In animals with a tapetum lucidum, the elastic and collagenous elements over the tapetum are absent; in the intercapillary zone the normal structure prevails. In the cow, which has a tapetum fibrosum, the usual structure is evident (Nakaizumi, 1964a, b; Nakaizumi et al., 1964).

Bruch's membrane can be measured more accurately in electron micrographs than with the optical microscope. The membrane varies in thickness

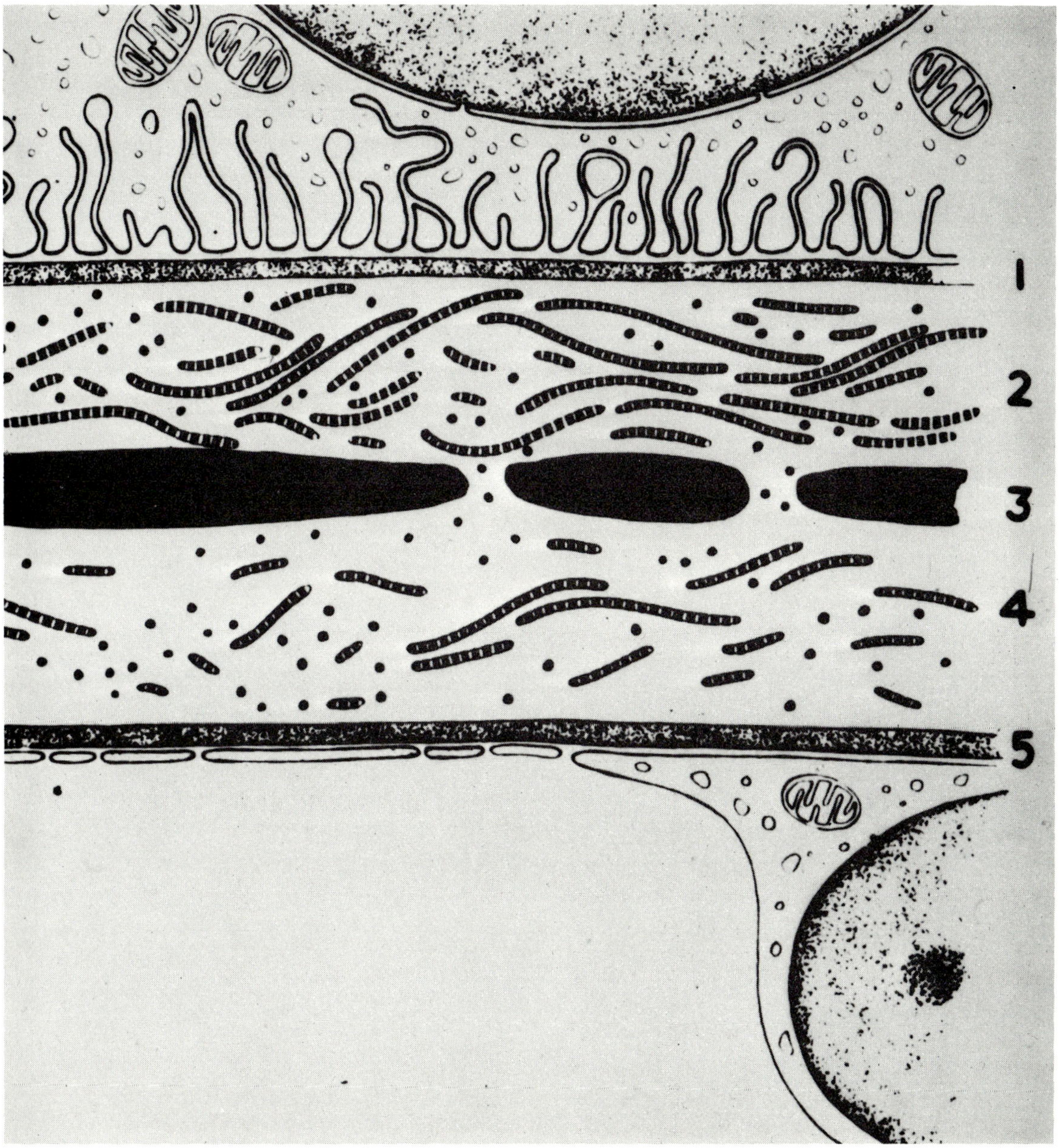

Figure 8–6. The layers of Bruch's membrane are shown as outlined in the text, based on electron microscopic studies.

in different portions of the eye; it measures 2 to 4 μm. thick near the disc, and gradually thins to 1 to 2 μm. in the periphery. Generally Bruch's membrane becomes thicker with increasing age, as a result of an accumulation of as yet unidentified substances in the collagenous areas and the intercapillary region. It is useful to subdivide Bruch's membrane into the following parts to describe its ultrastructure (Figs. 8–6 to 8–8 and 8–18): (1) basement membrane of the retinal pigment epithelium; (2) inner collagenous zone; (3) elastic layer; (4) outer collagenous zone; and (5) basement membrane of the choriocapillaris. Layer number 5 is absent in the intercapillary zone. Layer 1 belongs to the retina, since it is the basement membrane of the pigment epithelium; similarly, layer 5 actually belongs to the choriocapillary endothelium.

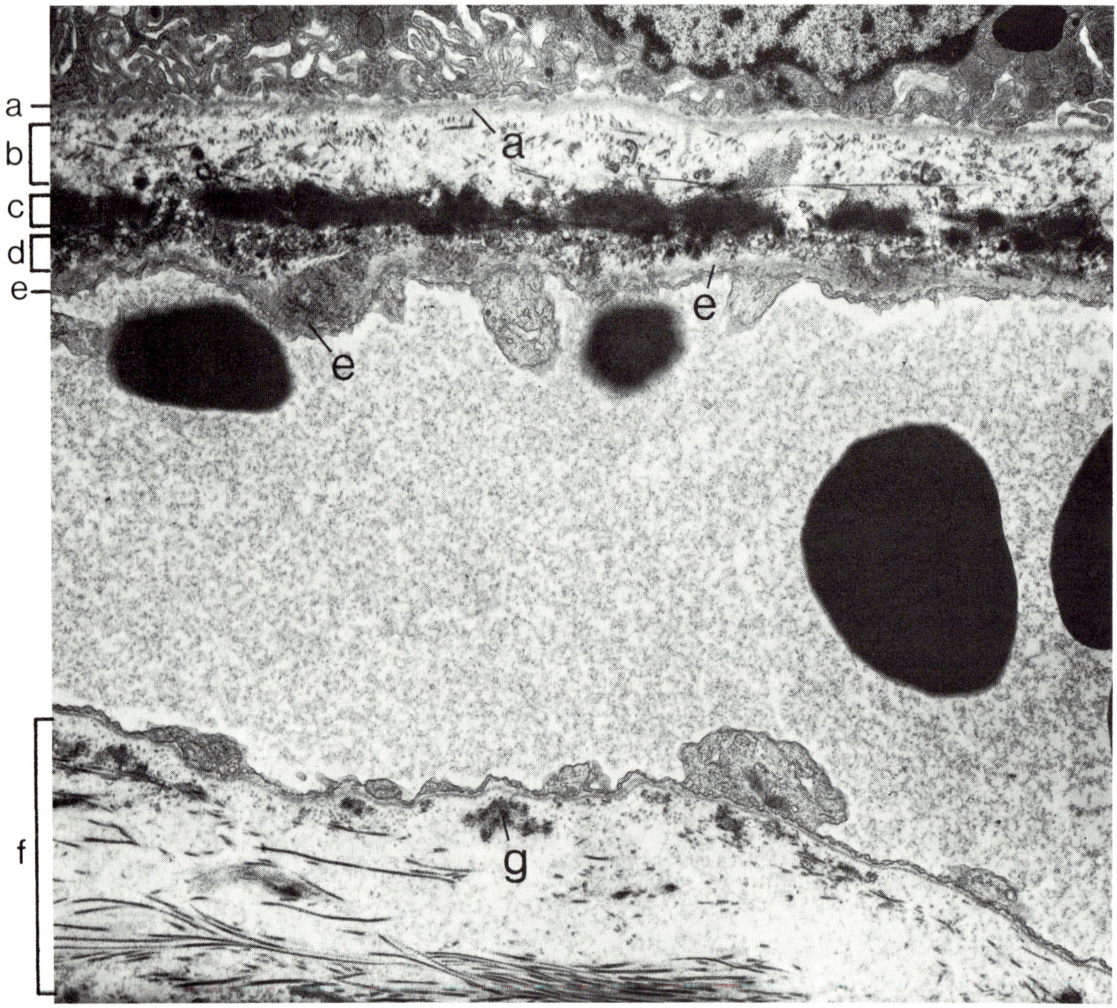

Figure 8–7. Bruch's membrane and the choriocapillaris. The five layers of Bruch's membrane are formed by the basement membrane of the retinal pigment epithelium (a); the inner collagenous zone (b); the elastic layer (c); the narrow outer collagenous zone (d); and the basement membrane of the choriocapillaris (e). The subcapillary collagen (f) is abundant; it contains clumps of elastic tissue (g). (× 9900.)

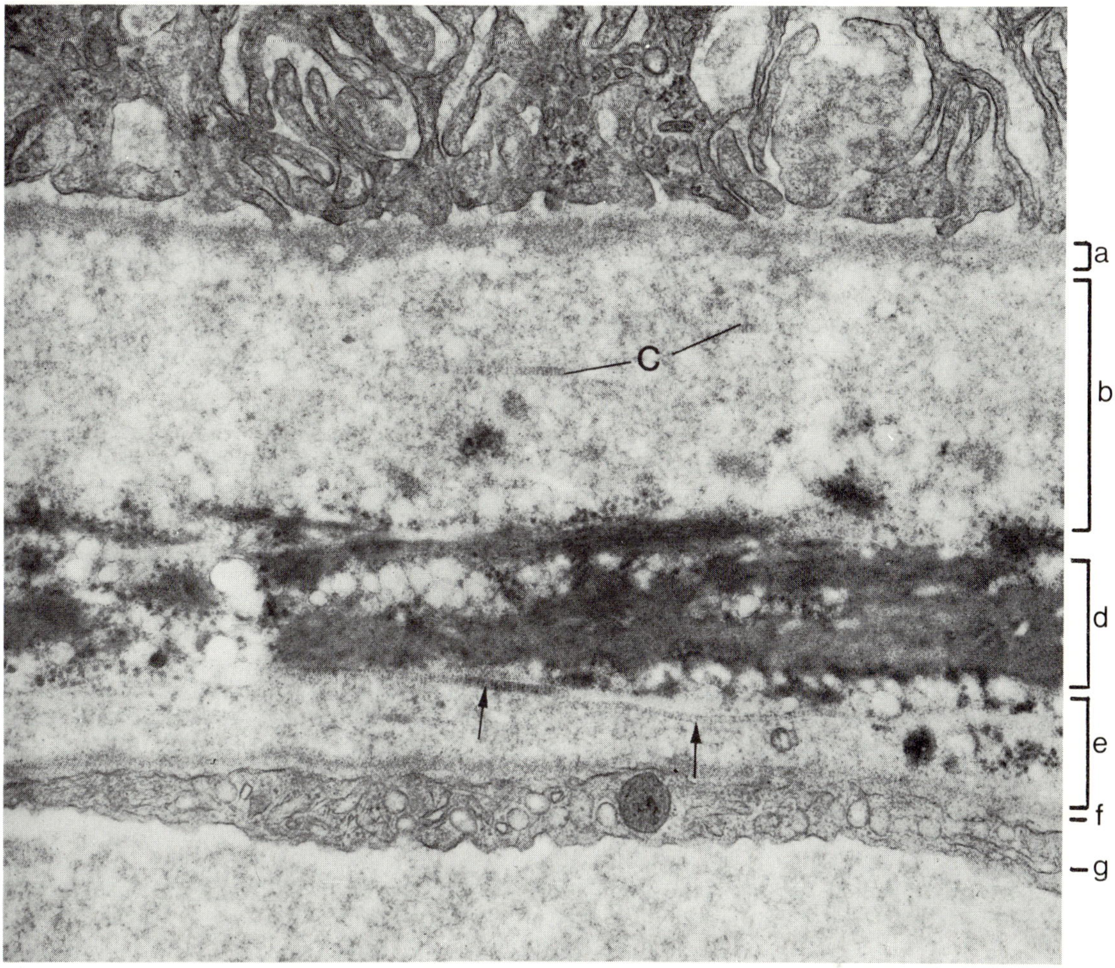

Figure 8–8. Bruch's membrane in the posterior choroid. The basement membrane of the pigment epithelium (a) which is the innermost part of Bruch's membrane measures 0.3 μm. in thickness and is composed of a light internal layer and a darker, finely granular external lamina measuring 0.1 μm. in thickness. The inner collagenous zone (b) measures 1.5 μm. in thickness. In this specimen it has only a few collagen fibrils (c) embedded in a finely granular ground substance. The elastic layer (d) is 0.8 μm. thick and shows areas of discontinuity. The narrower outer collagenous zone (e) measures 0.7 μm. in thickness and contains collagen fibrils (arrows) and a mucoprotein ground substance. The basement membrane (f) of the choriocapillary endothelium (g) is much thinner than that of the retinal pigment epithelium; it measures 0.14 μm. in thickness. (× 22,000.)

Basement Membrane of the Retinal Pigment Epithelium (Fig. 8-8). This thin membrane is composed of very fine filaments which extend from its inner and outer surfaces to join the cell membrane of the pigment epithelium and adjacent collagen (Garron, 1963). Its thickness is about 0.3 μm., and it is separated from the cell membrane by a space measuring 1000 A. It is continuous from the disc to the pupillary margin in the iris. The cell membrane at the base of the pigment epithelial cells shows marked infolding, but the basement membrane does not enter these folds.

Inner Collagenous Zone (Figs. 8-9 *A*, *B*, *C*, and *D* and 8-18). The inner collagenous zone is about 1.5 μm. thick and is composed of clearly

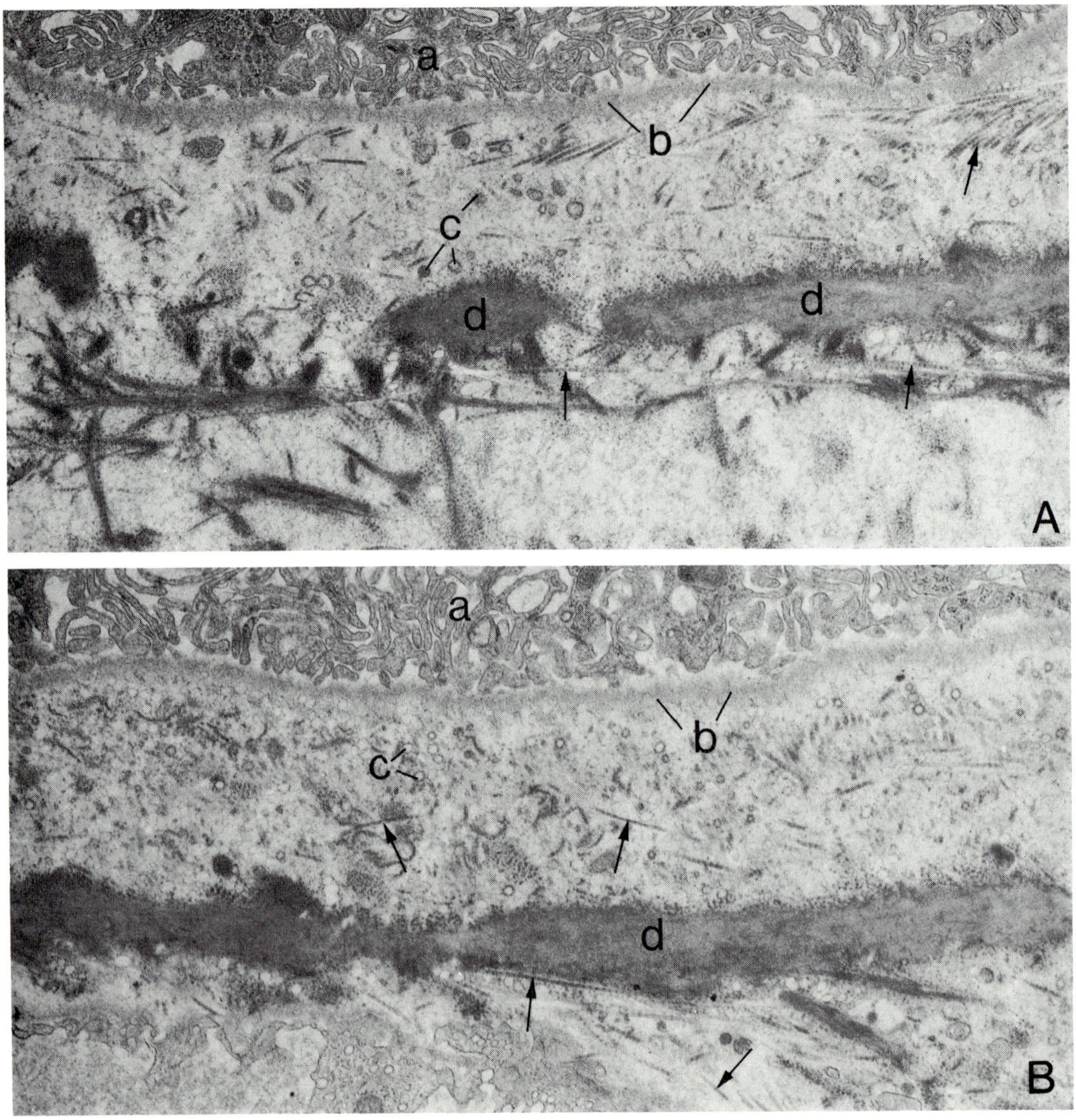

Figure 8–9. Electron micrographs of Bruch's membrane. *A* and *B*, There are numerous basal infoldings of the retinal pigment epithelial cells (a), and a thin basement membrane (b) is adjacent to the infoldings but does not enter into the folds. The inner and outer collagenous zones show a considerable number of collagen fibrils (arrows) and numerous vesicles (c) which appear to be coated with a granular material. The elastica (d) in *A* is interrupted, while in *B* it is continuous. The capillary endothelium in *B* has several pinocytotic vesicles. (× 9000.)

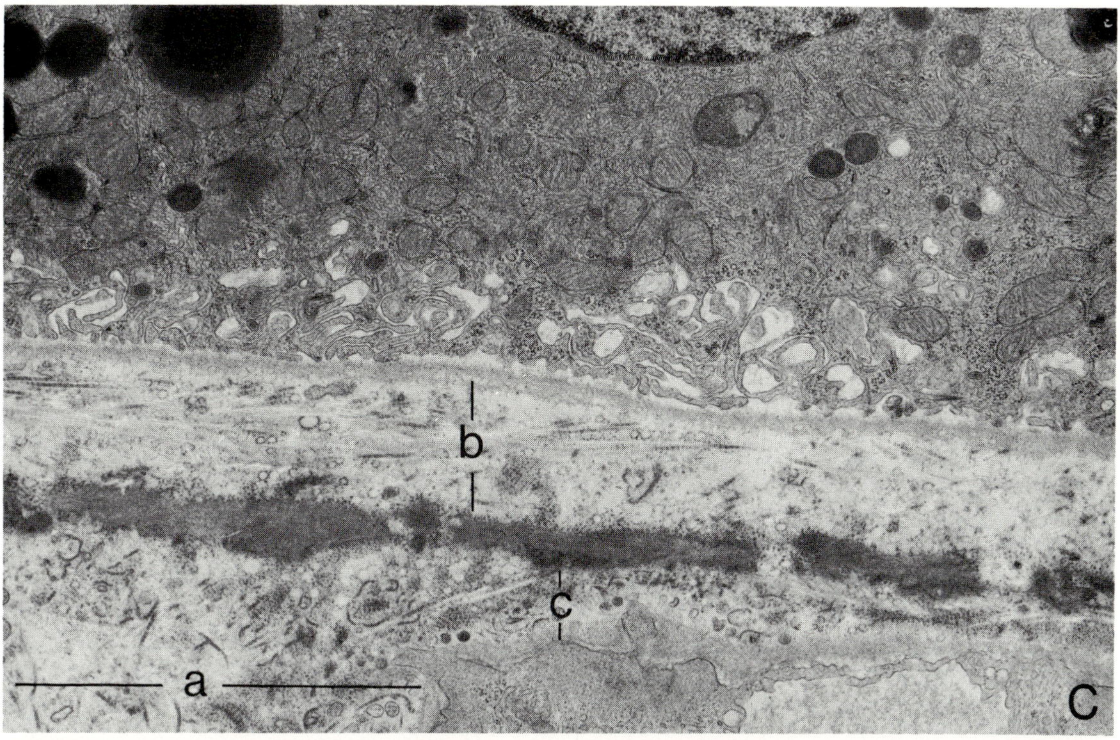

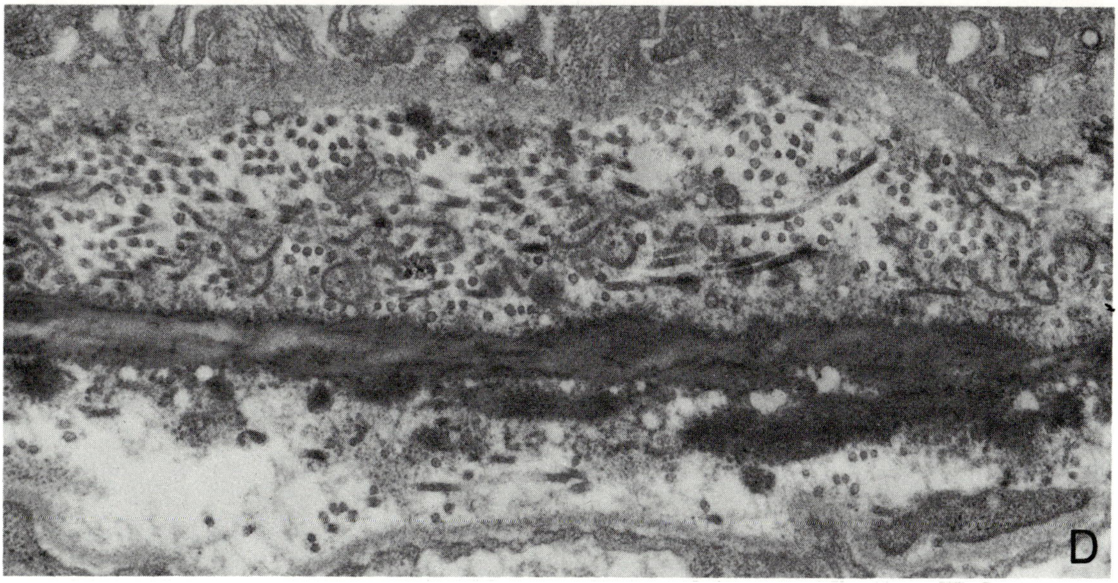

Figure 8–9. *Continued.*

C, The intercapillary region (a) appears on the left and the retinal pigment epithelium is across the top. The elastica is separated from the pigment epithelium by a rather regular distance, even in the intercapillary zone. The inner collagenous zone (b) is wider than the outer one (c). (× 9000.)

D, A large number of collagen fibrils are seen in the inner collagenous zone of this specimen. (× 15,000.)

interwoven but loosely arranged collagen filaments that are oriented in all directions, but in general they are parallel to the outer retina. The collagen fibrils are in close proximity to the basement membrane of the pigment epithelial cells. The fine filaments of the basement membrane, which merge with the collagen and the cell membrane of the pigment epithelium, probably are responsible for the strong bond between the epithelium and the choroid. This collagen is continuous through the meshes of the elastic zone with that in the outer collagenous zone. These fibrils produce the brush-like pattern observed by Wolter with the light microscope. The collagen fibrils are similar to those of the ciliary body, measuring 600 A. in diameter, with a periodicity of around 640 A.; they are embedded in a granular ground substance which is probably a mucopolysaccharide-protein complex. There are no cells or cell processes in this layer or in the outer collagenous layer, and no nerve fibers have been identified here.

Elastic Layer (Figs. 8–10 to 8–14 and 8–18) This layer is the "backbone" of Bruch's membrane; it lies closer to the choriocapillaris than to the retinal pigment epithelium. The layer is continuous from the optic disc into the pars plana of the ciliary body (p. 303) and has a fairly regular structure and pattern. In light micrographs, meridional sections show the layer to be interrupted, with gaps between the interruptions that vary considerably in size and shape. Oblique and flat sections, however, show the elastica to be formed of long, thin, straight fibers. These fibers form a grillwork two to four fibers thick; irregular spaces are formed by the criss-crossing fibers. Many fibers may meet at certain points, forming very dense nodes with only a few small oval openings. Collagen fibers pass randomly back and forth through the openings in the elastic layer.

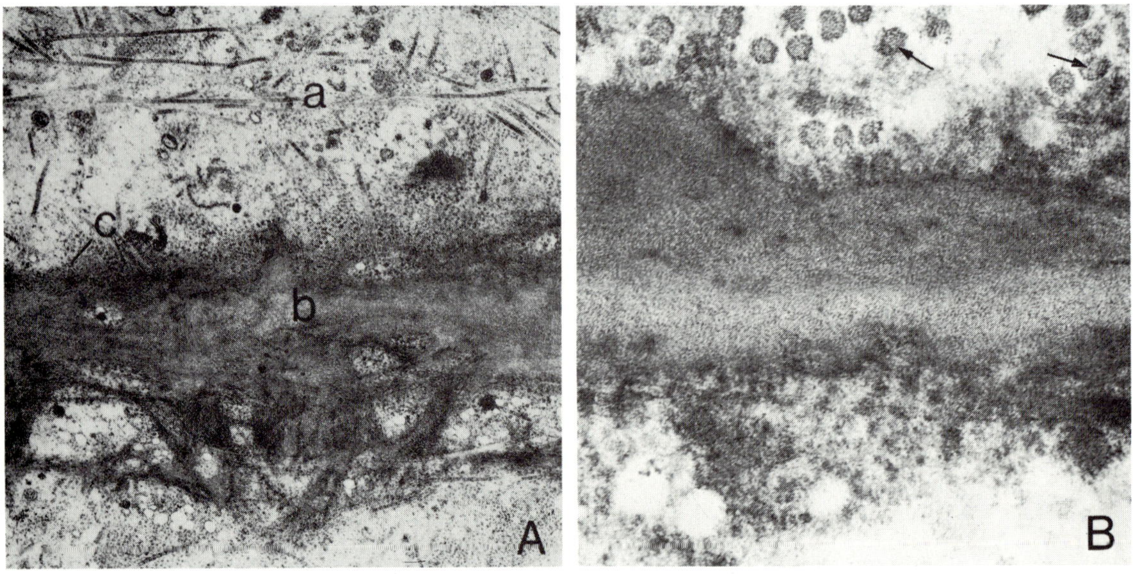

Figure 8–10. Elastic layer of Bruch's membrane. *A*, The inner collagenous zone appears at (a). The elastic fibers have a light homogeneous core (b) and a denser cortex (c). Numerous fine fibrils are associated with the cortex; they are cut in cross-section. (× 9300.)

B, Higher magnification of the elastic layer. It has a homogeneous core and dense cortex; collagen fibrils (arrows) of the inner collagenous zone are cut in cross-section. (× 45,000.)

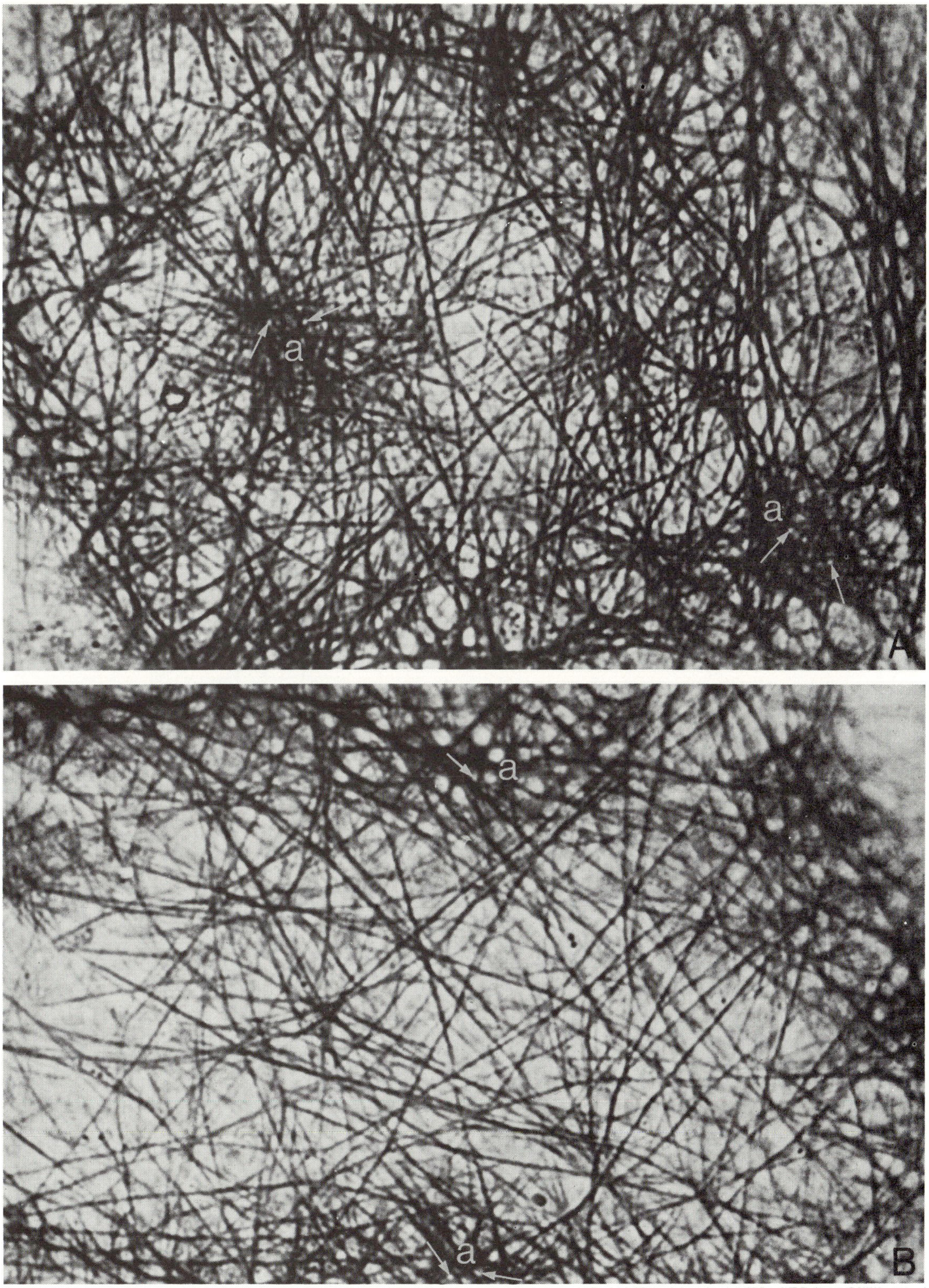

Figure 8–11. Flat sections of the elastic layer of Bruch's membrane. *A* and *B*, These light micrographs show the multilayered arrangement of the elastica and the rod-like structure of its elements. The elastica is extremely dense where its fibers intersect (a), and in these areas there are very few small openings (arrows). Elsewhere the elastic fibers form wide polygonal openings. Most of the elastic fibers have a long and rather straight course. (× 2600.)

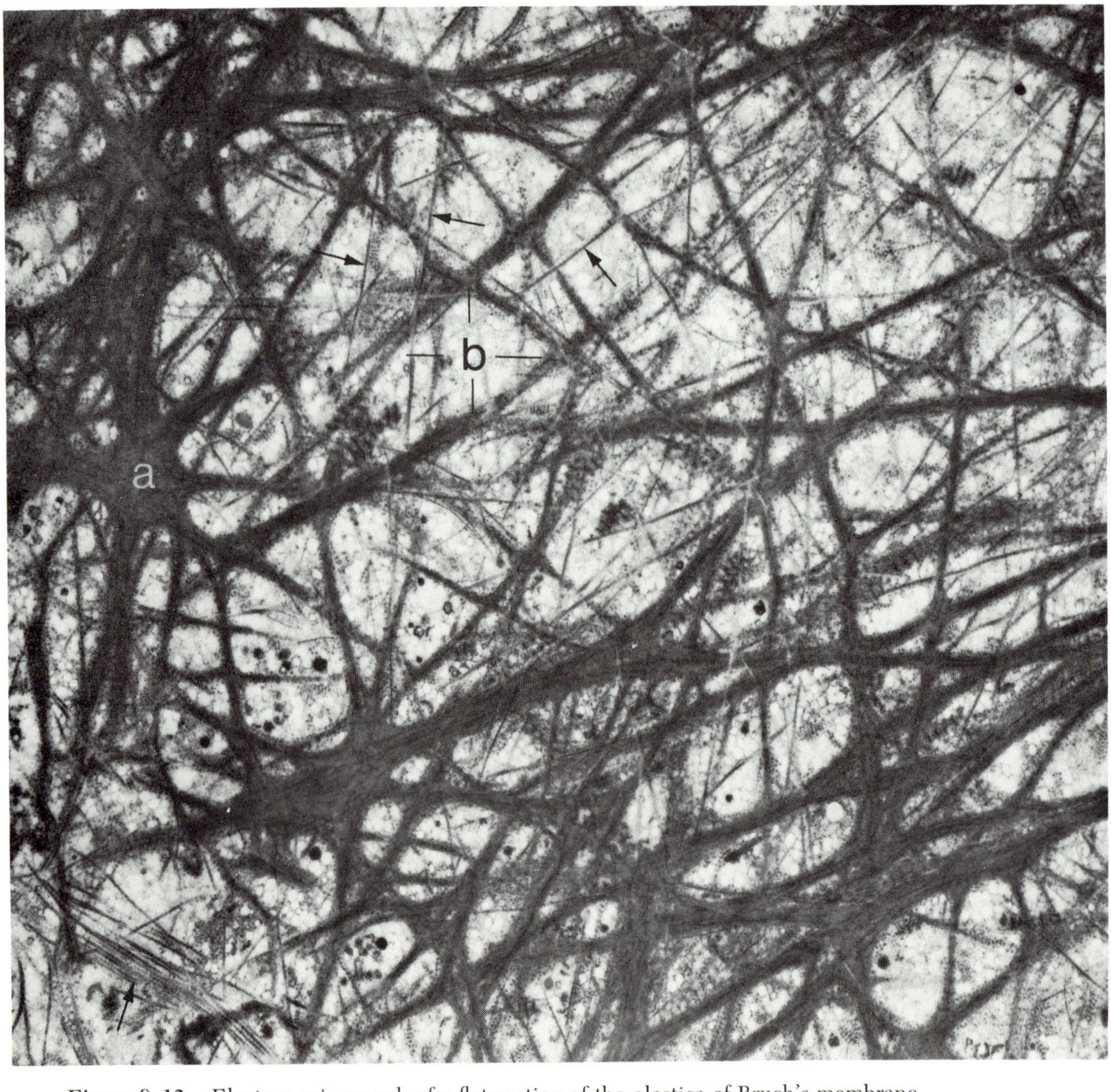

Figure 8–12. Electron micrograph of a flat section of the elastica of Bruch's membrane. The elastic fibers form large nodes (a) where they intersect. Elsewhere they form wide polygonal spaces (b) that are traversed by collagen fibrils (arrows). (× 8890.)

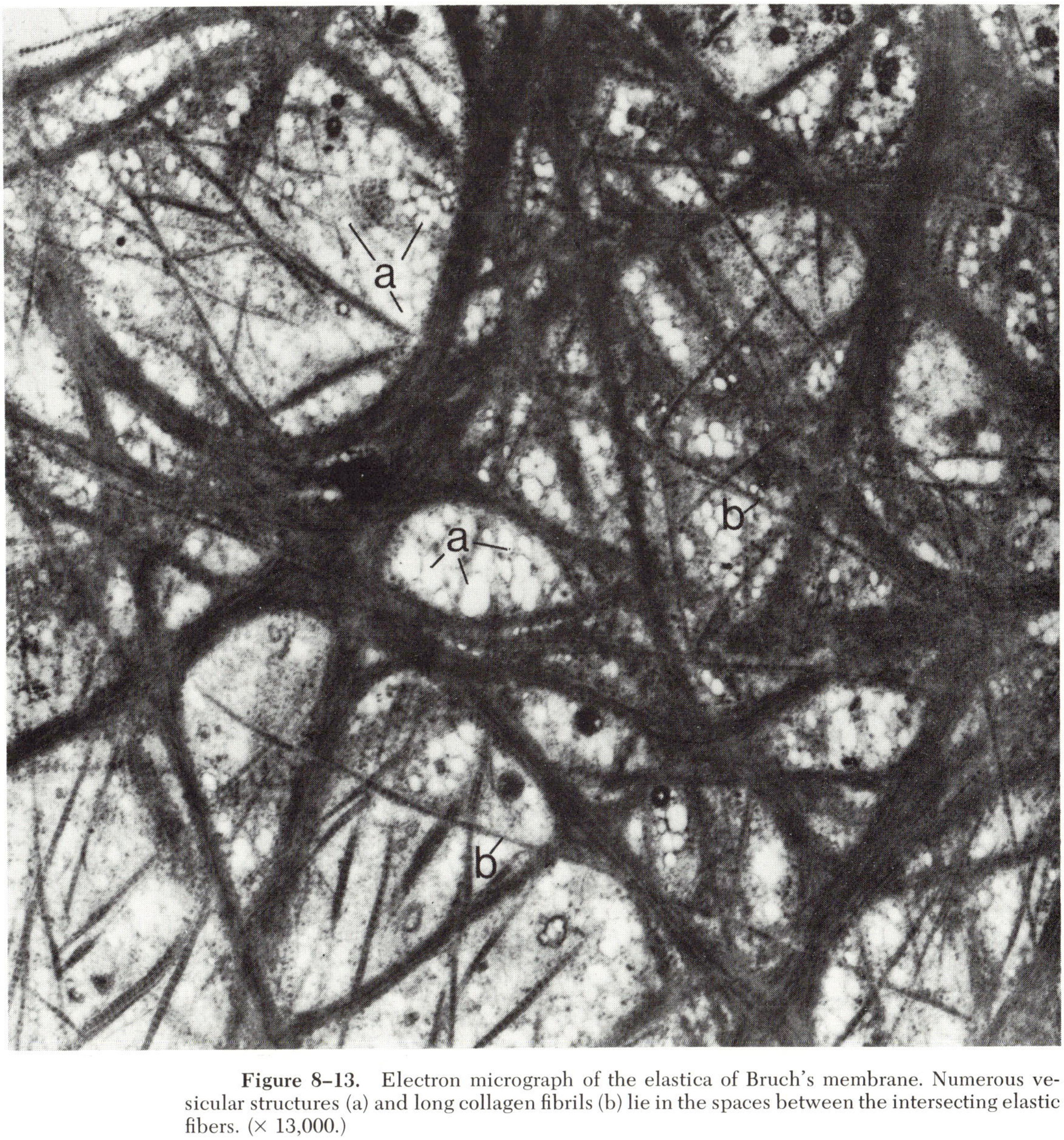

Figure 8–13. Electron micrograph of the elastica of Bruch's membrane. Numerous vesicular structures (a) and long collagen fibrils (b) lie in the spaces between the intersecting elastic fibers. (× 13,000.)

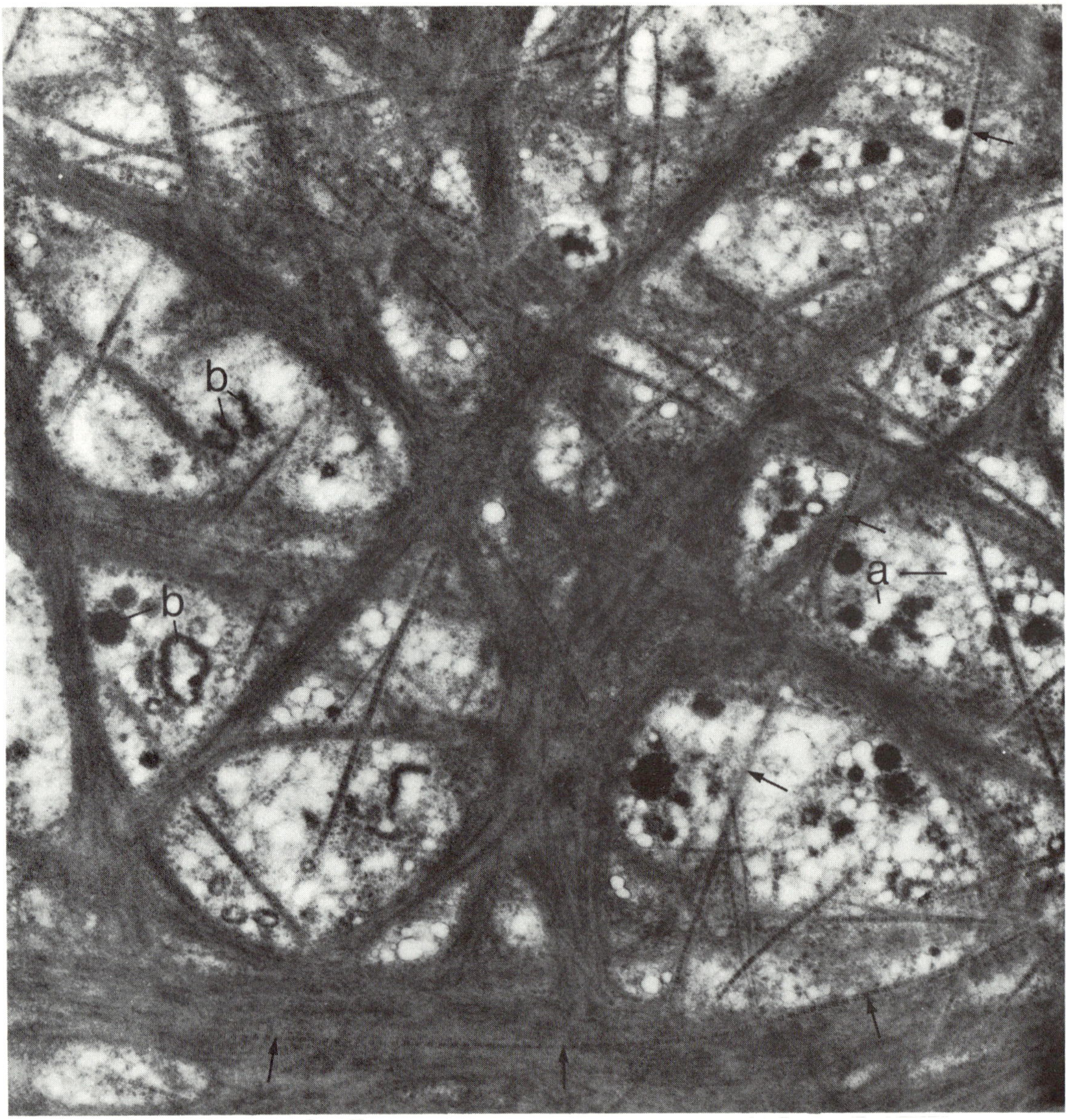

Figure 8–14. Electron micrograph of the elastica of Bruch's membrane. There is a close association between the collagen and elastic fibers. The collagen fibers are very long (arrows). Numerous vesicles (a) and electron-dense structures (b) occupy the spaces formed by the elastic fibers. (× 22,000.)

Outer Collagenous Zone (Figs. 8–9 *A* and *B*, 8–15 and 8–18) This layer is thinner than the inner collagenous zone, measuring about 0.7 μm. in thickness. It has the same structure as the internal collagenous layer, except in the intercapillary region, where it becomes continuous with the stroma of the choroid and subcapillary connective tissue. Fibroblasts and other wandering cells occasionally are seen at the ora serrata and posterior to it, but nerves have not been identified in the outer part of Bruch's membrane.

Basement Membrane of the Choriocapillaris. The outermost layer is

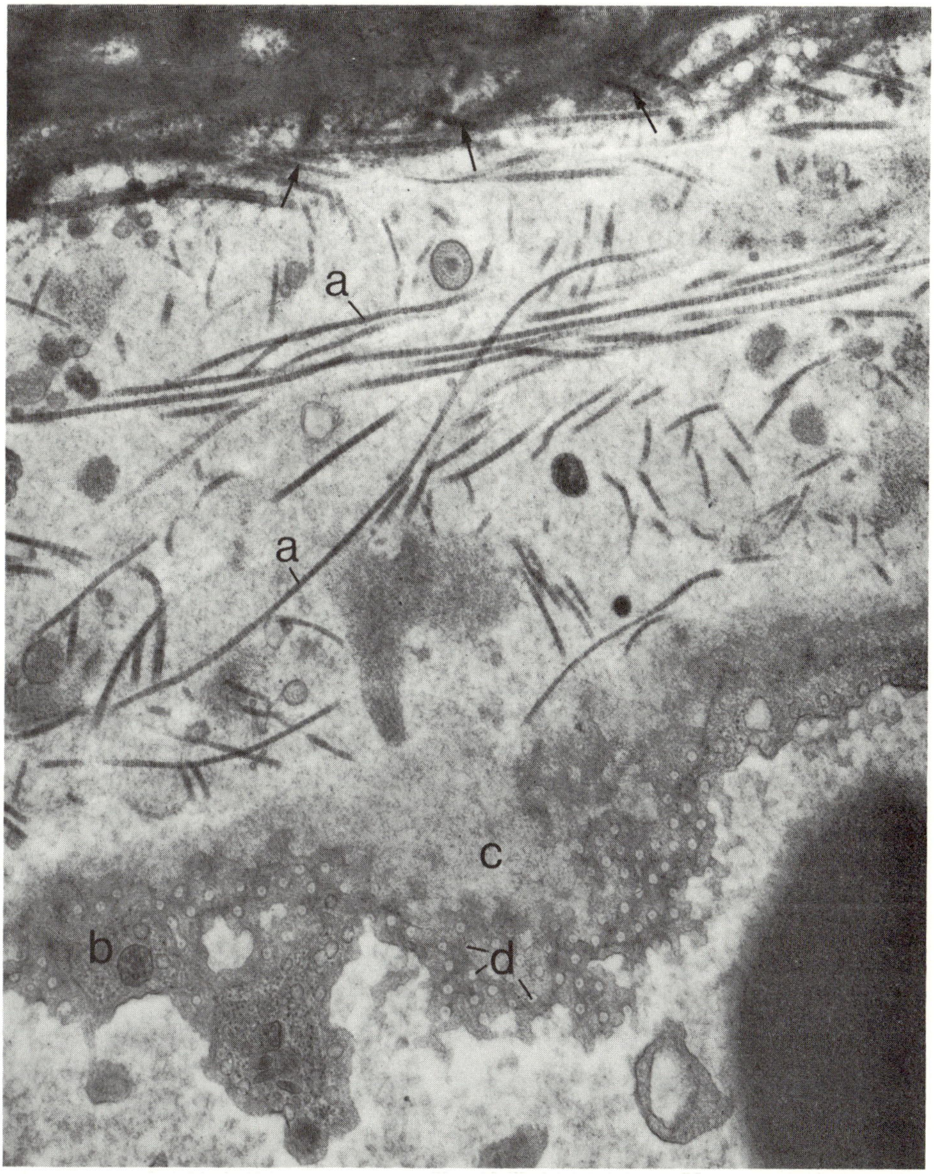

Figure 8–15. The outer collagenous zone of Bruch's membrane. The elastica appears at the top of the photograph. The collagen fibrils (arrows) merge with the elastica. Long, narrow collagen fibrils (a) and a finely granular ground substance occupy this zone. The choriocapillary endothelium (b) and its basement membrane (c) are sectioned on the bias. The pores (d) are fenestrations in this endothelial layer. (× 19,200.)

the basement membrane of the endothelium of the choriocapillaris; this layer is thinner than the basement membrane of the retinal pigment epithelium. It measures 0.14 μm. in thickness.

Intercapillary Region (Figs. 8-9 *C*, 8-18). One or two microns external to the elastic layer, the intercapillary collagen becomes more dense than that in the outer collagenous zone. Much of the collagen is oriented circularly around the capillary wall. There appears to be less ground substance in this region.

Termination of Bruch's Membrane

Papillary Region (Fig. 8–16) (See Optic Nerve, Fig. 10–12). The collagenous layers blend with the tissues at the edge of the optic nerve, some becoming oriented circularly, so that in meridional sections the collagen bundles are cut in cross-section. The elastic layer splits into three or four portions which gradually decrease in size; finally the parts become oriented circularly around the periphery of the optic nerve canal.

Ora Serrata Region (Figs. 8-2 *B*, 8-17 *A*, *B* and *C*). The basement membrane of the retinal pigment epithelium maintains its relationship with the pigmented epithelial cells of the ciliary body anterior to the ora serrata

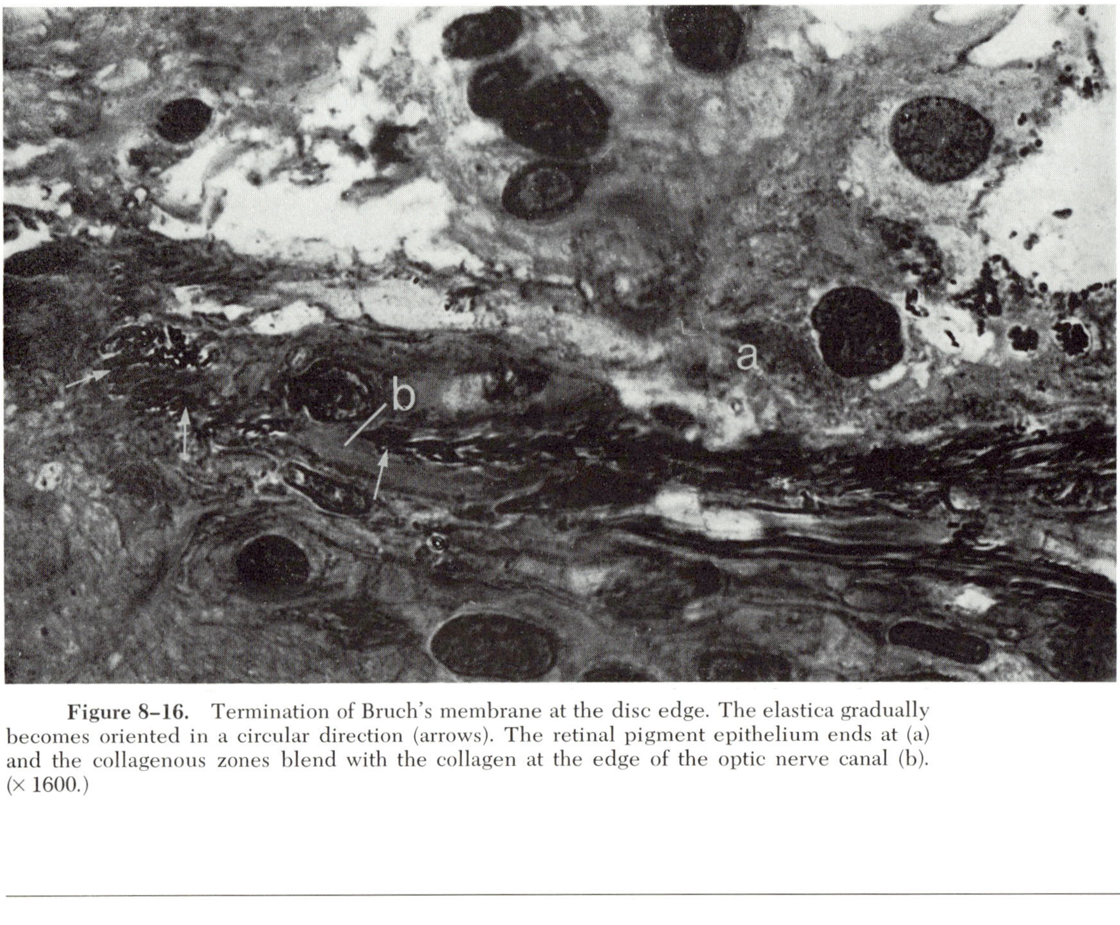

Figure 8–16. Termination of Bruch's membrane at the disc edge. The elastica gradually becomes oriented in a circular direction (arrows). The retinal pigment epithelium ends at (a) and the collagenous zones blend with the collagen at the edge of the optic nerve canal (b). (× 1600.)

Figure 8–17. *A*, Just posterior to the anterior termination of the choroid the inner collagenous zone (a) becomes widened and the elastica (b) gradually becomes more and more separated from the retinal pigment epithelium. The basement membrane of the pigment epithelium (c) often is thickened in this region. There are numerous collagen fibrils (d) and electron-dense circular particles (e). (× 11,500.)

B, There is splitting of the elastica (a), the two portions of elastic tissue being separated by collagen and fibroblasts (b). (× 13,200.)

C, Two fibroblasts (a) lie in the inner collagenous zone close to the retinal pigment epithelium (b). The elastica is beginning to split (c). (× 12,000.)

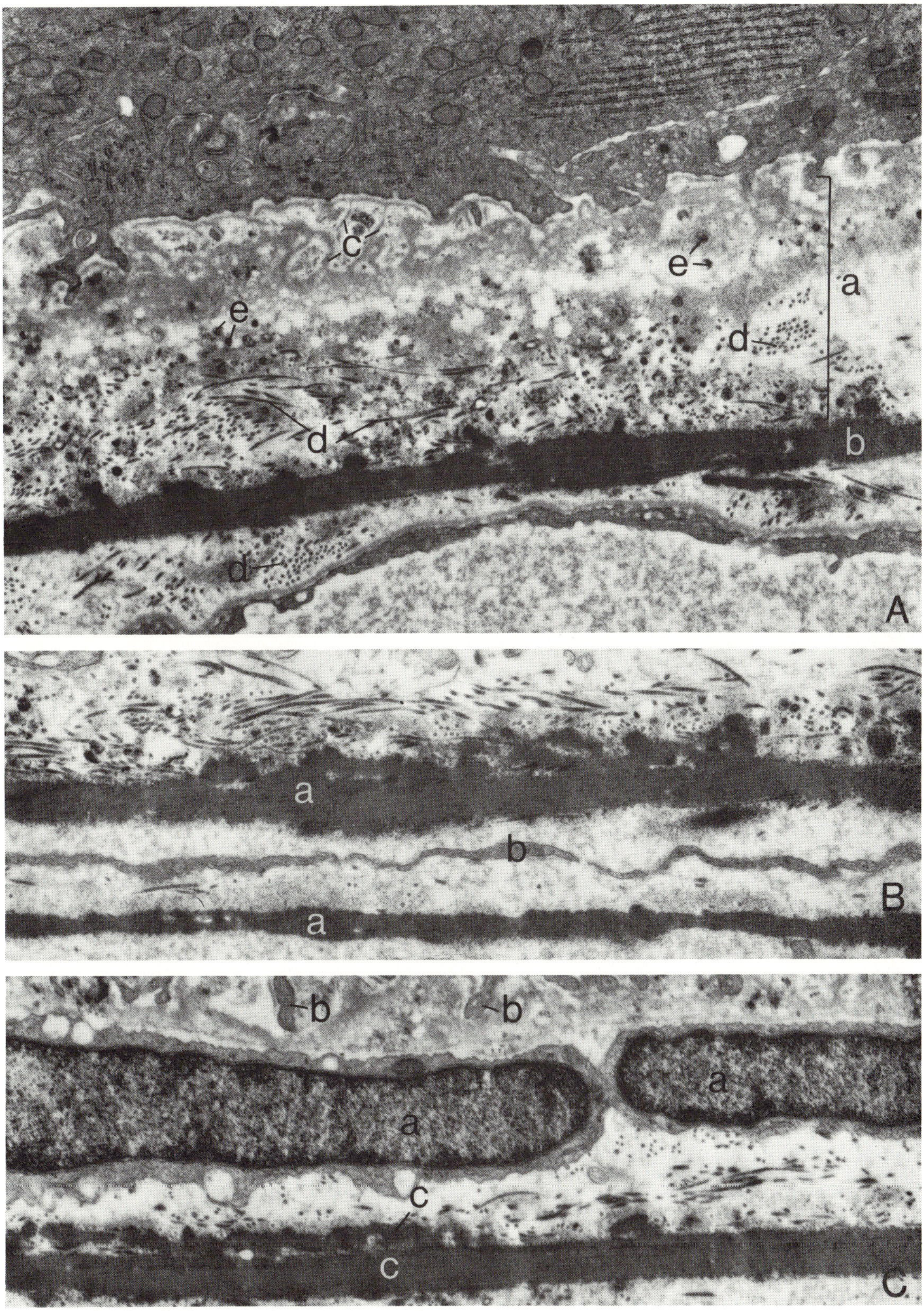

Figure 8–17. *See legend on opposite page.*

(see Ciliary Body, p. 303). The choriocapillaris ceases to be a pure capillary layer just posterior to the ora serrata because of the infiltration of venules in this layer. The elastic portion of Bruch's membrane is displaced externally by an increased amount of collagen and some fibroblasts in the inner collagenous zone.

Aging (Figs. 8–19 to 8–35). Bruch's membrane, of all the tissues of the choroid, undergoes prominent changes with aging. At about age 20 changes begin to occur in the inner collagenous zone and later include the elastica, the outer collagenous zone and the intercapillary connective tissue. The alterations progress throughout life, so that in the eyes of many elderly persons, Bruch's membrane shows extensive changes. It is not certain whether these changes precede development of senescent changes in the macular retina, nor is it clear whether the changes result from an accumulation of material from the choriocapillaris or from the retinal epithelium, or whether they develop from the collagen and ground substance in situ. The changes are associated with an increased PAS-positivity. The initial change is an accumulation of vesicular granular and filamentous material in the inner collagenous zone. This material appears in various forms, such as granular, amorphous, ring-like and even linear. The amount of this substance increases, finally occupying a good part of both collagenous zones. In persons over age 40 banded fibers of various lengths, widths and shapes appear in the collagen, most of them resembling the wide-spacing fibers found in the periphery of Descemet's membrane and trabecular sheets; the bands of these fibers are separated by a space measuring .12 μm. Long, dense, twisted osmiophilic fibrils with the diameter of collagen also appear, but these do not have continuous bandings. They appear to be altered collagen fibrils with a deposit of electron-dense substances on them.

The elastic zone also shows aging changes, characterized by development of a moth-eaten appearance, increased density around the central core and deposition of long, needle-like crystals. All these changes are associated with the increasing basophilia of the membrane. Such changes are more prominent in the macular and peripapillary regions, becoming less intense toward the equator. By electron microscopy changes can be detected which precede drusen formation. Deposits of amorphous granular material appear external to the basement membrane of the pigment epithelium or within its basal infoldings. This material contains round or oval globules of varying size. As drusen formation occurs, the material accumulates in the inner

Text continued on page 363

Figure 8–18. Three-dimensional drawing of the inner choroid and retinal pigment epithelium. The villi of the pigment epithelium (a) extend internally to enclose the outer segments of the rods and cones (b). The intercellular junctions are characterized by a zonula occludens (c) and a desmosome (d); otherwise, the cell relations are of the usual type. The cytoplasm of the pigment cells contains a nucleus (e), mitochondria (f), a Golgi apparatus (g), pigment granules (h), phagosomes (i), and it is characterized by a large amount of smooth-surfaced endoplasmic reticulum (j). The external cell membrane shows complex infoldings (l) and a basement membrane (m). Bruch's membrane shows an apparently interrupted elastic zone (n) in meridional section, but the elastica is layered and continuous in flat section (o). Collagen fibrils (p) that form the inner and outer collagenous zones have a random orientation around the elastic zone. The choriocapillaris (q) shows a fenestrated endothelium internally, laterally and, to a lesser extent, externally (r). The intercapillary zone shows considerable collagen (s). The lumen of the capillary contains two red blood cells.

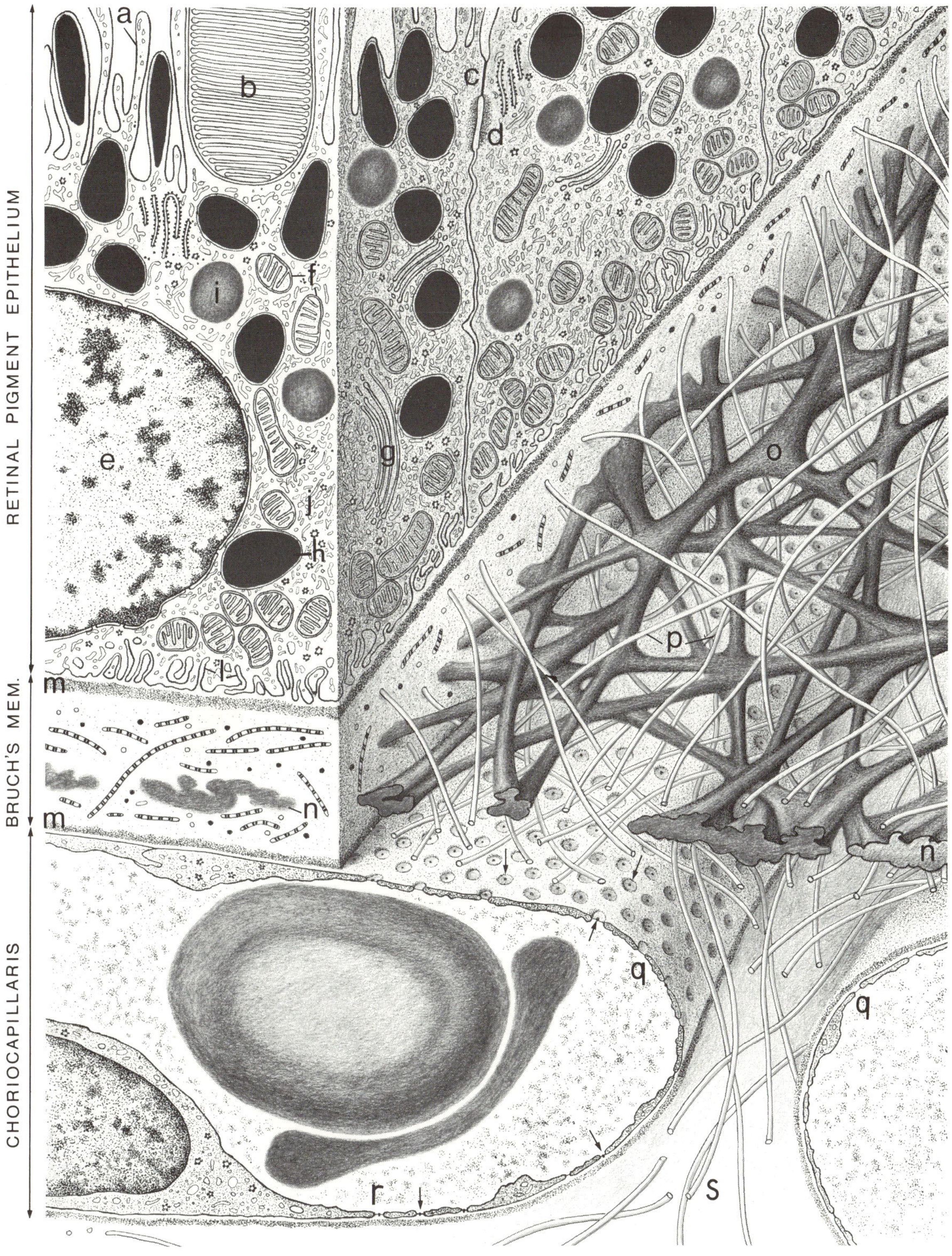

Figure 8-18. *See legend on opposite page.*

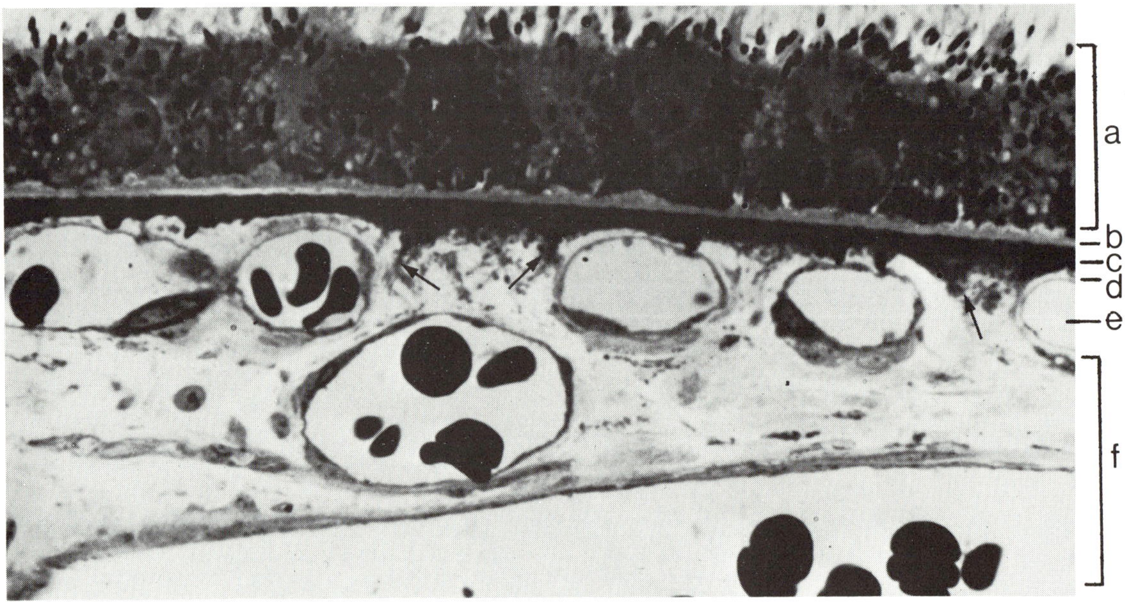

Figure 8–19. Light micrograph of aging changes in Bruch's membrane. The retinal pigment epithelium is seen at (a), the inner collagenous zone at (b), and the elastica is obscured by a dense material (c) that partially occupies the outer collagenous (d) and intercapillary zones (arrows). The choriocapillaris is shown at (e) and the choroidal stroma and a vortex vein are at (f). (× 1200.)

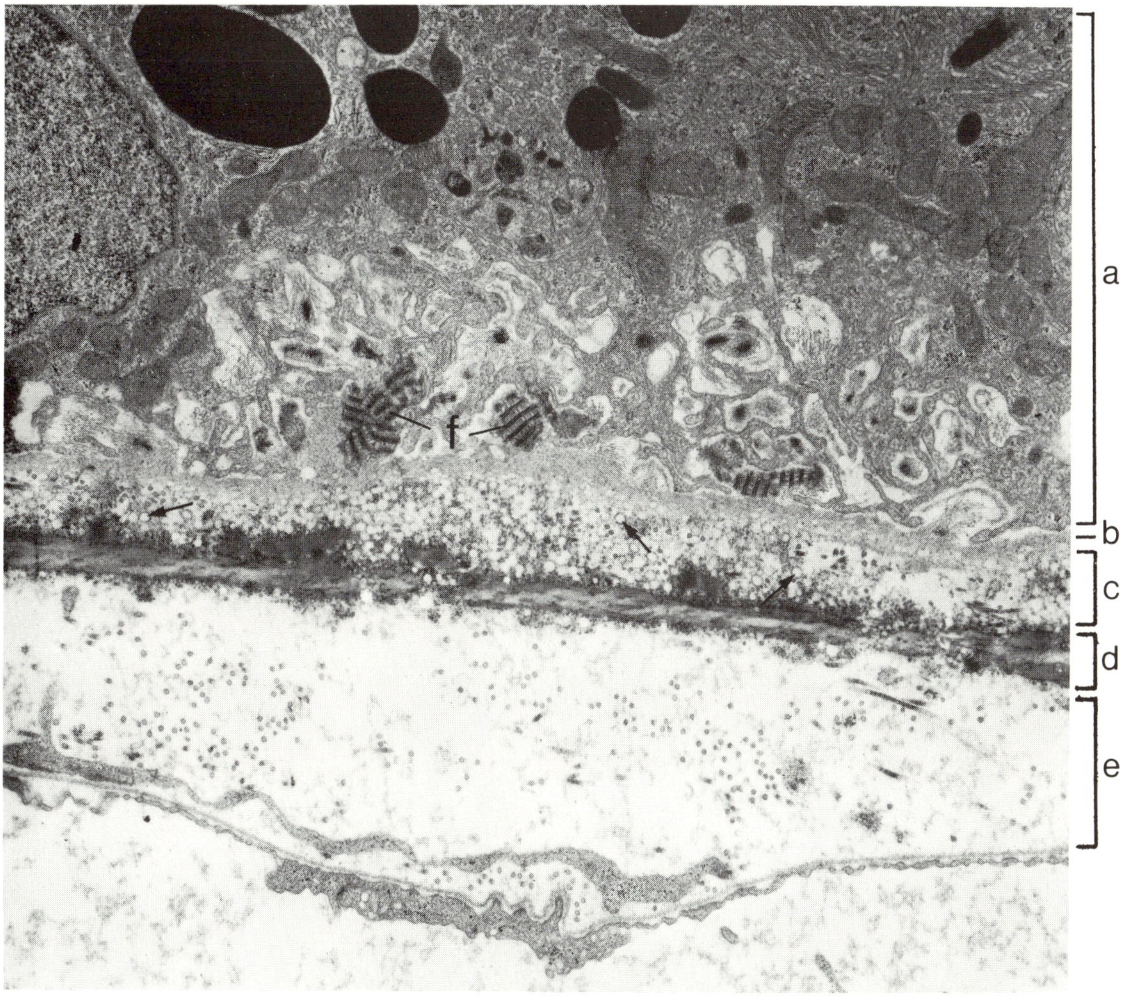

Figure 8–20. Electron micrograph of early aging changes in Bruch's membrane. The pigment epithelium (a), its basement membrane (b), the inner collagenous zone (c), the elastica (d) and the outer collagenous zone (e) are indicated. The early signs of aging are found internal to the elastica. In this specimen a large number of vesicular structures (arrows) occupy the inner collagenous zone. There is also an unusual accumulation of structures with widely spaced striations (f) internal to the basement membrane of the retinal pigment epithelium. The outer collagenous zone is normal. (× 11,200.)

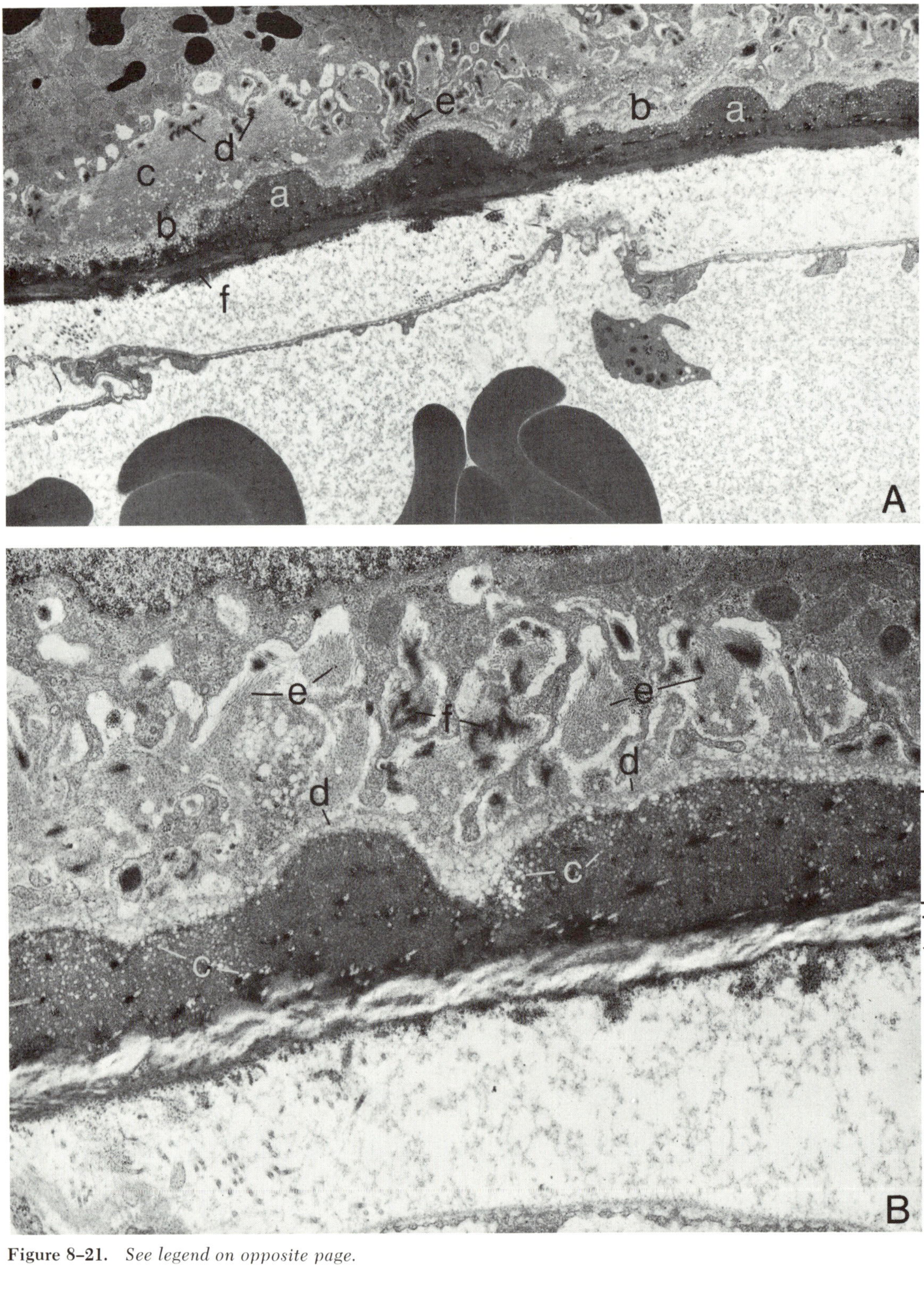

Figure 8–21. *See legend on opposite page.*

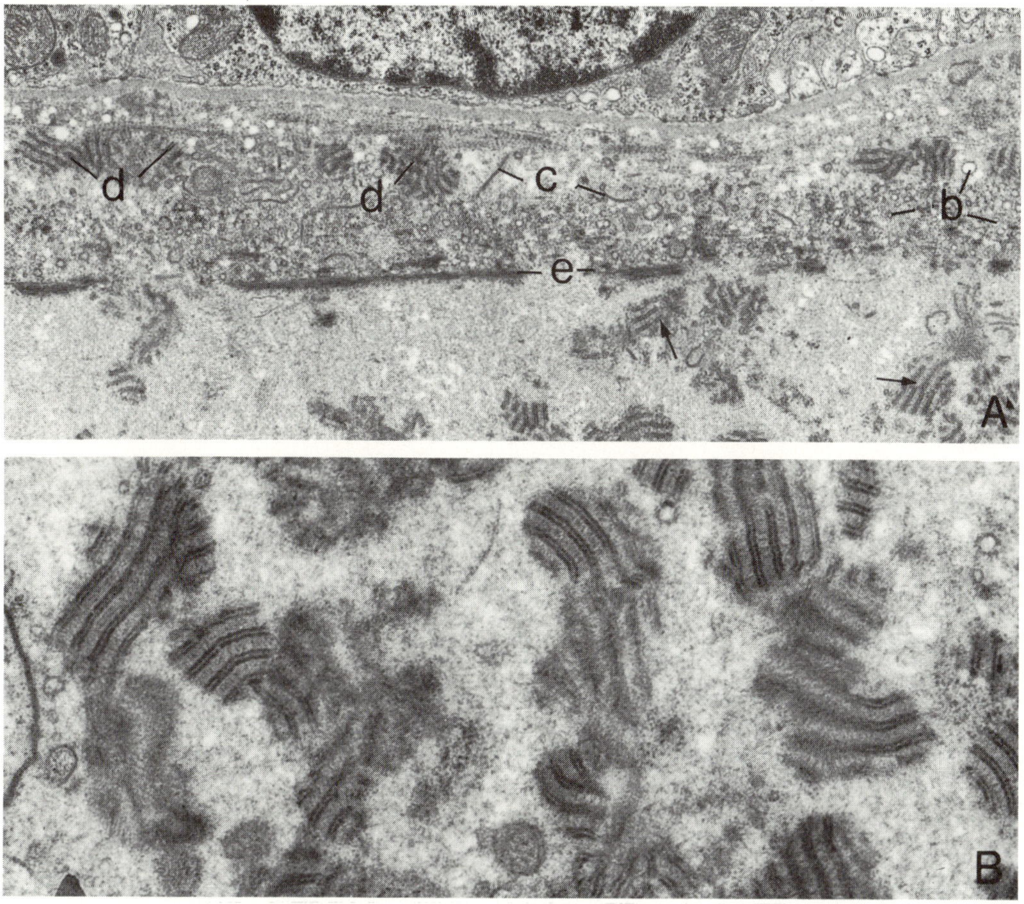

Figure 8–22. Aging changes in Bruch's membrane. *A*, The inner collagenous zone (a) is filled with vesicles (b), electron-dense fibrils (c), and structures with widely spaced striations (d), presumably of collagenous origin. The elastica (e) appears unaltered, while the outer collagenous zone also shows aging changes (arrows). (× 7500.)

B, The striations of banded material are spaced 1100 A. apart and resemble in vitro preparations of short-segment, long-spacing (SSLS) collagen, as well as similar banded material already described in the limbus and sclera. (× 18,000.)

Figure 8–21. Early aging changes in Bruch's membrane. *A*, The inner collagenous zone is filled with an electron-dense material (a) and vesicles (b). Internal to the basement membrane of the pigment epithelium is a finely granular material (c) containing clumps of an electron-dense substance (d) and structures with widely spaced striations (e). The elastica is barely discernible (f), and the outer collagenous zone is free of aging change. (× 7500.)

B, Higher magnification of the right portion of *A*. A finely granular, electron-dense material (a) rests on the elastica. A number of electron-lucent vesicles are found in the dense material (c). The basement membrane of the pigment epithelium is seen at (d), and internal to it is a fine fibrillar material (e) containing a few clumps of an electron-dense structure (f). (× 10,000.)

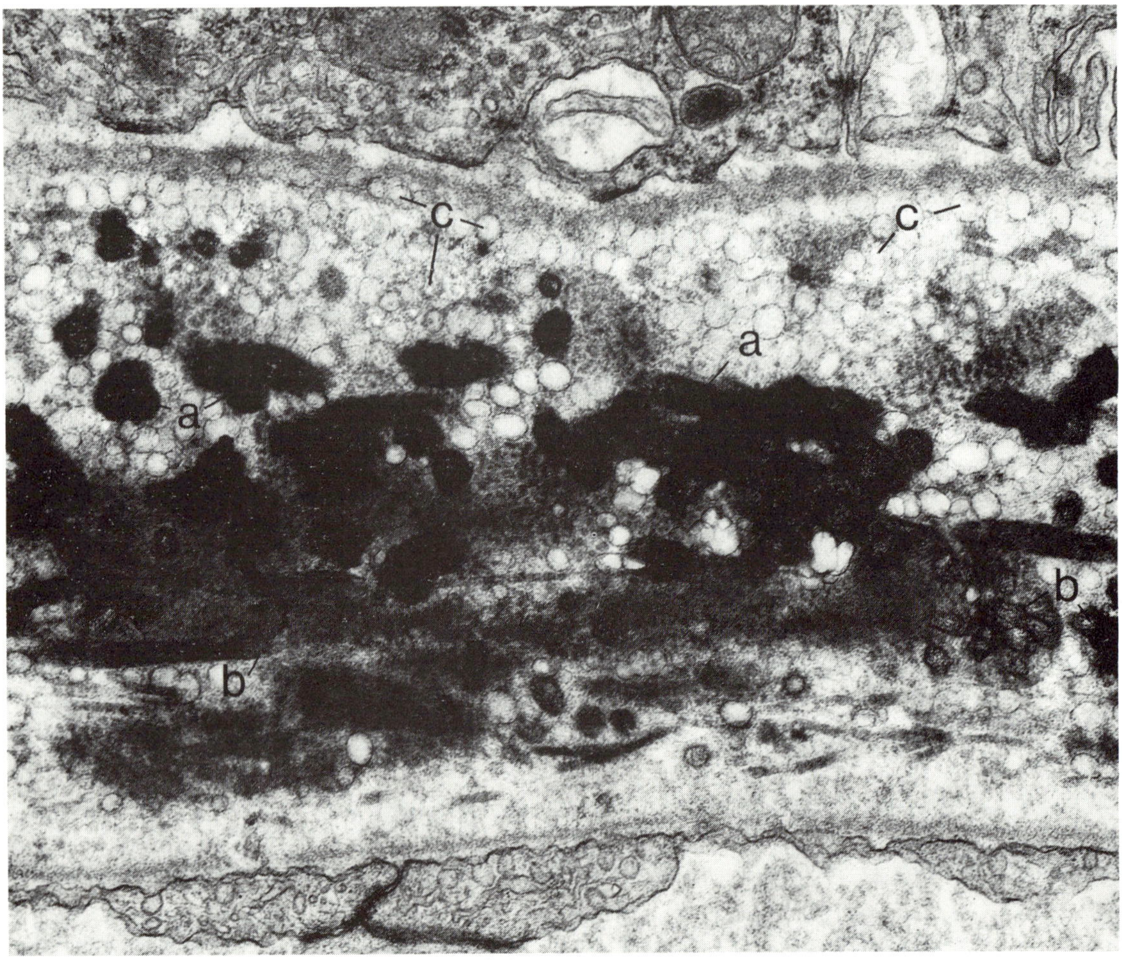

Figure 8-23. Aging changes in the elastica of Bruch's membrane. Newly formed elastic fibers (a) appear mainly in the inner collagenous zone. They are very electron-dense. Similar fibers (b) form in the elastica. Many vesicles (c) are seen internally in the membrane. (× 30,000.)

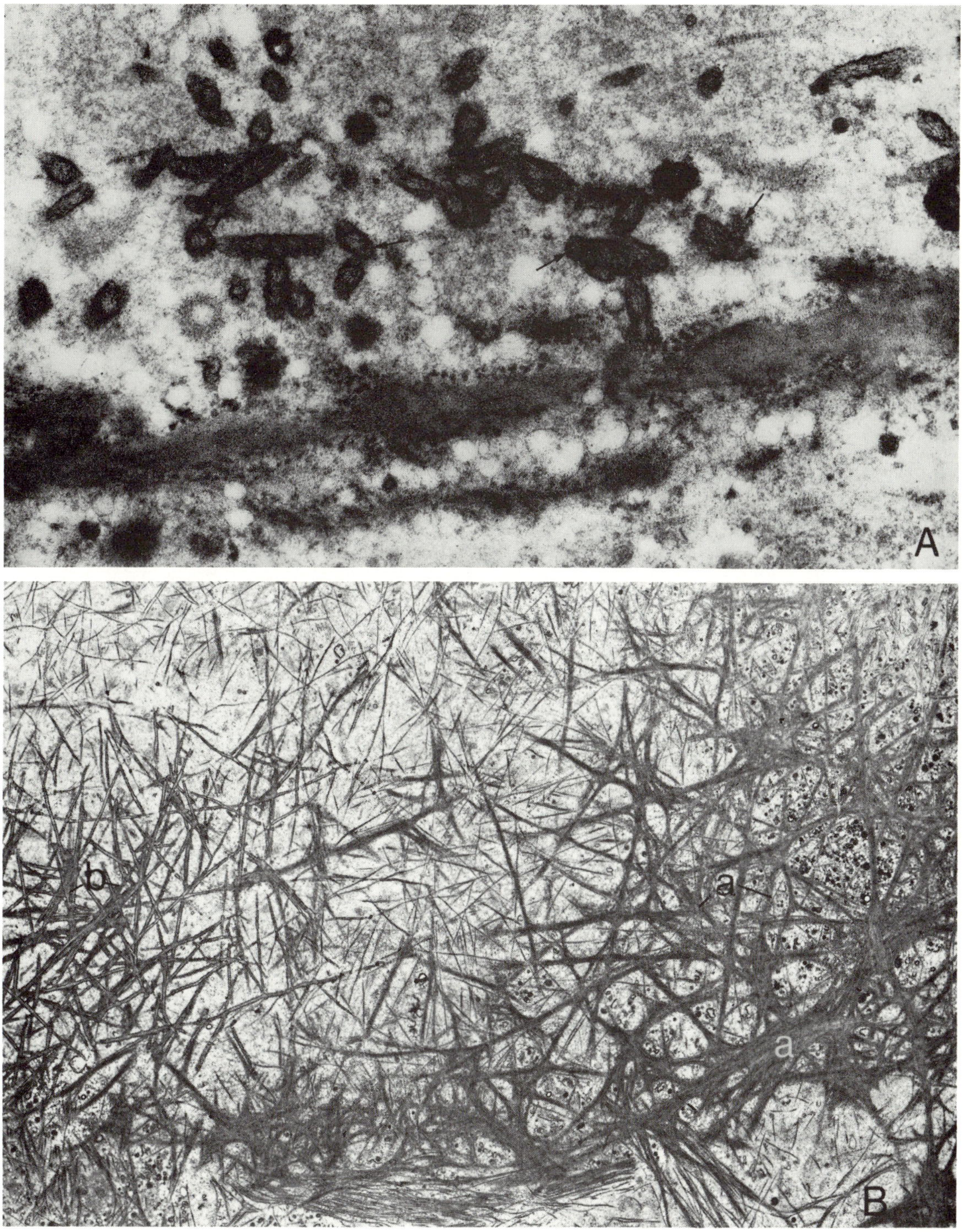

Figure 8-24. Aging changes in the elastica of Bruch's membrane. *A*, Crystal formation and calcification of the elastica frequently occur during aging. Newly formed thinner elastic fibers also appear in the inner collagenous zone (arrows). The cortex of these fibers is very electron-dense and appears to be crystallized. (× 30,000.)

B, This almost flat section shows both the normal elastica (a) and the newly formed thinner elastic fibers (b) which appear with aging in the inner collagenous zone. (× 4000.)

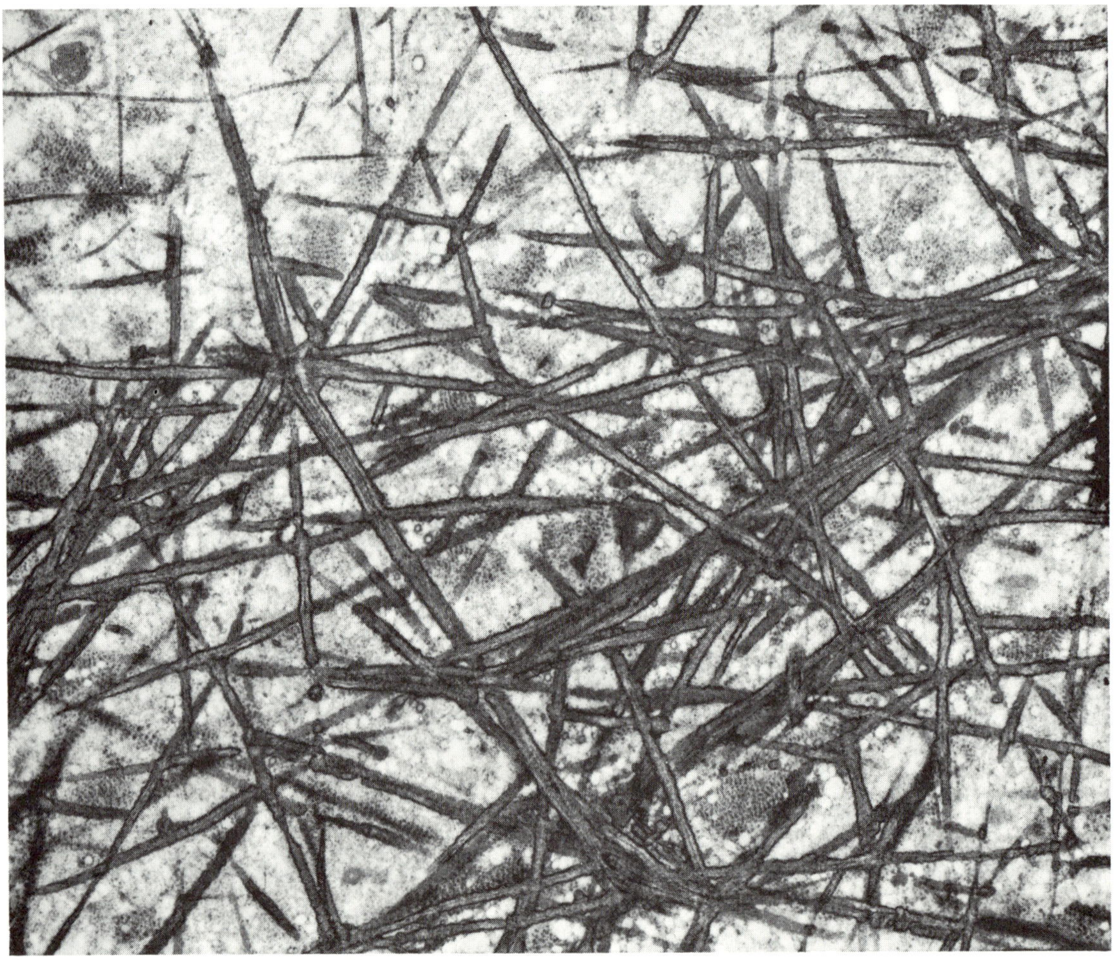

Figure 8-25. Aging changes in the elastica of Bruch's membrane. The light core and dense cortex of the elastic fibers are clearly seen. These fibers measure 1500 Å. in width and form a grillwork internal to the location of the normal elastic zone. (× 12,900.)

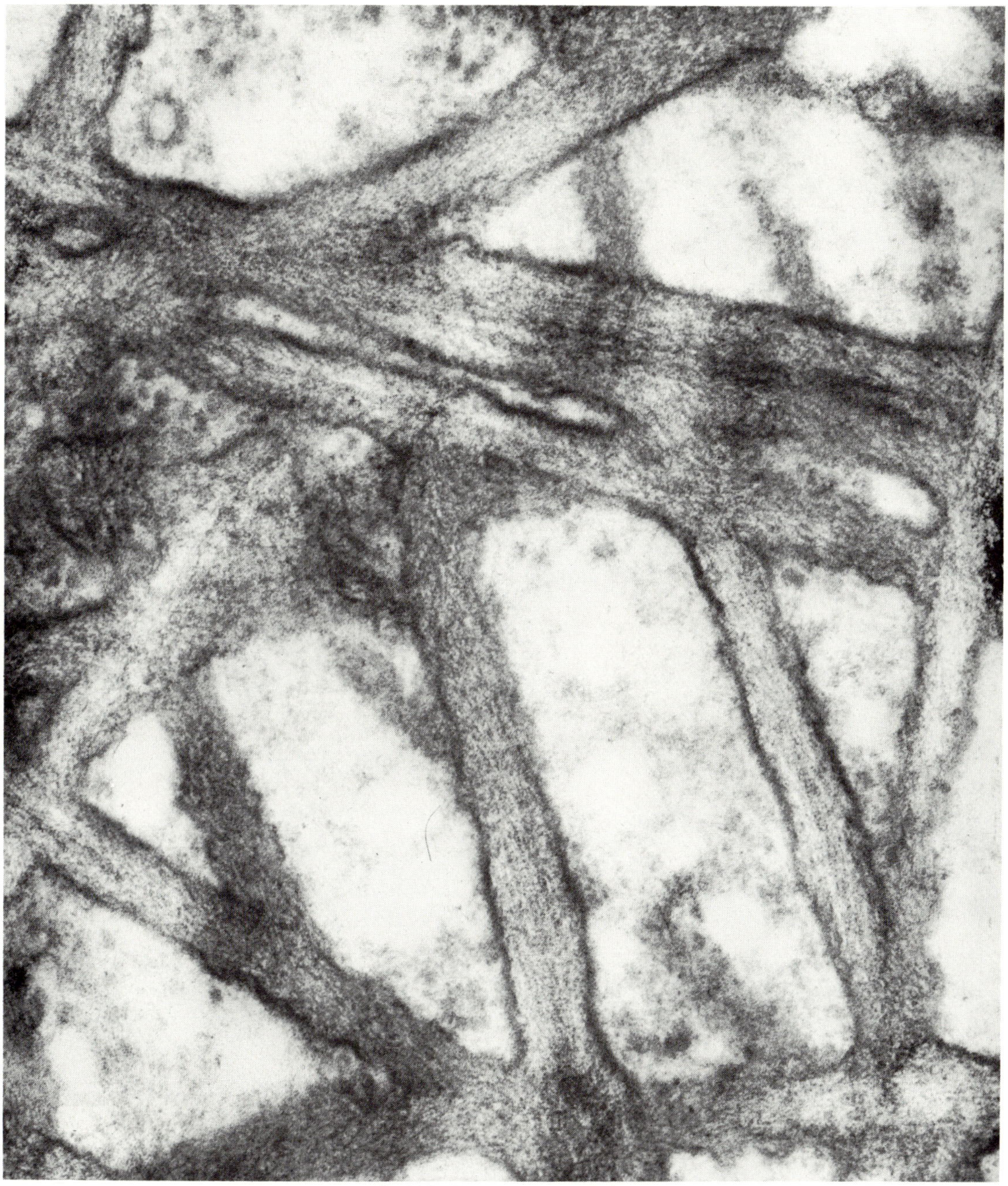

Figure 8–26. Higher magnification of the newly formed elastic fibers seen in Figure 8–25. The fibers have a lighter core and a dense cortex. (× 72,000.)

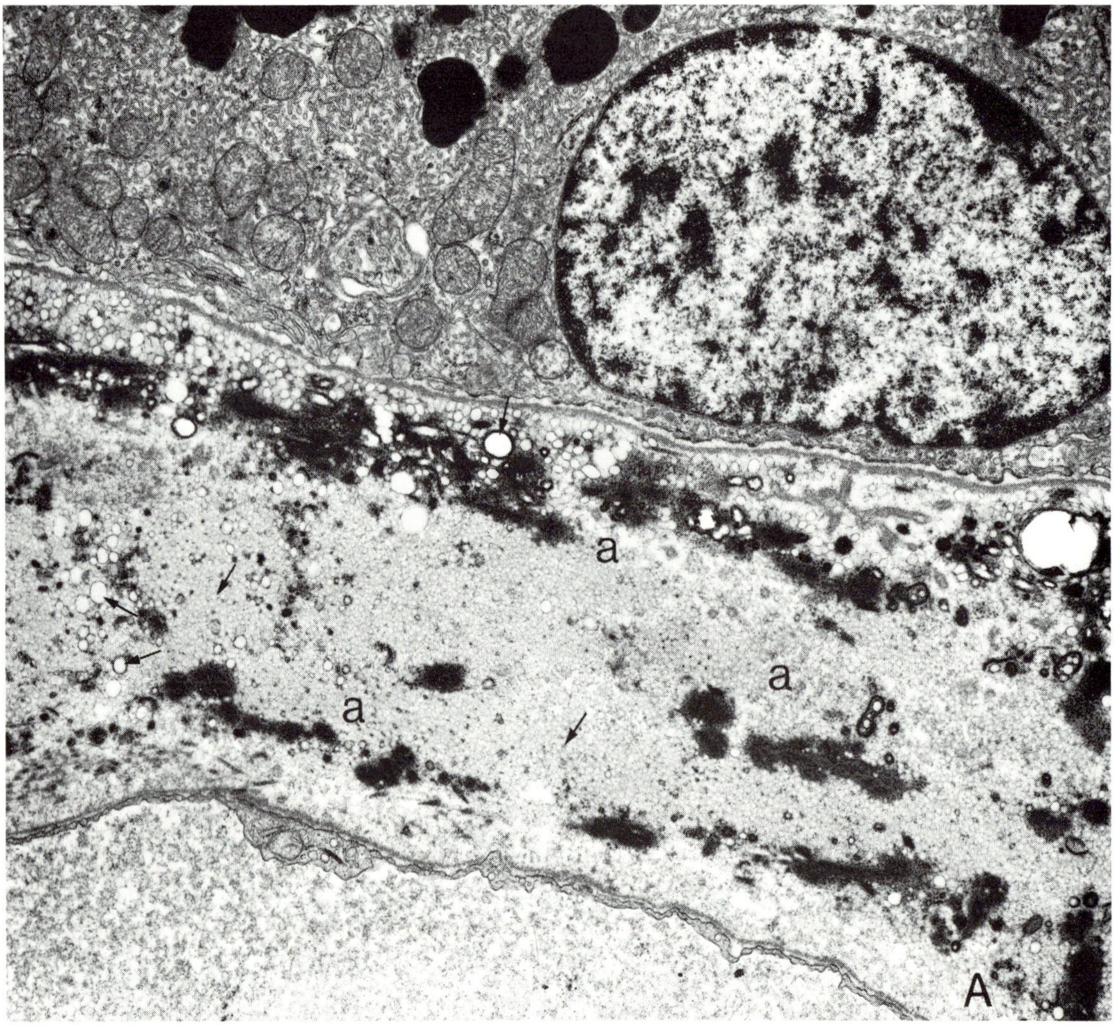

Figure 8-27. Aging changes in Bruch's membrane in the peripapillary region. *A*, The entire thickness of Bruch's membrane is occupied by varying sized vesicular structures (arrows). The splitting of the elastica of Bruch's membrane into layers is a constant finding in this region. (× 9800.)

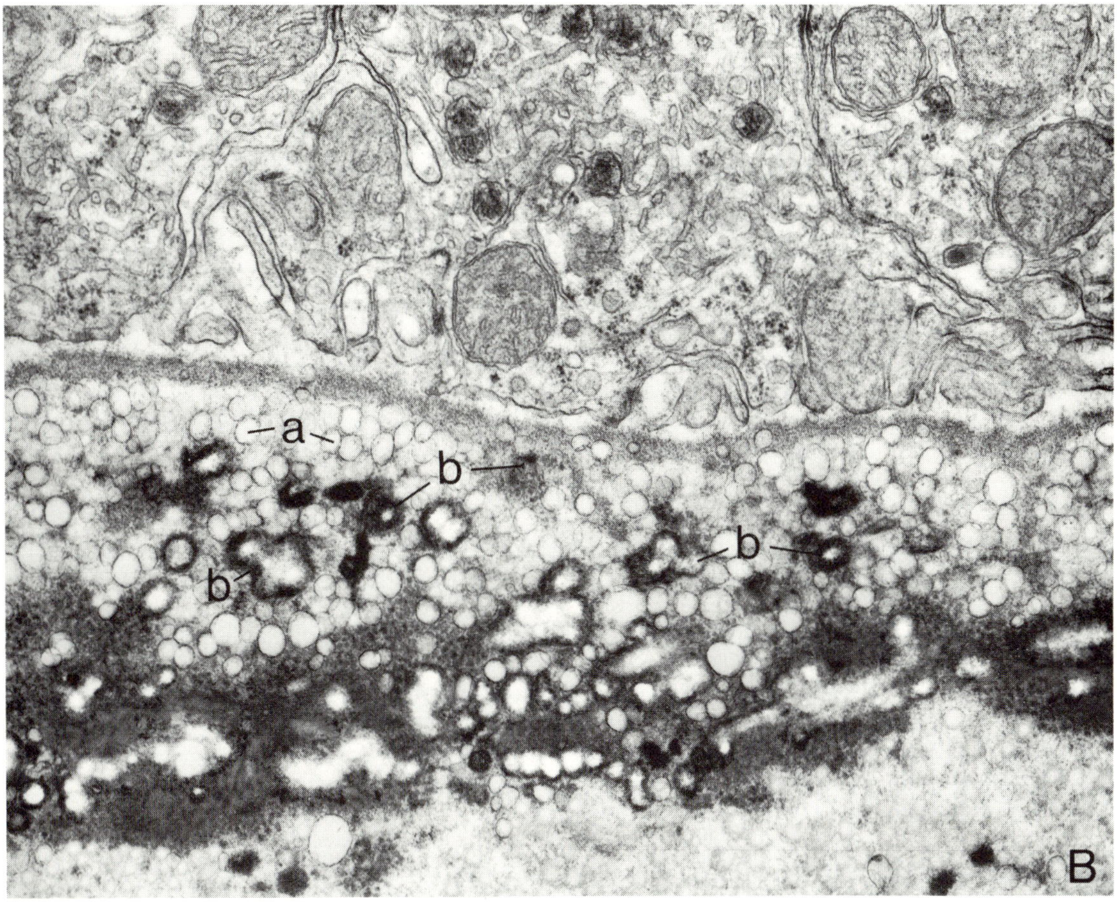

Figure 8–27. *Continued.*

B, Higher magnification of the vesicular structures (a) shown in *A.* Cross-sections (b) of crystallized elastic fibers are seen. (× 26,700.)

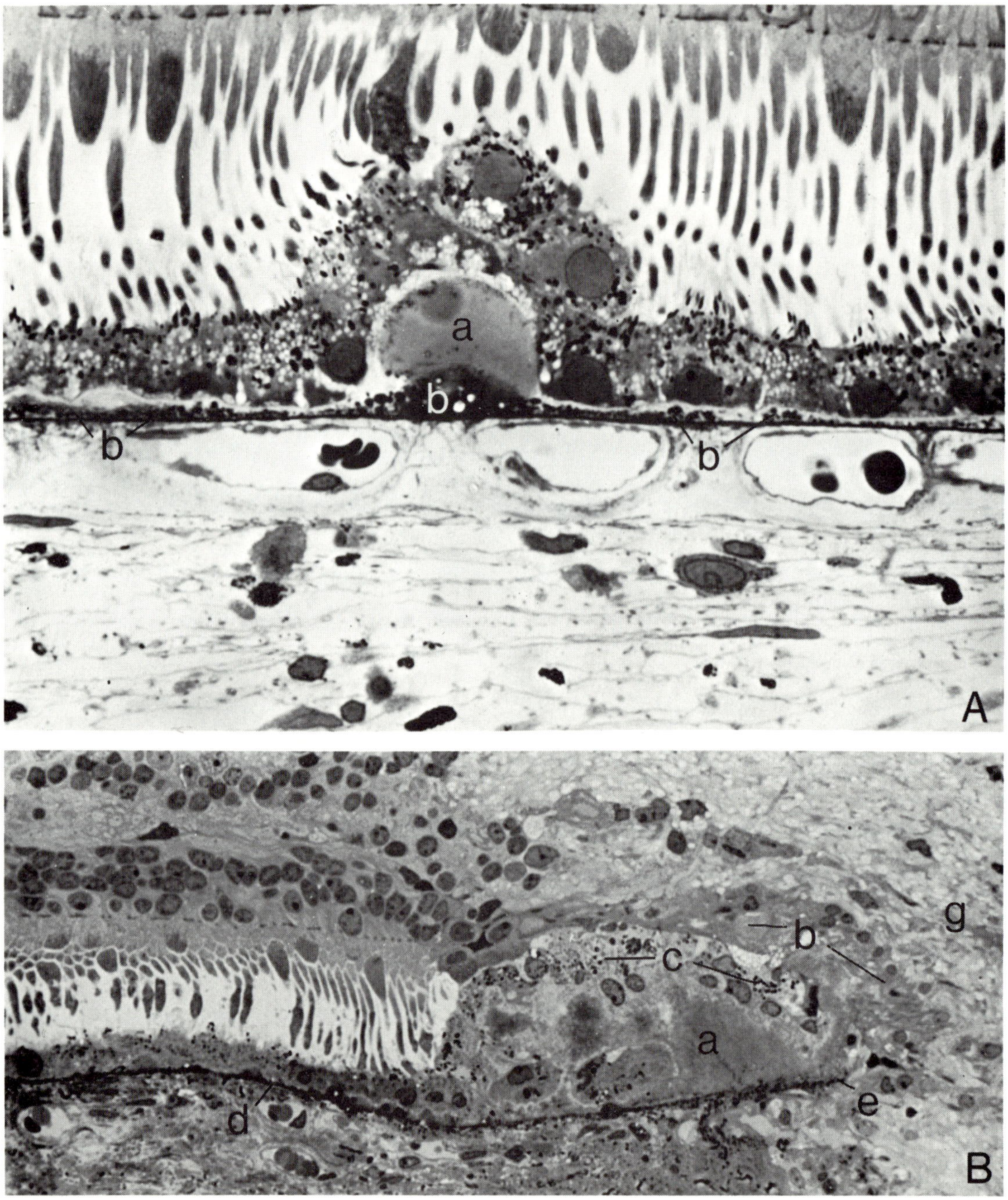

Figure 8-28. Drusen formation in Bruch's membrane. *A*, Drusen are formed in the inner collagenous zone (a), displacing the pigment epithelium internally. The external portion of the drusen (b) contains heavier staining material. This same material is also present elsewhere in the inner collagenous zone. The outer collagenous zone and the intercapillary zone are unaffected. (Approx. × 1000.)

B, Drusen (a) are frequently found at the posterior termination of Bruch's membrane. The astrocytes (b) forming the border tissue of the optic nerve are shown. The pigment epithelium (c) is internal to the drusen. The elastica of Bruch's membrane (d) terminates at (e) against the astrocytic border tissue. (× 425.)

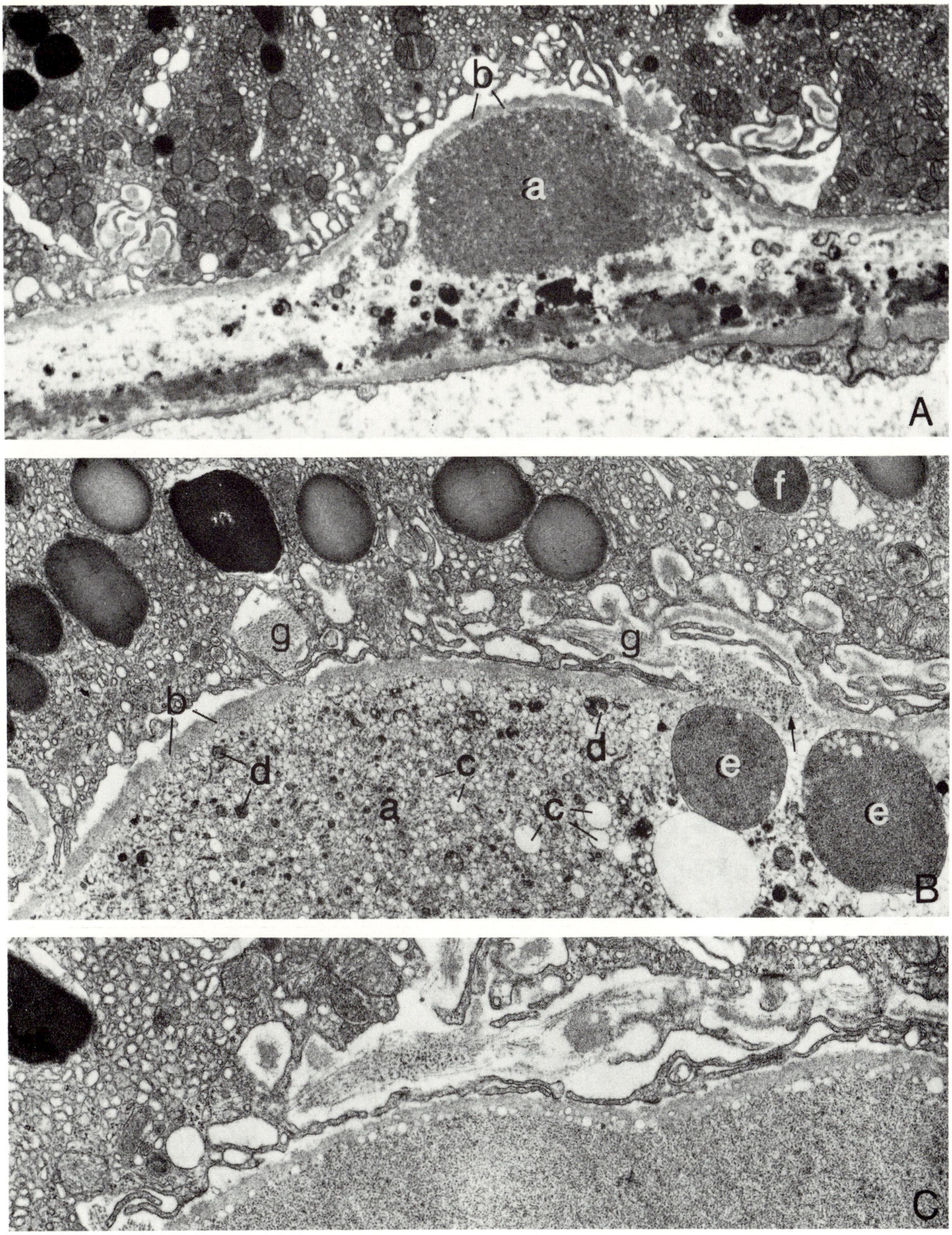

Figure 8–29. Electron micrographs of drusen. *A*, Low-power view of a small drusen (a), which is external to the basement membrane (b) of the retinal pigment epithelium. It occupies the inner collagenous zone. (× 11,000.)

B, Higher magnification of the more common form of drusen (a), under the retinal pigment epithelium (b). The drusen is composed of vesicular (c), electron-dense (d) and large enclosed masses (e), resembling residual bodies seen in the retinal pigment epithelial cytoplasm (f). The basement membrane of the pigment epithelial cells is interrupted (arrows) by a filamentous material, which is also seen between the basal infoldings. (× 13,600.)

C, Higher magnification of another type of drusen composed of a finely granular material. A fibrous material is seen internal to the basement membrane. (× 14,400.)

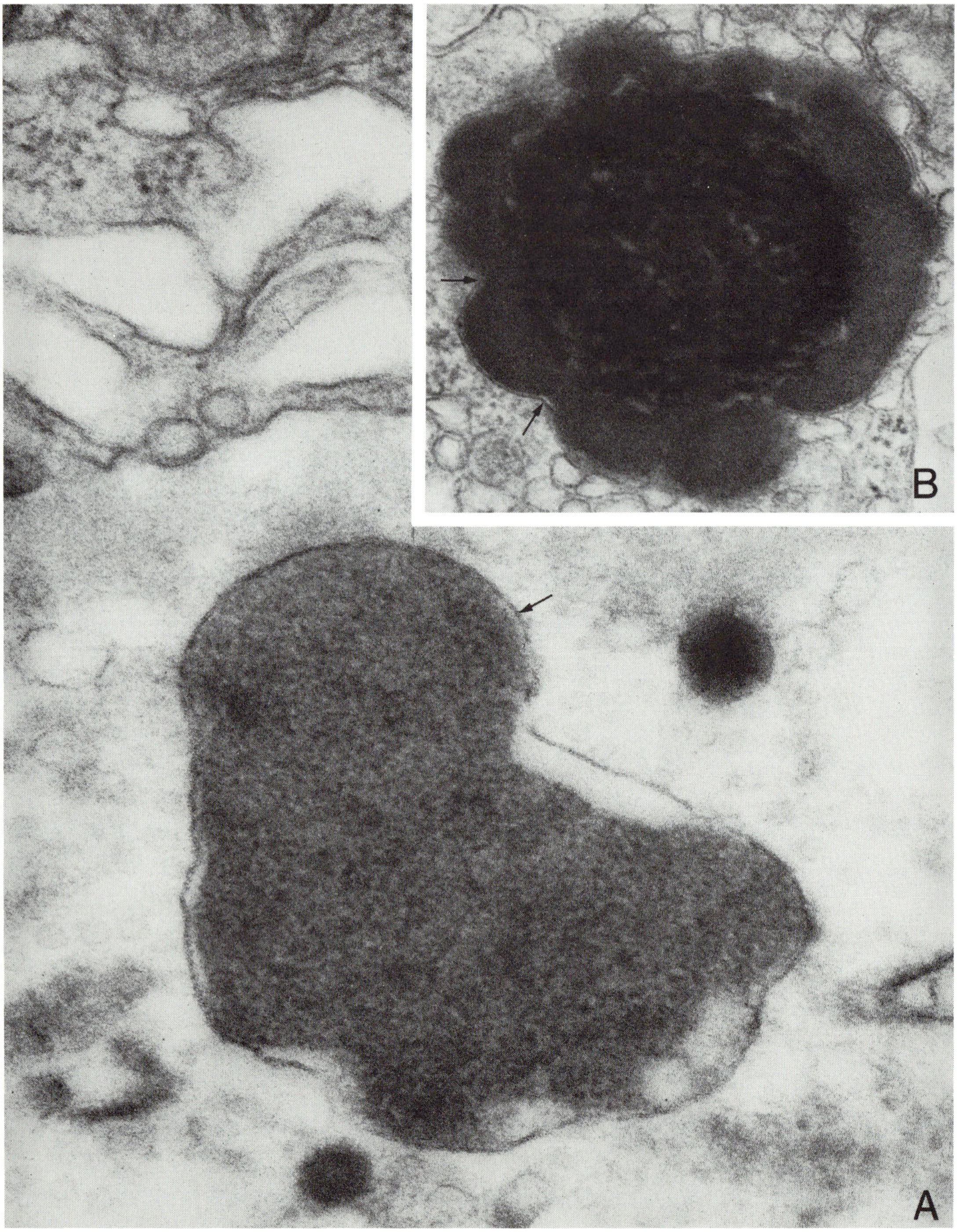

Figure 8-30. Aging changes in Bruch's membrane. *A,* Large membrane-bound structures (arrow) are commonly found near the basement membrane of the retinal pigment epithelium. These structures may be extruded by the pigment epithelium; they resemble residual bodies found within the pigment epithelium. (× 68,000.)

B, A structure like that shown in *A* is seen in the basal cytoplasm of the pigment epithelium. Note the scalloped edges (arrows) of this structure and its resemblance to the discs of the photoreceptors. These are probably residual bodies that are discharged from the pigment epithelium into Bruch's membrane. (× 61,200.)

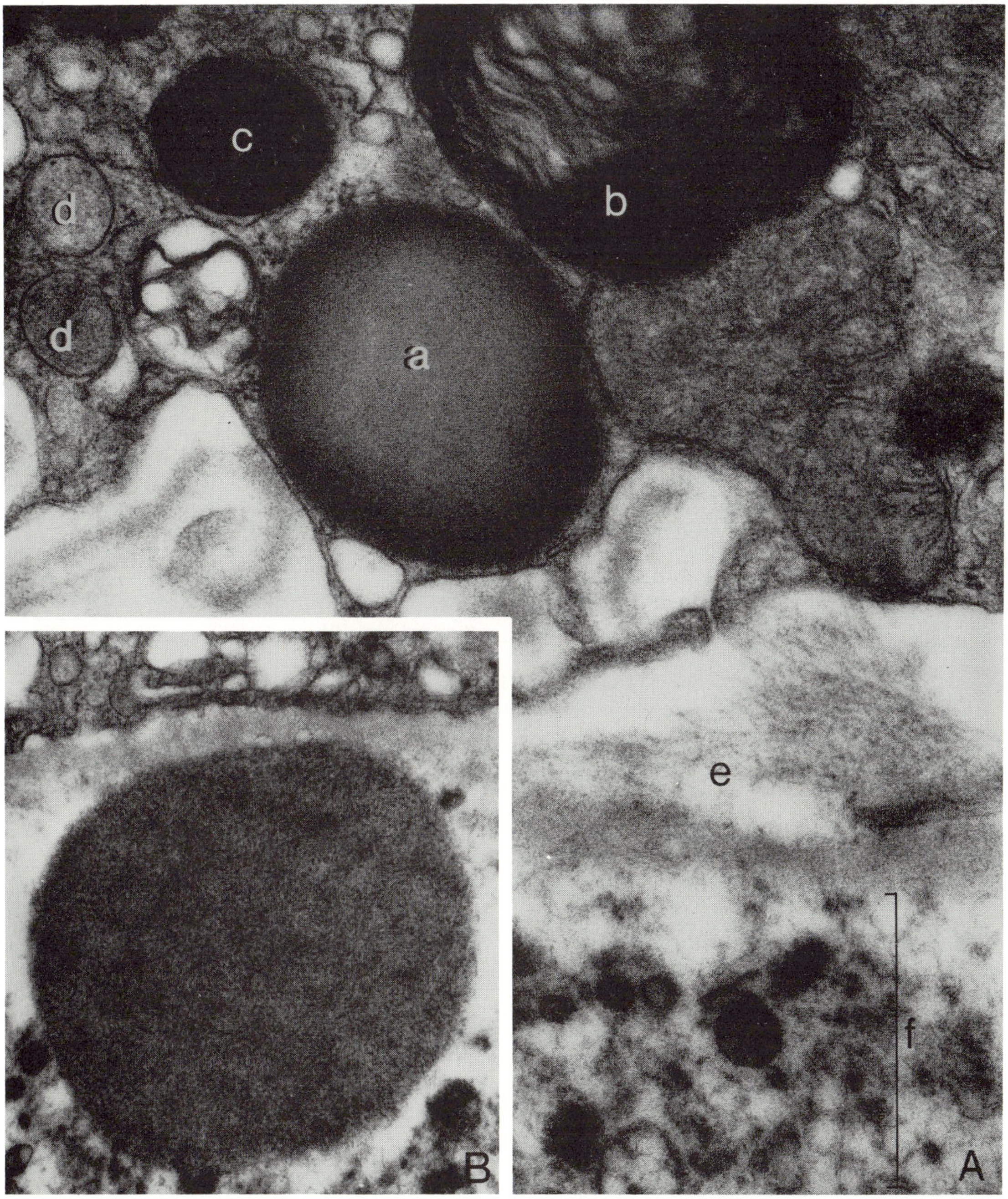

Figure 8–31. Aging changes in the retinal pigment epithelium and in Bruch's membrane. *A*, The basal cytoplasm of the retinal pigment epithelium shows a large, amorphous electron-dense vesicle (a), a membranous vesicle (b), a homogenous extremely electron-dense body (c) and two finely granular membrane-bound vesicles (d). The basement membrane (e) and a number of vesicles occupying the inner collagenous zone (f) are also shown. (× 48,000.)

B, An osmiophilic rounded structure is shown in the inner collagenous zone of Bruch's membrane; compare it with those shown above in the basal cytoplasm of the pigment epithelium. (× 3400.)

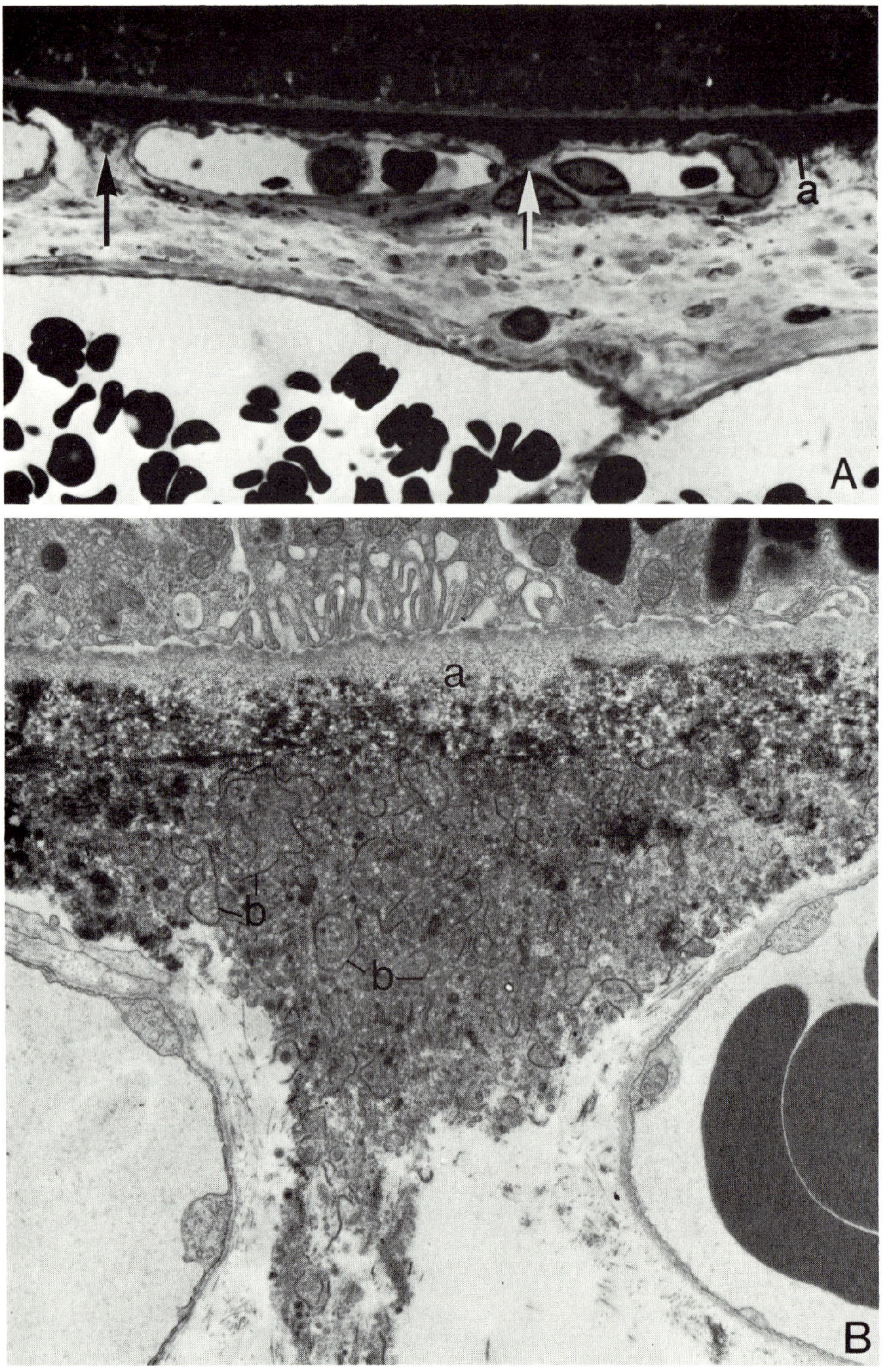

Figure 8–32. Light micrograph of late aging changes in Bruch's membrane. *A*, The inner and outer collagenous zones of Bruch's membrane are filled with a dense-staining material (a). The material is basophilic and PAS-positive. It also occupies the intercapillary zone (arrows). The choroidal stroma is normal. (Approx. × 1200.)

B, Electron micrograph of Bruch's membrane in the intercapillary zone. There is an accumulation of vesicular material (a) and electron-dense filaments (b). The filaments may represent crystallized collagen fibrils. (× 14,800.)

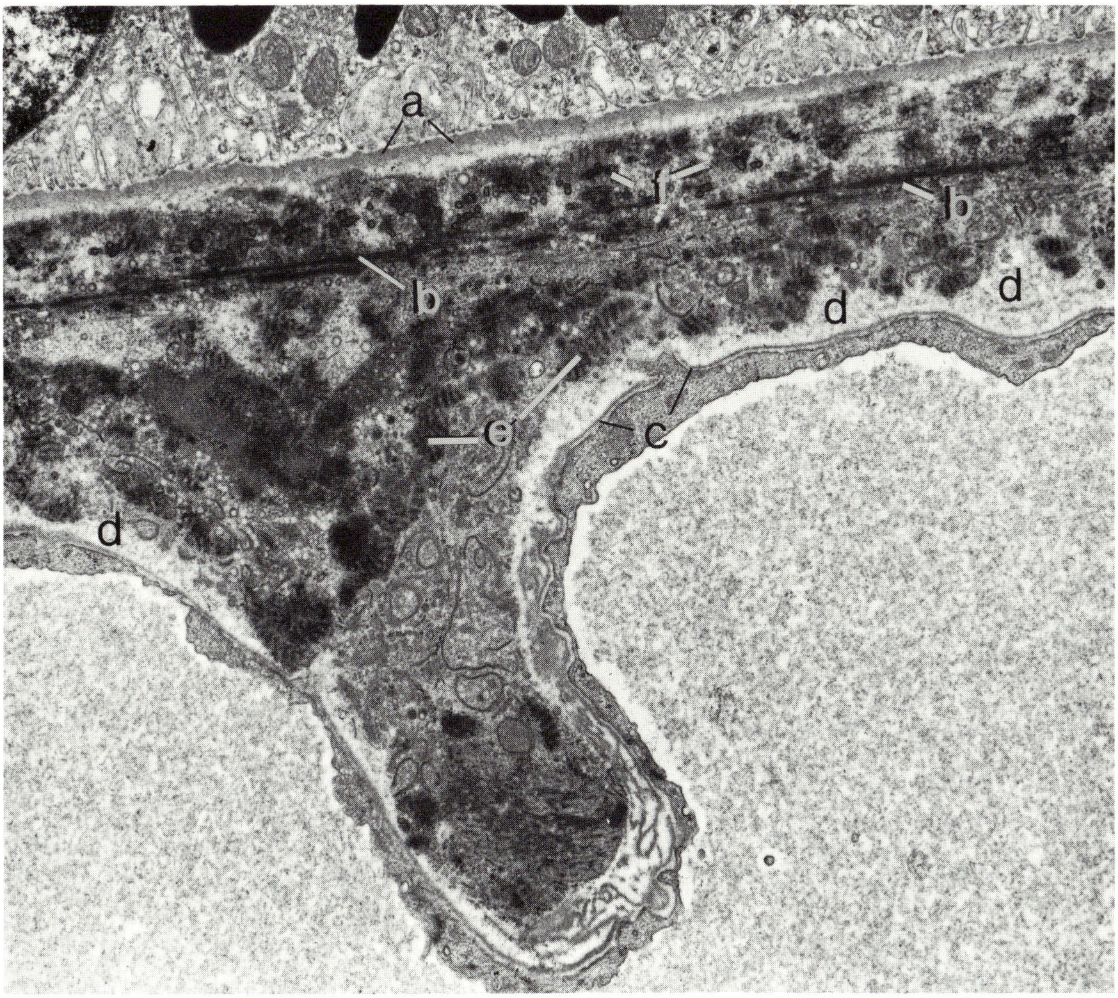

Figure 8–33. Late aging changes of Bruch's membrane. The basement membrane of the retinal pigment epithelium (a), the elastica (b) and the basement membrane of the choriocapillary endothelium (c) are shown. All of Bruch's membrane appears to be occupied by vesicles and filamentous material except for a narrow zone (d) near the endothelium. There is a considerable amount of wide-spacing collagen (e) and some crystallized elastic tissue (f). (× 7200.)

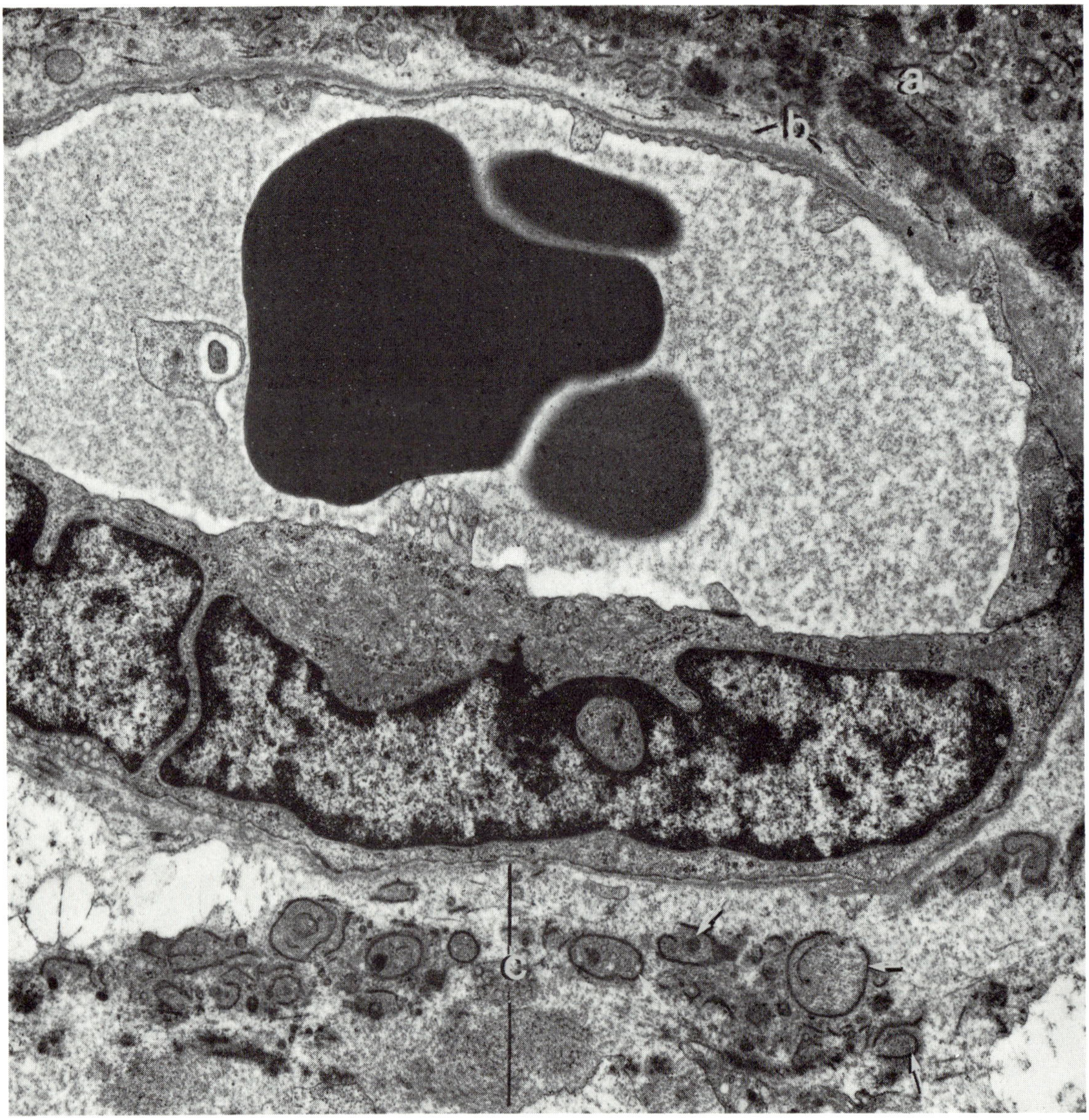

Figure 8-34. Late aging changes of Bruch's membrane and the choriocapillaris. The outer collagenous zone (a), the basement membrane of the capillary endothelium (b) and the subcapillary connective tissue (c) are shown. The changes in advanced age finally involve the subcapillary tissues (arrows). Very electron-dense filaments, which are curved, and widespacing collagen often accumulate in considerable amount. (× 6400.)

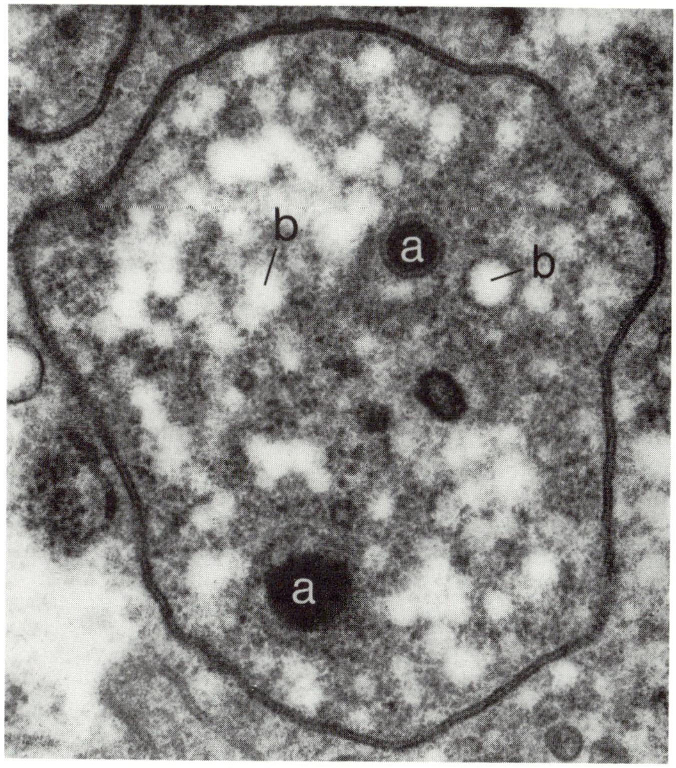

Figure 8–35. Enlargement of a mass of electron-dense vesicles (a) and electron-lucent material (b) which are enclosed in a dense calcified fiber. (× 47,600.)

collagenous zone, displacing the overlying epithelium internally; crystals are commonly seen in this granular material. The cytoplasm of the retinal pigment epithelial cells often shows structures exactly like those accumulated in the drusen.

Other drusen have been observed in which the material accumulated in the inner collagenous zone is finely fibrillar. When the fibrils are cut in cross-section this material appears to be finely granular. These fibrils first appear internal to the basement membrane of the pigment epithelium, but similar structures cannot be recognized in the epithelial cytoplasm.

The intercapillary region of older eyes shows pronounced changes. There is an increase in the amount of vesicular material, clumps of wide-spacing fibers, long, coiled osmiophilic fibers and dark, granular ground substance. These changes frequently extend into the subcapillary connective tissue in a less pronounced form.

Choriocapillaris (Figs. 8–36 to 8–43)

The capillaries of the choroid are located *solely* in the internal portion of the choroid. Their afferent arterial supply is from three sources: mainly from the short posterior ciliary vessels, which enter the choroid around the optic disc and branch extensively as they pass forward and internally in the choroid; from recurrent branches of the long ciliary vessels which pass back from the ora region to supply part of this tissue as far back as the equator;

Text continued on page 369

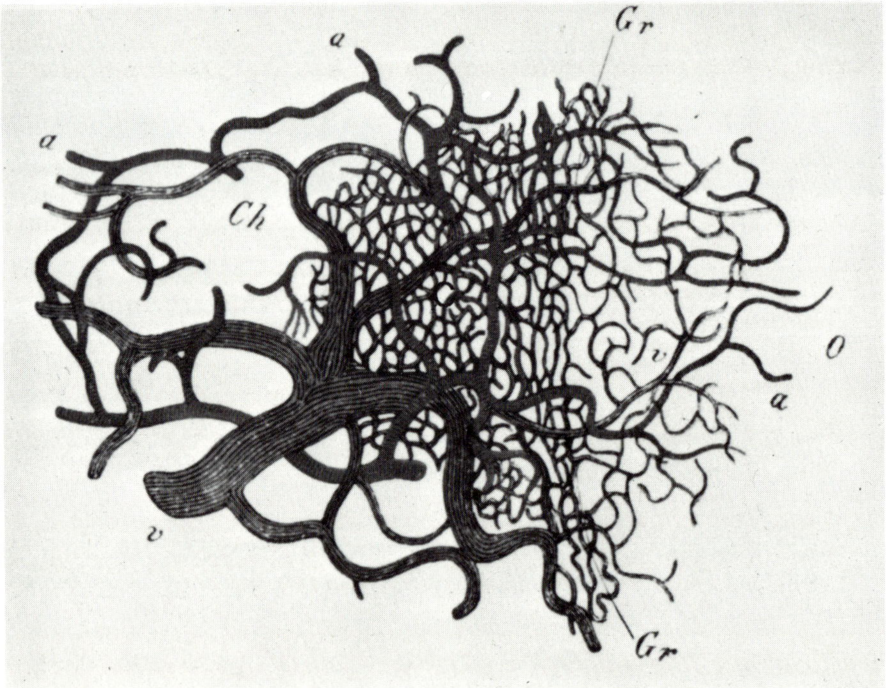

Figure 8–36. Circulation of the choroid. In the center is the choriocapillaris (c), which is formed rather suddenly by the branching of the posterior ciliary arteries (a). Venules and veins (v) collect blood from the choriocapillaris. The choriocapillaris forms a single layer along the inner choroid. (From Leber, Graefe Saemisch Handbuch ges. Augenheilk., 2nd ed., Leipzig 2 (2), 1903.)

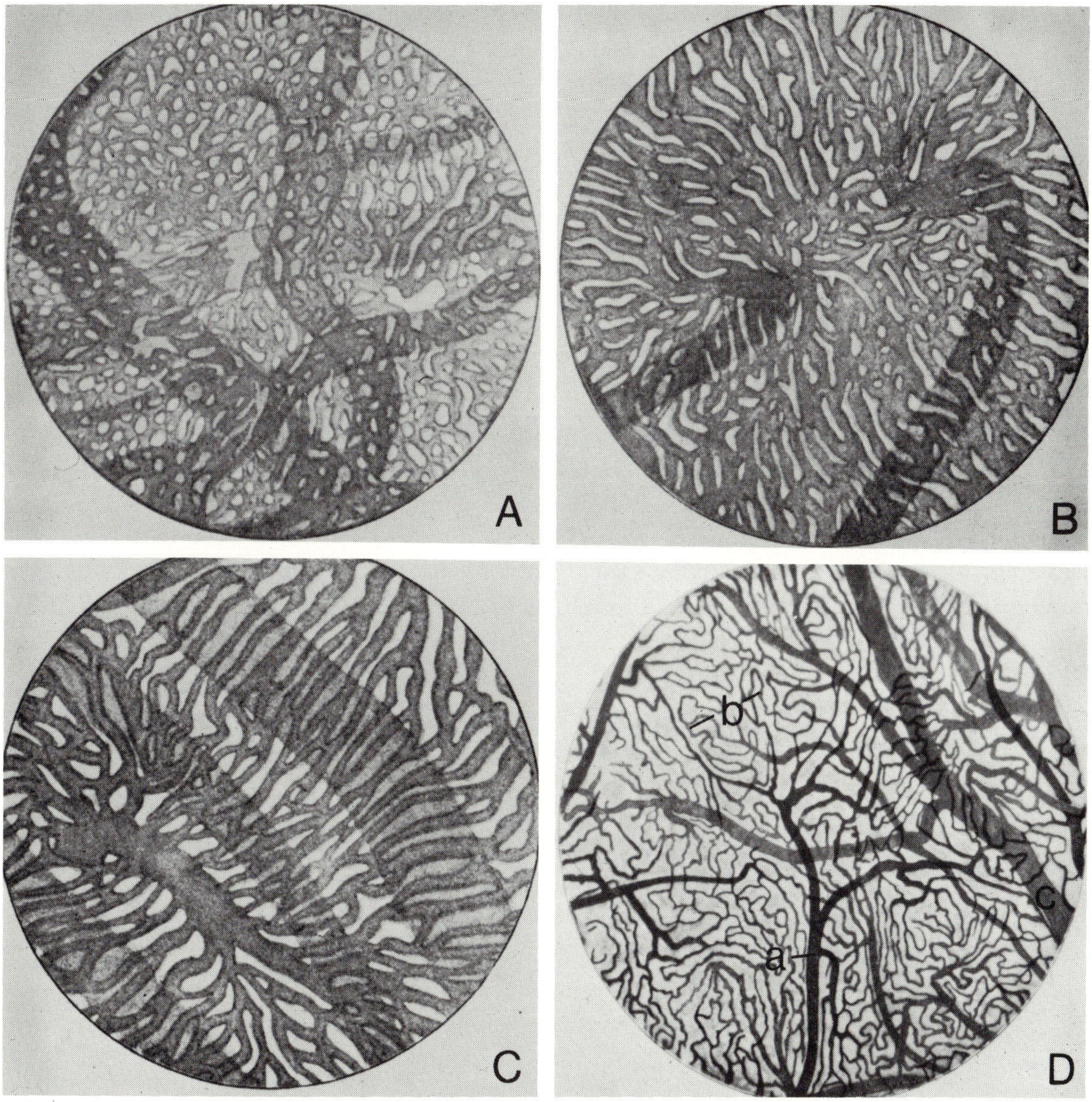

Figure 8–37. Circulation of the choroid. Regional differences in the pattern of the choriocapillaris. *A*, Macular capillary bed. The capillaries have a fairly uniform caliber and they branch frequently to form a net with small meshes.

B, Equatorial capillary bed. The meshes are wider and longer than in the posterior eye.

C, Peripheral choroid. In this region the meshwork is quite open, the branching is less frequent and the caliber of the vessels is more variable.

D, Detail of the distribution of the arterial and venous circulation of the choroid. The short posterior ciliary artery (a) enters the choroid around the optic nerve and quickly sends branches to the choriocapillaris (b). Venules in the inner choroid collect arterial blood and return it to the vortex system (c). (From Leber, Graefe Saemisch Handbuch ges. Augenheilk., 2nd ed., Leipzig 2(2), 1903.)

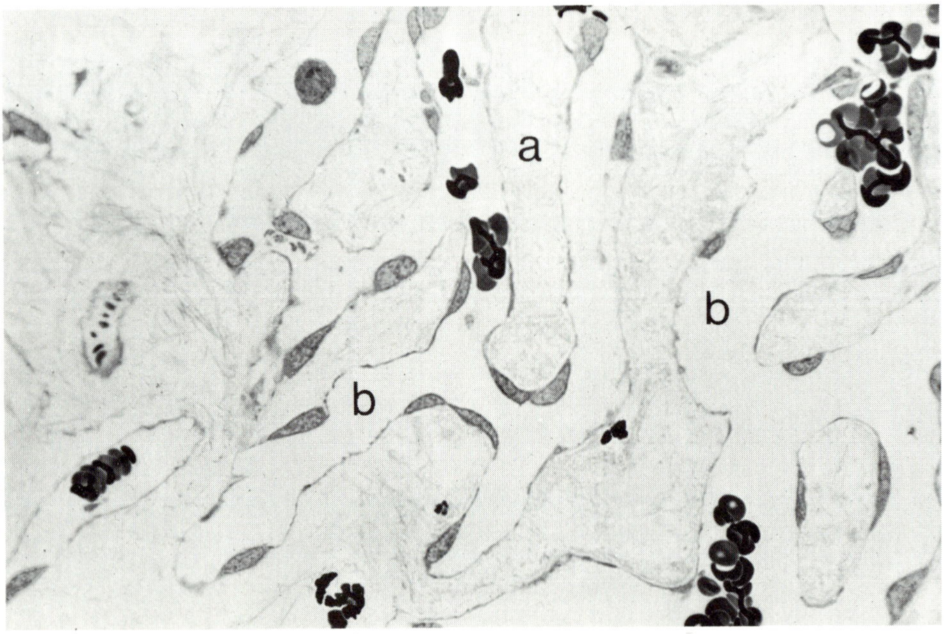

Figure 8–38. Choriocapillaris sectioned on the flat to show the fine meshes (a) formed by these vessels in the posterior choroid. The pattern is formed by the capillary lumina (b). (× 560.)

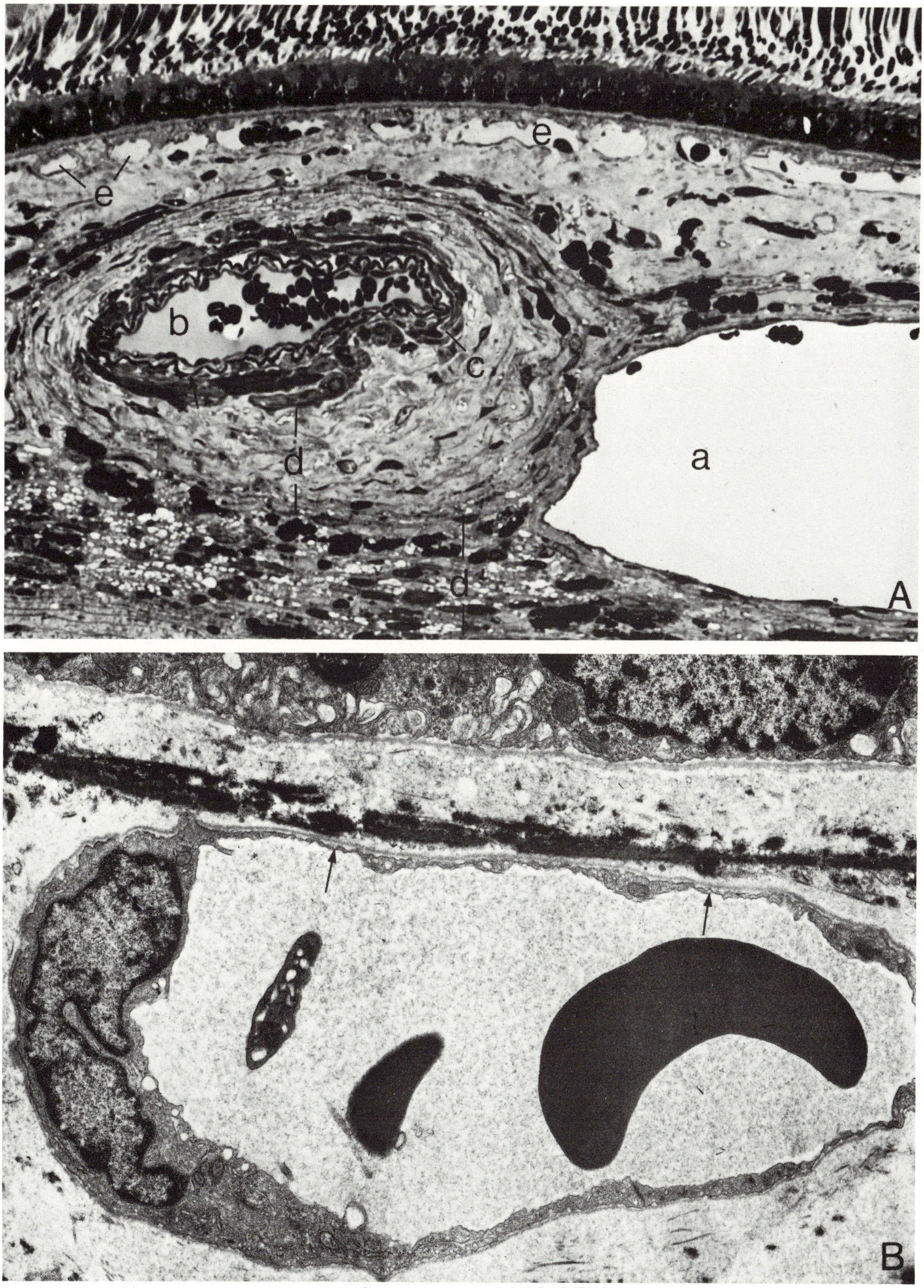

Figure 8–39. Light micrographs of the choroidal vessels. *A*, The thin wall of a vein (a) and its companion artery (b) are seen. The muscularis (c) and adventitia (d) of the artery are well developed. The suprachoroidea is at (d) and the choriocapillaris is at (e). (× 480.)

B, Electron micrograph of the choriocapillaris. The internal endothelial wall is very thin and contains numerous pores (arrows). (× 5000.)

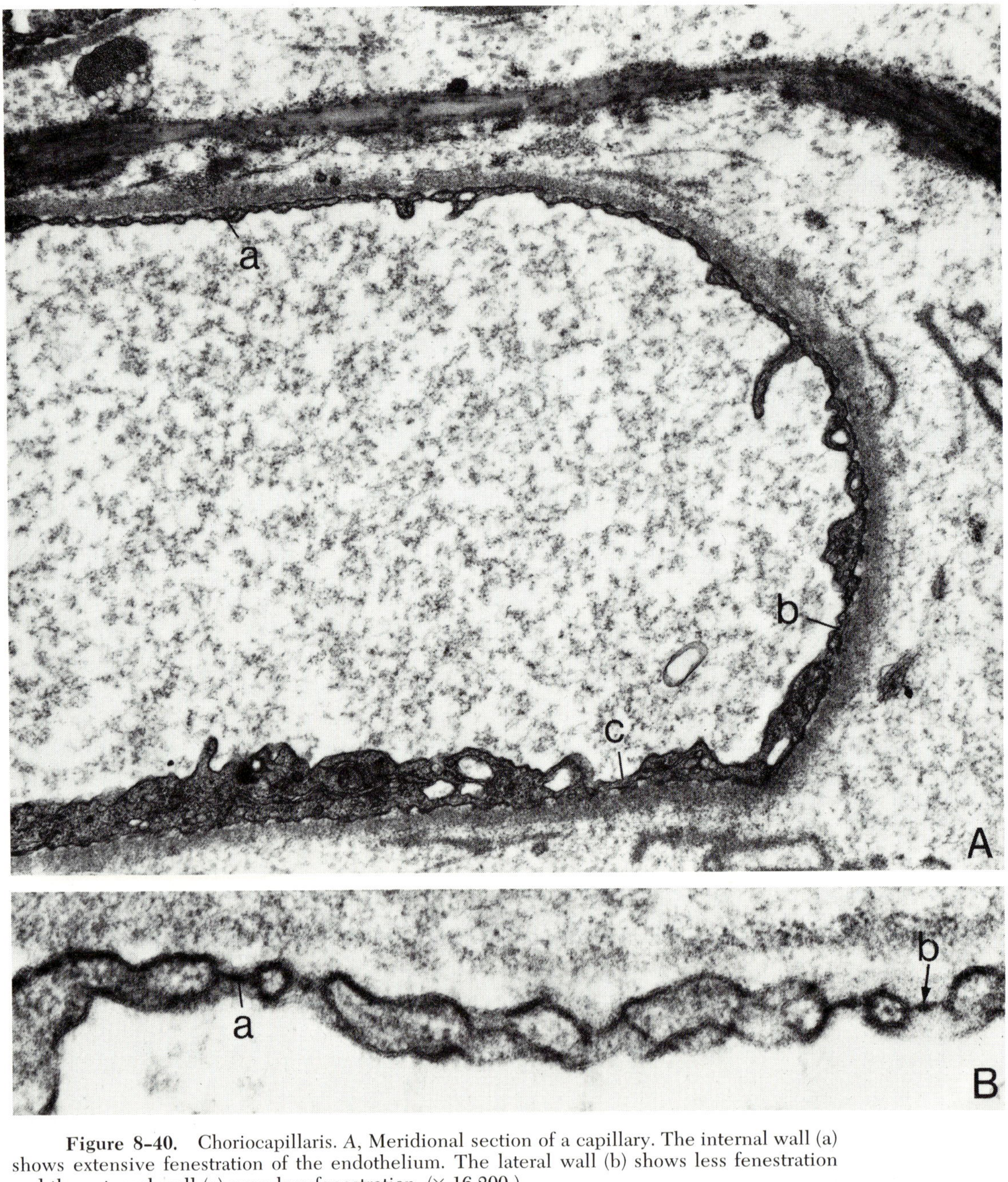

Figure 8–40. Choriocapillaris. *A*, Meridional section of a capillary. The internal wall (a) shows extensive fenestration of the endothelium. The lateral wall (b) shows less fenestration and the external wall (c) even less fenestration. (× 16,200.)

B, Higher magnification of the internal wall. There are numerous fenestrations (a) in the endothelium; they show a diaphragm that contains a central density (b). (× 82,800.)

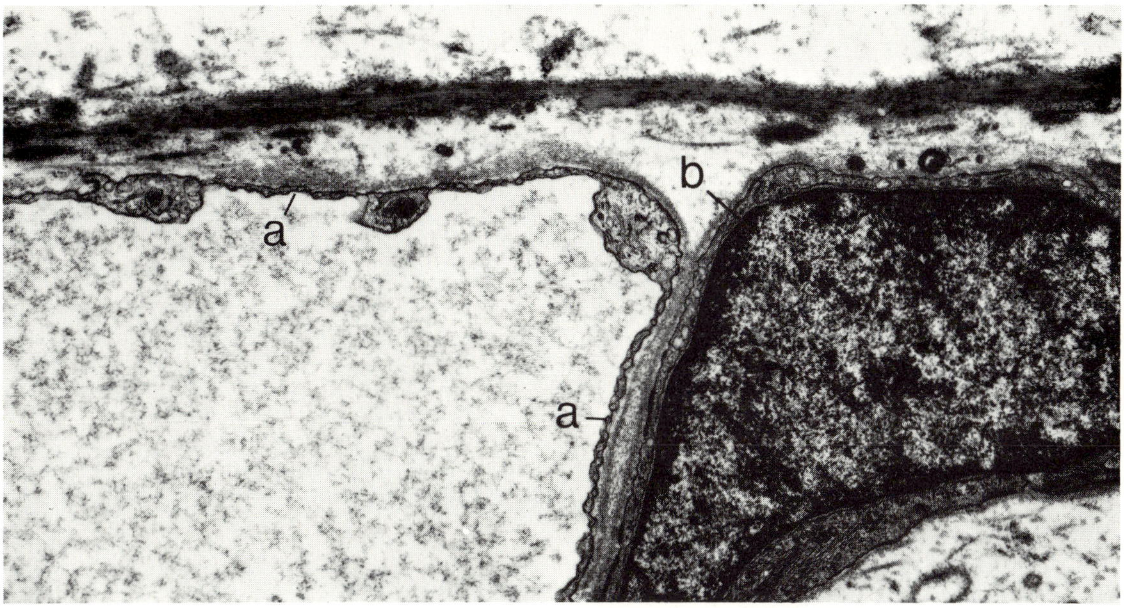

Figure 8–41. Choriocapillaris. Meridional section of the internal and lateral walls of the choriocapillaris to show the endothelial fenestrations along both walls (a), and a pericyte (b) along the lateral wall. This pericyte is surrounded by a thin basement membrane that is continuous with that of the endothelial cell. (× 15,000.)

and from a number of branches of the anterior ciliary arteries which pass back in the ciliary muscle, then enter the choriocapillaris. There are extensive anastomoses between the anterior and posterior arterial systems. The venous return is to venules lying external to the capillary zone, then into the vortex system. The meshes of the choriocapillaris are very small and somewhat oval in the posterior eye, where they measure about 3 by 18 μm. in diameter. The meshes become slightly wider and longer in the equatorial region, where they measure 6 to 36 μm. wide by 36 to 400 μm. long. In the peripheral third of the choroid the meshes become very irregular because of the entrance of arterioles and venules into the choriocapillary layer. Flat or tangential sections of the capillaries show sac-like or local widenings along their course, and their afferent and efferent vessels often enter the layer at somewhat oblique angles.

The choriocapillary vessels differ from those in other organs as well as those of the retina by the greater diameters of their lumina. In most capillaries the red blood cells traverse the lumen in single file or are deformed during their passage. In the choriocapillaris they can pass through at least two to three abreast. In the macular region the capillary diameter is about 20 μm., and elsewhere it varies between 18 and 50 μm.

Fibroblasts and some nerve fibers are found in the connective tissue of the subcapillary zone (see Figs. 8–4 *A* and *B* and 8–5 *A*.). Pericytes have been seen only occasionally in our preparations. The entire collagenous network around, between and beneath the capillaries is important not only because it provides a rigid framework for the support of this vascular layer, but also because it helps to support the retina. This collagen also develops profound changes in some eyes as a result of aging.

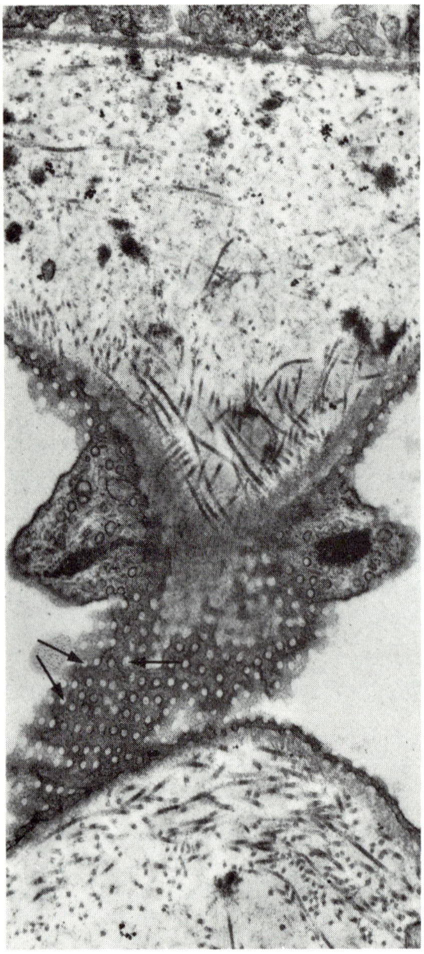

Figure 8–42. Grazing section of the internal and lateral walls of two adjoining capillaries. The circular fenestrations (arrows) containing small central densities are very regularly distributed along the wall. (× 18,200.)

The ultrastructure of these capillaries shows them to be of the visceral type, with fenestrae similar to those in the renal glomerulus and other organs (Fig. 8–18). The endothelial cells have numerous circular fenestrations measuring 800 A. in diameter. Unlike the fenestrations of the renal glomerular capillaries, those of the choriocapillaris have a diaphragm covering them. In flat sections these fenestrae clearly show a central density; meridional sections occasionally show a corresponding density. The endothelial cells are joined by sloping, somewhat folded borders, the intercellular space measuring 100 A. An occluding junction is seen between the cells near the lumen, and marginal folds are common.

External to the endothelium is a well developed basement membrane which is thinner than that of the retinal epithelium. The subcapillary connective tissue is dense, with marked imbrication of the fibrils. Cell processes are seen in the outermost of these fibrils, but this area is not too cellular. Just external to the capillary zone, nerve plexuses are seen frequently and ganglion cells are not rare. Unmyelinated nerve filaments extend into the subcapillary region from these plexuses, but no specific type of innervation has been observed.

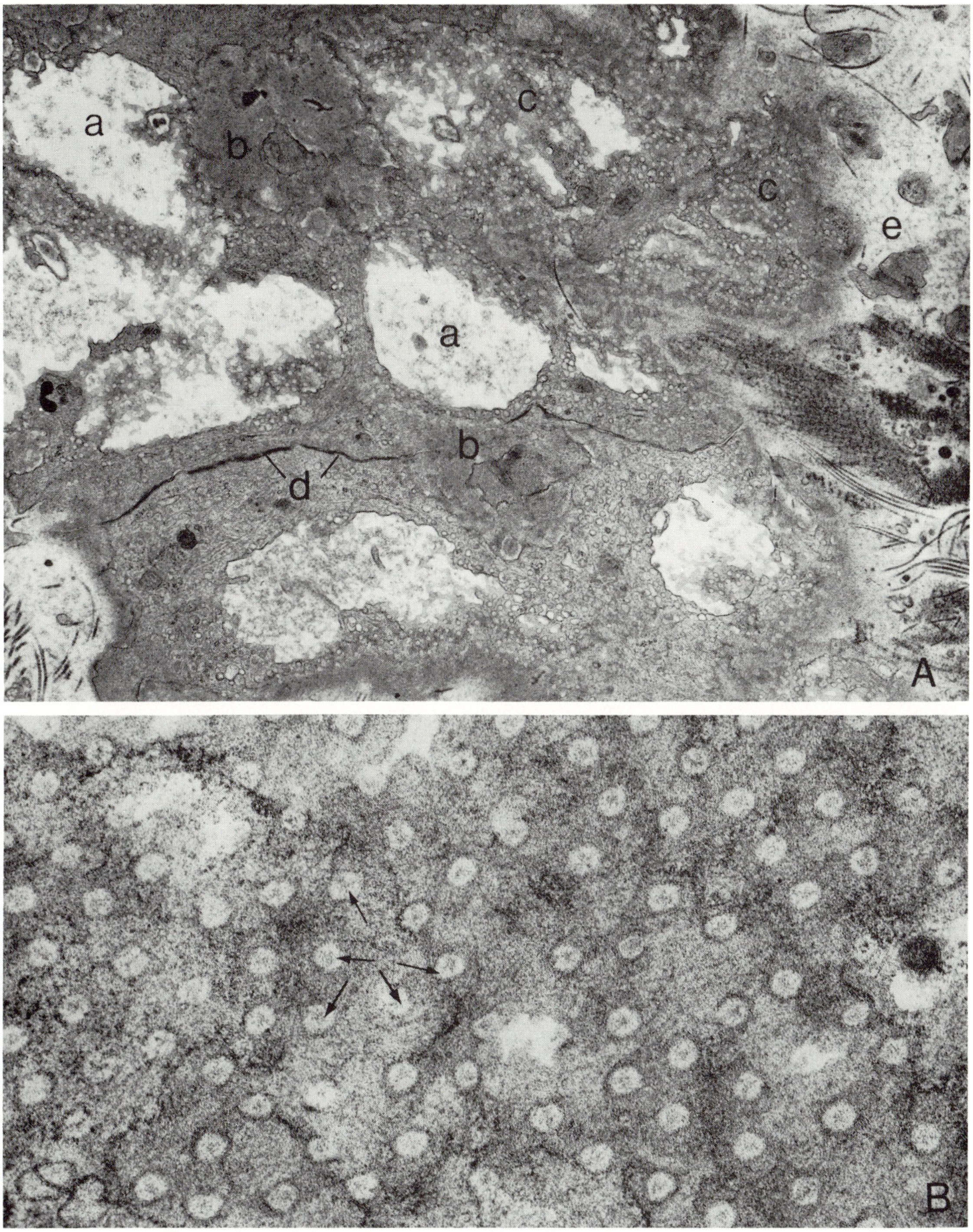

Figure 8-43. Choriocapillaris. *A*, Low-magnification electron micrograph of the internal wall of a capillary. The capillary lumen is at (a), the basement membrane at (b), and the endothelium with its fenestrations is seen at (c). Part of a zonula occludens is seen at (d), and the outer collagenous zone is at (e). (× 12,300.)

B, Higher magnification of a flat section of the internal endothelium of the choriocapillaris to show the regular disposition of the fenestrations. The diaphragm of each fenestration has a central density (arrows). (× 57,500.)

Stroma

Blood Vessels (Figs. 8–3, 8–44 to 8–47). The short ciliary arteries are small vessels which originally lie in the outer choroid and are distributed to the choriocapillaris. Their branches pass into the choroid and extend forward to the equator, where they anastomose with recurrent branches from the long posterior and anterior ciliary arteries. Extensive anastomoses exist between the various branches of all the short ciliary arteries, so that occlusion of one vessel ordinarily does not produce infarction of the choroid. These vessels do not form a large number of branches in the choroid, however, the apparent frequency of their branching is related to their tortuous courses. In meridional section the arteries are seen in cross-section, oblique section and longitudinal section. They become arteriolar in caliber in the connective tissue beneath the capillaries, then pierce this layer as they form the capillaries. With van Gieson stain and connective tissue stains, the arterial walls are typical of small arteries, with an endothelium, a folded internal elastic lamina, and an average of two muscle layers in the media. The adventitia is collagenous and is oriented circularly about the muscularis. Anterior to the macular region the arteries possess a single layer of muscle, and beyond the equator they are almost all of arteriolar caliber. The recurrent vessels from the ciliary body are almost all of arteriolar

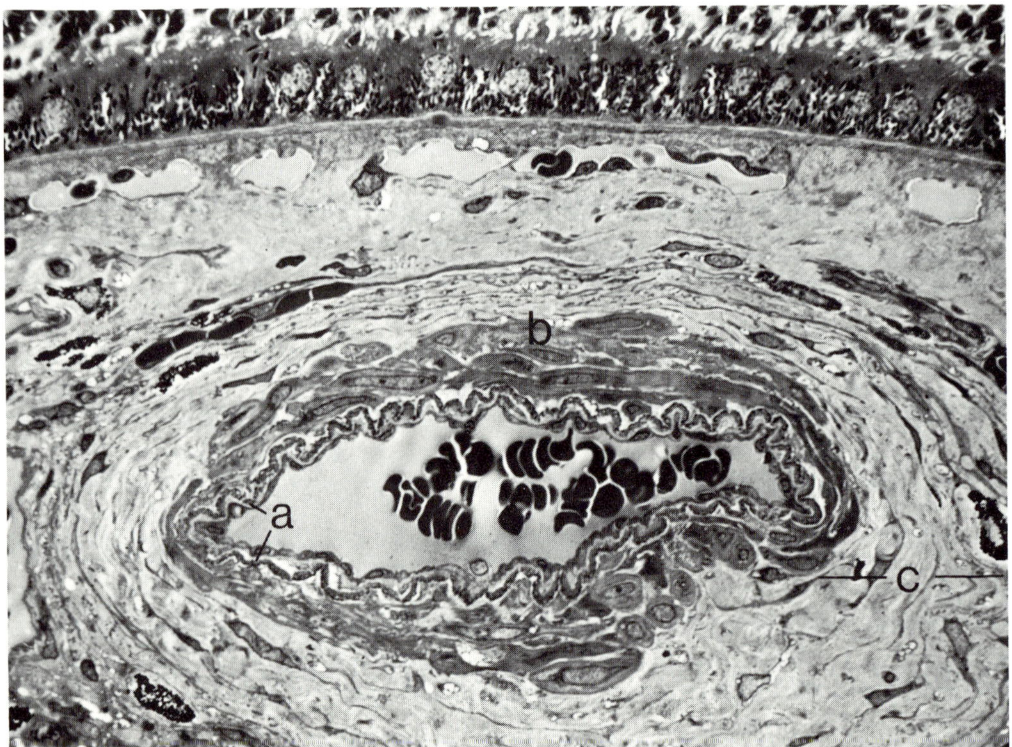

Figure 8–44. Phase-contrast light micrograph of a short posterior ciliary artery. The internal elastic lamina is thick and quite tortuous (a). There are two to three layers of muscle tissue in the media (b). The adventitia is thick and cellular, with the collagen being oriented circularly around the vessel (c). In its outer portion are numerous fibroblasts and melanocytes. (× 1700.)

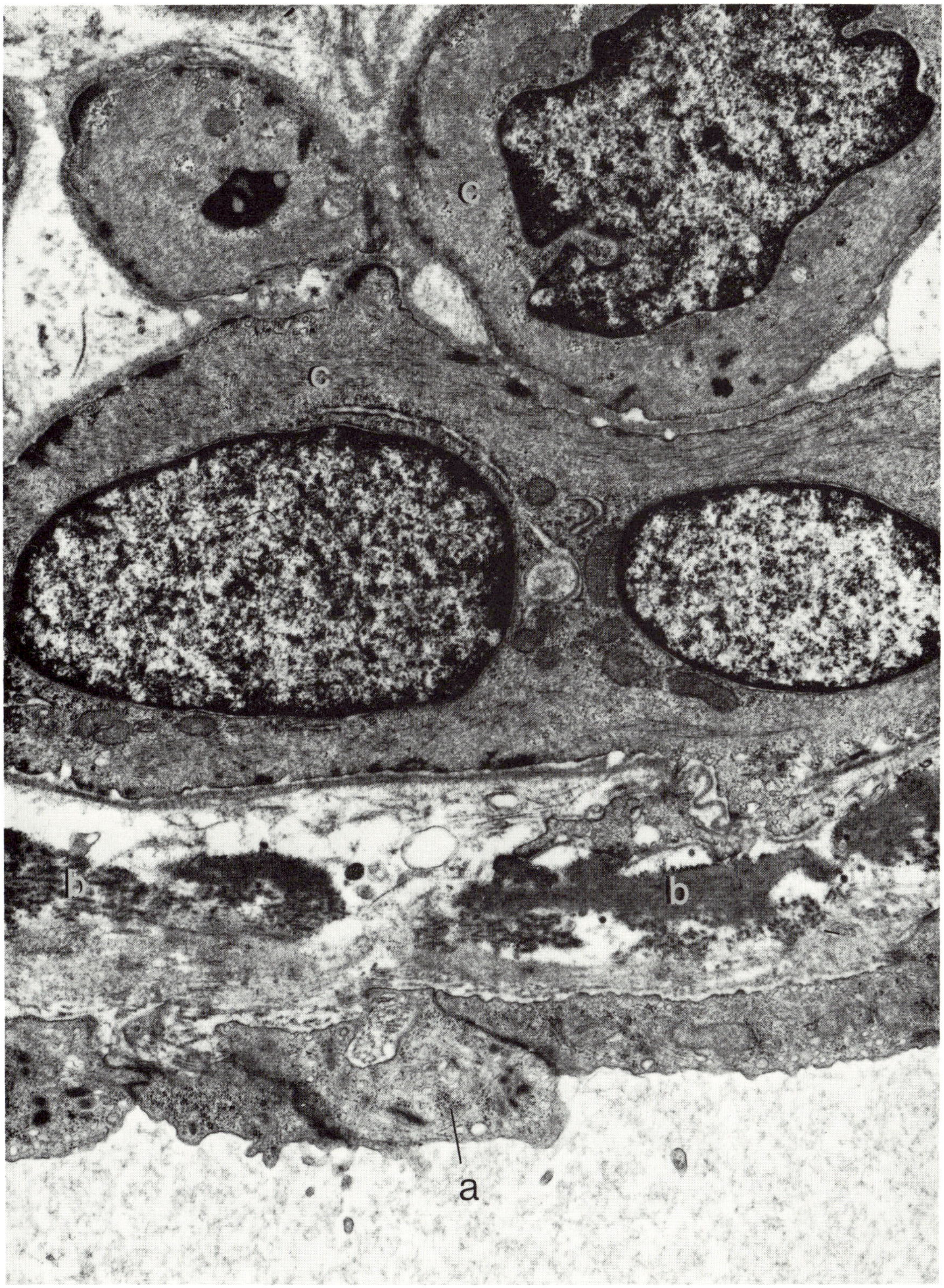

Figure 8-45. Electron micrograph of a short posterior ciliary artery. The endothelium (a) has a thin basement membrane along its outer surface. This membrane is continuous with the elastica (b), which appears to be formed of layers of elastic fibers surrounded by a granular ground substance. Two layers of typical arterial smooth muscle are seen (c). (× 10,800.)

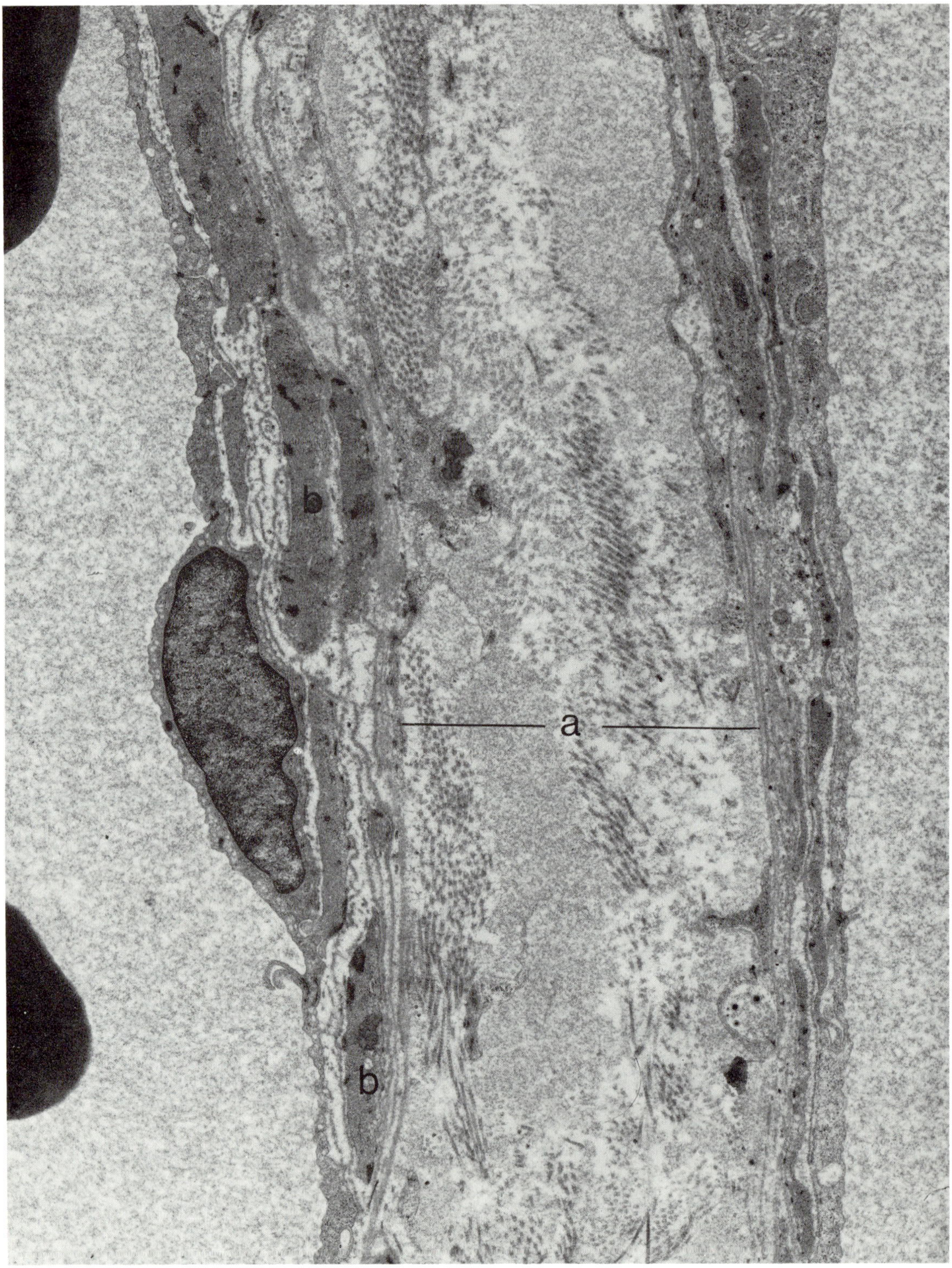

Figure 8-46. Electron micrograph of the walls of two choroidal veins, cut longitudinally. The adventitia (a) of these two vessels is continuous. The vein on the left shows a more prominent thin layer of muscle cells (b). There is no elastic tissue in the intima, and the endothelium is thick. (× 9000.)

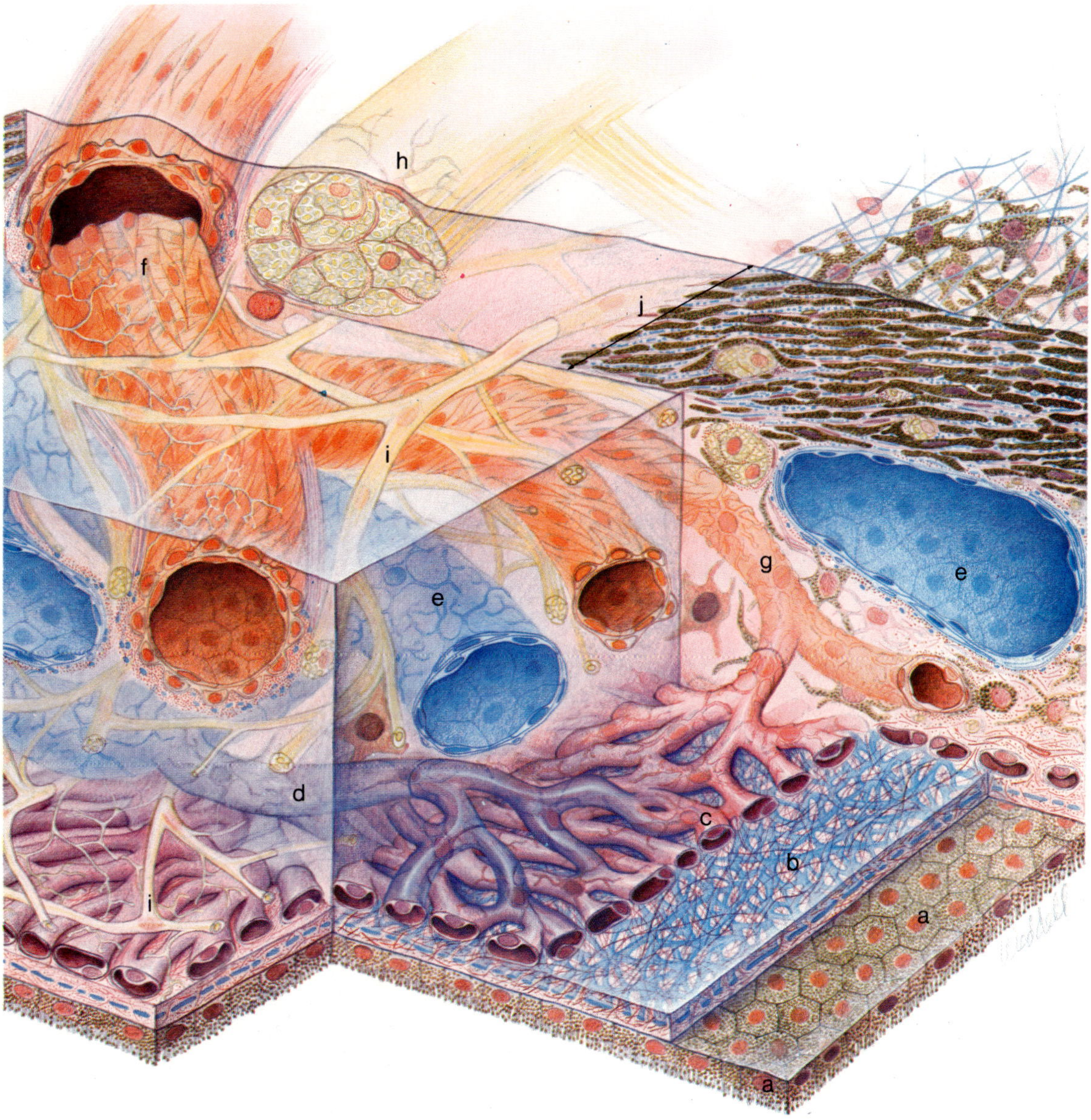

Figure 8–47. Drawing of the choroidal blood supply and innervation and Bruch's membrane. The pigment epithelium of the retina (a) is in close contact with Bruch's membrane (b). The elastica of Bruch's membrane is blue, and the meshes contain collagen fibrils. The choriocapillaris (c) forms an intricate network along the inner choroid. Venules (d) leave the choriocapillaris to join the vortex system (e). The short ciliary artery is shown at (f), prior to its branching (g) to form the choriocapillaris. A short ciliary nerve enters the choroid at (h) and sends ramifying branches into the choroidal stroma (i). The suprachoroidea with its star-shaped melanocytes is at (j).

caliber, with an intermittent muscularis, a weak internal elastic lamina and thin adventitia. The small arteries posteriorly have a diameter of 40 to 90 μm., the arterioles being reduced to 20 to 40 μm., which is about the size of the adjacent capillaries.

When studied by electron microscopy, the short posterior ciliary arteries have the structure of small arteries. Associated with the endothelium is a basement membrane often containing clusters of fine osmiophilic particles. The adjacent internal elastic membrane is composed of typical elastic fibers, arranged continuously around the endothelial basement membrane. The elastic membrane most often shows numerous folds resulting from fixation of the vessel in the contracted state. Reticulin fibers are seen in the outer part of the membrane. In the principal arteries there are two to three muscle layers, an internal one arranged circumferentially, and an external one arranged obliquely or longitudinally.

The muscle cells are separated from each other by basement membranes but their membranes often are contiguous. These membranes enclose clumps of reticulin and some collagen fibrils. The smooth muscle cells have the usual structure, the cytoplasm containing numerous myofilaments oriented parallel to each other. Among the long bands of filaments are dense osmiophilic structures resembling Z-bands, which probably represent fixation areas for the filaments. Other filaments are oriented toward thickenings along the cell membrane; the filaments attach to these thickenings in the manner of half-desmosomes. Many pinocytotic vesicles are located along the surface of the cell membrane. The nucleus is round, with one or two nucleoli. The cytoplasm contains elongated mitochondria, with the cristae oriented at a right angle to the long axis. Smooth and rough-surfaced endoplasmic reticulum are present in moderate amounts.

External to muscle layers is a circularly oriented adventitia of collagen, but there is no external elastic membrane. The adventitial collagen often contains portions of melanocytes and fibrocytes. Outside the adventitia, the collagen has a random distribution. The arterioles in the subcapillary region have a continuous endothelial lining, a well developed basement membrane beneath the endothelium, and no internal elastic lamina. They also contain an intermittent muscle layer. The endothelium and muscularis are surrounded by a thin, circular collagenous mantle.

The venous system accounts for most of the blood vessels that can be seen in the choroid with the ophthalmoscope. Such an abundant system is necessary because it drains all parts of the uveal tract, except for a small amount which exits out through the anterior ciliary veins and the region of the circle of Zinn. Except for their very small size, the veins have the same structure as veins elsewhere in the body. The wall shows an endothelial lining and a thin media composed of some muscle, fibroblasts and collagen; the adventitia is poorly developed. Salzmann (1912) described a second "protoplasmic tube," provided with flat nuclei, external to the endothelial lining, especially in the smaller veins. With thin sections and special stains, however, this layer is seen to contain collagen and reticulin, and the cellular lining is quite incomplete. The larger veins have diameters of 100 to 300 μm., the medium sized ones measure 50 to 100 μm., and the venules measure 10 to 40 μm. in diameter. The large vortex veins have the same structure as small veins, with an endothelial lining, an endothelial basement membrane, one or two layers of muscle cells and a surrounding collagenous adventitial layer.

Nerves (Figs. 8–48 to 8–53). The short posterior ciliary nerves supply most of the choroid. Approximately 20 of these nerves enter the sclera around the optic nerve. Initially they are myelinated, but after entering the choroid the nerves become unmyelinated. They branch and anastomose frequently, supplying filaments to the blood vessels and the stroma. Wolter (1960), employing a modification of the del Rio Hortega stain, found two types of nerve fibers: intervascular and perivascular. The perivascular branches course along the vessel, sending branches into the wall, where they end as small filaments without end-plates. He also found them to be closely connected to the melanocytes. Some of the nerve supply to the anterior choroid comes from the branches derived from the long ciliary nerves, which begin to branch in this region. It is not certain whether the short ciliary nerves carry all types of sensation, but it seems most likely that they contain many autonomic nerves to the blood vessels. Along their courses, these nerves branch and reunite with other branches, frequently forming ganglia, particularly in the suprachoroidea and middle layers. Numerous multipolar ganglion cells of the sympathetic type are seen, probably vasomotor cells.

Castro-Correia (1967) made an intensive study of the choroidal nerves in man, as well as in the rabbit, guinea pig and rat. He found the nerve plexuses to be diffusely distributed and not arranged in layers, as had been postulated by previous observers. Moreover, he found no special termination in the vessel walls. He observed nerve cells of a ganglionic type, indicating the existence of an intraocular autonomic supply. These ganglia were widely dispersed, but at times formed nests. He believed they might have some relation to the regulation of the ocular temperature, as well as the intraocular pressure. There is a highly organized nervous system in the peripheral suprachoroidal and supraciliary regions, containing bipolar and multipolar types of ganglion cells and many nerve filaments (Kurus, 1955). This system also extends into the meridional part of the ciliary muscle.

Almost all the nerves within the choroidal stroma are unmyelinated; they are wrapped with only a few layers of Schwann cell membranes and cytoplasm. The nerve bundles may contain 50 to 100 axons, all individually wrapped. Some nerves terminate in a ganglion cell which is usually multipolar, with terminals leaving in many directions to supply the choroidal components. Their abundant cytoplasm contains numerous fibrils, mitochondria, and both smooth and rough-surfaced endoplasmic reticulum. Nerve endings frequently are found around the walls of the arterial blood vessels, but no specialized endings have been seen. Nerves frequently end near the surface of choroidal melanocytes, but they show no specific endings.

Cells (Figs. 8–48 *A* and *B*, 8–54 to 8–60). A very large number of cells are found in the choroidal stroma, particularly in the outer two thirds. The melanocyte and the fibroblast are the principal cells of choroidal stroma; next most numerous are macrophages and mast cells, plasma cells and lymphocytes.

Melanocytes (Fig. 8–54). These cells are most numerous near the suprachoroidea, but they are frequently seen in other layers. They have a star shape, with numerous long, branching processes, and are like those of the iris and ciliary body.

Fibroblasts (Figs. 8–48 *A* and *B*, 8–55, 8–60). These cells have elongated bodies and long, branching processes which contact most of the choroi-

Text continued on page 385

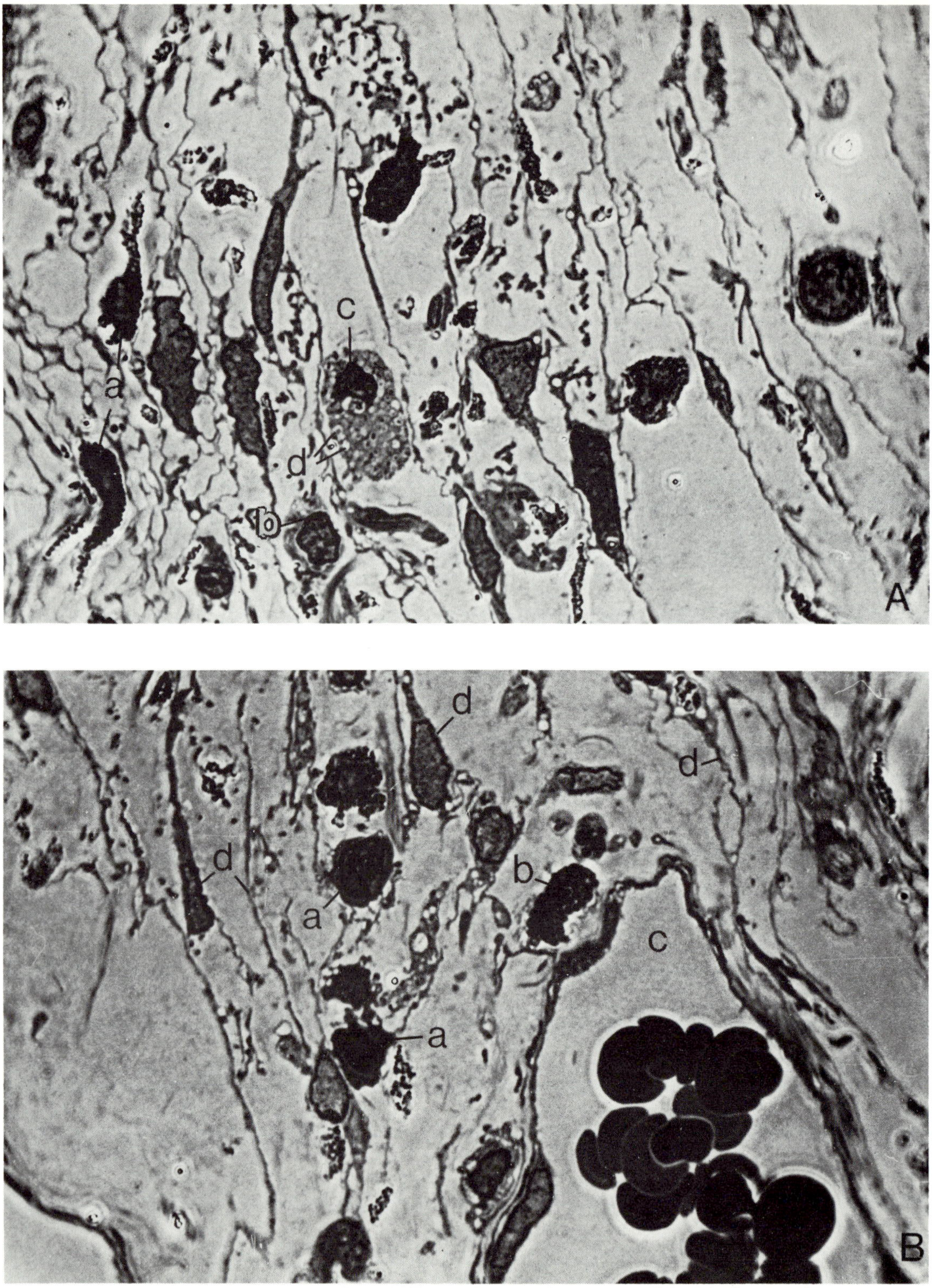

Figure 8-48. Phase-contrast light micrograph of the cells of the choroidal stroma. *A*, Melancoytes (a) and fibroblasts (b) comprise most of the cells found in the choroid. Unmyelinated nerve bundles with their Schwann cell wrapping are common in the outer choroidal stroma and in the suprachoroidea. The nucleus of a Schwann cell is shown at (c) and the nerve axons at (d). (× 1600.)

B, Plasma cells (a) and a mast cell (b) are shown in the choroidal stroma near a vein (c). The fibroblasts (d) have long processes and their perinuclear cytoplasm is scanty. (× 1600.)

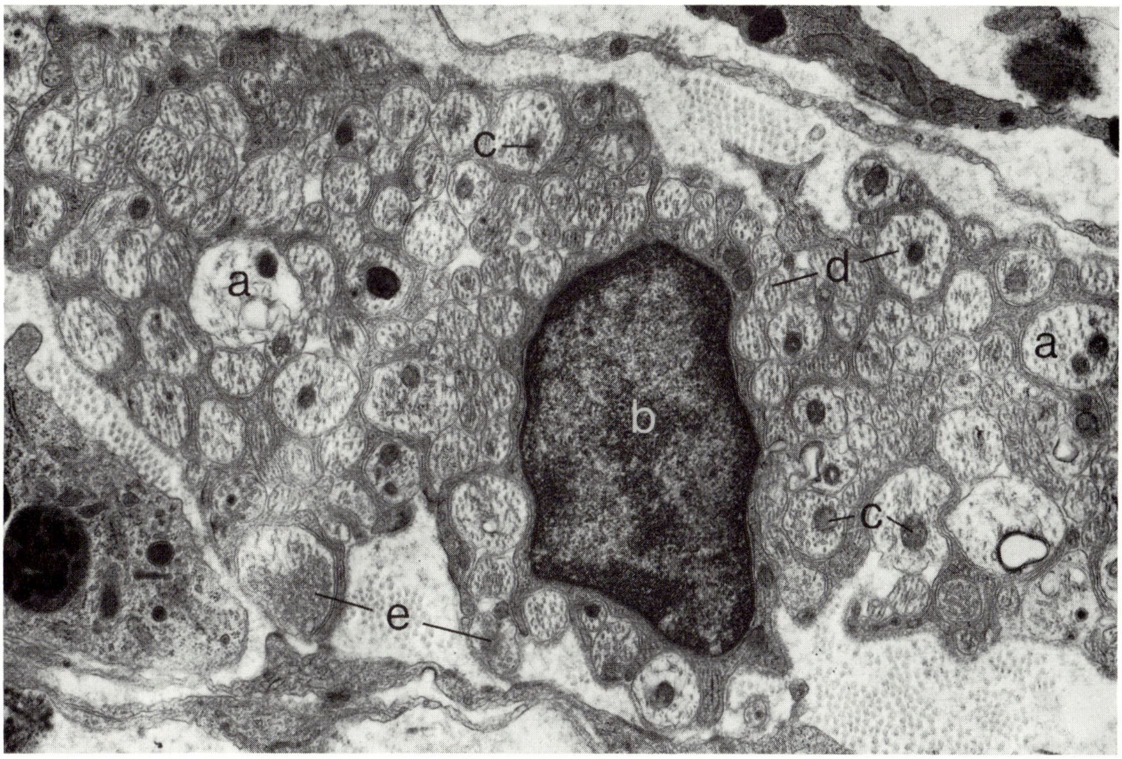

Figure 8-49. An unmyelinated nerve bundle in the external choroidal stroma and suprachoroidea. It contains more than 100 unmyelinated axons (a) and the nucleus of a Schwann cell (b). The axons have small, dense mitochondria (c) and numerous microtubules (d). Synaptic vesicles are present in two axons (e) found in the outer portion of the bundle. (× 12,900.)

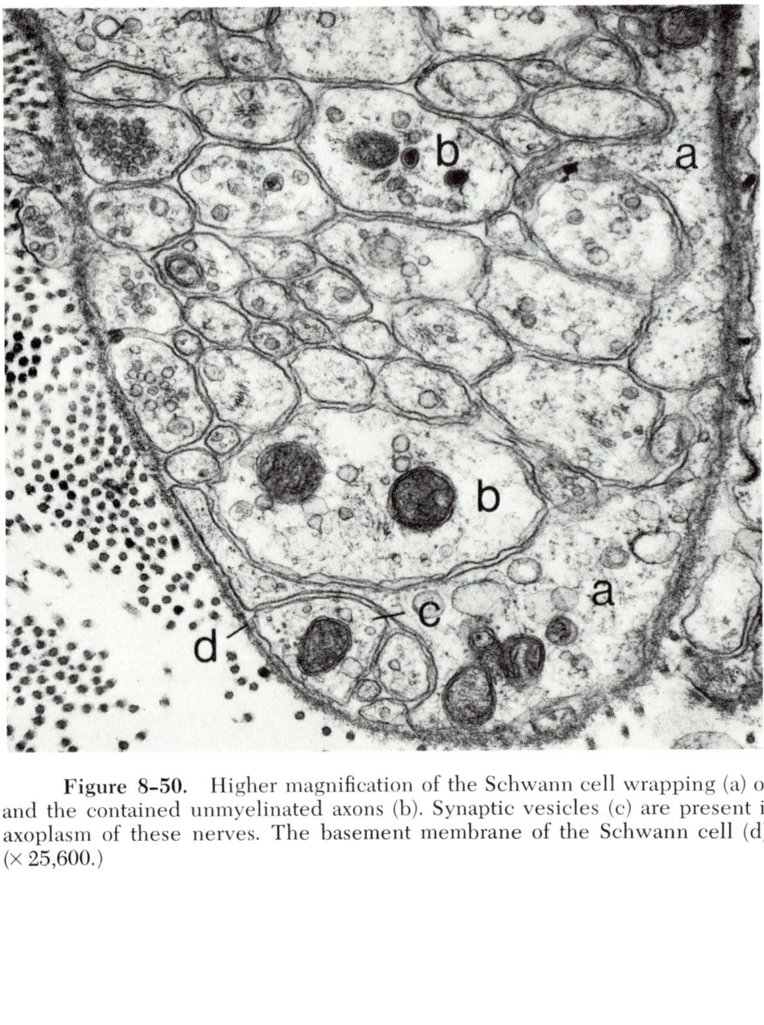

Figure 8-50. Higher magnification of the Schwann cell wrapping (a) of a nerve bundle and the contained unmyelinated axons (b). Synaptic vesicles (c) are present in the peripheral axoplasm of these nerves. The basement membrane of the Schwann cell (d) is clearly seen. (× 25,600.)

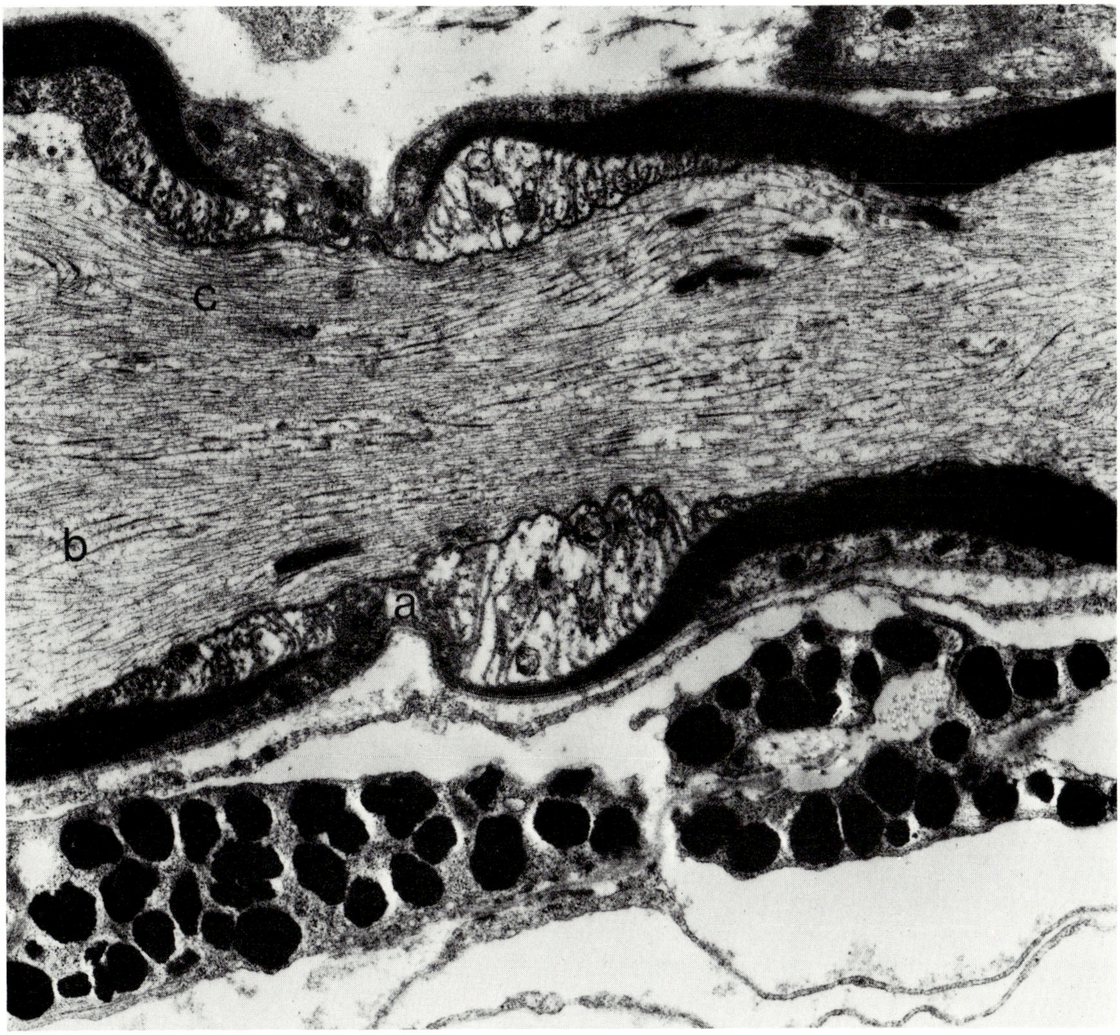

Figure 8–51. Electron micrograph of the myelinated long ciliary nerve in the suprachoroidea. These are the only myelinated nerves found in the choroid; they lose their myelin sheaths as they approach the ciliary body. A node of Ranvier (a), longitudinally sectioned microtubules (b) and neurofilaments (c) are shown. (× 10,500.)

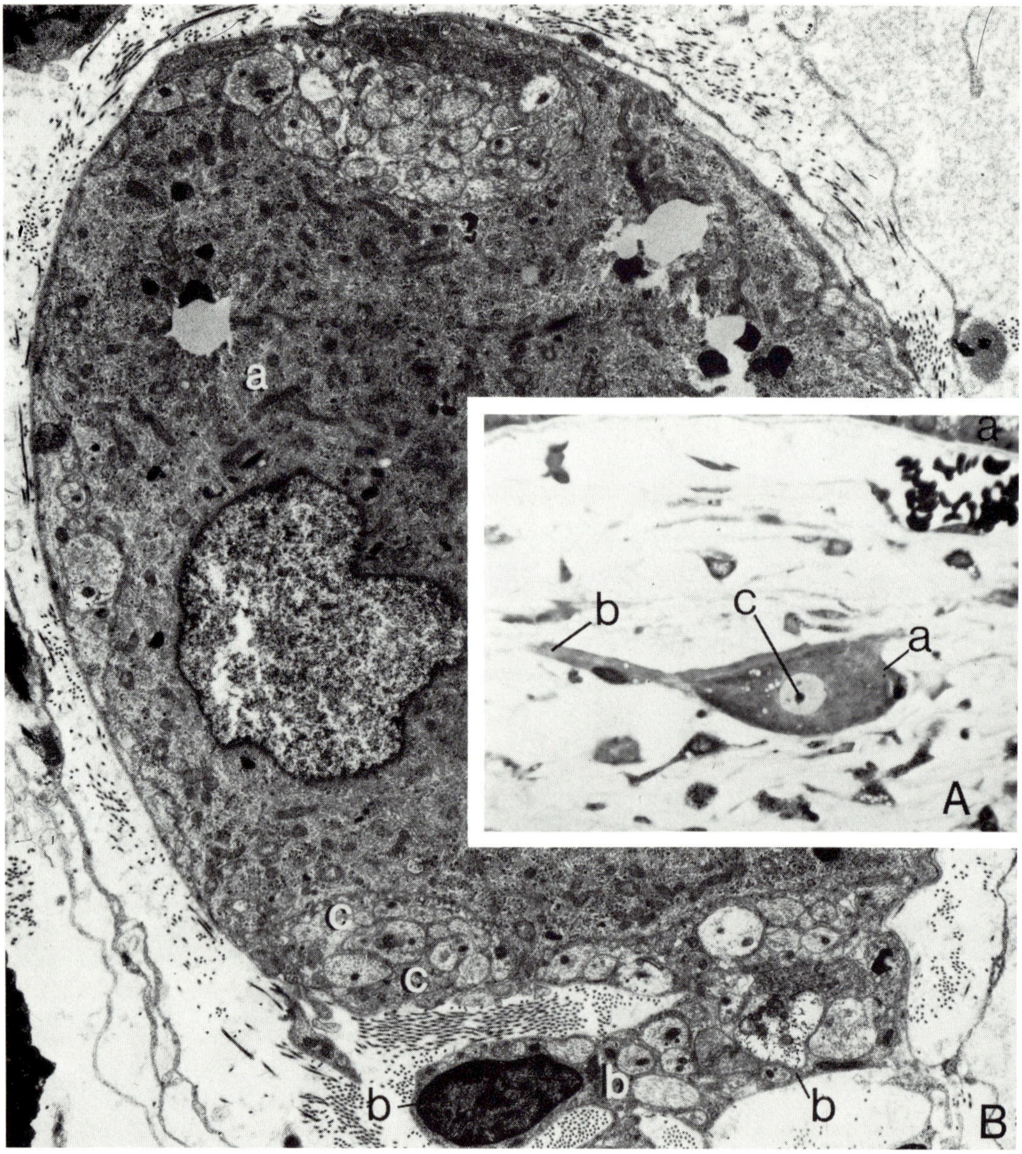

Figure 8-52. *A*, Light micrograph of a choroidal ganglion cell (a) and a nerve bundle with its Schwann cell (b). The unmyelinated nerve bundle comes in contact with the ganglion cell. These cells are much longer than other choroidal cells, measuring 40 μm. or more. Their nucleus has a prominent nucleolus (c). (× 400.)

B, Electron micrograph of a ganglion cell (a) and a bundle of unmyelinated nerves wrapped by a Schwann cell (b). The large size of the ganglion cell relative to the Schwann cell is striking. Two bundles of unmyelinated axons (c) are indented into the cytoplasm of the ganglion cell. (× 5600.)

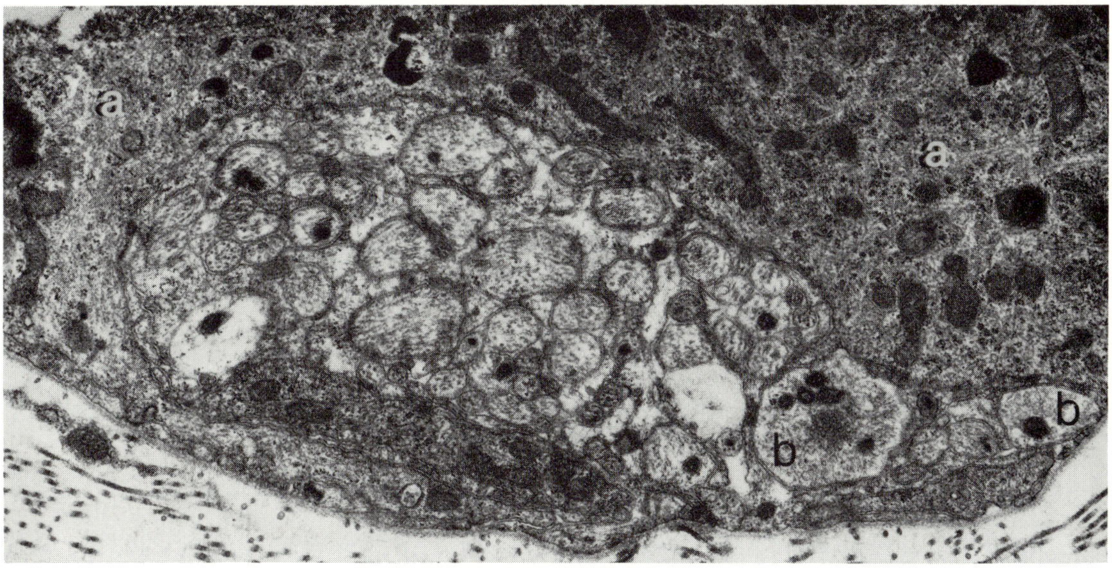

Figure 8–53. Higher magnification view of the nerve bundle seen on top of Figure 8–52*B*. The cytoplasm of the ganglion cell is shown at (a). It contains numerous mitochondria and ribosomes. Two of the unmyelinated axons (b) contain numerous synaptic vesicles; presumably this represents an area of synaptic contact between these axons and the ganglion cell. (× 12,000.)

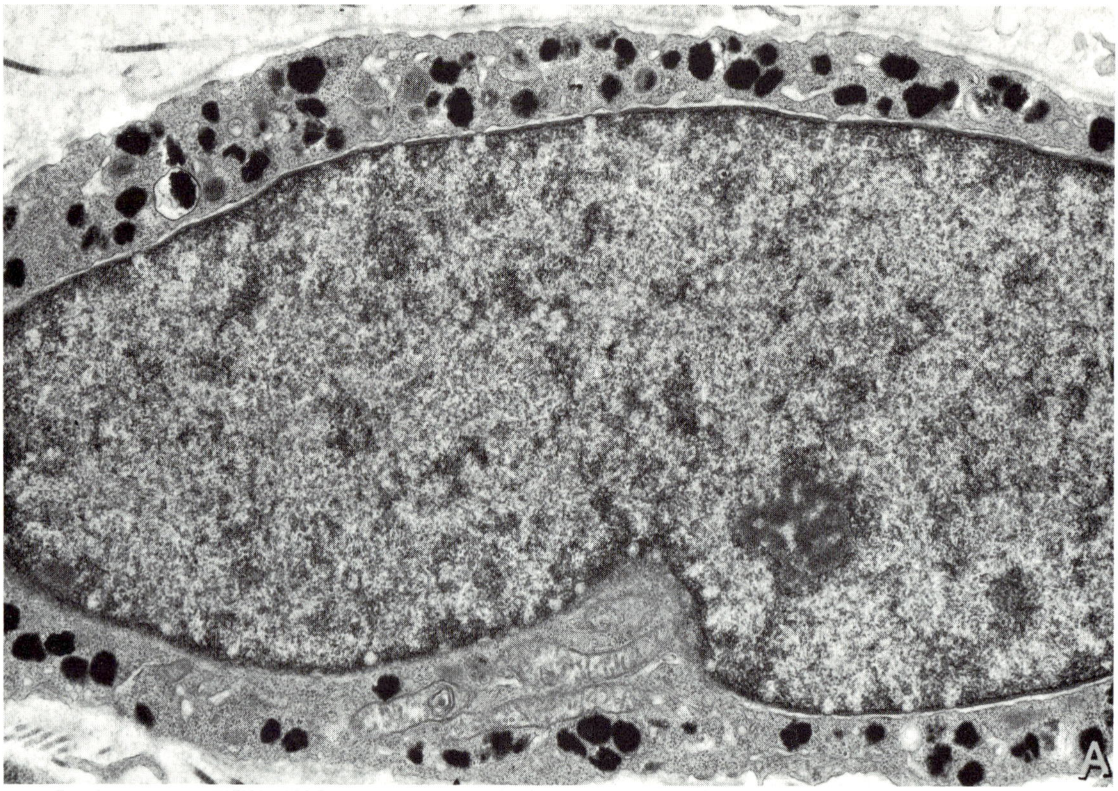

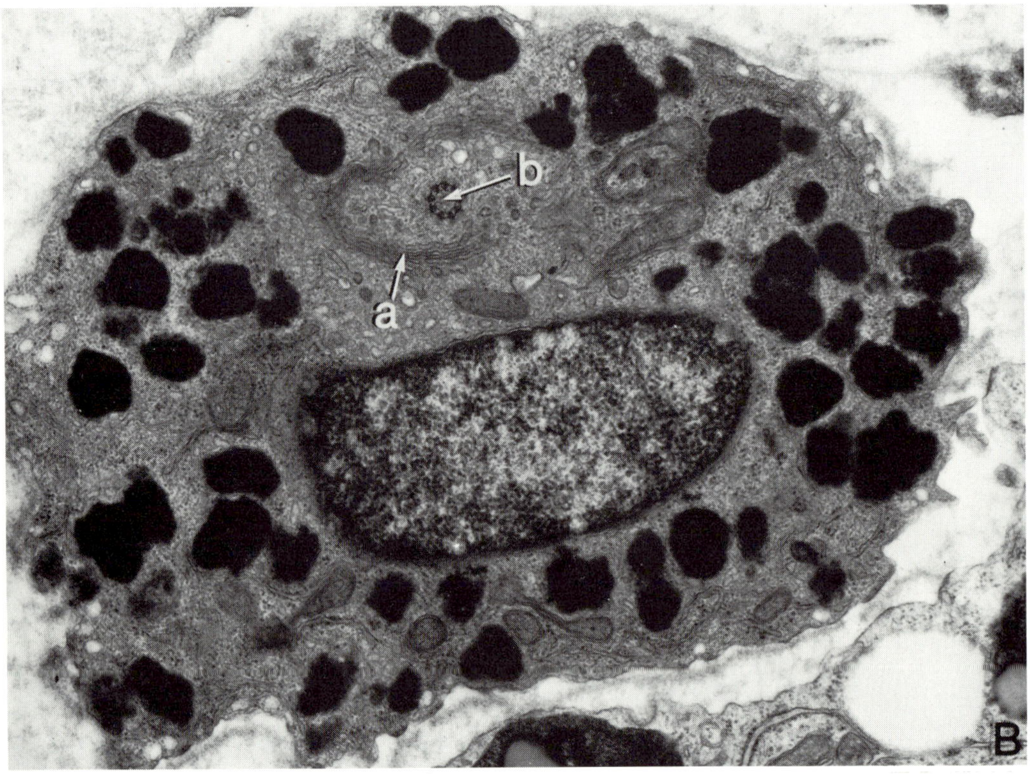

Figure 8–54. *See legend on opposite page.*

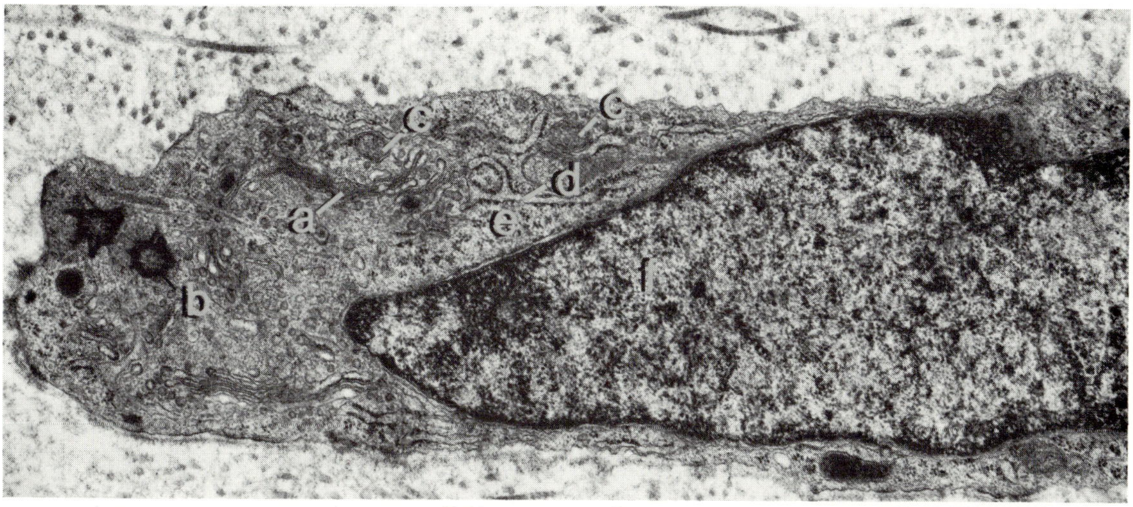

Figure 8–55. Perinuclear cytoplasm of a choroidal fibroblast. The scanty cytoplasm usually contains all the common cell organelles. The Golgi complex (a), two centrioles (b), small mitochondria (c), cisternae of the rough-surfaced endoplasmic reticulum (d), free ribosomes (e) and the nucleus (f) are indicated. (× 13,800.)

dal structures as well as other fibroblasts. They are oriented around the blood vessels and nerves, usually being arranged in a circumferential direction around these structures. They are freely mixed with processes and cell bodies of the melanocytes. The fibroblasts are like those described in the iris and ciliary body.

Macrophages (Fig. 8–56). Most of these cells contain phagocytosed material, mainly pigment from the melanocytes. They can be recognized by their large size, villous surface processes and cytoplasmic inclusions, which often are huge. Macrophages seen in the choroid resemble the "clump" cells of the iris.

Lymphocytes (Fig. 8–57). These cells are found wandering throughout most tissues, having escaped from the blood. Lymphocytes in the stroma have the same appearance as the circulating lymphocytes, with large nuclei and a scanty cytoplasm.

Mast Cells (Fig. 8–58). The mast cells of the choroid are of one type, unlike those of the iris, which show several morphologic features. Their granules are dense, strongly osmiophilic and measure 1500 A. in diameter. These cells closely resemble mast cells of other organs.

Figure 8–54. Melanocytes. *A*, Longitudinal section through the nuclear region of a choroidal melanocyte. The nucleus contains dispersed chromatin and a nucleolus. The melanin granules in the cytoplasm are all mature and are diffusely distributed. There are some mitochondria in the cytoplasm. (× 16,800.)

B, Cross-section of a choroidal melanocyte. There are many mature melanin granules in the cytoplasm. A portion of the nucleus is seen. The Golgi apparatus (a) is prominent and partially surrounds a centriole (b). (× 16,800.)

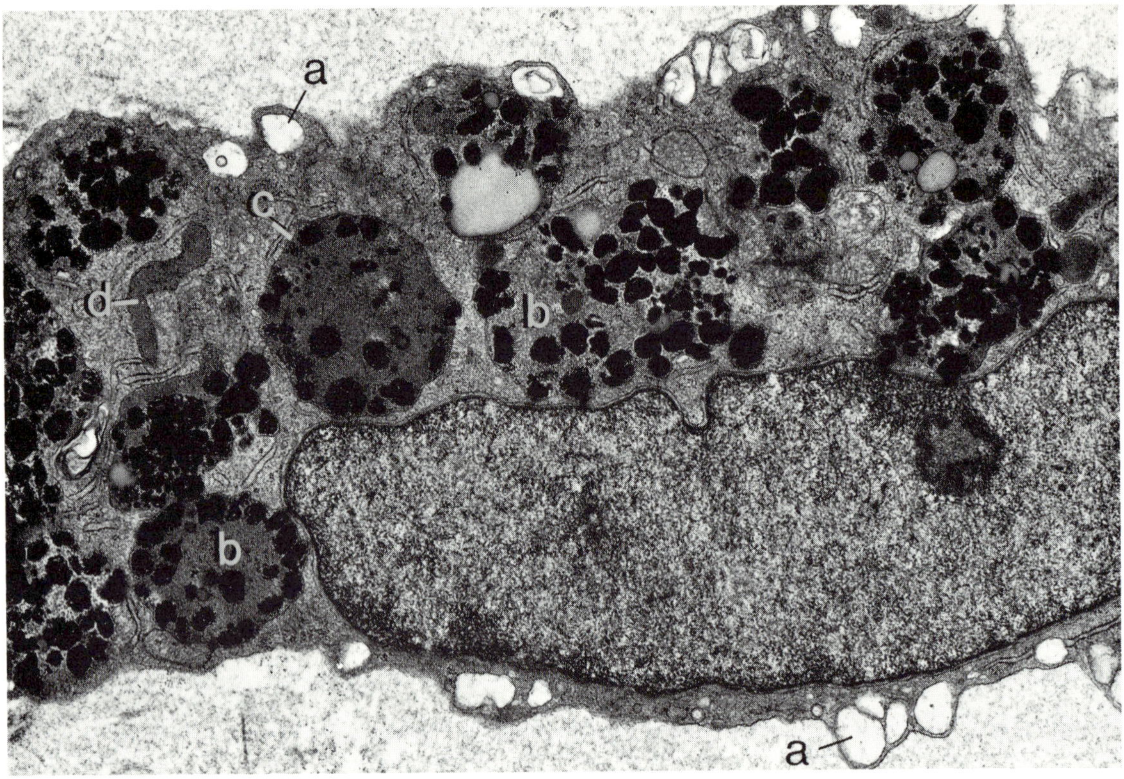

Figure 8–56. Macrophage in the choroidal stroma. Vesicle-like structures (a) are probably produced by enclosed villous projections. The cytoplasm shows large membrane-bound residual bodies (b) containing undigested melanin granules and other substances. Endoplasmic reticulum (c) and mitochondria (d) are shown. (× 6200.)

Plasma Cells (Fig. 8–59). Plasma cells are frequently encountered in the normal choroid. They have the characteristics of plasma cells found in other tissues of the eye and elsewhere.

Supporting Tissue (Figs. 8–1 *A* and *B*, 8–4 *A* and *B*, 8–39 *A*, 8–44, 8–46). The supporting tissue of the choroid is not voluminous because of the large space occupied by vessels, cells and nerves. The collagenous framework loosely encloses these vessels, nerves and cells. As the suprachoroidea is approached, the collagen becomes aggregated into bundles oriented parallel to the inner surface of the sclera. It is not possible to study the ground substance in light microscopic sections. With appropriate stains, reticulin fibers can be seen adjacent to the fibroblasts.

SUPRACHOROIDEA (Figs. 8–1 *A* and *B*, 8–4 *A* and *B*, 8–60)

The suprachoroidea lies between the choroid and the sclera and appears to be derived partly from each tissue. It is about 30 μm. thick and forms a transition zone composed of layers of long, ribbon-like processes that branch and are interconnected. The processes are heavily pigmented and are composed of collagen. Numerous fibroblasts, melanocytes, ganglion cells and nerve plexuses are enmeshed in the collagen.

Text continued on page 392

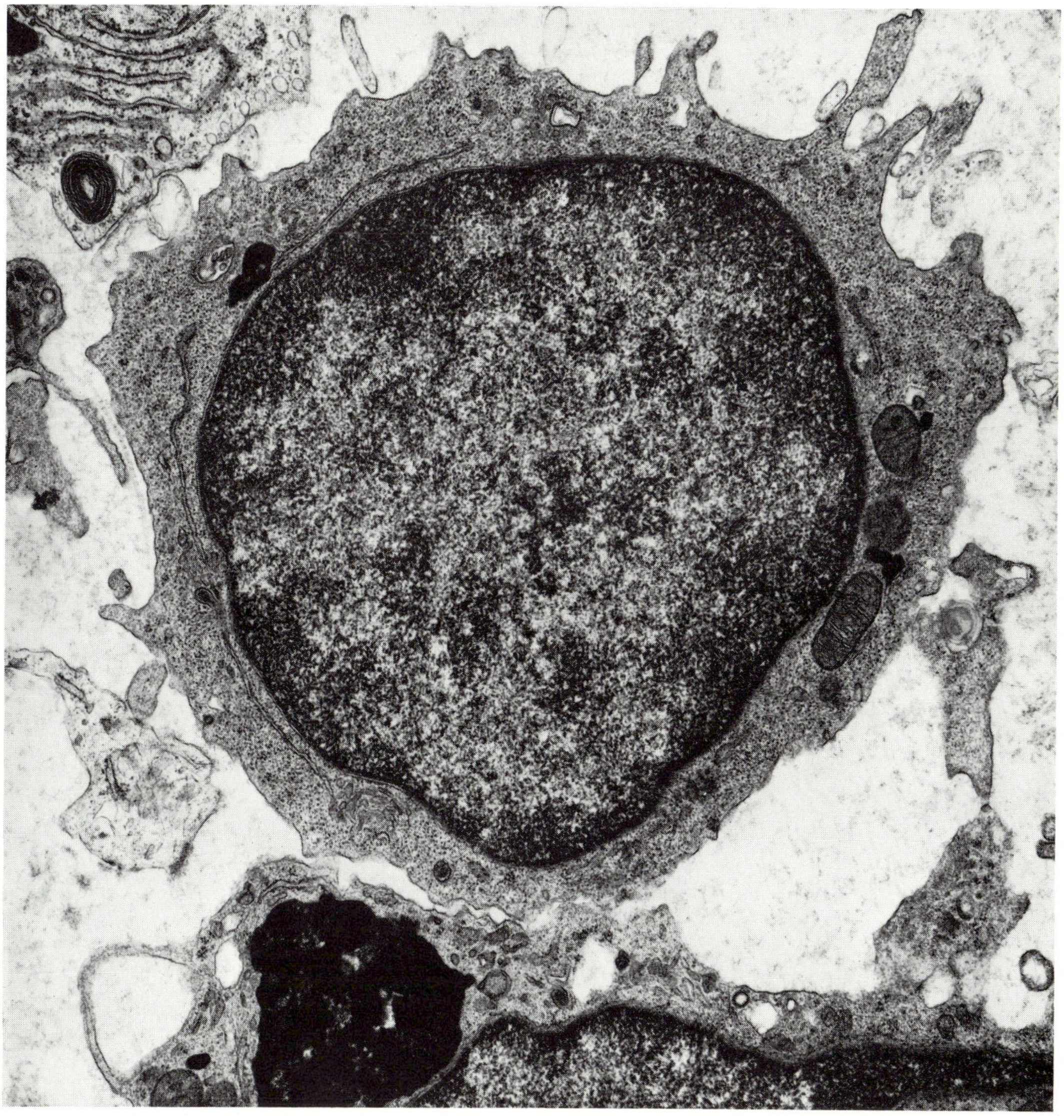

Figure 8-57. Lymphocyte in the choroidal stroma. The nucleus is large and shows peripherally placed heterochromatin. The cytoplasm is very dense owing to the large content of free ribosomes. Some small mitochondria and long profiles of endoplasmic reticulum are seen at the left. The surface shows numerous villous processes. (× 15,000.)

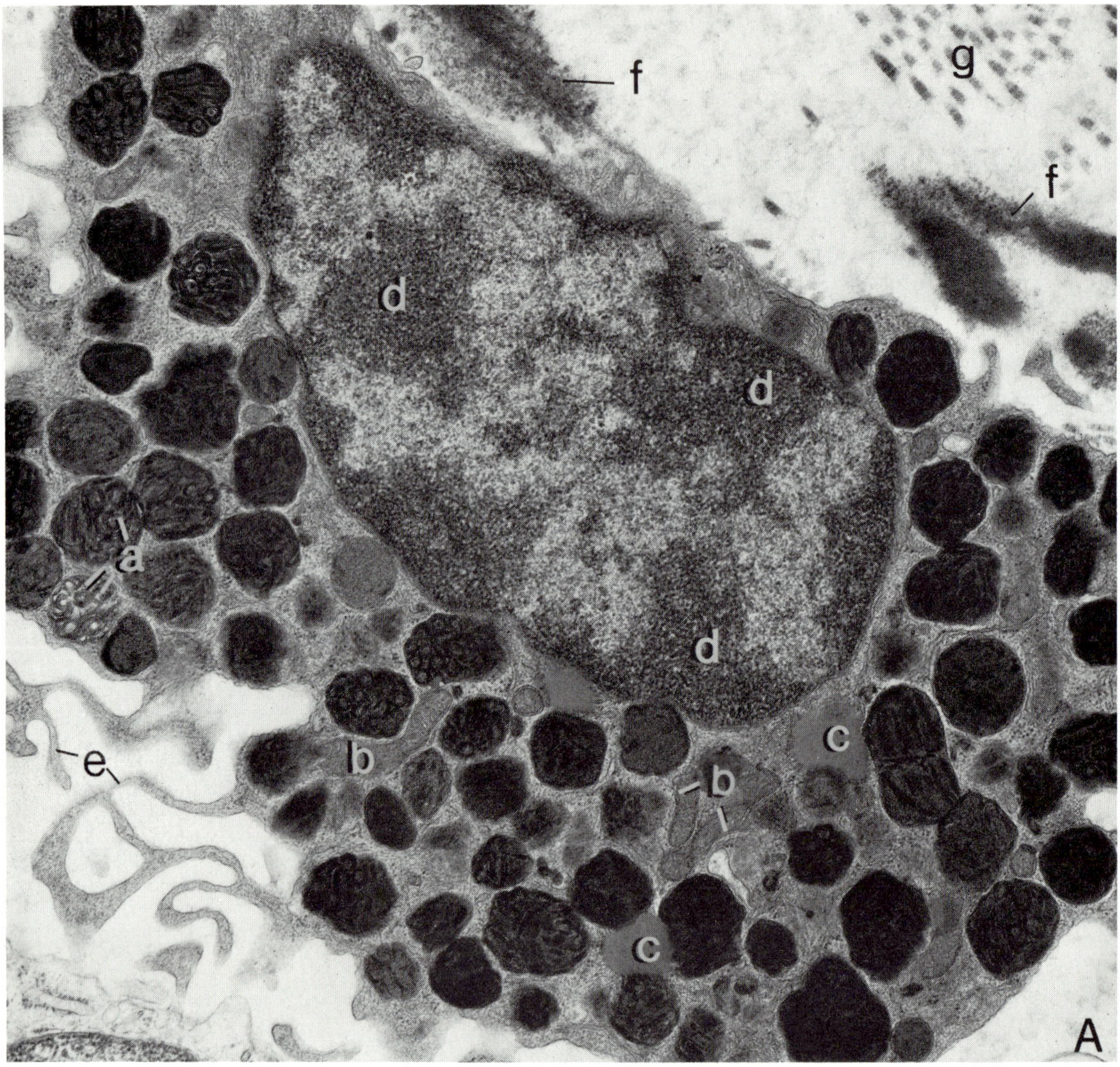

Figure 8-58. Electron micrographs of a choroidal mast cell. *A*, Unlike the mast cells of the iris and limbus, the choroidal mast cells contain only granules of one morphologic type. These granules measure 1500 A. in diameter and are filled with tightly packed scroll-like structures (a). The cytoplasm also has mitochondria (b) and lipid vacuoles (c). The nucleus has several patches of heterochromatin (d) and is oval in shape. Villous processes (e) extend into the choroidal stroma where elastic (f) and collagen fibrils (g) are shown. (× 18,000.)

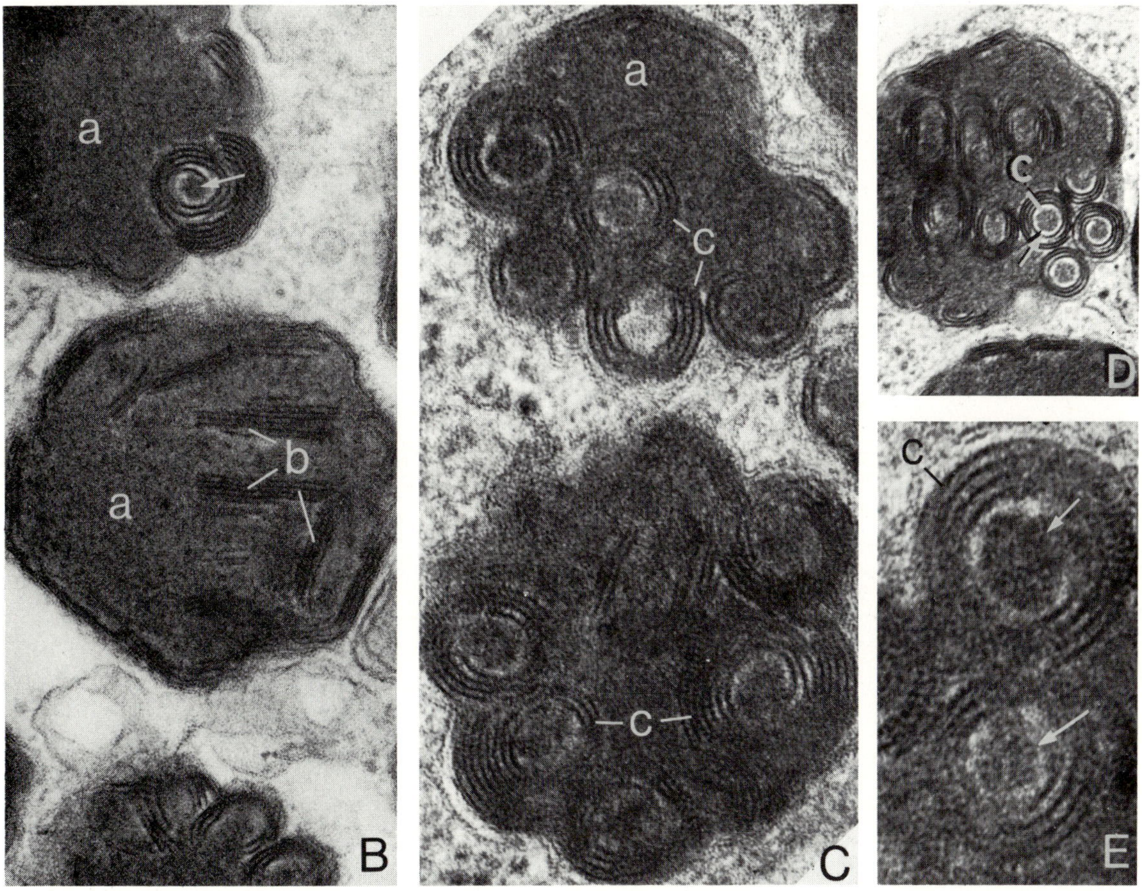

Figure 8–58. *Continued.*

B, C, D and *E,* The mast cell granules are filled with unorganized, finely granular electron-dense material (a) and scroll-like structures. The scrolls are seen sectioned longitudinally at (b) and in cross-section at (c). The center of the scroll contains a granular, less dense substance (arrows). The scrolls measure 3000 A. in length and 1500 A. in cross-section. The sheets forming the scrolls are 75 A. thick and are separated from each other by a space measuring 150 A. (*B,* ×93,500; *C,* ×91,500; *D,* ×60,000; *E,* ×210,000.)

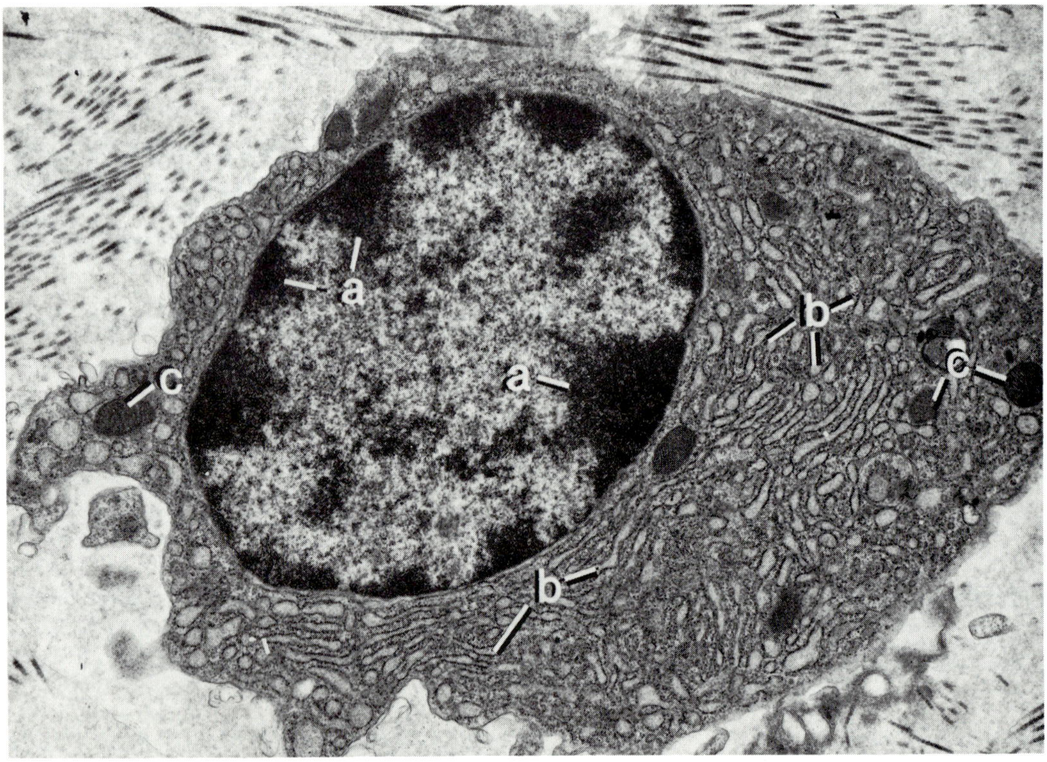

Figure 8-59. Electron micrograph of a choroidal plasma cell. The characteristic clock-shaped nucleus of these cells is displaced to one side; the "hours" of the clock are marked by patches of heterochromatin (a). The cytoplasm is largely occupied by the cisternae of the rough-surfaced endoplasmic reticulum (b) that is, presumably, filled with gamma globulins. Mitochondria are seen at (c). (× 10,750.)

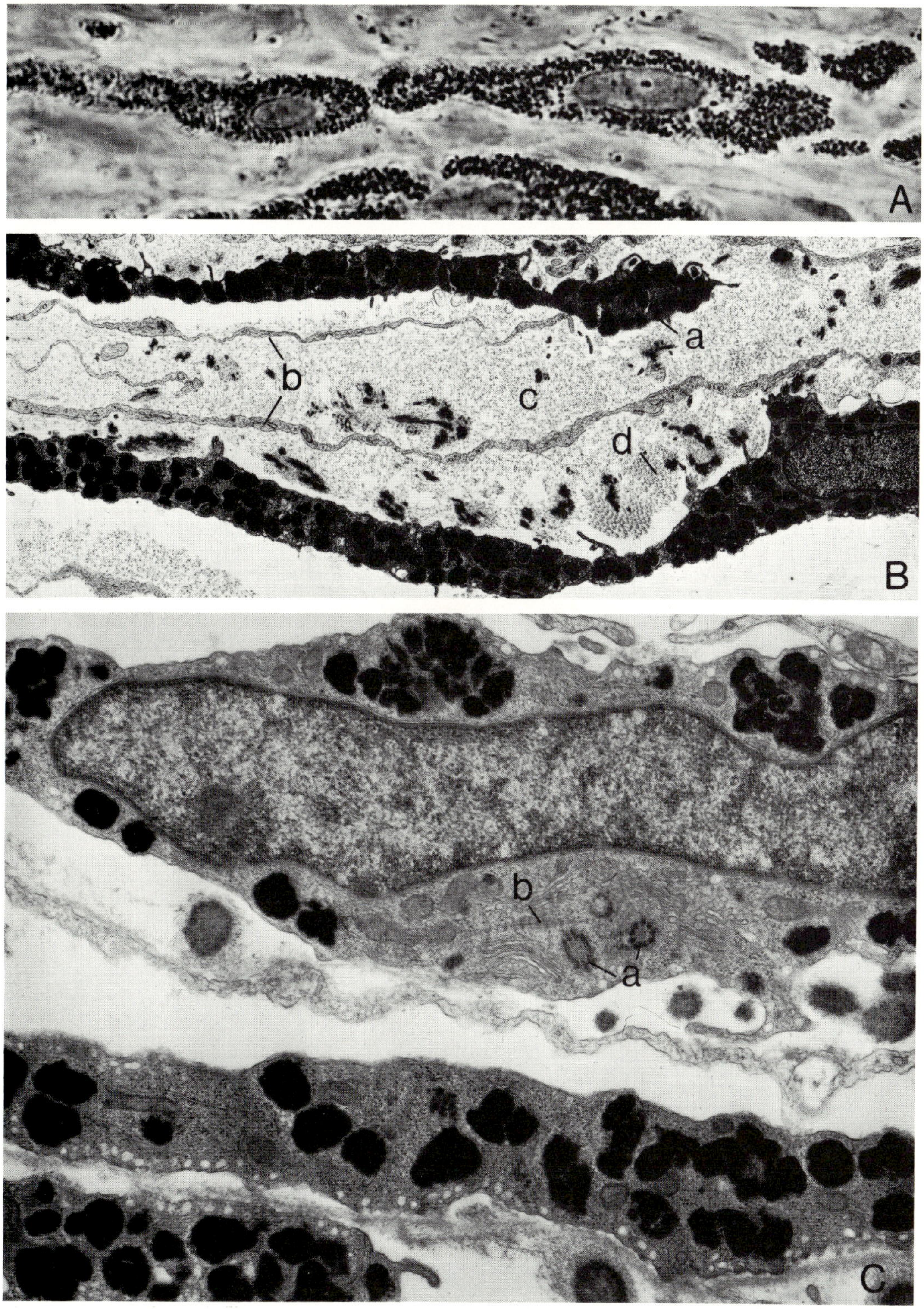

Figure 8-60. Suprachoroidea. *A*, Light micrograph of the suprachoroidea. The collagen here is more closely packed and contains long, heavily melanized melanocytes. (× 1600.)

B, Electron micrograph of the suprachoroidea containing long strips of melanocytes (a) and fibroblasts (b). The ground substance in which these cells are embedded is granular (c). Cross-sections of some collagen fibrils are seen (d). (× 6500.)

C, The melanocytes and fibroblasts are narrow and long. Most of the melanin granules are mature. The upper melanocyte contains a pair of centrioles (a). A striated body leads into the cytoplasm (b) from the vicinity of the centrioles. (× 15,600.)

The ultrastructure of the suprachoroidal tissues and lamina fusca show no special organization. The layers of collagen which fill out this area are not remarkable, except for their fairly regular orientation. This area is characterized by its pigmentation from the numerous melanocytes, which have long processes.

REFERENCES

Bernstein, M. H., and Hollenberg, M. J.: Fine structure of the choriocapillaris and retinal capillaries. Invest. Ophthal. *4*:1016, 1965.

Bill, A.: Ocular circulation. *In* Moses, R. A. (ed.): Adler's Physiology of the Eye. 5th ed. St. Louis, The C. V. Mosby Co., 1970, pp. 278–296.

Castro-Correia, J.: Studies on the innervation of the uveal tract. Ophthalmologica *154*:497, 1967.

Collier, R. G.: Experimental embolic ischemia of the choroid. Arch. Ophthal. *77*:683, 1967.

Fehér, I., and Valu, L.: Aging changes of collagenous fibres of the choroid. Investigation by polarisation optics. Graefes Arch. Klin. Ophthal. *172*:249, 1967.

Friedman, E., and Oak, S. M.: Choroidal microcirculation in vivo. Bibl. Anat. *7*:129, 1965.

Garron, L. K.: The ultrastructure of the retinal pigment epithelium with observations on the choriocapillaris and Bruch's membrane. Trans. Amer. Ophthal. Soc. *61*:545, 1963.

Gray, A. J., Goldor, H., and Smith, M.: Chorioretinal vascular occlusions with latex spheres. Invest. Ophthal. *3*:647, 1964.

Hogan, M. J.: Ultrastructure of the choroid. Its role in the pathogenesis of choroidal diseases. Trans. Pac. Coast Oto-Ophthal. Soc. *42*:61, 1961.

Kurus, E.: A system of ganglion cells in the human choroid. Klin. Mbl. Augenheilk. *127*:198, 1955.

Leopold, I. H.: Autonomic drugs and their influence on choroidal blood vessel capacity. Trans. Amer. Ophthal. Soc. *49*:625, 1951.

Lerche, W.: Electron microscopic observations of Bruch's membrane in the human eye. Ber. Dtsch. Ophthal. Ges. *65*:384, 1963.

Lerche, W.: Electron microscopic observations on the histogenesis of Bruch's membrane in man. Z. Zellforsch. *65*:163, 1965.

Nakaizumi, Y.: The ultrastructure of Bruch's membrane. I. Human, monkey, rabbit, guinea pig and rat eyes. Arch. Ophthal. *72*:380, 1964a.

Nakaizumi, Y.: The ultrastructure of Bruch's membrane. II. Eyes with a tapetum. Arch. Ophthal. *72*:388, 1964b.

Nakaizumi, Y., Hogan, M. J., and Feeney, L.: The ultrastructure of Bruch's membrane. III. The macular area of the human eye. Arch. Ophthal. *72*:395, 1964.

Salzmann, M.: The Anatomy and Histology of the Human Eyeball. Chicago, Deuticke, 1912.

Sumita, R.: The fine structure of Bruch's membrane in the choroid. Acta. Soc. Ophthal. Jap. *65*:1188, 1961.

Wolfrum, M.: Contributions to the anatomy and histology of the choroid in man and higher animals. Graefes. Arch. Klin. Ophthal. *67*:307, 1908.

Wolter, J. R.: Histologic character of the connection between Bruch's membrane and choriocapillaris of the human eye. Arch. Ophthal. *53*:208, 1955.

Wolter, J. R.: Nerves of the human normal choroid. Arch. Ophthal. *64*:120, 1960.

Wudka, E., and Leopold, I. H.: Experimental studies of the choroidal blood vessels. Arch. Ophthal. *55*:857, 1951.

Chapter Nine

RETINA

The retina and optic nerve are derivatives of the forebrain; consequently their morphology and physiology are very much like that of the brain. The neuroretina is connected to the brain by the optic nerve through the optic chiasm and optic tracts. The receptor cells of the retina comprise a complex layer of specialized cells, the rods and cones, which contain photopigments that change on exposure to light to produce chemical energy. This energy is converted to electrical energy, which is then transmitted to the visual cortex in the occipital lobe of the brain. The retinal pigment epithelium furnishes important metabolites to the receptors; it is also engaged in the removal of the outermost ends of the external segments of the photoreceptors as they are replaced during the aging of the eye.

In humans, primates and many other species the two eyes are oriented to facilitate binocular single vision in most of the visual field. Binocular vision is achieved by the forward position of the eyes in the head and by the chiasmal crossing of all the axons derived from the ganglion cells of the nasal portions of the retinas, and the absence of crossing of those from the temporal portions (Fig. 9–1). In this way, axons carrying impulses from the right visual field form the left optic tract, and vice versa.

In the normal eye the macular area of the retina is the center of the posterior focal point of the optical system. The cornea and lens are so placed and constructed that they focus light on the photoreceptors.

PHYSIOLOGY AND BIOCHEMISTRY

The retina receives almost all its nutrition from the retinal and choroidal capillaries, but a small amount probably is derived from the vitreous. The retina has one of the highest rates of metabolism of any tissue in the body, and its dual blood supply is adequate for the ordinary retinal requirements. If either source of nutrition is interrupted, ischemia occurs. This is poorly tolerated by the retina and may lead to complete loss of retinal function.

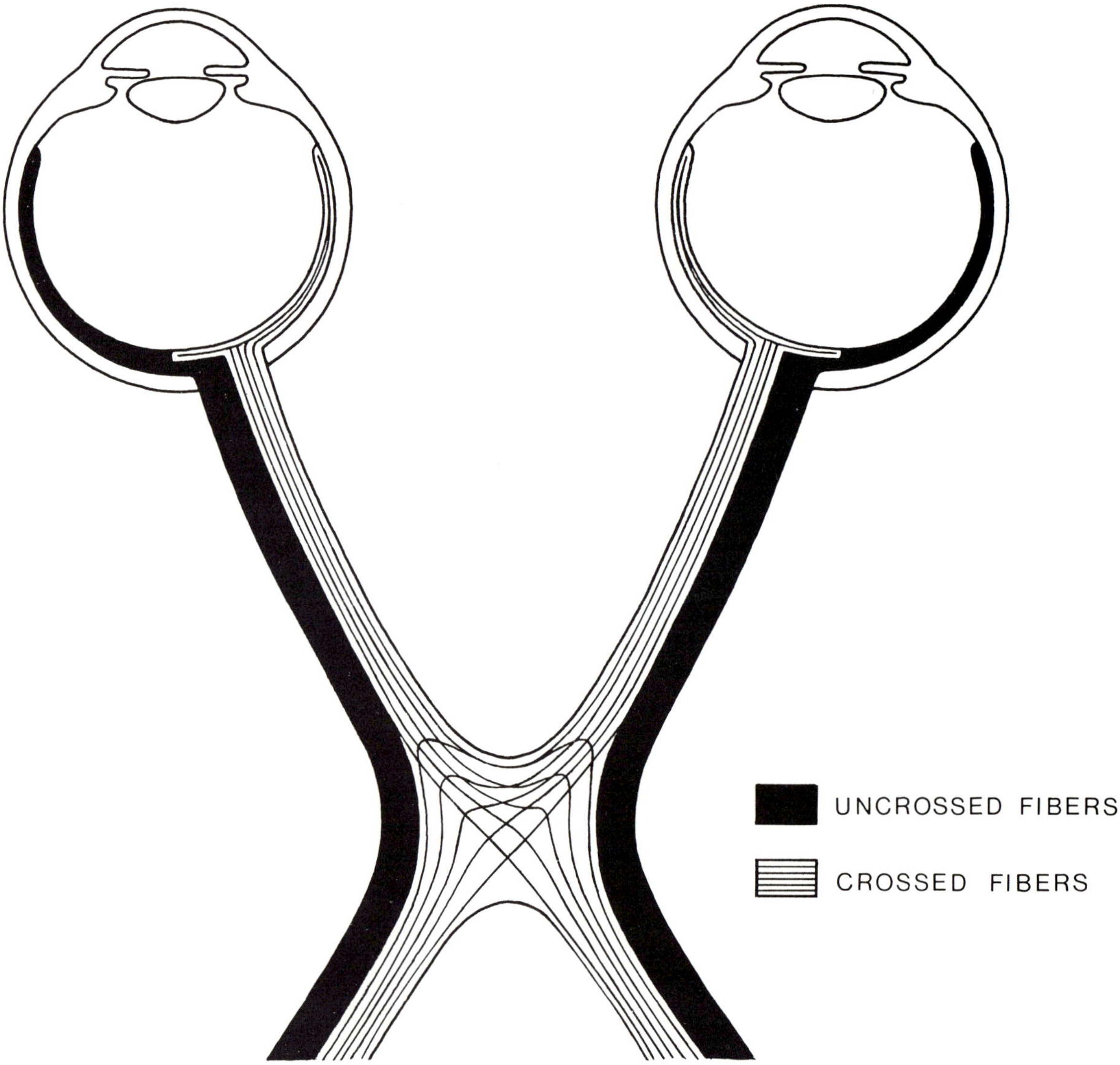

Figure 9–1. The axons from the retinal ganglion cells nasal to the macular center extend toward the brain through the medial portion of the optic nerve, then cross in the chiasm to enter the opposite optic tract. The axons from ganglion cells temporal to the macular center do not cross in the chiasm but pass directly into the homolateral tracts.

Exposure to light seems to have no effect on oxygen consumption; on the other hand, there is an increase in metabolic activity of the enzyme succinic dehydrogenase in the light- compared to the dark-adapted retina; this activity is predominantly found in the ellipsoids of the photoreceptors. The oxygen and glucose needed for its metabolism come directly from the capillaries, but it has been shown that the Müller cells store glycogen, which is readily available, and also possess such glycolytic enzymes as lactic acid dehydrogenase for the breakdown of glucose. The retina appears to be able to synthesize glycogen from glucose, but not from any other substrate. Glucose seems to be broken down in the retina mainly by the Embden-Meyerhof pathway. The oxidation of lactate and pyruvate occurs through the citric acid cycle, and many of the enzymes of this cycle, such as citric acid dehydrogenase, have been found in the retina. Histochemical studies have shown that glycolytic enzymes are more abundant in the outer retina, while the enzymes of the citric acid cycle are localized mainly in the inner retina.

The blood-retina barrier is not completely understood but it probably is formed by the capillary endothelial cells and their basement membrane. Since there is very little extracellular space in the retina, the astroglia and Müller cells probably play an important role in transporting solutes directly to the neurons.

Amino acids apparently are obtained directly from the blood for synthesis into proteins by the retina. Glucose can also be converted into amino acids in the retina, glutamic acid being an early product of this pathway. Radioactively labeled amino acids have been shown to be incorporated into proteins at all levels of the retina, especially in the ganglion cell layer.

Mucopolysaccharide is present in the retina, particularly around the outer segments of the rods and cones and in the inner limiting membrane. The mucopolysaccharide around the rods and cones appears to be manufactured by the retinal pigment epithelium.

PHOTOCHEMISTRY

The initial impulses for vision arise in the photoreceptor layer of the retina, which is composed of rods and cones. It has been known for many years that the rods and cones differ in function, giving rise to the *duplicity theory* of retinal photoreceptor function. According to this theory, the cones function in daylight to provide sharp visual acuity and color perception, while the rods are more sensitive in dim illumination and are used for night vision; the rods do not discern color and cannot detect fine detail. The highest degree of cone function is found in the macular region, where the cones are concentrated. The ratio of cones to ganglion cells is greater than that of rods to ganglion cells, and the better acuity of the cone portion of the retina probably is related to the nearly equal cone-ganglion cell ratio. Rod synapses cover greater areas of the retina, which probably explains why they are more efficient at gathering light in dim illumination. The sensitivity of the retina to light varies with the wavelength of the light, the spectral sensitivity of the retina being within the range of 4000 to 7000 A. The photopic spectral sensitivity is shifted slightly more toward the longer wavelengths (5550 A.) than the scotopic (5070 A.), producing what is known as the Purkinje shift.

The visual pigments associated with the photoreceptors are colored substances that occupy the discs in the outer segments of the rods and cones. These pigments break down to colorless products on absorbing light energy. Each pigment varies in its facility to absorb light, depending on the wavelength of the light. The wavelength that each pigment absorbs best is known as its absorption maximum. This characteristic is used to classify the pigment; for example, rhodopsin 498 absorbs best in the 498 nm. (nanometer) band and rhodopsin 502 absorbs best at 502 nm.

Each visual pigment is formed by the combination of one of a number of water insoluble proteins collectively termed opsin, and a fat soluble hydrocarbon related to beta-carotene, the alcohol of which is vitamin A.

Opsin is a lipoprotein with a molecular weight of 30,000 to 40,000 (Krinsky, 1958).

Vitamin A may be modified at three important sites, each of which is labeled as A, B, or C, in Figure 9–2. If the end-group on the side chain is an alcohol (Fig. 9–2, A) the vitamin A is known as retinol; if the end-group is an aldehyde it is known as retinal.

If the side-chain of retinol or retinal is straight the arrangement is called *all-trans*. If the side chain is twisted at site B in Figure 9–2, the vitamin is called *11-cis* retinol or *11-cis* retinal. If the bond on the ring (at C) of the vitamin A molecule is saturated it is called retinol$_1$ or retinal$_1$. If this bond is unsaturated it is called retinol$_2$ or retinal$_2$. 11-*cis* retinal$_1$ is the chromatophore of most vertebrate visual pigments. 11-*cis* retinal$_2$ is found in fresh water fish and amphibians in certain phases of their development. The cone pigment extracted from chicken retina has been called iodopsin and that from fresh water fish has been termed porphyropsin.

Rhodopsin, the rod pigment, has been extracted and studied extensively. Its breakdown and regeneration are diagrammed in Figure 9–3. The first step is triggered when a molecule of rhodopsin containing *11-cis* retinal$_1$ absorbs a single photon that changes it to the more stable *all-trans* form, which then becomes separated from opsin. The first step results in the formation of prelumirhodopsin, which is unstable. Following this, the breakdown is exothermic and proceeds spontaneously. Further light absorption can, however, reverse the process with the re-formation of rhodopsin.

Once *all-trans* retinal is free from opsin it may be isomerized to 11-*cis* retinal to re-form rhodopsin (Fig. 9–4), or it may be reduced by a dehydrogenase and NAD to *all-trans* retinol, and then esterified. The ester is stored in the pigment epithelium until needed for dark adaptation. After the *all-trans* ester has been de-esterified, oxidized and isomerized, 11-*cis* retinal is once again available for spontaneous regeneration of rhodopsin in the dark. Vita-

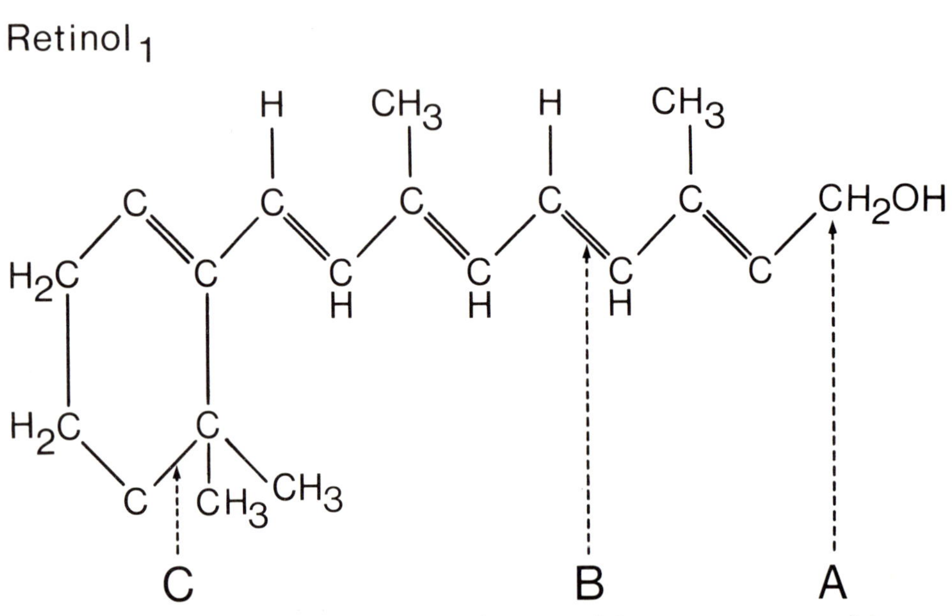

Figure 9–2. The structure of vitamin A. The A, B, and C sites represent areas of change in the structure of vitamin A that are important in photoreception. These changes are discussed in the text.

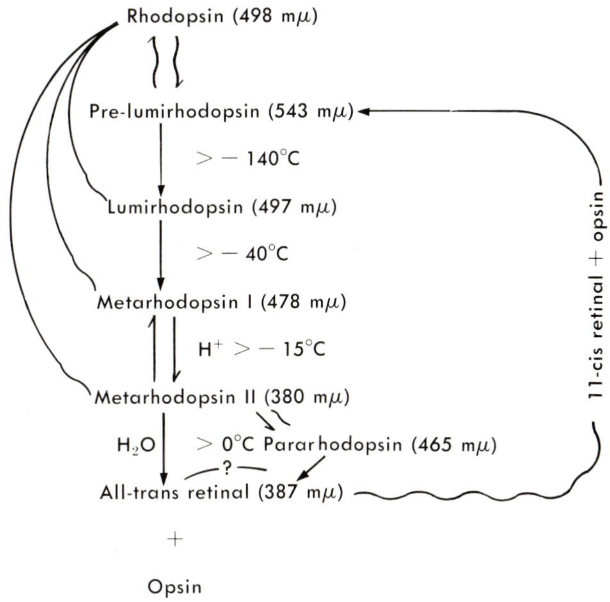

Figure 9–3. Intermediates in bleaching and regeneration of rhodopsin: wavy arrows indicate photoreactions; straight arrows indicate thermal ("dark") reactions. Interrelationships of pararhodopsin with final products of bleaching still present problems. (From Wald, G.: Science *162*:230–239, 1968. © Nobel Foundation 1968.)

min A in the eye has a fairly slow turnover with the other body supplies of vitamin A, and only a small fraction of ingested vitamin A reaches the eye.

Droz (1963) provided the first evidence that a protein, possibly opsin, is formed continuously in the ellipsoids of the rods and cones, after which it is found in the outer segments of the retinas of rats and mice. Young (1967) used radioactive methionine to show that the outer segments in the retinas of the frog, rat and mouse are being renewed constantly. The labeled protein first accumulated in the inner segments at the junction with the outer segments. Over a period of days the label moved as a discrete band into the outer segment toward the pigment epithelium and disappeared in the apical part of the outer segment; this process took nine days in the rat and 30 days in the frog retina. Young also showed that this renewal occurs more quickly in the light- than in the dark-adapted eye. These findings are interpreted to

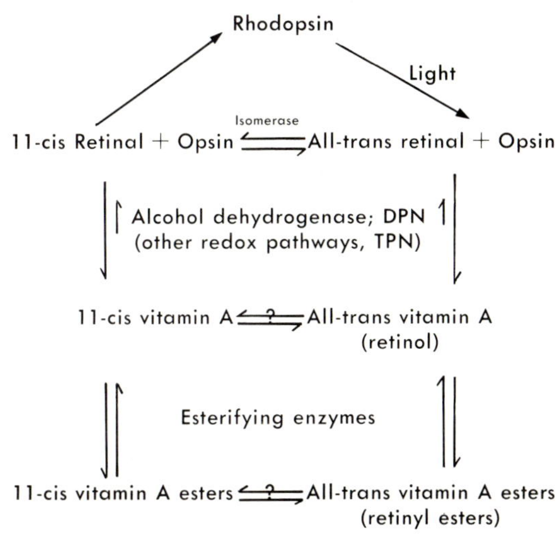

Figure 9–4. All-trans retinal may be isomerized to re-form rhodopsin or it may be reduced to all-trans retinol. Following esterification it can be stored in the retinal pigment epithelium until needed for dark adaptation. (From Wald, G.: Science *162*:230–239, 1968. © Nobel Foundation 1968.)

indicate that as new outer segment discs are formed from the region of the ellipsoid, the apical ends of the outer segments are being removed continuously by the retinal pigment epithelial cells.

The earliest electrical event after light exposure is the *early receptor potential* that has no lag time and is presumably caused by the isomerization of the retinal moiety. Just how this electrical change is amplified and propagated to the optic nerve is unknown, but three theories have been advanced, of which the ionic is most currently favored.

Wolken (1963) has proposed a structural model for vertebrate retinal rods based on their geometry and rhodopsin content. Cattle rods were calculated to contain 4×10^6 rhodopsin molecules. If the number of discs and their surface areas are known, the space occupied by the rhodopsin molecule can be determined. The cross-sectional areas calculated for cattle rhodopsin were found to be 2500 A., and the diameter of the rhodopsin molecule would be approximately 50 A. Figure 9-5 shows the molecular stacking of retinene with opsin in the retinal rod discs. There is one retinene molecule for every opsin molecule. The area available indicates that there would be sufficient space for all the pigment (rhodopsin) to cover all lamellar surfaces of the discs.

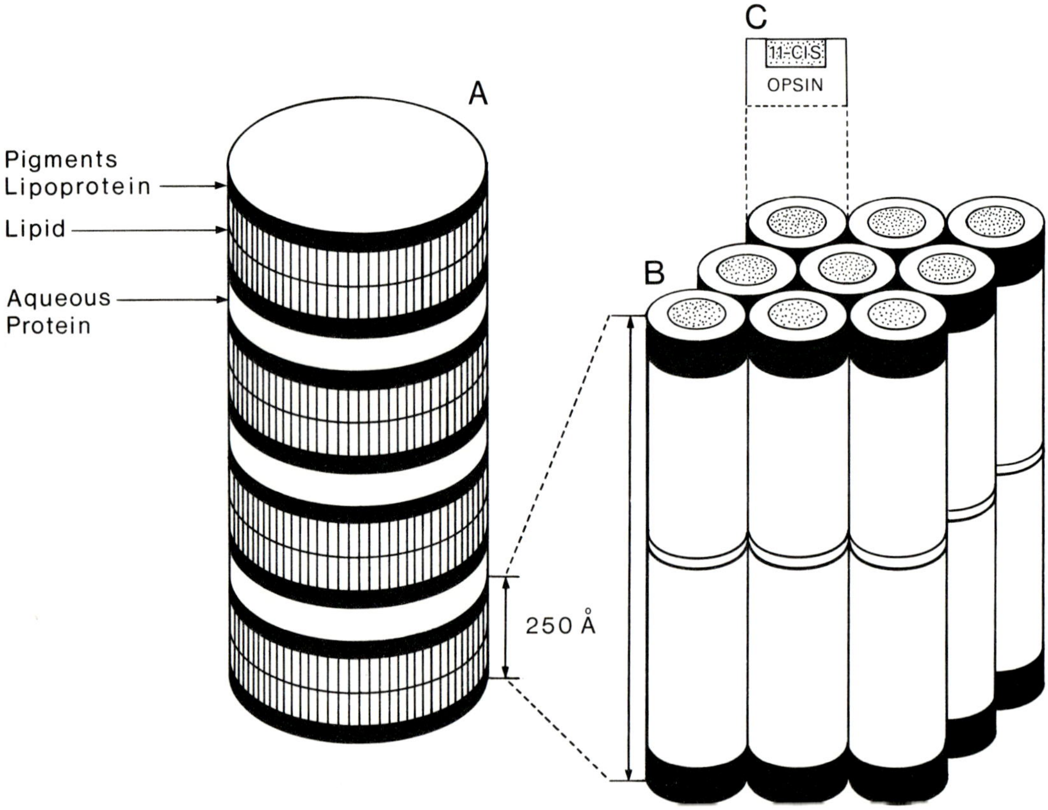

Figure 9–5. Schematic model of the molecular structure of a retinal rod as postulated by Wolken. The photopigments lie in the double membrane of the disc associated with lipoproteins. An aqueous protein medium separates the discs (A). A detailed view of the disc is shown at (B), and the location of 11-cis retinal$_1$ and opsin are shown at (C). (Modified from Wolken, J. J.: J. Optical Soc. Amer. 53:1–19, 1963).

Cone Pigments

We have seen that the photopic and scotopic spectral sensitivity of the rods and cones is different. Some pigment must be present in the cones whose absorption spectrum matches the photopic spectral sensitivity curve. Wald and associates (1955) extracted a photosensitive pigment from the cones of the chicken retina similar to rhodopsin but having an absorption maximum of 5400 A. Apparently the $retinal_1$ of the cones is identical to that of the rods, but their opsin moiety is different. Rushton and Campbell (1954, 1955) have identified at least two pigments in the retinal cones by using a technique which measures the reflection of light from the foveal cones. One of the pigments was found to be sensitive to red light and the other to green. Three absorption maxima at 440, 540 and 570 nm. have been found, however, in different primate cones in vitro. This observation would seem to confirm Young's trichromatic theory of color vision.

EMBRYOLOGY

The optic vesicle has developed prior to the fourth week of embryonic life, and during the fourth week it invaginates to form the optic cup. This results in the formation of two layers of neuroectodermal cells which contact each other at their apices; the base of the cells of the inner layer faces the vitreous and those of the outer layer face the choroid. The outer layer of neuroectoderm differentiates into a single layer of pigmented epithelium, and the inner layer of cells forms the sensory retina.

Prior to the fourth week the epithelium of the optic vesicle in the region of the future lens divides to form approximately eight to nine layers of cells. The cell layers occupy nine tenths of the thickness of this part of the developing retina, while only a thin non-nucleated zone, the marginal zone, separates the cells from the ectoderm. After formation of the cup during the fourth week (4.0 to 7.5 mm. stage) a thin capillary net appears in the region of the fetal fissure and extends outward to cover most of the entire optic cup. This net atrophies on the internal side of the cup by the 7 mm. stage. Pigment granules appear in the neuroepithelial layer, which forms the outer wall of the cup during this stage.

During the fifth week (4 to 12 mm. stage) the cells of the inner layer of the cup differentiate into an inner and an outer neuroblastic layer, these two layers being separated by the non-nucleated transient fiber layer of Chievitz. The cells of the inner and outer neuroblastic layers eventually develop into the retinal neurons and glia, and the outer layer also will form the rods and cones. Müller cells have formed the inner limiting membrane of the retina. During the seventh week (17 to 24 mm. stage), axons arise from the retinal ganglion cells and extend through the marginal zone toward the optic stalk.

Vrabec (1966) has shown that the neuroblastic layers of the macular region develop first in the human retina and that the more peripheral axons must arch around these layers and their axons in order to reach the disc. The fibers from the temporal macula, being more numerous than the peripheral ones, must arch around the fovea to reach the disc. At the same time they are forced to curve toward the disc by all the approaching peripheral fibers.

At this time the retina has reached its definitive thickness and subsequently increases only in area. Prior to the seventh week cilia have projected through the outer retina toward the pigment epithelium; they disappear late in the seventh week and are replaced by primitive rod and cone inner segments, with the outer segments forming soon thereafter. The inner neuroblastic layer differentiates into an outer layer composed of five or six rows of cells which will become Müller, amacrine and horizontal cells, and an inner two or three layers of cells which will become the ganglion cell layer.

During the eighth week retinal cellular differentiation extends from the posterior cup forward toward its periphery. Pigmentation of the cells in the outer layer of the cup increases in intensity and spreads both anteriorly and posteriorly. By the tenth week (50 mm. stage) rod and cone nuclei can be distinguished from each other, and the external limiting membrane is seen clearly. The anterior margin of the cup grows forward at this time to form the neuroectodermal epithelium of the future ciliary body and iris. By the end of embryonic life (twelfth week, 70 mm. stage) the inner plexiform layer separates the ganglion cell layer from the inner nuclear layer in the posterior retina; the plexiform layers then extend forward into the anterior retina. During the fourth month (70 to 110 mm. stage) the outer plexiform layer appears between the rods and cones, and the cells of the inner nuclear layer and bipolar, amacrine, Müller and horizontal cells can all be recognized. About this time the transient fiber layer of Chievitz almost completely disappears. The retinal pigment epithelial cells of the macular region begin to enlarge at the fourth month, and by the eighth month these cells are larger than those in most adult paramacular areas.

The final arrangement of cells and their processes becomes complete during the sixth month (160 to 200 mm. stage); thereafter the rods and cones differentiate further; the final form of the rods is evident early in the seventh month. The nerve fiber layer is present in the peripheral retina shortly after the seventh month. The ora serrata is at a level of the midciliary body at the seventh month, and it slowly recedes to the posterior border of the ciliary body during the final six weeks before birth.

Some retinal differentiation occurs after birth, especially in the macular region. An increase in cell density of the retinal pigment cells occurs between birth and two years of age, when the adult range is achieved (Streeten, 1967).

The first retinal vessels appear in the fourth month, when solid endothelial cords sprout from the nerve head to form the future central retinal artery (Cogan, 1963, b). By the sixth fetal month, these vessels have extended 1 to 2 mm. from the disc, and their endothelial cells show many mitoses. A great number of retinal blood vessels arranged in a "chicken-wire" pattern are found in the peripapillary region; they form the anlagen of the definitive retinal vessels. Around the fifth to sixth month the vessels form solid cords, but they soon develop a faint lumen that occasionally contains a red blood cell. By the seventh to eighth month vessels extend almost to the ora serrata nasally, and to the equator temporally; their chicken-wire mesh pattern persists through the ninth month but it is less uniform and has larger meshes, particularly in the posterior retina. Pericytes or mural cells (see p. 518) are not evident up to this time, and they do not appear until about two months after birth; however, these cells have been observed within human fetal capillaries (Mutlu and Leopold, 1964). The retinal vasculature achieves the adult pattern by the fifth month after birth. At this time the chicken-wire mesh is gone, but the peripheral vessels still have no mural cells. After the fifth postnatal month the capillaries differ from those of the adult retina only by their greater cellularity and weaker staining properties.

GROSS ANATOMY

The retina is a very thin, delicate, transparent tissue which lines the inner eye and is attached to the choroid through its pigment epithelium. The neural retina is loosely attached to the retinal pigment epithelium, this connection being particularly evident during retinal detachment when the separation occurs between the layer of rods and cones and the pigment epithelium, rather than between the pigment epithelium and Bruch's membrane. In the living eye the retina is completely transparent and can be recognized by the column of blood in the retinal vessels; after death it becomes milky and somewhat opaque.

Externally the retinal pigment epithelium is in contact with the collagen and elastic tissue of Bruch's membrane of the choroid. Bruch's membrane provides an elastic, yet unyielding layer that probably helps to stabilize the positions of the pigment epithelium and photoreceptors. *Internally* the retina is next to the vitreous body; the two structures are in intimate contact at the internal limiting membrane of the retina, especially around the ora serrata and in a 4 mm. zone posterior to the ora. *Anteriorly* the retinal pigment epithelium extends into the ciliary body. *Peripherally* the neuroretina ends at the ora serrata, but it is continuous with the unpigmented layer of epithelium over the ciliary body. *Posteriorly* all retinal layers except the nerve fiber layer terminate at the optic disc, being separated from the disc tissues by a layer of glial tissue, the intermediary tissue of Kuhnt. At the disc edge the retinal pigment epithelium ends slightly before the termination of Bruch's membrane.

The retina is thickest near the optic disc, where it measures 0.56 mm. It thins to 0.18 mm. at the equator and 0.1 mm. at the ora serrata (Fig. 9–6)

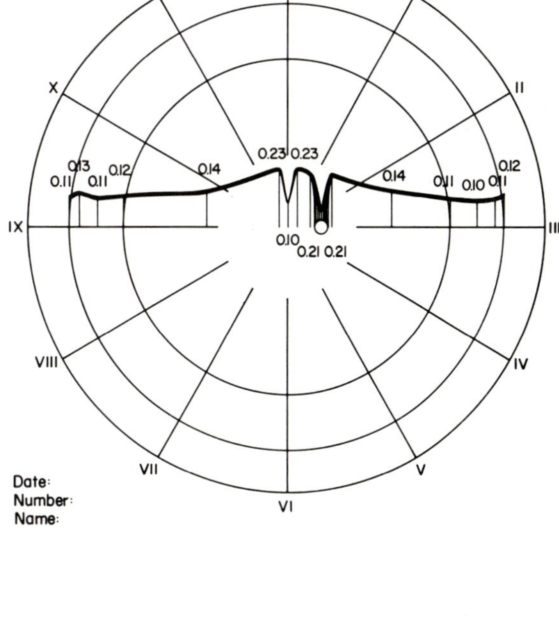

Figure 9–6. Profile of the thickness of the retina. The thinnest portion is in the foveola, and the thickest portion is in the parafoveal region. There is gradual thinning from the posterior to the peripheral retina. (From Straatsma, B. R., Foos, R. Y., and Spencer, L. M.: The retina—topography and clinical correlations. *In* New Orleans Academy of Ophthalmology: Symposium on Retina and Retinal Surgery. St. Louis, The C. V. Mosby Co., 1969.)

(Thomson, 1912). Peripherally the retina terminates at the ora serrata, where it forms dentate processes (teeth) that extend forward into the ciliary body. Deep bays occupy the intervals between the teeth, their convexities being directed posteriorly. Just posterior to the ora serrata the retina often shows cystoid degeneration (Iwanoff's cysts). This process commences early in youth, and with increasing age extends posteriorly from the ora serrata into the peripheral retina. This cystoid degeneration is uniformly found in adult eyes, so that it can be considered to be physiologic (see p. 498).

The retina can be subdivided into two general portions; the distinguishing features of each area are discussed here.

Central Retina

The central part of the retina is 5 to 6 mm. in diameter and contains the macula, the fovea and the foveola. Within the central retina is a zone known as the *macula lutea;* it measures about 2.0 mm. horizontally and 0.88 mm. vertically and is slightly yellow in color. With red-free light, the yellowish color is enhanced, and excised retinal tissue or very fresh tissue viewed with the dissecting microscope also shows this same yellow color in an area about 3 mm. in diameter around the fovea. The diameter of the yellow macula lutea area, however; is less than half that of the central area of the retina. The yellow color, which does not appear in the foveola, is believed to be due to the presence of the carotenoid, xanthophyll, which is found in the ganglion cells as well as in the bipolar layer cells in this region (Wald, 1946). Fine (1963) has suggested that the yellow color results from the numerous cytoplasmic inclusions found in these cells. (The central area of the retina will be discussed in more detail in the final pages of this chapter.)

Peripheral Retina

The peripheral retina may be subdivided into four regions: (1) near periphery, (2) midperiphery, (3) far periphery, and (4) ora serrata.

The *near periphery* is an area 1.5 mm. wide around the macula. Henle's fiber layer is absent in this zone. The cones are thick here, with about nine to ten cones per 100 μm., and they are surrounded by a collar of rods. The *midperiphery* is about 3 mm. wide. The ganglion cells are discontinuous here and the cones, which number eight to ten per 100 μm., are separated from each other by at least three rods. The *far periphery* is 9 to 10 mm. wide on the temporal side and 16 mm. wide on the nasal side. The ganglion cells here are spaced more widely, and some are quite large. The cones are reduced to six or seven per 100 μm., and their outer segments are shortened. The *ora serrata* is 2 mm. wide temporally and 0.7 to 0.8 mm. wide nasally. The rods gradually disappear in this region and are replaced by malformed cones. The rod and cone nuclear layers fuse as the outer plexiform layer disappears. The ganglion cells, the nerve fibers and the rods and cones cease about 0.5 mm. before the retinal termination. (A more detailed discussion of the structure of the ora serrata will be given later in this chapter.) The equator of the eye has been discussed in Chapter Two. The *retinal equator* conforms to the descriptions given there.

Blood Supply

The retina receives its blood supply from two sources: the external portion, which includes the retinal layers from the epithelium externally to the inner nuclear layer internally, is nourished by the choriocapillaris of the choroid. The remainder of the retina is supplied by the central retinal blood vessels. These vessels are distributed to the four quadrants of the retina, an artery and a vein passing from the disc within the nerve fiber layer of the retina into each quadrant. Arteriovenous crossings are frequent in the retina; they are more numerous in the temporal quadrants, especially the upper one, probably because the temporal retina has a greater area. The vein usually lies deeper than the artery at these crossings. The central macular region of the retina is avascular.

The blood flow through the retinal vessels is slower than through the choroidal vessels. In the human eye the retinal rate of flow has been estimated at 1.6 to 1.7 ml. per mm. per gm. of the retina (Anderson and Saltzmann, 1964). The mean retinal circulation time in man has been determined to be 4.7 ± 1.1 sec. (Hickman and Frayser, 1965); the mean transit time is 3 to 4 seconds (Friedman et al., 1964). The structure of the retinal vessels is discussed subsequently in this chapter, p. 508.

MICROSCOPIC ANATOMY

The retina customarily is subdivided into ten well defined layers that can be identified easily with the light microscope. These layers are (Figs. 9–7 and 9–8): (1) retinal pigment epithelium, (2) rod and cone layer, (3) outer limiting membrane, (4) outer nuclear layer, (5) outer plexiform layer, (6) inner nuclear layer, (7) inner plexiform layer, (8) ganglion cell layer, (9) nerve fiber layer, and (10) inner limiting membrane.

Prior to discussing the individual layers, the general organization of the retina is emphasized. There are three neurons and some receptor cells in the visual pathway. The first of these neurons is the bipolar cell that is completely within the retina. The second neuron is the ganglion cell that lies in the inner retina; its axons extend through the optic nerve to the chiasm and end in the lateral geniculate body. The third neuron extends from the geniculate body to the occipital cortex. The rods and cones are the sensory receptors in this pathway, and their outer segments contain photopigments which initiate the excitatory visual responses to light. The cell bodies of the rods and cones are in the outer nuclear layer of the retina, and their axons synapse with the dendrites of the first neuron in the outer plexiform layer. The bipolar cells lie in the inner nuclear layer. Dendrites of the bipolar cells extend into the outer plexiform layer to synapse with the axons of the rods and cones, and their axons extend into the inner plexiform layer to synapse with dendrites of the ganglion cells. Ganglion cells' axons form the nerve fiber layer of the retina. There is considerable horizontal integration of the cells of all parts of the retina through the horizontal and amacrine cells. The horizontal cells have extensive connections in the outer plexiform layer, while the amacrine cell connections are in the inner plexiform layer.

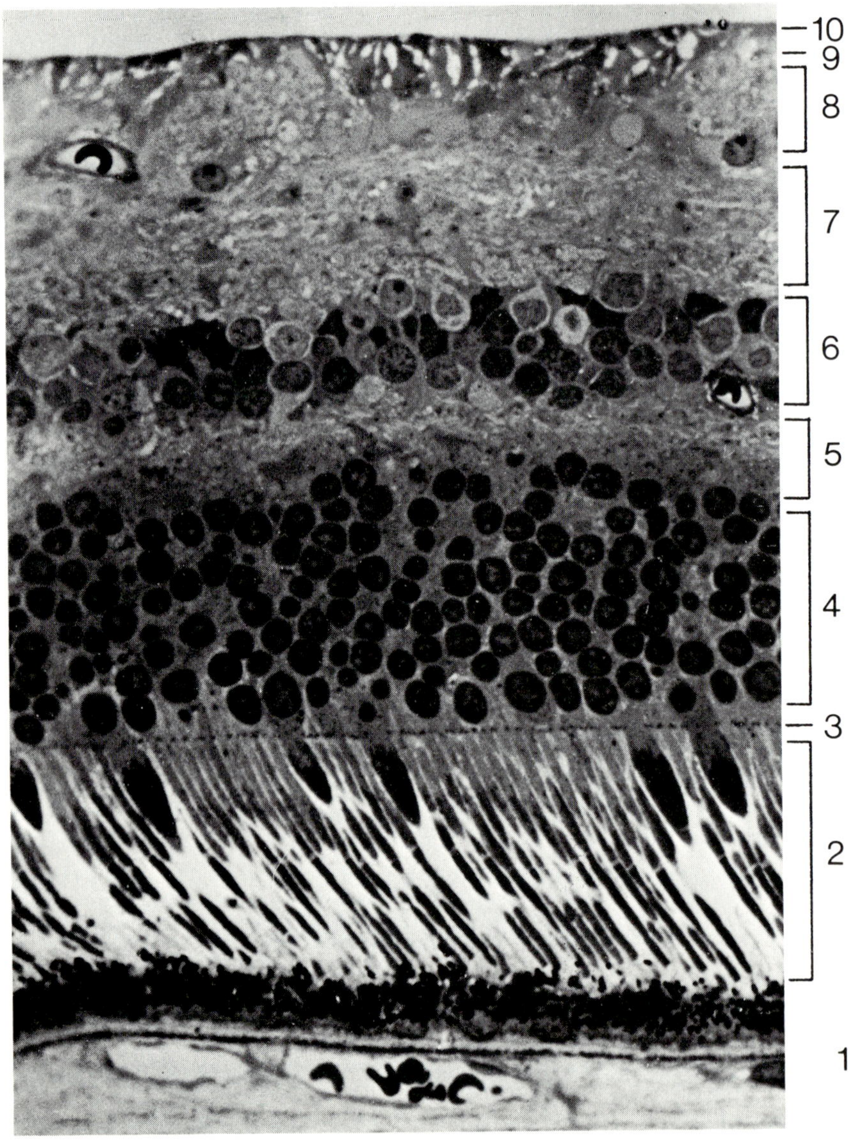

Figure 9–7. Light micrograph of a plastic-embedded, thin section of the full thickness of the retina. The layers are identified by numbers corresponding to those on page 403 of the text. (× 720.)

The Retinal Pigment Epithelium

The retinal pigment epithelium is a fairly uniform single layer of cells around the outer circumference of the retina, extending from the edge of the optic disc to the ora serrata (Figs. 9–8 to 9–21). These cells are hexagonal in shape and form a remarkably regular pattern in all species (Figs. 9–9 and 9–10). The estimated number of pigment epithelial cells per eye is 4.2 to 6.1 million, with greater numbers in older eyes. The pigment epithelium has a brown color, but the density of the pigment varies in different parts of the retina, as well as within individual cells. For example, the cells are more pigmented in the macular region in an area measuring 4 to 5 mm. in diameter than elsewhere in the retina. The cells in the macular region measure about 14 μm. in diameter by 10 to 14 μm. tall (Salzmann, 1912; Ts'o and Friedman, 1967). At the ora serrata they are flatter and wider, measuring up to 60 μm. in diameter, while cell size and shape are more irregular in the peripheral retina than elsewhere.

The nucleus of a typical retinal pigment epithelial cell in the human eye is located in the basal portion of the cell; it measures 5 to 12 μm. in diameter. Many of the cells are multinucleated, particularly in the ora serrata region; the ratio of mononucleate to binucleate cells is approximately 30 to 1 (Ts'o and Friedman, 1967). The large cells in the ora serrata region frequently contain up to three or four nuclei (Ts'o and Friedman, 1968). Mitoses have not been observed in the retinal pigment epithelial cells and it is generally believed that they are not replaced if they die, but adjacent cells slide laterally to fill the space left by a dead cell. It is possible that the multinucleated cells seen peripherally result from amitotic division.

Growth. In fetal and postnatal eyes, the entire pigment epithelium gradually increases in size. A disproportionate, nonuniform enlargement of cells occurs in the ora serrata region from infancy into adolescent life in a zone that gradually enlarges from 1 to 4 mm. wide. By the time the eye has achieved a sagittal diameter of 23 mm. (three to six years of age), growth is largely confined to the oral-equatorial region (Streeten, 1967). Between the second and third years of life, the surface area of the retina increases by 37 per cent, with the total number of retinal pigment epithelial cells increasing only slightly (Ts'o and Friedman, 1968). Only a 20 per cent increase was found in the number of equatorial cells, but the area covered by the pigment epithelial cells in the periphery was found to be doubled as a result of thinning and stretching of the cells. The area covered by the pigment epithelial cells in the macular region, however, actually decreased in the same eyes.

Aging. Some aspects of aging of the retinal pigment epithelium and Bruch's membrane have been discussed in the chapter on the choroid. A considerable number of studies have involved senescent changes in the human retinal pigment epithelial cells, especially in eyes showing senile degenerative changes. A significant degree of pleomorphism occurs as an aging phenomenon, involving the size and shape of the cells, their nuclei and the pigment granules (Friedman and Ts'o, 1968). A distinguishing feature of senile eyes is the presence of many normal-appearing cells with smaller and more basophilic nuclei. According to these authors the macular cells were found to increase in height and to become narrower with increasing age from fetal and infantile life to adulthood, whereas the op-

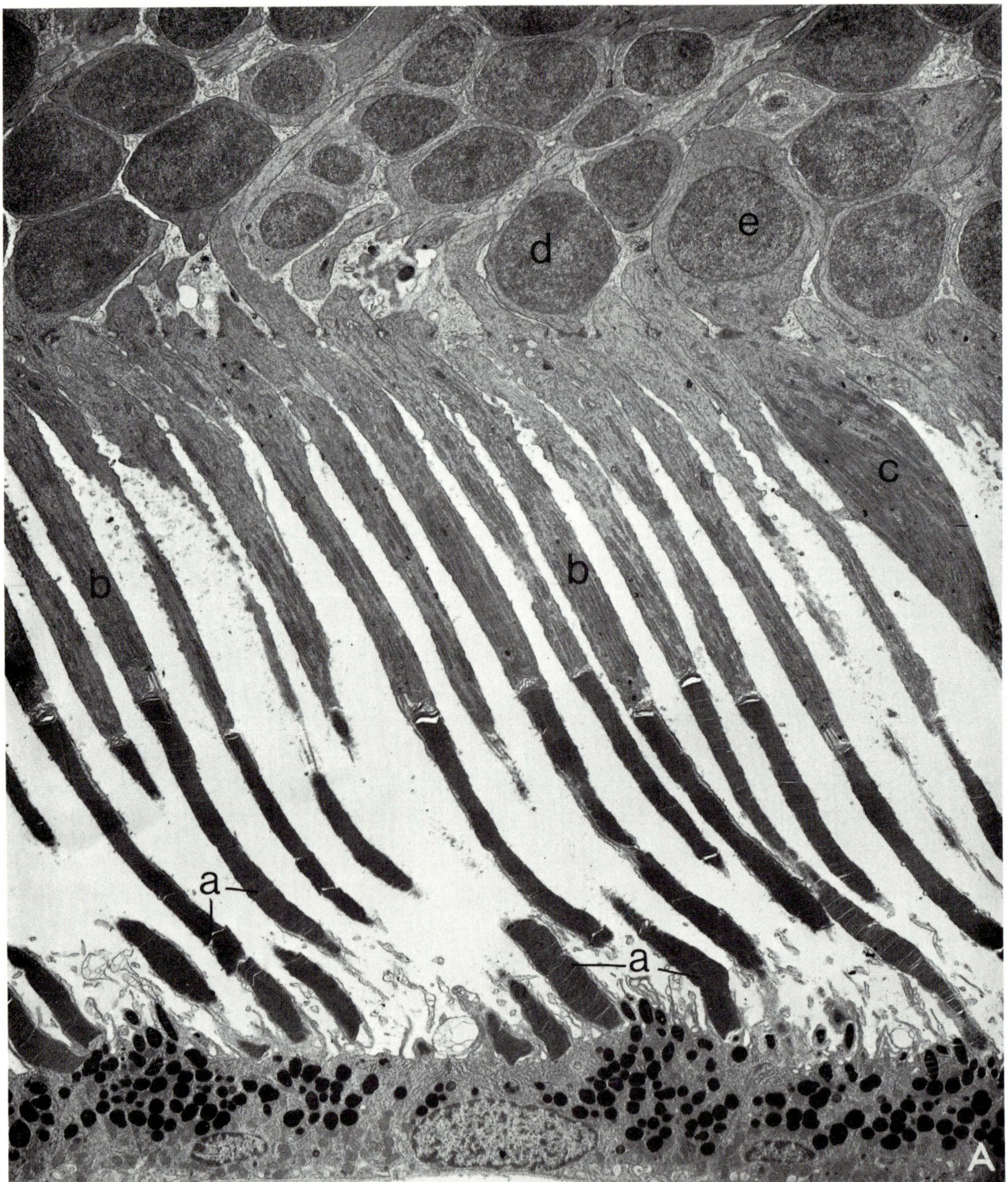

Figure 9–8. Electron micrographs to identify the retinal layers as they are seen with the light microscope in Figure 9–7. *A*, The external retina. The outer segments (a) of the receptors are intimate with the pigment epithelium. The rod inner segments are at (b) and those of the cones at (c). A rod nucleus is at (d) and a cone nucleus at (e). (×2400.)

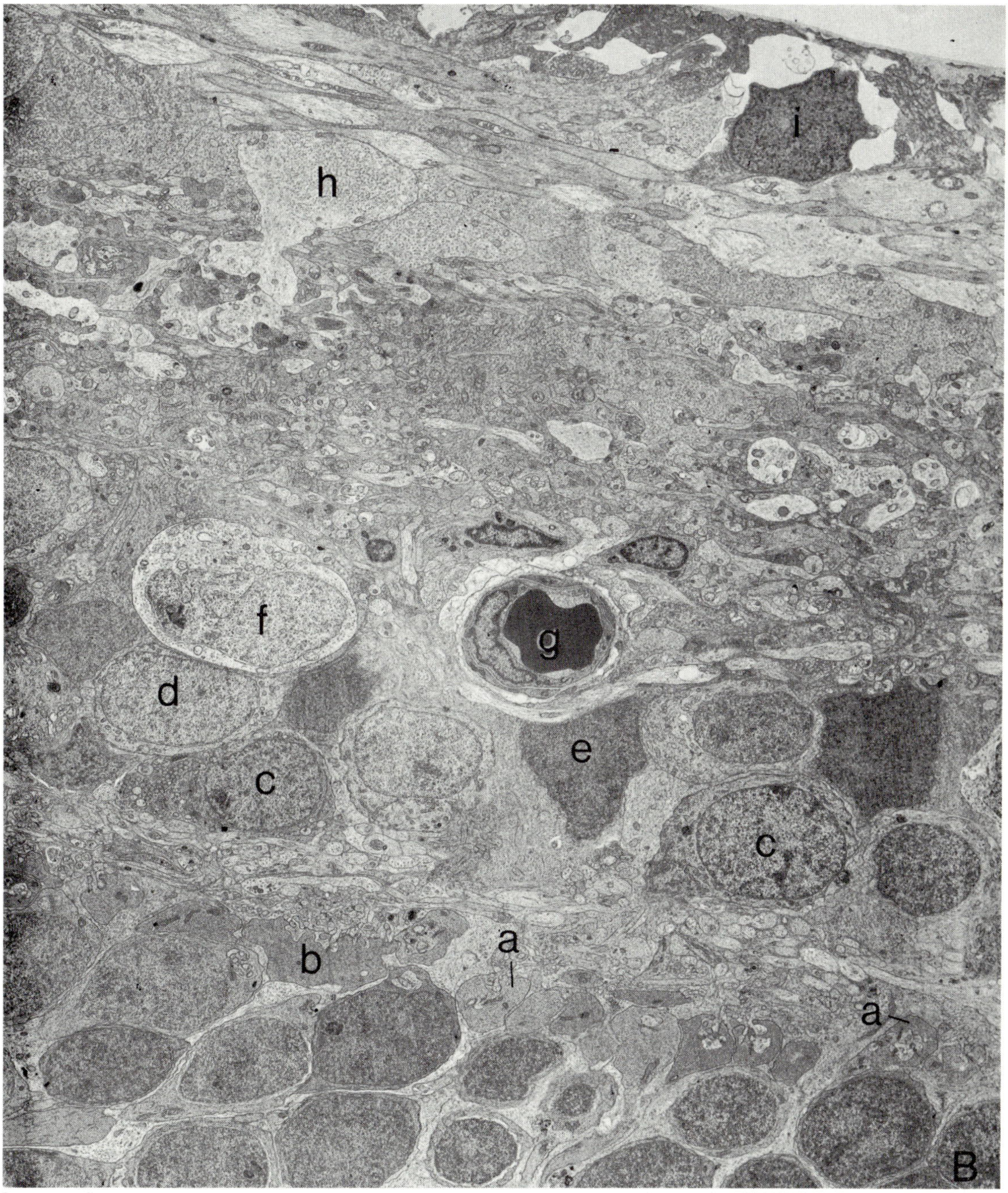

Figure 9–8. *Continued.*

B, The internal portion of the retina, adjacent to that shown in *A*. A rod synapse (a) and a cone synapse (b) are seen in the external plexiform layer. The horizontal cell nuclei of the internal nuclear layer are at (c), and a bipolar nucleus is at (d). Other identifiable structures are a Müller cell nucleus (e), an amacrine cell nucleus (f), a capillary (g), a ganglion cell (h) and a glial cell nucleus (i). The inner retina is seen at the top of the photograph. (× 2800.)

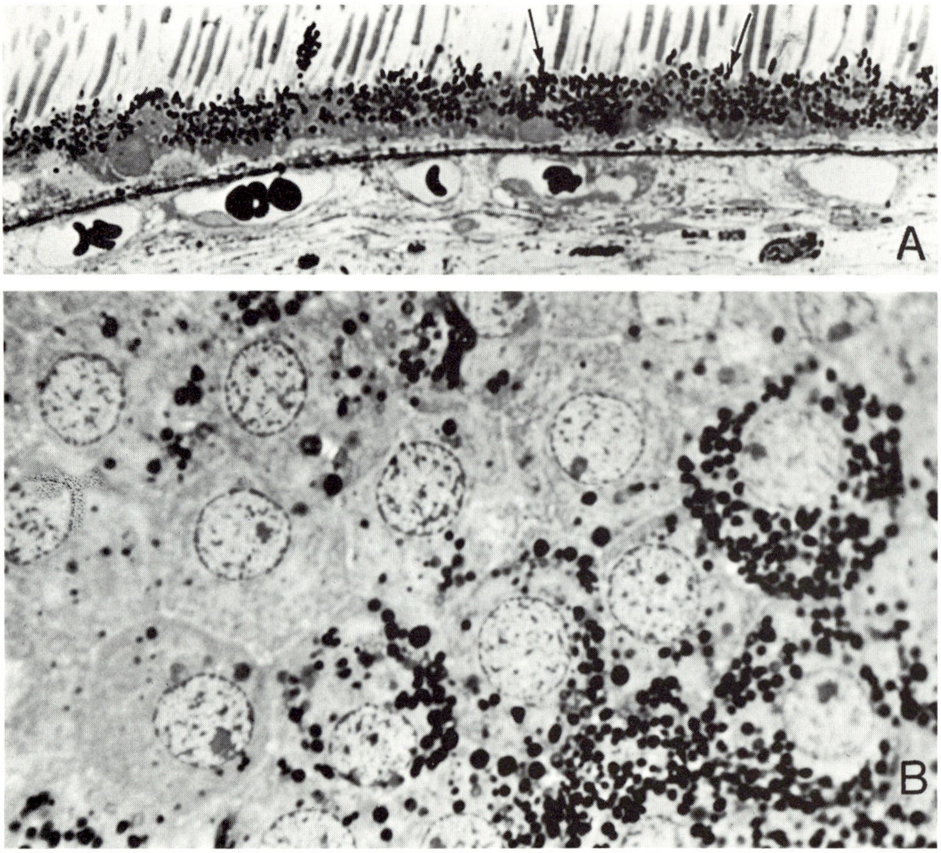

Figure 9–9. Meridional and tangential light micrographs of the retinal pigment epithelium. *A*, The pigment granules occupy the apical part of the cell and the nuclei are found in the basal region. The outer segments of the rods and cones meet and are surrounded by the processes of the apical pigment epithelium (arrows).

B, This flat section shows the hexagonal shape of the pigment epithelial cells. Those cells that are sectioned close to the apical portion are heavily pigmented while others that are sectioned through the basal portion show no pigment. (× 1700.)

posite was found in the peripheral cells. The degree of pigmentation was found to be less in the cells of young eyes than in older eyes, and again the reverse was found in the periphery. The degree of pleomorphism exhibited by the macular cells with increasing age was no different from that at the equator. In the periphery, however, the cells became broader, lower, more vacuolated, and markedly pleomorphic. Friedman and Ts'o found that the retinal pigment cells were displaced by drusen (see p. 344, Choroid) but were otherwise normal in appearance. Degeneration or loss of cells occurred in areas where large drusen were present, however. The drusen were randomly distributed in most specimens, but in some they were organized in patterns resembling those of the underlying choriocapillaris. The cytoplasm of the pigment epithelial cells accumulates lipid and a granular material as it ages. This material leaves the cells and is deposited in the inner collagenous zone of Bruch's membrane, frequently producing masses which are called drusen. Thinning and atrophy of the pigment cells frequently occurs over these drusen (Hogan, 1963).

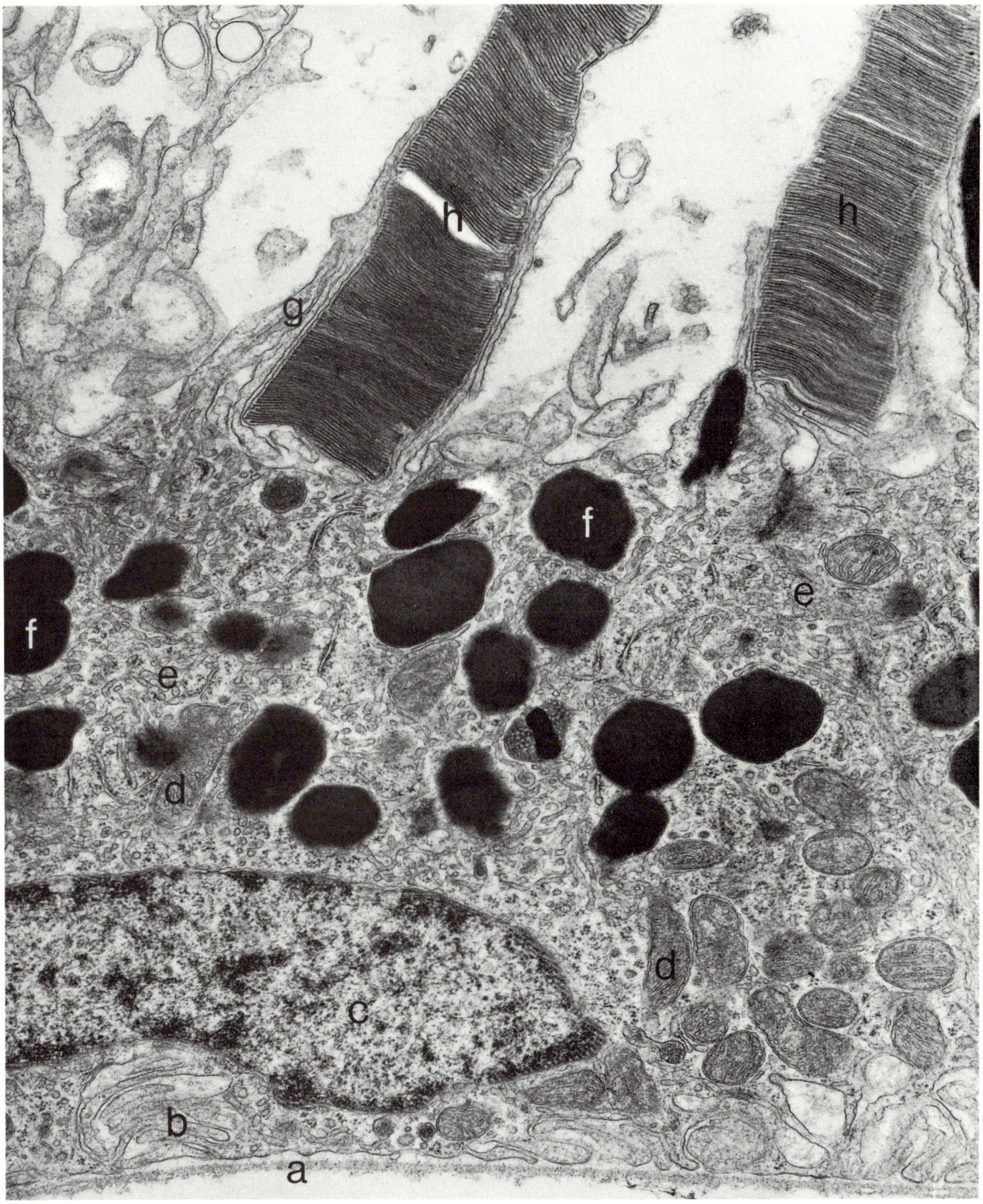

Figure 9–10. Electron micrograph of the retinal pigment epithelium to show its relation to the rod outer segments. The pigment epithelial basement membrane is at (a), the basal infoldings of its cell membrane are at (b), the nucleus is at (c), and the external cytoplasm contains numerous mitochondria (d). Characteristically there is a large amount of reticulum (e). The pigment granules (f) are located mainly in the apical portion of the cell. Microvilli (g) along the apical surfaces of these cells extend internally to surround the outer segments of the photoreceptors (h). (× 18,000.)

Cell Membrane. The membrane enclosing the cytoplasm and organelles of the pigment epithelial cells is a typical unit membrane. The cell membrane at the *base of the cell* facing Bruch's membrane shows marked complex infoldings which extend 1 μm. or more into the cytoplasm (Fig. 9–11). Infolding of this type is usually found in cells involved in absorption of substances from adjacent cavities or blood vessels. The infoldings extend along the entire basal surface of the cells. External to the cell membrane is a space of low electron density separating the cell membrane from an adjacent basement membrane (Figs. 8–8 and 9–10). The basement membrane is faintly fibrillar, some of the filaments extending to the inner part of Bruch's membrane. These connections may account for the greater cohesion between the pigment epithelium and Bruch's membrane than between the epithelium and the receptors. This basement membrane is PAS-positive. There are no half-desmosomes along the retinal pigment epithelial cell membrane at its base, as are seen in the corneal epithelium. The basement membrane disappears at the optic disc concurrently with the epithelial cells; at the ora serrata it continues as the basement membrane of the pigment epithelium of the ciliary body.

The *lateral cell membranes* are only slightly interdigitated. The cells are separated from each other along their lateral walls by a normal space of variable width (Fig. 9–12). The intercellular spaces are sealed off from the apical lumen by zonulae occludentes, and zonulae adherentes are regularly found external to the zonulae occludentes. Desmosomes are found inconstantly along the lateral cell membranes. By light microscopy these junctional complexes along the lateral cell membranes produce the effect of a continuous membrane, which was first described by Verhoeff (1903) and has come to be called Verhoeff's membrane.

The *apical cell membrane*, facing the rod and cone receptors, shows many microvilli which are of two types, fine ones about 5 to 7 μm. in length that lie principally between the outer segments of the receptors, and shorter ones about 3 μm. in length that form a sheath around the terminations of the outer receptors. These microvilli surround the external third of the outer processes of the rods and cones (Figs. 9–13 to 9–15). Junctional complexes do not unite the receptor outer segments to the pigment epithelium.

A viscous ground substance surrounds these villi as well as the outer and inner segments of the rods and cones. When stained with the alcian blue

Text continued on page 415

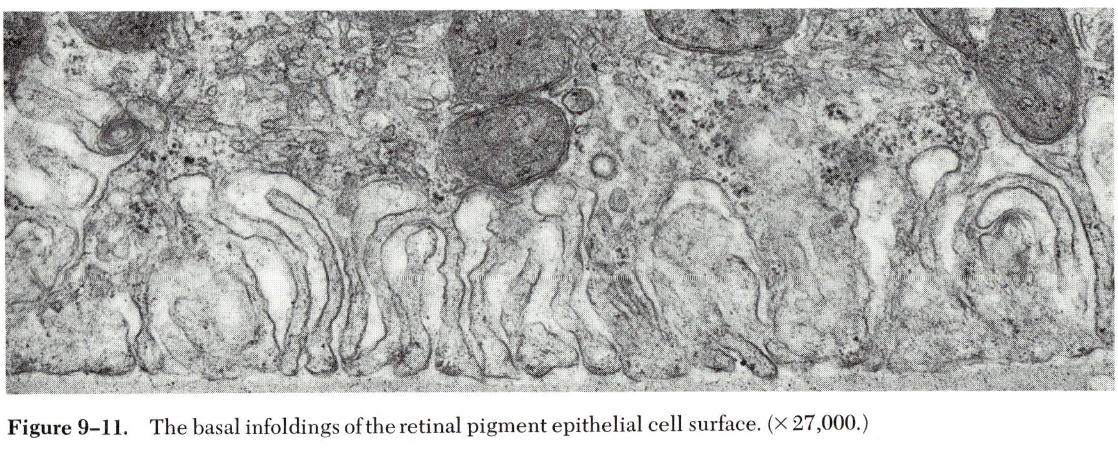

Figure 9–11. The basal infoldings of the retinal pigment epithelial cell surface. (×27,000.)

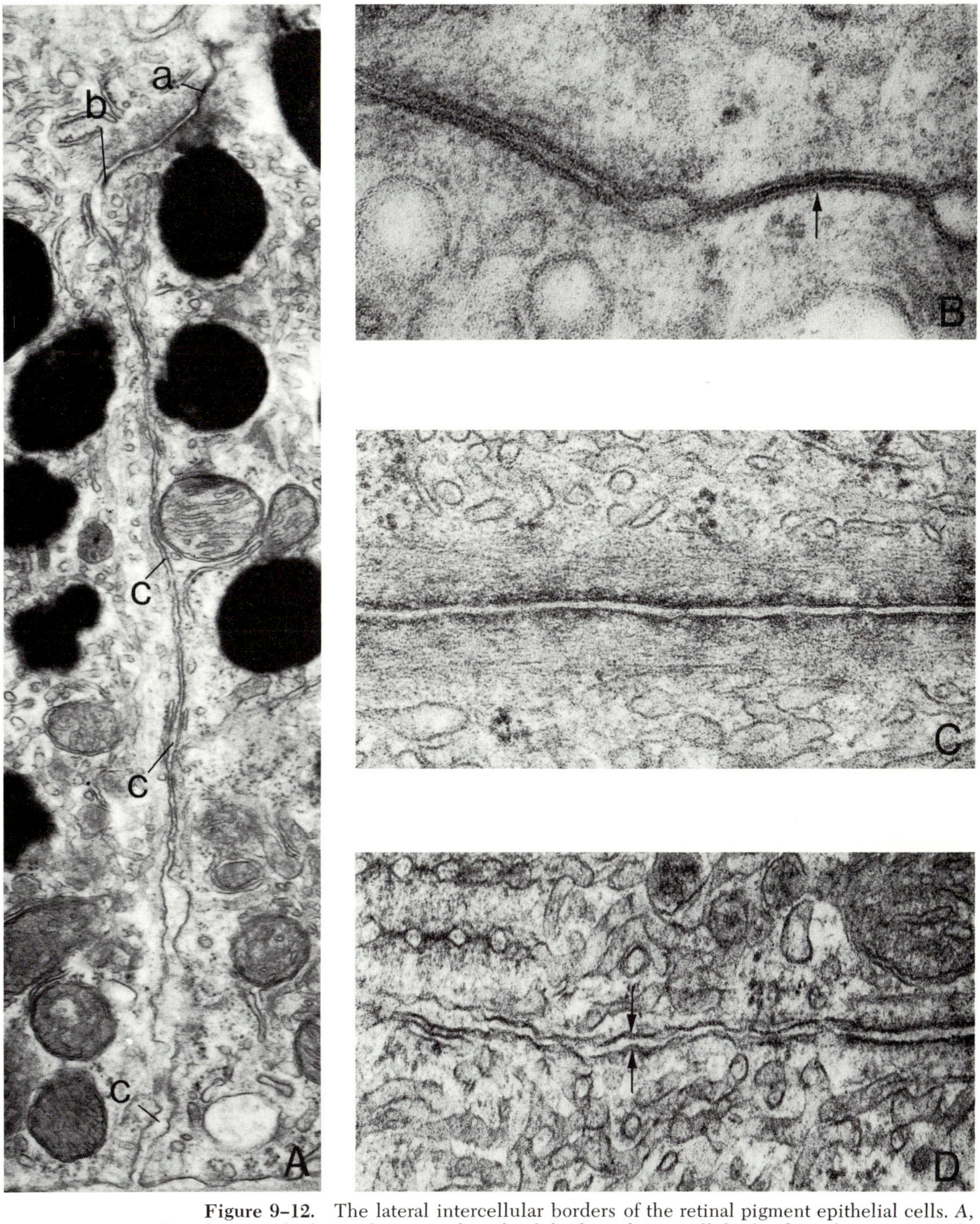

Figure 9–12. The lateral intercellular borders of the retinal pigment epithelial cells. *A*, This photograph shows the entire length of the lateral intercellular border. There is a zonula occludens (a), a zonula adherens (b) and the remainder of the intercellular space (c). (× 26,100.)

B, Zonula occludens (arrow). (× 132,000.)

C, Zonula adherens. (× 60,000.)

D, Intercellular space near the basal portions of these cells. The continuous cell membranes are shown (arrows). (× 60,000.)

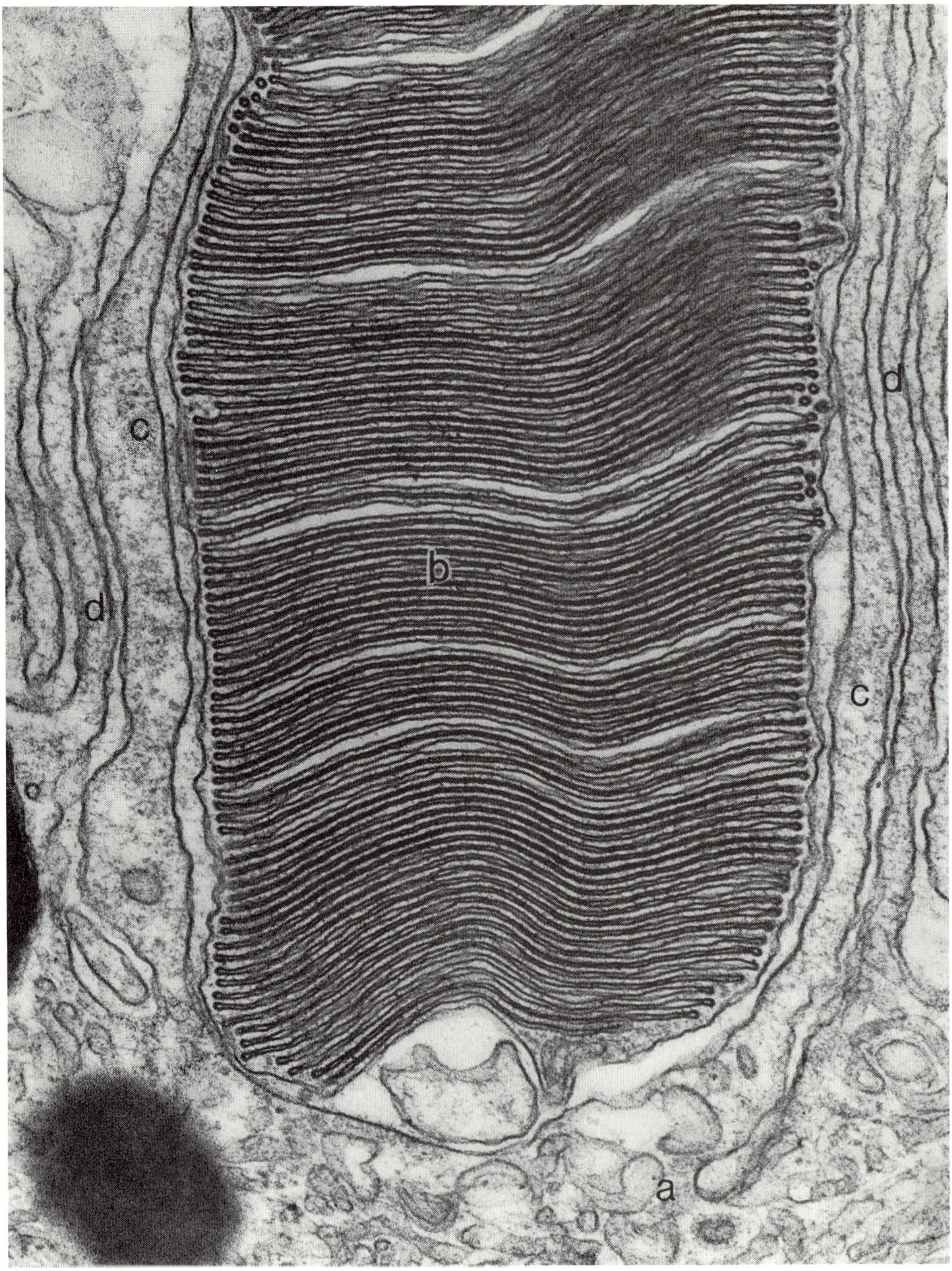

Figure 9–13. Meridional section of the apical portion of the retinal pigment epithelium showing its villi and an enclosed outer segment of a rod. The pigment epithelial cytoplasm is seen at (a) and the rather thick sheaths (c) encompass the photoreceptor (b). The thinner fringe-like villi between the photoreceptors are at (d). (× 60,000.)

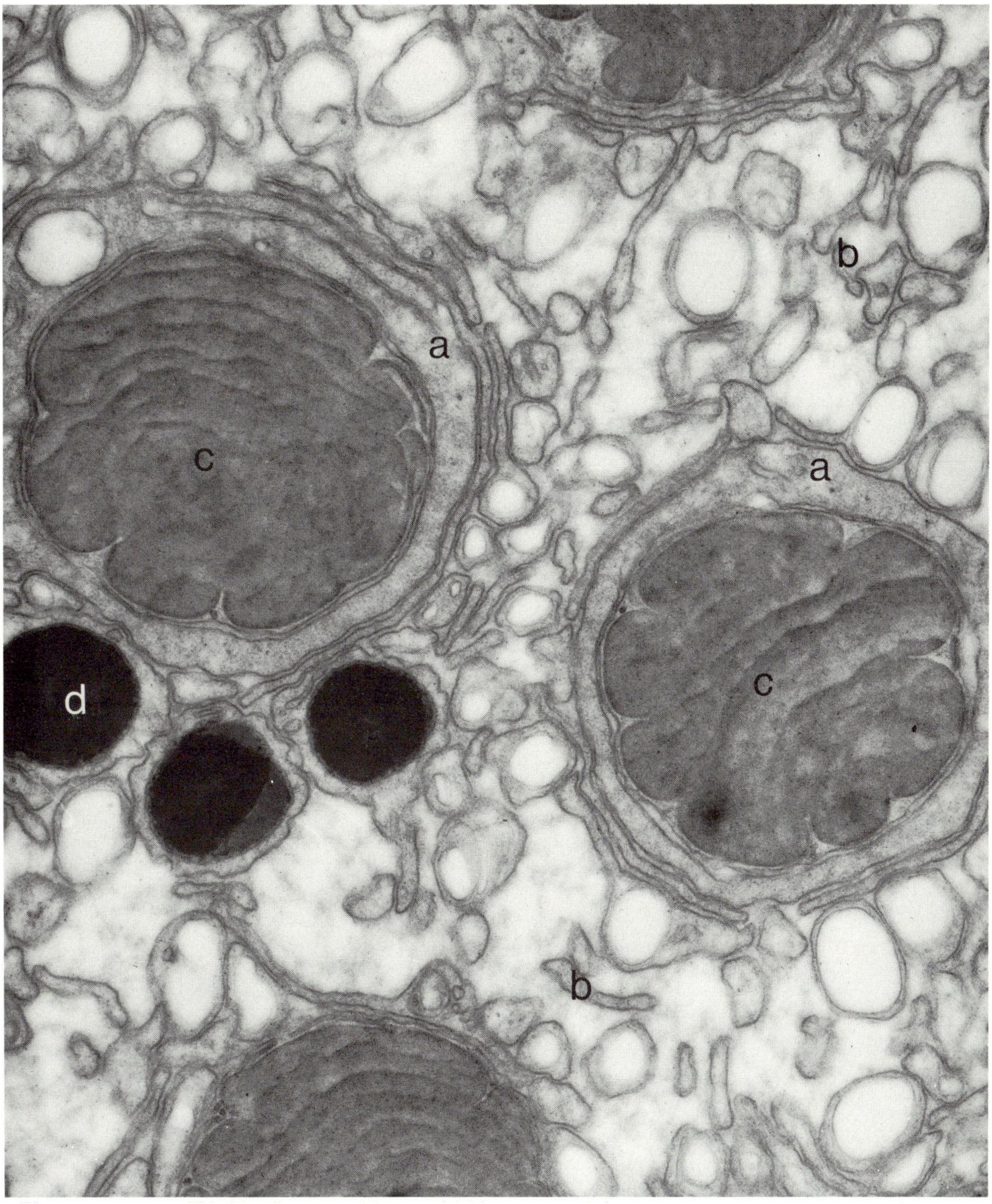

Figure 9–14. A cross-section of the same pigment epithelial receptor area as shown in Figure 9–13. The sheaths around the receptors (a) are thicker and heavier than the interreceptor villi (b). A cross-section of a rod disc is seen at (c). Pigment granules (d) are found in the cytoplasm of the cell. (× 40,000.)

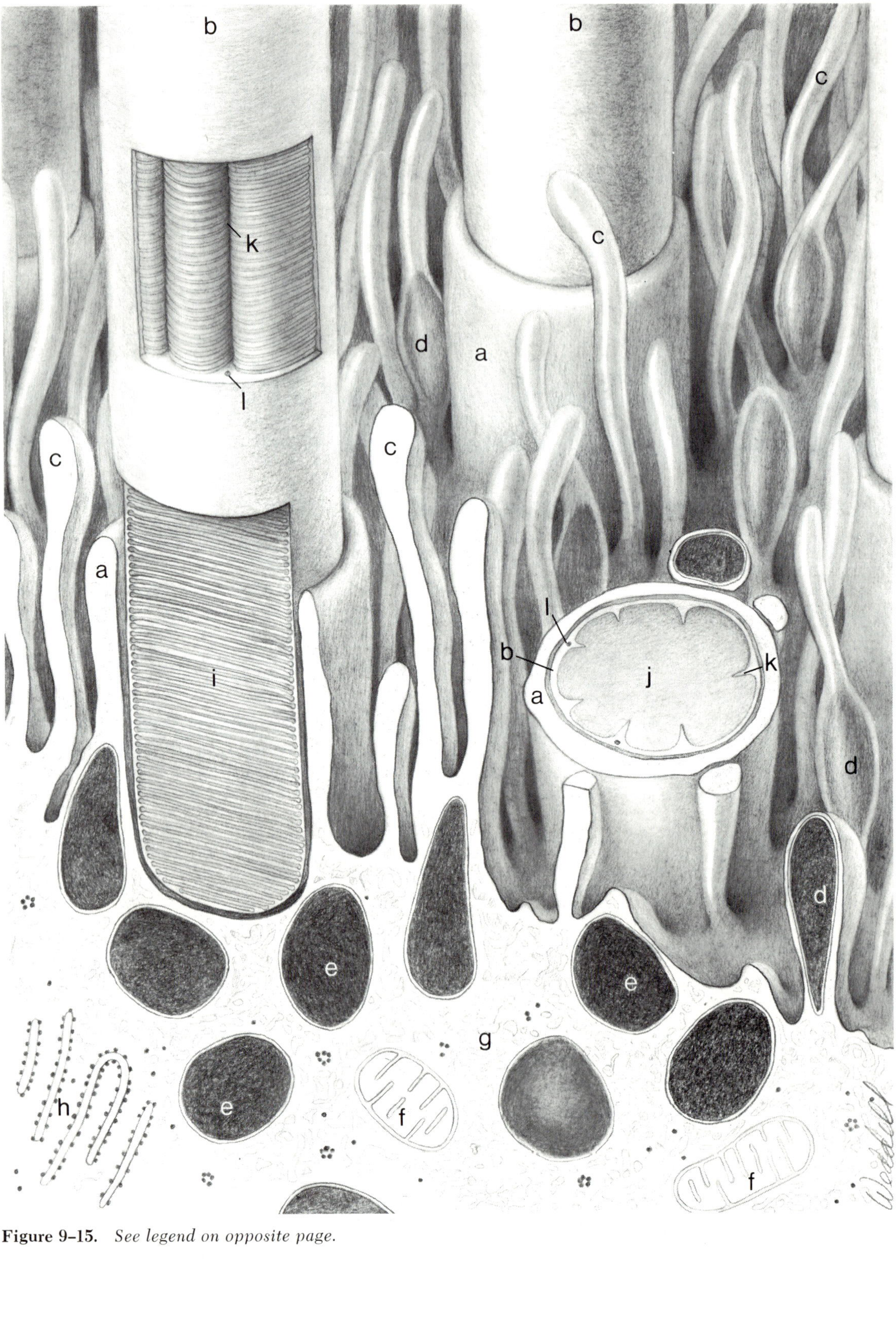

Figure 9–15. *See legend on opposite page.*

and AMP stains the substance is strongly positive for mucopolysaccharide, but it is not soluble in testicular or streptococcal hyaluronidase (Zimmerman, 1958). Berman and Bach (1968) identified two polysaccharides in the interstitial matrix surrounding the photoreceptor cells of cattle retina. Two thirds of the polysaccharide was a hyaluronidase-sensitive, "half-sulfated" chondroitin sulfate, and the other third was a hyaluronidase-resistant, nonsulfated heteropolysaccharide for which the name sialoglycan was proposed.

Cytoplasm. The cytoplasm of the pigment epithelial cells contains a rather large nucleus and numerous large pigment granules in addition to the usual organelles. Most of the mitochondria are located between the nucleus and the basal cell membrane (Fig. 9–10). Mitochondria are also seen easily in ordinary hematoxylin- and eosin-stained sections, probably because this part of the cytoplasm has less pigment. The high pigment content of the cytoplasm elsewhere obscures cytoplasmic detail under the light microscope. The nucleus is displaced slightly toward the base of the cell; it is somewhat oval, with the long axis parallel to Bruch's membrane. It contains one or two nucleoli and its chromatin is diffuse.

When viewed by electron microscopy the cytoplasmic structure is dense and complex. It contains many free ribosomes and numerous small mitochondria, which are rod-shaped in longitudinal section and round in cross-section; they measure about 0.5 to 1.0 μm. in length (Fig. 9–16). Their cristae are arranged transversely. The smooth-surfaced endoplasmic reticulum occupies the greater portion of the cytoplasm; such development of this reticulum is not seen elsewhere in the eye except for the Müller cells. The reticulum is formed by tubular, vesicular and lamellar structures. In the peripheral retina the amount of smooth-surfaced endoplasmic reticulum diminishes and the rough-surfaced endoplasmic reticulum becomes more prominent; cytoplasmic fibrils are also more abundant, giving the cytoplasm a more compact, dense appearance. Another organelle characteristically found in the pigment epithelium consists of a stack of annulate lamellae, usually located in the basal portion of the cell (Fig. 9–16 *D*). Such lamellae have been identified with active protein synthesis. The rough-surfaced endoplas-

Figure 9–15. A three-dimensional drawing of the relation of the outer segments of the rods to the retinal pigment epithelial cells. Thick sheaths (a) of the pigment epithelium enclose the external portions of the rod outer segments (b). Numerous finger-like villous processes (c) are found between the photoreceptors; they contain pigment granules (d). The apical portion of the pigment epithelial layer of cells is seen at the bottom. It contains numerous pigment granules (e), mitochondria (f), a well developed, smooth-surfaced endoplasmic reticulum (g), a poorly developed, rough-surfaced endoplasmic reticulum (h) and scattered free ribosomes. The stacks of the rod outer segment discs are depicted in meridional section at (i) and in cross-section at (j). There is scalloping of the periphery of the discs (k). Microtubules originating in the basal body of the rod cilium extend externally into the outer segment; one such microtubule is shown in cross-section at (l).

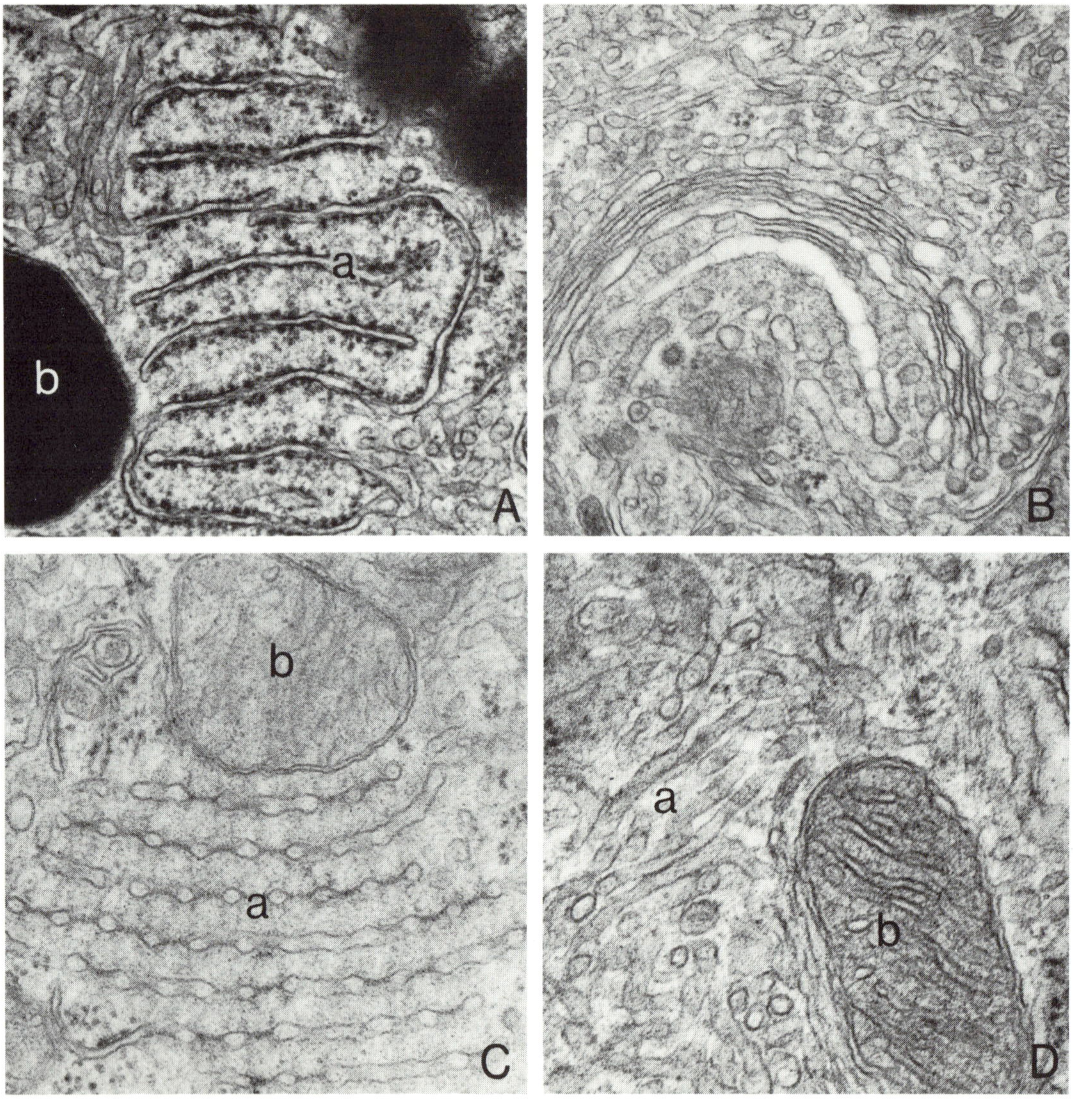

Figure 9–16. Cytoplasmic organelles in the retinal pigment epithelium. *A*, Rough-surfaced endoplasmic reticulum (a) and a pigment granule (b). (× 36,000.)

B, Golgi apparatus. (× 36,000.)

C, Annulate lamellae (a) and a mitochondrion (b). (× 54,000.)

D, Smooth-surfaced endoplasmic reticulum (a) and a mitochondrion (b). (× 60,000.)

Figure 9–17. Melanin formation. The synthesis of melanin granules starts with the formation of the enzyme tyrosinase in the rough-surfaced endoplasmic reticulum (1). This enzyme is then presumably transferred to the Golgi apparatus (2) where it is segregated into discrete membrane-bounded vesicles (3) which are known as premelanosomes (4). The tyrosinase of the premelanosomes is associated with a finely striated protein framework. Once tyrosine is polymerized into melanin on this striated protein framework, the granules become known as melanosomes (5). Melanin formation continues until the granule is completely filled with melanoprotein, at which time the granules are called melanin granules. Such granules do not have demonstrable tyrosinase activity (6). (Modified from Seiji, M.: Subcellular particles and melanin formation in melanocytes. *In* Montagna, W. (ed.): Advances in Biology of the Skin. New York, Pergamon Press, 1967, p. 189.)

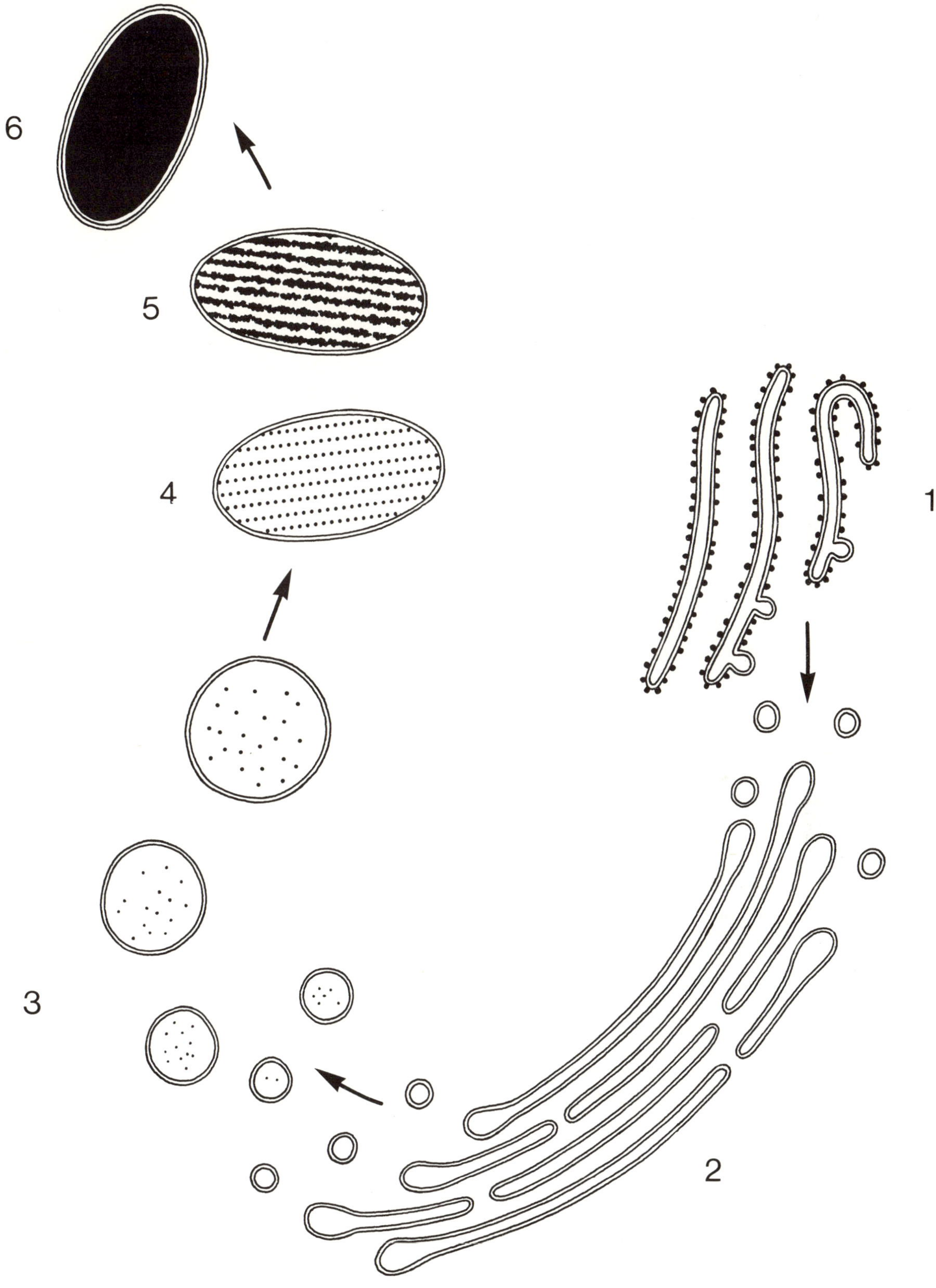

Figure 9–17. *See legend on opposite page.*

mic reticulum is poorly developed in the posterior retina, but it becomes more prominent near the ora serrata. It is found in the apical portion of the cells and most often forms parallel arrays of five to 10 cisternae.

Pigment granules measuring up to 1 μm. in diameter and 2 to 3 μm. in length are a prominent feature of the cytoplasm of these cells. The granules are found in the apical and midportions of the cell, but the basal cell cytoplasm is almost free of them. Classically the pigment granules have been considered to have a football or needle shape, and some reports indicate that those granules in the apex of the cell are needle-like, whereas those in the perinuclear cytoplasm are oval or round.

Pigment develops in these epithelial cells at an early stage in embryonic life, so that the pigment granules presumably become "mature" long before birth. Miyamoto and Fitzpatrick (1957) found the granules to be tyrosinase-negative in the adult eye, but in the developing chick eye and in a 6 month old human fetus, the granules were found to be tyrosinase-positive. In the chick no tyrosinase activity was found after the fourteenth day of development, indicating maturity of the granules. According to the stage of development of the individual melanin granules, they can be recognized in various forms, as follows (Fig. 9–17) (Seiji, 1967):

Premelanosome. A cytoplasmic organelle containing oriented fibrils without melanin or tyrosinase activity.

Melanosome. An organelle having some melanin and tyrosinase activity.

Mature Melanin Granule. A heavily pigmented particle without tyrosinase activity.

Melanin granules are found in the retinal pigment epithelial cells at about the fifth week of gestation, and between the eighth and fourteenth weeks granules of all stages can be observed (Fig. 9–18) (Feeney et al., 1965; Breathnach and Wyllie, 1966). The premelanosomes and melanosomes found at these stages correspond to those seen in the skin. Between the fifth month of fetal life and two years of age, polymerization of melanoprotein occurs in these granules and they finally become tyrosinase-negative.

With the electron microscope the pigment granules are seen to be surrounded by a thin membrane, the internal surface of which is in direct contact with the melanoprotein that fills the space. The granules are polymorphic, some being round and others elliptical, the pleomorphism being mainly the result of the plane of sectioning. The majority of the pigment granules lack an internal structure (Fig. 9–19).

Lipofuscin, another pigment, has also been described in the cytoplasm of the retinal pigment epithelial cells (Streeten, 1961; Feeney et al., 1965). This pigment is considered to be formed as a result of "wear and tear" and is like that found in neural cells and other tissues. Lipofuscin granules probably are *residual bodies*, representing the end product of phagosomal activity (see p. 33). With the light microscope, Streeten found the lipofuscin granules to appear for the first time at the age of 16 months. After age 20 they increased in number and in size. These granules are sudanophilic and contain unsaturated fatty acids, probably in a phosphatid complex. The sudanophilic granules and rod outer segments show the same histochemical staining qualities. Stains for "myelin-like" substances such as lipofuscin myelins and lipid of the retinal rod outer segments are positive in these granules, suggesting that they may be derived from the rod discs.

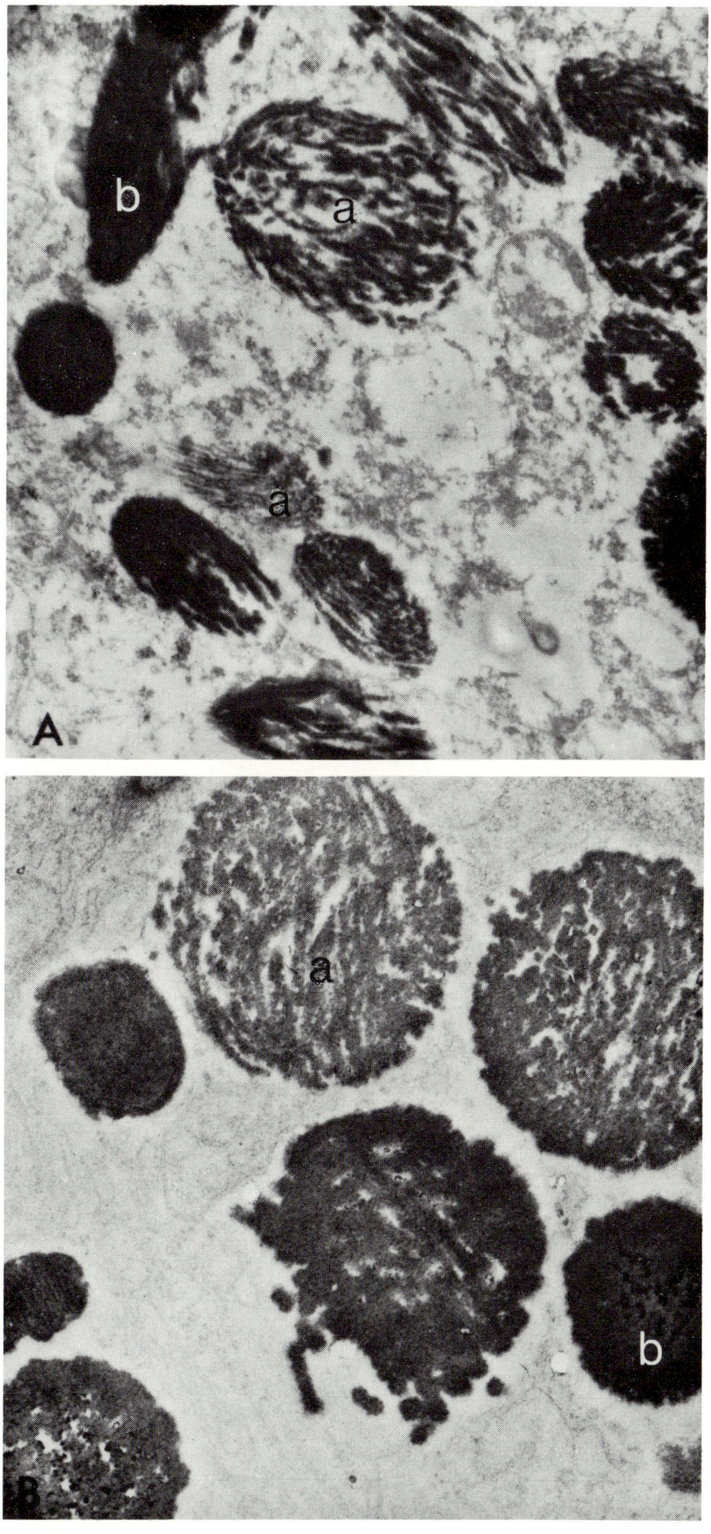

Figure 9–18. Melanin granules in the retinal pigment epithelium of a 10 week old embryo eye and in the eye of a 20 week old fetus. *A*, Ten week old embryo. Different stages of melanin granule formation are seen. The immature granules (a) are incompletely melanized. The mature granules (b) show much greater melanization. (× 15,500.)

B, Twenty week old fetal eye. An incompletely melanized granule is seen at (a) and a melanized one at (b). (× 15,500.) (From Feeney, L., et al.: Studies on human ocular pigment. *In* Rohen, J. W. (ed.): The Structure of the Eye. Stuttgart, Schattauer, 1965.)

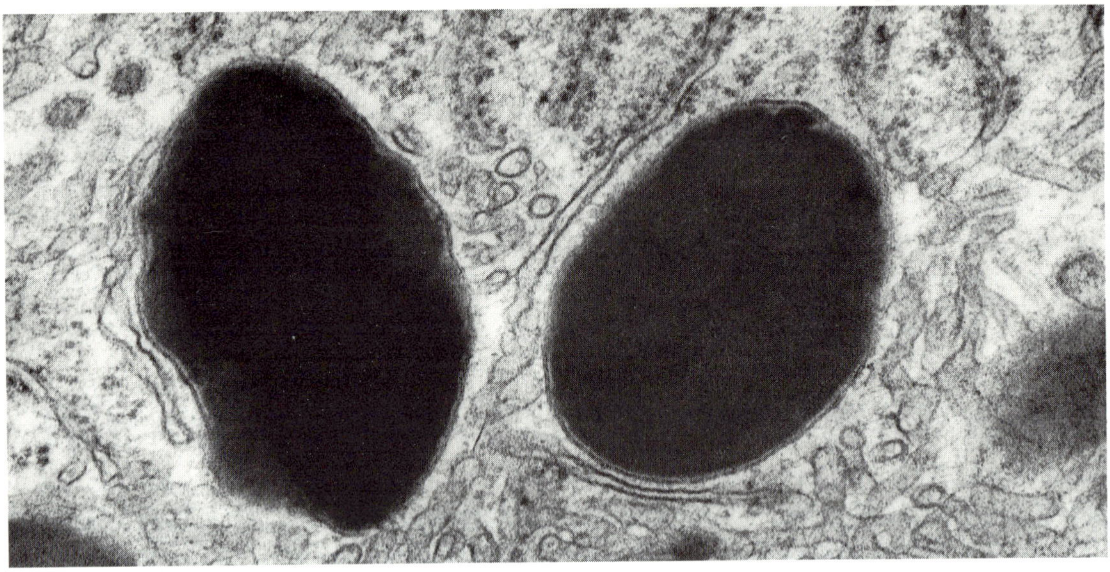

Figure 9–19. Two pigment granules in the cytoplasm of a retinal pigment epithelial cell. They are surrounded by a single membrane and have very little internal structure. (× 60,000.)

Lipid granules not enclosed by a membrane are also seen occasionally in the basal cytoplasm.

A number of observers have described lamellar inclusions in the cytoplasm of the retinal pigment epithelial cells. They were first described in human pigment epithelial cells by Bairati and Orzalesi (1963). Since the membranes of these lamellae greatly resemble those of the outer segments of the photoreceptors, they have been believed to represent portions of photoreceptors ingested by the pigment cells (see p. 422). Autoradiographic studies confirm the idea that the pigment epithelium constantly "nibbles" away segments of the outer ends of the photoreceptors (Young, 1967). This process also can be demonstrated in the human eye with the electron microscope (Spitznas and Hogan, 1970).

Two types of villous processes arise from the apices of the pigment epithelial cells that face the photoreceptors: (1) a slender process which is fringe-like and of variable thickness and length, occupying the space between the outer segments of the photoreceptors (Figs. 9–13 to 9–15). (2) Broad rampart-like villi which encompass the external 4 μm. of the tips of the outer segments (Figs. 9–13 to 9–15). These villi form bowl-like sheaths around the photoreceptors and are important in the phagocytosis of their tips. They form cytoplasmic protrusions that extend in from all sides to sequester 30 or 40 discs (Fig. 9–20). The protrusions fuse to enclose the discs and their surrounding cell membrane in the epithelial cell cytoplasm. These cytoplasmic inclusions are known as *phagosomes* (Young and Bok, 1969); they measure 1.5 to 2.0 μm. in length and are surrounded by the cell membrane of the photoreceptor. This, in turn, is surrounded by another cell membrane that is derived from the pigment epithelial cell. This process, then, is a true example of phagocytosis. The phagosome is displaced deeper and deeper into the cytoplasm and exhibits progressive disintegration (Fig. 9–21).

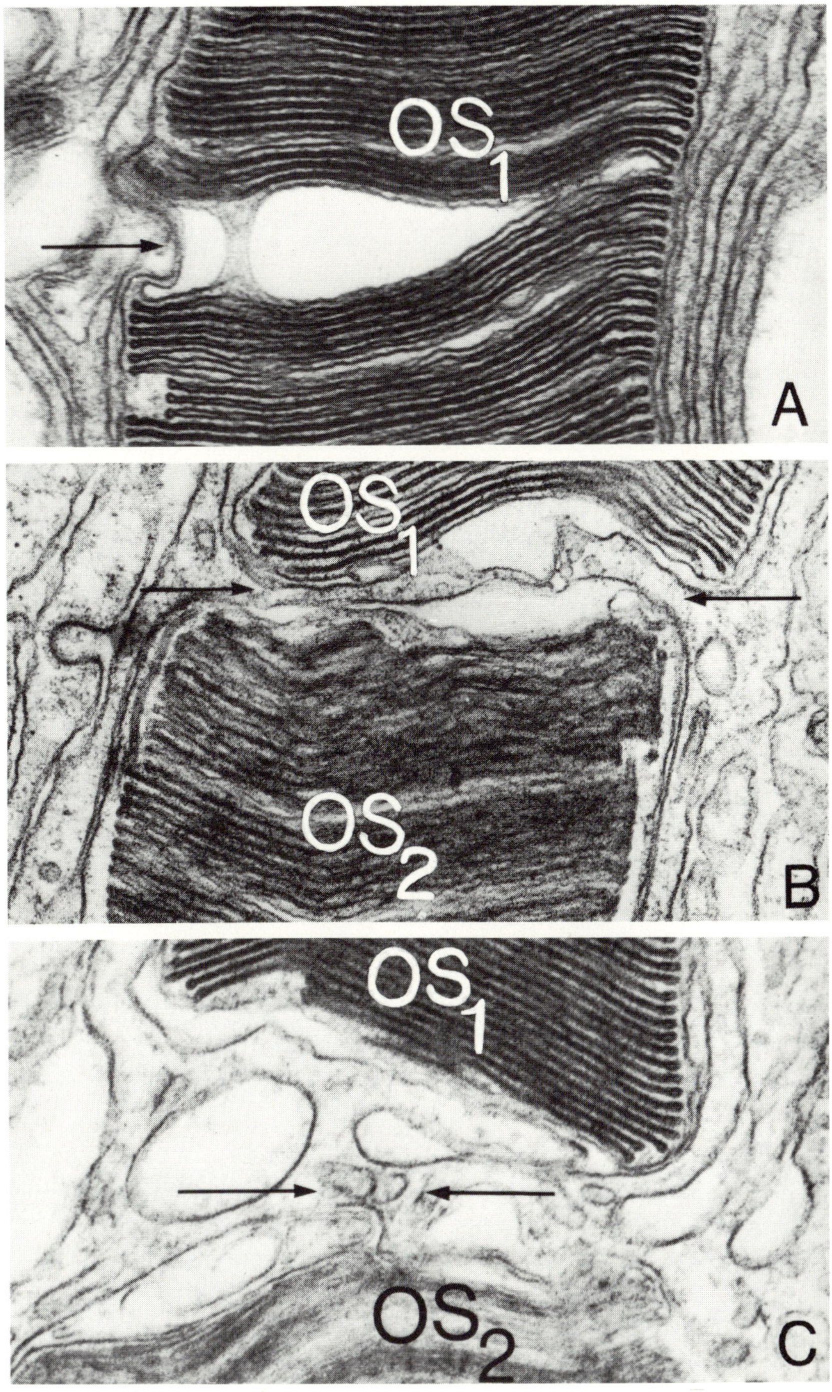

Figure 9–20. Different stages in the phagocytosis of the rod outer segment discs by the retinal pigment epithelium. *A*, Separation of a group of discs by protrusions from the thick surrounding rampart-like villi (arrow). The outer segment with its discs is seen at OS_1.

B, The villi have accomplished separation of a group of external segment discs (arrow). The sequestered discs are seen at OS_2.

C, Later stage of the same process. The segregated discs (OS_2) are now separated by a wide interval from OS_1 (arrows). (× 48,000.)

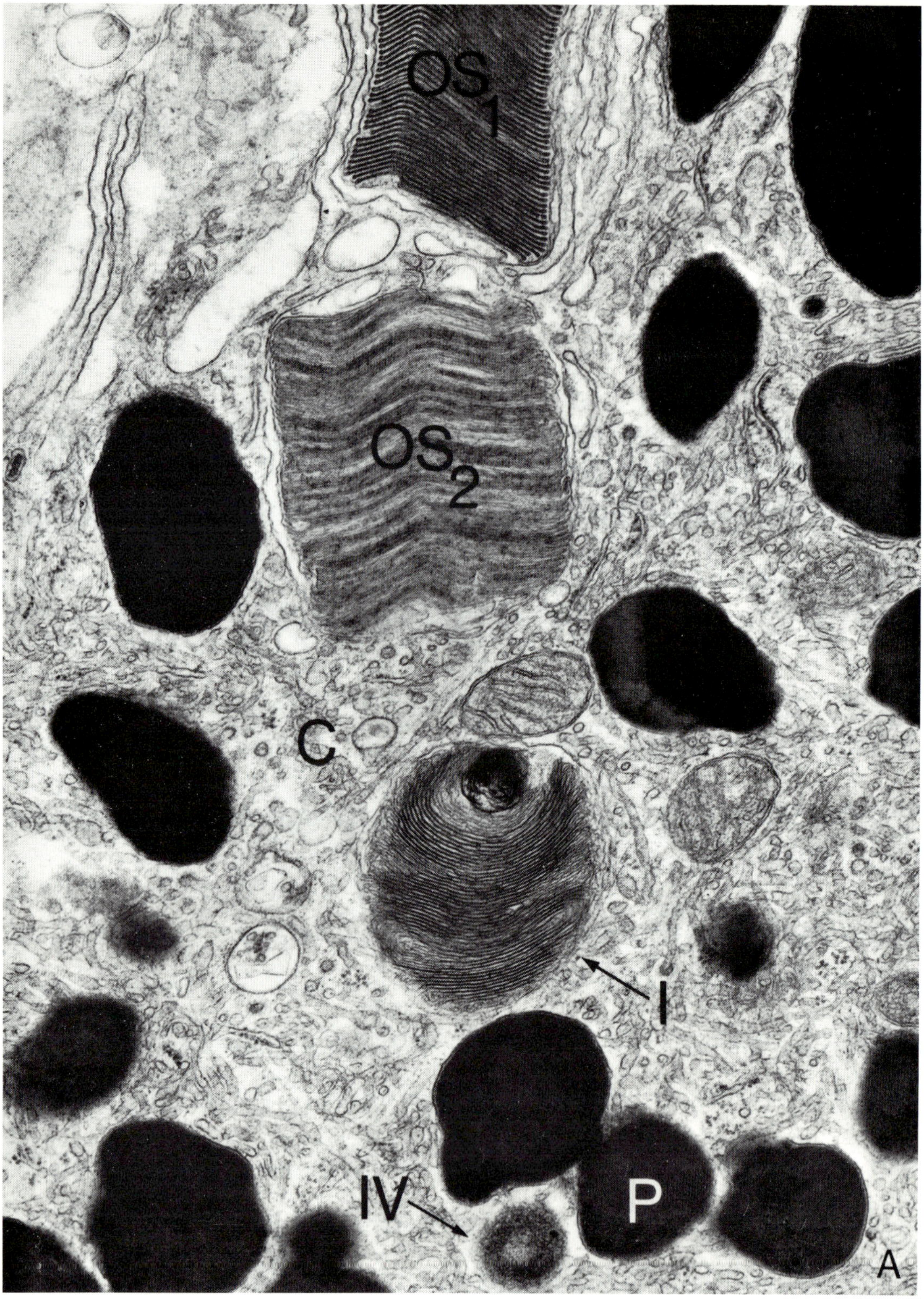

Figure 9–21. *A*, A follow-up on the stages of digestion of the outer segment discs that were seen in Figure 9–20. The pigment epithelial cell cytoplasm is at (c) and a pigment granule at (P). A recently formed phagosome (I) contains rod discs. IV is a phagosome in the end-stage of hydrolytic digestion. (× 28,800.)

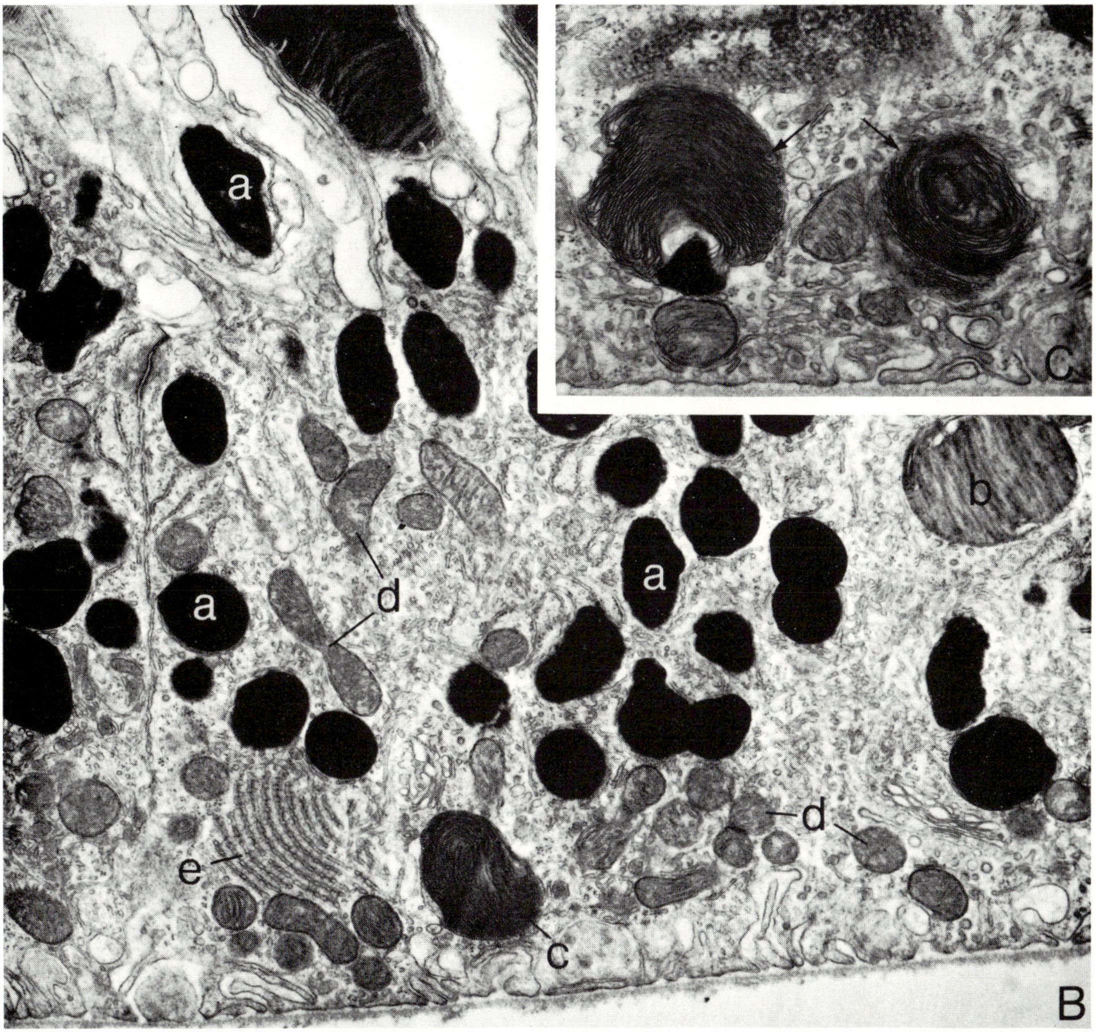

Figure 9–21. *Continued.*

B, The pigment epithelial cell contains many pigment granules (a), one phagosome (b), near its apex and a relatively intact phagosome (c) close to its basal surface. Mitochondria (d) and a stack of annulate lamellae (e) are also shown. (× 13,500.)

C, Two phagosomes (arrows) containing relatively intact (discs) presumably derived from rod outer segments are shown close to the basal surface of the pigmented epithelium. (× 24,300.)

Rod and Cone Layer (Receptor Layer)

External to the outer limiting membrane the rods and cones are composed of a thick inner segment and a thin outer segment (Figs. 9–7, 9–8 and 9–23). The transition of the outer and inner segments lies about halfway between the retinal pigment epithelium and the outer limiting membrane of the retina. The inner and outer segments of both the rods and the cones are joined by a slight constriction, but the cell membrane is continuous between the two parts. A cilium arises in the apical portion of the inner segment and connects the inner to the outer segment of the receptor.

With the low power of the light microscope the outer segments of these cells form a fibrillar layer of parallel processes which are short and coarse (cones) or long and thin (rods). The length of the combined outer and inner segments is 58 to 67 μm. in the middle of the fovea, approximately 40 μm. about 1 mm. from the fovea, and beyond the equator the length is reduced to 37 to 40 μm. (Salzmann, 1912). In freshly fixed human retinas, the measurements are greater, the length of the cones being up to 75 μm. and the rods up to 120 μm. (Eichner, 1957). The foveal cones are more like rods, their thickness being only about 2.5 μm. The central fovea contains only cones in an area measuring about 0.5 mm. At the edge of the central fovea the cones are thicker and arranged in oblique rows. Toward the periphery the cones decrease in length, especially their outer segments, so that at the ora serrata they are only about 6 μm. long. The inner segment also becomes shorter and broader toward the periphery, but the inner and outer segments of the rods retain their form until the far periphery.

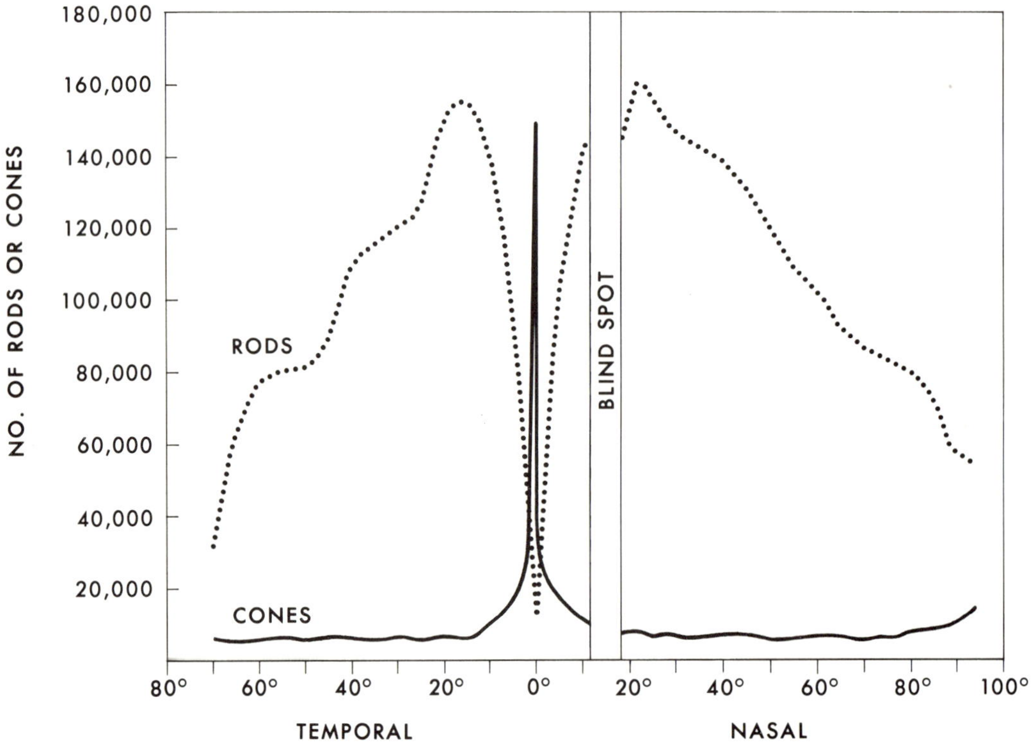

Figure 9–22. The distribution of rods and cones in the retina. (From Østerberg, G. A.: Acta Ophthal. 6:1, 1935.)

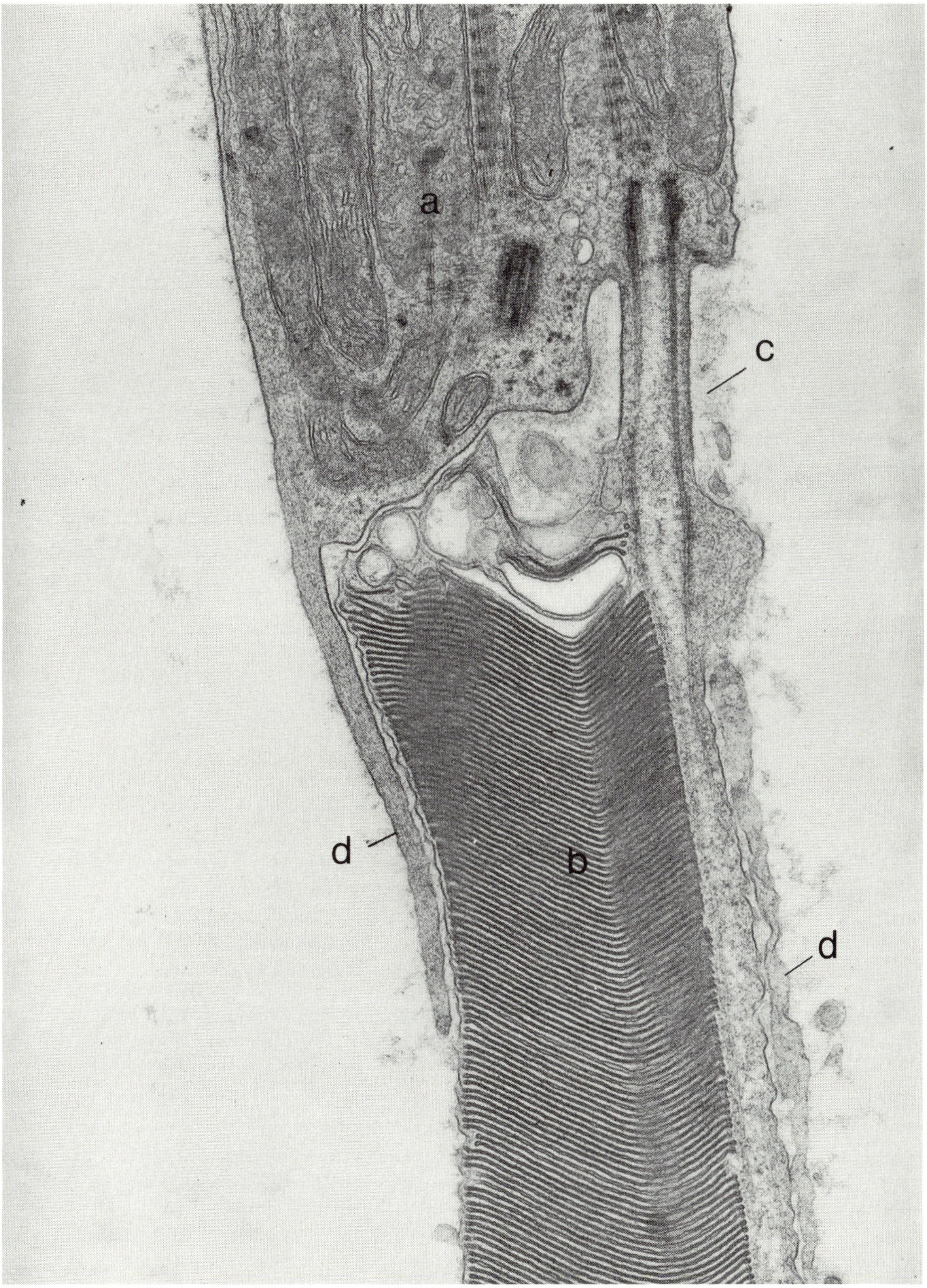

Figure 9–23. A rod showing the inner (a) and outer (b) segments and a connecting cilium (c). Thin cytoplasmic extensions of the inner segments (d) surround part of the outer segments. (× 36,000.)

Østerberg (1935) made flat sections of a complete retina, counting the number of photoreceptors in different regions. Figure 9–22 shows the number and disposition of the retinal receptors oriented outward from the fovea. He found a total of 110 to 125 million rods and 6.3 to 6.8 million cones in the retina. The highest density of cones was in the center of the fovea, where there were 147,300 cones per sq. mm. The number decreased rapidly in the first 10 degrees from the foveal center and leveled off at about 5000 per sq. mm. in the periphery. A slight increase was found again near the ora serrata. The foveola was free of rods, the first rods appearing 130 μm. from the foveal center, increasing to a ring with a maximum density of 160,000 per sq. mm. at a distance of 5 to 6 mm. from the fovea. The number diminished continuously toward the ora serrata, where they amounted to 23,000 to 50,000 per sq. mm.

Rod Outer Segments. The rod outer segments are composed of a series of superimposed discs or plates, stacked on each other like poker chips and surrounded by a cell membrane (Figs. 9–23 to 9–32). The outer segment has a peculiarly brilliant refractility and positive birefringence. It is also PAS-positive. Schmidt (1935), on the basis of polarization studies, found that the outer segment discs behave like an uniaxial crystal, and that they are formed of alternating layers of protein and lipid. Schmidt also demonstrated that the visual purple is in the protein layers, and he advanced the hypothesis that the process of decolorization of visual purple is accomplished by the action of light on the molecules to modify their orientation along the axis of the outer segment discs.

The rod outer segments, as seen with the electron microscope, consist of a pile of discs varying in number from 600 to 1000, depending on the species studied (Sjöstrand, 1953; Missotten, 1960). In the human and primate retina the discs are not connected to the cell membrane, whereas in some lower vertebrates they are. The discs are stacked at right angles to the length of the outer segment. Each disc is composed of two unit membranes that are continuous at the ends. The unit membranes enclose a less dense narrow space, the intradisc space, which has a uniform thickness except at the edges, where it widens. Each of the double membranes of the discs has an average thickness of 55 to 65 A. in the central portion and 70 to 80 A. at the edge (Fig. 9–24). The intradisc space measures about 100 A. thick. Therefore, the entire thickness of each disc is about 225 to 245 A. (Fig. 9–25) (Cohen, 1965). The space between two discs, called the interdisc space, measures about 210 A.

Flat sections show lobulation of the outer segment discs of the rods (Fig. 9–26). In the human eye Cohen (1965) found about 33 discs to occupy 1 μm. and Missotten (1964) found about 24 to 28 discs per micron. The cell membrane of the rod surrounds all the discs, being continuous with that of the connecting cilium and the inner segment. It does not enter into the crypts between the lobulations of the outer segment. At times cross-sections of the discs show tubules in the crypts between the disc lobules and the cell membrane; these may be microtubules from the connecting cilium. The discs "float" in some type of watery protein within the cell membrane. The inner segments have tongue-like prolongations which extend externally around the inner one third of the outer segment (Fig. 9–27). The microvilli of the pigmented epithelial cells also form enveloping processes around the external portions of the outer segments. Only the central portions of the outer segments are without a cytoplasmic wrapping. The cementing mucopro-

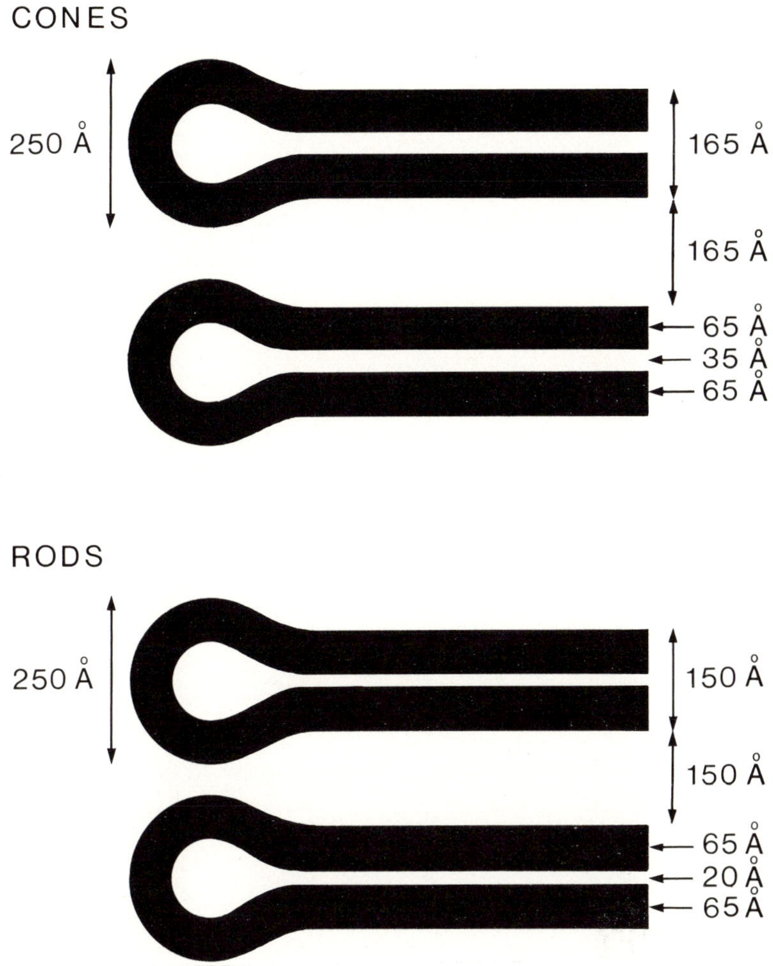

Figure 9–24. Drawing of the rod and cone discs to show the thickness of their membranes, as well as the width of the intradisc and interdisc spaces.

tein that separates the outer segments surrounds these receptors. The prolongations of inner segment cytoplasm along the surface of the outer segments were termed calyces by Cohen (1965).

Connecting Cilium. Fürst (1904) demonstrated a diplosome having the characteristics of a cilium in the inner segments of the receptors. With the phase-contrast microscope a thread can be seen to connect the outer and inner segments. Sjöstrand (1953) found "connecting fibrils" between the outer and inner segments with the electron microscope, and DeRobertis (1960) was the first to describe the connecting cilium by electron microscopy. The cilium originates in the basal body, which is located in the cytoplasm of the ellipsoid slightly to one side of its central axis, facing the outer segment (Fig. 9–28).

There is condensation of the cytoplasm around the basal body. Spokelike prolongations that extend radially into the cytoplasm from the midportion of the basal body probably serve as roots or stabilizing devices for the cilium. The cilium contains nine doublets of tubules arranged in a ring which measures 0.2 to 0.5 μm. (Missotten, 1961). The central pair of fila-

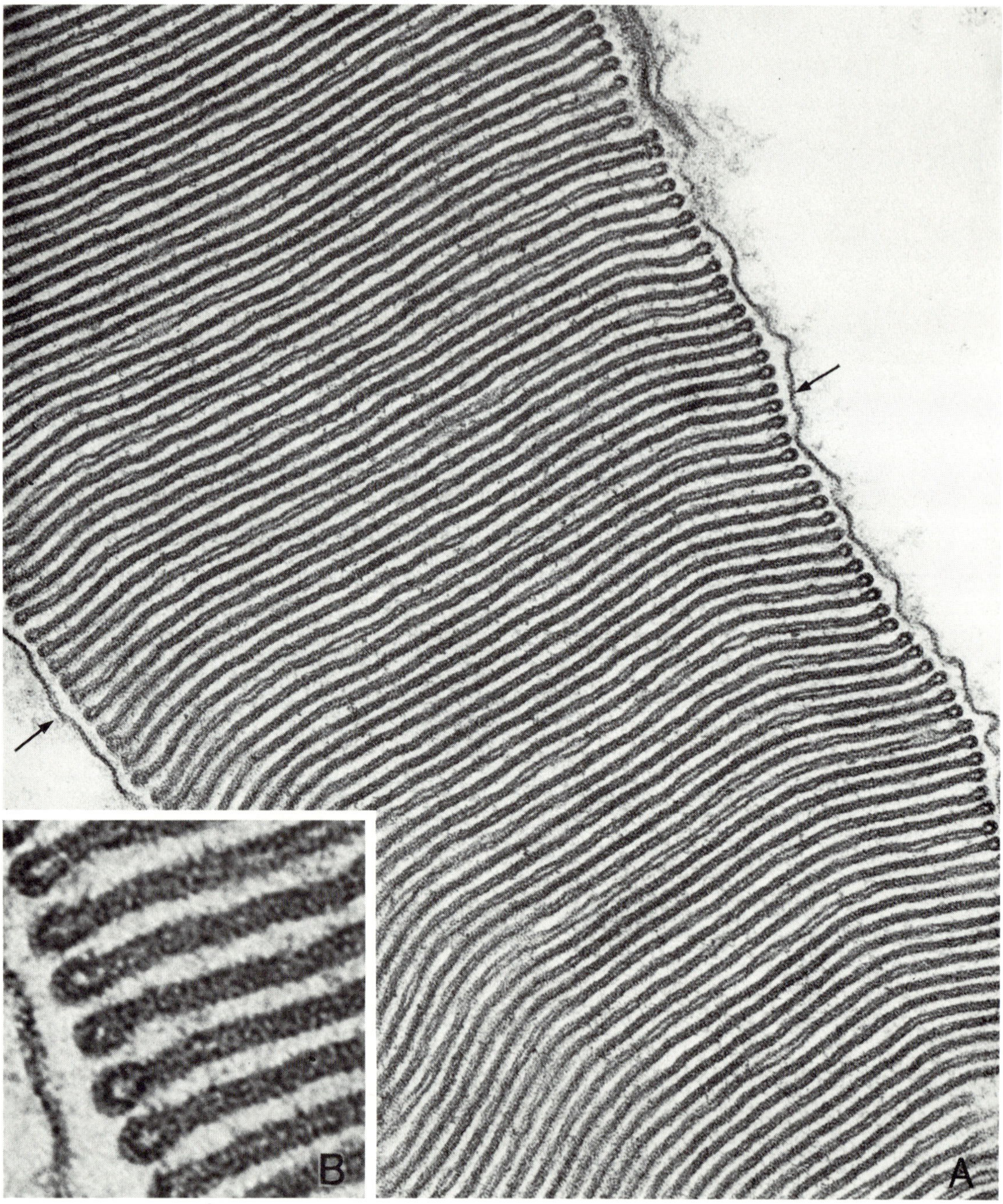

Figure 9–25. The disc of the rod outer segment. *A*, The arrows show the cell membrane surrounding the discs. (× 90,000.)

B, Magnified view of the edges of the discs and the cell membrane. There is an enlargement of the intradisc space at the edges of the discs. (× 300,000.)

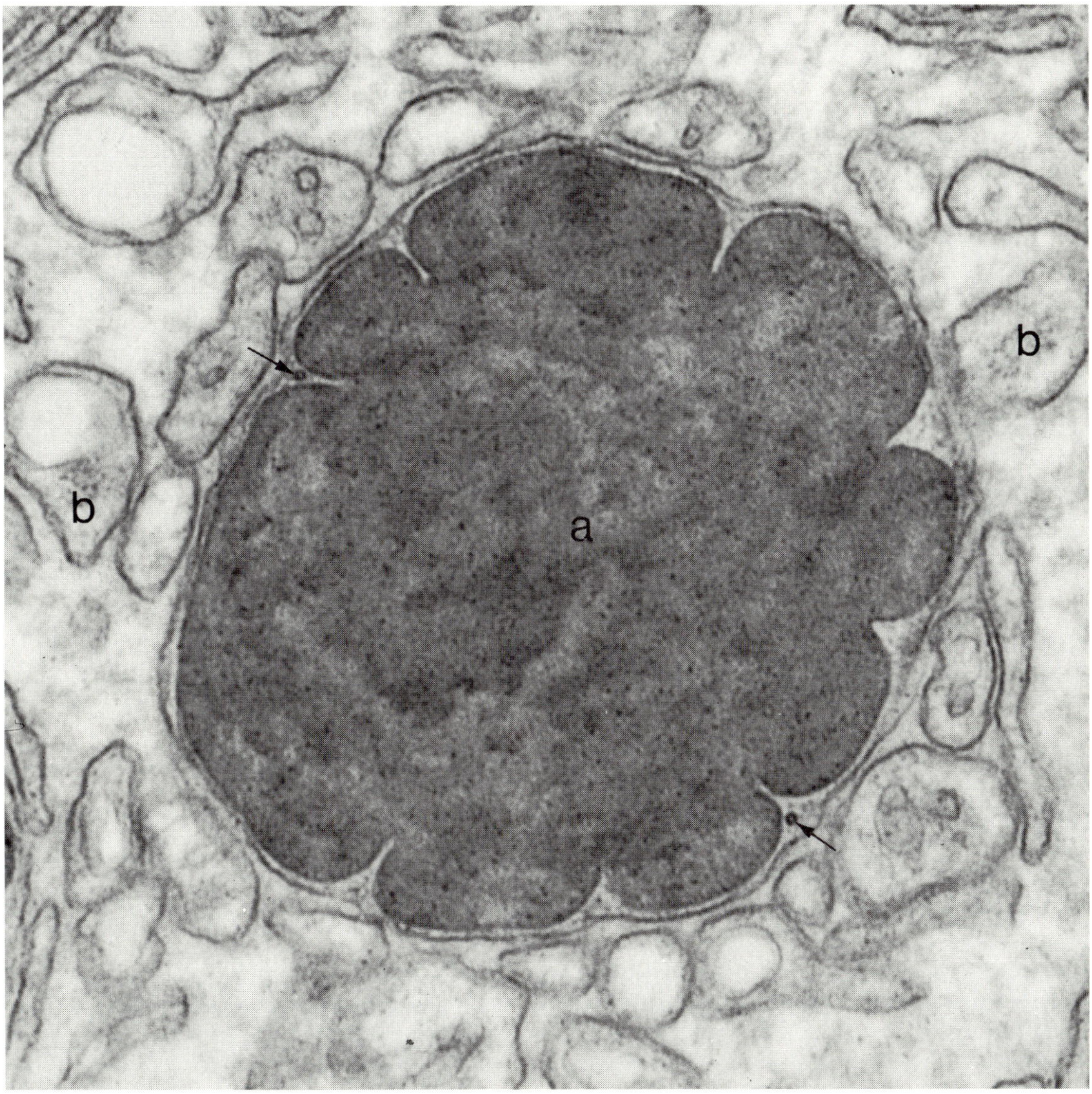

Figure 9–26. A tangential section of a rod disc (a) to demonstrate its lobulated surface. Villi (b) of the retinal pigment epithelium surround the outer segment at a level internal to the outermost portion of the outer segment. For this reason the heavier sheath-like enclosures of the photoreceptors by the retinal pigment epithelium are not seen. The arrows point to cross-sections of the microtubules of the connecting cilium. (× 60,000.)

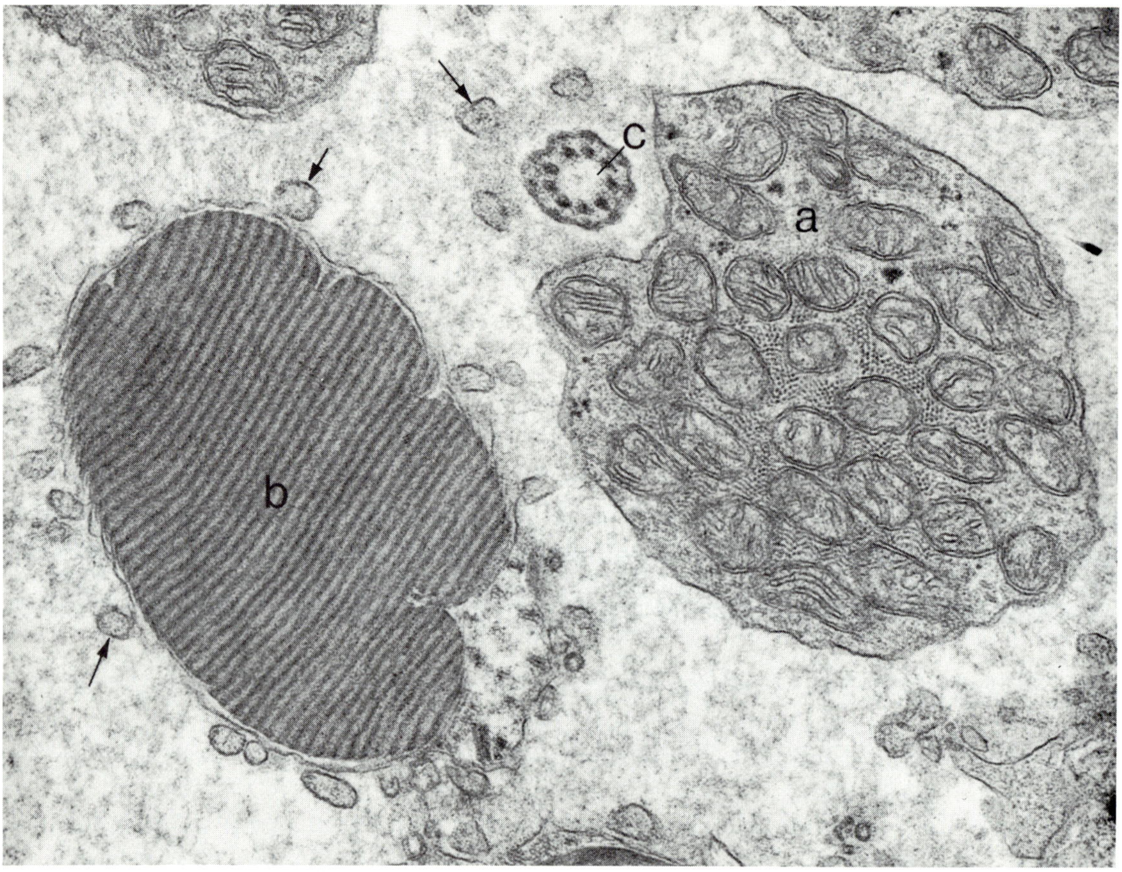

Figure 9–27. An oblique section through the transition zone between the outer and inner segments of a rod. The inner segment (a) contains numerous mitochondria, while the outer segment (b) is composed of a stack of discs. Because of the sectioning the connecting cilium (c) appears to be separated from the receptor. The arrows show cross-sections of the tongue-like processes from the inner segments that extend externally around the outer segments. (× 31,500.)

ments, which are characteristic of *motile* cilia, are absent here (DeRobertis, 1956). The core of the cilium is less dense than the surrounding cytoplasm. The nine pairs of tubules become a ring of nine singlets soon after leaving the basal body (Cohen, 1965). The tubules gradually become more attenuated as they extend into the outer segment. Some are observed to end close to the tip of the outer segment, while others end sooner (Fig. 9-26). Bundles of root filaments originate from the two centrioles of the basal body in the rod inner segments. These filaments traverse the ellipsoid and enter the myoid where they terminate freely in the cytoplasm. The bundles of root filament exhibit a weak striation of about 700 A. (Fig. 9–23) (Sjöstrand, 1953; Cohen, 1960, 1961).

In the area where the cilium connects the outer and inner segments, the width of the photoreceptor is decreased to 0.3 μm. in an area measuring 1 μm. in length. The cilium, a small amount of surrounding cytoplasm and the cell membrane provide the only connection between the rod outer and inner segments.

The method by which electrical energy generated in the rod and cone discs is transmitted to the first neuron has been studied intensively.

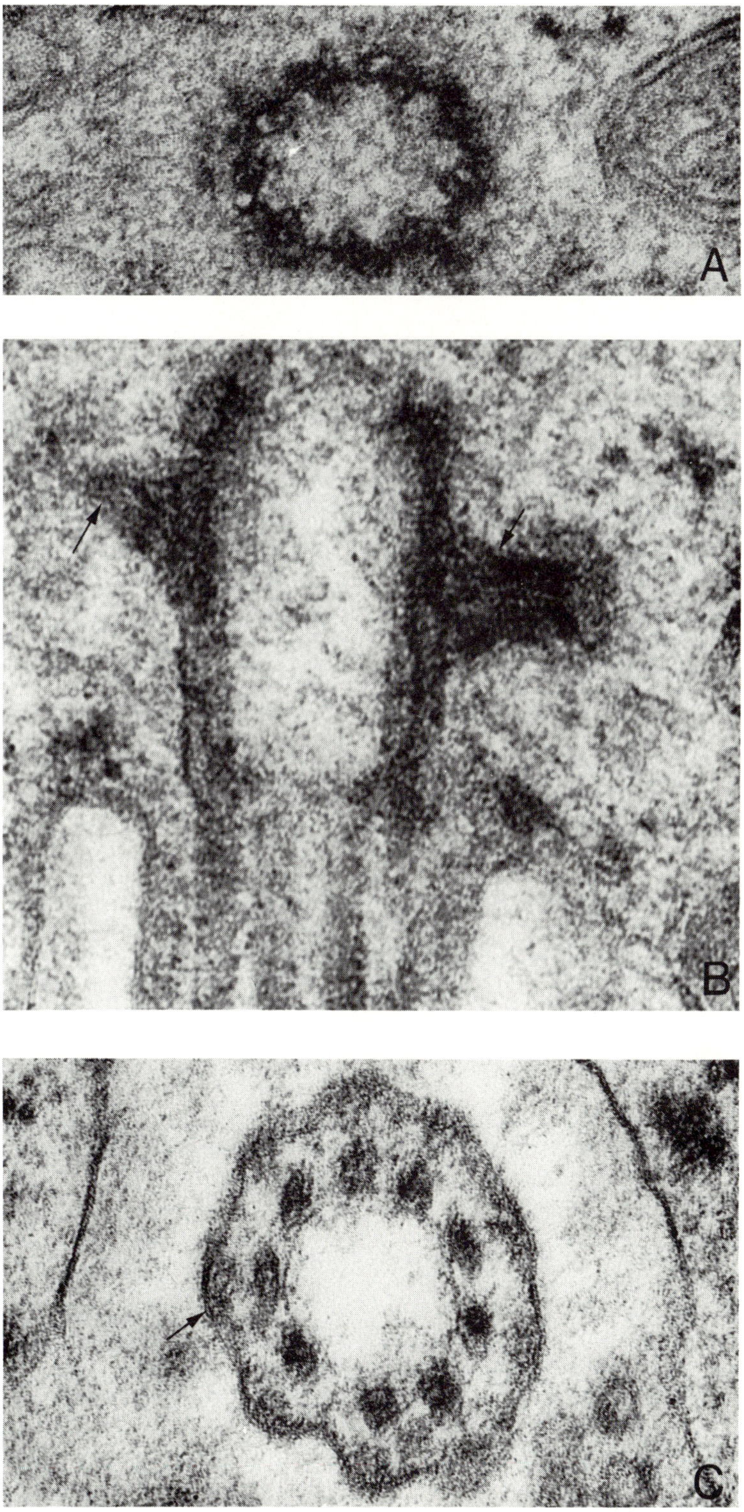

Figure 9–28. A connecting cilium of a rod at high magnification. *A*, A cross-section of the basal body with its triplets. (× 120,000.)

B, A longitudinal section of the basal body; spoke-like prolongations extend from it into the cytoplasm (arrows). (× 132,000.)

C, A cross-section of the connecting cilium. The nine doublets arranged in a ring are characteristic. The cilium is surrounded by the rod cell membrane (arrow). (× 120,000.)

These discs have been compared to a photomultiplier tube in their ability to intensify the electrical energy produced by the photochemical reaction in their membranes. There is no direct connection between the individual rod discs in human and primate outer segments, however, and this makes it difficult to explain the mechanism for transmission of the energy produced. Except for stabilization of the receptors, the function of the cilium is unknown, and its role in the transmission of electrical impulses is uncertain. Not all tubules of the cilium traverse the length of the outer segment, but this may not be necessary for them to play an important part in energy transmission.

Rod Inner Segments. The inner segments are elongated, barrel-shaped structures containing a finely granular cytoplasm. They are subdivided into two elements, an outer *ellipsoid* that joins the outer segment, and an inner *myoid*, which is continuous with the soma of these cells in the outer nuclear layer. The ellipsoid is acidophilic and shows the enzyme reactions characteristic of mitochondria. The myoid contains much glycogen and is basophilic because of its high content of ribosomes.

By electron microscopy the rod ellipsoid contains a remarkable number of mitochondria, a cross-section usually showing 30 to 50 (Fig. 9-29). The mitochondria generally measure about 0.15 to 0.30 μm. in thickness and 3.0 μm. in length (Missotten, 1964). The cytoplasm contains some glycogen and some of the vesicles of smooth-surfaced endoplasmic reticulum, neurotubules, many wavy neurofibrils and free ribosomes. The cell membrane of the inner segment is continuous with that of the outer segment.

The myoid (Fig. 9–30) contains a considerable amount of the randomly oriented, smooth-surfaced endoplasmic reticulum which is arranged in round or oval vesicles. Some rough-surfaced endoplasmic reticulum also is present. Many vesicles of the Golgi apparatus are usually seen close to the outer limiting membrane of the retina. Free ribosomes, which often form polyribosomes, are found in the cytoplasm, and a small number of mitochondria are present here also. The ribosomes account for the basophilia of the myoid by light microscopy. Some electron-dense bodies, which are probably lipid, are also found here. There are many neurotubules in the cytoplasm, mostly oriented in the direction of the axis of the rod. The inner segments are not in direct contact with adjacent receptor cells but are separated from each other by thin villous extensions of Müller cells, so-called *fiber baskets*, beyond the external limiting membrane (Figs. 9-31 and 9-32). These villi extend externally along the surface of the myoid, the cell membranes being separated by a space of about 100 A. The cytoplasm of the Müller cells in these extensions is very homogeneous and dense. In light microscopy there is an intensely basophilic zone just inside the external limiting membrane of the retina between the nucleus and the myoid; it is almost linear at low magnification and is characteristic for cone-containing retinas.

Cone Outer Segments (Figs. 9-33 to 9-36). The structure of the cone outer segments is essentially the same as that of the rods, but the inner portion is somewhat wider than the outer, producing the characteristic cone shape (Fig. 9–33). These segments are shorter here in the rod, and they appear to have only loose contact with the long, finger-like villi of the retinal pigment epithelium. The basic structure of double membrane discs is the same in the cone outer segment as in the rods. There are about 1000 to 1200 discs in the

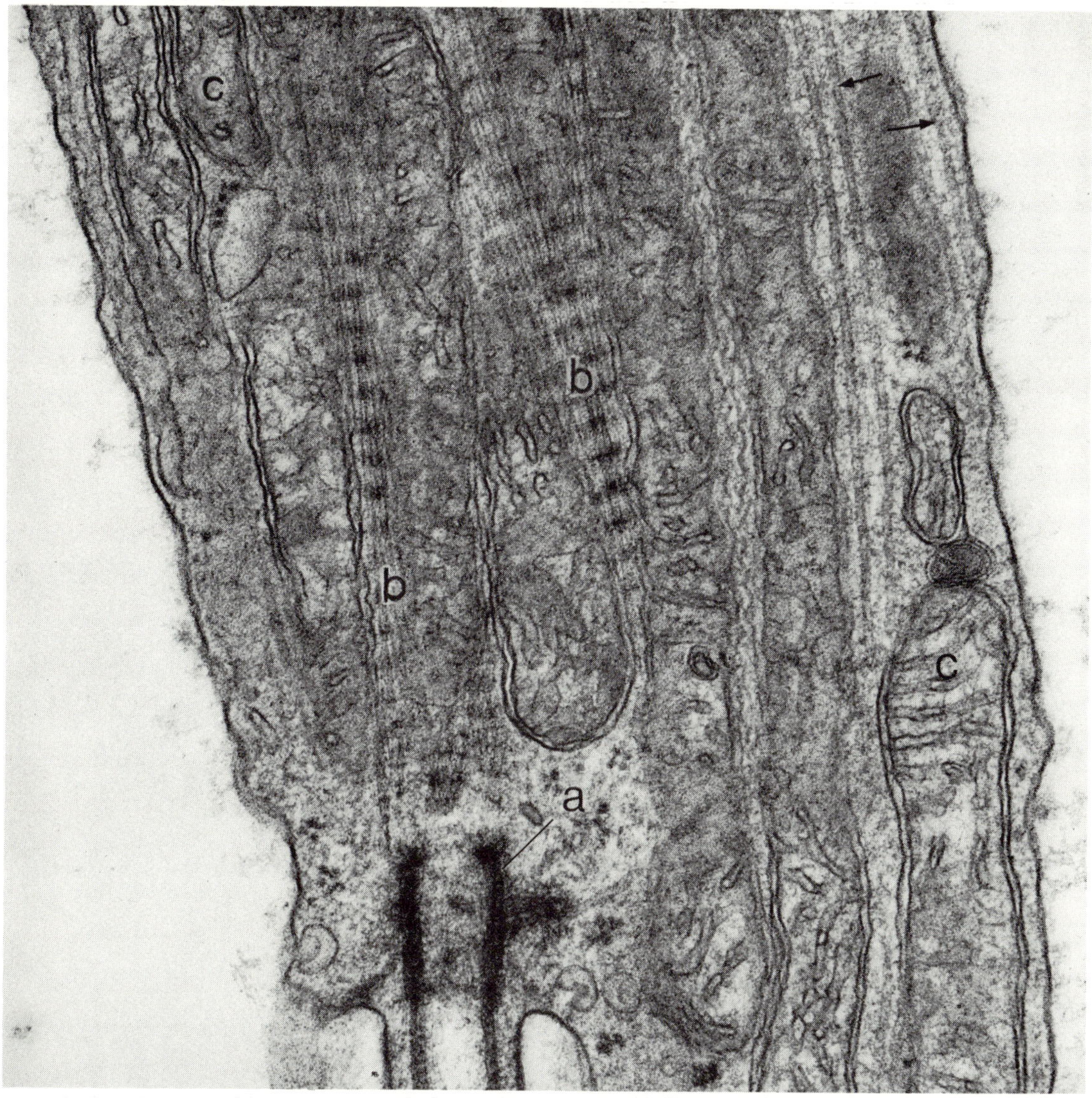

Figure 9–29. The rod ellipsoid and connecting cilium. The basal body of the cilium is at (a) and the root filaments that extend toward the myoid are at (b). There are numerous long mitochondria (c). The arrows indicate the cytoplasmic microtubules. (× 60,000.)

outer segment of the foveal cones in the rhesus monkey, and there are about the same number in the human. The discs are narrower (50 A.) than those of the rods, and the clear central intradisc space measures about 40 A. The disc membranes are 50 A. in thickness, and the interdisc space measures about 180 A., so that the distance between two discs is about 310 A., making about 30 discs per micron (Fig 9–34) (Dowling, 1965). The cone discs differ from those of the rods by the wider intradisc space and interdisc space. In flat sections the cone discs do not show the incisions or lobulations that are found in the rod discs.

Connecting Cilium. The cilium of the cone receptors has the same structure and arrangement as in the rods, except for its reduced length.

Cone Inner Segments. This portion of the cone is also composed of an ellipsoid and a myoid; the cone inner segments are wider and more

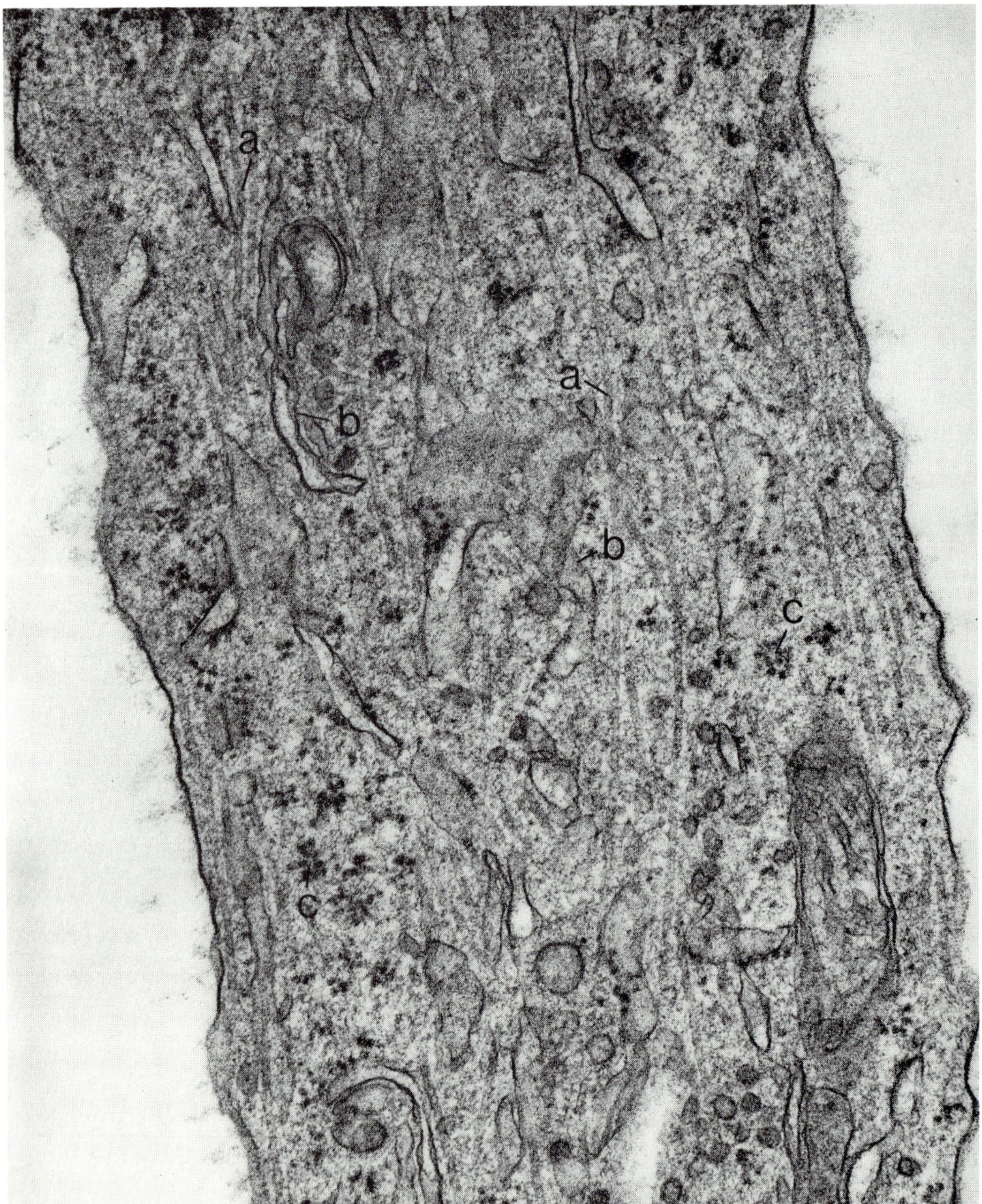

Figure 9–30. The myoid of this rod contains microtubules (a), smooth-surfaced endoplasmic reticulum (b) and clusters of free ribosomes (c). (× 60,000).

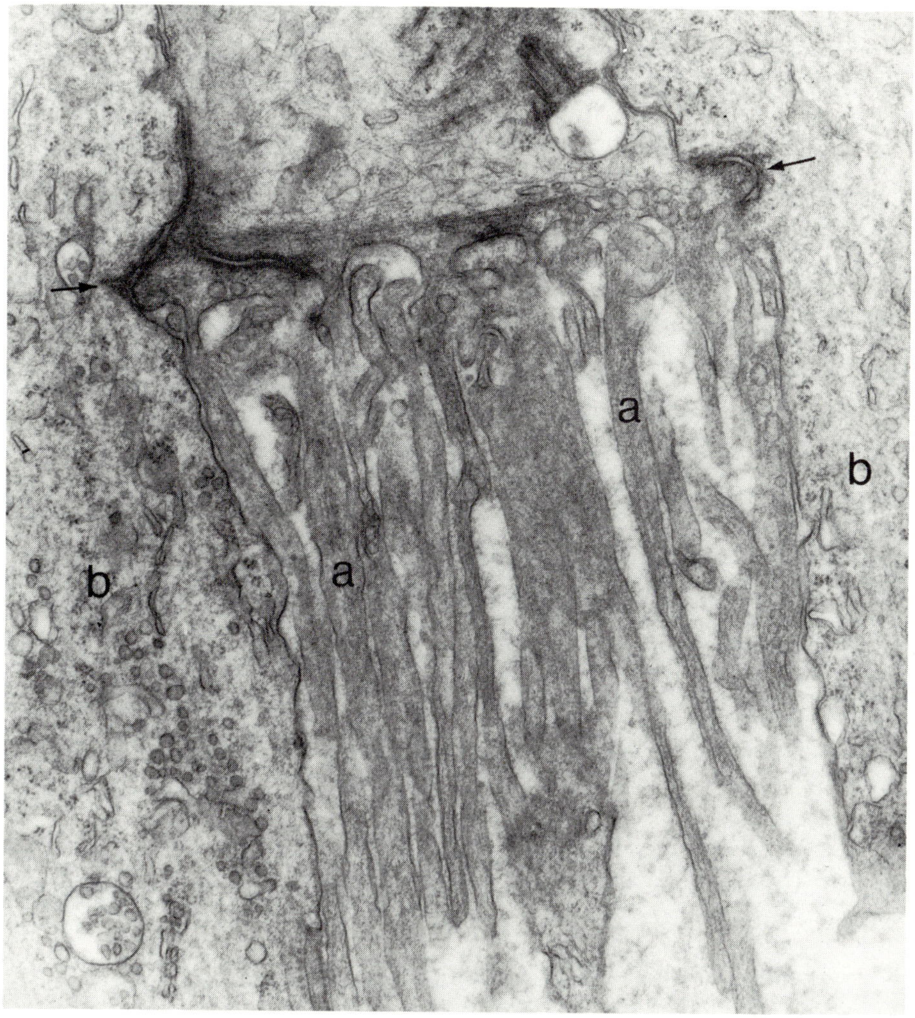

Figure 9–31. The fiber baskets of Müller cells as they extend beyond the external limiting membrane (arrows). All these long villous cellular processes (a) occupy spaces between the inner segments of the photoreceptors (b). (× 24,000.)

conical than those of the rods. The cone ellipsoid is more plump because of its higher content of mitochondria. By electron microscopy the foveal cone receptors have long, tapering inner segments, whereas the extrafoveal ones are distinctly cone-shaped. The many long mitochondria of the ellipsoid are generally oriented in the axis of the cell and occupy about 45 per cent of the volume of the ellipsoid (Figs. 9-35 and 9-36). A cross-section often shows 200 to 300 mitochondria, and Missotten (1964) has estimated that there are about 200 in each cross-section viewed. They are more dense than those of the rod ellipsoid, the cristae being oriented mostly in a longitudinal direction.

The myoid has about the same structure as that of the rod (Fig. 9-37). The inner segments of the cones are also surrounded by microvilli of the Müller cells, which project beyond the outer limiting membrane. Some observers believe that these projections are important for the metabolism of the inner segments of the photoreceptors. *Text continued on page **442***

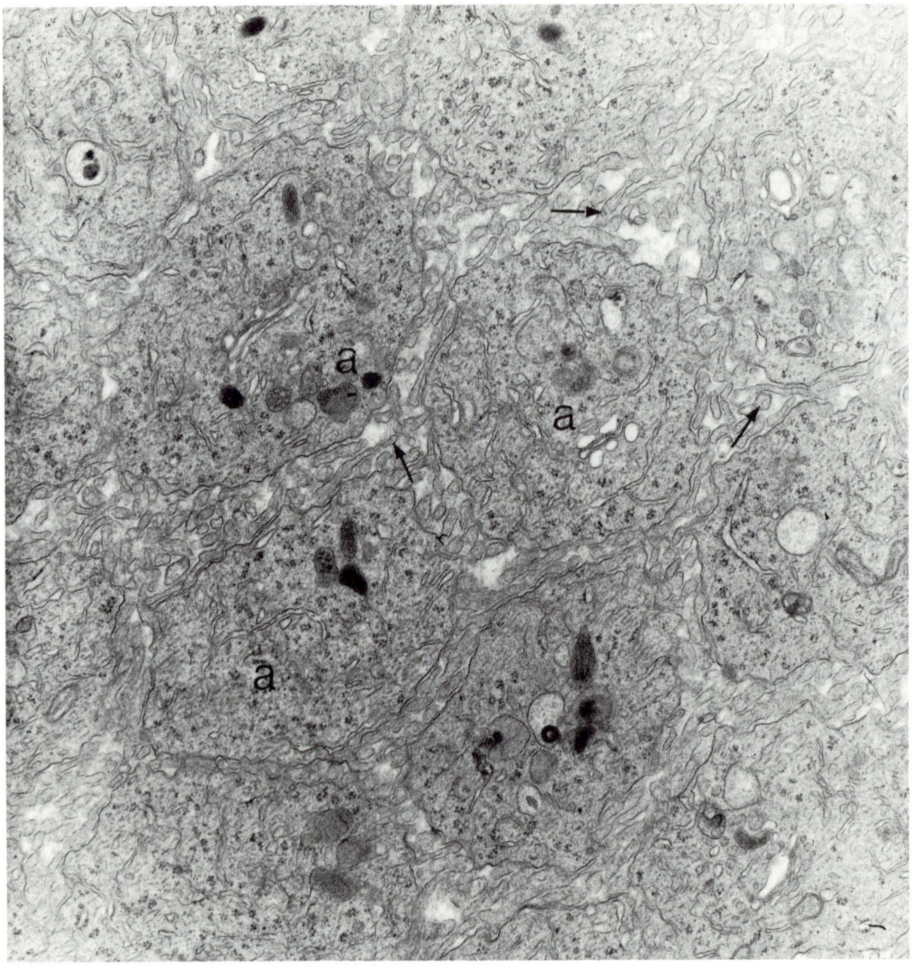

Figure 9–32. Tangential sections of Müller cell fiber baskets (arrows) that surround the inner segments of the photoreceptors (a). (× 13,000.)

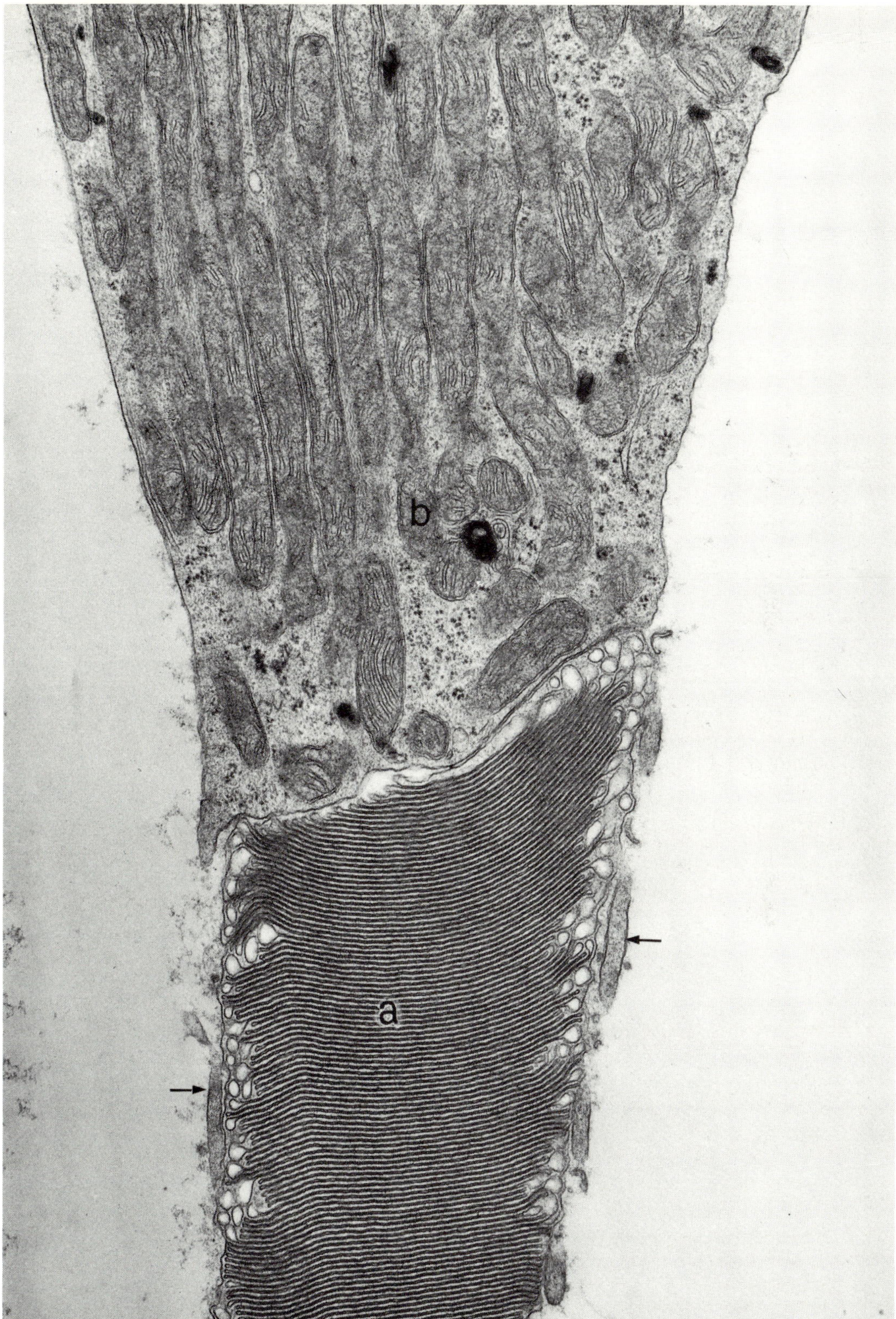

Figure 9–33. A retinal cone; electron micrograph of the outer (a) and inner (b) segments. The section does not traverse the plane of the connecting cilium. The arrows show the tongue-like processes of the inner segment that surround the outer segment. Mitochondria are more numerous in the ellipsoid of the cone than in the rod. (× 36,000.)

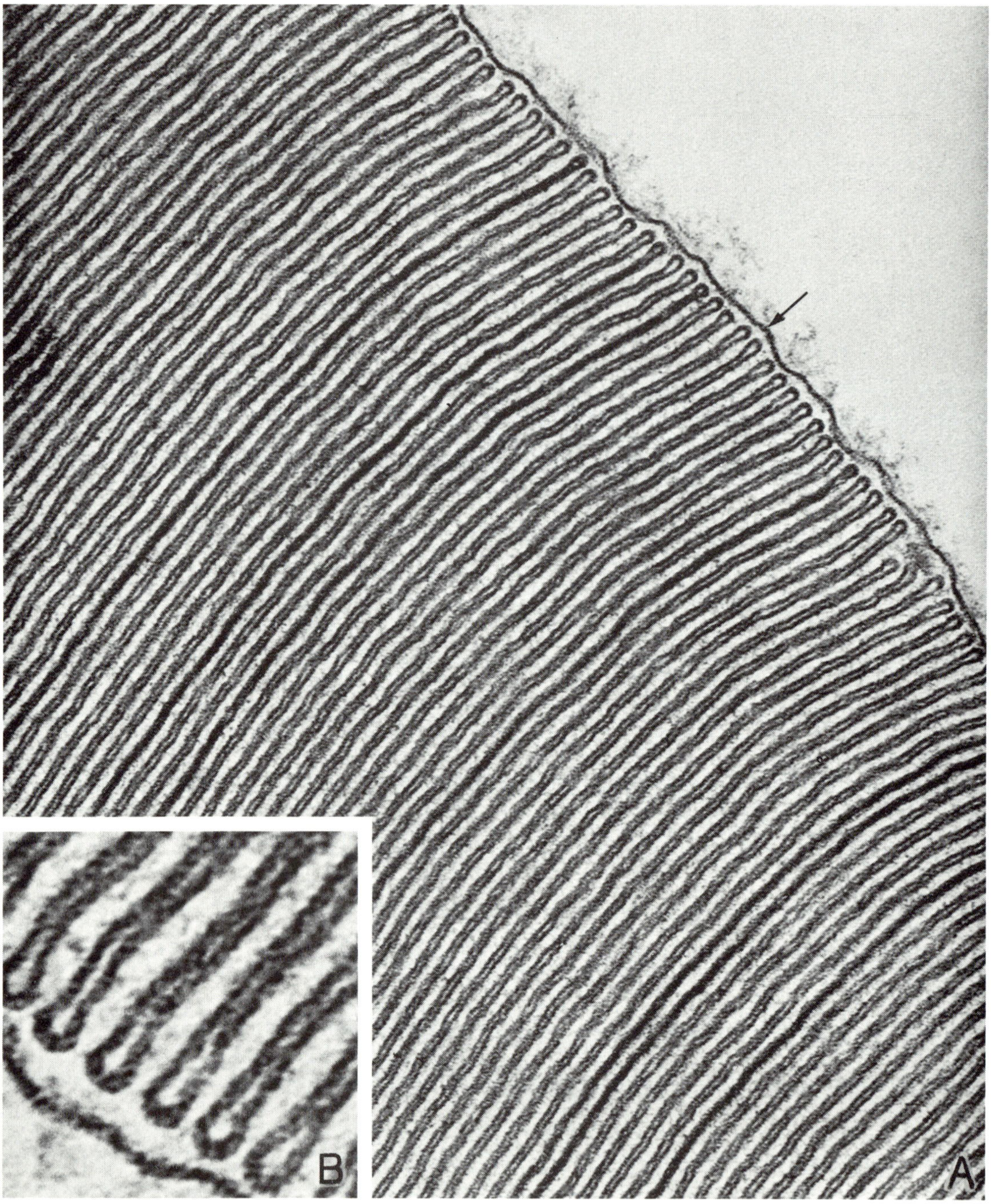

Figure 9–34. Meridional view of the outer segment of a cone. *A*, The arrow shows the cell membrane that surrounds the discs. (× 90,000.)

B, Magnified view of the edges of the discs and the cell membrane. The intradisc and interdisc spaces are wider than those of the rod. (See Figs. 9–24 and 9–25.) (× 300,000.)

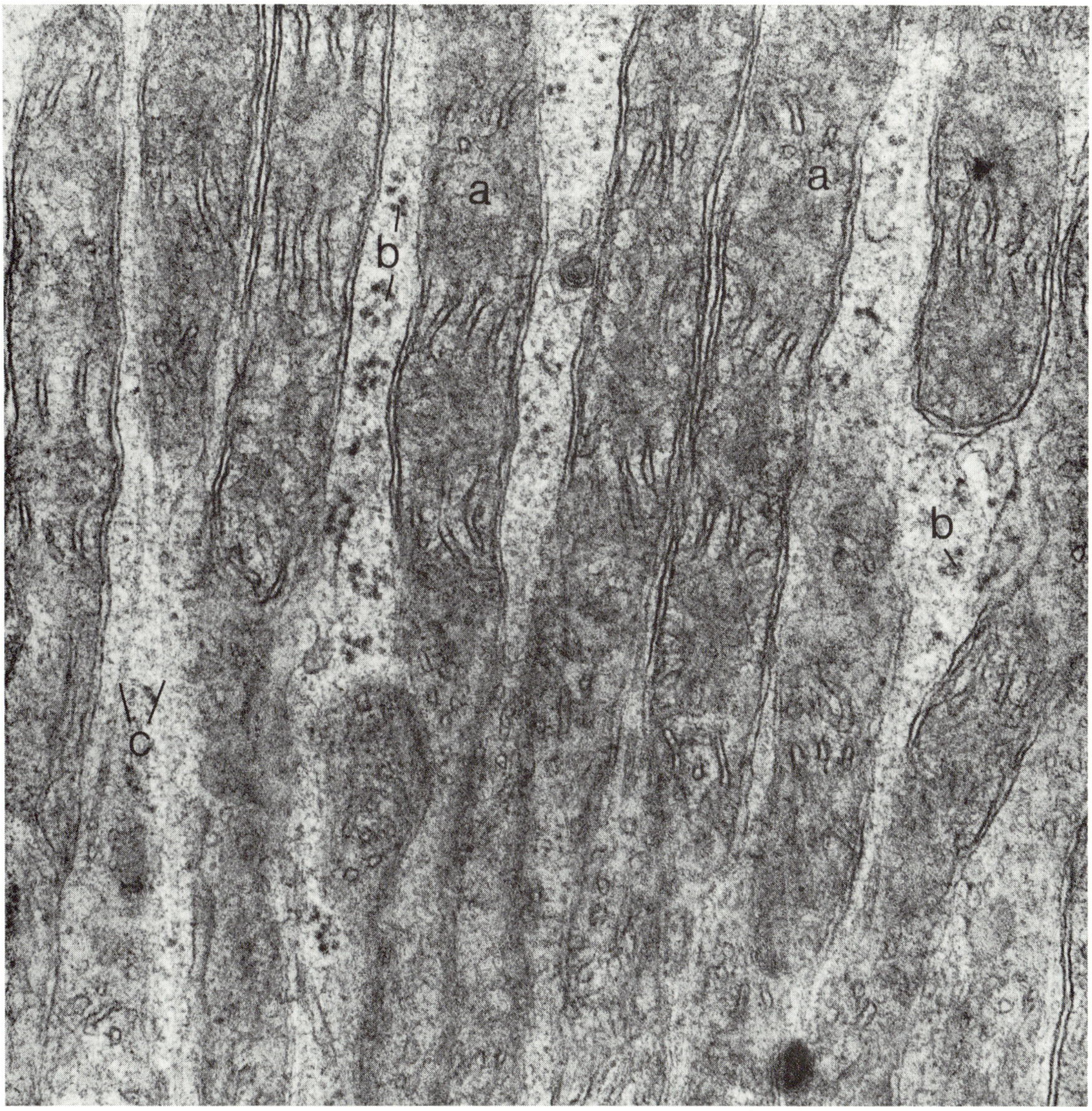

Figure 9–35. A cone ellipsoid that contains numerous long mitochondria (a), free ribosomes (b) and neurotubules (c). (× 90,000.)

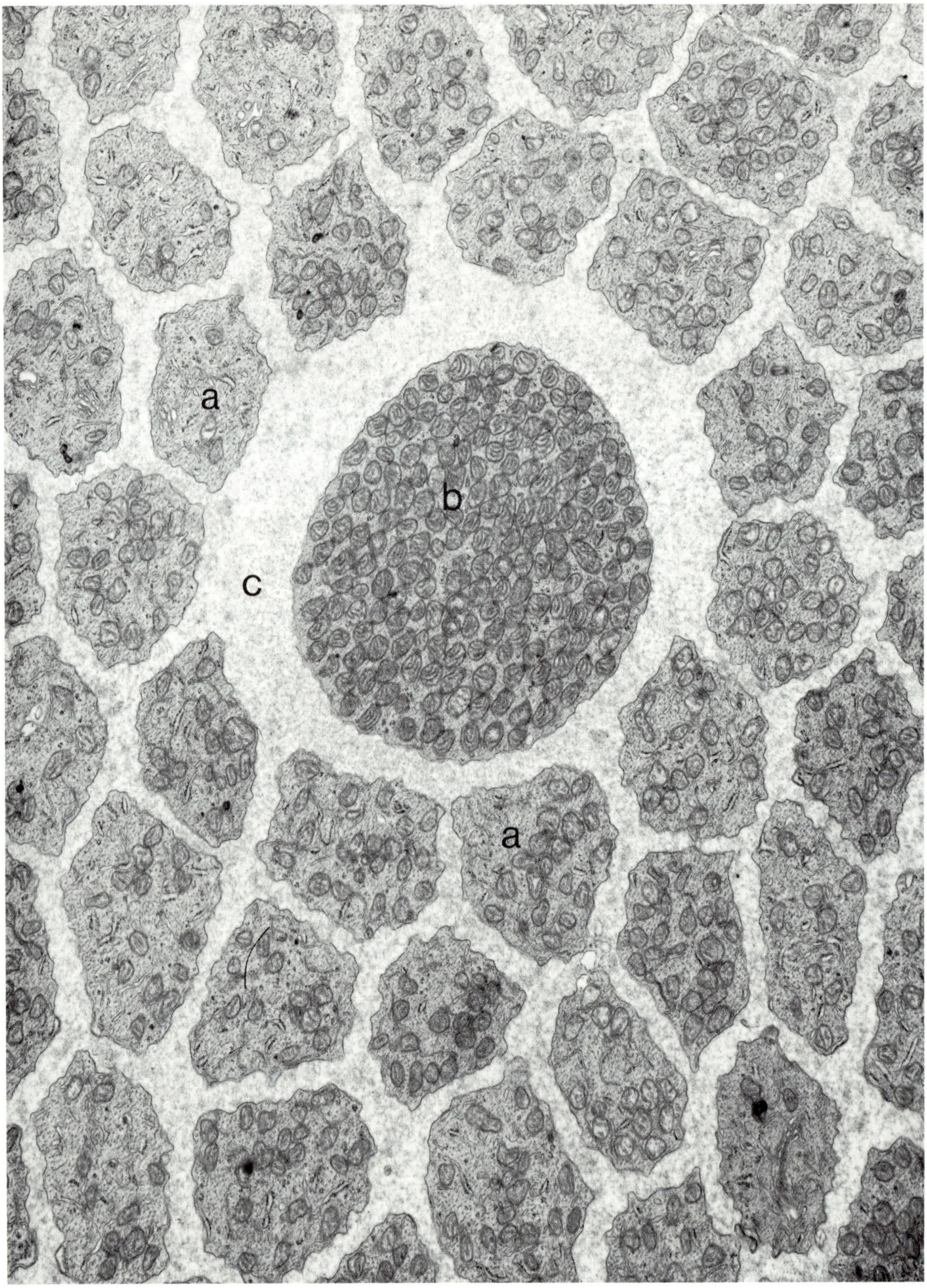

Figure 9–36. A tangential section of rod (a) and cone (b) ellipsoids. The spaces between them are filled with a mucopolysaccharide-protein complex (c). The larger diameter and number of mitochondria in the cone compared to the rod ellipsoid is evident. (× 7200.)

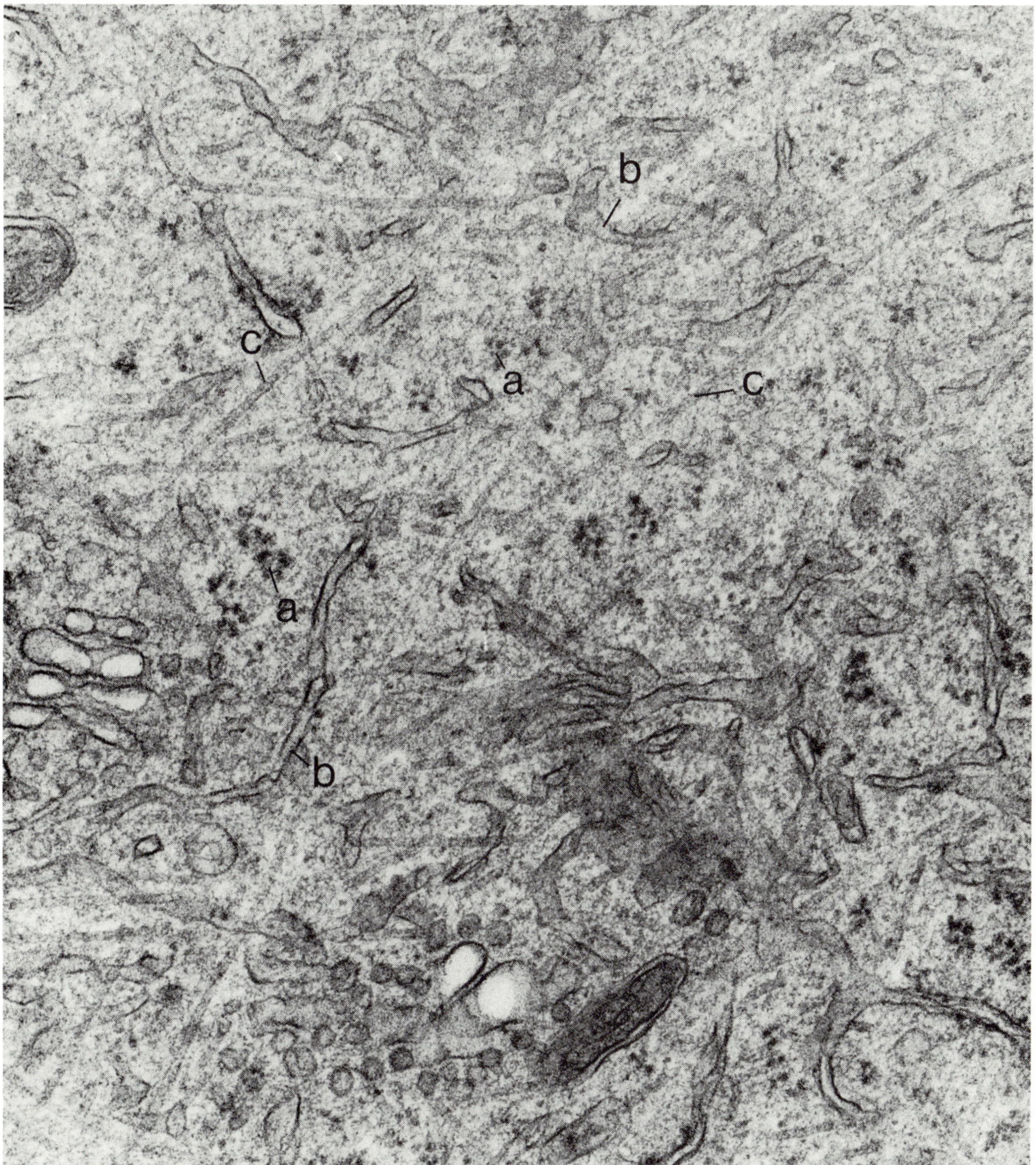

Figure 9–37. The cytoplasm of a cone myoid. There are clusters of ribosomes (a), profiles of smooth-surfaced endoplasmic reticulum (b), and neurotubules (c). (× 50,000.)

The Outer Limiting Membrane

By light microscopy the limiting membrane of the outer retina appears as an extremely thin, fenestrated membrane extending from the disc edge to the ora serrata (Figs. 9–7, 9–31, 9–40). At the edge of the optic disc the external limiting membrane ceases concurrently with the outer segments of the receptors. At the ora serrata the external limiting membrane becomes closely related to the retinal pigment epithelium shortly posterior to the termination of the neuroretina. This transition will be discussed in more detail subsequently. For the most part the membrane has the same curve as the eye, except for an anterior convexity in the macular region due to the greater length of the foveal cones.

Early histologists believed the external limiting membrane was formed by apposition of the terminal expansions of Müller fibers (Greeff, 1899). Verhoeff (1903) considered it to be elaborated by the rods and cones. Early observers also noted that the fenestrations of this layer are produced by extensions of the inner segments of the rods and cones through it. For this reason the external limiting membrane was believed to have the

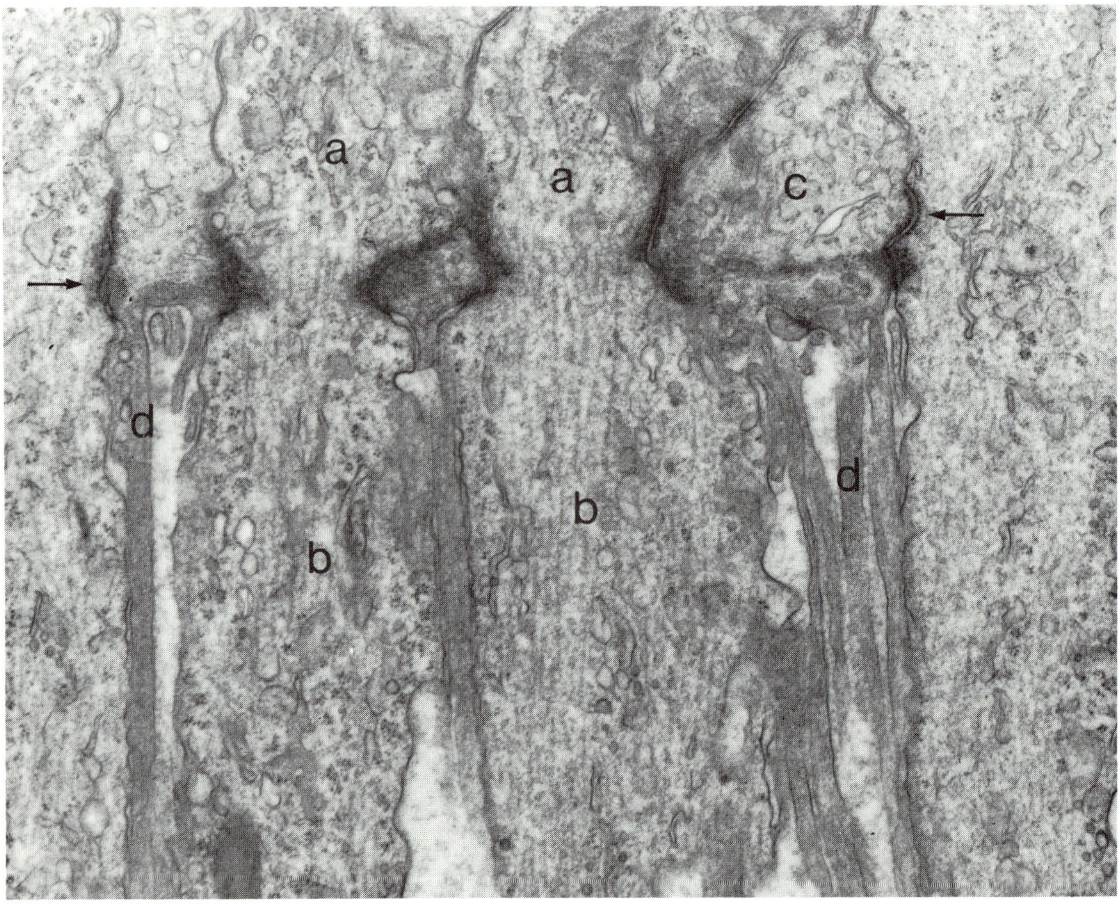

Figure 9–38. The external limiting membrane (arrows) in meridional section. The external receptor fibers (a) of the rods and cones are continuous with the inner segments of the photoreceptors (b). These fibers are separated from each other by Müller cell processes (c) that are continuous with the Müller cell fiber baskets (d) that continue beyond the external limiting membrane. (× 18,000.)

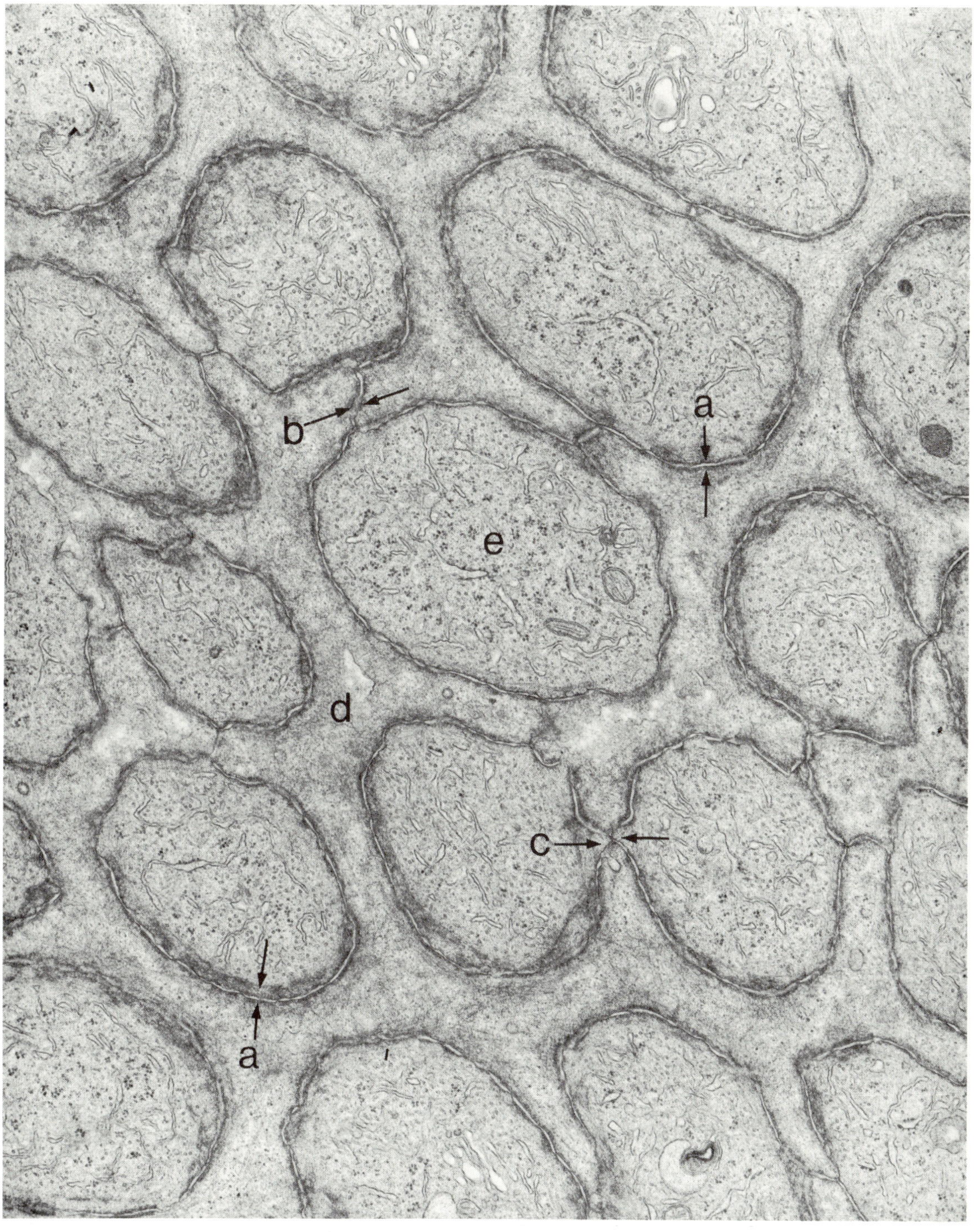

Figure 9–39. A tangential section through the region of the external limiting membrane. A junction between a photoreceptor and a Müller cell is seen at (a); a junction between two Müller cells is at (b); a photoreceptor-to-photoreceptor contact is seen at (c); Müller cell cytoplasm is at (d); and inner segment cytoplasm is at (e). (× 15,000.)

structure of a sieve. Salzmann (1912) considered the external limiting membrane to be connected to Müller cells of the retina on one side and believed that fine fiber baskets extend from the membrane on the other side. Salzmann believed the membrane to be derived from remnants of cement substance of fetal retinal cells.

Arey (1932) was the first to show that the external limiting membrane is not a membrane in the ordinary sense, but that it is produced by "terminal bars" uniting the cell membranes of the rods and cones to the Müller cells. A number of electron microscopic studies between 1958 and 1960 confirmed Arey's opinion (Sjöstrand, 1958; Yamada et al., 1958; Porter and Yamada, 1960; Cohen, 1960; Missotten, 1960; Fine, 1961; Fine and Zimmerman, 1962, 1963). Most of these observers described cytoplasmic densities in the photoreceptor inner segment (Fig. 9-38) and Müller cell cytoplasm at the level of the membrane and applied different names to these areas, the name changing from year to year and depending on electron microscopic concepts. The names "terminal bar" or "desmosome" have been used most often. Cohen (1965), in a study of primate eyes, correctly interpreted the structure forming the "membrane" as "zonulae adherentes." His work recently was confirmed and amplified in the human eye by Spitznas (1970). In flat sections the "outer limiting membrane" consists of zonulae adherentes which more often join the inner segments of the rods and cones to the Müller cells, also Müller cell to Müller cell, and, rarely, photoreceptor to photoreceptor (Fig. 9–39).

Outer Nuclear Layer

The outer nuclear layer contains the cell bodies of the rods and cones with their nuclei and cytoplasm (Figs. 9-40 to 9-42). The axons of these cells synapse in the outer plexiform layer with the bipolar and horizontal cells.

Close to the *nasal* edge of the disc the outer nuclear layer measures about 45 μm. thick and contains eight or nine rows of nuclei. The rows of nuclei and, accordingly, the thickness of the layer diminish perceptibly toward the periphery. On the *temporal* side of the disc, the outer nuclear layer is thinner; here it measures about 22 μm. thick and has only four rows of nuclei. It then increases to a thickness of about 50 μm. in the fovea, containing about 10 rows of nuclei, which belong exclusively to the cones. This area is discussed in detail in the section on the central retina (p. 493). In the remainder of the retina, with the exception of the ora serrata region, the outer nuclear layer is approximately 27 μm. thick and consists of a single layer of cone nuclei close to the outer limiting membrane; internal to the cone nuclei are about four rows of rod nuclei (Fig. 9-40). The rod nuclei are round or slightly oval with a diameter of approximately 5.5 μm. Their chromatin is dispersed, and a nucleolus is frequently seen. The cone nuclei are also slightly oval in shape and larger than those of the rods, measuring approximately 5 by 7 μm. They contain less heterochromatin than the rod nuclei, which accounts for their fainter staining seen with the light microscope. Occasionally, as a normal variation most commonly seen in the macular region, cone nuclei are found to be displaced external to the outer limiting "membrane."

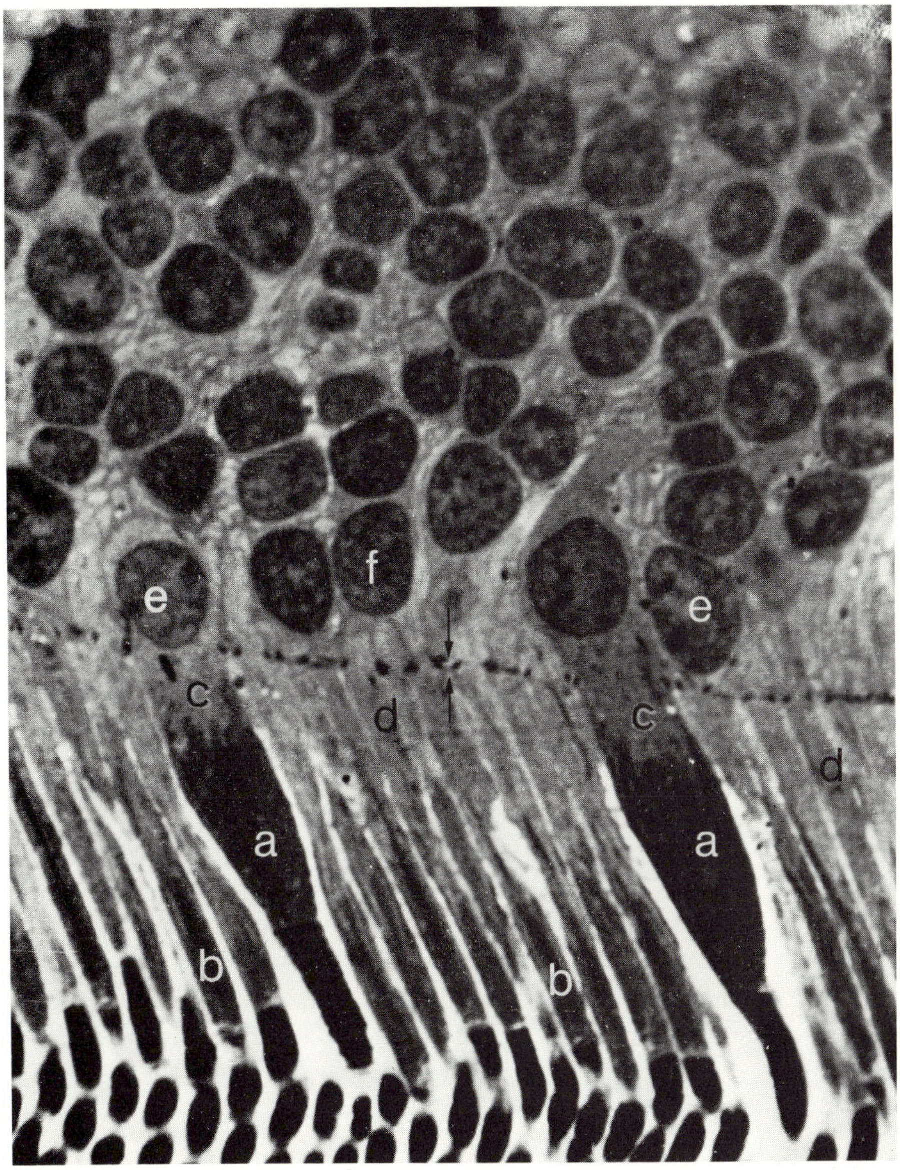

Figure 9–40. Light micrograph of the outer retina. The cone (a) and rod ellipsoids (b) are continuous with the cone (c) and rod (d) myoids. The cone nucleus is at (e) and the rod nucleus at (f). Arrows indicate the outer limiting membrane. (× 1480.)

The structure of the cytoplasm of the rod and cone cell bodies is essentially the same. After passing the outer limiting membrane, it is called the "outer rod fiber" or "outer cone fiber" (Figs. 9-41 and 9-42). It contains some elongated mitochondria and vesicles of smooth-surfaced endoplasmic reticulum which vary in size. Occasionally parallel arrays of rough-surfaced endoplasmic reticulum are also seen, and free ribosomes are present in moderate amounts. Many neurotubules are aggregated around the nucleus, which occupies much of the cell body and extends into the axon.

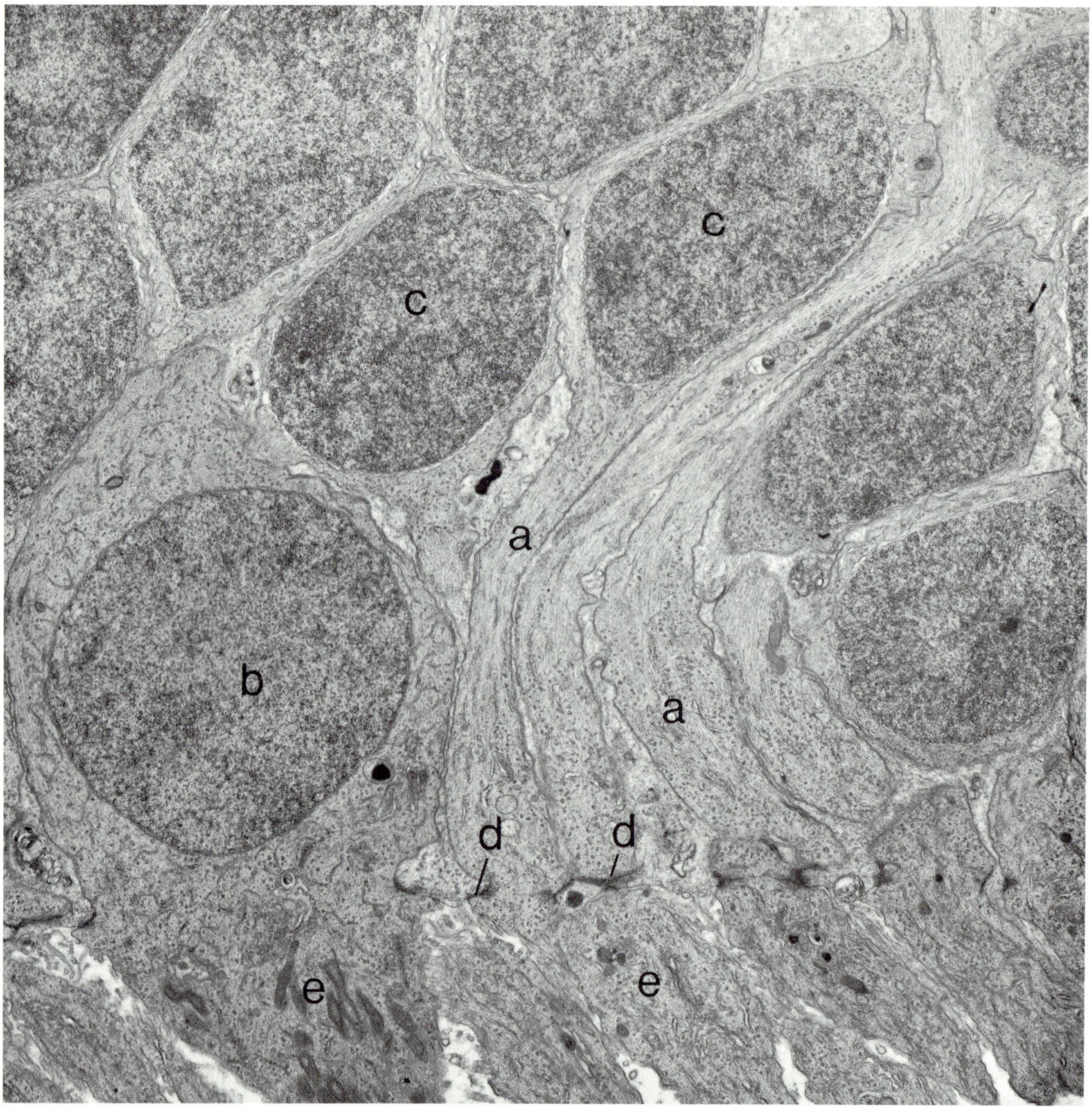

Figure 9–41. Electron micrograph of a meridional section of the outer nuclear layer. An outer rod fiber is at (a), a cone nucleus at (b), and rod nuclei are seen at (c). The external limiting membrane (d) is internal to the inner segments of the rods and cones (e). (× 3000.)

Figure 9–42. Outer nuclear layer showing the receptor fibers in cross-section. *A*, Internal receptor fibers (a) showing neurotubules. The nuclei of the receptors are seen at (b). (× 16,000.) *B*, The external receptor fibers are at (a) and the Müller cell processes at (b). (× 16,000.)

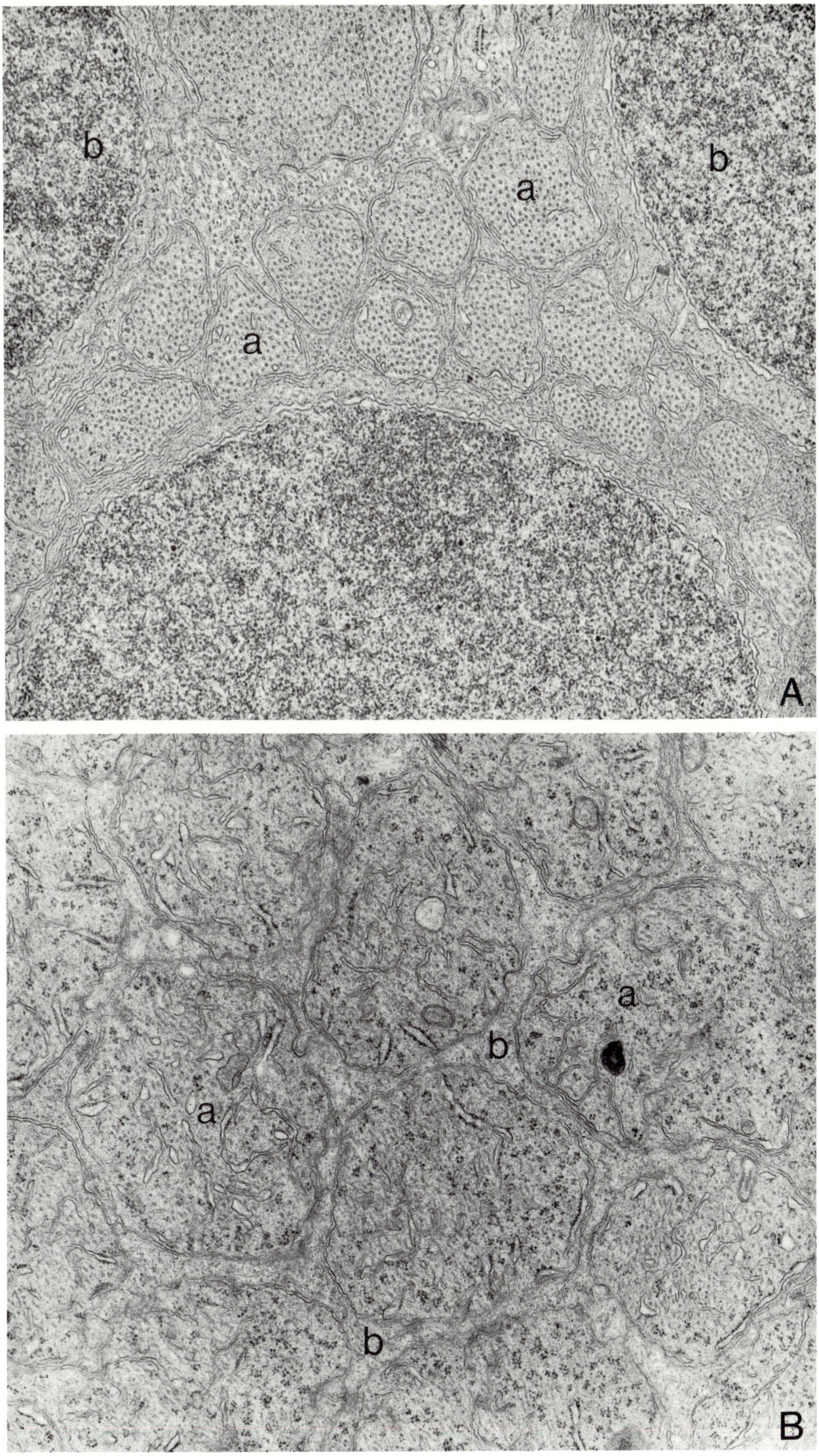

Figure 9–42. *See legend on opposite page.*

Outer Plexiform Layer

The outer plexiform layer measures 2 μm. in the extrafoveal region; it is the transition zone from the receptors (neuroepithelial) to the first order neurons. It becomes much thinner anterior to the equator because of the diminishing number of receptors.

The outer plexiform layer has a reticular structure; its texture is thick and looser in the outer two thirds than the inner third. Even with the low power of the light microscope, the axons of the rods and the cones can be traced into the outer plexiform layer in specially stained specimens. The rods end in an oval structure known as a "spherule," and the cones end in a broad conical swelling, the "pedicle." At the transition of the outer two thirds and the inner third, the cone pedicles are arranged in a row. They are much larger than the rod spherules and increase in size toward the periphery (Fig. 9-43).

In the macular region the outer plexiform layer is thicker and more fibrous in an area measuring approximately 51 μm. wide because the axons of the rods and cones become more oblique and longer as they deviate away from the fovea. In this zone the external plexiform layer is known as the fiber layer of Henle. At the edge of the foveola the cone fibers lie almost parallel with the external limiting membrane.

The outer plexiform layer can be divided into three zones: (1) an *external zone* containing the meridionally oriented fibers of the rods and

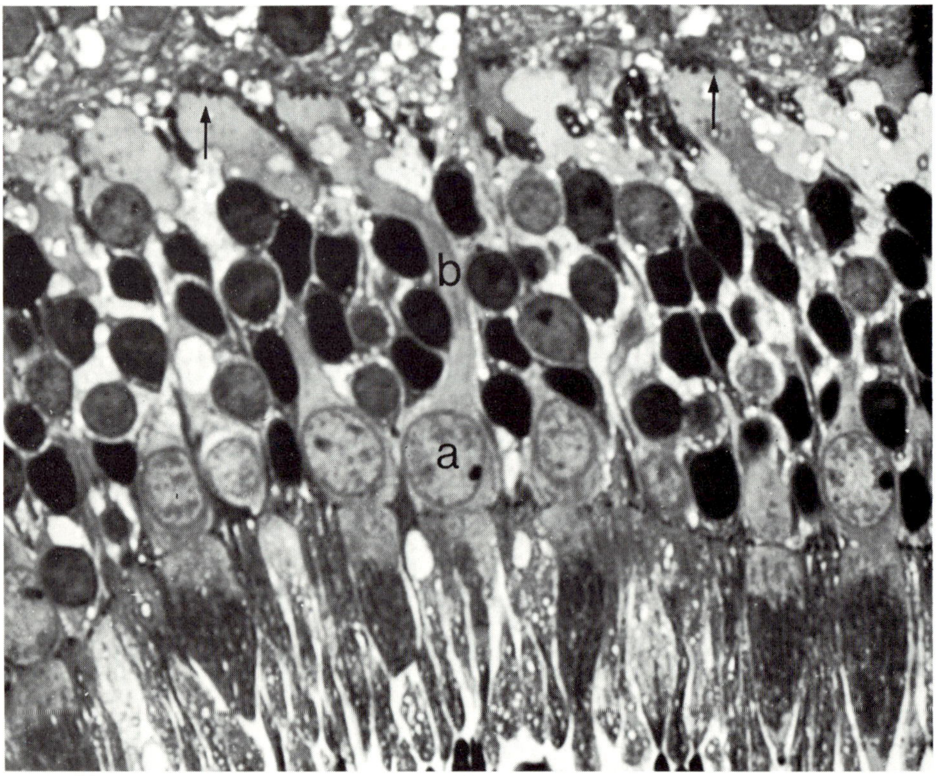

Figure 9–43. A light micrograph of the outer plexiform layer showing the pedicles of the cone synapses (arrows). A cone cell (a) and its internal receptor fiber (b) extend toward the pedicle. (× 1280.)

cones and many branching processes of the Müller cells; (2) a *middle zone* marking the terminations of the receptor cell fibers in the pear-shaped spherule and the broad, flat cone pedicles; and (3) an *internal zone* composed almost exclusively of the arborizing processes of the bipolar and horizontal cells and the many processes of the Müller cells, which fill the areas not occupied by neural cells.

When studied by electron microscopy, the axons of the photoreceptor cells are narrow, those of the rods being one fourth the diameter of the cones (Fig. 9-44). The rod axon is known as the *internal rod fiber* and it contains occasional mitochondria, a few vesicles and some free ribosomes and neurotubules. The neurotubules are microtubules, which are found in nerve and glial cells throughout the central nervous system. They measure 150 to 250 A. in diameter, their walls are about 50 A. thick, and their length is uncertain but often greater than 1 μm. (Fig. 9-45). The exact function of the neurotubules has not been determined; they play an important role in mitosis and they may be involved in conduction of stimuli, intracellular transportation of fluid, rigidity and elasticity and in the function of the cilia (Kuwabara, 1965). The cytoplasm of the cone axon has the same organelles but contains more neurotubules.

Rod Spherule. The rod spherule (synaptic ending) is the dilated oval termination of the axon; it is found in the middle part of the external plexiform layer (Figs. 9–46 and 9–47). Generally the rod endings lie external to

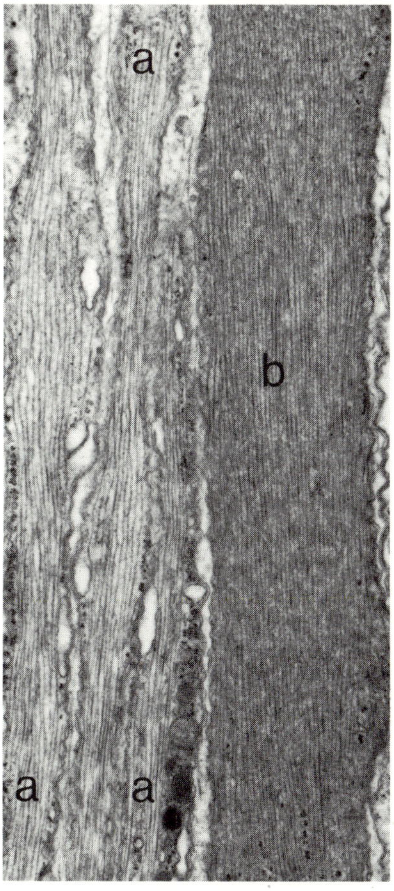

Figure 9–44. Internal receptor fibers of a rod (a) and of a cone (b). (× 9000.)

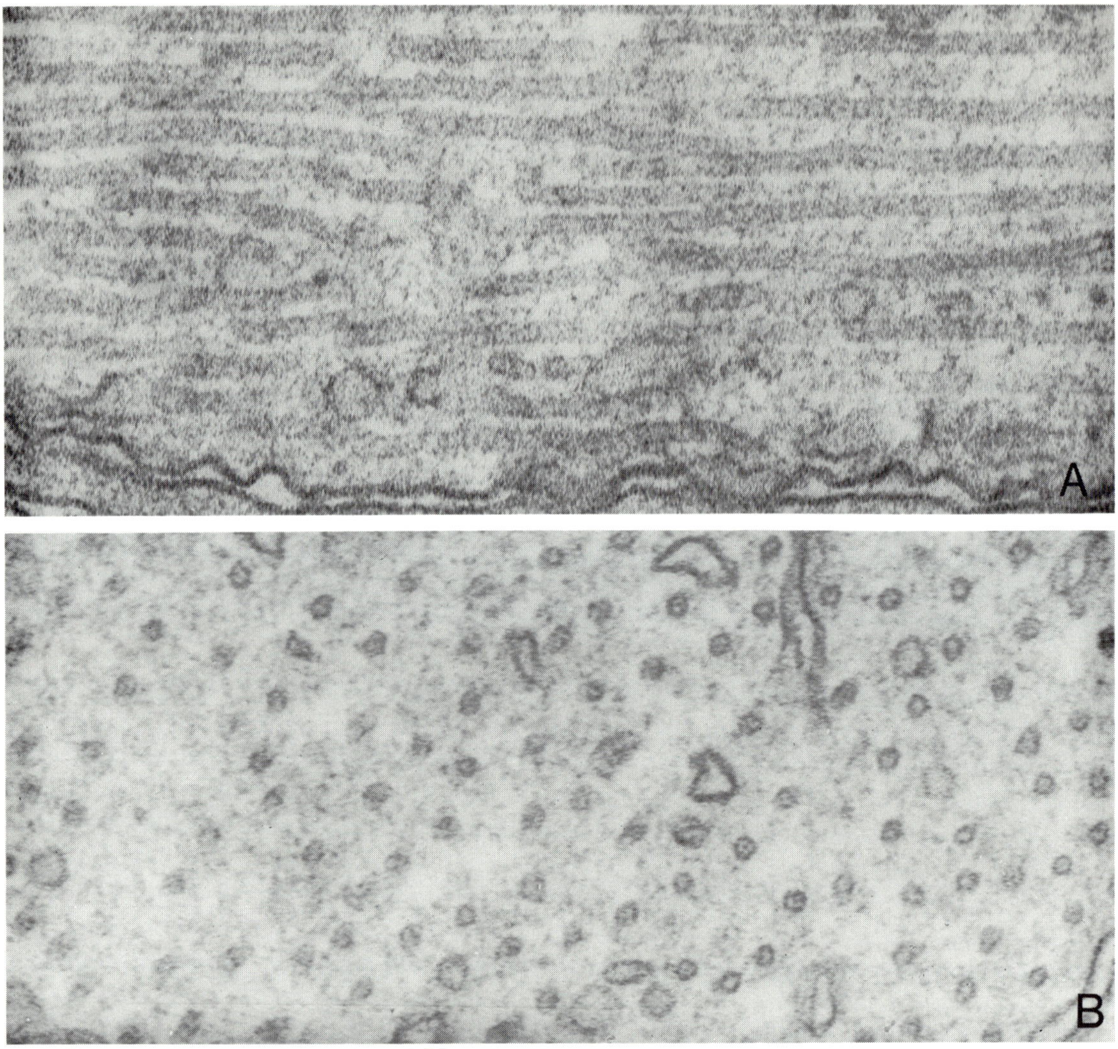

Figure 9–45. *A* is a tangential and *B* is a longitudinal section to demonstrate the neurotubules of an internal receptor fiber. The cross-sections of neurotubules frequently show a central dense opacity. (× 120,000.)

the cone endings, but spherules may even be found close to the cell body in the external part of the layer. The internal surface of the spherule is invaginated by several nerve fibers, which are derived from cells in the inner nuclear layer; the cell wall of the spherule encloses the terminations of these fibers. The unit that comprises the rod spherule and its enclosed nerve fibers represents the synaptic complex. Its function is to transmit impulses generated in the photoreceptors. The synaptic complex is composed of three parts—presynaptic (the spherule); synaptic (spherule-bipolar and spherule-horizontal cell contacts); and postsynaptic (bipolar dendrites, horizontal cell processes).

The presynaptic portion is the rod spherule itself, which contains large numbers of presynaptic vesicles, mitochondria and some neurotubules and ribosomes. The presynaptic vesicles are scattered throughout the spherule but are more dense in the region of the cell membrane adjacent to the enclosed nerve fibers. The cell membranes at the synapse of the rods with the bipolar and the horizontal cells are not thickened like typical synaptic endings. There is a synaptic cleft about 150 A. wide between the cell membranes of the spherule and the enclosed processes. Fine threads or other structures are not found in the cleft as elsewhere in the central nervous system. The portions of the cell membranes which participate in formation of the synapse are known as the presynaptic (rod) and postsynaptic (bipolar and horizontal cell) membranes (Fig. 9-46). Within the rod spherule is an osmiophilic, sickle-shaped lamellar structure, the *synaptic ribbon*, which is about 500 A. in thickness and 0.5 μm. long. This ribbon is composed of three dense layers approximately 120 A. in thickness, separated from each other by two less electron-dense layers of 40 A. in thickness (Fig. 9-47). It is oriented at a right angle to the surface of the cell and faces the enclosed nerve processes. Interposed between the end of the synaptic ribbon and the cell membrane is a dense curved structure, the *arciform density*. Each spherule may contain two to seven such synaptic ribbons, depending on the number of enclosed nerve fibers. The function of both the synaptic ribbon and the arciform density are not known; they are believed to have something to do with nerve transmission. This type of specialized structure is also found in the inner plexiform layer of the retina, as well as in the hair cells in the organ of Corti and the vestibular system. Numerous synaptic vesicles surround the synaptic lamella and the arciform density. Sometimes they form straight lines parallel to the synaptic ribbons but usually they are separated from it by a distance of about 200 A.

Missotten and co-workers (1963) reconstructed rod spherules with serial sections, showing that two to seven dendrites may make contact with the spherules, but commonly only two to four contacts are observed. It is known that both bipolar and horizontal cells make contact with the spherules. According to Missotten (1965) and Dowling and Boycott (1966), it is most likely that the lateral and more deeply inserted processes of the invaginations represent horizontal cell endings, whereas the centrally placed processes belong to rod (mop) bipolar cells. The largest of the bipolar and horizontal cell processes in the spherule usually contain numerous postsynaptic vesicles and some mitochondria.

The lateral surfaces of the rod spherules are frequently in close relation to lateral expansions from the pedicles of the cones. No synaptic ribbons or synaptic vesicles are found in the rod or cone cytoplasm at these sites.

Cone Pedicle. The cone pedicle has a pyramidal shape, the cone axon forming the apex and the synaptic surface forming its base (Figs. 9-48 and 9-49). Each pedicle contains grouped mitochondria, microtubules and synaptic vesicles, found here in much the same arrangement as in the rod spherule. The synaptic ribbons are smaller and more numerous than those of the spherule, but they are oriented in the same way with respect to the synaptic membranes.

A large number of dendrites make contact with the synaptic surface of the pedicle. Missotten and associates (1966) reconstructed pedicles with serial sections and arranged the contacts into three groups: (1) endings making deep invaginations and grouped in symmetric triads, with each pedicle containing about 25 units; (2) about 500 endings making light depressions in the surface of each pedicle; and (3) interreceptor contacts through lateral expansions to adjacent cones or rods. It is difficult to identify the cell

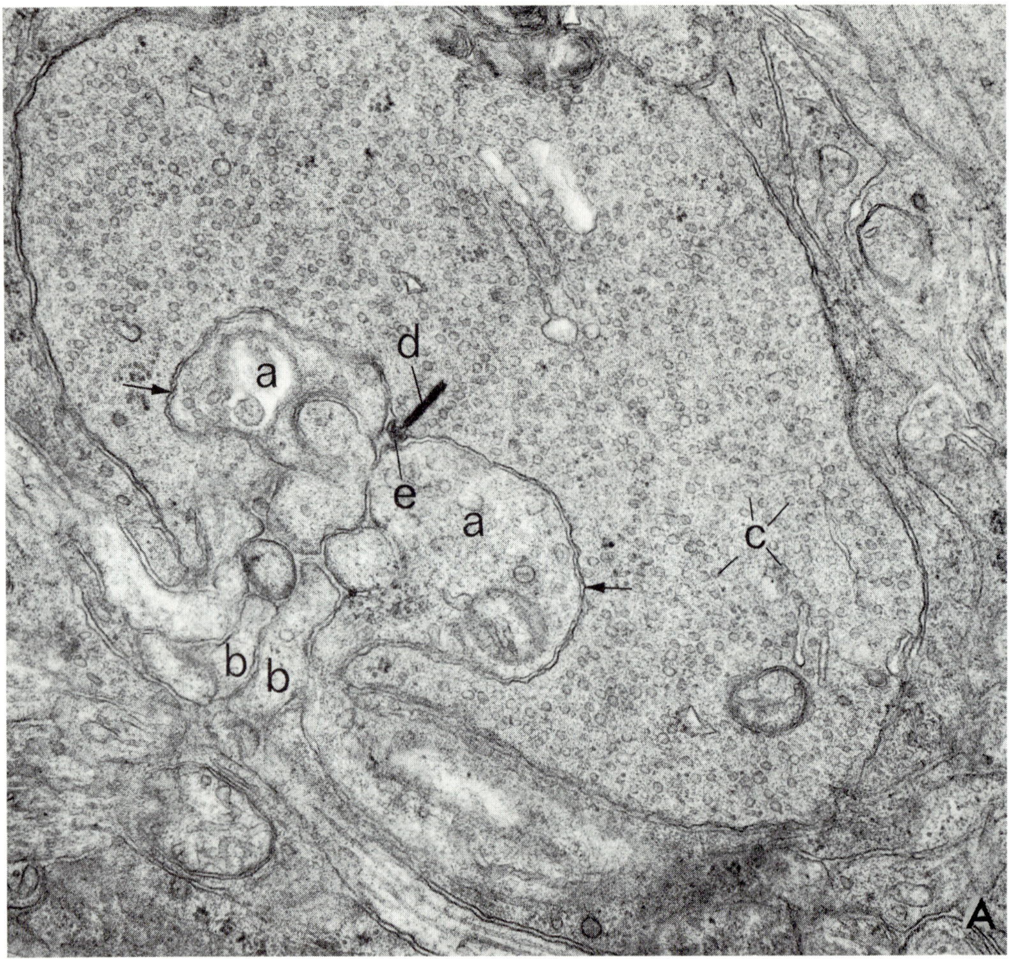

Figure 9–46. *A*, Rod spherule showing the lateral horizontal cell processes (a) and the central bipolar cell processes (b). The spherule contains numerous synaptic vesicles (c), a synaptic ribbon (d), and the arciform density (e). Arrows point to the synaptic cleft. (× 50,000.)

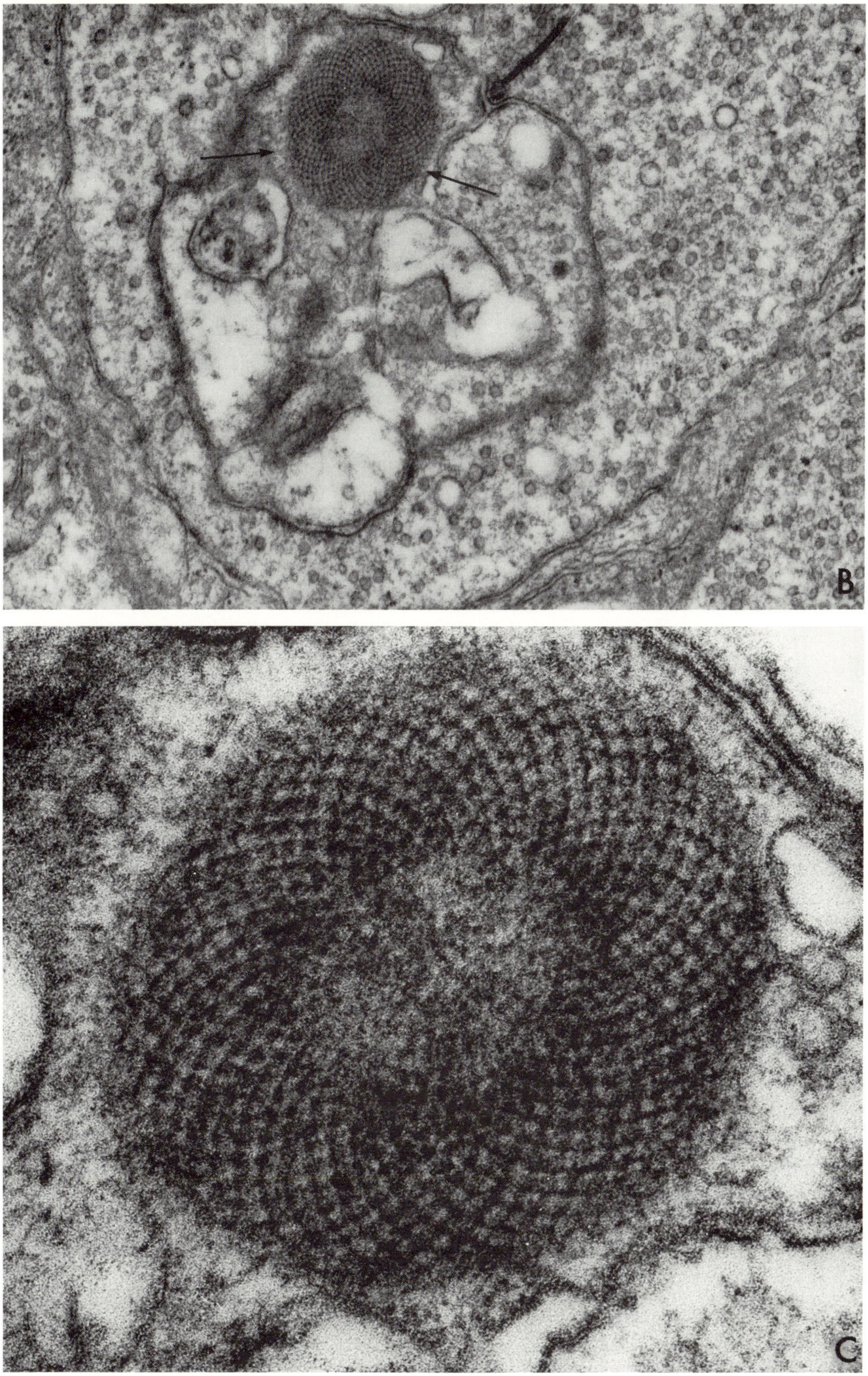

Figure 9–46. *Continued.*

B, Rod spherule showing a crystal-like structure (arrow) in the lateral cell processes. (×46,000.)

C, Higher magnification of the postsynaptic crystal-like structure present in the lateral cell processes. This structure presumably belongs to a horizontal cell. (× 170,000.)

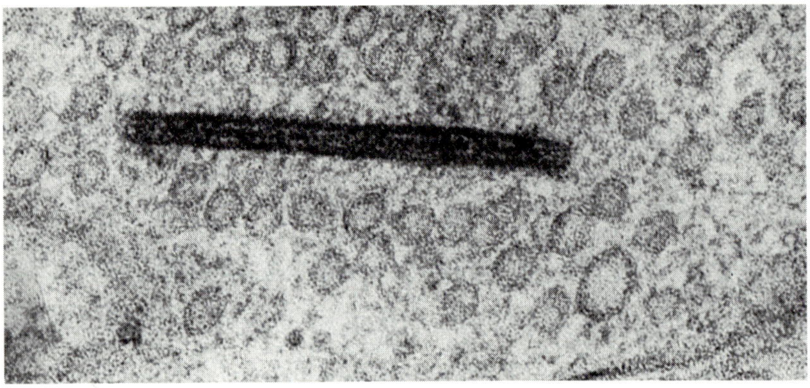

Figure 9–47. The synaptic ribbon possesses five layers, three dark and two light. The ribbon is surrounded by synaptic vesicles. (× 128,000.)

processes as they pass toward their contacts with the pedicles, because the processes of the bipolar and horizontal cells have such an even contour and are only 0.2 to 0.4 μm. in diameter. The small amount of cytoplasm in these processes also makes their identification difficult, but differences in the processes are evident at their terminations.

Deep Invaginations. The two lateral processes of the triads are invaginated further into the pedicle and are larger than the central dendrite, which is small and has a shallower invagination. The lateral processes often contain scattered synaptic vesicles, which produces an axonal appearance, whereas the small central dendrite is more like a postsynaptic fiber in that it does not have these vesicles. The central process may contain some endoplasmic reticulum, neurotubules and a few ribosomes, structures which are characteristic of dendrites. As a result of the work of Missotten (1965), it is widely accepted today that the lateral processes of the triads represent horizontal cell axons and that the central processes can be either horizontal cell dendrites or midget bipolar endings (see later). According to Dowling and Boycott (1966), however, the central processes in the triads belong exclusively to midget bipolar cells, and the horizontal cell processes that end in the triads have no definite characteristics of either dendrites or axons. Their morphology in this respect resembles the structure of amacrine cell processes. This resemblance suggests that the horizontal cell may be analogous to the amacrine cell in its ability to receive and transmit stimuli in a horizontal direction, thus creating interretinal cross-connections and probably feedback information or regulation of function in this layer. In the triads the cell membranes of the three processes are closely related, but as in the spherule, there is no thickening of the membranes or bridging of the synaptic cleft. The synaptic ribbon faces the triad at a right angle, and the arciform density lies between the synaptic ribbon and the cell membrane. As in the spherule, there are numerous synaptic vesicles around the synaptic ribbon, the arciform density and in the region of the cell membrane.

The bipolar termination is more than 800 to 1000 A. from that of the cone pedicle cell membrane, whereas the terminations of the horizontal cells are close to the membrane. Dowling and Boycott suggest this as a mechanism whereby the horizontal cells can regulate the function of the bipolar cell. There appear to be no obvious horizontal cell contacts flanking

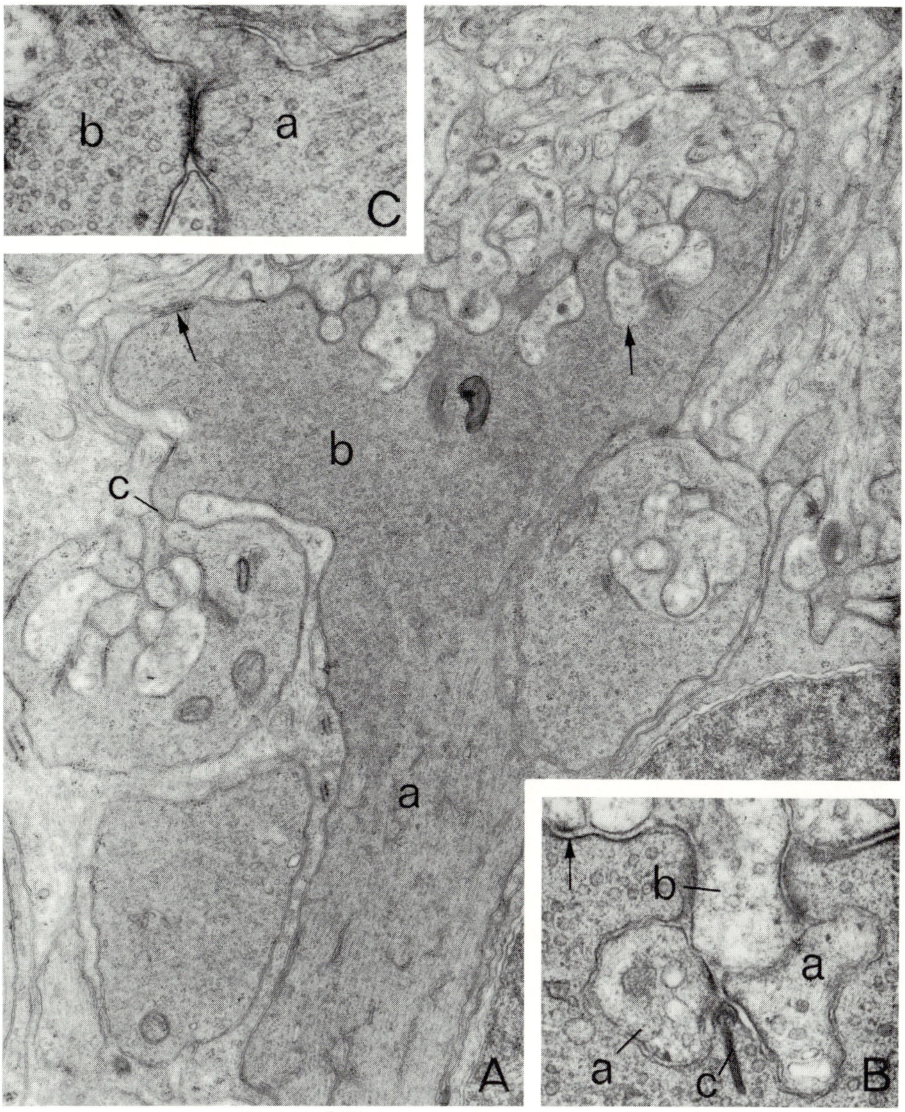

Figure 9–48. A cone pedicle with its connections. *A*, The cone internal receptor fiber (a) terminates in the pyramidal cone pedicle (b). Horizontal cells, flat bipolar cells and midget bipolar cells make contacts with the pedicle (arrows). A rod spherule makes a contact with the pedicle at (c). (× 10,000.)

B, A triad formed by lateral horizontal processes (a) and a central midget bipolar process (b). The synaptic ribbon is at (c). The arrows indicate surface contacts with flat bipolar cells. (× 40,000.)

C, A lateral contact between a cone pedicle (a) and a rod spherule (b). (x 40,000.)

the superficial contacts of the flat bipolars on the base of the cone pedicles, however; therefore it seems possible that the horizontal cell contacts regulate transmission to the bipolar cells regardless of the site of contact.

Surface Contacts. The numerous processes synapsing with the cones in shallow indentations on the basal surfaces of the pedicles resemble the central dendrites of the triads and have been found to belong to flat bipolar cells. There is only a slight thickening of the pedicle and bipolar membranes in these areas, and neither synaptic vesicles nor ribbons are present. As described previously, the cones make contact with two types of bipolar cells,

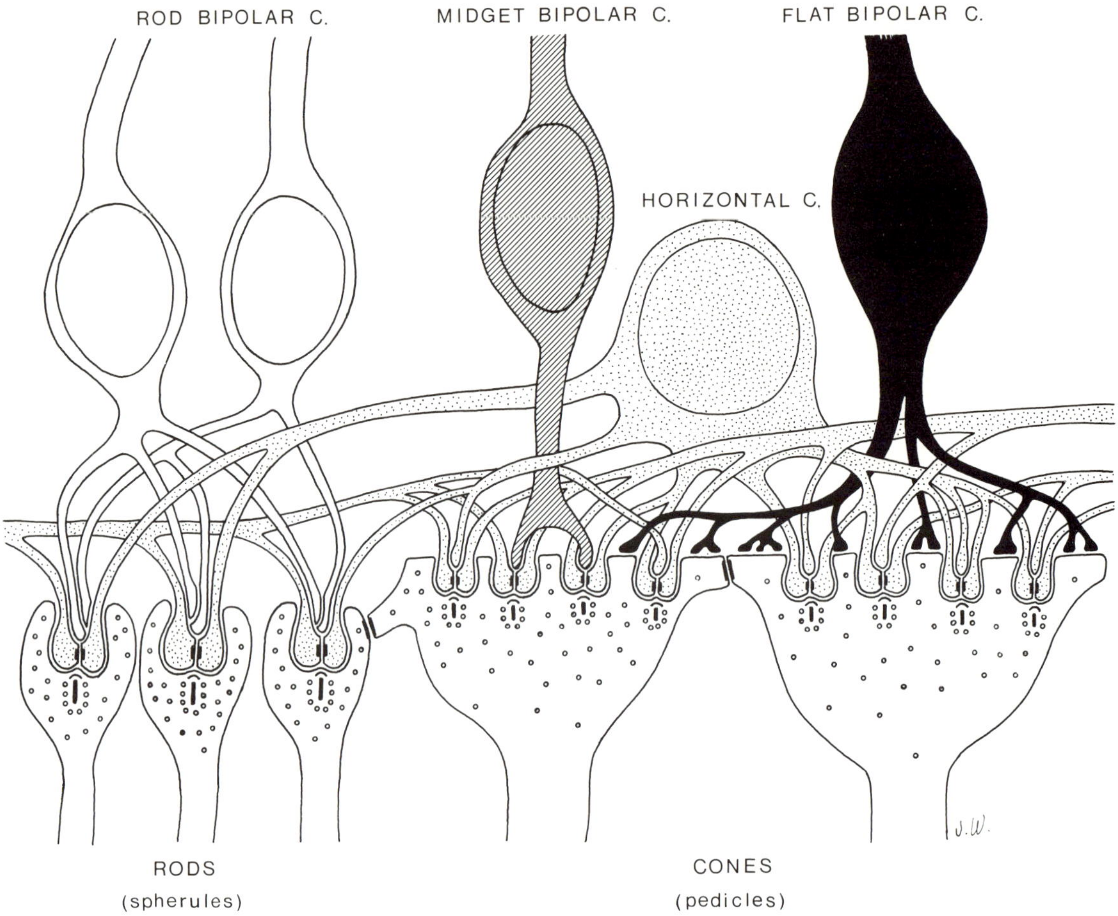

Figure 9–49. A schematic representation of a rod spherule and a cone pedicle with their synapses. Rod and cone bipolar cells show extensive contacts. The horizontal cells also make synapses with both the rods and the cones. Interconnections are also shown between rod spherules and cone pedicles. (Modified from Dowling, J. E., and Boycott, B. B.: Proc. Roy. Soc. London Biol. *166*:80, 1966.)

the midget and the flat cells. The midget bipolars appear to contact only one cone, although they may make contact with that cone many times through multiple processes. The flat bipolar cells, however, make contact with the surface of numerous pedicles. (See Fig. 9–49.)

Interreceptor Contacts. Each pedicle demonstrates six to 12 extensive lateral expansions, all containing neurotubules. These expansions extend a considerable distance horizontally toward the extremity of the lateral expansions of an adjacent cone or the lateral surface of a rod spherule. There are no synaptic vesicles on either side of the contact. Occasionally the intercellular space narrows in these areas, and some observers have found tight junctions here (Dowling and Gibbons, 1962; Cohen, 1965). These tight junctions are more readily demonstrated in glutaraldehyde-fixed material than with osmium. It is not certain whether these lateral expansions are sites of conduction or of transmission of nerve impulses.

Up to now we have been concerned mainly with the neurons of the retina. An extensive system of Müller cell branches exists in this and all

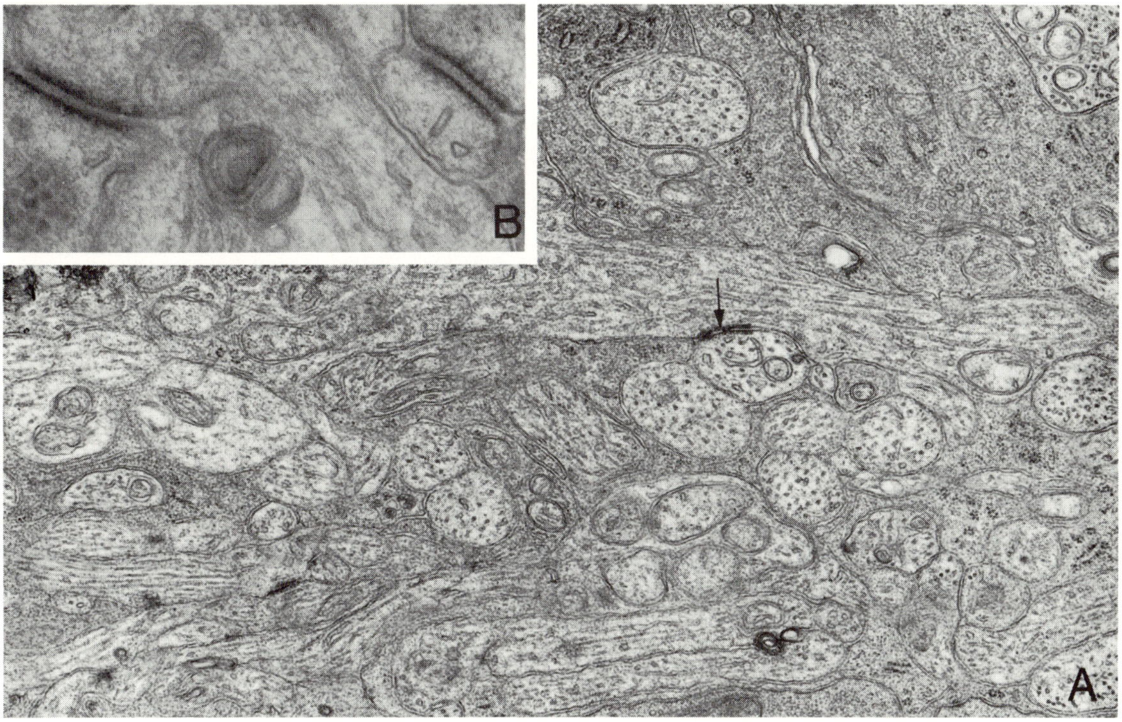

Figure 9–50. Inner zone of the external plexiform layer. *A*, The nerve processes are oriented in various directions. They contain neurotubules and often show desmosome-like junctions (arrow). (× 20,000.)

B, Two desmosome-like junctions at higher magnification. (× 80,000.)

other layers of the retina. The branches are thin and flat, interposing themselves around and between the nerve cells to provide support and nutrition. They are recognized by their increased cytoplasmic density compared to that of adjacent neurons.

The inner zone of the outer plexiform layer is a dense meshwork of branches and arborizations of bipolar, horizontal and Müller cells. With the exception of Müller cell processes, it is virtually impossible to determine the cell type to which these fibers belong without preparing serial sections (Fig. 9-50). Occasionally contacts that are morphologically similar to desmosomes can be found between adjacent fibers; the functional significance of these contacts is unknown.

Inner Nuclear Layer

Four types of cells can be identified in the inner nuclear layer: *horizontal cells, Müller cells, bipolar cells* and *amacrine cells* (Figs. 9–51 to 9-63). The amacrine and horizontal cells have long branches that make many contacts with other cells, probably for the purpose of integrating retinal functions. The bipolar cells comprise the first order neuron in the conducting system, and the Müller cells have a supporting and nutritive function. The cells in this layer generally are arranged in sublayers, but there is some intermingling of the cells within these layers. The outermost sublayer, adjacent to the outer plexiform layer, is composed of somata of the horizontal cells.

Horizontal Cells (Figs. 9–51 to 9–53). The horizontal cells occupy one to two levels. In flat sections examined with the light microscope, these cells can be seen to have a number of relatively short processes, which radiate fairly symmetrically from the perikaryon, and one long process, which arises either at the side of the perikaryon or from the base of one of the short processes. This long process does not branch within 200 to 300 μm. from the parent cell and is often up to 1 mm. long. There seems to be no preferred direction for these processes to extend across the retina. No process of this kind has been observed to cross the foveal pit.

Two different kinds (types A and B) of horizontal cells were demonstrated recently by light microscopy (Boycott and Dowling, 1969). The type A horizontal cells represent *"cone horizontals,"* and the type B cells probably are *"rod horizontals."* The short processes of every cell of *type A* break up into seven groups of endings which go to seven cone pedicles, where they take part in the formation of several triads. Each pedicle is in contact with the endings of two to four horizontal cells. The short processes of *type B* cells form 10 to 12 groups of endings. As yet it has not been possible to determine how many rods might come into synaptic relationship with a single type B horizontal cell (Fig. 9-51).

It is probable that the horizontal cell processes are not true axons or dendrites and that the horizontal cell should be considered as being able to send as well as to receive information along its branches. The number and length of their branchings increase from the central retina toward the periphery. In the central retina they are more concentrated and comprise most of the outermost row in the external plexiform layer.

The horizontal cells are quite angular, and their cytoplasmic content is similar to that of the bipolar cells (Fig. 9-52) except for the presence of a rather unique cytoplasmic inclusion, Kolmer's crystalloid. This inclusion is so large it can also be seen with the light microscope, and it stains directly with basic dyes because of its heavy ribosome content. Its function is not known. It measures approximately 0.4 μm. in diameter and 5.0 μm. in length. It is formed by parallel rows of varying numbers of tubes with membranous walls (Fig. 9-53). Many ribosomes are found in the area of the organelle, especially on the inner surface of the tube walls. The lumen of the tubes contains cytoplasm in which there are vesicles of smooth-surfaced endoplasmic reticulum.

The *outer intermediate* sublayer is composed principally of a variety of bipolar cells. According to Cajal (1911) and Boycott and Dowling (1969), who performed elaborate studies on the identification of the cellular elements of the retina in humans and other vertebrates, the following types of bipolar cells can be identified with the light microscope.

Rod Bipolar Cells (Mop Bipolar Cells) (Fig. 9–54). These cells are the only bipolar cells to contact the rods; they have a large cell body and a vast, abundantly branching dendritic system which extends into the outer plexiform layer to contact the *rod spherules*. Their dendritic arborizations are bulkier in the peripheral retina. The axons of these cells are unbranched and end in knot-like terminations in the inner plexiform layer. They make contacts not only with the soma of one or more of the outer ganglion cells, but also with the inner ganglion cells in such a way that each rod bipolar is related to one to four ganglion cells.

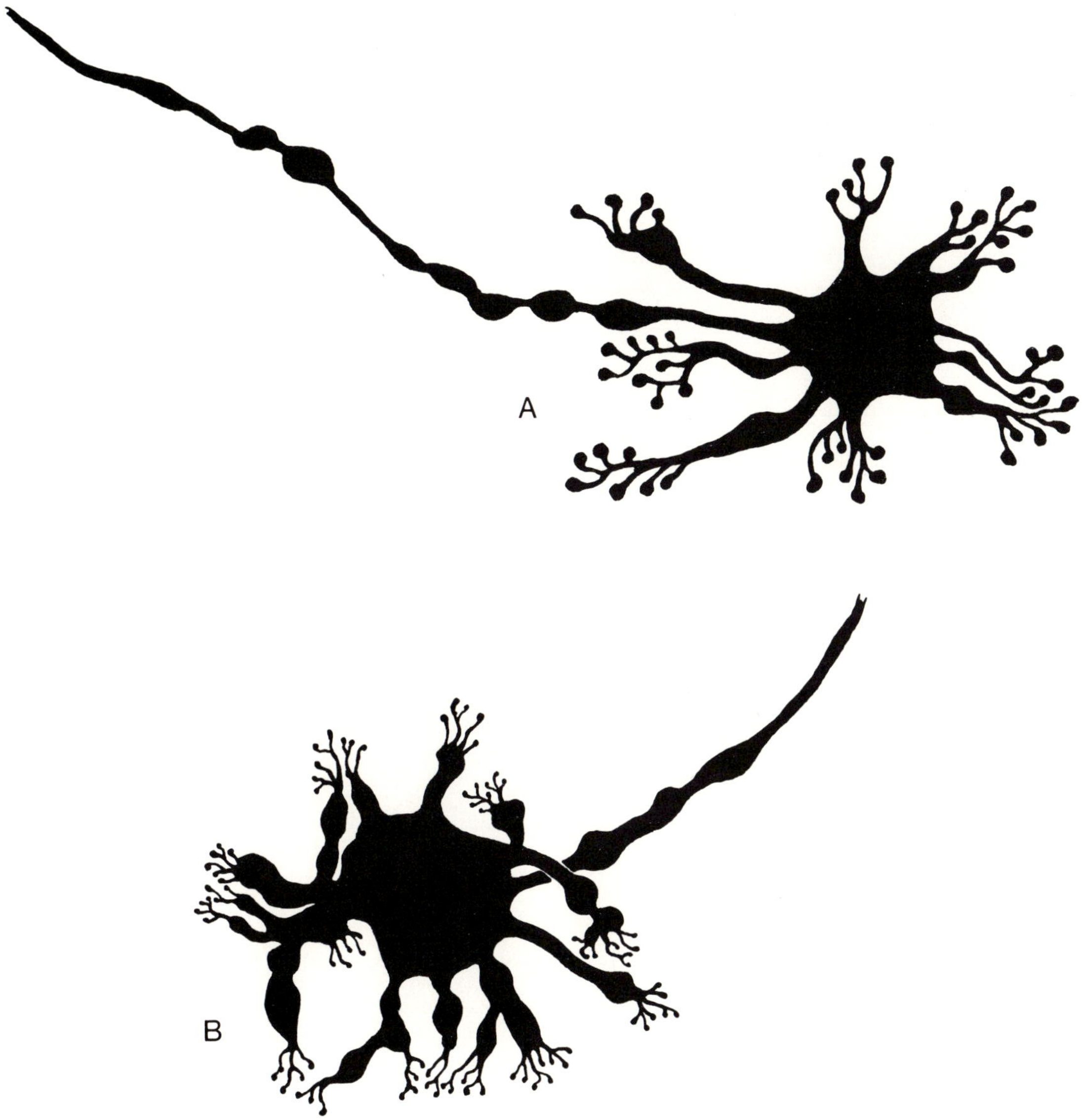

Figure 9–51. Horizontal cells. (A) cone horizontal; (B) rod horizontal.

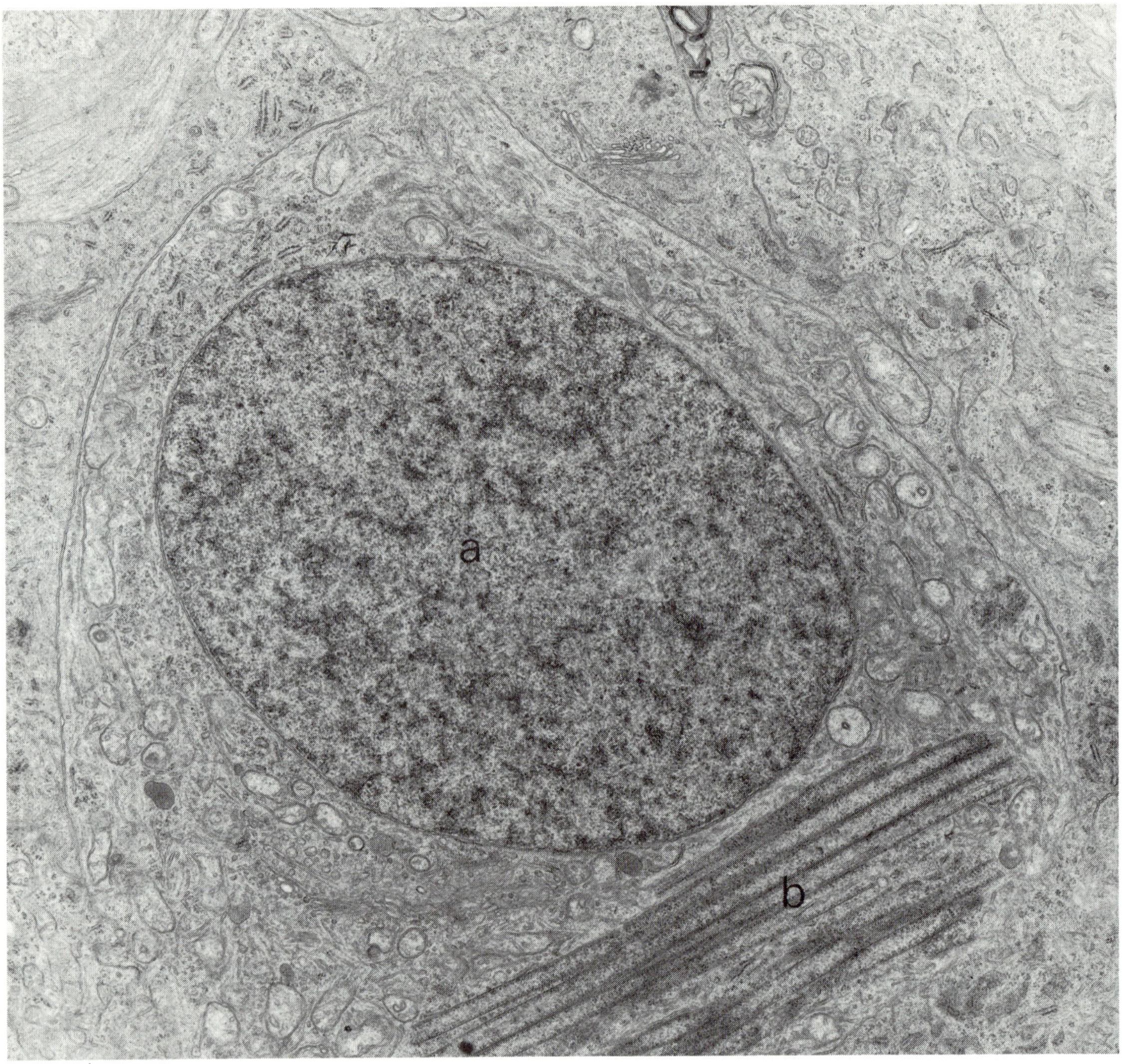

Figure 9–52. A horizontal cell with its nucleus (a) and Kolmer's organelle (b). (× 20,000.)

Midget Bipolar Cells (Fig. 9–54). These monosynaptic cells are relatively small and lie very close to the outer plexiform layer. They are the *true cone bipolars,* which come into contact with the cone pedicles in the triads. There is no apparent direct contact between the dendrites of adjacent bipolar cells. The midget bipolar axons extend into the inner plexiform layer where they synapse with a single *midget ganglion cell.*

Flat Bipolar Cells (Brush Bipolar Cells) (Fig. 9–54). The chief dendritic contact of these polysynaptic cells is with the cones. When viewed with the light microscope, they are characterized by the flat, cut-off appearance of their dendritic expansions. Their many endings make synapses with the dendrites of all types of ganglion cells.

Little work has been done on the ultrastructure of these cells except for that of Missotten (1965). With the electron microscope the different types of bipolar cells are difficult to distinguish. Their perikarya contain numerous mitochondria, many free ribosomes, smooth-surfaced endoplasmic reticu-

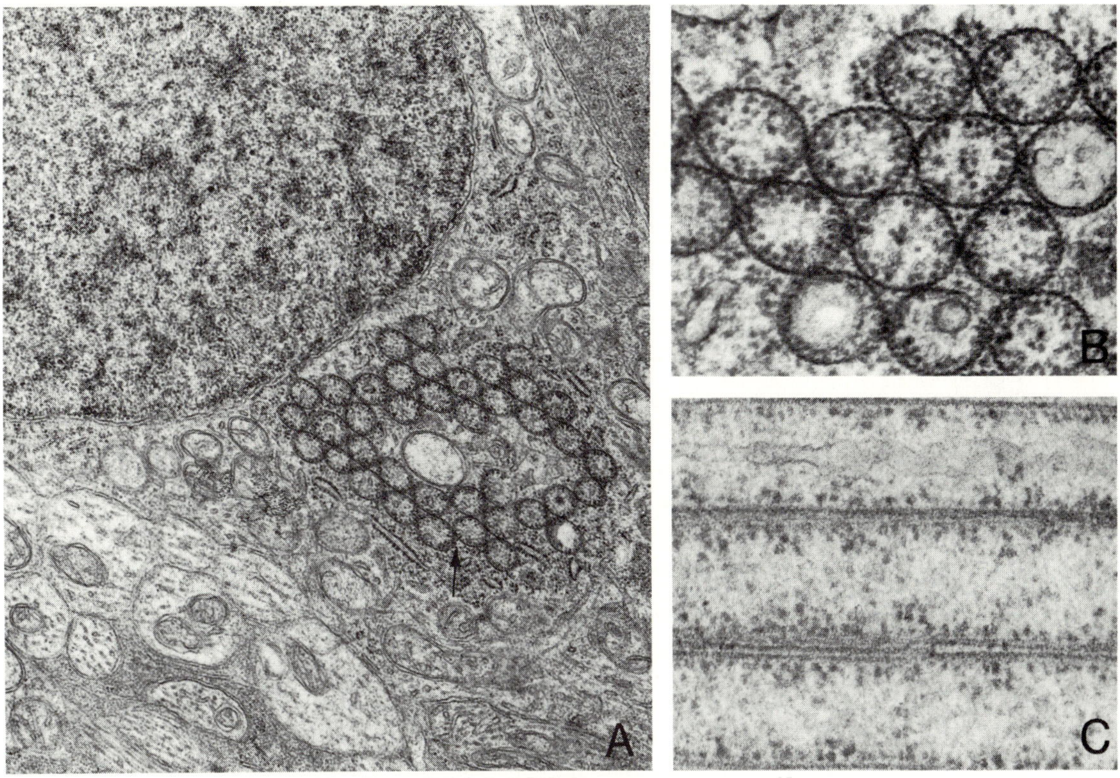

Figure 9–53. Kolmer's organelle of the horizontal cell. *A*, The organelle (arrow) is composed of an array of tubes that are seen in cross-section. (× 20,000.)

B, A magnified cross-section through the tubules of the organelle. (× 60,000.)

C, A longitudinal section through three tubules that are parallel. They contain many ribosomes. (× 60,000.)

lum, scattered cisternae of rough-surfaced endoplasmic reticulum and neurotubules. The content of neurotubules is more pronounced in the cone (midget and flat) bipolar cells and increases in their axons (Fig. 9-55). The axon of the rod (mop) bipolar cells is characterized by many vesicles close and parallel to the cell membrane. In serial or tangential sections these vesicles can be determined to be cross-sections of a long tubular organelle oriented helically in the cytoplasm close to the cell membrane of the axon (Missotten, 1965). In the perikaryon of the rod bipolar cells the elements of this organelle are less clearly visible (Fig. 9-56).

The *inner intermediate* layer is composed mainly of the cell bodies of the Müller cells. *Müller cells* are giant cells which occupy the full thickness of the retina from internal to external limiting membrane and even extend beyond the external limiting "membrane" as villous processes (Fig. 9–57). They are recognized by their increased cytoplasmic density compared to the adjacent neurons. These cells are important because they furnish glucose to the nerve cells, and they have been shown to contain a considerable amount of lactic acid dehydrogenase activity and an ability to synthesize and store glycogen (Cogan and Kuwabara, 1967). Since their cell bodies and nuclei are located in the inner nuclear layer, they are described here. Their extensions enclose most of the neurons and insulate the nerve fibers. Müller cells also can be considered as "space-occupying" cells, since their extensions fill out

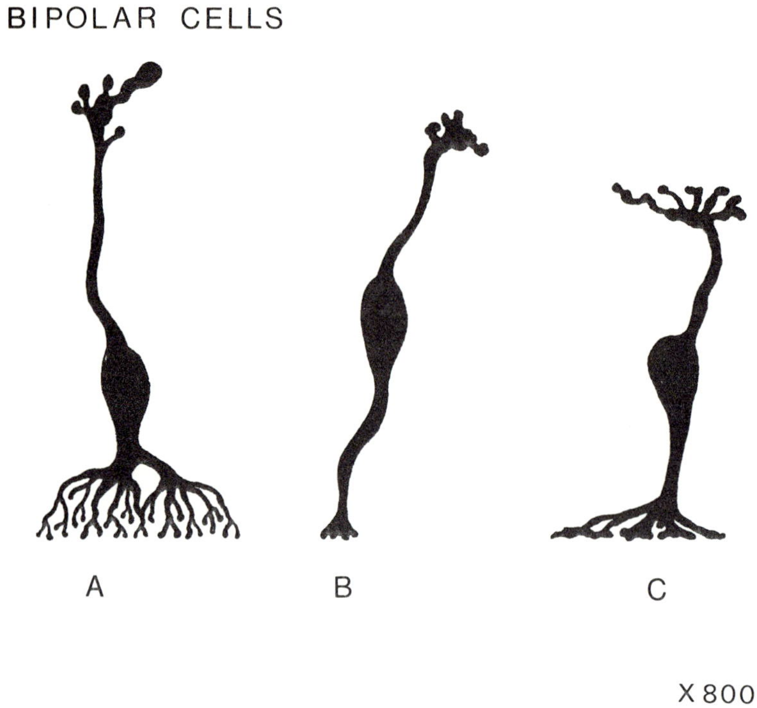

Figure 9–54. The differences between three types of bipolar cells in the synaptic region. A is a rod bipolar, B is a midget bipolar and C is a flat bipolar.

all the retinal areas not occupied by neurons, except in the inner retina, where the astrocytes also participate in this process.

The nuclei of the Müller cells are found almost exclusively in the inner intermediate portion of the internal nuclear layer; they are angular and have a dense chromatin. Embryologically Müller cells are derived from the inner layer of the optic cup, their apices facing the pigment epithelium and their bases facing the vitreous.

The mature Müller cell is complex in shape and distribution as follows (Figs. 9-57 and 9-58):

Radial Processes. Arising on both sides of the cell body in the internal nuclear layer, these stout main processes pass radially through the retinal layers. In the nerve fiber layer they terminate in large conical expansions (Fig. 9–71), which participate in the formation of the internal limiting membrane.

Honeycomb Meshwork. In the nuclear layers, including the ganglion cell layer, the lateral cell processes form cytoplasmic lamellae around the perikarya. Neighboring lamellae fuse to form a meshwork which encloses the somata of the cells.

Horizontal Fibers. These fine processes extend laterally in the two plexiform layers and in the nerve fiber layer to embrace the retinal dendrites, axons and synapses and send small branches to the surfaces of the retinal vessels. They are best developed in the external plexiform layer, where they insinuate themselves around the spherules, pedicles and other processes.

Fiber Baskets. These thin, villous prolongations extend beyond the

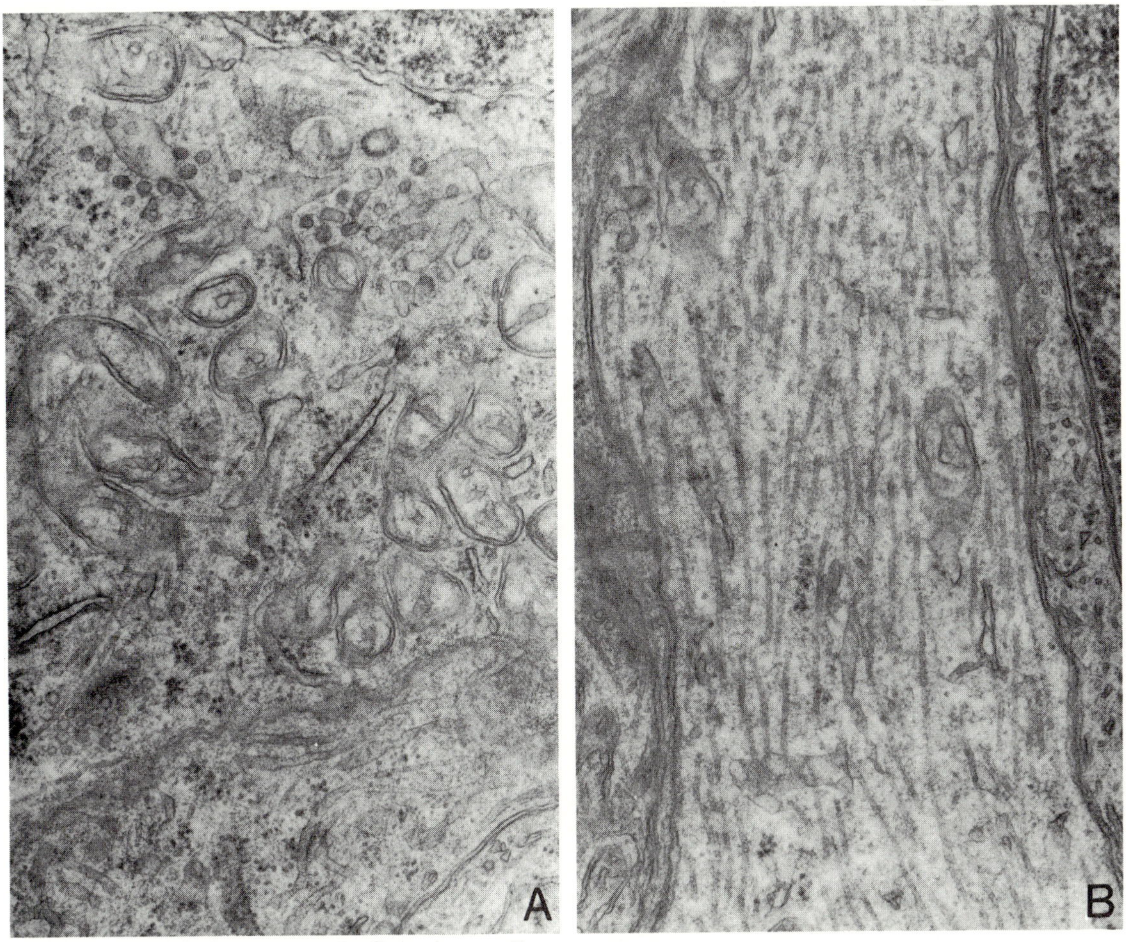

Figure 9–55. The perikaryon and axon of a cone bipolar cell. *A*, Perikaryon. The cytoplasm contains numerous mitochondria, smooth- and rough-surfaced endoplasmic reticulum and a few neurotubules. (× 32,000.)

B, Axon. The cytoplasm contains an abundance of neurotubules. (× 32,000.)

external limiting membrane and embrace portions of the inner segments of the photoreceptors. (See Figures 9–31 and 9–32.)

Morphologic studies of Müller cells have shown their composite structure (Cohen, 1961; Fine and Zimmerman, 1962; Pedler, 1963; Hogan and Feeney, 1963; Villegas, 1964; and Inomata, 1965). The *nucleus* varies in shape, depending on the arrangement of the surrounding tissues. It often is flattened in comparison to the uniformly round nuclei of the bipolar cells. The nucleoplasm and the perinuclear cytoplasm are darker than that of surrounding cells (Fig. 9-59). Near the inner retinal boundary the cells branch extensively, their processes spreading out in umbrella shape, their vitreal surfaces forming blunt villous processes along the inner retina. The cytoplasm contains numerous well developed fibrils measuring 100 A. in diameter. These fibrils are randomly oriented except near the cell membrane, where they lie parallel to the inner surface. They are especially abundant near the inner limiting membrane. The smooth-surfaced endoplasmic reticulum of these cells exhibits a degree of development not seen in any other cell layer of the ocular tissues except for the pigment epithelium.

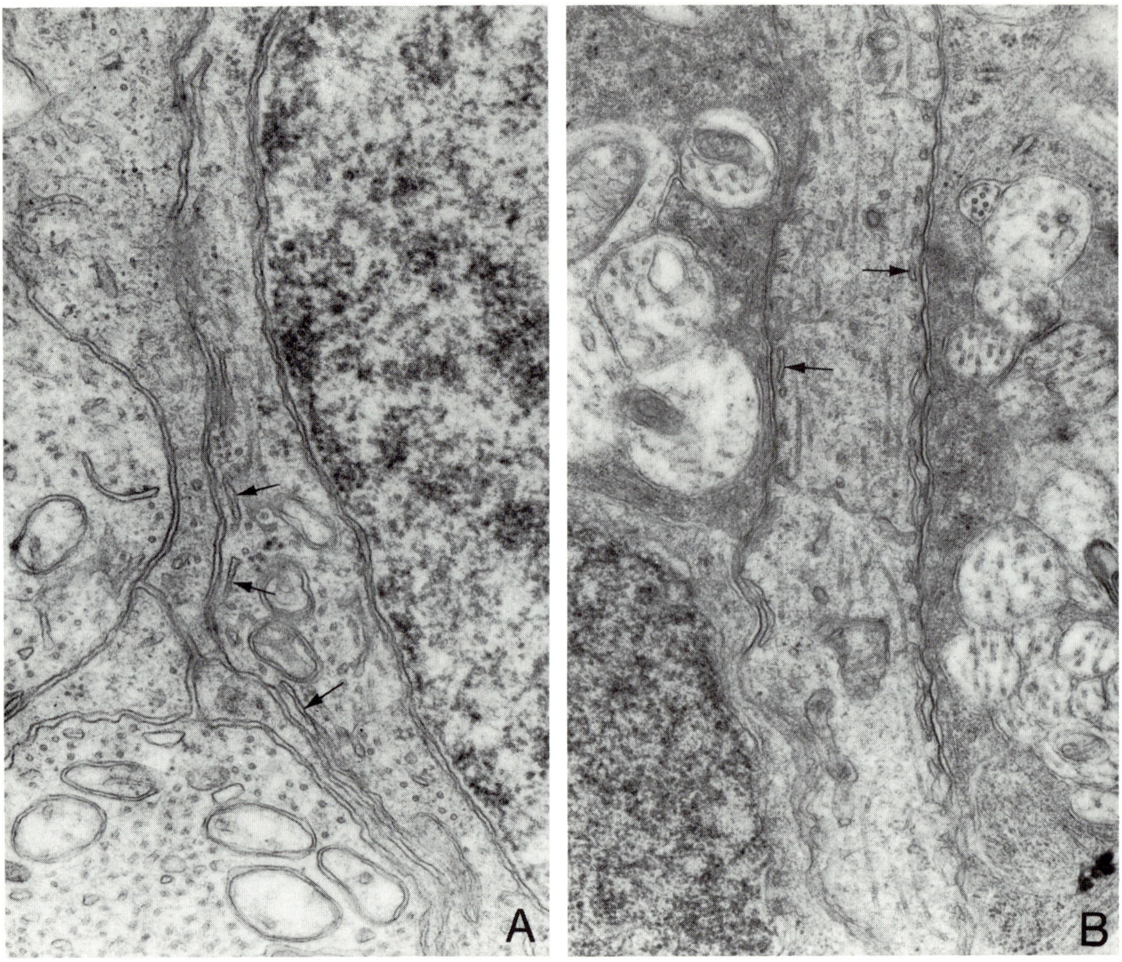

Figure 9–56. The perikaryon and axon of a rod bipolar cell. *A*, Perikaryon. The section shows the helical organelle (arrows) that is in proximity to the cell membrane; it appears to be comprised of smooth-surfaced endoplasmic reticulum. (× 32,000.)

B, Axon. The helical organelle (arrows) is more visible here than in the perikaryon. There are scattered neurotubules. (× 32,000.)

Figure 9–57. A schematic drawing to show the structure of the Müller cell. The various portions are labeled according to the description in the text.

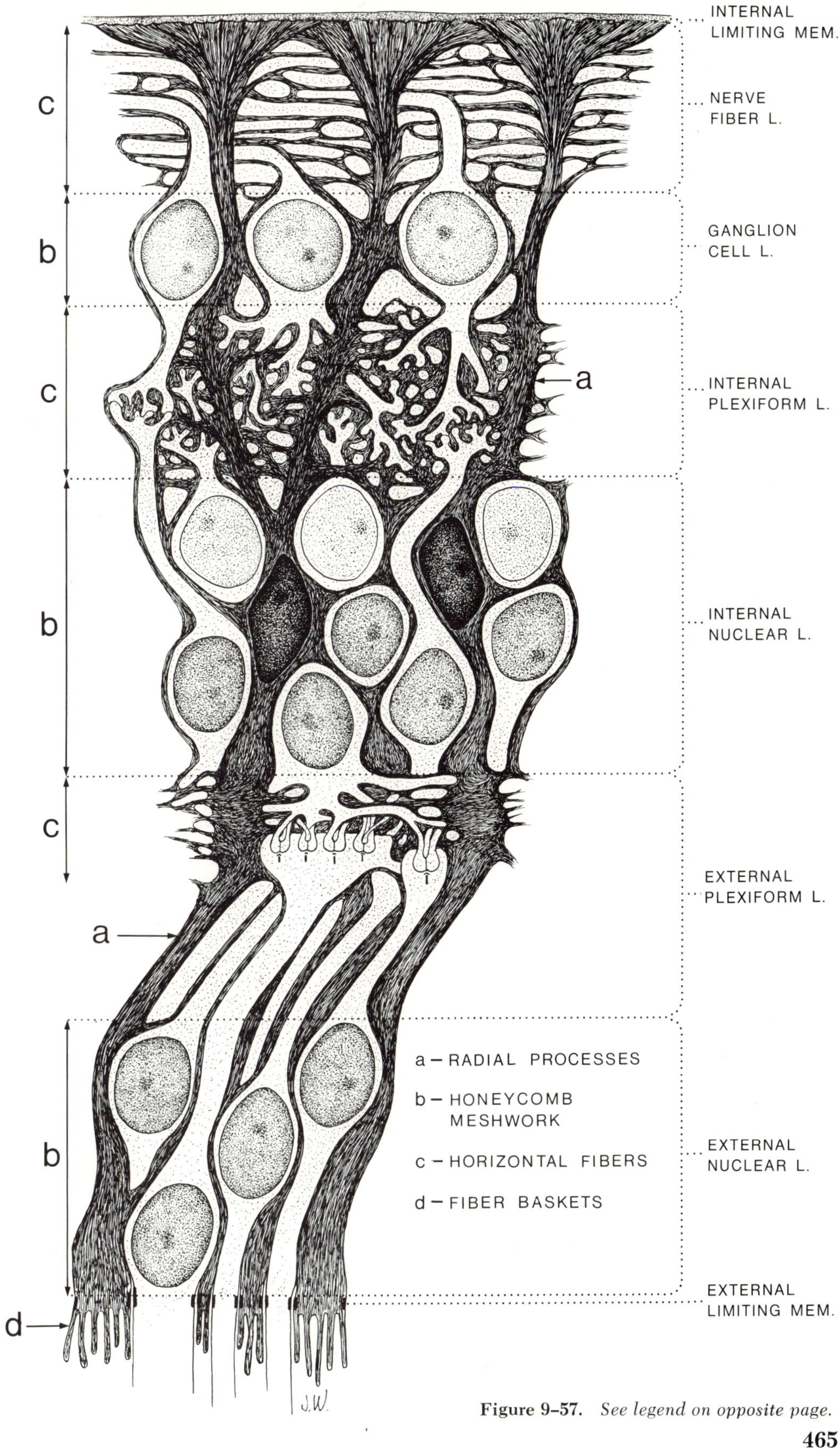

Figure 9–57. *See legend on opposite page.*

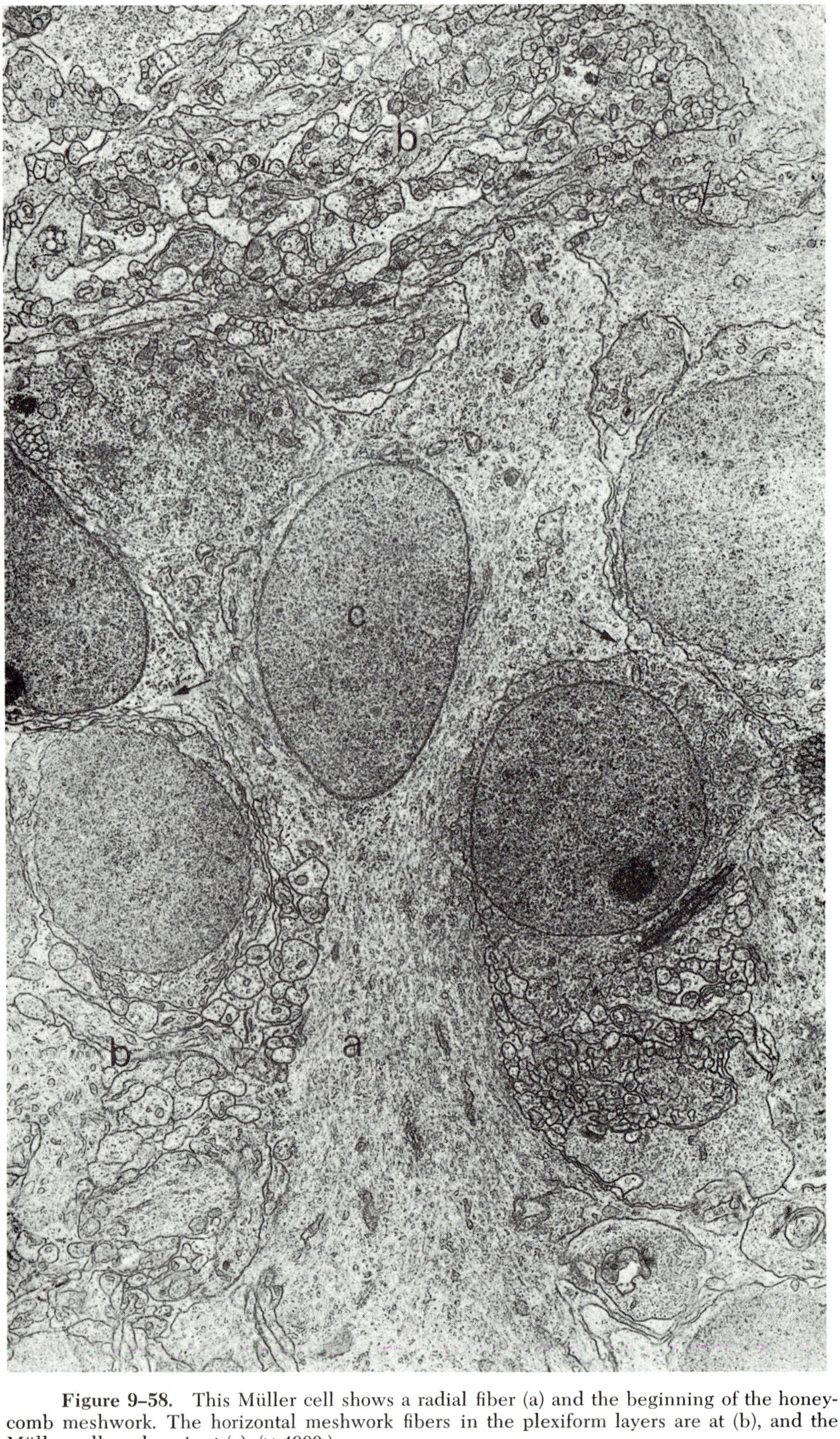

Figure 9–58. This Müller cell shows a radial fiber (a) and the beginning of the honeycomb meshwork. The horizontal meshwork fibers in the plexiform layers are at (b), and the Müller cell nucleus is at (c). (× 4000.)

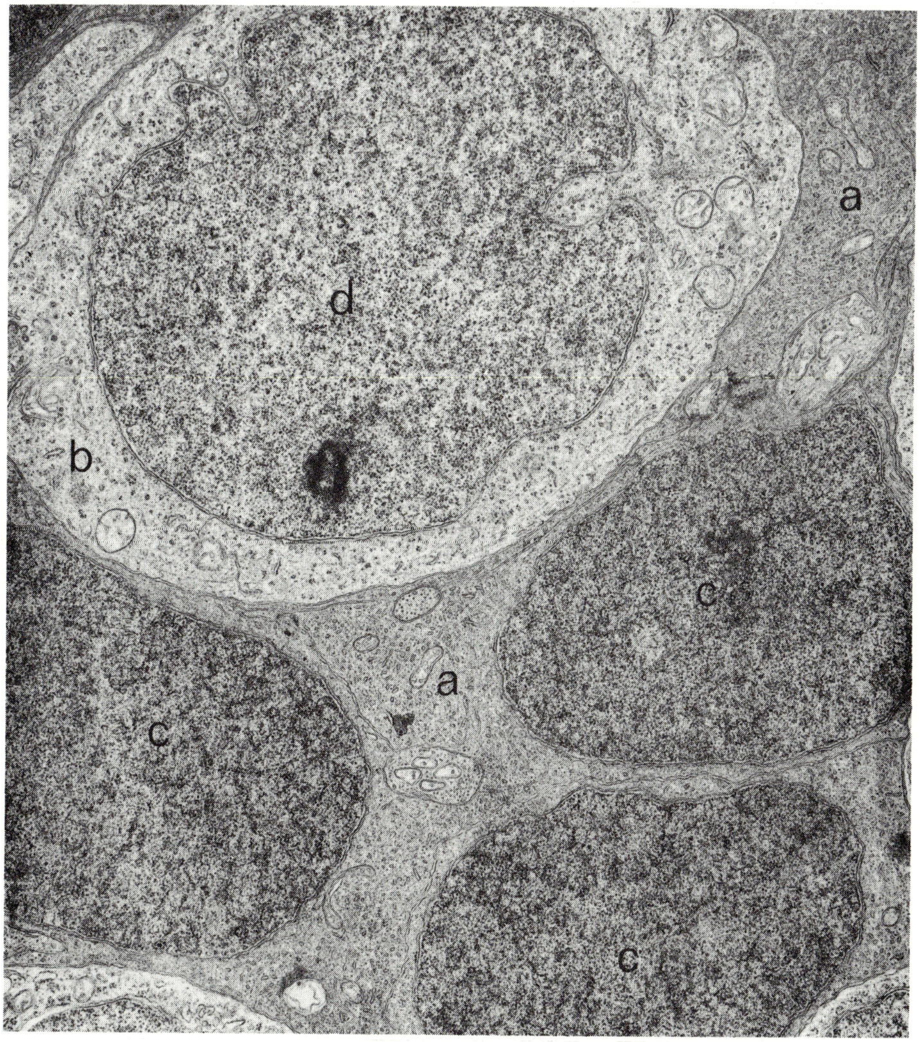

Figure 9–59. A Müller cell perikaryon (a) and an adjacent amacrine cell (b). The nuclei of the Müller cells are at (c), and an amacrine cell nucleus is at (d). (× 8000.)

It is formed of vesicles of irregular size and shape distributed in the cytoplasm; they may appear empty or contain a finely granular material. Glycogen granules measuring 250 to 300 A. in diameter are widely distributed in the cytoplasm, frequently lying on the cytoplasmic fibrils. Ribosomes also are abundant in the cytoplasm and are either free or associated with endoplasmic reticulum. Mitochondria are scattered and are of the usual type, with transverse cristae. Müller cells are often wrapped many times around the processes in the nuclear and plexiform layers. Thin strips of cytoplasm are present between each layer of wrapping, however, so that fusion of the cell membranes into a myelin-type sheath does not occur (Fig. 9-60). In the retinal layers that contain blood vessels, Müller cell processes surround large areas of the capillary walls. Arterioles and venules and, to a considerable extent, some of the surface area of large vessels are also surrounded by Müller cell extensions. A basement membrane is always found under those portions of the Müller cell cytoplasm which cover the vessel wall. The

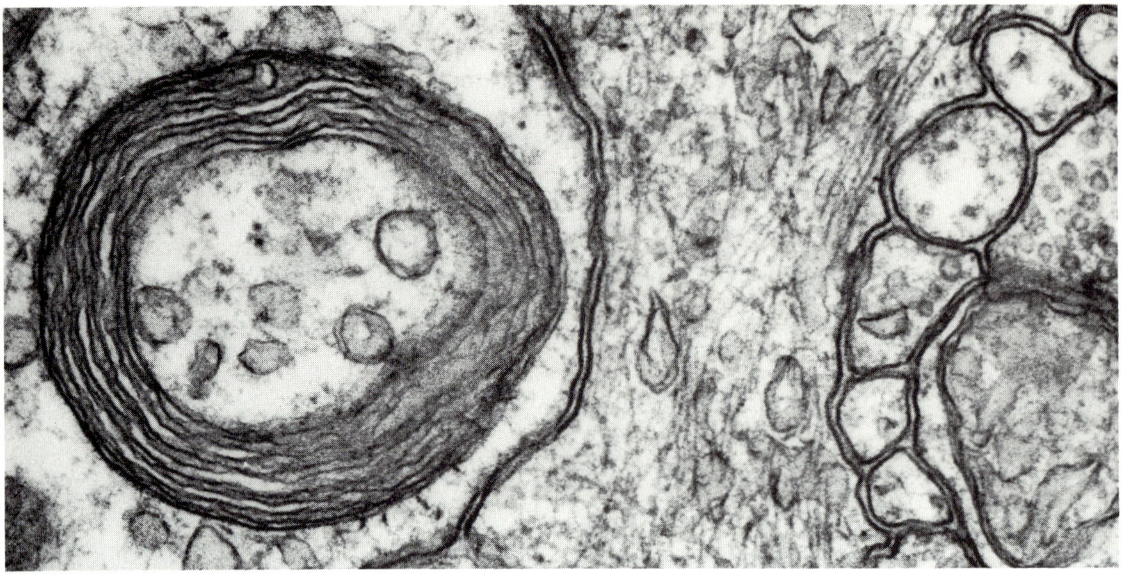

Figure 9–60. Müller cell process forming wrappings around a bipolar cell process. (× 60,000.)

basement membranes of the perivascular Müller cells merge with the adventitial ground substance of the vessel walls without leaving a perivascular space. Smaller vessels, which lack an adventitia, show fusion of the Müller cell basement membrane with that of the adjacent smooth muscle cells, pericytes or endothelial cells.

Because of the close contact of the Müller cells with the other retinal cells, it is evident that there is little extracellular space in the retina. Intercellular attachments are common between adjacent Müller cell membranes as the branches approach the inner limiting membrane.

The *inner sublayer* of the inner nuclear layer contains almost all the cell bodies and primary processes of the amacrine cells. Toward the fovea it gradually thins out, and it is completely absent in the foveal center. The amacrine cells form an important part of the inner plexiform layer, their processes intermingling and synapsing with the bipolar and ganglion cells. They have long processes which radiate out in all directions from the cell body into the inner plexiform layer and along the inner nuclear layer.

Using light microscopic techniques on human retina, Boycott and Dowling (1969) recently proposed the following classification:

Stratified Amacrine Cells (Fig. 9–61)

Unistratified Amacrine Cells. There are two types of unistratified amacrine cells. The first is smaller and sends processes to the external half of the internal plexiform layer; the branches cover a field about 100 to 200 μm. in diameter. The second is larger and possesses three main processes, which lie at the junction of the internal nuclear layer with the internal plexiform layer. The diameter of spread of these processes probably measures up to 1 μm.

Bistratified Amacrine Cells. The processes of these cells divide in a plane immediately adjacent to the internal nuclear layer, where they spread out over a field of about 100 μm. in diameter. Their fine processes extend

AMACRINE CELLS

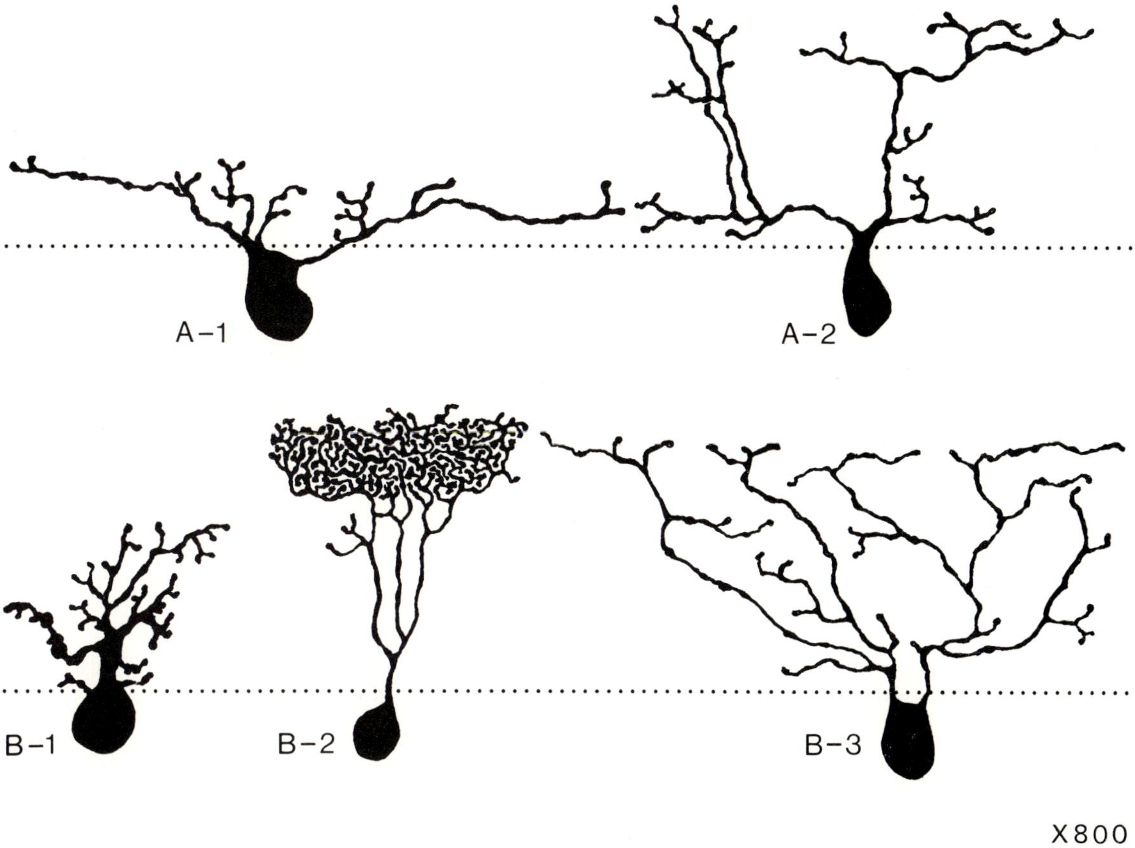

Figure 9–61. Drawings of the various types of amacrine cells. Unistratified amacrine cell (A-1), bistratified (A-2), narrow-field diffuse amacrine cells (B-1), stratified diffuse (B-2) and wide-field diffuse amacrine cell (B-3).

through the internal plexiform layer to the ganglion cell layer, where they branch frequently.

Diffuse Amacrine Cells (Fig. 9-61)

Narrow Field Diffuse Amacrine Cells. These probably correspond to Polyak's "knotty amacrine." Their tufted expansions extend more horizontally, with a large number of branches throughout the whole thickness of the inner plexiform layer, the field of each cell being rather narrow. They make contacts with the unistratified ganglion cells (probably Polyak's small diffuse ganglion cells).

Stratified Diffuse Amacrine Cells. These cells resemble the narrow field diffuse amacrine cells, and their branches are found only in the outer middle or inner thirds of the internal plexiform layer.

Wide Field Diffuse Amacrine Cells. These cells possess several branches which cross unbranched through the internal plexiform layer and run parallel to the ganglion cell layer for up to 500 μm., branching loosely near the perikarya of the ganglion cells.

Centrifugal bipolar cells (Polyak's "i-type" cells), which have been included classically among the amacrine cells, were not found by Boycott and Dowling. They are now believed to represent developmental stages of different amacrine cells.

With the electron microscope amacrine cells are characterized by an indented nucleus with dispersed nucleoplasm (Figs. 9-62 and 9-63). Their perikarya can be recognized easily along the inner margin of the inner nuclear layer, and they are larger than those of the bipolar cells because of their more abundant cytoplasm. The cytoplasm of the perikaryon contains many cisternae of rough-surfaced endoplasmic reticulum, free ribosomes, a well developed Golgi apparatus, profiles of smooth-surfaced endoplasmic reticulum and scattered microtubules. Isolated cilia are a common finding in these cells. Occasionally crystalline structures can be seen in the cytoplasm. As yet it has not been possible to identify with the electron microscope the subtypes described by Boycott and Dowling.

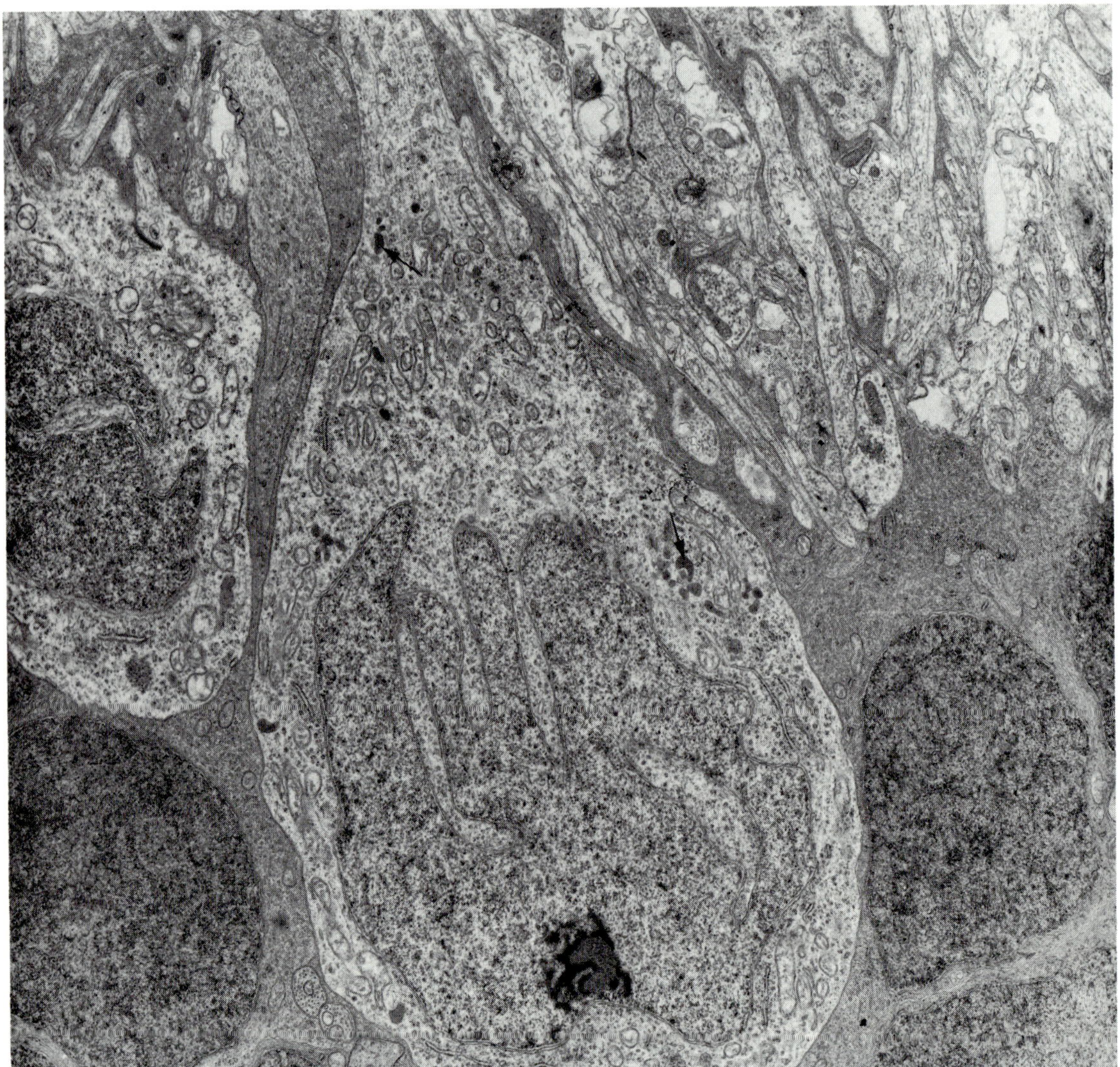

Figure 9–62. An amacrine cell. The nucleus is indented and shows a distinct nucleolus. The cytoplasm is less dense than that in the processes of the surrounding neural cells. Electron-dense bodies (arrows) are scattered through the cytoplasm. (× 5000.)

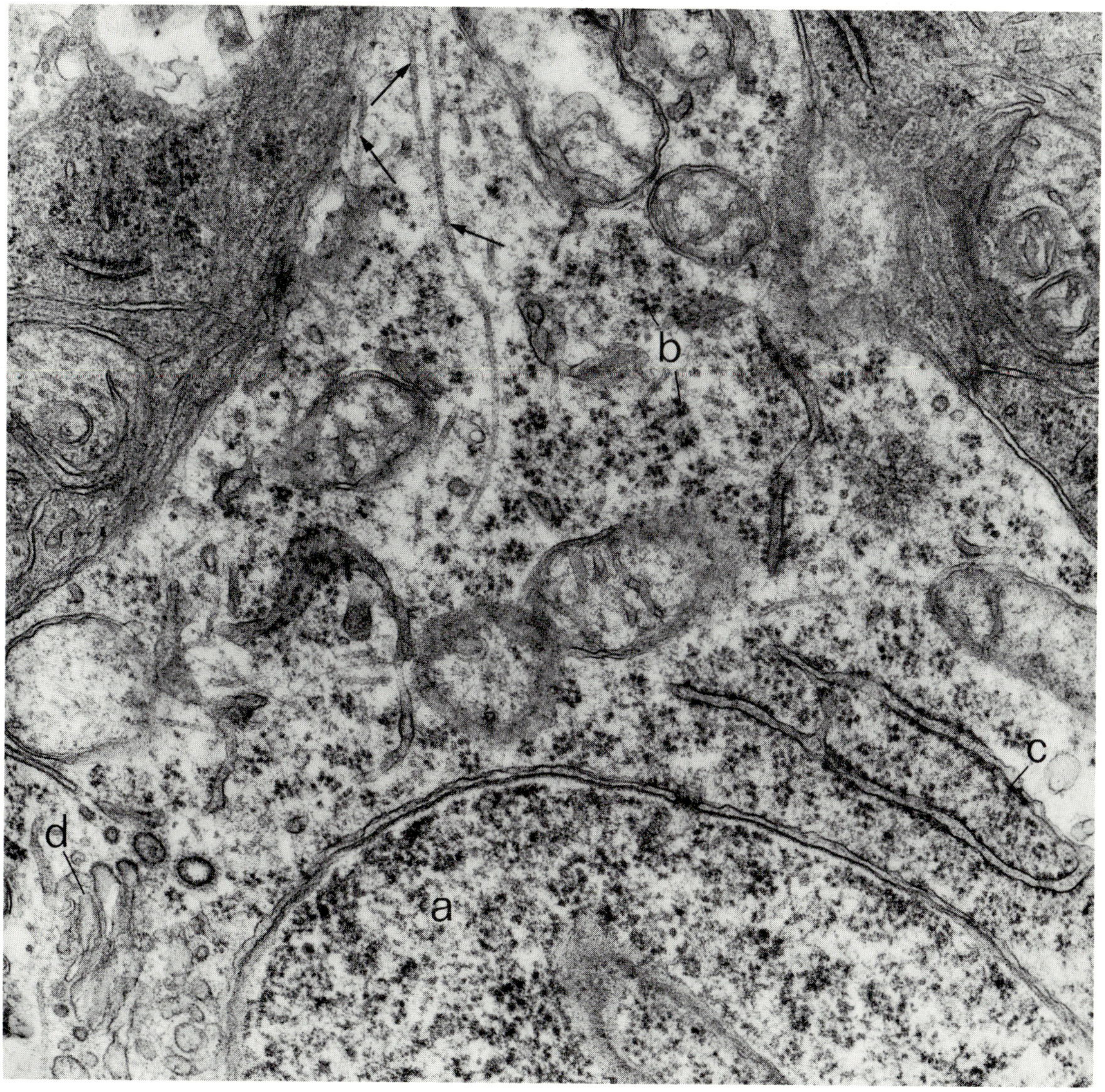

Figure 9–63. The perikaryon of an amacrine cell. The nucleus is at (a) and there are numerous free ribosomes (b). Rough-surfaced endoplasmic reticulum is seen at (c) and the Golgi apparatus is at (d). Neurotubules extend into the process (arrows). (× 35,000.)

Internal Plexiform Layer

The internal plexiform layer marks the junction between the first order and second order (cerebral) neuron of the retina (Figs. 9-64 to 9-68). It is formed by the many processes of the cells of the inner nuclear and ganglion cell layers and is the site of synapses between the *bipolar, amacrine* and *ganglion* cells. Nuclei occasionally seen in this layer are mostly displaced ganglion or amacrine cells. The remaining space is filled by the processes of Müller cells, leaving only the extracellular space, which has a maximum width of 200 A., between the cell membranes. Rare astroglial cells found in this layer are distinguished by clumped cytoplasmic filaments, vesicular endoplasmic reticulum, a few mitochondria and clusters of ribo-

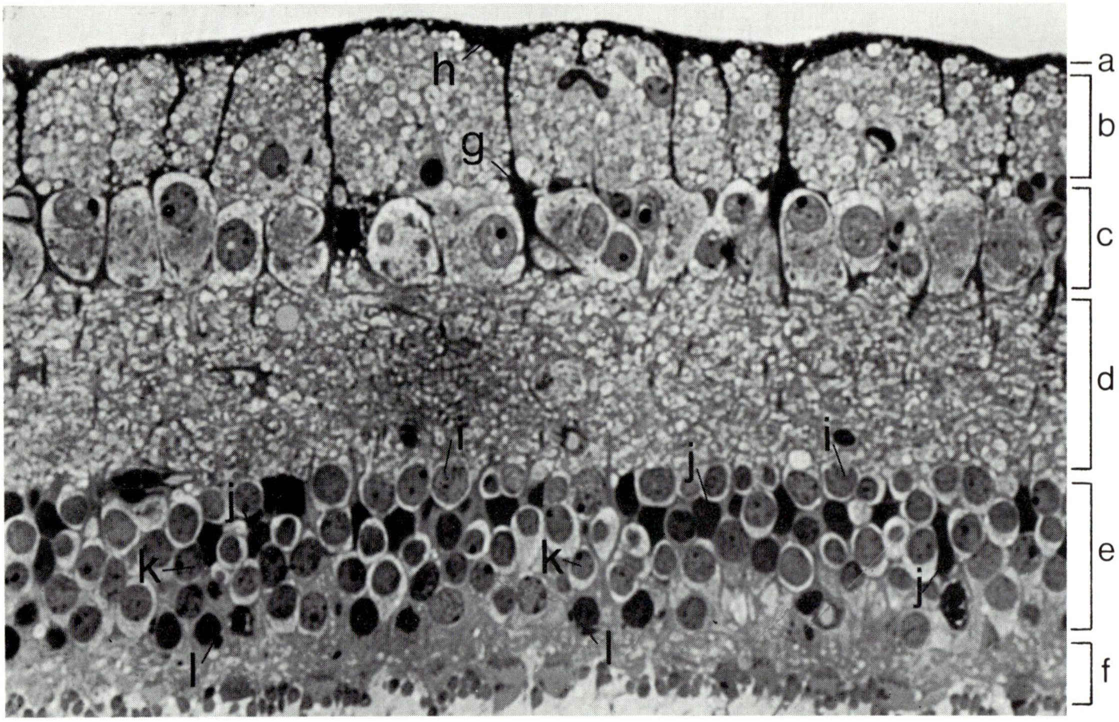

Figure 9–64. A light micrograph of the inner retina. The internal limiting membrane (a), nerve fiber layer (b), ganglion cell layer (c), internal plexiform layer (d), internal nuclear layer (e), and external plexiform layer (f) are seen. The radial fibers (g) and the umbrelliform terminations (h) of the Müller cells are seen. Amacrine cell nuclei are seen at (i), Müller cell nuclei at (j), bipolar nuclei are at (k), and horizontal cell nuclei are at (l). (× 160.)

somes. This layer, particularly the amacrine cell processes, contains a considerable amount of acetylcholinesterase, which is considered to be important in neurotransmission (Nichols and Koelle, 1967).

The internal plexiform layer varies in thickness between 18 and 36 μm., but it is quite uniform in many parts of the retina, especially on the nasal side of the eye. It is absent in the middle of the fovea. This layer has a finely reticular appearance and a faint horizontal striping, revealing the principal course taken by the nerve processes in this layer. Capillaries form a network here and are continuous with those of the inner nuclear layer.

Only a few electron microscopic studies have been made of the internal plexiform layer (Missotten, 1960; Kidd, 1962; Fine, 1963; Cohen, 1965; Dowling and Boycott, 1966; Allen, 1969). It is difficult to unravel the complex arrangement of the branches that participate in the formation of this layer. In addition to the glial cells, three morphologically distinct types of processes corresponding to the *bipolar, amacrine* and *ganglion* cells can be identified with the electron microscope. With the light microscope and silver staining, several subtypes of each of these cells and their processes can be distinguished, but so far it has not been possible to distinguish these subtypes with the electron microscope.

Bipolar Axons. These have a rounded appearance, the cytoplasm containing numerous neurotubules, neurofilaments and, occasionally, mitochondria oriented parallel to the course of the axon (Fig. 9-66). The synaptic

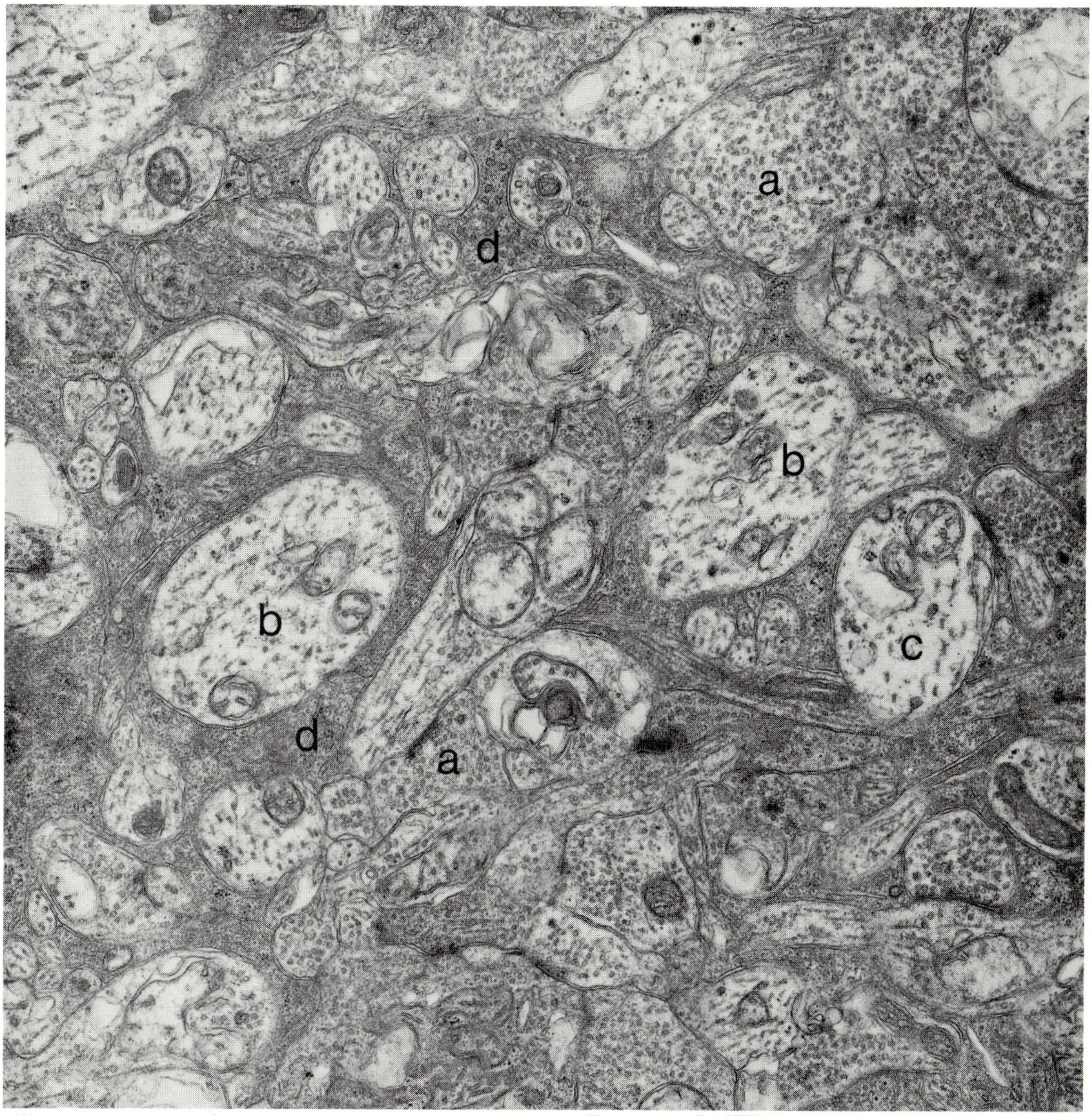

Figure 9–65. Electron micrograph of the internal plexiform layer. Bipolar axons (a), amacrine processes (b) and a ganglion cell process (c) are shown. Müller cell processes are seen at (d). (× 15,000.)

terminations of these processes are found throughout the inner plexiform layer as large, bag-like structures containing numerous evenly distributed synaptic vesicles, a few mitochondria and synaptic ribbons. Synaptic ribbons are found to occur *only* in the bipolar terminals; therefore, they provide reliable means of identifying the bipolar cell endings. They differ from the synaptic ribbons of the rods and cones in their smaller size and are usually surrounded by a halo of synaptic vesicles that are denser than those of the photoreceptor endings. Between some of the synaptic ribbons and the cell membrane is a semicircular area of increased density, the arciform density, which has been described previously in the rod and cone terminals. The

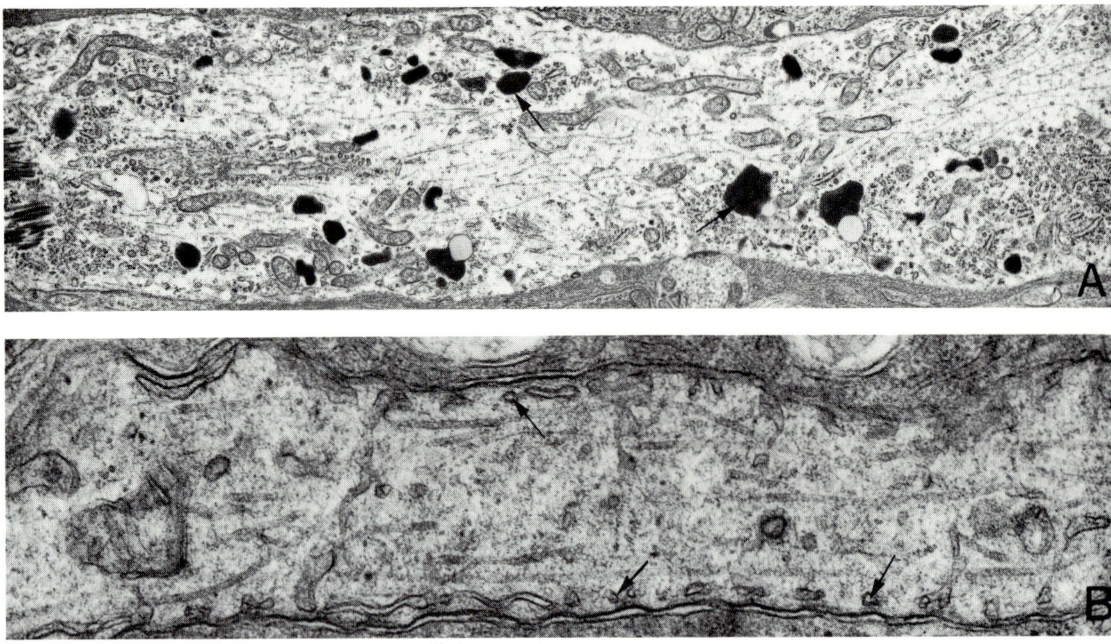

Figure 9–66. Electron micrographs of an amacrine process and a rod bipolar axon. *A*, An amacrine process contains mitochondria, neurotubules, some rough-surfaced endoplasmic reticulum, and a number of dense bodies (arrows). The cytoplasm is much less dense than that of the rod bipolar cell in B. (× 6000.)

B, A rod bipolar axon. The cytoplasm contains mitochondria, neurotubules and the helical organelle (arrows). (× 36,000.)

ribbons most often are positioned at right angles to the cell membrane at the terminal.

Amacrine Cell Processes. These processes, which have characteristics of both axons and dendrites, can be distinguished from the bipolar axons and ganglion cell dendrites by their relatively clear cytoplasm and uniform size along their entire length, their paucity of ribosomes and endoplasmic reticulum, and a large but variable amount of scattered synaptic vesicles, microtubules and mitochondria. Large vesicles, multivesicular bodies, some dense bodies and subsurface cisternae are also found. The ribosomes and the endoplasmic reticulum present are located near the soma. The amacrine endings do not contain synaptic ribbons. They show dense aggregations of synaptic vesicles at presumed sites of synaptic contact and this, along with otherwise unevenly scattered synaptic vesicles in a process containing few other cytoplasmic organelles, best characterizes an amacrine cell process.

Ganglion Cell Dendrites. These are difficult to identify, except in the central retina, where the dendrites that make synaptic contacts are thick and can be traced back to the cell body. Most characteristic of these dendrites is their content of grouped ribosomes, which differentiates them from other processes. They also contain mitochondria and irregularly shaped vesicles. In the central retina the dendritic cytoplasm is identical to that in the ganglion cell soma, being characterized by grouped ribosomes, vesicular endoplasmic reticulum, mitochondria and granular structures surrounded by membranes which are similar to lysosomes. Some ganglion cells are often displaced into the internal plexiform layer or even into the adjacent inner nuclear layer. The displaced cells are like those of the ganglion cell layer in structure. A variety of synaptic contacts are formed by these cells in the internal plexiform layer (Fig. 9-67).

Bipolar Synapses

Axodendritic Contacts. These contacts are characterized by a synaptic ribbon in the bipolar ending, which faces two postsynaptic processes. There is thickening of the presynaptic and postsynaptic cell membranes, particularly the latter, in glutaraldehyde-fixed material. This type of synapse is called a "dyad" (Dowling and Boycott, 1966). The postsynaptic nerve fiber processes forming the dyads are found most often to be a ganglion cell dendrite and an amacrine cell process.

Axosomatic Contacts. *Bipolar Cell-Ganglion Cell Contacts.* This type of contact occurs between the bipolar axon and the ganglion cell soma outside the central area of the retina and is therefore presumed to be a rod bipolar synapse. No synaptic ribbons or vesicles appear at these axosomatic junctions. However, tight junctions of the zonula or macula occludens type are scattered along the areas of contact, suggesting that they are areas of impulse transmission.

Bipolar Cell-Amacrine Cell Contacts. These contacts are found between bipolar cell terminals and amacrine cell somata, with an occasional synaptic ribbon at the contact.

Amacrine Synapses. Amacrine cells do not have axons in the ordinary sense (Cajal, 1911), their uniform processes appearing to be both axonic and dendritic. Dowling and Boycott (1966) refer to the branches of these cells as processes, but for convenience they termed the synaptic contacts as "axoaxonic" or "axosomatic."

Axoaxonic Contacts. In addition to the previously described axodendritic contacts in the dyads, amacrine cells make numerous other contacts, primarily with bipolar cell terminals or axons. Their morphology is like that of other synapses in the central nervous system. There are aggregations of synaptic vesicles along the presynaptic membrane, a slightly widened synaptic cleft, and some membrane thickening along the presynaptic and postsynaptic surface. There is no synaptic ribbon. In the dyad synapses there is an occasional synaptic contact by the amacrine process back onto the bipolar terminal within about 0.5 to 1.0 μm. of its postsynaptic relationship in the dyad, a so-called reciprocal synapse.

Axodendritic Contacts. Occasional amacrine processes that contact ganglion cell dendrites have synapses similar to axoaxonic contacts.

Axosomatic Contacts. Amacrine processes also contact ganglion cell somata; they are similar to axoaxonic contacts.

To emphasize the complexity of the intercellular contacts in the inner plexiform layer, Dowling and Boycott (1966) made montages of sections of the retina in the parafoveal region. The greatest number of contacts in both montages were the dyads and the axoaxonic amacrine-bipolar synapses (Fig. 9-68). These authors calculated that the total number of synapses in the inner plexiform layer in the parafoveal retina would be approximately 2,100,000 contacts per sq. mm. Because the amacrine processes spread widely throughout the inner plexiform layer for up to 0.5 to 1.0 mm., a much greater spread than that of the bipolar cells, it seems likely that amacrine cells contact more than one bipolar cell.

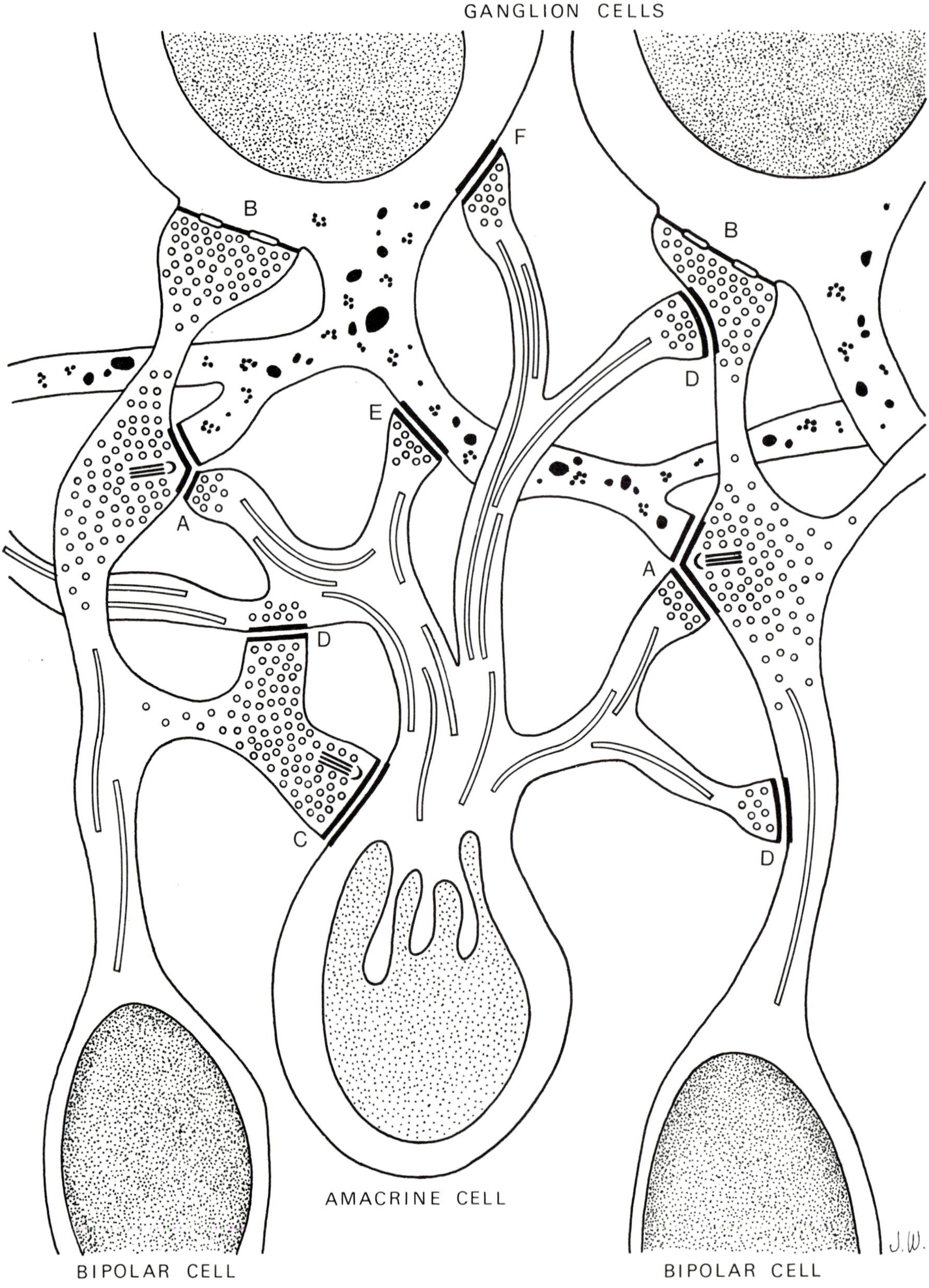

Figure 9–67. *See legend on opposite page.*

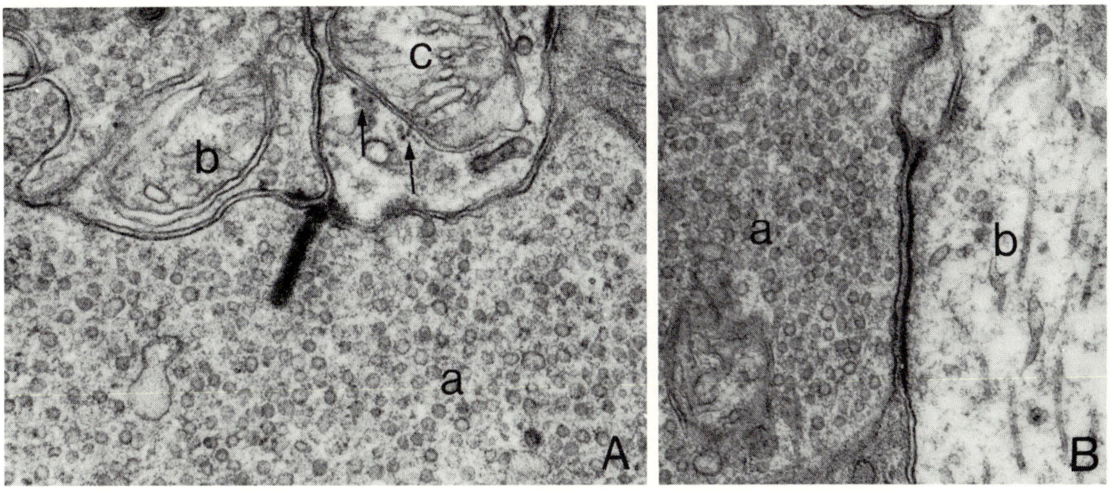

Figure 9–68. The main synapses in the internal plexiform layer. *A*, Dyad (a) is a bipolar axon containing numerous synaptic vesicles and a synaptic ribbon. An amacrine cell process is at (b), and (c) is a ganglion cell dendrite with clusters of ribosomes in its cytoplasm (arrows). (× 40,000.)

B, An axoaxonic synapse between a bipolar axon (a) and an amacrine cell process (b) showing an electron density along the synaptic membranes.(× 36,000.)

Ganglion Cell Layer

This layer contains the cell bodies of the second retinal (cerebral) neuron, the ganglion cells (Figs. 9-64, 9-69 and 9-70). It has a general thickness of 10 to 20 μm. in the nasal retina and increases in thickness to 60 to 80 μm. in the macular region. The cells are closely spaced in the posterior eye, but the distance between cells becomes greater toward the retinal periphery. Throughout most of the retina the ganglion cells form a single row, but on the temporal side of the disc they form two layers. In the macular region the cells increase to eight to 10 layers, and they diminish in number toward the fovea, where they disappear entirely.

The ganglion cell bodies vary in size and are generally rounded. Some are quite large, with a diameter of 25 to 30 μm., and a clear round or slightly oval nucleus 10 μm. in diameter with a prominent nucleolus. Most of the cells are smaller, however, measuring 12 μm. in size and having a nucleus of 8 to 9 μm. in diameter. Only the smaller cells are found in the macular region. These nerve cells vary in size and resemble those of the central system.

The ganglion cells are multipolar, with dendrites extending laterally as well as into the inner plexiform layer. Their axons, which do not branch

---

Figure 9–67. Schematic drawing of the synaptic contacts between bipolar, amacrine and ganglion cells in the internal plexiform layer. *A*, *B* and *C* depict bipolar axonic endings: *A*, Axodendritic endings at a dyad; *B*, Axosomatic ending on a ganglion cell; *C*, A bipolar axon-amacrine soma contact. *D*, *E* and *F* represent amacrine cell contacts with the other cells: *D*, An axoaxonic contact between bipolar and amacrine cell processes; *E*, An axodendritic contact between an amacrine and a ganglion cell; *F*, An axosomatic contact between an amacrine cell process and the soma of a ganglion cell. (Modified from Dowling, J. E. and Boycott, B. B.: Proc. Roy. Soc. London (Biol.) *166*:80, 1966.)

and vary considerably in size, run internally and then become parallel to the inner surface of the retina. Here they form the nerve fiber layer and later the optic nerve fibers. The large axons arise from large ganglion cells and the smaller ones from small ganglion cells. The ganglion cell cytoplasm is fibrillar and contains Nissl granules, which are rounded or irregularly shaped areas of increased density in the cytoplasm. They stain prominently with basic dyes and extend into the dendrites but not into the axon. Müller cells and neuroglial cells that insinuate themselves between and around the ganglion cells can be recognized in this layer; their characteristics will be discussed in the section on the nerve fiber layer.

Boycott and Dowling (1969) amplified the original work of Cajal (1911) and Polyak (1941) and distinguished the following types of ganglion cells (Fig. 9-69).

Monosynaptic Ganglion Cells

Midget Ganglion Cells. These cells are the most common ganglion cells in the central retina and are believed to represent cone ganglion cells (Fig. 9-69). They are characterized by a single dendrite, which extends straight and unbranched into the inner plexiform layer; its tip forms a few short branches that embrace the terminals of a midget bipolar cell. The branching of the midget ganglion cells tends to be either in the inner or outer third of the inner plexiform layer. As illustrated in Figure 9-54, there is some difference in the shape of the midget bipolar cells in the central compared to the peripheral zones of the retina. The diameter of the dendrites of the midget ganglion cells varies, those with a narrower diameter being nearer the fovea. Even in the periphery, however, the diameter of the dendrite of a midget ganglion cell is rarely wider than 10 μm. The axonal terminals of the midget bipolar cells and the dendritic terminals of the midget ganglion cells come into virtually exclusive contact with each other. With the electron microscope a large number of axodendritic contacts can be seen between midget bipolar endings and the dendrites of midget ganglion cells. These synapses are usually paired with another process, mostly that of an amacrine cell, thus forming the so-called "dyad."

The frequent appearance of midget bipolar axonal endings in the close embrace of midget ganglion cell dendrities, especially in the foveal area, shows that many midget ganglion cells are connected to only one midget bipolar cell. Because the midget bipolar cell is in postsynaptic contact with only one cone and because of the synaptic relationship described previously, it is probable that a single midget ganglion cell could be specific for a single cone. This arrangement, however, does not mean that a single cone is only specific for a single ganglion cell for, as we have seen (p. 451, pedicles), every cone is connected to at least one flat bipolar cell (possibly more), as well as to at least one midget bipolar cell. Amacrine contacts of these units through the dyads and the reciprocal contacts furnish interconnections to other fields throughout the retina.

As yet it has not been possible to determine whether other types of bipolar cells synapse with the midget ganglion cell or if midget bipolar cells synapse with other kinds of ganglion cells. The sharp change in visual acuity beyond the fovea suggests that midget bipolar and midget ganglion cells have wider connections the further they are from the fovea.

Polysynaptic Ganglion Cells. These cells increase from the center toward the periphery of the retina (Fig. 9-69).

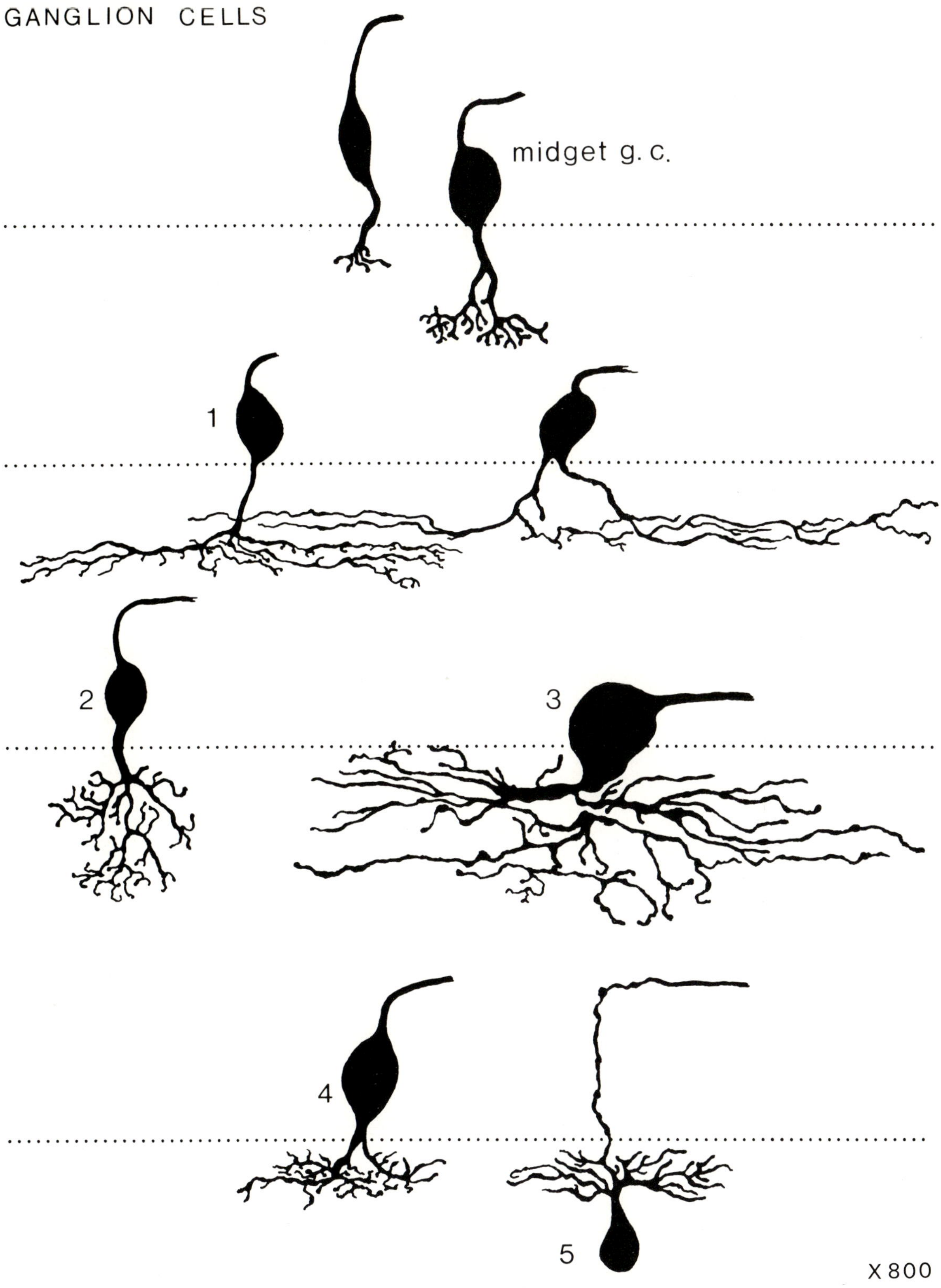

Figure 9–69. Drawings of the various types of ganglion cells in the human retina. They are numbered according to the description in the text. A midget ganglion cell is shown at the top. Unistratified (1), diffuse (2), large diffuse (3), stratified diffuse (4), and displaced ganglion cell (5).

Unistratified Ganglion Cells. Two different kinds of unistratified ganglion cells can be distinguished; the dendrites of both types branch in a plane. The first type of cell is most numerous in the central part of the retina and corresponds to Polyak's "small diffuse" ganglion cells. The smooth, long and thin dendrites of these cells mainly branch, mostly near the inner nuclear layer, whereas the spiny dendrites of the second type, which Polyak termed "garland" ganglion cells, spread near the ganglion cell layer. They divide into a small number of rather thin but very long secondary fibers, which have additional branches. These dendrites are the largest of all the ganglion cell varieties, spreading out for great distances and making contact with hundreds of bipolar cells. The exact plane of branching probably differs for individual cells of the same type; therefore, dendrites of unistratified ganglion cells may be found at any level of the inner plexiform layer.

Diffuse Ganglion Cells. These cells usually possess one thick dendrite arising from the perikaryon in the outer portion of the ganglion cell layer and branching at all levels of the inner plexiform layer (Fig. 9-69). The branches ascend and descend toward or away from the inner nuclear layer, and their tips are split into branches that end in fine terminals. The dendritic distribution is analogous to that of the narrow field amacrine cells. The perikarya have a diameter of 16 μm., whereas the dendritic fields increase from about 30 μm. to about 75 μm. in the periphery. According to Polyak (1941), the diffuse ganglion cells which correspond to his "shrub" type may be postsynaptic to all types of bipolar cells.

Large Diffuse (Giant) Ganglion Cells. The perikaryon of these cells is about 30 μm. in diameter, and the branches cross the inner plexiform layer in all directions (Fig. 9-69). The dendritic spread is approximately 250 to 300 μm. This type of ganglion cell is especially characteristic of the area surrounding the central portion of the retina.

Stratified Diffuse Ganglion Cells. The perikarya of these cells usually form the innermost row of the cells in the ganglion cell layer of the posterior retina (Fig. 9-69). They do not fit neatly into the classifications of stratified and diffuse cells that are commonly found. With the exception of the edge of the central area of the retina, where they may have several dendrites, these cells have a single dendrite of about 3 to 4 μm. in diameter. This dendrite goes directly to one of three levels in the internal plexiform layer, where it branches frequently. As with the diffuse stratified amacrine cells, these finer dendritic branches lie in a horizontal plane in the internal plexiform layer. Most often the branching occurs in the external third of this layer, but there is also some branching in its middle and internal thirds. Near the fovea the field diameter of the branches is 40 μm., and it increases to twice this size toward the retinal periphery.

Polyak (1941), who named these cells "parasol" ganglion cells for the flat-topped appearance of their branchings, supposed them to synapse with any type of bipolar except those of the rods.

Displaced Ganglion Cells. The perikarya of these cells have the characteristics of ganglion cells; they lie in the inner portion of the internal nuclear layer (Fig. 9-69). Their dendrites form a field of about 50 μm. in diameter. One of the dendrites bears a long unbranched process that is presumed to be an axon; it traverses the inner plexiform and ganglion cell layer into the nerve fiber layer. It is not known whether this axon goes on to the brain or whether it loops in the nerve fiber layer to re-enter the internal plexiform layer.

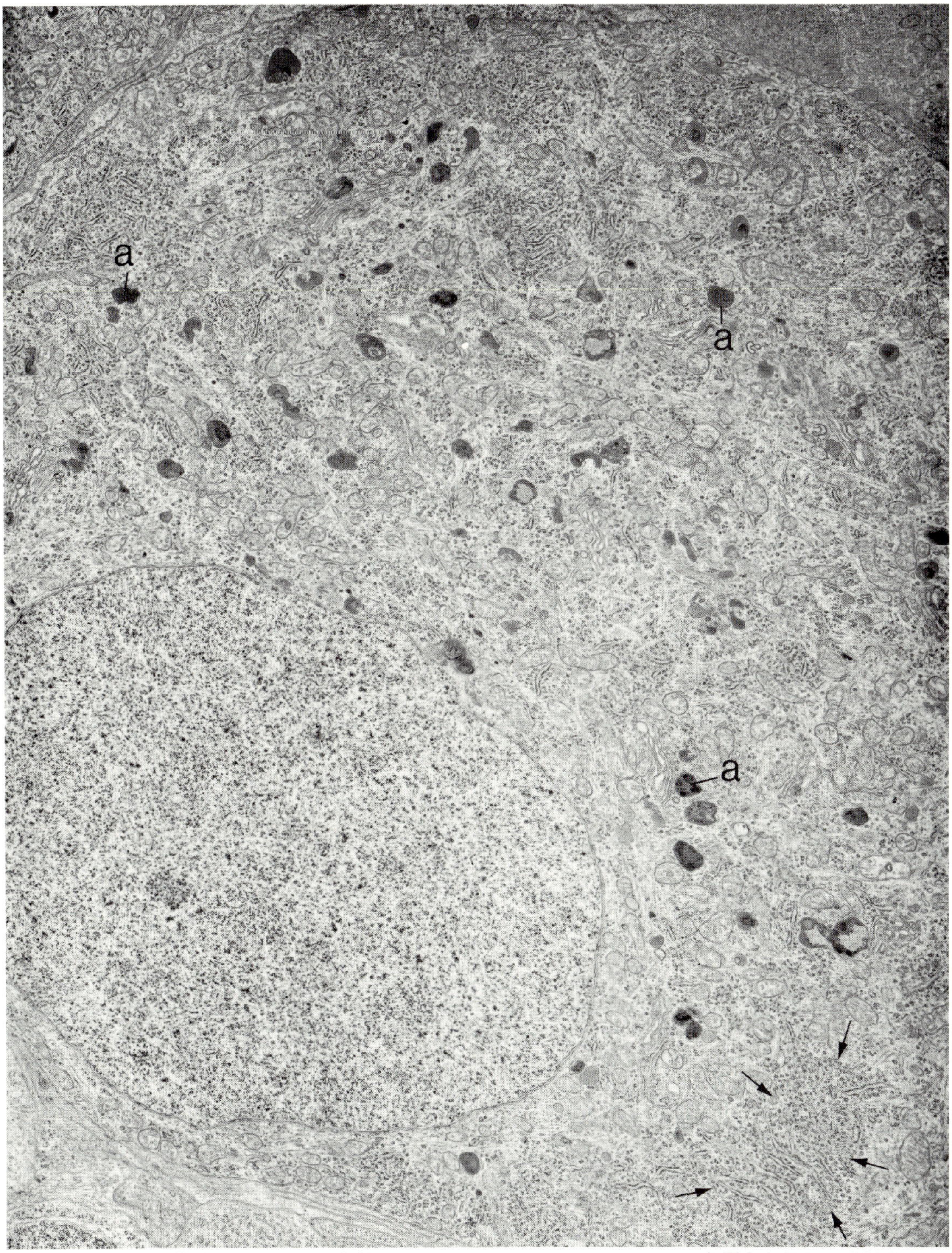

Figure 9–70. Electron micrograph of a retinal ganglion cell. Arrows point to rough-surfaced endoplasmic reticulum that forms the Nissl substance. Numerous dense bodies (a) are distributed in the cytoplasm. These are believed to produce the yellow color of the macula lutea. (× 5400.)

It is not possible by electron microscopy to differentiate the various types of ganglion cells that can be seen with the light microscope in silver-stained sections. The dendritic processes of these cells and their ultrastructural characteristics and connections have been discussed under the internal plexiform layer (p. 471). The ganglion cells of the retina have the same cell structure as those which have been studied elsewhere in the central nervous system (Fig. 9-70). They have an abundant cytoplasm in which there are large cluster-like aggregates of many short, randomly oriented cisternae of rough-surfaced endoplasmic reticulum. Under the light microscope these clusters are identical to the Nissl substance. This substance may be more abundant in the peripheral cytoplasm, but it can be distributed throughout the cell. Free ribosomes are also numerous in the cytoplasm, which contains much smooth-surfaced endoplasmic reticulum as well. Scattered mitochondria, a Golgi apparatus and many microtubules are randomly distributed in the cytoplasm, especially in that of the dendritic processes and axons. Delicate unoriented cytoplasmic filaments are also seen, and lipofuscin granules are found, particularly in older eyes. Other dense membrane-bound bodies measuring 0.25 to 0.50 μm. in diameter are seen as well. Fine (1963) proposed that the accumulation of dense bodies in the cytoplasm might account for the yellow color observed at the macula.

Nerve Fiber Layer

The nerve fiber layer is composed of the axons of the ganglion cells, which extend from all parts of the retina toward the optic disc to form the optic nerve (Figs. 9–71 to 9–73). (See also Fig. 10–8.) They are surrounded by glial cell and Müller cell processes. A well developed vascular system is a prominent feature of this layer. The neurons of the nerve fiber layer consist primarily of two types of fibers: *centripetal* (afferent) fibers, which carry impulses from the retinal ganglion cells to the brain; and *centrifugal* (efferent) fibers, which would transmit impulses from the brain to the retina. Their existence, however, is in doubt, even up to the present time. Dowling and Boycott (1966) recently stated that they were not able to identify fibers of this type in the human or primate retina or in other vertebrates, but that they could show them in the pigeon retina. Cajal (1911) originally described them, but Polyak (1941) expressed doubt as to their existence. Wolter (1956, 1957a, 1965), Granit (1947), Dodt (1956), and Cowan and Powell (1963) all claimed to have demonstrated these fibers. Those who believe they exist insist that their nuclei are located in the brain, particularly in the region of the nucleus isthmo-opticus (Mukai, 1970). The axons of these cells have been described as having endings in the internal plexiform layer or in the innermost part of the inner nuclear layer. They are believed to have close connections to the amacrine cells and to the walls of capillaries, since some of these fibers may have vasomotor functions.

The nerve fiber layer is thickest around the optic nerve entrance, where it measures about 20 to 30 μm. thick. Its thickness diminishes in the peripheral retina, and in the extreme periphery the nerve fiber and ganglion cell layers blend into a single layer. The axons from the retinal ganglion cells are arranged in a direction that is radial to the optic nerve entrance. The axons from the nasal retinal ganglion cells maintain this radial direction throughout their course, whereas those of the temporal retina are less direct; the ones arising from the retina, temporal to the fovea, arch above and below the macula to approach the disc at its upper and lower edges. The fibers which pass from the macula and retina between the disc and macula course directly toward the temporal disc as the *papillomacular bundle*. Because of the divergence of the temporal bundles toward the upper and lower disc, the thickness of the nerve fiber layer at the temporal edge of the disc is reduced to about 10 μm. (Fig. 10–8).

The nerve axons from the retinal ganglion cells are grouped into bundles. They are surrounded by astroglial and Müller cell processes, which most often form branches that enclose individual axons. The diameters of the nerve fibers vary widely according to the ganglion cells from which they come. Occasionally disc-like or globe-shaped nervous end-bulbs are seen along the fibers; their significance is unknown.

Ultrastructurally the axons of the nerve fiber layer are unmyelinated and have a variable size when viewed in cross-section, the variation being between 0.6 and 2.0 μm. (Figs. 9-71 and 9-72) (Villegas, 1964). Only occasionally are small myelinated fibers seen. The cytoplasm contains many fine fibrils, microtubules, mitochondria and disoriented vesicles of smooth endoplasmic reticulum. The axons more often are separated by strips of glia or

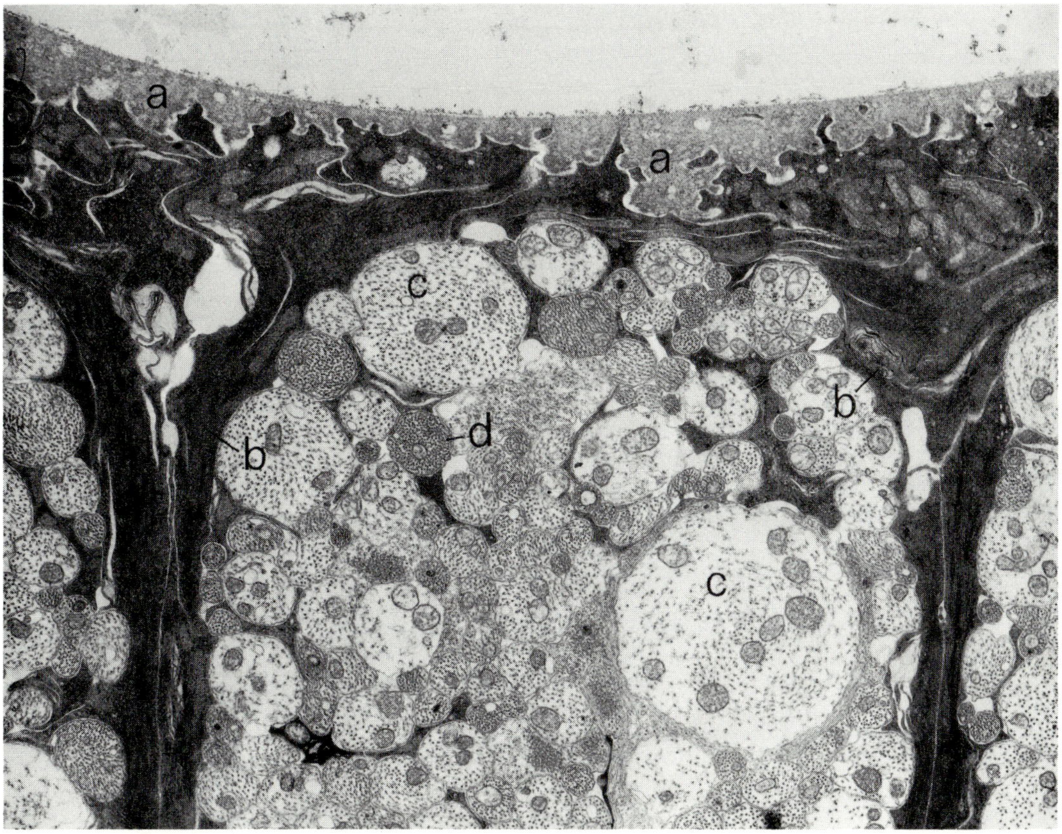

Figure 9–71. Nerve fiber layer of the retina. The inner limiting membrane (a) is lined by fine particles that represent sections of vitreous collagen filaments. Two Müller cells (b) partly form the inner limiting membrane. Their radial fibers enclose bundles of nerves. Axons in the nerve fiber layer are large (c), while others are small (d). (× 4000.)

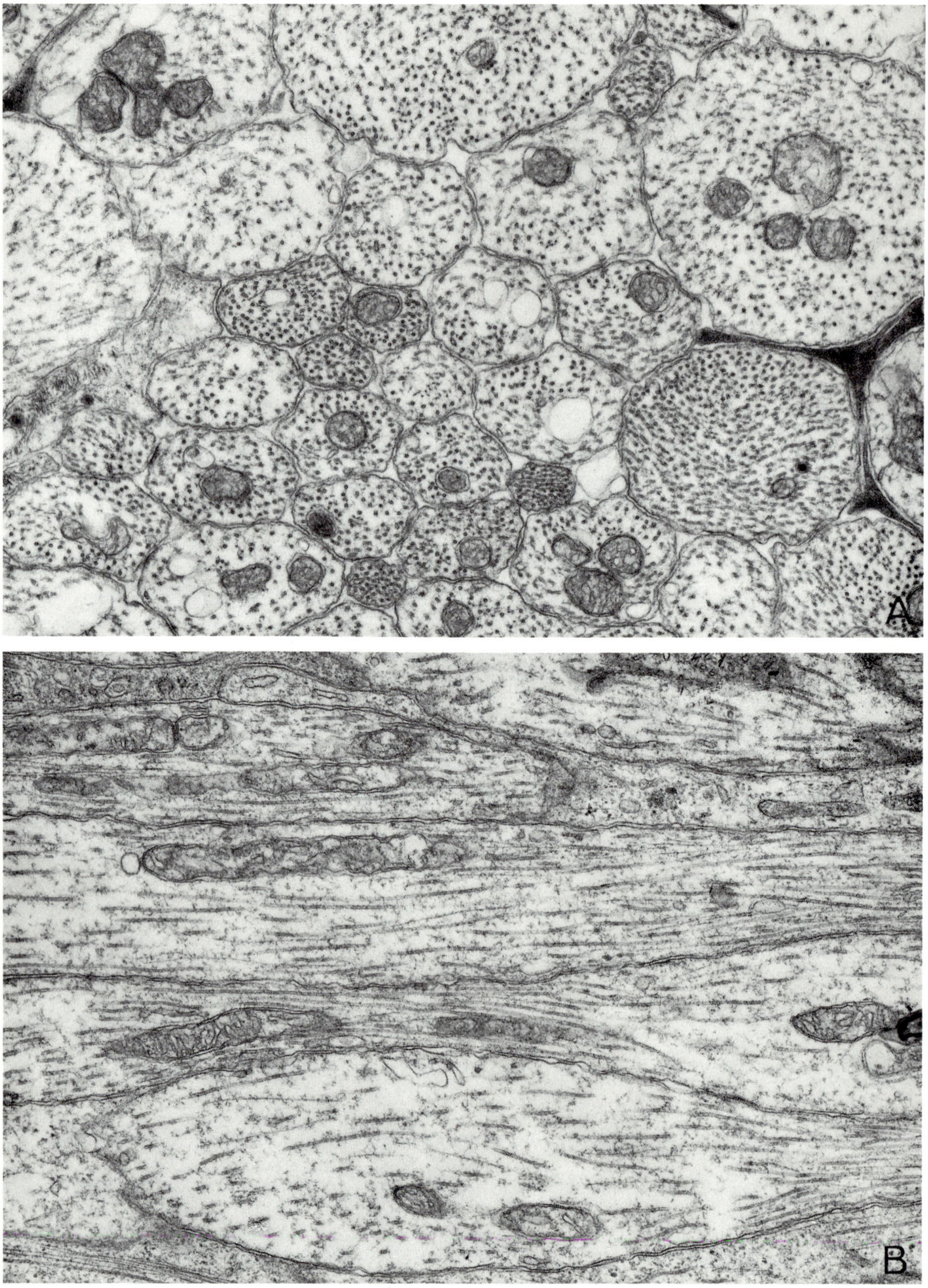

Figure 9–72. Sections of retinal nerve fiber layer axons. *A*, A cross-section of an axon that shows numerous neurotubules. (× 15,000.)

B, A longitudinal section showing both mitochondria and neurotubules. (× 24,000.)

Müller cells. Not all axons are surrounded by glial tissue, however, and in some bundles many of the axons are close to each other without intervening glial tissue (Fig. 9-72). The cell membranes of some axons are joined to each other by junctions. The neurofibrils are seen most easily in longitudinal sections which show periodic enlargements that are probably the result of adjustment of the axon to its surrounding or to a change in its course. Near the inner limiting membrane, the nerve fibers are separated from the membrane by branching portions of the Müller cells and by occasional glial processes.

Retinal Glia. With silver stains the glial cells (astrocytes) and their processes can be demonstrated easily (Figs. 9-74 to 9-76). The astrocytes are star-shaped cells with flattened oval nuclei; they lie in the nerve fiber layer, ganglion cell layer, inner plexiform layer, and, to a limited extent, the inner nuclear layer. Extensive studies have been made of the retinal glial cells to show their supportive and nutritive role for the retinal tissues. Their wide foot-processes lie close to the surfaces of blood vessels (Wolter, 1955 a and b;

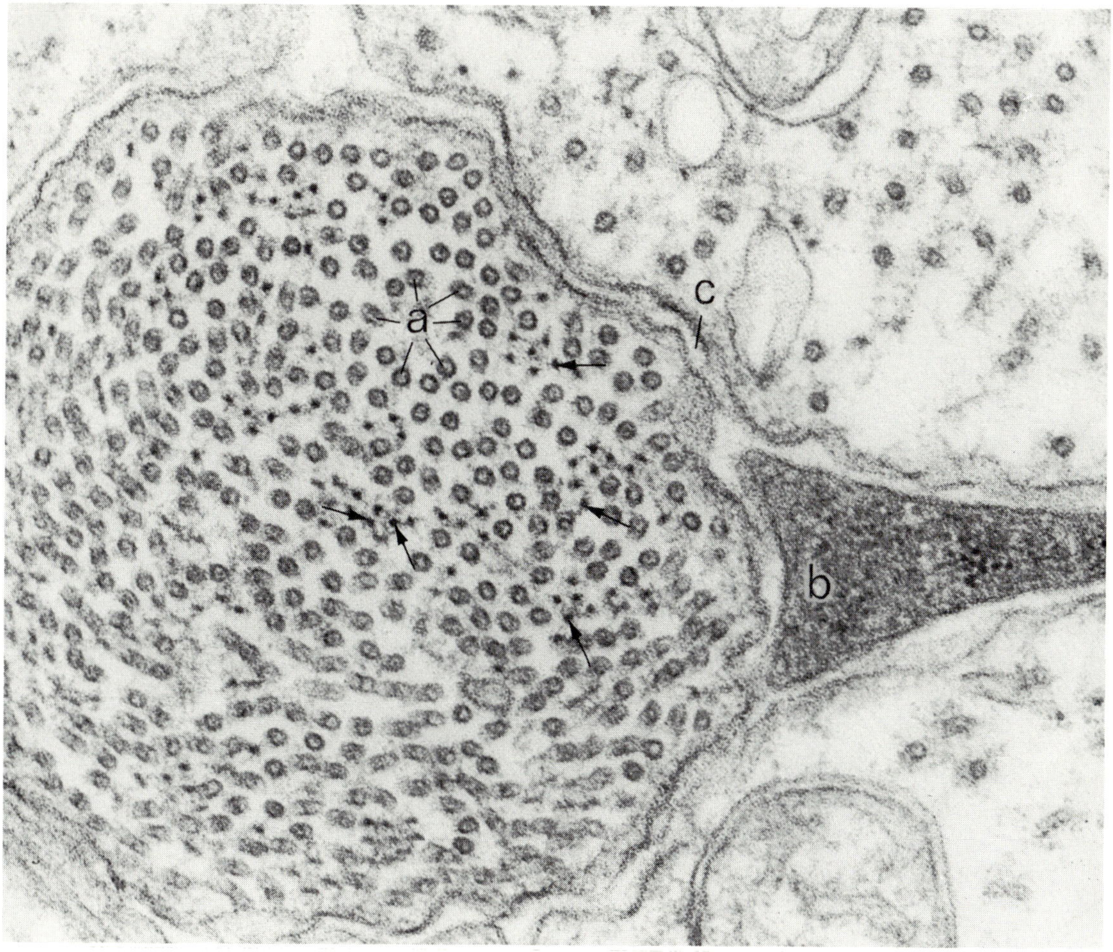

Figure 9–73. An axon in the nerve fiber layer shows cross-sections of neurotubules (a) and neurofilaments (arrows). A Müller cell process is at (b), and (c) is an intercellular space between two neurons that does not contain an interposed astrocyte process. (× 95,000.)

1957 a and b; 1959; 1961). The inner nuclear layer contains no glial cells of its own, but glial cell processes extend from the inner plexiform layer a short distance into its inner portion.

When studied with the light microscope the retinal glia has been subdivided into four types of cells: astrocytes, perivascular glia, Müller cells and microglia.

Astrocytes. Astrocytes have long, branching processes which form an irregular network in the inner retina around nerve cells and their processes, as well as sending branches to the blood vessels. Typical star-shaped astrocytes, like those of the central nervous system, are found in the ganglion cell and inner plexiform layers. Some of the astrocyte processes contact ganglion cells, while others lie close to the capillary surfaces.

In the nerve fiber layer, astrocytic cells most often are bipolar, and their axes generally are parallel to the courses of the axons. They have elongated nuclei and two long, straight processes; one process is oriented around the nerves, and the other meets the wall of a blood vessel. These bipolar astrocytes are identical to the co-called "elements of Remak" or "lemmocytes" in the central nervous system. Not all astrocytes in the nerve fiber layer are bipolar, however, and transition forms are common.

Perivascular Glia. The second system of specialized glial cells found in the retina is the perivascular glia, originally described by Liss (1956; 1958) in the olfactory bulb and the neurohypophysis. They were later identified in the retina by Wolter (1959). These glial cells are found around the retinal capillaries. The cell body is star-shaped and has many long processes that wind around the walls of the blood vessel, but there are few extensions around the adjacent retinal nerve fibers. These cells probably have an insu-

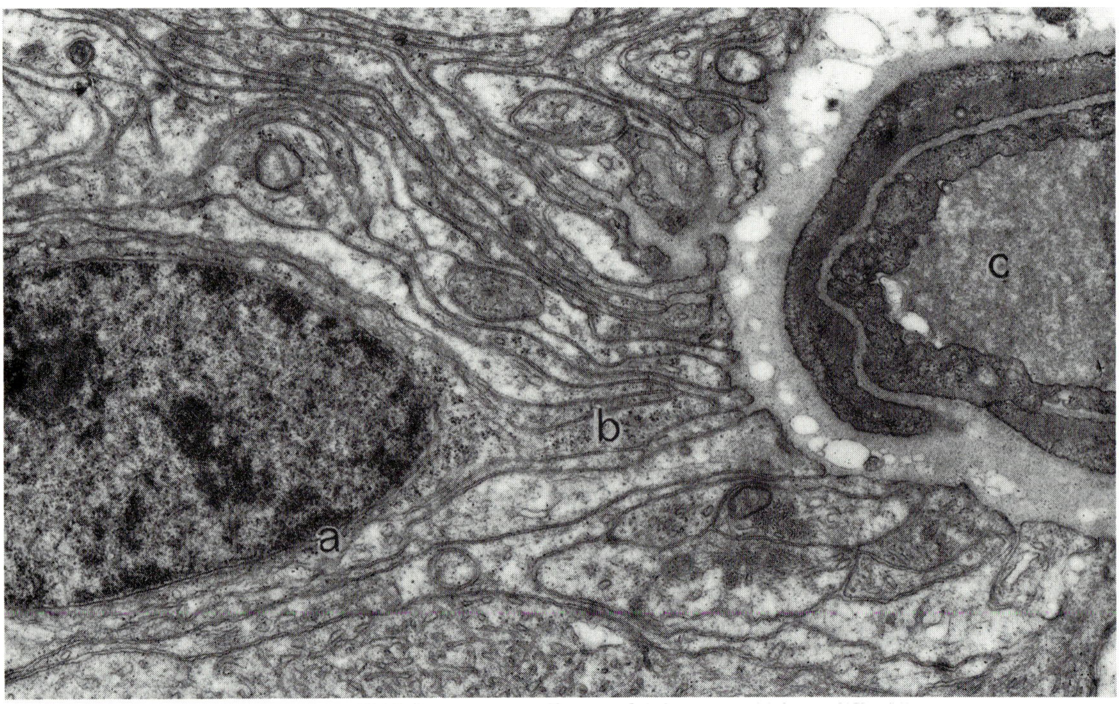

Figure 9–74. Retinal glial cells. An astrocyte (a) and its processes (b) that contact a capillary (c). (× 12,000.)

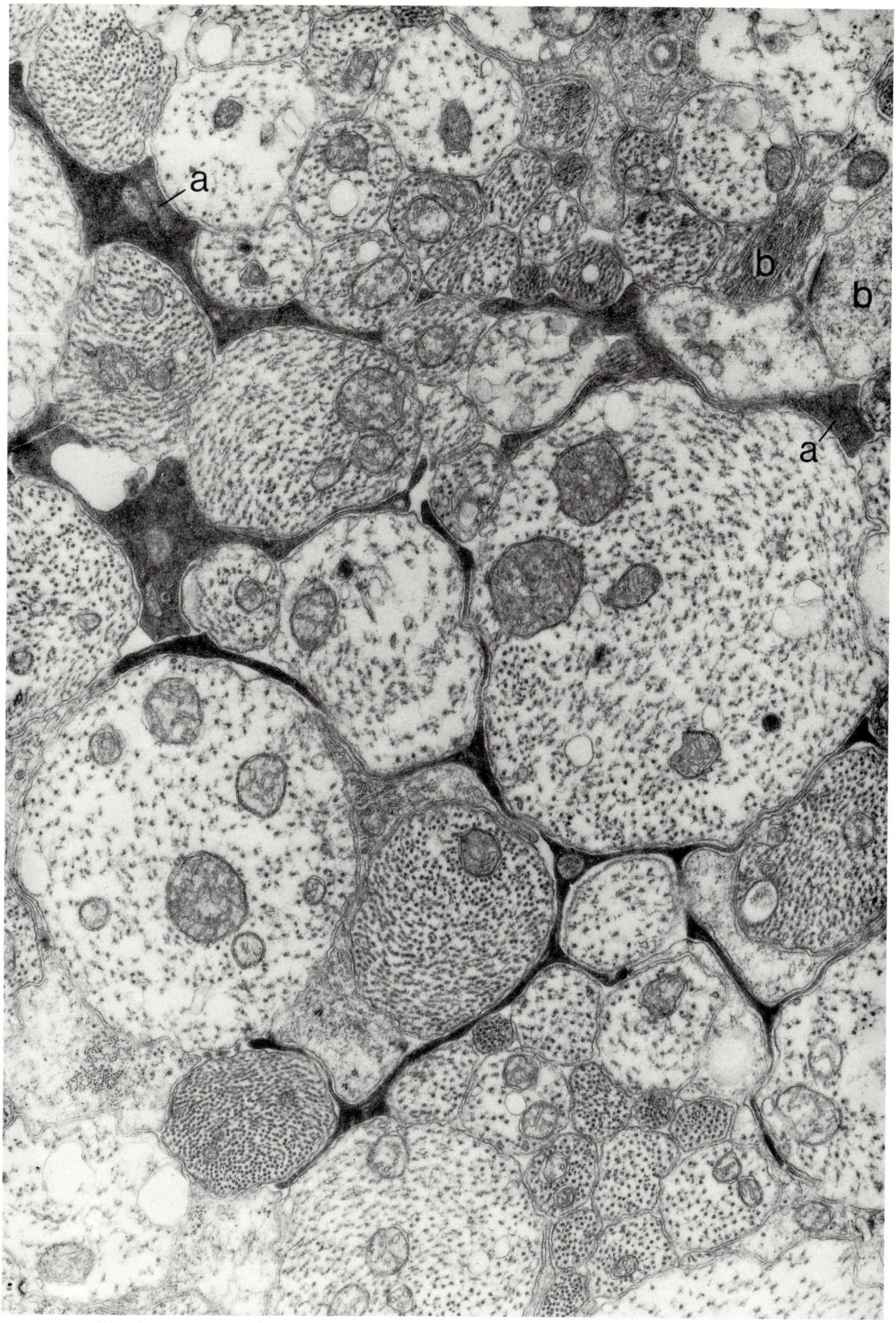

Figure 9–75. Nerve fiber layer showing Müller cell (a) and astrocyte processes (b). (× 12,000.)

lating action because they fill out the spaces not occupied by astrocytic sucker feet and Müller cells.

Müller Cells. These have been discussed previously (p. 461).

Reticuloendothelial Microglial Cells. These cells are found in the inner retina, especially in the nerve fiber layer. They are not numerous and are identical to the wandering phagocytes that are found in all tissues.

Several astrocyte types have been described by electron microscopy, but it is probable that they represent variations in the shape of the astrocyte to conform to the disposition of the surrounding tissues. They are found most often in the inner part of the internal plexiform layer in relation with the blood vessels of the retina. They are also found in relation to the nerve cells and their processes.

Astrocytes have an oval nucleus containing much heterochromatin (Figs. 9-74 and 9-75). The relatively clear cytoplasm contains mitochondria, cisternae of rough-surfaced endoplasmic reticulum, some profiles of smooth-surfaced endoplasmic reticulum and clusters of free ribosomes. There are numerous fine fibrils, which are more pronounced in the many slender, irregularly shaped processes. These processes extend for varying distances to the walls of the blood vessels, where they form blunt terminations. Other processes invest the neurons, particularly in the nerve fiber layer.

By electron microscopy the *perivascular glial cells* are fairly typical astrocytes and they have no distinctive ultrastructural characteristics.

Those glial cells facing the external surface of a blood vessel have a basement membrane. A few astrocytes often lie under the inner limiting membrane of the retina, occasionally sending processes to it. In such instances they contribute to the structure of this membrane.

INNER LIMITING MEMBRANE

For many years before and after the studies of Salzmann (1912) were published, there was disagreement as to the existence of an inner limiting membrane in the retina. Some observers believed that there was no such structure but that the so-called "membrana hyaloidea," the limiting membrane of the vitreous also served as a limiting membrane of the retina. Others believed that there was a definite limitans interna in the retina and that a hyaloid membrane did not exist. Salzmann handled the situation nicely by stating, "In any case, one must say that this membrane has just as much relation to the vitreous as it has to the retina, and that it looks like the inner glass membrane of the retina in one preparation and like the outer border membrane of the vitreous in another." He actually preferred the name "membrana limitans interna," because of the presence of an analogous membrane over the inner surface of the ciliary epithelium.

The classic light microscopic concept of the structure of the inner retinal limiting membrane is that it is formed by the terminations of the conical branching processes of the Müller cells. Polyak (1941), for example, endorsed the view that the internal limiting membrane is formed by the Müller cells. Wolff (1968) demonstrated that the branching processes of the Müller cells were inserted into, but did not actually form, the membrane. He observed that with the Mallory triple stain the internal limiting membrane was deep blue like collagen, while the processes of Müller cells stained red like neuroglia.

Some recent light and electron microscopic studies have shown that a membrane measuring 1 to 2 μm. in thickness does exist on the inner surface of the retina (Pedler, 1961; Fine, 1961; Gärtner, 1962; Matsuo and Kitajima, 1961; Hogan, 1963). It is PAS-positive, and its external surface is irregular because of the branching basal processes of the Müller cells, which cover irregular polygonal fields (Fig. 9-76). It continues uninterrupted over the fovea and is gradually lost at the optic disc edge.

By electron microscopy the Müller and some glial cell processes comprise the inner cellular termination of the retina proper, their vitreal surfaces exhibiting a basement membrane that averages 0.5 μm. in thickness (Figs. 9-76 and 9-77). It has a moderate electron density and a fine filamentous character. Over the retina the basement membrane is smooth on the vitreal side, whereas on the retinal side it is undulating because it follows the Müller cell contours. This membrane, which thickens with age, is located either close to the cell membrane of the Müller cells or is separated from it by a narrow space containing a "cement" substance. Vitreous collagen fibrils and amorphous material are seen to merge with this basement membrane and to contribute to its thickness. Oblique sections show these vitreous collagen fibrils to penetrate about half the thickness of the membrane but not to pass the space between basement membrane and adjacent cell membranes. The actual union between the vitreous gel, its fibrils and the basement membrane is probably at a structural level below the resolution of the electron microscope, that is, at a chemical bond level.

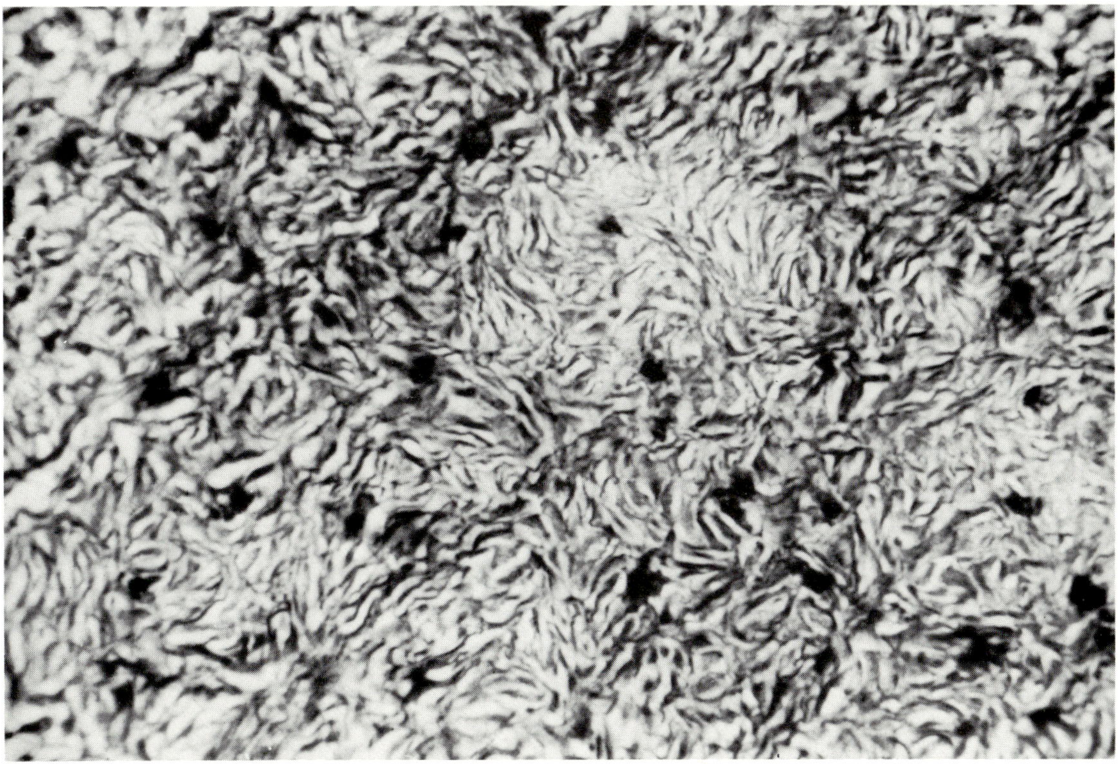

Figure 9–76. A flat section through the inner limiting membrane that depicts the arborizing processes of the Müller cells. (× 900.)

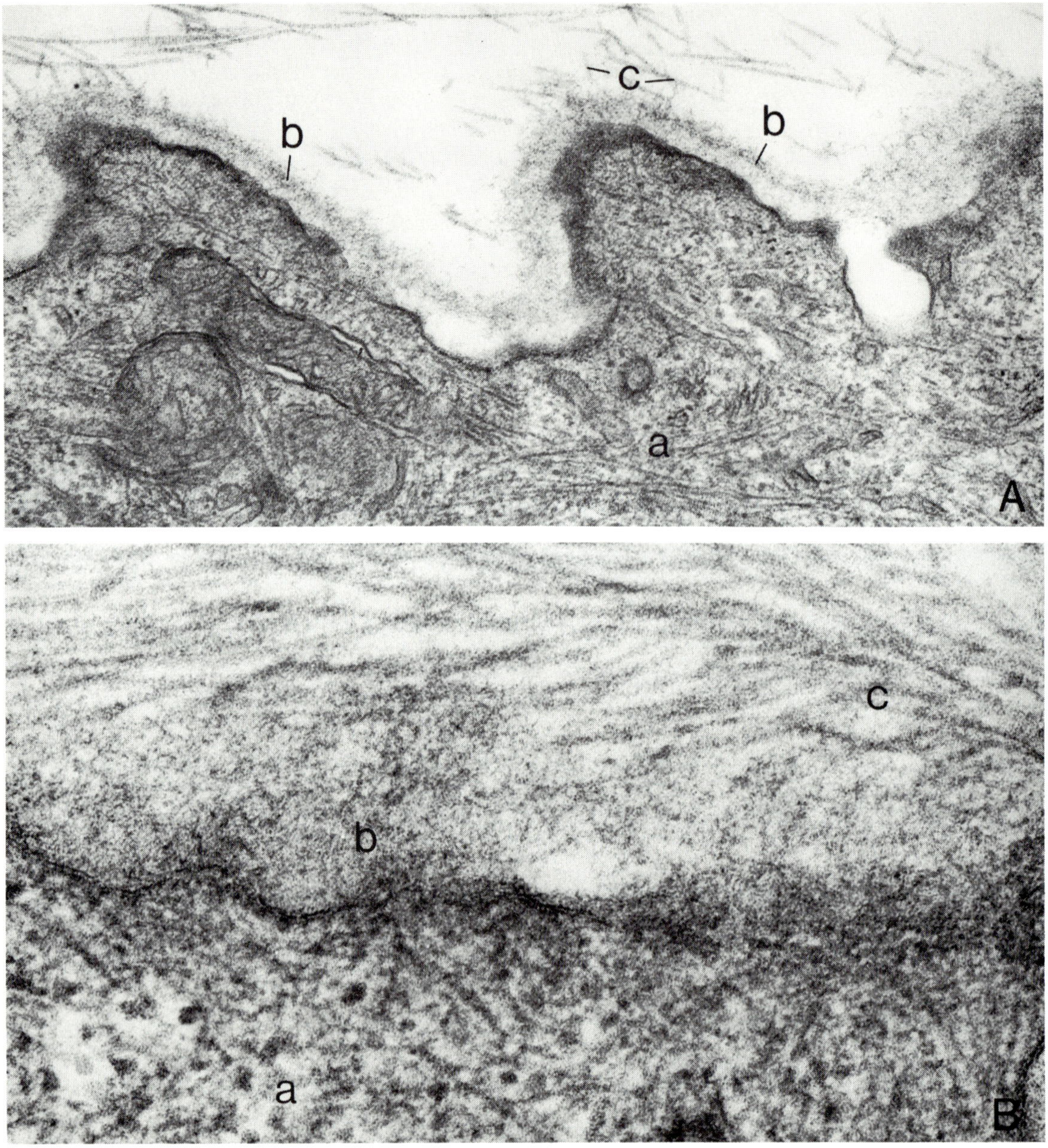

Figure 9–77. Inner limiting membrane of the retina. *A*, Equatorial retina. The Müller cell (a) has a rather well defined basement membrane (b) that is continuous with vitreous fibrils (c). (× 48,000.)

B, Peripheral retina. The Müller cell cytoplasm is at (a). The basement membrane (b) of these cells is closely related to the vitreous fibrils (c). (× 120,000.)

Wolff (1968) appears to have been correct about the nature of the inner limiting membrane. The basement membranes of the Müller and glial cells form the principal part of the membrane, which stains like glia. The remainder of the inner limiting membrane is formed by vitreous fibrils and mucopolysaccharide, which join with the basement membrane. Since the vitreous fibrils are collagenous, this portion stains blue with the Mallory stain.

THE MACULAR REGION

The central retina (area centralis), with a diameter of 5.5 mm., has rather specific histologic limits which are based on the number of rows of cells in the nuclear layers, as well as on the orientation of the fibers in the outer plexiform layer and the presence of cones alone in the receptor layer. The peripheral limit of the macula is at the site where the ganglion cells are reduced to a single layer (Fig. 9-78). The ophthalmoscopic and gross anatomic limits of this central area are less clearly defined.

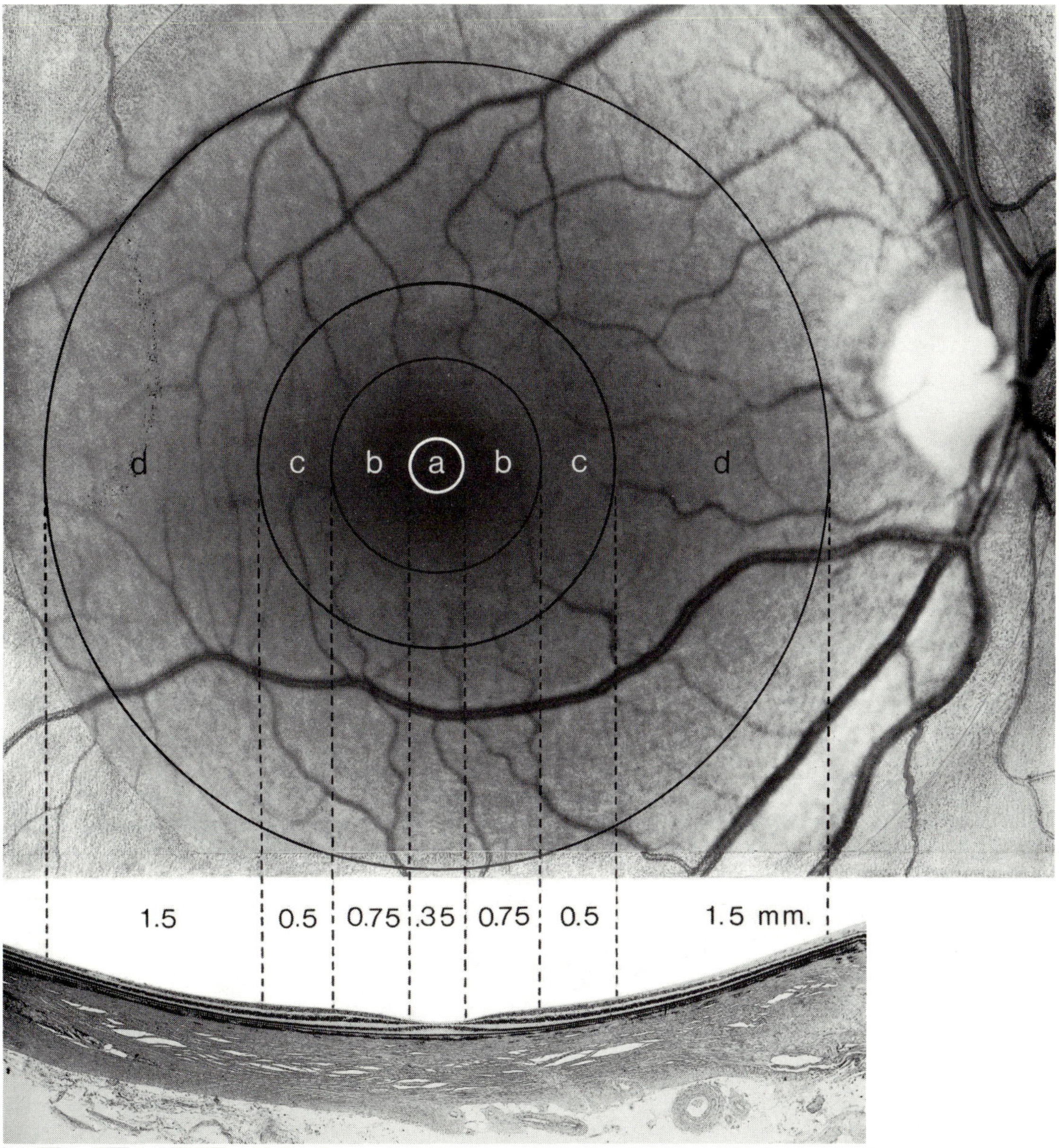

Figure 9-78. This fundus photograph is matched with a meridional light micrograph of the macular region. The fundus photograph shows the foveola (a), fovea (b), parafoveal area (c) and perifoveal region (d).

The macular area is subdivided into the following portions (Figs. 9-79 to 9-84): (1) fovea, (2) parafovea, and (3) perifovea.

Fovea

The central fovea (fovea centralis) is a small depression or excavation in the internal or vitreal surface of the retina. Its center is located 4.0 mm. temporal and 0.8 mm. inferior to the center of the optic disc. The floor of the fovea is slightly curved, and its center contains a concavity; this portion is known as the *clivus*. The entire fovea measures 1.5 mm. in diameter, and its floor is approximately 0.4 mm. wide. The foveola is 0.35 mm. across (Figs. 9-79 to 9-81). There is a variation in depth of the fovea, but on the average it is 0.25 mm. deep in the human eye. The fovea is about one half the thickness of the normal retina, which is about 0.37 mm. In the very center of the fovea the thickness of the retina is reduced to about 0.13 mm.

The photoreceptor layer of the foveal region is comprised entirely of cones. The thickness of this layer increases from the foveal periphery toward its center because of the progressive increase in length of the cones to about double that of the photoreceptors at the periphery. This increase in length causes the outer limiting membrane to be displaced vitreally, creating a curve in its contour, the external fovea (fovea externa), which has concavity facing the retinal pigment epithelium. The external fovea has a diameter about one third that of the inner central fovea. The increased length of the cones is associated with a diminished diameter, so that the cones are like elongated rods. The rods at the periphery of the central fovea also have this elongated form. The central rod-free area of the fovea measures about 0.57 mm. in diameter. In the human fovea the central cones are approximately 80

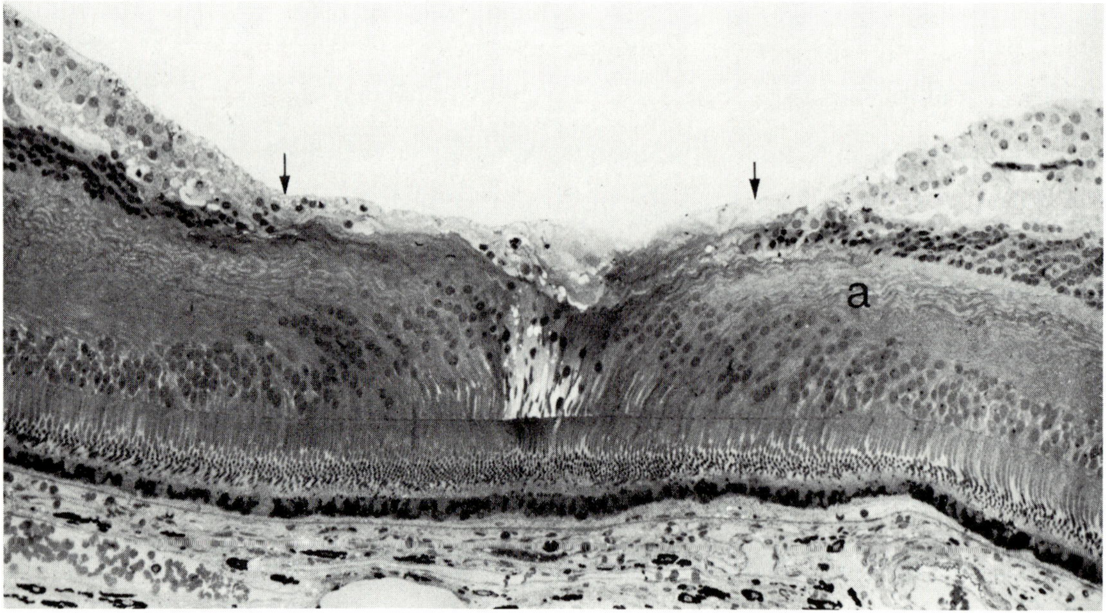

Figure 9–79. Light micrograph of the foveal region. The foveola is included in the area between the arrows. Only the photoreceptors, glial cells and Müller cells are present in this area. Henle's fiber layer is seen at (a). (× 85.)

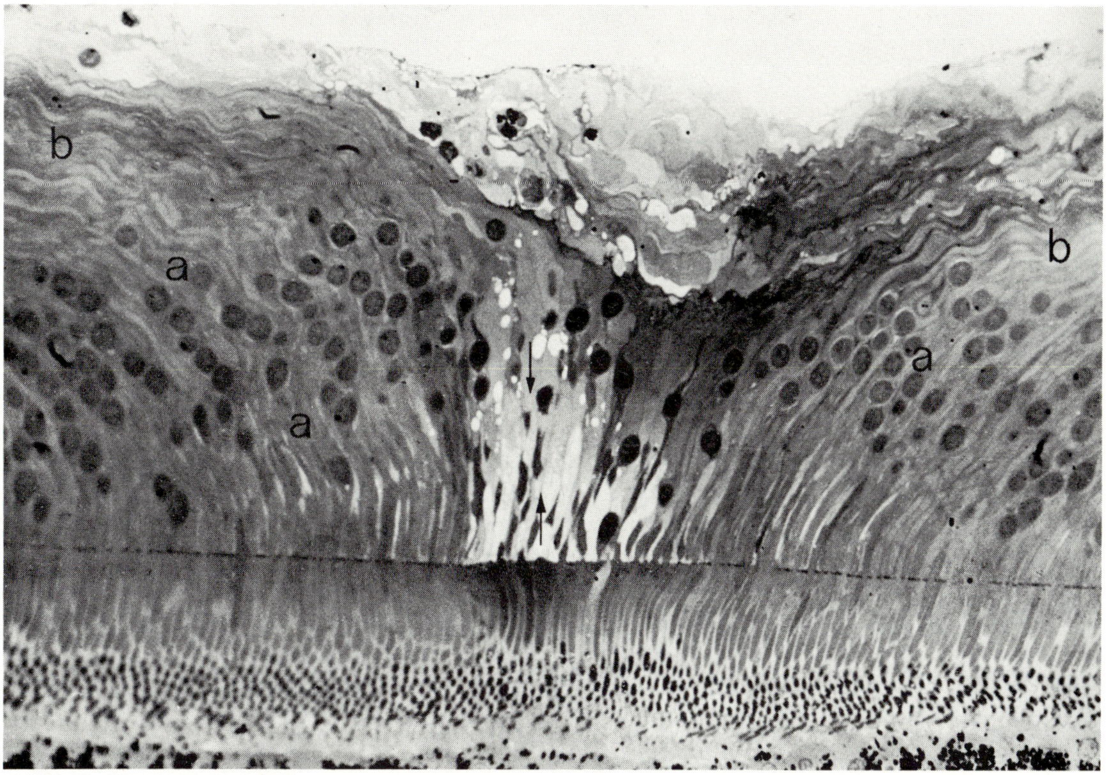

Figure 9–80. An enlargement of Figure 9–79 showing the details of the foveola. The nuclei of the photoreceptors are displaced internally (a), and the curving internal receptor fibers are seen at (b). The lighter cytoplasm of the Müller cells (arrow) is seen in the center of the fovea. (× 425.)

μm. long, and the inner segments are 3 μm. thick at the base and 2 μm. thick at the tip, with a length of 20 to 30 μm. The outer segments are 2 μm. in thickness by 45 μm. long (Yamada, 1969). Along the clivus the thickness of the inner segments increases. The mitochondria of the inner segments are widely dispersed in the cytoplasm, and the dense aggregation of mitochondria seen in the normal ellipsoid is lacking in the foveal region. The nucleus of these central cells is quite large, measuring 7 μm. in diameter. At the edge of the fovea the cone inner segments become 3.5 to 4.0 μm. thick, while the outer segments remain at 1.3 μm. Those rods approaching the outer fovea are approximately 1 μm. thick in their inner segments.

In the rod-free central fovea there are approximately 35,000 cones, and within the total foveal surface area of 1.75 sq. mm. there are approximately 100,000 cones. Within the central fovea the foveola contains 2500 closely packed cones. Meridional sections of this region show the cones to be perfectly straight and oriented vertically with respect to the retinal surface. Their axes are parallel to each other. Flat sections show them to form an evenly distributed mosaic, the inner segments being separated from each other by Müller cells. The cones here are 0.3 μm. apart. Electron microscopic study of a central foveal area measuring 50 μm. in diameter reveals only long, fine cone fibers, separated from each other by Müller cells (Fig. 9–81).

The outer nuclear layer is slightly thinner in the parafoveal region than in the rest of the retina. Along the foveal slope, the number of rows of nuclei increases to eight or 10, but these decrease again to two or three loosely arranged rows in the center of the fovea. The nuclei of this layer are

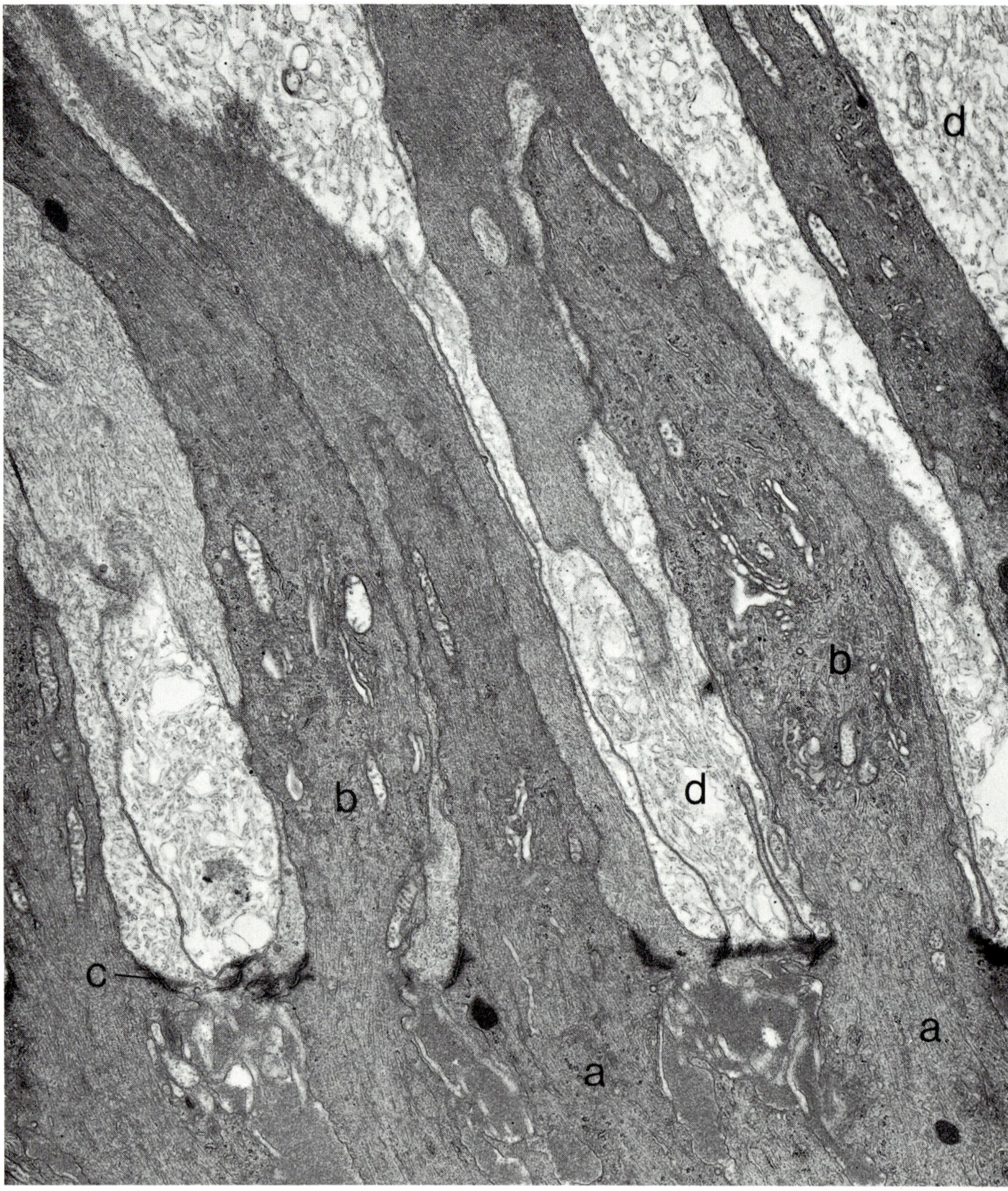

Figure 9–81. Center of the foveola. The myoids of the cones (a) are continuous with the outer cone fiber (b). The external limiting membrane is at (c). Müller cell processes (d) are interposed between the outer cone fibers. (× 6000.)

displaced away from the outer limiting membrane, so that they are closer to the inner limiting membrane. This displacement is the opposite of that seen along the slopes of the fovea, where the inner nuclear and ganglion cell layers are displaced somewhat toward the outer limiting membrane. The nuclei in this layer are typical of cone nuclei, but nuclei belonging to the Müller cells are also seen here on occasion. The nuclei of this layer are oriented in slanting columns, away from the central fovea.

The course of the fibers in the outer plexiform layer is almost parallel to the surface of the retina. In the foveolar area the external cone fibers have a meridional course, and the internal fibers make an almost right angle turn away from the foveola. The inner and outer fibers of the other foveal cones as well as the rod and fibers in the parafoveal and perifoveal regions pursue similar courses. The aggregate of all these horizontally oriented fibers produces *Henle's fiber layer* in the macular region (Figs. 9-82 to 9-84). All these

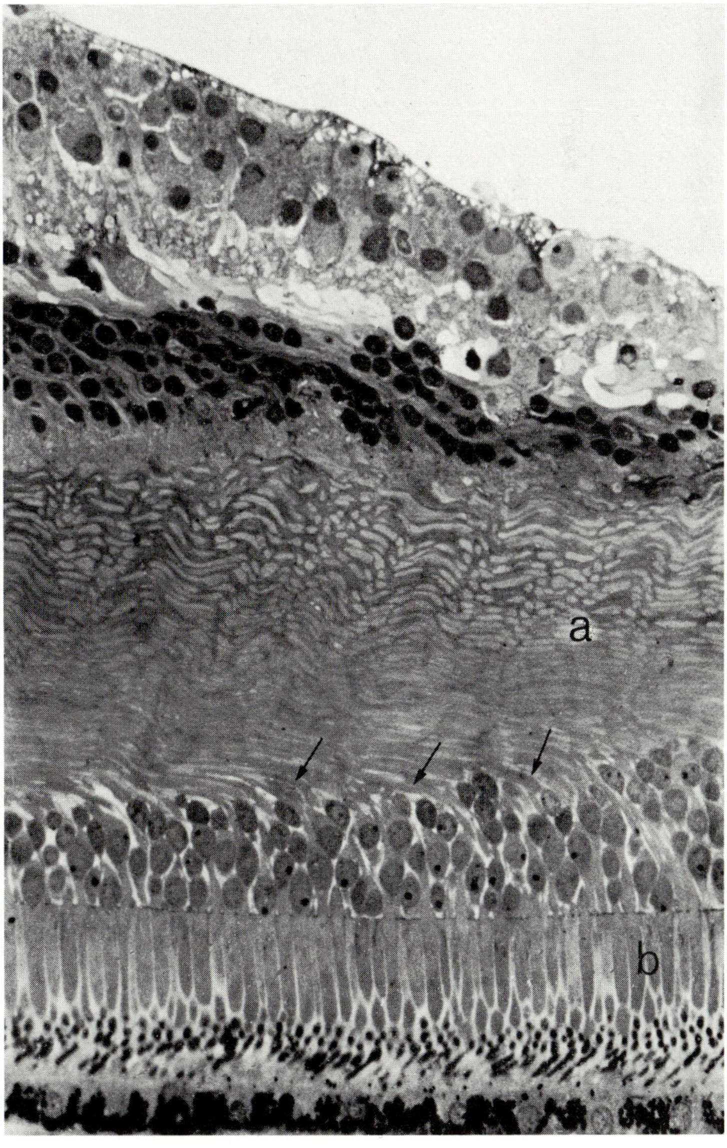

Figure 9-82. Light micrograph of Henle's fiber layer (a). The inner cone fibers (arrows) arise from the perikarya of the cells in the outer nuclear layer. The rod-like inner segments of the cones are seen at (b). (× 425.)

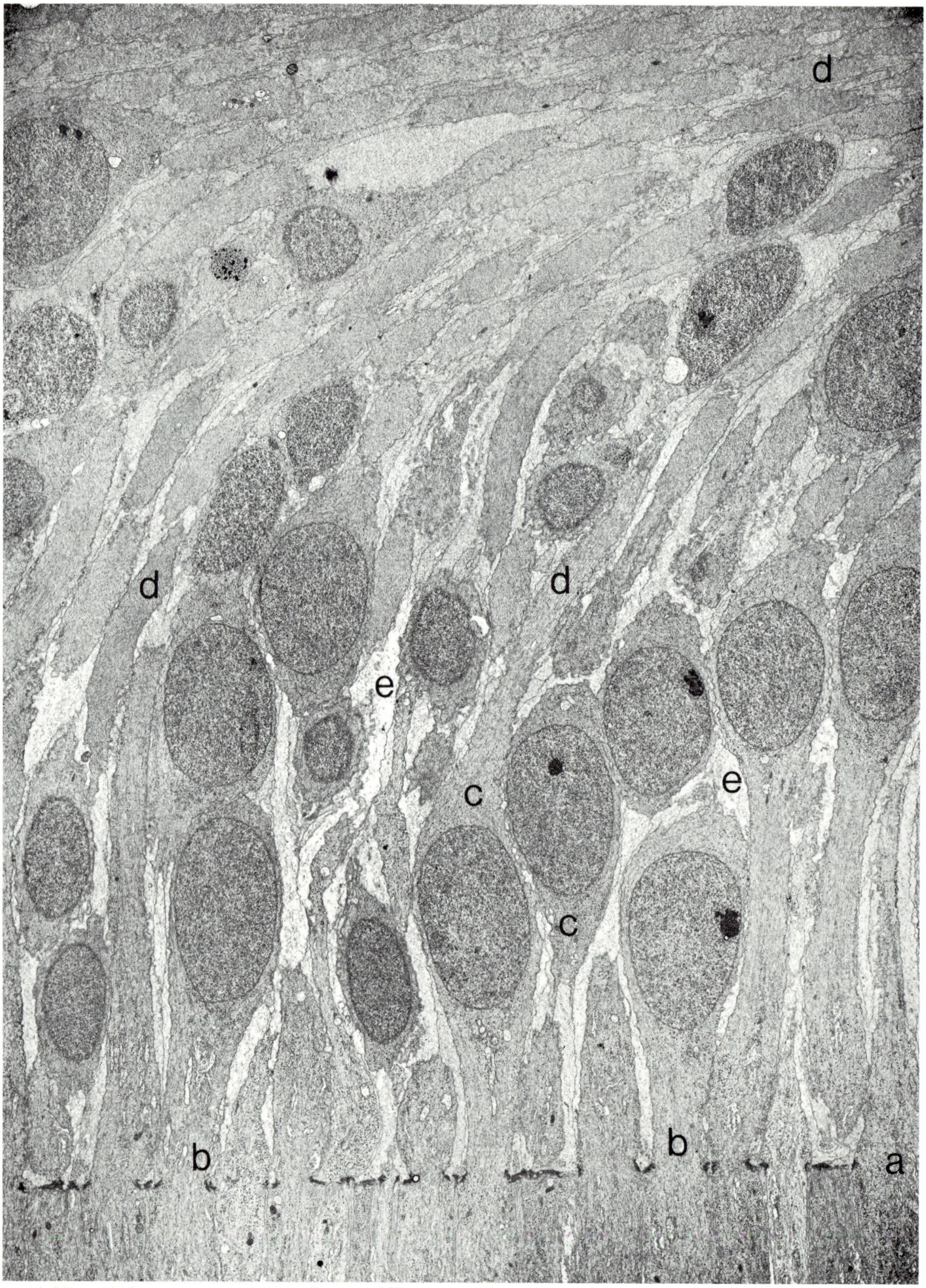

Figure 9–83. Electron micrograph of Henle's fiber layer of the fovea. The external limiting membrane is at (a). The outer cone fibers are at (b), and the cone perikarya are at (c). The internal cone fibers (d) form the fiber layer of Henle. Müller cells are seen at (e). (× 3600.)

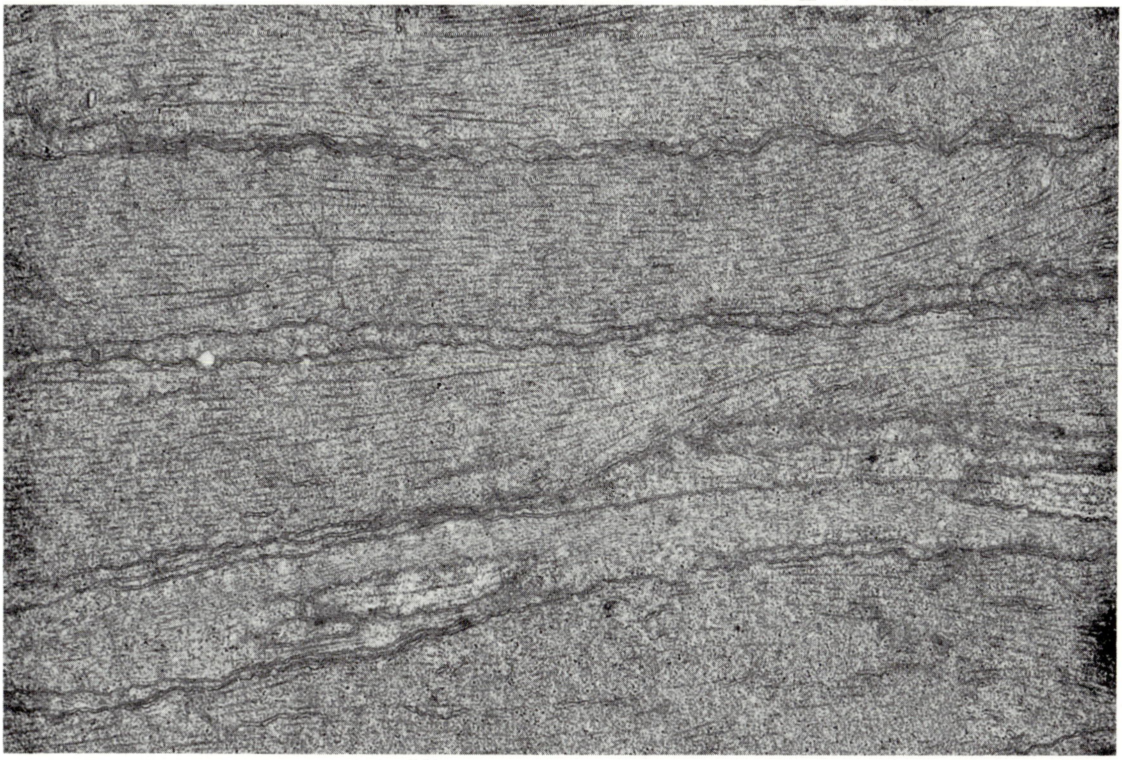

Figure 9–84. Henle's fiber layer, showing the parallel arrangement of the inner cone fibers and their numerous neurotubules. (× 10,500.)

fibers turn again to become meridional in the parafoveal and perifoveal regions and synapse with the cells of the inner nuclear layer. No spherules or pedicles are seen in an area with a diameter of 0.2 mm. from the central fovea. The entire course of these fibers is that of an S-shaped curve. The middle zone of the outer plexiform layer ends short of the fovea, and the inner portion of the outer plexiform layer becomes thinner at the junction of the parafoveal and foveal regions and extends in this attenuated form into the slope of the fovea.

The inner nuclear layer is reduced to a double row of cells at the edge of the fovea and is absent within the fovea. The internal plexiform, ganglion cell and nerve fiber layers are also absent from the fovea. The processes of the Müller cells occupy most of the inner fovea. They also form the inner limiting membrane, which is 0.4 μm. thick in the peripheral fovea, but in the foveal center the membrane is reduced to 100 to 200 A. in thickness (Yamada, 1969). By electron microscopy a central area about 200 μm. in diameter, composed exclusively of cones, can be identified. This area probably corresponds to the foveolar area that was observed by the light microscopists (Yamada, 1969).

The blood vessels of this part of the retina are mostly capillaries. They are present in the inner retinal layers up to the edge of the fovea. Capillaries and small arterioles are seen in the ganglion cell layer in the foveal edge and along the foveal slope. The capillary-free zone in the macula is about 0.4 mm. in diameter.

Parafoveal Central Retina

This portion of the retina has a width of about 0.5 mm. and with the foveal region measures approximately 2.5 mm. in diameter (Fig. 9-78). It is characterized by the largest accumulation of nerve cells in the entire retina, especially those of the ganglion cell and inner nuclear layers. The parafoveal area is also characterized by the thick outer plexiform layer, known as the layer of Henle in this region.

The rod and cone receptor layer here has a thickness of 40 to 45 μm. The thickness of the cone inner segments is 4 to 5 μm., and the outer segments are 1.5 to 2.0 μm. thick. The average distance between inner cone segments is 1 to 3 μm., and there are about 100 cones per 100 μm. in this region. The intervening space between adjacent cones contains one rod. Four to five rows of nuclei are seen in the outer nuclear layer, and in the outer part of this zone they become mostly rod nuclei. The layer of Henle is two to three times the thickness of the external plexiform layer elsewhere in the retina, and both rod spherules and cone pedicles appear here. The inner nuclear layer contains up to 12 rows of cells. The ganglion cell layer is composed of small cells of fairly uniform size, packed closely together; they form seven rows at the foveal edge. The cells increase in size but decrease in number toward the periphery of this region. The nerve fiber layer is thickest in the region of the papillomacular bundle, nasal to the fovea, and is much thinner on the temporal side in the parafoveal area.

Perifoveal Central Retina

This portion of the retina measures 1.5 mm. in width, its outer boundary being 2.75 mm. from the foveal center (Fig. 9–78); the entire macular area, therefore, measures 5.5 mm. in horizontal width. In the visual field this corresponds to 18 degrees 20 minutes. It commences at the point where the ganglion cell layer has four rows of nuclei and ends where the layer is reduced to the single layer that is seen elsewhere in the retina.

The thickness of this layer is unchanged from that of the parafoveal central retina, but the average distance between inner cone segments increases to 3 to 5 μm. There are 12 cones to each 100 μm., and the space between adjoining cones contains an average of two rods. The outer nuclear layer contains five to six rows of nuclei, the innermost being cone nuclei. The outer plexiform layer is half the thickness of that in the perifoveal region. The inner nuclear layer is reduced to six or seven rows of nuclei having the same thickness here as in the peripheral retina. The inner plexiform layer has increased slightly in thickness. The ganglion cells are somewhat larger, but vary in size.

ORA SERRATA

The extreme periphery of the retina is known as the ora serrata (Figs. 9-85 through 9-95). It is so named because the retinal termination is serrated, forming dentate processes or teeth that encroach on the pars plana of the ciliary body, and bays that lie between the teeth and have their convexities posterior. This area measures 2.1 mm. wide temporally and 0.7 to 0.8 mm. wide nasally.

The size and distribution of the teeth varies from eye to eye and even within the quadrants of the same eye. Straatsma and co-workers (1969) observed the meridional distribution of dentate processes and oral bays in 200 human eyes. The highest incidence of processes and bays occurred in the nasal ora region, especially the upper nasal. A progressive decrease in the number of these topographic features of the ora region was found in the inferior nasal and superior and inferior temporal meridians. For the most part this pattern was remarkably consistent, but in some eyes the ora was extremely smooth; in others it was irregular. There was remarkable symmetry in a pair of eyes from a single individual. The teeth may be long and pointed or short and blunted. Generally the dentate processes extend forward toward the valleys between the ciliary processes, and their number varies from 20 to 30. They are more evident on the nasal side, especially in the upper nasal quadrant. Meridional folds of the retina may exist at the bases of the teeth and consist of long, narrow elevations of the retina itself above the general level of the surrounding retina. The oral bays have some variation in number and size, generally being more evident in the portions of the ora serrata, with prominent dentate processes. They may be shallow or absent and occasionally are enclosed within an area of normal retina adjacent to the ora serrata proper.

Straatsma and associates list the morphologic features of the ora serrata (total in 200 eyes) as follows:

Feature	*Number*
Dentate processes	2573
Oral bays	2037
Doubled oral bays	185
Retinal tags in oral bays	174
Giant dentate processes	109
Meridional folds	80
Large dentate processes	64
Large oral bays	63
Meridional folds with posterior abnormalities	25
Enclosed oral bays	16
Partly enclosed oral bays	10

The peripheral retina gradually becomes attenuated as it approaches the ora serrata (Fig. 9–85). In the very young eye the entire retina gradually thins as a result of loss of the nerve fiber and ganglion cell layers in the peripheral 0.5 to 1.0 mm. of retina, as well as thinning of the plexiform layers. The outer nuclear layer is reduced to two to three layers, and gradually there is displacement of nuclei into the outer plexiform layer, so that the inner nuclear and outer nuclear layers are fused. Neuroglia and Müller cells replace the absent neural cells. The collagen fibrils of the vitreous base insert into the inner limiting membrane of the retina in a zone 4 mm. wide posterior to the ora serrata, so that the inner limiting membrane becomes thicker. The rod photoreceptors disappear about 1 mm. posterior to the ora and are replaced by malformed cones (Fig. 9–86). The external limiting membrane continues forward between the two epithelial layers of the ciliary body, but not in the form in which it appears in the retina.

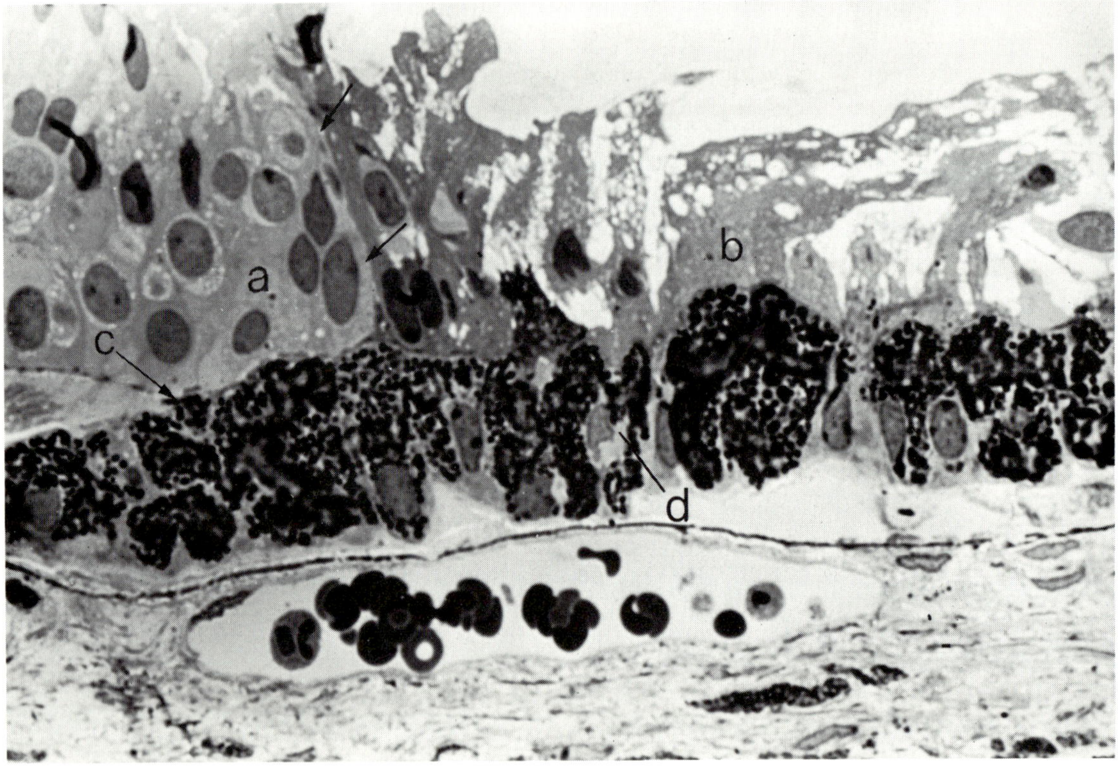

Figure 9–85. Ora serrata showing the transition between retina (a) and ciliary body (b). The outer limiting membrane of the retina and Verhoeff's membrane fuse at (c). The pigmented epithelium of the ciliary body is at (d). The two arrows indicate the area of transition from retina to ciliary body. (× 700.)

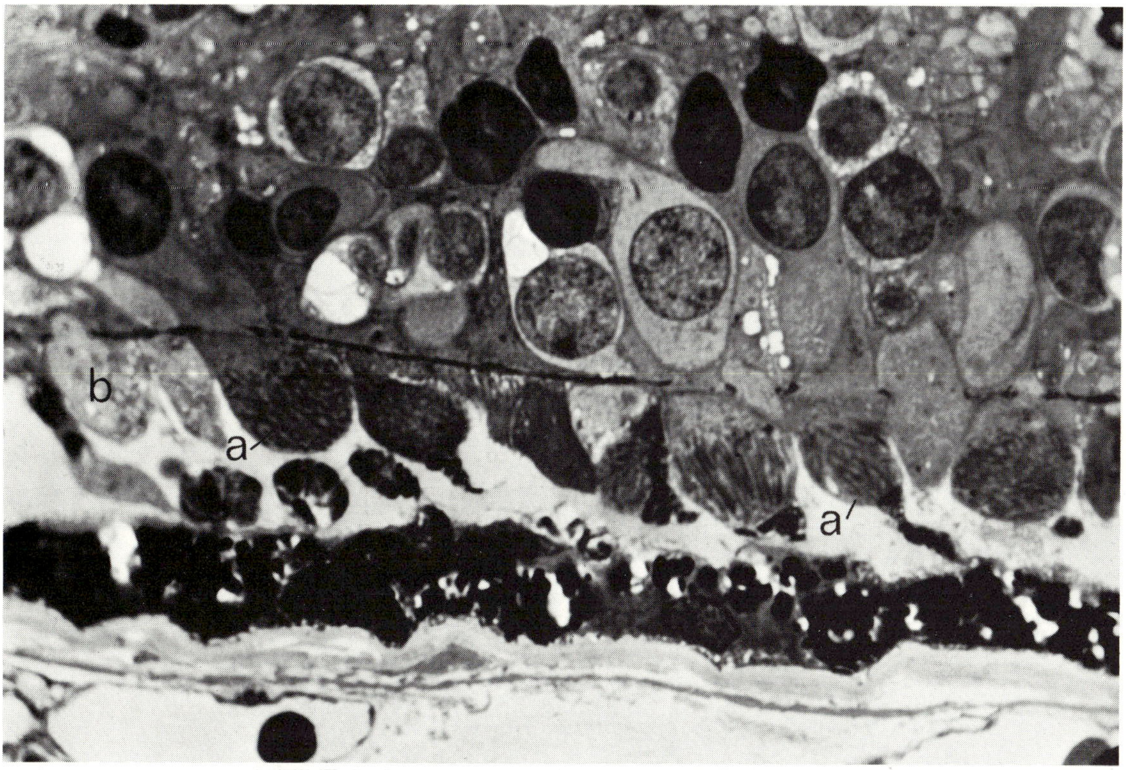

Figure 9–86. Peripheral retina in the ora serrata region to show the malformed photoreceptors (a). There is a degenerating photoreceptor at (b). (× 1400.)

With increasing age the normal architecture of the retina is altered at and posterior to the ora serrata for a considerable distance. The inner limiting membrane increases in thickness and often shows areas of vacuolation. The retinal stroma exhibits the formation of two types of cystoid spaces, typical and reticular, one arising in the outer plexiform layer and the other in the inner plexiform layer (Fig. 9–87). These spaces are surrounded by glial cells and are filled with acid mucopolysaccharide. Frequently the cystoid spaces open directly into the adjacent vitreous cavity in the extreme retinal periphery.

When viewed with the electron microscope the transition of ciliary body epithelium to retinal neuroepithelium is fairly abrupt (Fig. 9–88). Junctional complexes join both ciliary epithelium and retinal neuroepithelium to the pigmented epithelial layer. There are no photoreceptor outer or inner segments adjacent to the ora serrata; the inner segments first appear 0.28 mm. from it (Pei and Smelser, 1968). Cysts can be seen within the neural retina close to the ora serrata. The first cells on the retinal side of the ora serrata appear to be undifferentiated; posterior to them are Müller cells. The Müller cells are attached to each other and to the pigment epithelium by desmosomes, but no zonulae occludentes can be identified in this peripheral area. Small spaces or lacunae are found in the short attachment zone between the pigment epithelium and the neuroretina. These increase in complexity posteriorly and first contain only processes derived from the pigment epithelium and Müller cells (Fig. 9-89). The zonulae adherentes

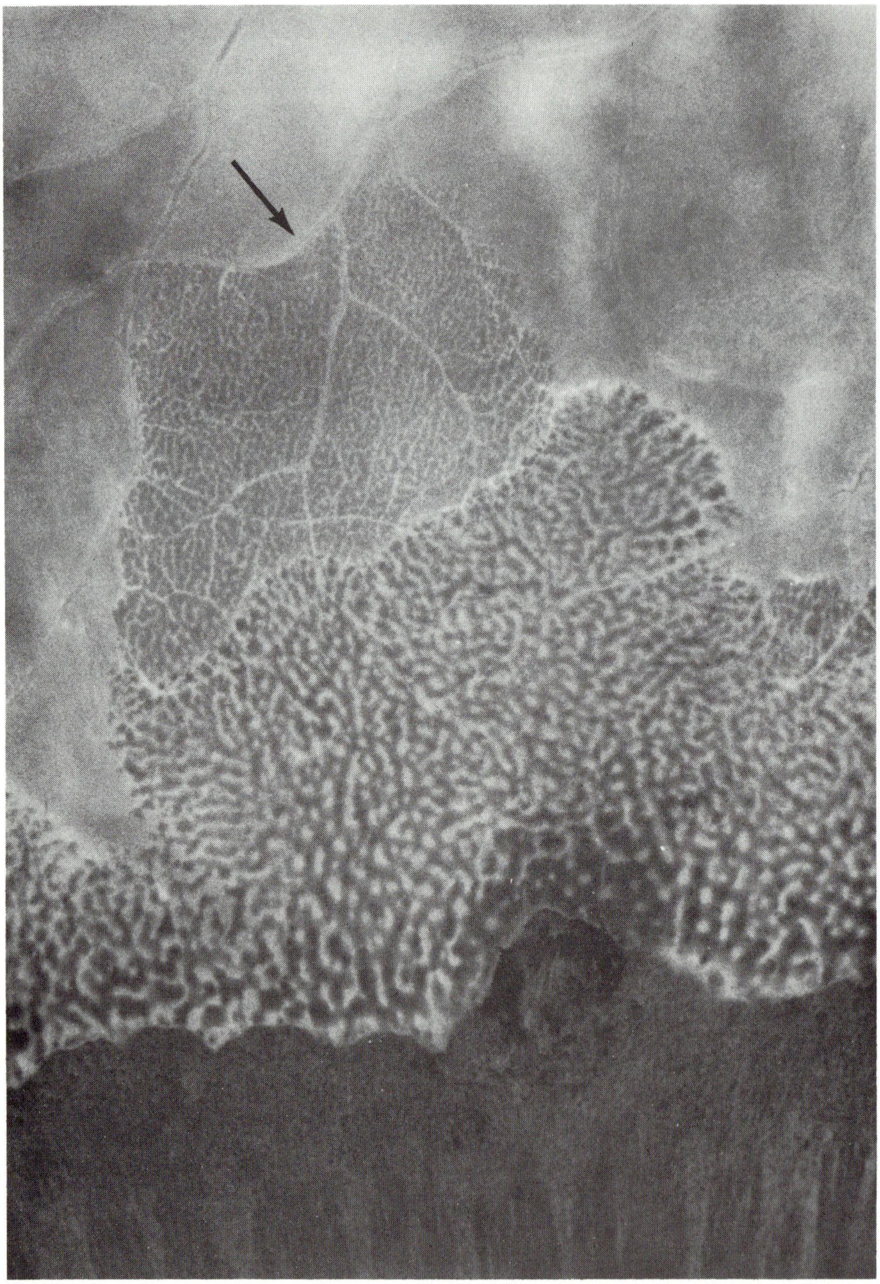

Figure 9–87. Cystoid degeneration, typical (anterior) and reticular (posterior), in inferotemporal quadrant showing usual contiguous relationship. When compared with its normal (typical) counterpart, reticular cystoid degeneration is notable for its conspicuous vascular pattern and gray background, delicate (reticulated) surface pattern and its free margins, limited by vessels (arrow). A deep, pigmented bay is a common developmental anomaly of ora serrata inferiorly. (× 20.) (Kindly furnished by Dr. Robert Foos, Jules Stein Eye Institute, University of California at Los Angeles.)

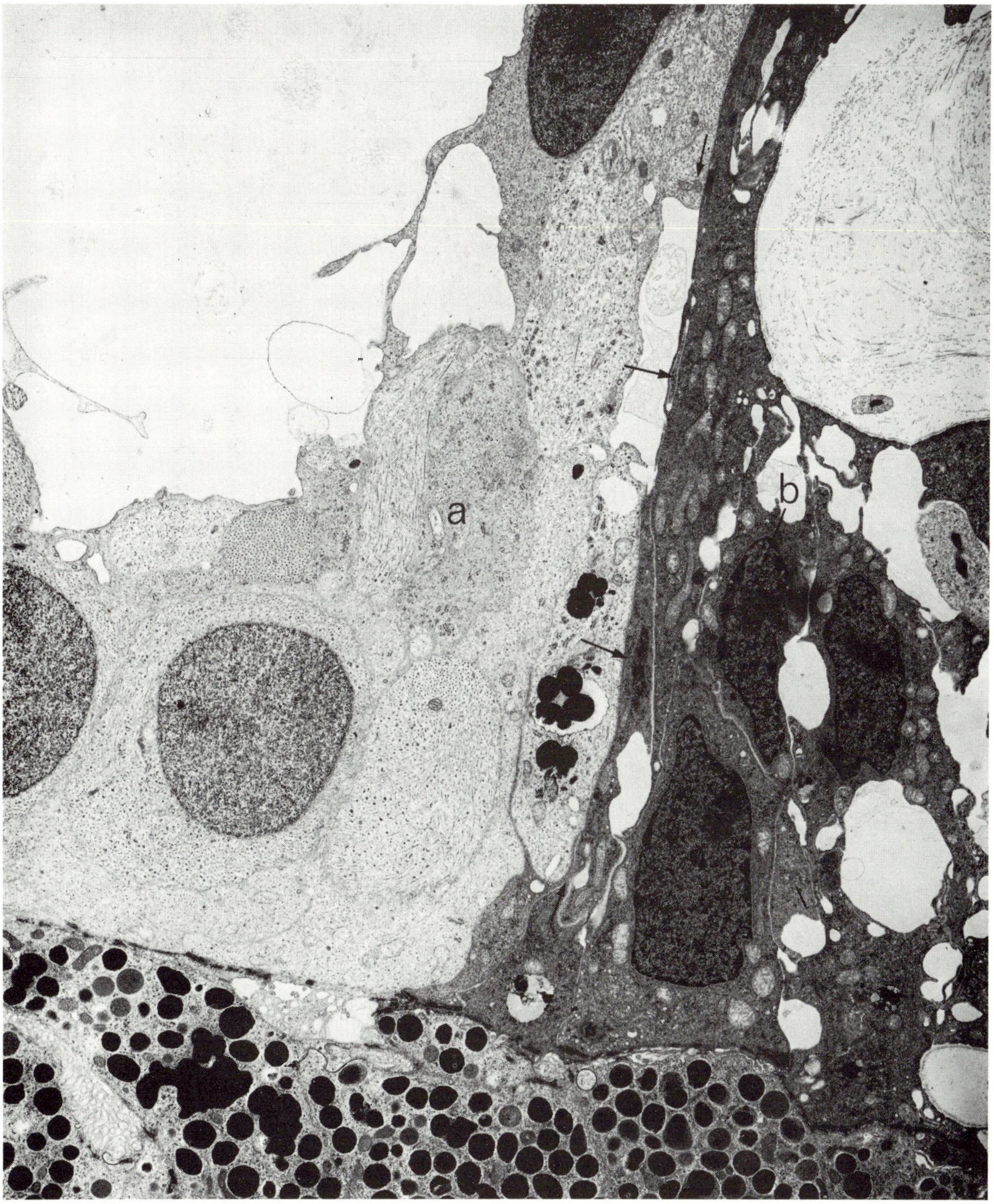

Figure 9–88. Ora serrata showing the terminal retinal cells (a) and beginning of ciliary body cells of the pars plana (b). The transition is at the arrows. (× 3000.)

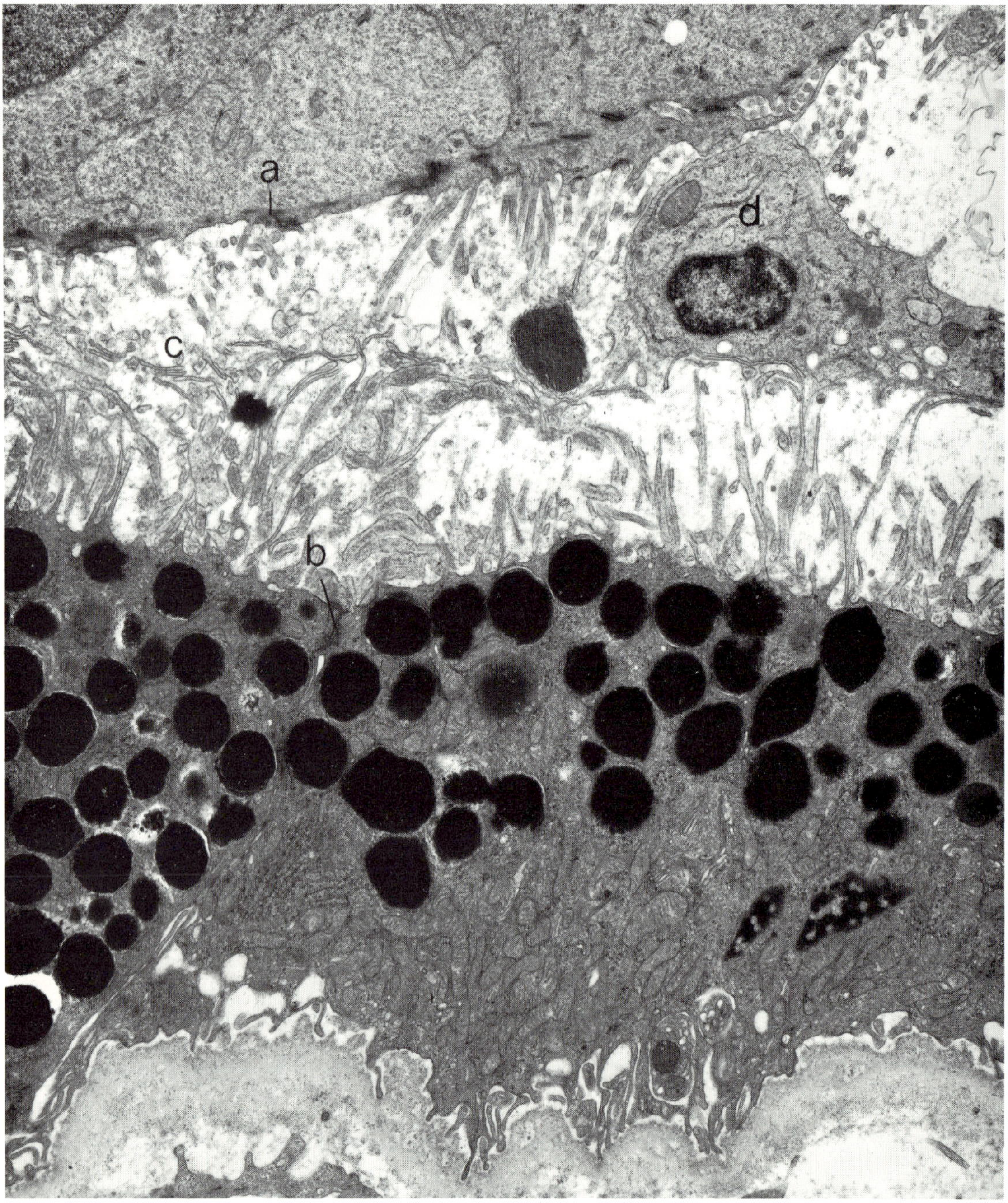

Figure 9–89. The most peripheral retina at the ora serrata immediately before the fusion of the outer limiting membrane (a) and Verhoeff's membrane (b). There are no photoreceptors in the lumen of the former optic vesicle (c). A displaced glial cell is seen at (d). (× 6000.)

which form the external limiting membrane in the posterior retina are also found between the Müller cells in this region.

More posteriorly, where the first malformed photoreceptors appear, their inner segments project as mushroom-like structures external to the limiting membrane (Fig. 9-90).

Abortive outer segments of the photoreceptors are a frequent finding in this area (Fig. 9-91). The gradual evolution of the primitive neuroretinal cells at the ora serrata into mature cells posterior to this zone seems to duplicate the embryonic development of the retinal cells (Pei and Smelser, 1968). The inner retina near the ora serrata provides a firm attachment for the collagen fibrils of the vitreous base. These fibrils insert into the inner limiting membrane. They often enter into lacunae formed by the Müller cells of the inner retinal surface (Figs. 9–92 and 9–93).

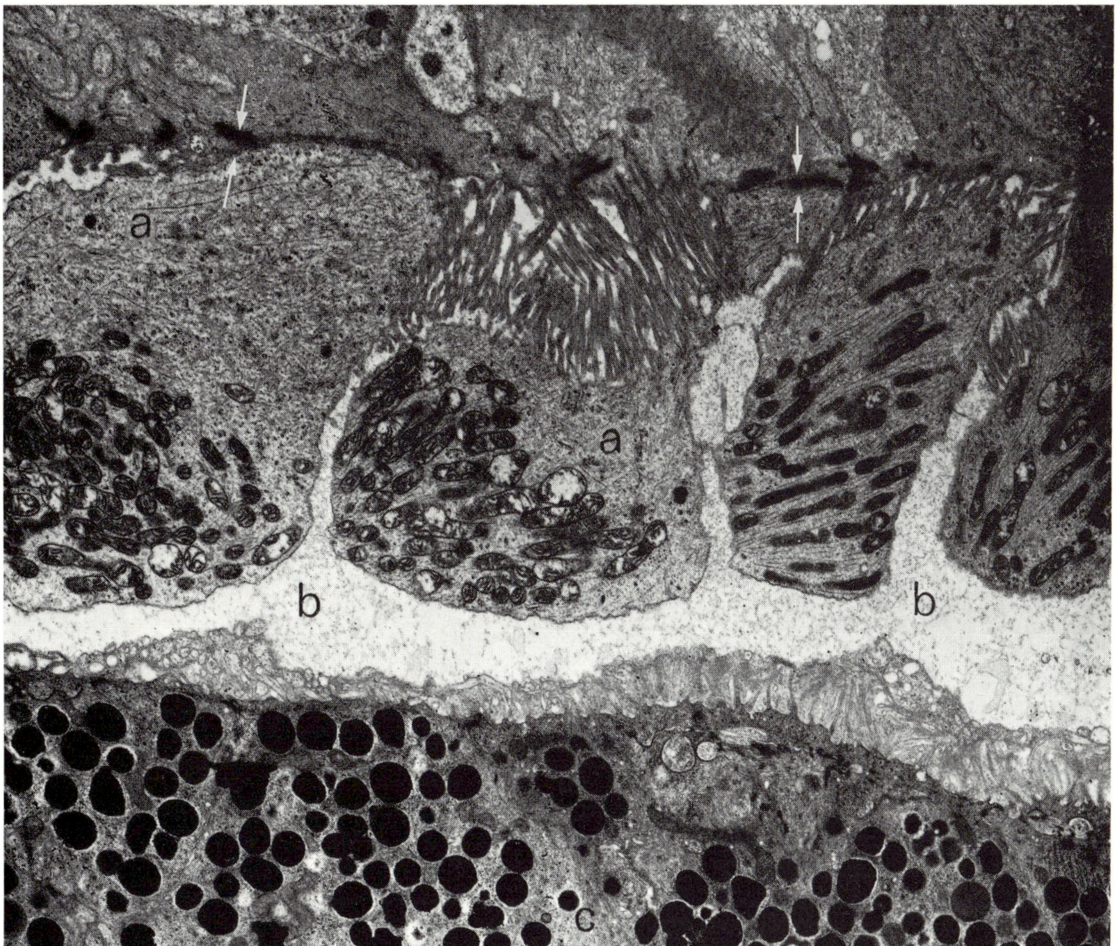

Figure 9–90. The mushroom-like processes (a) of the inner segments of the photoreceptors near the ora serrata. The outer segments are absent. Mucopolysaccharide surrounds the inner segments (b), and the pigment epithelium is at (c). Arrows indicate the outer limiting membrane. (× 2160.)

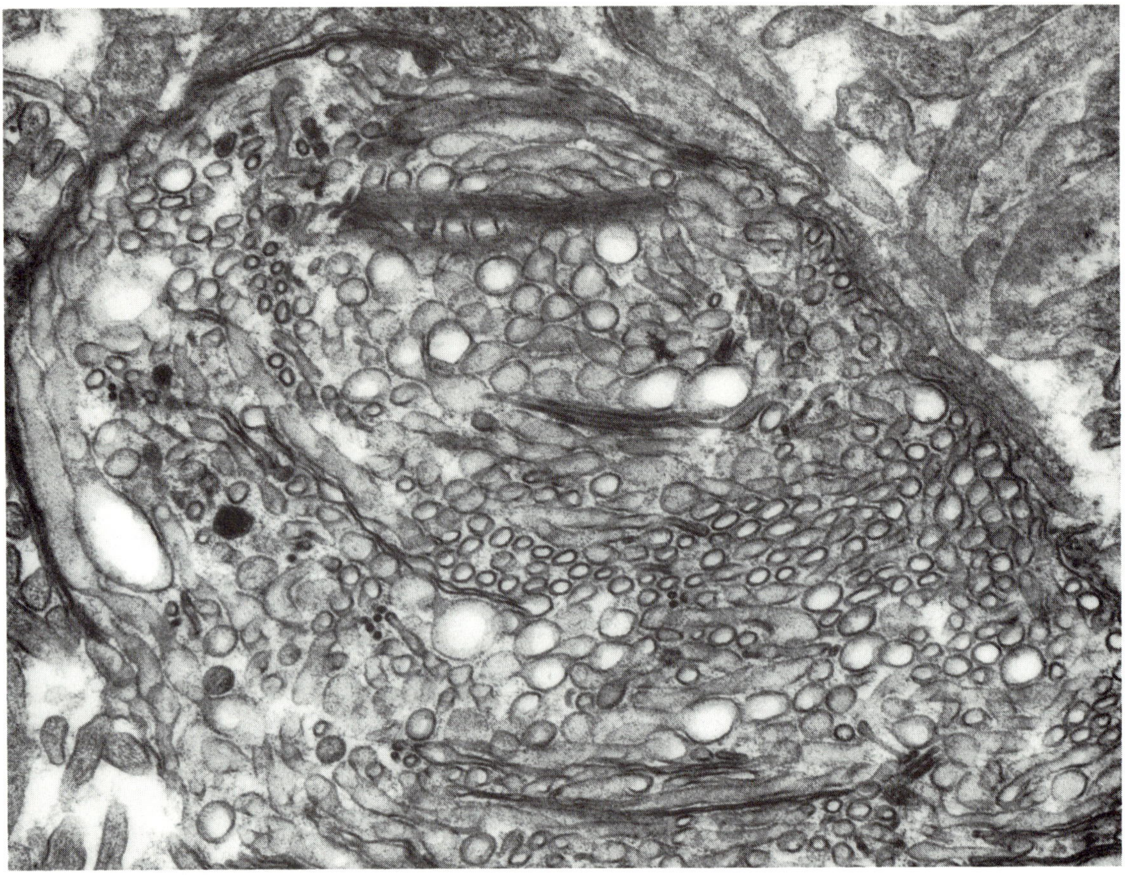

Figure 9–91. A degenerating outer segment of a photoreceptor at the ora serrata. The small circular structures are remnants of the discs. (× 48,000.)

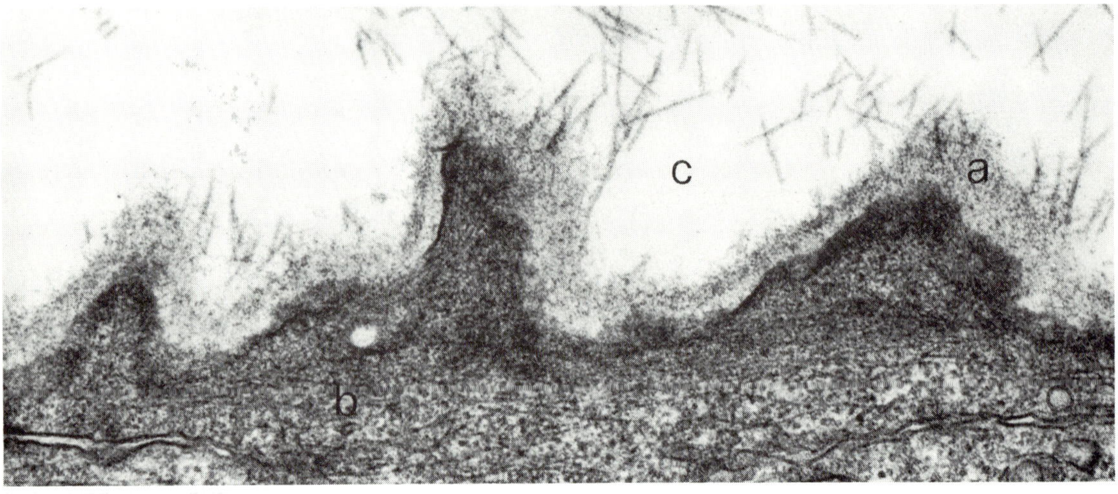

Figure 9–92. Inner limiting membrane (a) and Müller cells (b) at the vitreous base in the ora serrata area (c). (× 48,000.)

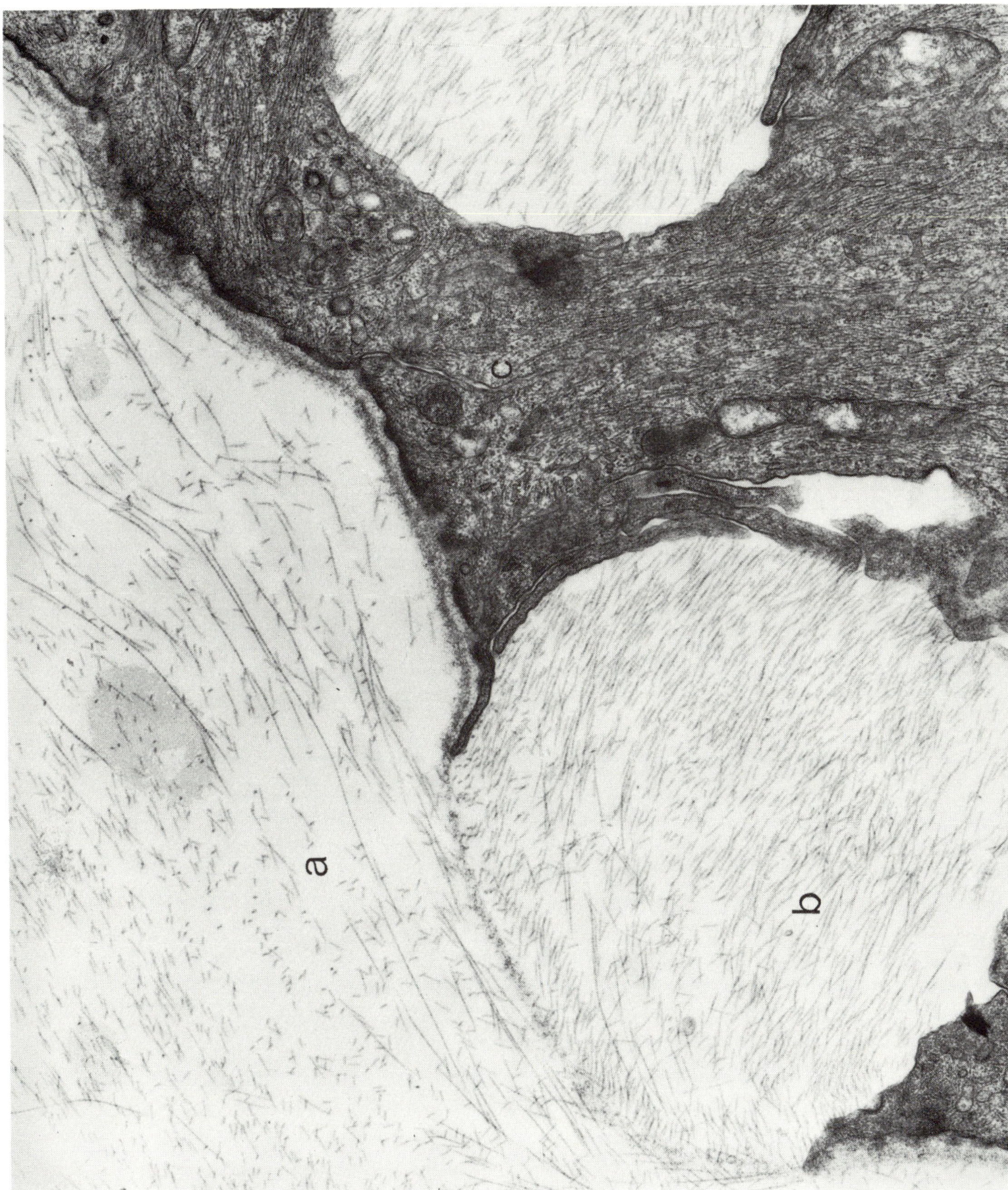

Figure 9–93. Vitreous base (a) showing numerous fibrils arising from the crypts (b) formed by the Müller cells (c). (×23,000.)

Blood Supply

The central retinal artery forms two main branches in the optic nerve (Figs. 9-94 to 9-99). Each of these branches further divides in the nerve into a superior nasal and temporal, as well as inferior nasal and temporal branches that supply the four quadrants of the retina. The corresponding retinal venous branches have roughly the same distribution as the arteries. In the eyes of about 15 to 20 per cent of individuals, cilioretinal arteries, derived from the choroidal vessels, enter the retina around the edge of Bruch's membrane (Hayreh, 1963). The amount of retina they supply varies considerably; they can supply the macular region or portions of the upper or lower temporal retina. In about 15 per cent of eyes having cilioretinal arteries the branches supply the macula alone.

The principal arterial and venous branches lie in the nerve fiber layer close to the internal limiting membrane. The successive principal divisions of these vessels are at the same level. As they extend toward the periphery they give off arterioles, or receive venules as they return toward the disc. The retinal arteries branch either dichotomously or at right angles to the length of the main trunks. Right-angle branchings are more common posteriorly, whereas dichotomous branchings are formed at and anterior to the equator. The retinal arterial circulation in the human eye is truly terminal, so that ordinarily there is no direct communication between the retinal and any other system of vessels, nor are there any arteriovenous anastomoses. The retinal artery and vein to a quadrant supply most of that quadrant alone, so that if the arterial supply to a quadrant is interrupted, infarction of its retina occurs. Between the arteries and the veins in each quadrant, the arterioles and venules run toward each other and break up into an extensive capillary network in the inner retina. This capillary network lies in all the inner retinal layers as far externally as the external border of the internal nuclear layer.

Arteries. Adjacent to the optic disc the arteries have a luminal diameter of 0.1 mm. and their walls are about 18 μm. thick. All the branches of the main arteries have the structure of small arteries, and their arterial character persists into the peripheral retina. Near the disc the arterial wall has five to seven layers of smooth muscle cells, which diminish to two or three layers at the equator and to one or two peripherally. The endothelial cells are oriented circumferentially or obliquely along the axis of the vessel, their cell walls interdigitating or overlapping somewhat. Their basic structure is like the endothelium of other vessels. There is an endothelial basement membrane, measuring 0.1 to 0.5 μm. in thickness, that is continuous with the basement membrane of the adjacent smooth muscle cells. There is no internal elastic lamina in any of the retinal arteries. The basement membrane often is interrupted by small bundles of collagen and reticulin, but there is no elastin. The muscle cells are oriented both circularly and longitudinally, each layer being surrounded by a basement membrane that contains an increasing amount of collagen toward the adventitia. Each muscle layer is apparently discontinuous, although intercellular attachments of cytoplasmic processes are seen occasionally.

An unusual feature of these vessels is the frequent displacement of typical muscle cells into the adventitia, these cells being separated from the media by a laminated basement membrane with a thickness of 1 μm. The muscle cells in the media are typical for vascular smooth muscle. The

Text continued on page 513

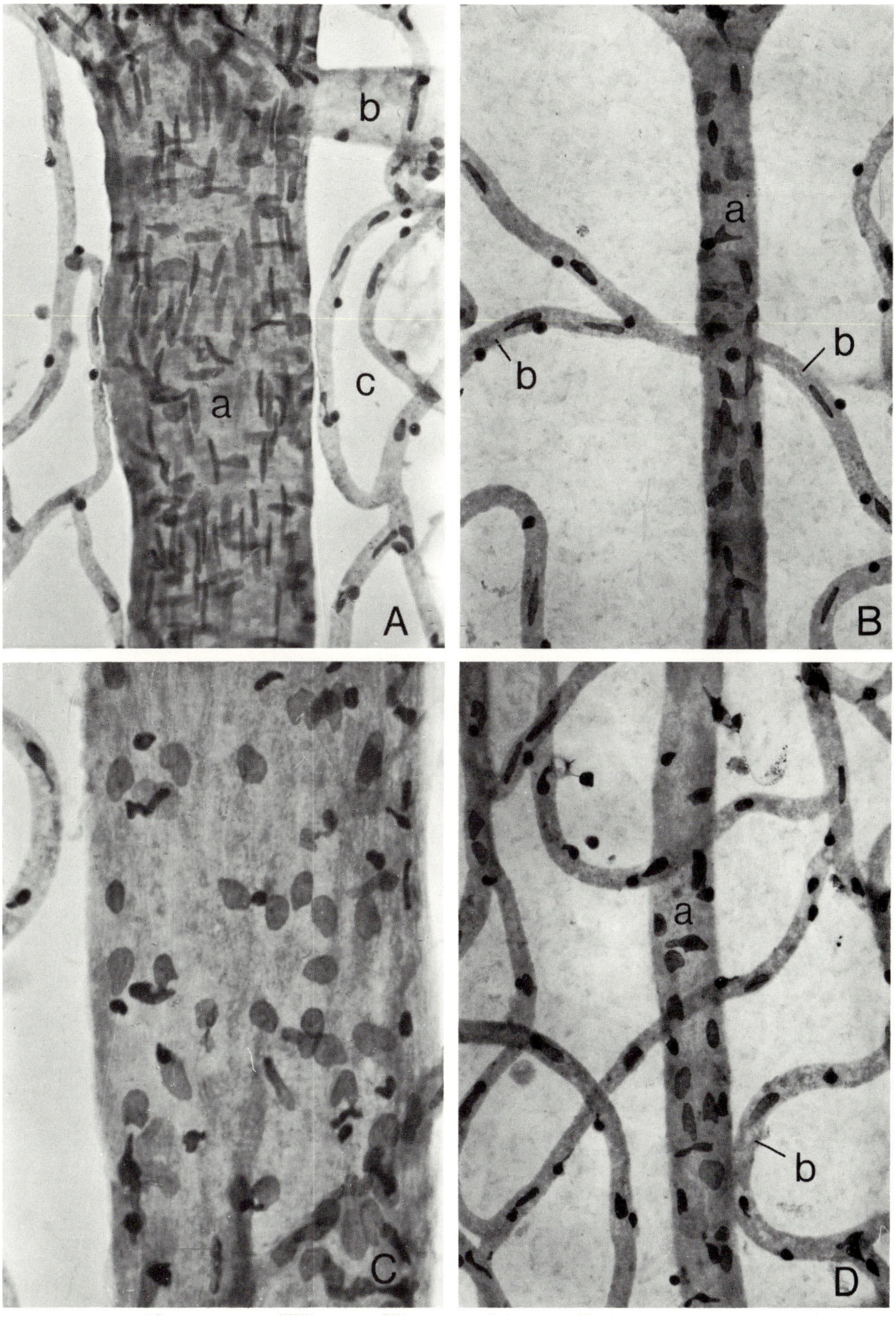

Figure 9–94. A trypsin-digested specimen to show the character of the arterial and venous channels in the retina. *A*, An artery (a) with an outer circular muscular layer gives off an arteriole (b); this in turn becomes a capillary (c). (× 280.)

B, An arteriole (a) with connecting capillaries (b). (× 430.)

C, A vein. (× 280.)

D, A venule (a) with connecting capillaries (b). (× 430.)

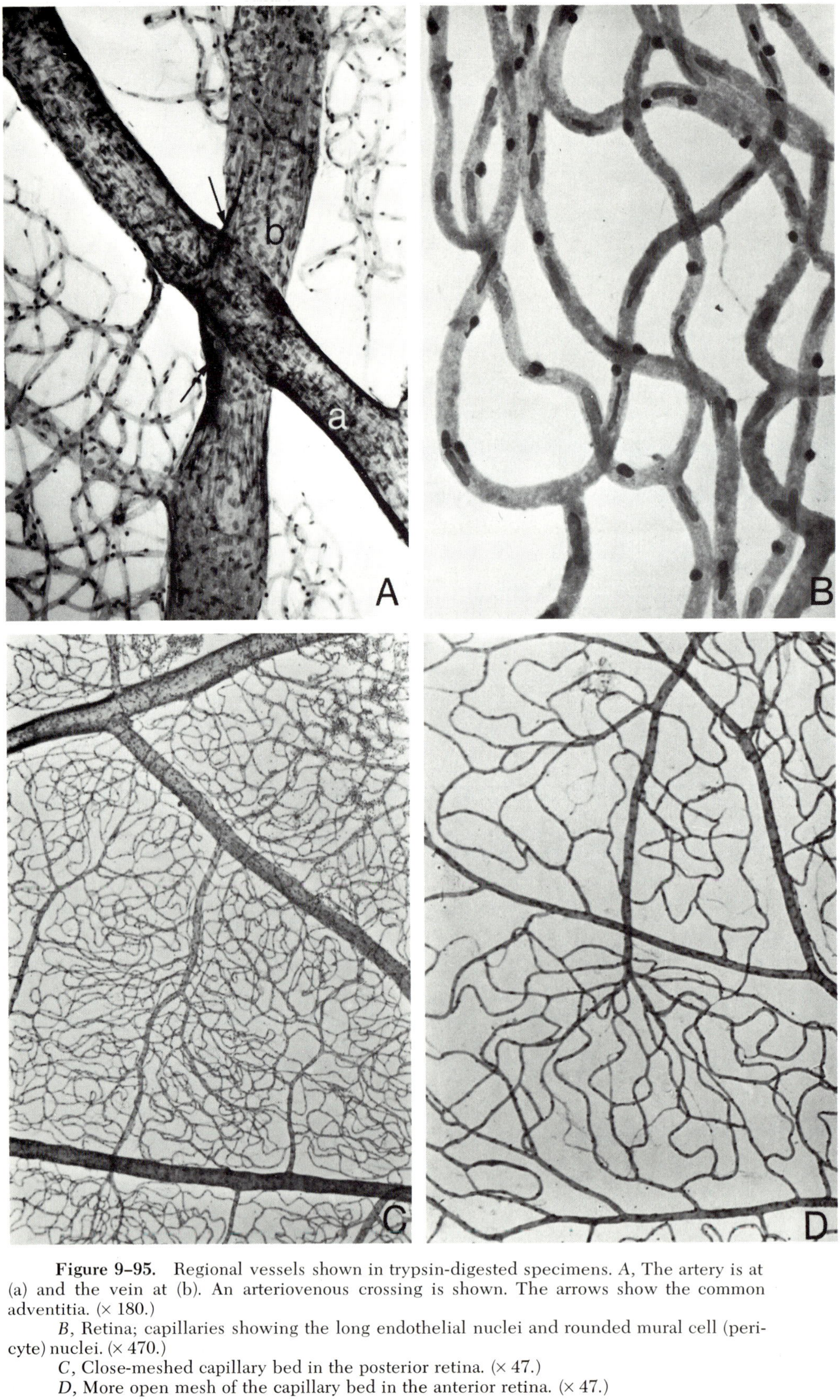

Figure 9–95. Regional vessels shown in trypsin-digested specimens. *A*, The artery is at (a) and the vein at (b). An arteriovenous crossing is shown. The arrows show the common adventitia. (× 180.)

B, Retina; capillaries showing the long endothelial nuclei and rounded mural cell (pericyte) nuclei. (× 470.)

C, Close-meshed capillary bed in the posterior retina. (× 47.)

D, More open mesh of the capillary bed in the anterior retina. (× 47.)

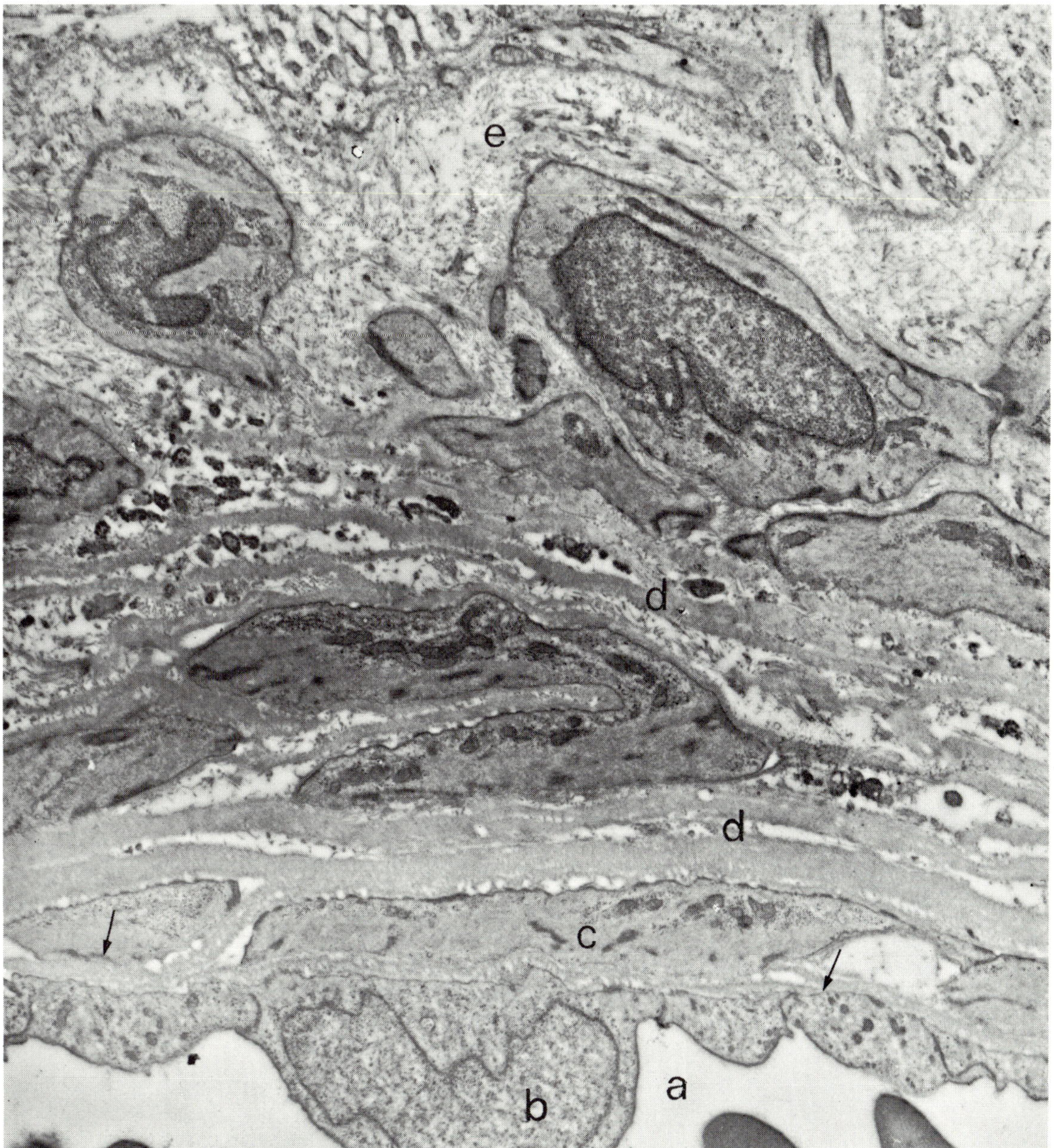

Figure 9–96. Retinal artery. The lumen is at (a). The endothelium (b) has a basement membrane (arrow) that is continuous with the adjacent muscle cell (c). There is no internal elastic lamina. All the muscle cells in the media have thick basement membranes (d). The adventitia is at (e). (× 8000.)

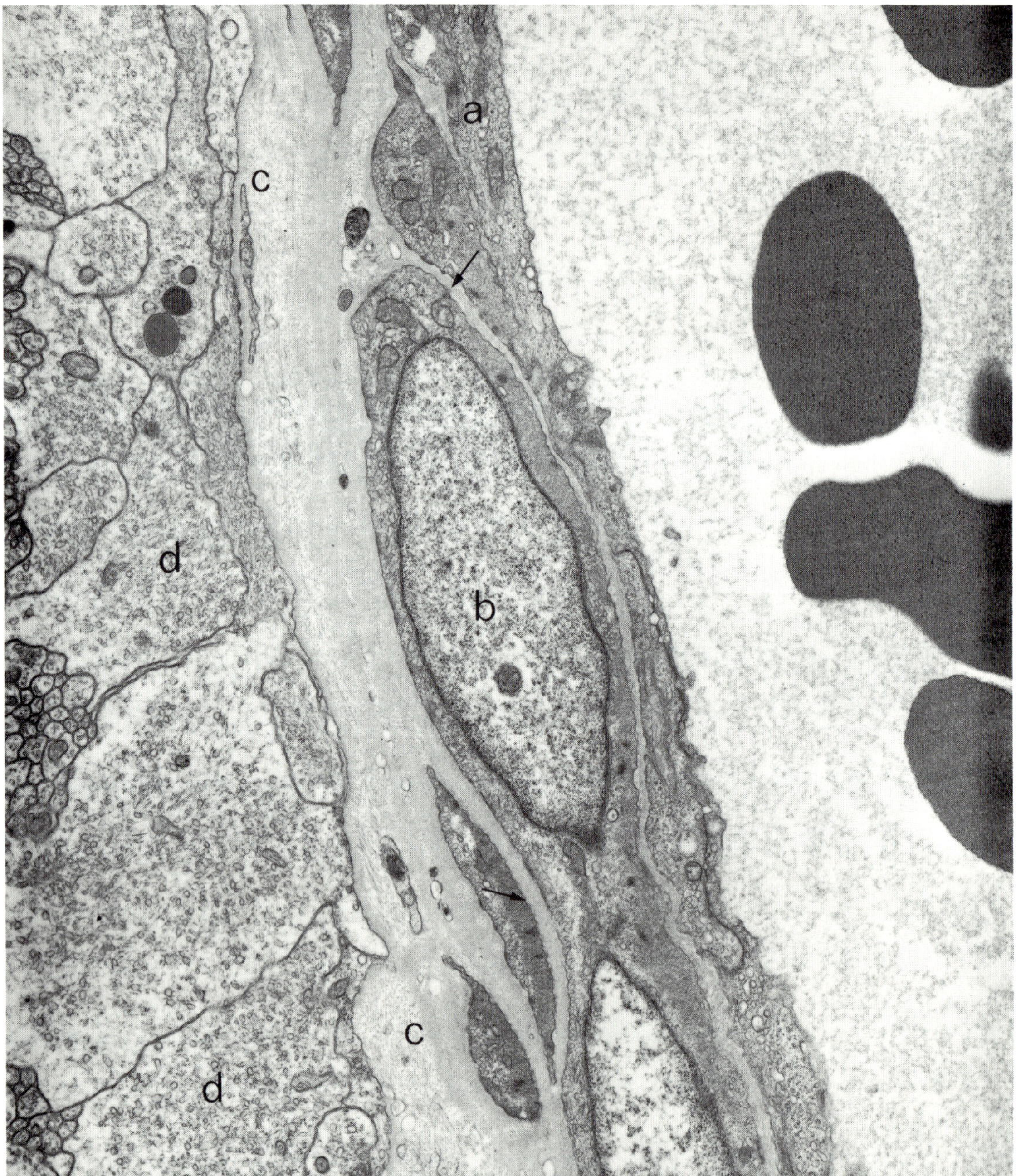

Figure 9–97. Branch of the central retinal vein in the retina. The lumen and some red blood cells are at the right. The endothelium (a) and a muscle cell (b) join each other. The basement membrane (arrows) of the muscle and endothelial cells varies in thickness. The adventitia is at (c). Müller cell processes (d) contact the adventitia. (× 6250.)

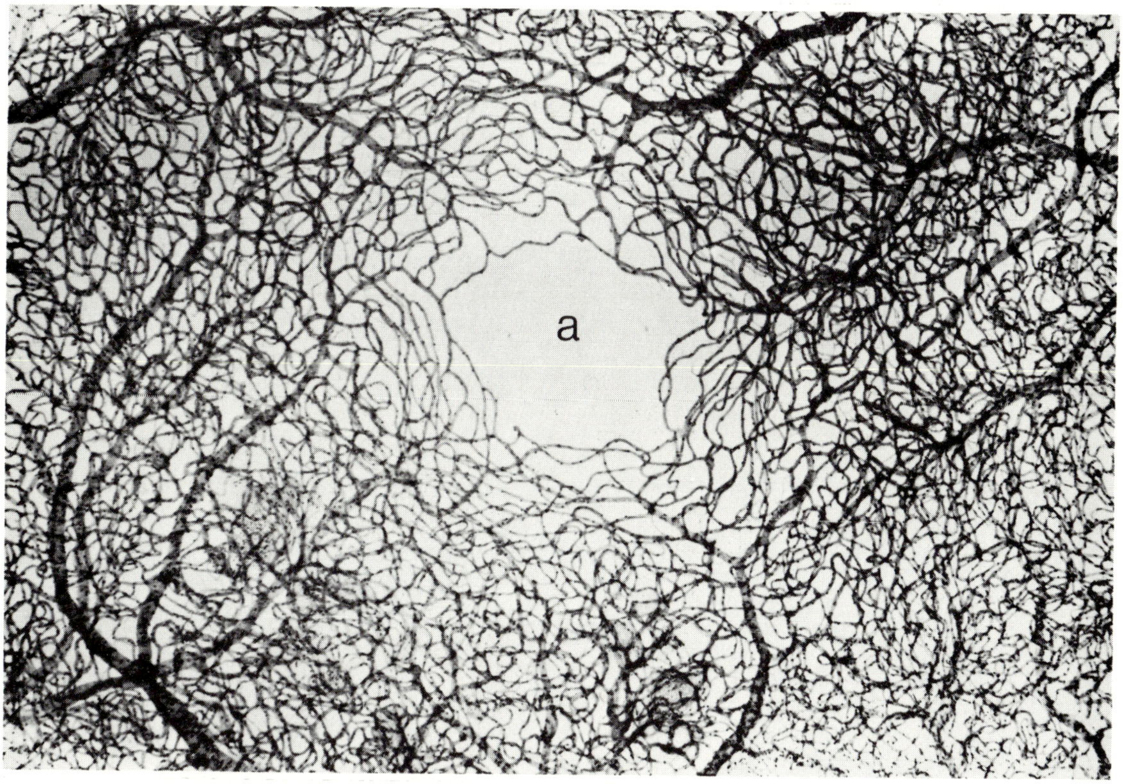

Figure 9–98. Capillary bed of the macular region. There is a capillary-free zone in its center (a). (× 42.5.)

cytoplasm contains numerous myofibrils, usually oriented in the long axis of the cell. Some bundles of myofibrils are attached to the cell membrane at zones of increased density. The arterial adventitia contains a moderate amount of collagen, which is mainly oriented circularly. The adventitial collagen is separated from the axons in the nerve fiber layer by the basement membranes of the glial and Müller cells.

The retinal arteries differ from muscular arteries of the same size in other organs in their lack of an internal elastic lamina and an unusually developed muscularis. Most texts describe the retinal arteries as arterioles after the first branching in the retina, but electron microscopic studies show them to be arterial beyond the equator.

Veins. The principal branches of the central vein near the disc have a luminal diameter of about 0.2 mm. The veins in the peripheral retina are venules. The endothelial cells of the retinal veins are like those of the arteries, but their basement membrane is only 0.1 μm. thick and it is continuous with that of the adjacent muscle cells. A thick basement membrane containing scattered bundles of collagen surrounds the muscle cells and, on their external surfaces, it often increases to 0.5 μm. in thickness. The larger veins in the posterior retina have three to four layers of muscle cells in their walls, but these cells disappear from the vessel wall within a short distance from the disc and are replaced by fibroblasts. The outermost cells along the entire length of the vein probably are fibroblasts; they have a flattened nucleus, rough-surfaced endoplasmic reticulum and pinocytotic vesicles.

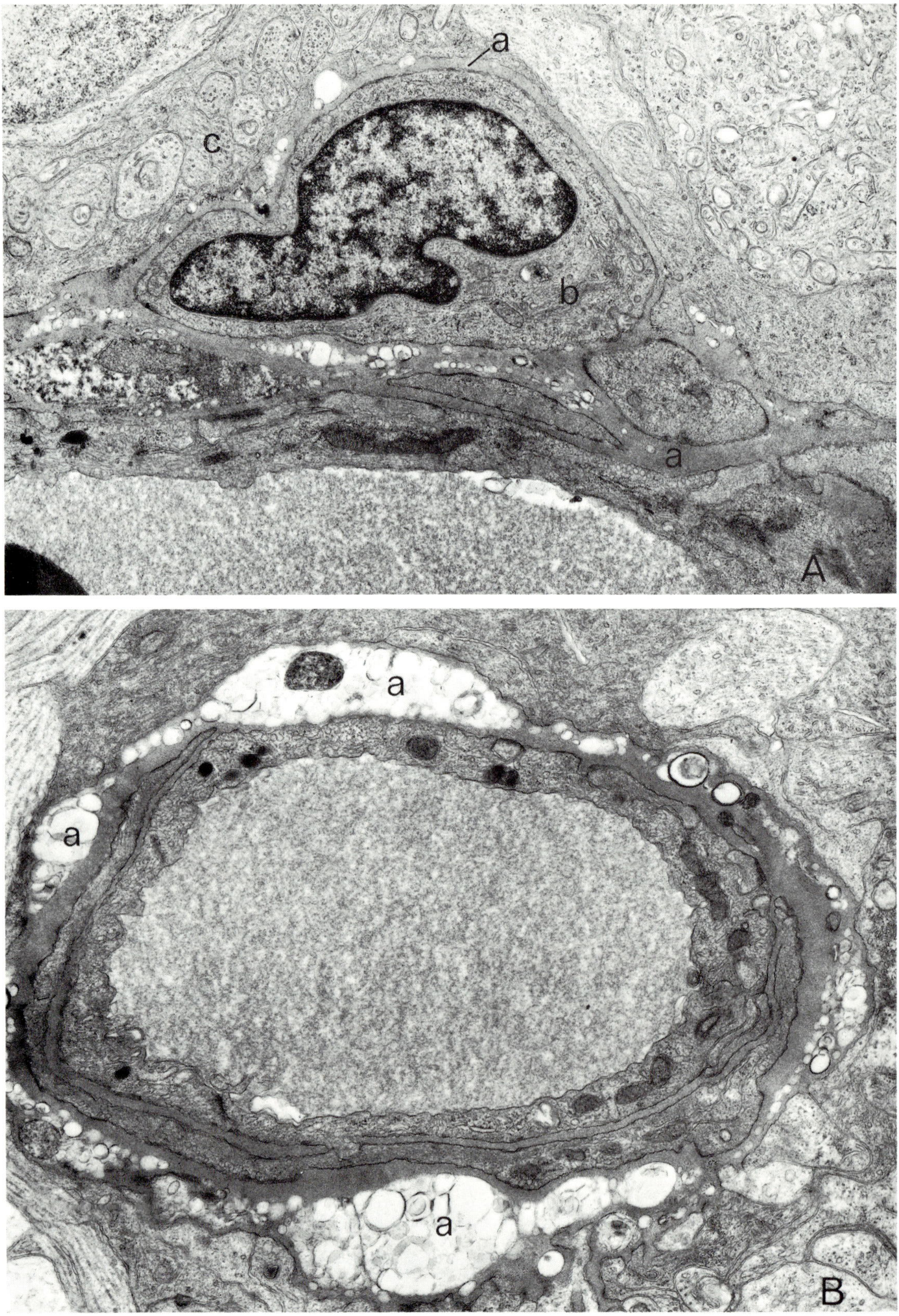

Figure 9–99. *See legend on opposite page.*

Arterioles. The arteriolar lumen is about 8 to 15 μm. in size, and the wall is like that of other arterioles. The cells in the walls of larger arterioles are easy to distinguish because they have all the characteristics of smooth muscle cells. The endothelial basement membrane joins the basement membrane of the adjacent smooth muscle cell, which is oriented in a circular direction near the major arterial branches and obliquely elsewhere. External to the muscle is a thin layer containing scattered bundles of collagen that are in contact with the basement membranes of adjacent glial cells. The basement membrane of the muscle cells of the smaller arterioles may show the same type of vacuolation as that of the capillary mural cells.

Venules. Venules have a diameter of 8 to 20 μm. The endothelium, basement membranes and mural cells are indistinguishable from those of the capillary. Collagen appears in the outer wall of the vessel after it is beyond 8 μm. in size. Many venules show a thickening of the basement membrane as the vessel enlarges, with little or no change in collagen content. The basement membranes of the mural cells of these vessels may also show vacuolation with increasing age. The mural cells become widely spaced as the vessel changes from venule to small vein.

Capillaries. (Figs. 9–94; 9–95; and 9–98 through 9–101.) Recently important observations have been made on the retinal vascular system by investigators utilizing flat preparations of the human retina after trypsin digestion and staining with various substances (Kuwabara and Cogan, 1961; Toussaint et al., 1961; Cogan, 1963, a and b). By this method the distribution of all the retinal vessels can be studied in a three-dimensional pattern. The retinal capillaries are diffusely distributed between the artery and vein of a quadrant, and they do not form laminae in the various retinal layers. There is a capillary-free zone along the arteries, especially in the more peripheral retina, but the zone is less apparent around the macula. There is no unusual concentration of capillaries around the retinal veins. The arterial capillaries which arise from the arterioles in the innermost retinal layers pass directly into the retina, often at right angles to the vessel of origin. They connect with the venous capillaries at all levels of the inner retina. In the area between the disc and the macula, the capillaries often emerge directly from the exterior surfaces of the main vessels and join with deeper capillary plexuses. The space between the arteries and veins contains the capillary plexus, suspended like a hammock between its feeding arterioles and draining venules. This arrangement of capillaries is like the blood supply of the renal glomerulus, as there is a one-to-one relationship between a relatively large arteriole and a venule, the two being connected by a rich capillary plexus without the intervention of shunt mechanisms that are present in other microcirculatory systems. *Intercapillary bridges,* however, are found to arise from one capillary wall and extend to that of another. These bridges stain with PAS and eosin, but they have no lumina; their function is not known.

Figure 9–99. Retinal capillaries of a young (*A*) and an old (*B*) individual. *A*, The basement membrane (a) of the endothelial cell is mostly intact. The pericyte (b) also is surrounded by basement membrane on the side facing the internal plexiform layer at its transition to the internal nuclear layer (c). (× 9000.)

B, The capillary shows the same basic structure as in *A*. The basement membrane around the mural cell, however, shows extensive cavitation (a). (× 10,000.)

The meshes of the capillary plexus have a uniform diameter, especially around the macular region, but they become increasingly wide peripherally. The capillaries in the peripheral retina of older eyes may show widespread acellularity. This cellular loss commences at about 50 years of age and is characterized initially by the loss of an individual endothelial cell, which is followed by the loss of pericytes. Individual capillaries in the posterior or equatorial retina may show a similar loss of cells, and acellular vessels are often found to connect two normal capillaries. The capillary walls of these acellular vessels often stain less intensely with PAS and other stains and show a ragged outline; such vessels do not contain red blood cells (Kuwabara et al., 1961; Kornzweig et al., 1966).

There are three retinal areas that show distinctive capillary patterns: the peripapillary retina, the macular area, and the peripheral retina.

Radial Peripapillary Network. As with the retina generally, the peripapillary capillaries ramify extensively in the inner retina without stratification (Figs. 9-100 and 9-101). In addition to this capillary network, the peripapillary retina also has a distinct group of capillaries, which arise in the region of the disc to form a capillary network in the nerve fiber layer. This network has the distribution of the Bjerrum scotoma of glaucoma in man and

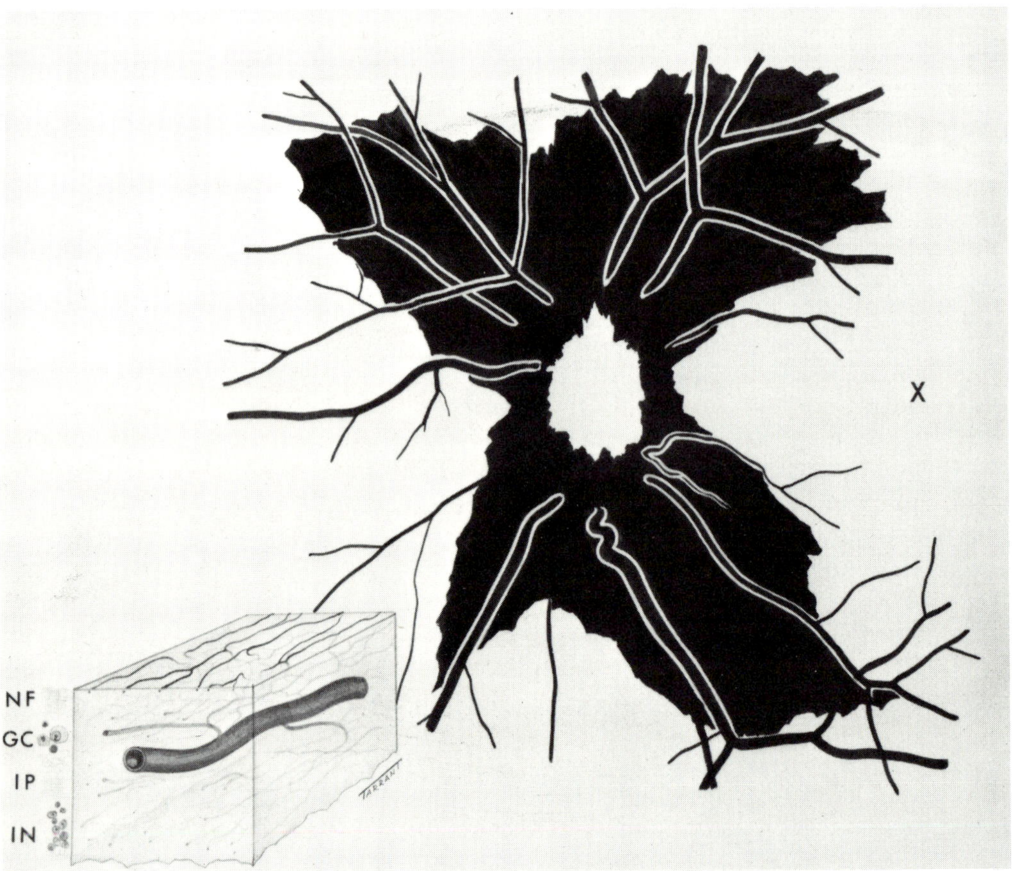

Figure 9-100. The radial peripapillary network. The distribution of these capillaries is shown in the blocked-out area. The inset shows the location of the radial capillaries in the internal retina. NF = nerve fiber layer; GC = ganglion cell layer; IP = internal plexiform layer; In = inner nuclear layer. (From Henkind, P.: Invest. Ophthal. 6:103–108, 1967.)

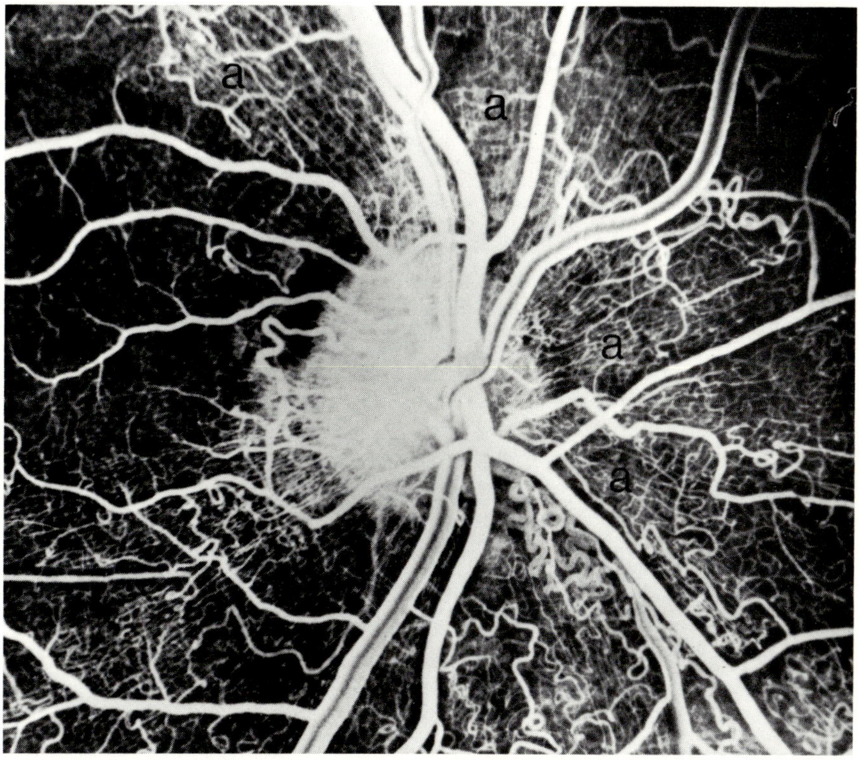

Figure 9–101. Fluorescein angiogram to show the radial peripapillary network (a). (From Henkind, P.: Invest. Ophthal. *6*:103–108, 1967.)

primates (Henkind, 1967 a). This layer of capillaries is arranged along the vessels and nerve bundles, following the arcuate course of the nerve bundles above and below the macula. These capillaries arise from the arterioles on either side of the principal arteries and supply the nerve fiber layer directly, particularly the bundles arising in the peripapillary region of the temporal retina in human eyes. The capillaries of this layer are long and approximately parallel to each other. Interanastomosis of these capillaries occurs to some extent with those in the deeper network (Michaelson, 1954; Toussaint et al., 1961; François and Neetens, 1962; Henkind, 1967 a and b). Henkind found the radial peripapillary network of capillaries to exist not only in the human eye, but also in the eyes of monkeys, cats and pigs. The long courses and infrequent anastomoses of these capillaries would suggest their vulnerability in eyes with ocular hypertension.

Macular Capillaries. The macular capillaries arise from the arteriolar branches of the superior and inferior temporal arteries and form arcades without stratification, dividing and subdividing at all levels of the inner retina. They are especially numerous in the perimacular region, diminish rapidly in number toward the central macula, and are absent in the fovea in an area measuring 0.5 mm. in diameter (Fig. 9–98). Because of the thickness of the ganglion cell layer and the radial orientation of the fibers in the external plexiform layer, the capillaries are more numerous in the ganglion cell layer and lie closer to the fovea in this layer than in the external plexiform layer.

Peripheral Retina. In the peripheral retina there is a much less dense capillary network, and the capillaries occupy a very narrow zone in the retina because of its thinness. There are no capillaries in the peripheral 1.5 mm. of the retina.

In flat preparations of whole trypsin-digested retina, two types of cells are identified with the capillaries, an endothelial cell and a mural cell or pericyte. There is almost a one-to-one ratio of endothelial cells to pericytes in the retinal capillaries. Only the brain capillaries have a similar cellular relation. The mural cells have been found in the capillary walls of all species of animals that have intraretinal blood vessels, but they do not appear in the capillaries of the conjunctiva, choriocapillaris, hyaloid system, mesentery and granulation tissue (Cogan and Kuwabara, 1967). The endothelial cells are oriented along the axis of the capillary and have long, pale-staining nuclei, whereas the mural cells lie in the capillary wall, outside the endothelium, and have a small, round, dark-staining nucleus. Cogan and Kuwabara proposed the name mural cell for these cells because they lie within the capillary wall, encased in basement material, which is continuous with the basement membrane of the endothelial cells. Histochemically and by electron microscopy, the mural cells cannot be distinguished from endothelial cells, but they are distinct from the muscle cells on the arterioles.

The endothelial cells behave in a special way in some eyes. They disappear from some capillaries after experimental ischemia. The mural cells, however, persist for a long time. The opposite effect is seen in the posterior and central retina in diabetes, in which there is a specific loss of mural cells and the endothelial cells are spared or even proliferate to form cellular masses.

A number of studies of the ultrastructure of the retinal capillaries and other small vessels have been made (Yamada et al., 1958; Maeda, 1958, 1959; Missotten, 1961, 1964; Kuwabara and Cogan, 1963; Ikui and Tominaga, 1965). These studies have revealed that the retinal capillaries of young children are different from those of adult eyes (Fig. 9–99). They are more cellular and have delicate basement membranes which are fibrillar or granular. Mural cells are found in these vessels, but they are surrounded by a much thinner basement membrane than those of the adult eye. The basement membranes of the endothelium and mural cells are much thicker in the adult eye, the mural cells are considerably more numerous and they are completely surrounded by a basement membrane. The endothelial cells are not fenestrated. A lip-like fold and moderate interdigitation is common at their edges, and they are joined near their luminal surfaces by a zonula occludens. The basement membrane of these cells measures about 500 A. in thickness but varies in thickness and density, depending on the proximity of the cell body of the adjacent mural cells. The basement membrane is double or triple its usual thickness if the mural cell is at a distance from the area under study. In tangential sections the basement membrane is somewhat fibrillar.

The mural cells form an integral part of the capillary wall, so that their axes are parallel to the length of the vessel and their long branches are wrapped circumferentially around the wall. Their thick basement membrane is continuous with the endothelial cell basement membrane. Externally, along the wall, the basement membrane of the mural cell measures up to 0.4 μm. in thickness and is in contact with glial and Müller cells. Because the long, branching processes of these cells extend along and encircle the vessel wall, only thin strips of cells surrounded by a basement membrane are seen in most electron micrographs.

The cytoplasm of mural cells greatly resembles that of the smooth muscle cells of arterioles, except for the absence of myofilaments. There are no attachments between these cells in areas where they come into close relation with each other. After age 20 the basement membrane on the external side of the mural cell contains a system of spaces of various sizes, which creates a curious Swiss-cheese effect. These spaces or cavitations are often continuous for a considerable distance. The largest vesiculations are greater than 1 μm. in diameter and are usually found in capillaries of persons over age 65. The significance of these cavities is not known, but they appear to be a result of aging. They probably contain material that is extracted in fixation and preparation of the specimens. Capillaries with a diameter of 8 to 10 μm. may have some reticulin fibrils in the outer part of the basement membrane which faces the glial cells. These fibrils mark the transition zone between capillary and venule or capillary and arteriole.

REFERENCES

Allen, R. A.: The retinal bipolar cells and their synapses in the inner plexiform layer. *In* Straatsma, B. R., Hall, M. O., Allen, R. A., and Crescitelli, F. (eds.): The Retina; Morphology, Function and Clinical Characteristics, Los Angeles, University of California Press, 1969.

Anderson, B., Jr., and Saltzmann, H. A.: Retinal oxygen utilization measured by hyperbaric blinkout. Arch. Ophthal. *72*:792, 1964.

Arey, L. B.: Retina, choroid and sclera. *In* Penfield, W. (ed.): Cytology and Cellular Pathology of the Nervous System. New York, Paul B. Hoeber, Inc., 1932, Vol. 2, p. 743.

Bairati, A., Jr., and Orzalesi, N.: The ultrastructure of the pigment epithelium and of the photoreceptor-pigment epithelium junction in the human retina. J. Ultrastruct. Res. *9*:484, 1963.

Berman, E. R., and Bach, J.: The acid mucopolysaccharides of cattle retina. Biochem. J. *108*:75, 1968.

Boycott, B. B., and Dowling, J. E.: Organization of the primate retina: Light microscope. Proc. Roy. Soc. London (Biol.) *255*:109, 1969.

Breathnach, A. S., and Wyllie, L. M. A.: The ultrastructure of retinal pigment epithelium of the human fetus. J. Ultrastruct. Res. *16*:584, 1966.

Cajal, S.: Histologie du Systeme Nerveux de l'Homme et des Vertebrés. Vol. II. Paris, Librairie Maloine, 1911.

Cogan, D. G.: Retinal architecture and pathophysiology. (The Sanford R. Gifford lecture.) Amer. J. Ophthal. *54*:347, 1963a.

Cogan, D. G.: Development and senescence of the human retinal vasculature. Trans. Ophthal. Soc. U. K. *83*:465, 1963b.

Cogan, D. G., and Kuwabara, T.: The mural cell in perspective. Arch. Ophthal. *78*:133, 1967.

Cohen, A. I.: The ultrastructure of the rods of the mouse retina. Amer. J. Anat. *107*:23, 1960.

Cohen, A. I.: The fine structure of the visual receptors of the rhesus monkey. Exp. Eye Res. *1*:128, 1961.

Cohen, A. I.: New details of the ultrastructure of the outer segments and ciliary connectives of the rods of human and Macaque retinas. Anat. Rec. *152*:63, 1965.

Cowan, W. M., and Powell, T. P. S.: Centrifugal fibres in the avian visual system. Proc. Roy. Soc. London (Biol.) *158*:232, 1963.

DeRobertis, E.: Electron microscope observations on the submicroscopic organization of the retinal rods. J. Biophys. Biochem. Cytol. *2*:319, 1956.

DeRobertis, E.: Some observations on the ultrastructure and morphogenesis of photoreceptors. J. Gen. Physiol. *43*:1, 1960.

Dodt, E.: Centrifugal impulses in rabbit's retinae. J. Neurophysiol. *19*:301, 1956.

Dowling, J. E.: Foveal receptors in the monkey retina. Science *147*:57, 1965.

Dowling, J. E., and Boycott, B. B.: Organization of the primate retina: Electron microscopy. Proc. Roy. Soc. London (Biol.) *166*:80, 1966.

Dowling, J. E., and Gibbons, I. R.: The fine structure of the pigment epithelium in the albino rat. J. Cell Biol. *14*:459, 1962.

Droz, B.: Dynamic condition of proteins in the visual cells of rats and mice as shown by radioautography with labeled amino acids. Anat. Rec. *145*:157, 1963.

Eichner, D.: Über Histologie und Topochemie der Sehschicht in der Netzhaut des Menschen. Mikr-anat. Forsch. *63*:82, 1957.

Feeney, L., Grieshaber, J., and Hogan, M. J.: Studies on human ocular pigment. *In* Rohen, J. W., (ed.): The Structure of the Eye. Stuttgart, Schattauer-Verlag, 1965.

Fine, B. S.: Limiting membranes of the sensory retina and pigment epithelium. Arch. Ophthal. *66*:847, 1961.

Fine, B. S.: Ganglion cells in the human retina, with particular reference to the macula lutea: An electron microscopic study. Arch. Ophthal. *69*:83, 1963.

Fine, B. S., and Zimmerman, L. E.: Müller cells and the "middle limiting membrane" of the human retina. Invest. Ophthal. *1*:304, 1962.

Fine, B. S., and Zimmerman, L. E.: Observations on the rod and cone layer of the human retina. Invest. Ophthal. *2*:446, 1963.

François, J., and Neetens, A.: Comparative anatomy of the vascular supply of the eye in vertebrates. *In* Davson, H. (ed.): The Eye. New York, Academic Press, Inc., 1962, pp. 369–416.

Friedman, E., Smith, T. R., and Kuwabara, T.: Retinal microcirculation in vivo. Invest. Ophthal. *3*:217, 1964.

Friedman, E., and Ts'o, M. O.: The retinal pigment epithelium. II. Histologic changes associated with age. Arch. Ophthal. *79*:315, 1968.

Fürst, C. M.: Zur Kenntnis der Histogenese und des Wachstrum der Retina. Acta Univ. Lund *40*:1, 1904.

Gärtner, J.: Histologische Beofachtungen über physiologische vitreovasculäre Adhärenzen. Klin. Mbl. Augenheilk. *141*:530, 1962.

Granit, R.: Sensory Mechanism of the Retina. New York, Oxford University Press, 1947.

Greeff, R.: Das Wesen der Fuchs'schen Atrophie im Sehnerv. IX Congres International d'Optalmologie d'Uttrecht 237, 1899.

Hayreh, S. S.: The central artery of the retina; its role in the blood supply of the optic nerve. Brit. J. Ophthal. *47*:651, 1963.

Henkind, P.: Radial peripapillary capillaries of the retina. I. Anatomy: Human and comparative. Brit. J. Ophthal. *51*:115, 1967a.

Henkind, P.: Symposium on glaucoma: Joint meeting with the National Society for the Prevention of Blindness. New observations on the radial peripapillary capillaries. Invest. Ophthal. *6*:103, 1967b.

Hickman, J. B., and Frayser, R.: A photographic method for measuring the mean retinal circulation time using fluorescein. Invest. Ophthal. *4*:876, 1965.

Hogan, M. J.: The vitreous. Its structure and relations to the ciliary body and retina. Invest. Ophthal. 2:5:418, 1963. (Proctor Gold Medal Award Lecture.)

Hogan, M. J., and Feeney, L.: The ultrastructure of the retinal blood vessels. J. Ultrastruct. Res. *9*:10, 1963.

Ikui, H., and Tominaga, Y. L.: Electron microscopic studies of the blood vascular system in the optic nerve and retina of the human eye. Trans. Asia-Pacific Acad. Ophthal. *2*:347, 1965.

Inomata, H.: Fine structure of cystoid degeneration in the peripheral retina. Acta Soc. Ophthal. Jap. *69*:1357, 1965.

Kidd, M.: Electron microscopy of the inner plexiform layer of the retina in the cat and the pigeon. J. Anat. *96*:179, 1962.

Kornzweig, A. L., Eliasoph, I., and Feldstein, M.: The retinal vasculature in macular degeneration. Arch. Ophthal. *75*:326, 1966.

Krinsky, N.: The lipoprotein nature of 688 rhodopsin. Arch. Ophthal. *60*:688, 1958.

Kuwabara, T.: Microtubules in the retina. *In* Rohen, J. W. (ed.): The Structure of the Eye. Stuttgart, Schattauer-Verlag, 1965.

Kuwabara, T., and Cogan, D. G.: Retinal glycogen. Arch. Ophthal. *66*:680, 1961.

Kuwabara, T., and Cogan, D. G.: Retinal vascular patterns. VI. Mural cells of the retinal capillaries. Arch. Ophthal. *69*:492, 1963.

Kuwabara, T., Carroll, J. M., and Cogan, D. G.: Retinal vascular patterns. III. Age, hypertension, absolute glaucoma, injury. Arch. Ophthal. *65*:708, 1961.

Liss, L.: The astroglia of the human optic nerve, chiasm and tract; a study with silver carbonate. J. Neurol. *105*:151, 1956.

Liss, L.: Nervous end-structures in the human neuropophysis; a study with silver carbonate. Acta Neuroveget. *17*:294, 1958.

Maeda, J.: Electron microscopy of the retinal vessels. Acta Soc. Ophthal. Jap. *62*:1002, 1958.

Maeda, J.: Electron microscopy of the retinal vessels. I. Human retina. Jap. J. Ophthal. *3*:37, 1959.

Matsuo, N., and Kitajima, S.: Electron microscopical studies on the internal limiting membrane of the retina. Folia Ophthal. Jap. *12*:760, 1961.

Michaelson, I. C.: Retinal Circulation in Man and Animals. Springfield, Ill., Charles C Thomas, 1954.

Missotten, L.: Étude des bâtonnets de la rétine humaine au microscope électronique. Ophthalmologica *140*:200, 1960.

Missotten, L.: Étude des synapses de la rétine humaine au microscope électronique. Proc. Europ. Reg. Conf. Elec. Microsc. Vol. II. Delft, 1961, pp. 818-821.

Missotten, L.: L'ultrastructure des tissue oculaires. Bull. Soc. Belg. Ophtal. *136*:1, 1964.

Missotten, L.: The synapses in the human retina. *In* Rohen, J. W. (ed.): The Structure of the Eye. Stuttgart, Schattauer-Verlag, 1965.
Missotten, L., Appelmans, M., and Michiels, J.: L'ultrastructure des synapses des cellules visuelles de la rétine humaine. Bull. Soc. France Ophtal. *76*:59, 1963.
Missotten, L., and Van den Dooren, E.: L'ultrastructure de la rétine humaine. Les contacts lateraux des pédoncules de cones de la fovea. Bull. Soc. Belg. Ophtal. *144*:800, 1966.
Miyamoto, M., and Fitzpatrick, T. B.: On the nature of the pigment in retinal pigment epithelium. Science *126*:449, 1957.
Mukai, N.: Axonal reaction of the optic nerve following heat coagulation. Canad. J. Ophthal. *5*:78, 1970.
Mutlu, F., and Leopold, I. H.: Structure of retinal vascular system of the dog, monkey, rat, mouse and cow. Amer. J. Ophthal. *58*:261, 1964.
Nichols, C. W., and Koelle, G. B.: Acetylcholinesterase: Method for demonstration in amacrine cells of rabbit retina. Science *155*:477, 1967.
Østerberg, G. A.: Topography of the layer of rods and cones in the human retina. Acta Ophthal. *6*:1, 1935.
Pedler, C.: The inner limiting membrane of the retina. Brit. J. Ophthal. *45*:423, 1961.
Pedler, C.: The fine structure of the radial fibres in the reptile retina. Exp. Eye Res. *2*:296, 1963.
Pei, Y. F., and Smelser, G. K.: Some fine structural features of the ora serrata region in primate eyes. Invest. Ophthal. *7*:672, 1968.
Polyak, S. L.: The Retina. Chicago, University of Chicago Press, 1941.
Porter, K. R., and Yamada, E.: Studies on the endoplasmic reticulum. V. Its forms and differentiation in pigment epithelial cells of the frog retina. J. Biophys. Biochem. Cytol *8*:181, 1960.
Rushton, W., and Campbell, R.: Measurement of rhodopsin in the living eye. Nature *174*:1096, 1954.
Rushton, W., and Campbell, R.: Measurement of the scotopic pigment in the living human eye. J. Physiol. *130*:131, 1955.
Salzmann, M.: The Anatomy and Histology of the Human Eyeball. Chicago, Deuticke, 1912.
Schmidt, W. J.: Doppelbrechung, Dichröismus und Feinbau des Aussengliedes der Schzellen vom Frosch. Z. Zellforsch. *22*:485, 1935.
Seiji, M.: Subcellular particles and melanin formation in melanocytes. *In* Montagna, W. (ed.): Advances in Biology of the Skin. New York, Pergamon Press, 1967, p. 189.
Sjöstrand, F. S.: The ultrastructure of the inner segment of the retinal rods of the guinea pig eye as revealed by electron microscopy. J. Cell Comp. Physiol. *42*:45, 1953.
Sjöstrand, F. S.: Ultrastructure of retinal rod synapses of the guinea-pig eye as revealed by three-dimensional reconstructions from serial sections. J. Ultrastruct. Res. *2*:122, 1958.
Spitznas, M.: Zur Feinstruktur der sog. Membrana limitans externa der menschlichen Retina. Graefes Arch. Ophthal. *180*:44, 1970.
Spitznas, M., and Hogan, M. J.: Interrelationship. Outer segments of photoreceptors and the retinal pigment epithelium. Interrelationship in the human eye. Arch. Ophthal. *84*:810, 1970.
Straatsma, B. R., Foos, R. Y., and Spencer, L. M.: The retina—topography and clinical correlation. *In* Symposium on Retina and Retinal Surgery. Trans. New Orleans Acad. Ophthal., 1969, pp. 1-26.
Streeten, B. W.: The sudanophilic granules of the human retinal pigment epithelium. Arch. Ophthal. *66*:391, 1961.
Streeten, B. W.: Development of the human retinal pigment epithelium and the posterior segment. Arch. Ophthal. *81*:383, 1967.
Toussaint, D., Kuwabara, T., and Cogan, D. G.: Retinal vascular patterns. II. Human retinal vessels studied in three dimensions. Arch. Ophthal. *65*:575, 1961.
Thomson, A.: The Anatomy of the Human Eye. Oxford, Clarendon Press, 1912.
Ts'o, M. O., and Friedman, E.: The retinal pigment epithelium. I. Comparative histology. Arch. Ophthal. *78*:641, 1967.
Ts'o, M. O., and Friedman, E.: The retinal pigment epithelium. 3. Growth and development. Arch. Ophthal. *80*:214, 1968.
Verhoeff, F. H.: A hitherto undescribed membrane of the eye and its significance. Boston Med. Surg. J. *149*:456, 1903.
Villegas, G. M.: Ultrastructure of the human retina. J. Anat. *98*:501, 1964.
Vrabec, F.: The temporal raphe of the human retina. Amer. J. Ophthal. *62*:926, 1966.
Wald, G.: Metamorphosis of visual systems in amphibia. Biol. Bull. *91*:239, 1946.
Wald, G., Brown, P., and Smith, P.: Iodopsin. J. Gen. Physiol. *38*:623, 1955.
Wolff, E.: Anatomy of the Eye and Orbit. 6th ed. Philadelphia, W. B. Saunders Company, 1968.
Wolken, J. J.: Structure and molecular organization of retinal photoreceptors. J. Opthal. Soc. Amer. *53*:1, 1963.
Wolter, J. R.: The astroglia of the human retina and other glial elements of the retina under normal and pathologic conditions. Amer. J. Ophthal. *40*:88, 1955a.
Wolter, J. R.: The cells of Remak and the astroglia of the normal human retina. Arch. Ophthal. *53*:832, 1955b.

Wolter, J. R.: Further evidence of the existence of the centrifugal nerve fibers in the human retina. Graefes Arch. Ophthal. *158*:235, 1956.

Wolter, J. R.: Über Endigungen zentrifugaler Nerrenfasern an den Blutgefässen der menschlichen Netzhaut. Graefes Arch. Ophthal. *158*:524, 1957a.

Wolter, J. R.: Perivascular glia of the blood vessels of the human retina. Amer. J. Ophthal. *44*:766, 1957b.

Wolter, J. R.: Glia of the human retina. Amer. J. Ophthal. *48*:370, 1959.

Wolter, J. R.: Silver carbonate techniques for the demonstration of ocular histology. *In* Smelser, G. K. (ed.): The Structure of the Eye. New York, Academic Press, Inc., 1961.

Wolter, J. R.: The reactions of the centrifugal nerves of the human eye: *In* Rohen, J. W. (ed.): The Structure of the Eye. Stuttgart, Schattauer-Verlag, 1965, pp. 85-95.

Yamada, E.: Some structural features of the fovea centralis in the human retina. Arch. Ophthal. *82*:151, 1969.

Yamada, E., Tokuyasum K., and Iwaki, S.: The fine structure of retina studied with electron microscope. III. Human retina. J. Kurume Med. Ass. *21*:1979, 1958.

Young, R. W.: The renewal of photoreceptor cell outer segments. J. Cell Biol. *33*:61, 1967.

Young, R. W., and Bok, D.: Participation of the retinal pigment epithelium in the rod outer segment renewal process. J. Cell Biol. *42*:392, 1969.

Zimmerman, L. E.: Applications of histochemical methods for the demonstration of acid mucopolysaccharides to ophthalmic pathology. Trans. Amer. Acad. Ophthal. Otolaryng. *62*:697, 1958.

Chapter Ten

OPTIC NERVE

The optic nerve transmits the information gathered by the retina to the occipital cortex in close to 1.2 million axons. The structure of the optic nerve is like that of the central nervous system, and because of this it differs greatly from the other cerebrospinal nerves. The optic nerve has the same organization as the white matter of the brain, particularly in regard to its glia and blood supply. The axons which form the optic nerve originate in the ganglion cell layer of the retina and extend through the optic nerves, the chiasm and the optic tracts to the medial and lateral geniculate bodies, superior colliculi, and pretectal nuclei. Most of these axons are concerned with vision: some provide a pathway for the pupillary light reflex, others relay general responses to light (eye, face, neck, trunk and limb muscles), and possibly some are centrifugal (efferent) fibers to the inner retina and its blood vessels.

The optic nerve is enclosed by its meningeal sheaths in the orbit and optic nerve canal; these sheaths are continuous with and have the same structure as those covering the brain.

The nerve axons in the optic disc are surrounded and segregated into bundles only by astrocytes; for this reason, the nerve bundles are easily separated from each other by edema. Beginning at the lamina cribrosa, however, the nerve bundles are enclosed in connective tissue septa, which prevent significant swelling by edema. In addition to the support given the nerve bundles by the glia and connective tissue septa, the glia also plays an important role in the nutrition of the axons. Other glial cells function like the Schwann cells of peripheral nerves in providing a myelin sheath for the nerve axons.

PHYSIOLOGY

Three neurons form the visual pathway from the retina to the occipital visual cortex. These neurons have been discussed in the chapter on the retina (p. 403). The second order neuron extends from the ganglion cell layer of the retina to the lateral geniculate body and forms most of the optic nerve in the first part of its course. In man about 80 per cent of the optic nerve axons decussate in the optic chiasm to the opposite side of the brain; the remaining 20 per cent pass to the homolateral cortex (see Fig. 9-1).

Conduction

The speed of conduction along large myelinated nerve fibers is 10 to 130 meters/second. Small autonomic fibers conduct at 7 to 15 meters/sec., while unmyelinated fibers conduct at 15 to 30 meters/sec. Little is known about the conduction rates of the optic nerve fibers of man.

Ogden and Miller (1966) studied the conduction properties of the ganglion cell axon along its intraretinal course as well as in its course through the optic nerve where the axons are myelinated. They found the average velocity of the fastest and slowest intraretinal fibers to be 1.2 meters/-sec. and 0.45 meters/sec., respectively. The myelinated axons in the optic nerve conduct impulses much more rapidly. The authors recorded velocities ranging from 3.3 meters/sec. to 10 meters/sec.

Light causes photochemical changes and excitation in the retinal receptors, which are transduced to electrical impulses that are transmitted to the cerebral cortex. Since each retina has about 130 million photoreceptors, and the optic nerve contains approximately one million axons, it follows that one ganglion cell transmits to its axon the information it has received from many receptors scattered over a wide area (the receptive field). The response in the optic nerve as a result of photic stimulation of the retina is a series of spike potentials of constant size and shape, which vary in frequency with the intensity of the stimulus.

Hartline (1925) identified three types of ganglion cell in the retina of the frog while recording in the optic nerve the ganglion cell response to flashes from a microbeam of light. He found that 20 per cent were fibers from *on* ganglion cells, these responding immediately to light and continuing to fire as long as the light was turned on; 50 per cent were found to be *on-off*, firing at the beginning of the light stimulus, then ceasing, and firing again when the light was turned off; 30 per cent were fibers from *off* ganglion cells, firing only when the light was turned off. The receptive fields of the retina appear to be smaller centrally than peripherally, but the field size may vary with the strength of the light stimulus. Hartline showed that *inhibition* plays a part in the response, so that an on response occurs in the optic nerve if the stimulus is displayed in the central part of the field; an off response is obtained if the peripheral field is stimulated; and an on-off response accompanied stimulation in the midperiphery. Numerous studies of animals with rod retinas, cone retinas and photosystems based on retinol and 3-d-retinol have indicated that each nerve axon merely transmits spikes of electrical activity, which have been analyzed by the retina to convey information on the intensity, wavelength, intermittency and movement of the stimulus, spatial relations and the state of adaptation of the eye.

Axon Degeneration

If an axon in the optic nerve is severed, it degenerates in both directions from the site of injury to the ganglion cell bodies in the retina and to the synapse in the lateral geniculate body. Transneuronal degeneration may also occur beyond the geniculate body synapse into the cerebral cortex. The difference between this type of optic nerve fiber degeneration from injury and the wallerian degeneration that occurs in the cerebrospinal and peripheral nerves substantiates the idea that the optic nerve is a central nervous system tract.

EMBRYOLOGY

The optic nerve develops from three sources: the retinal ganglion cell axons, which form the nerve proper; the neuroectodermal layers of the optic stalk, which form the glial system of the nerve; and the associated mesoderm surrounding the optic stalk, which forms the connective tissue and the vascular components of the optic nerve and its meninges. Two mesodermal components have been found: one produces a condensation on the outer surface of the nerve that becomes the meninges, the other is an ingrowth of vascular connective tissue that forms the nerve septa.

The optic stalk appears during the 4 mm. stage (third week) at the same time as the optic vesicle. The stalk is continuous with the forebrain, and a round constriction is formed at their junction. Invagination of the optic vesicle and stalk occurs at the 4.5 mm. stage, with the formation of a fissure along their ventral aspects. The invagination deepens as the stalk lengthens, but it disappears in the region of the forebrain. The primitive epithelial (neuroectodermal) papilla is present at the site where the stalk opens into the optic cup by the 7.5 mm. stage (fourth to fifth week), and the hyaloid artery appears within the recess of the optic fissure at about this time. The lips of the fissure in the optic stalk begin to close over the hyaloid artery by the 10 to 12 mm. stage (fifth week). The closure commences in the region of the prosencephalon and gradually extends distally toward the primitive epithelial papilla. The margins of the invaginated stalk fuse between the 12 and 17 mm. stages (sixth week), producing an external and an internal neuroectodermal layer. The fissure also closes at the optic disc; after this time only a tiny crescentic area remains in the region of the papilla as a remnant of the cavity of the optic cup. During the same period the axons from the retinal ganglion cells move toward the disc, reaching it at about the 16 to 17 mm. stage. As the axons enter the disc tissue, they split off a cone-shaped vascularized mass of glial cells at the disc surface (Bergmeister's papilla). The primitive epithelial papilla soon disappears, its epithelial cells being converted into glial tissue, so that the primitive optic disc is rich in neuroglia. This glia forms a thick mantle around the hyaloid artery at the disc. When the hyaloid vessel system regresses from the vitreous to the disc, a layer of glia is left between the internal surface of the disc and the connective tissue around the newly developing central retinal vessel system. This glial layer is the central connective tissue meniscus of Kuhnt; in late fetal life it undergoes a variable amount of regression to form the physiologic cup.

As the nerve axons grow back into the optic stalk, many cells in the inner layer of neuroectodermal epithelium become vacuolated and show marked irregularities in their contours. Many of these cells are eventually replaced by nerve axons, while those remaining become neuroglia. Simultaneously the outer layer of neuroectodermal epithelium in the stalk is completely transformed into neuroglia that supports and nourishes the nerve fascicles. During the 17 to 24 mm. stage (seventh week), there is condensation of the mesoderm around the stalk to form the optic nerve sheaths. By the end of the seventh week, the retinal axons have reached the recessus opticus and the early optic chiasm appears.

During the 24 to 40 mm. stage (eighth to ninth week) the nerve is formed, decussation occurs in the chiasm, and the optic tracts begin to develop. In the 60 to 70 mm. period (twelfth week), the orbital optic nerve becomes vascularized from vessels that have developed in the mesodermal septa, while the intraocular nerve is supplied from vessels of the hyaloid system. The circle of Zinn can be identified by the 110 to 160 mm. stage (fifth month), branches arising from the circle supply the distal optic nerve region. The nerve measures about 1.2 mm. in diameter and is 7 to 8 mm. long at the 65 to 70 mm. stage (twelfth week). Its diameter increases to 1.9 mm. by the seventh month (200 mm.). During the last month of fetal life the nerve increases in diameter to 2.7 mm. and its length to 24 mm. Medullation commences in the optic tracts at about the seventh month and extends forward to the chiasm about six weeks before birth. By this time the optic nerve is medullated anteriorly almost to the lamina cribrosa region.

The neuroectodermal basis of the lamina cribrosa is laid down at the 8 to 30 mm. stage (sixth to eighth week) by a condensation of glial cells from the outer layer of neuroectodermal epithelium of the stalk. These glial cells are oriented at right angles to the length of the stalk. At about the 140 to 160 mm. stage (fifth month), mesodermal elements from the adjacent sclera migrate into the canal region to form the lamina cribrosa, which is completely formed by the seventh month. The collagen initially forms a palisade along the scleral canal, then sends short and long septa into the nerve between the neuroglial tissue. The short septa extend only a short distance into the nerve and anchor it to the wall of the canal, whereas the long ones extend inward, either joining the connective tissue around the central retinal vessels or completely crossing the canal.

Postnatal Growth

The optic nerve is usually fully medullated within three months after birth, but continues to increase in size for six to eight years. Sylvester and Ari (1961) measured intracranial optic nerve dimensions in 210 patients and found that nerve thickness increases principally from birth to the age of four, with slight thickening until six to eight years of age.

GROSS ANATOMY

The optic nerve pierces the layers of the posterior eye about 3 mm. medial to and very slightly above the posterior pole of the eye. (See Figure 2-3.) The center of the nerve is 4 mm. medial and 0.1 mm. inferior to the center of the macula, 27 mm. from the nasal limbus, and 31 mm. from the temporal limbus. The optic nerve length varies between 35 and 55 mm. from the disc to the chiasm, and the right and left nerves may differ somewhat in length. The optic nerve may be subdivided into intraocular, intraorbital, intracanalicular and intracranial portions; the orbital and intraocular portions are discussed in detail. These parts vary in length, but generally the intraocular nerve is 1 mm. long; the intraorbital nerve length is 25 mm.; the intracanalicular nerve measures 4 to 10 mm.; and the intracranial nerve is 10 mm. long. There is some slack in the intraorbital portion, so that the nerve has two curves, an anterior one with a downward convexity and a posterior one with a lateral convexity.

The diameter of the intraorbital nerve portion is about 3 to 4 mm., while that of the intracranial portion is 4 to 7 mm. At the optic disc the nerve is slightly oval, with a greater vertical diameter. The intraocular portion measures 1.5 mm. in diameter at the disc; myelination of the nerve axons behind the lamina cribrosa increases this diameter to 3 mm., giving the posterior portion of the intraocular optic nerve canal a conical shape.

INTRAOCULAR PORTION

The intraocular optic nerve has three parts—retinal, choroidal and scleral (Figs. 10-1 and 10-2). The nerve may be cylindrical in shape as it passes through the ocular coats if the canal has parallel sides, but a conical shape is more common because the canal often becomes wider in the scleral portion. In rare instances the inner scleral portion of the canal is truncated, so that the canal widens both internally and externally; or the opposite may occur, giving the canal a diamond shape.

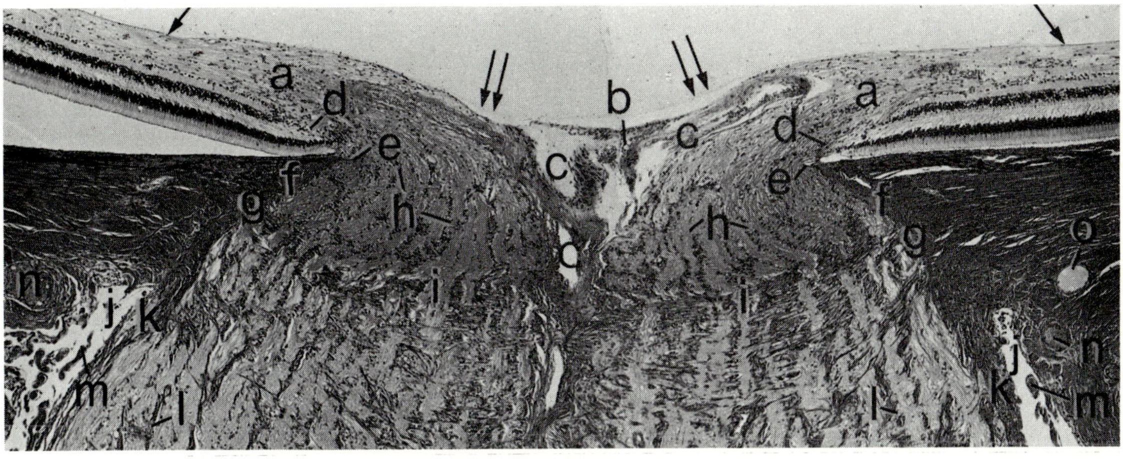

Figure 10–1. Meridional section of the optic disc, surrounding retina and the optic nerve canal. The internal limiting membrane of the retina ends at the single arrows. Internal to the disc surface, the vitreous is very loosely attached (double arrows). The nerve fiber layer becomes thicker at the disc edge (a). The inner limiting membrane of Elschnig and the central meniscus of Kuhnt (b) form the innermost layer of the disc. Beneath it are the central retinal blood vessels and their branches (c). At the edge of the disc, the retina and choroid are shielded from the disc tissues by glial tissue (d). The termination of Bruch's membrane is at (e), the choroidal portion of the canal is at (f), and the scleral portion at (g). The prelaminar glial septae that separate the nerve bundles are seen at (h). The lamina cribrosa (i) traverses the nerve canal and provides a sieve-like meshwork for passage of the optic nerve fibers. The subarachnoid and subdural spaces are seen at the edge of the nerve (j), and the nerve proper is clothed by pia mater (k). The septae of the orbital portion of the nerve (l) subdivide it into compartments. Arachnoidal trabeculae (m) lie outside the pia mater. Dural vessels (n) and the circle of Zinn (o) furnish part of the blood supply to the optic nerve. (× 60.)

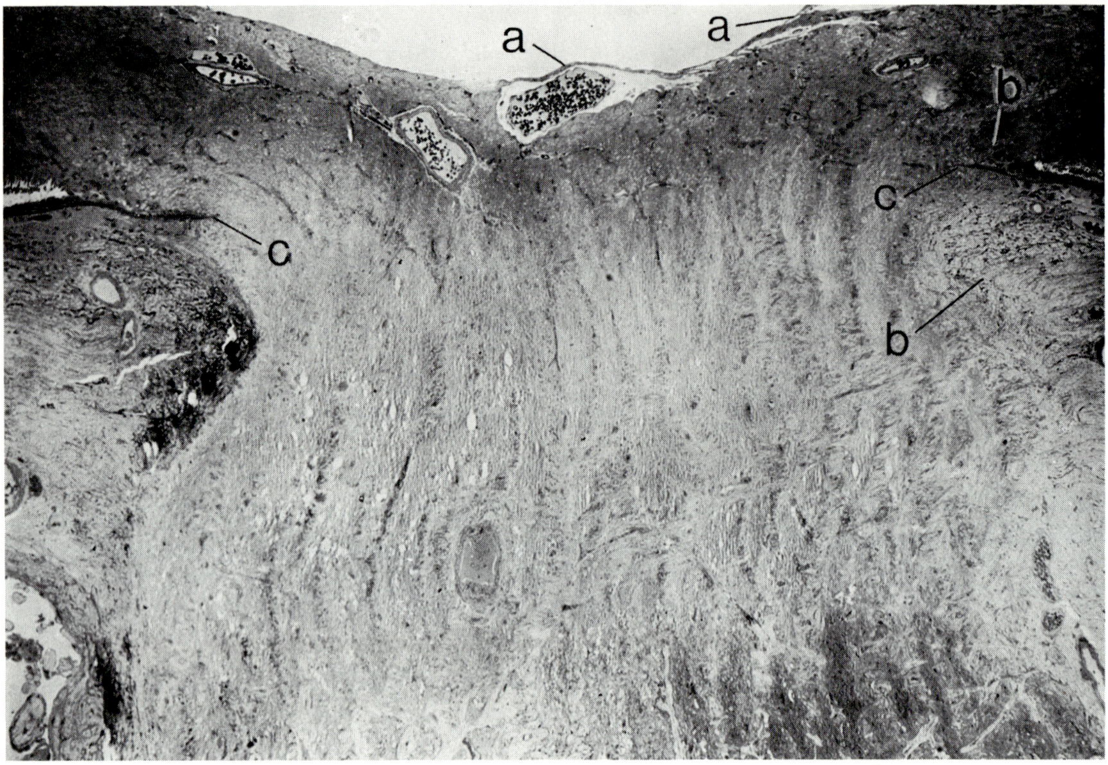

Figure 10-2. Light micrograph of the optic disc near its anterior surface. The inner limiting membrane (a) forms the inner disc and covers the retinal vessels. Glial tissue separates the nerve fiber layer (b) from the adjacent retinal tissue and the choroid. Bruch's membrane ends at (c). (× 75.)

The terms *nerve head, papilla* and *optic disc* have been used interchangeably to describe the retinal and choroidal portions of the optic nerve. *Optic disc* and *nerve head* can be used interchangeably, because they refer to all the tissues comprising the anterior termination of the nerve extending from the disc surface back to the lamina cribrosa. The disc tissues comprise a major part of the intraocular portion of the nerve. The term *papilla* is not exactly synonymous with optic disc and nerve head, however. The papilla is the elevation produced by the large number of nerve axons converging on the disc margin. This elevation can be pronounced or moderate, depending on such factors as the amount and persistence of connective and glial tissue, branching of the central retinal vessels and the size of the disc and cup. Elevation is greatest at the nasal and the superior edge, slightly less inferiorly, and least on the temporal side of the disc. The *internal* disc surface is in contact with the vitreous humor (Fig. 10-2). *Laterally* the nerve axons and their astrocytes are separated from the retina and the choroid by neuroglia. Adjacent to this glia is a layer of connective tissue that is continuous with the framework of the choroid. The *posterior* limit of the disc is at the level of the lamina cribrosa. The scleral portion of the optic nerve contains the lamina cribrosa, a sieve-like connective tissue that supports the nerve fascicles coursing through it.

Posterior to the lamina cribrosa the optic nerve becomes myelinated and the septal system first appears. The septal connective tissue is in continuity laterally with the pial connective tissue and with the lamina cribrosa internally.

Orbital Portion

Behind the eye the optic nerve and its sheaths are in contact with all the tissues within the muscle cone. The extraocular muscles are inserted into the orbital periosteum at the apex of the orbit. Several nerves are located between the optic nerve and the origin of the lateral rectus muscle: two divisions of the third cranial nerve, the nasociliary nerve, the sixth cranial nerve and sympathetic nerve fibers; the ophthalmic vein or veins also may be found here. The long and short ciliary arteries and nerves are closely related to the dural sheath near the posterior eyeball, and the ciliary ganglion lies at the lateral side of the nerve, between it and the lateral rectus muscle. The central retinal artery and vein are in close contact with the inferolateral aspect of the optic nerve and pierce the meningeal sheaths to enter the nerve about 12 mm. posterior to the eyeball.

Intracanalicular Portion

Within the optic nerve canal the dura directly contacts the bone, firmly anchoring the nerve to the canal wall. The dural sheath of the nerve splits into two portions at the orbital end of the optic nerve canal; one portion forms the periosteum of the orbit, and the other becomes the dural sheath of the nerve. For this reason patients with optic neuritis affecting the posterior portion of the nerve may feel pain on rotation of the eye because of traction by the muscles from the dura mater.

The optic nerve is invested with meninges throughout its intraorbital and intracanalicular course. In the intracanalicular portion, the arachnoid is attenuated, whereas in the intracranial portion the dura leaves the nerve to become continuous with the cranial dura. Anteriorly at the eyeball the dura merges with the outer two thirds of the sclera, and the pia-arachnoid ends in the optic nerve canal near the lamina cribrosa. The arachnoid layer is more closely related to the dura than to the pia mater because its trabeculae are closely connected to the dura. The subdural and subarachnoid spaces are continuous with those of the brain; spinal fluid occupies the subarachnoid space of the nerve.

Ophthalmoscopic Correlation

Much work has been done to correlate the ophthalmoscopic appearance with the microscopic structure of the optic disc. The red reflex of the fundus is produced by the reflection of light from the retinal pigment epithelium, plus a small amount of light which diffuses back from the choroidal pigment and blood vessels. The sclera and choroid become visible if the retinal pigment epithelium is missing in any part of the fundus, and for the same reason the optic nerve margin becomes visible where the retinal pigment epithelium ends. The ophthalmoscopic appearance of the disc also must be correlated with the refractive state of the eye and the angle the nerve pursues as it courses through the ocular layers. If the retinal pigment epithelium does not quite reach the edge of the optic nerve, the choroidal edge often becomes visible as a *choroidal crescent* between the border tissue of the canal and the edge of the pigment epithelium. If neither the retinal pigment epithelium nor the choroid reaches the disc edge, the ophthalmoscope shows a scleral *crescent* (Fig. 10-3). In some eyes a *pigment crescent* is seen at the nasal edge of the disc as a result of thickening or folding of the retinal pigment epithelium (Fig. 10-4); ophthalmoscopically this pigment appears as an incomplete pigmented ring (Figs. 10-3 and 10-4).

The course of the nerve through the optic nerve canal also affects the ophthalmoscopic appearance of the disc. Usually this course forms a right angle to the surface of the eye, but in some eyes the optic nerve canal may follow an oblique course (Fig. 10-5). If the nerve axis is oblique toward the temporal side, the ophthalmoscope shows the disc to be tilted; in this case the temporal side is flatter and the temporal optic nerve canal wall becomes visible (Fig. 10-5). In eyes with high myopia, for example, obliquity of the disc is almost always seen with the temporal edge flattened and the nasal edge raised. The tissues on the raised nasal side cover the disc margin, and the optic nerve canal wall is invisible on this side in contrast to its increased visibility temporally. Occasionally the course of the nerve is somewhat oblique nasally, so that ophthalmoscopic examination shows the nasal disc margin to be flatter and the temporal margin raised (Fig. 10–5). At other times an oblique angle inferiorly produces an inferior conus. Both nasal and inferior tilting of the optic disc are pathologic and often are associated with reduced visual acuity.

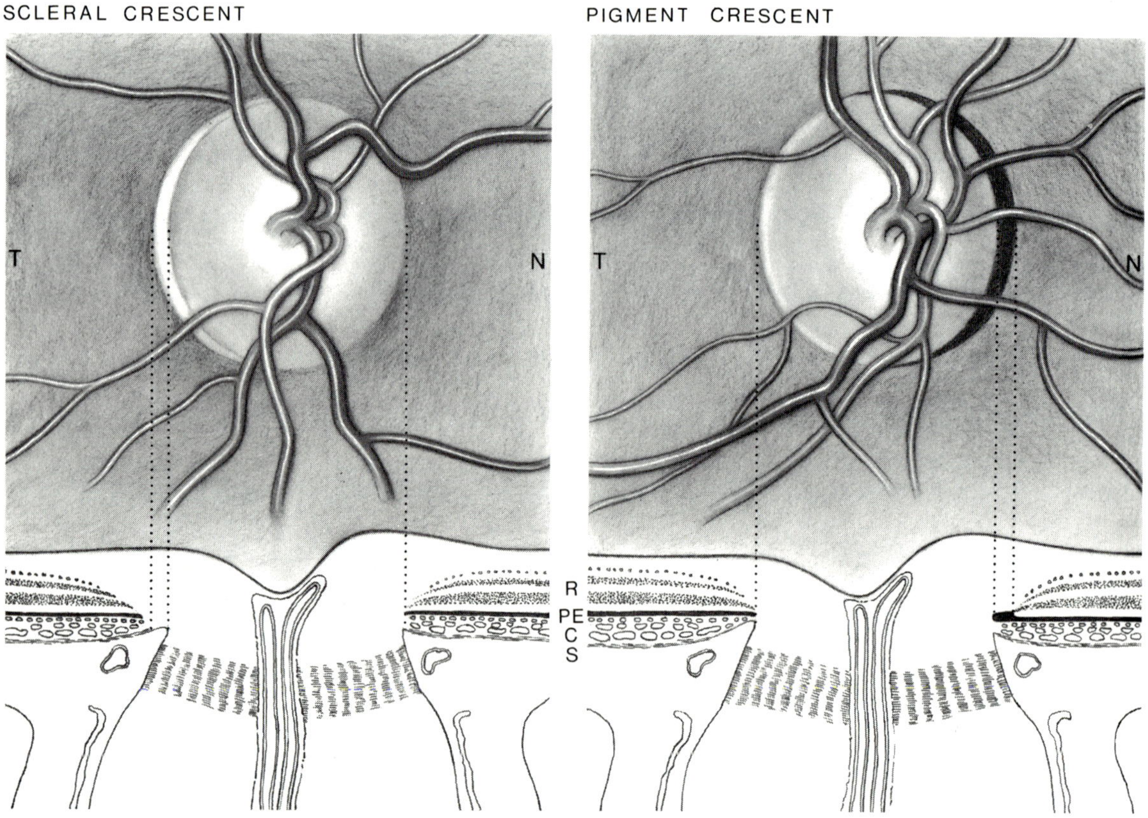

Figure 10–3. Drawing of a scleral crescent as seen ophthalmoscopically and correlated with a histologic section. The letters in this and subsequent drawings are the same. T = temporal; N = Nasal; R = retina; PE = pigment epithelium; C = choroid; S = sclera.

Figure 10–4. Pigment crescent.

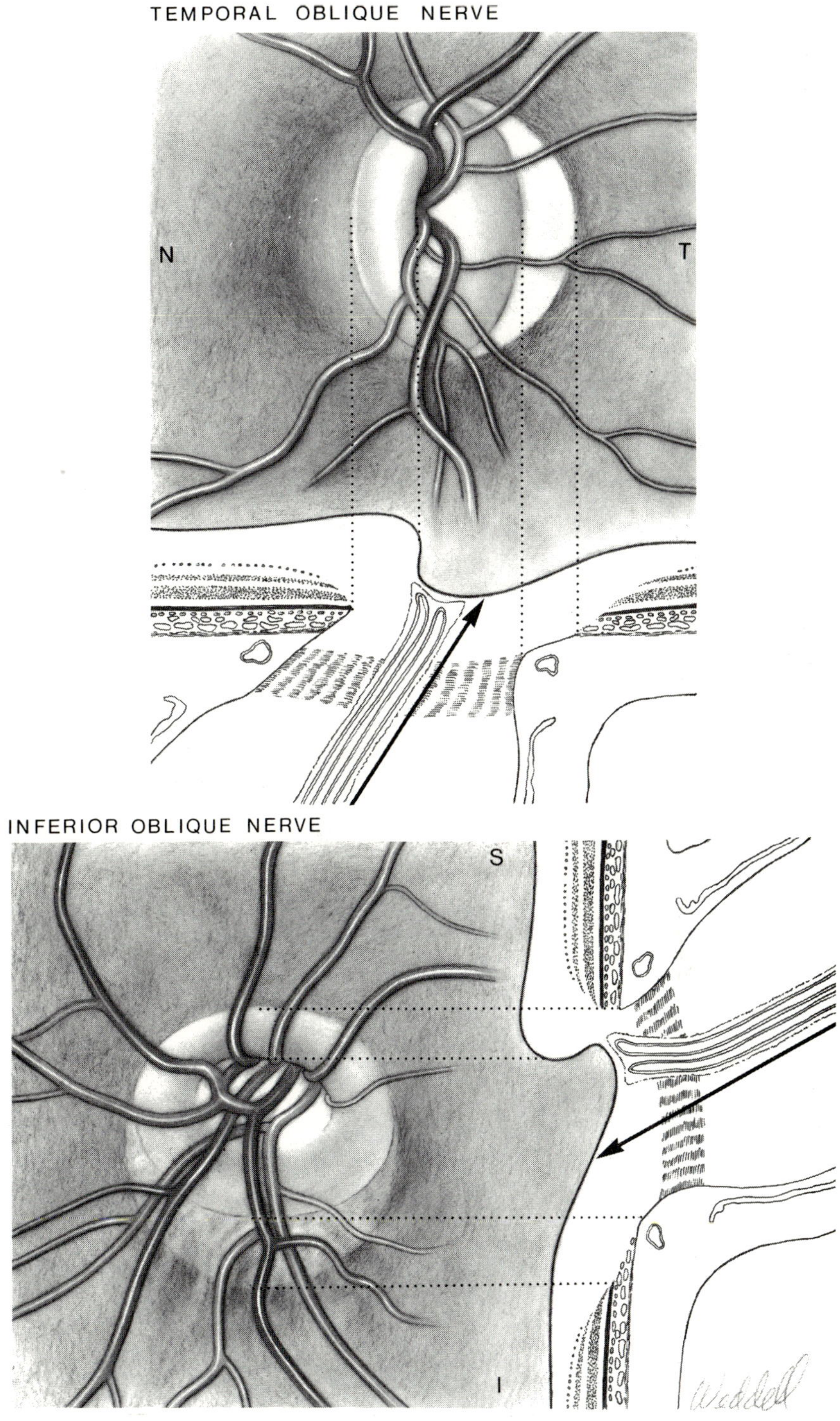

Figure 10–5. Drawings showing the varying direction of the optic nerve through the canal. The arrows depict the axis of the nerve. S = superior; I = inferior.

CYLINDRICAL CUP

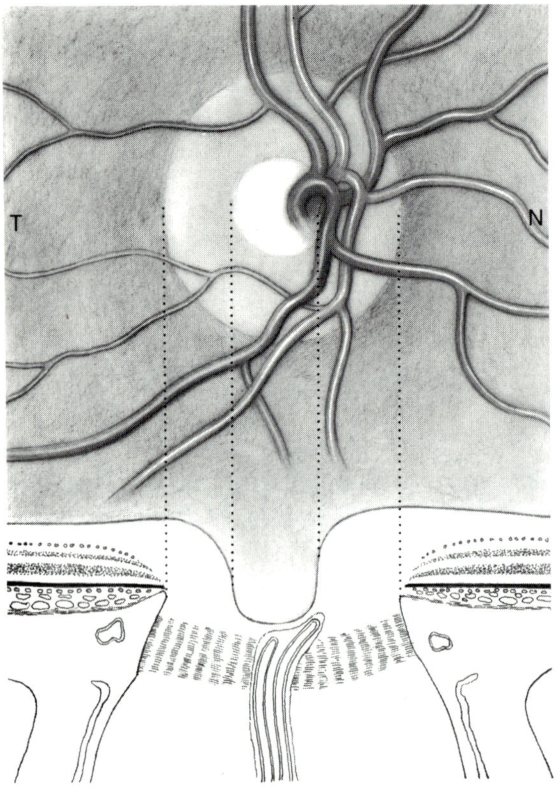

TEMPORAL CUP

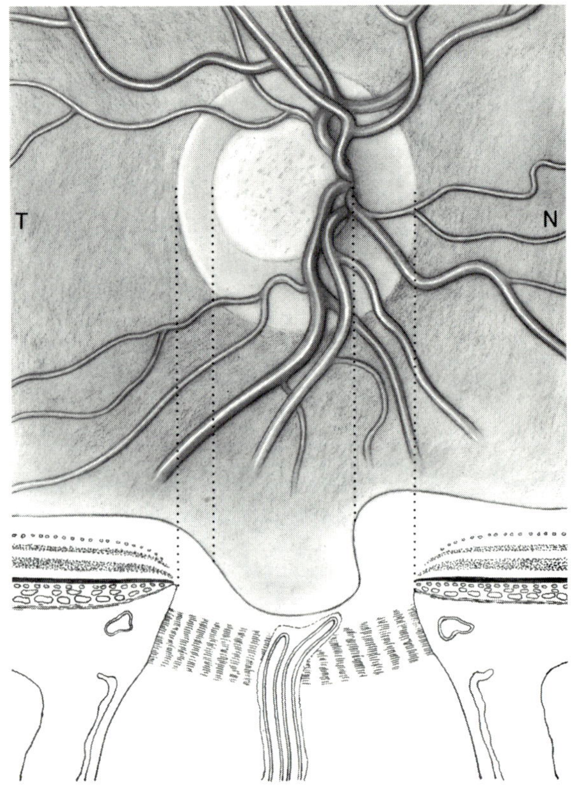

BOWL-SHAPED CUP

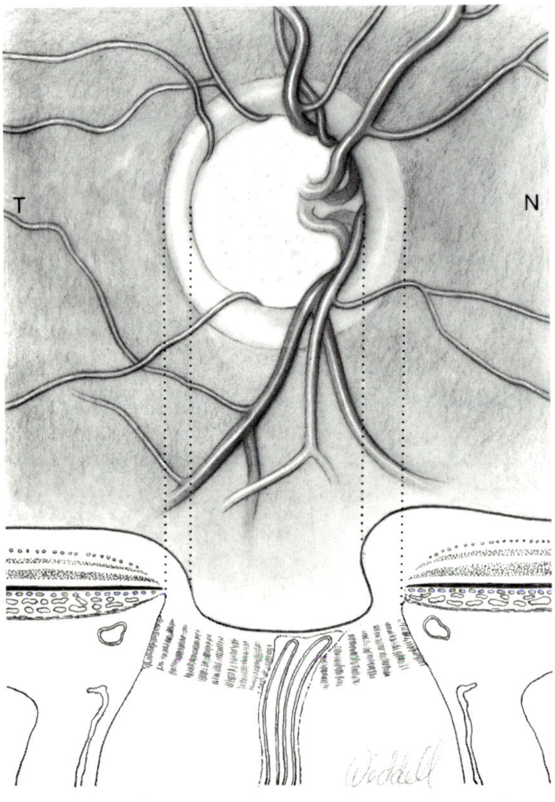

Figure 10–6. Types of physiologic cup in the optic disc.

Almost all eyes have some type of cup or physiologic excavation of the disc. Some of the factors that determine the shape and size of the physiologic excavation are the obliquity of the disc, its size, vessels, and the amount of glial and connective tissue (Fig. 10-6). A small disc in a nerve which courses at a right angle through the eye is associated with a central cylindrical vessel funnel or excavation. A bowl-shaped cup results when the course of the nerve is at a right angle to the sclera and there is less glial tissue within the disc. A larger disc associated with an oblique nerve course usually shows a cup that is larger on the side to which the disc is tilted; a temporal cup is most commonly observed.

Blood Supply

The detailed structure of vessels around and within the optic nerve is included in the descriptions of specific sections of the nerve. Some aspects of the afferent vascular supply to the optic nerve are discussed here.

The arterial branches to the intracranial part of the optic nerve come from the internal carotid artery inferiorly and from the anterior cerebral artery superiorly. The ophthalmic and anterior communicating arteries also furnish some afferent vessels.

In the orbit the ophthalmic artery sends branches to the dura, which then enter the pia mater. The central retinal vein and artery traverse the meningeal sheaths and usually enter the optic nerve on the inferior side, although they occasionally enter inferonasally (Fig. 10-7). Branches from the central retinal artery at its site of entrance into the optic nerve join the pial system; other branches from this artery within the nerve enter into the pial septa to supply the nerve fascicles.

Investigators have debated the source of the blood supply of the anterior optic nerve for many years; early concepts have been modified by development of new techniques for studying blood vessels. Researchers agree that the pial system of vessels contributes the principal blood supply to the optic nerve and that this system arises from branches of the ophthalmic and central retinal arteries. The main controversy recently has centered around the blood supply to the intraocular part of the nerve and the anastomoses between the retinal, pial and ciliary systems. There is disagreement as to the role of the central retinal artery in the nutrition of the intraocular portion of the nerve.

The present interpretation is that the entire intraorbital and intraocular optic nerve is supplied by the ophthalmic artery, primarily through branches arising directly from the artery, but also through branches from other vessels such as the central retinal artery, medial muscular arteries, medial posterior ciliary arteries, posterior ethmoid arteries, supraorbital arteries and other muscular arteries. No axial centrifugal vascular system is apparent in the posterior part of the intraorbital nerve, except for rare recurrent branches from the central retinal artery, which may run back in the center of the optic nerve for 2 to 3 mm.

Anterior to the entrance of the central retinal vessels into the nerve, the pial system of vessels receives its supply from the collateral branches of the ophthalmic artery, central retinal artery, recurrent pial branches from the circle of Zinn and some choroidal vessels. About 75 per cent of the optic

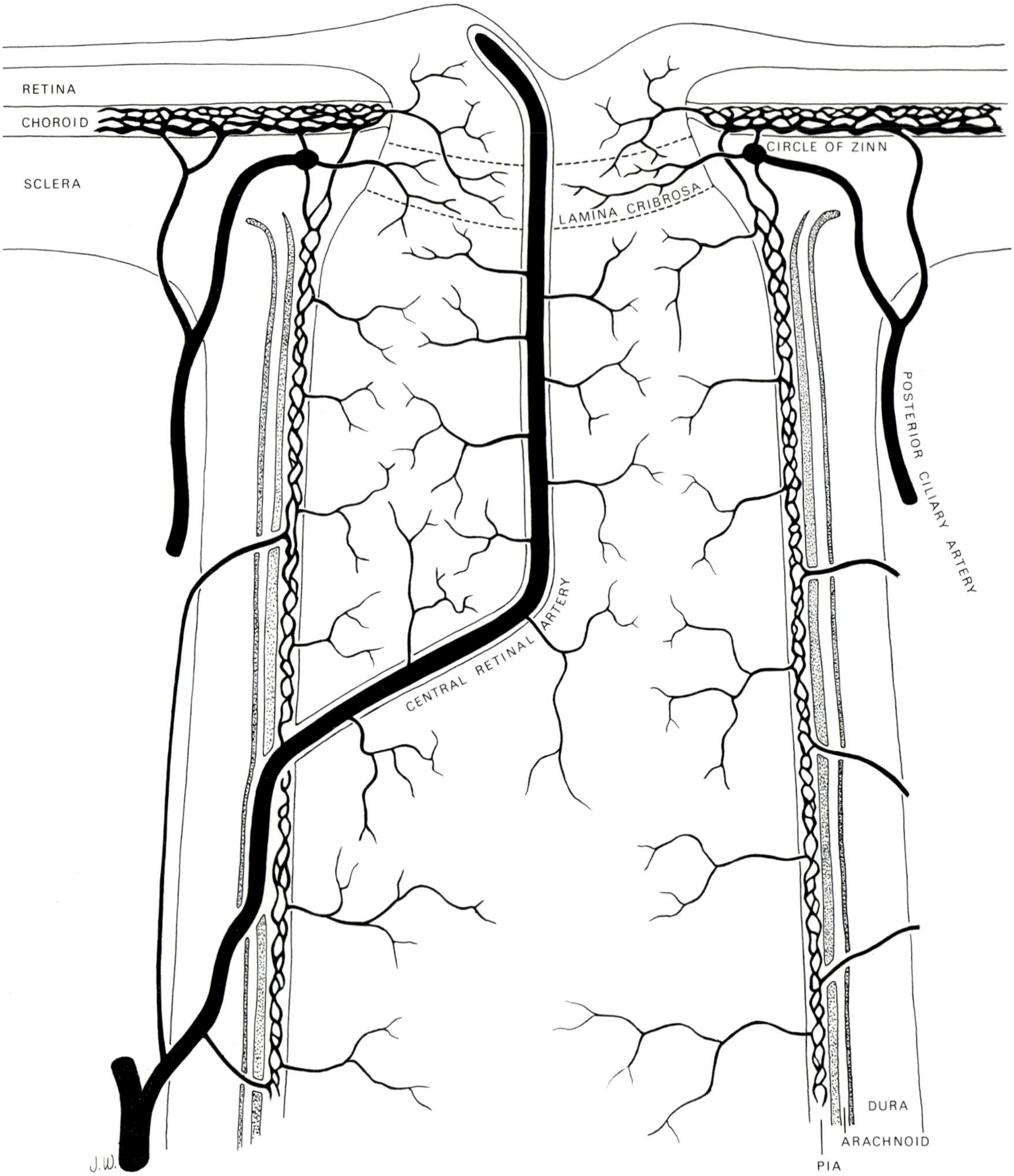

Figure 10–7. Blood supply to the optic nerve, based on the work of Hayreh, 1963. The central retinal artery, a branch of the ophthalmic artery, pierces the dura of the optic nerve approximately 10 to 12 mm. from the eyeball. It sends branches to the pial system of vessels and the central portion of the optic nerve. Some investigators believe the central retinal artery does not nourish the laminar and prelaminar optic nerve. This region is supplied by the circle of Zinn and some branches from the choroid vasculature. The peripheral optic nerve is largely supplied by the pial system of vessels.

nerves studied contain an axial vessel system derived from the central retinal artery, which supplies a variable amount of the central nerve. Some researchers believe that there is a "central artery of the optic nerve" that supplies the disc region (Behr, 1935; Francois et al., 1954, 1955, 1956; Wybar, 1956; Wolff, 1968). Others disagree with this concept after demonstrating the many anatomoses between the pial vessels and branches from the circle of Zinn in the disc region, as well as the absence of a specific artery to the disc tissues (Beauvieux and Ristitch, 1924; Steele and Blunt, 1956; Hayreh, 1963, 1966). The choroidal vessels have recently been shown to send branches to the prelaminar optic nerve. In the primate these vessels appear to be end arteries that supply segments of the nerve (Hayreh, 1969).

Current techniques cannot demonstrate every interconnection between the pial system, the central retinal artery branches and the circle of Zinn, but certainly many arteriolar and capillary interconnections exist among these vessels. In fact, the vessels are so closely related that it would seem odd if each did not participate in the nutrition of the intraocular nerve.

Retinal Source of the Optic Nerve Fibers

First it is important to review the general organization of the nerve and the distribution of its axons as they pass from the retina to form the nerve (Fig. 10-8). Many studies have been designed to evaluate the orientation of the retinal nerve axons as they cross the optic disc. Investigators have produced large and small retinal injuries near the disc, in the macular region, above and below the temporal raphé and in the peripheral retina, using either a sharp instrument or a light coagulator. Degenerative changes in the nerve were then evaluated with special staining techniques.

A vertical line through the center of the fovea divides the retinal ganglion cells into two groups: those related to the temporal hemiretina, and those related to the nasal hemiretina (including a temporal and a nasal hemimacula, respectively). This subdivision is important for the assessment of visual fields because axons arising in the nasal hemiretina cross in the chiasm, while axons arising in the temporal hemiretina do not cross. The ganglion cells in the retina can also be subdivided into an upper and lower hemiretina by a line passing horizontally through the center of the fovea and the optic disc. These vertical and horizontal lines divide the retinal ganglion cells into four quadrants. The ganglion cells in each quadrant are responsible for vision in that quadrant, including the macula and fovea. Most of the nerve fibers in the macular region and those of each quadrant of the retina of one eye have corresponding cells in the retina of the fellow eye, making binocular vision possible. Some cells in the peripheral nasal retina are concerned only with uniocular vision, however, because of the position of the eyes in the head.

The axons from the retinal ganglion cells converge on the optic disc in a fairly regular pattern. Those from the nasal, superior and inferior retina have a rather straight course, while the axons arising in the temporal retina follow a curved path toward the disc. Those axons which arise from ganglion cells in the retina temporal to the disc form the papillomacular bundles, which pass in gentle curves toward the temporal as well as the upper and lower disc. All the axons from the upper and lower macula peripheral to the

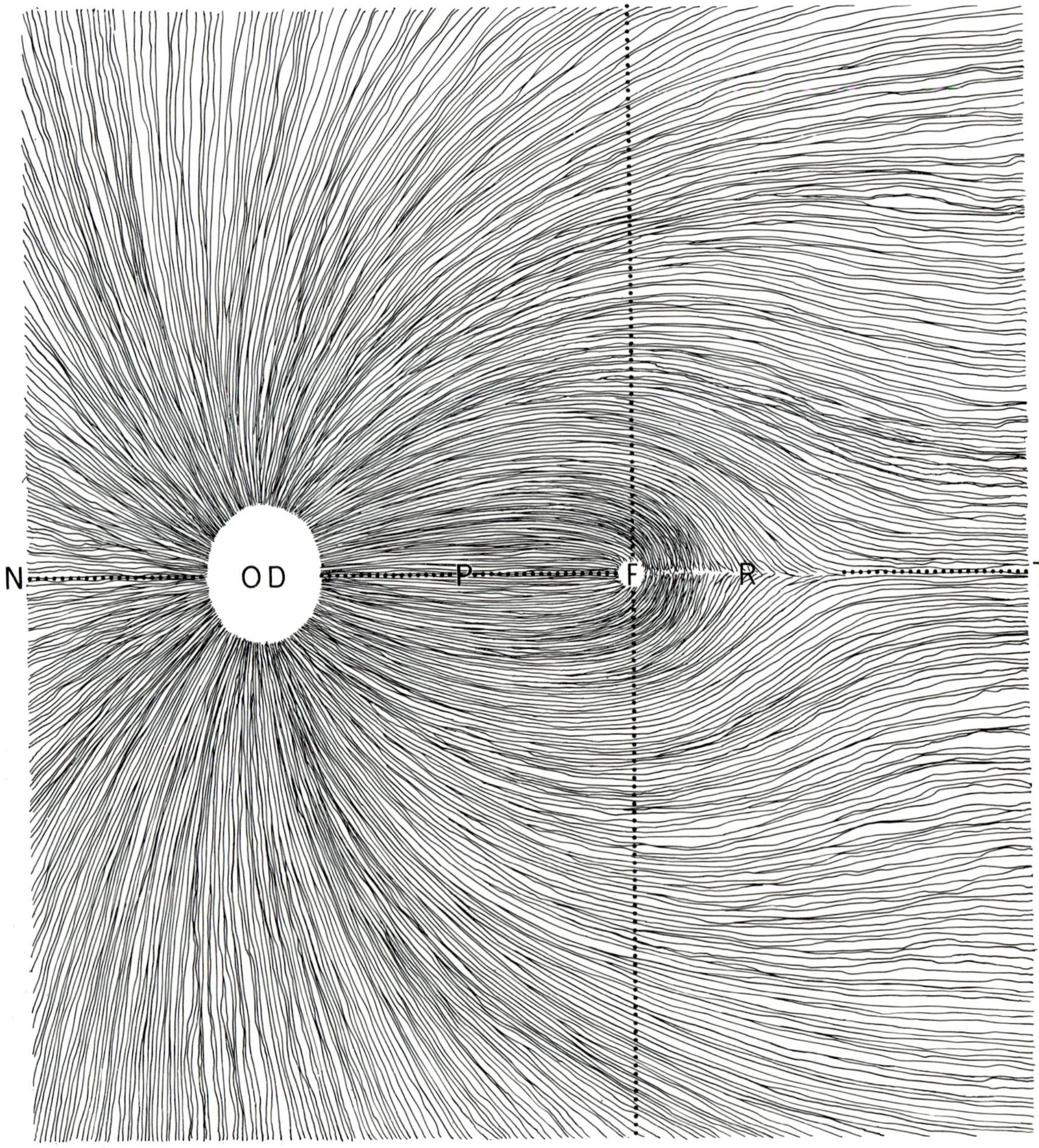

Figure 10–8. Drawing of the retinal nerve axons as they extend from the ganglion cells to the disc. The superior, inferior, and nasal axons are fairly straight. The course of the temporal axons is curved, and becomes increasingly greater in the macular region. The axons arising from the nasal macula extend directly toward the optic disc (OD) as the papillomacular bundle (P). Temporal to the fovea (F) is the horizontal raphé (R). In the region of the raphé the courses of the axons are of three types – vertical, oblique, and triangular. The vertical axons are more numerous. The dotted lines delineate the nasal, temporal, superior and inferior hemiretina. N = Nasal; T = Temporal.

fovea arch above and below the horizontal meridian to enter the upper and lower temporal disc. Axons arising in the temporal macula and retina that originate above the horizontal meridian (raphé) pass to the upper disc, while those arising below the horizontal raphé go to the lower disc. Vrabec (1966) showed that the horizontal raphé is confined to temporal fibers comprising the macular complex and does not include the axons arising in the temporal peripheral retina.

Axons from the peripheral retina enter the peripheral portion of the optic nerve, while those from the posterior retina enter the central nerve. The macular fibers lie along the temporal aspect of the disc. Hoyt and Tudor (1963) have shown that axons arising from the area between the disc and macula pass directly to the disc where they cross its temporal edge. Hoyt (1962), using the Nauta stain to detect axon degeneration after producing photocoagulative lesions in the retina, found that the arcuate papillomacular bundles pass through the disc and nerve in a stable way without rotation during their passage through the optic nerve and chiasm. The macular fibers were found to occupy the upper and lower temporal portions of the optic nerve. Hoyt and Luis (1962), using the same technique, confirmed that the peripheral retinal fibers occupy the peripheral portion of the optic nerve. They also found that the macular fibers are located temporally in the optic nerve immediately around the eye, but they are diffusely distributed in the nerve posteriorly. These authors, however, did not confirm the common assertion that there is rotation of the retinal quadrants about 45 degrees clockwise in the right eye and counterclockwise in the left eye between the eye and the chiasm.

Nerve Axons

Each optic nerve is composed of 800,000 to one million fibers (Polyak, 1941). The optic nerves contain 38 per cent of all the afferent fibers of the combined cranial nerves. In the orbital portion of the optic nerve, the fibers are organized into about 800 to 1200 fascicles, each surrounded by a pial sheath (Deyl, 1895). These fascicles interanastomose, often being incompletely segregated by the pial septa; they are segregated by neuroglial septa, however. The axons that form the nerve have been reported to vary in thickness between 0.7 and 10 μm., most of them measuring close to 1 μm. Polyak (1941) furnished statistical evidence that the smaller axons come from the midget bipolar and midget ganglion cells of the central part of the retina, and that the larger axons come from the ganglion cells of the peripheral retina.

Oppel (1963) examined the number and thickness of the myelinated nerve fibers of the human optic nerve. He found the nerve to have an area of 6.509 sq. mm., with the nerve fibers occupying 5.275 sq. mm. and the septa 1.234 sq. mm. of this area. He calculated the number of axons to be 1,186,172. Three sizes of nerve axons were described: larger (from the small diffuse and garland ganglion cells), which form 1.9 per cent of the axon types; intermediate size (from the parasol and shrub ganglion cells), which form 5.9 per cent of the axons; and small (from the midget ganglion cells), which compose 92.2 per cent of the myelinated fibers.

Kupfer and co-workers (1967) studied the optic nerves, chiasm, tracts and geniculate bodies in a patient who had undergone unilateral enucleation for a malignant melanoma of the choroid two years previously. They estimated the number of optic nerve axons to be between 1,060,100 and 1,126,268, and established the ratio of crossed to uncrossed fibers in the chiasm as 53:47. Most nerve axons measured 0.5 μm. or more in diameter and the authors believed that all these axons arise from the retinal ganglion cells, since silver stains did not reveal centrifugal nerve fibers in the optic nerve on the enucleated side. Cell counts in the lateral geniculate body showed the overall ratio of optic nerve axons to postsynaptic cells to be 1:1. The ratio of lateral geniculate cells in crossed laminae to those in uncrossed laminae was 58:42, a comparison favorable to the ratios in the chiasm.

MICROSCOPIC ANATOMY

Intraocular Optic Nerve

To facilitate the description of the intraocular part of the optic nerve we will use the classification of Hayreh and Vrabec (1966): *prelaminar, laminar* and *postlaminar.* (See Figure 10-1.) The *prelaminar* portion is composed of the nerve axons, the neuroglia and the blood vessels with their connective tissue anterior to the lamina cribrosa. The *laminar* portion includes the nerve axons and their neuroglia, the collagen of the lamina cribrosa, and the vessels with their supporting tissue in the scleral portion of the lamina cribrosa. The *postlaminar* portion includes a small part of the nerve and the sheath up to the point behind the lamina cribrosa where the nerve exits from the eye.

Prelaminar Portion (Figs. 10-9 to 10-30). The vitreal surface of the disc has no internal limiting membrane like that over the retina, containing instead a thin layer of astrocytes known as the *inner limiting membrane of Elschnig* (Fig. 10-11). This layer is often quite thick in the physiologic cup; the thickened tissue is called the *central meniscus of Kuhnt.* In eyes that have a large physiologic cup, the central meniscus of Kuhnt is attenuated as a result of resorption of the glial tissue associated with Bergmeister's papilla. In eyes with a small cup, this tissue is often much thicker.

Commencing at the margin of the optic disc, the retinal axons curve rather sharply across the disc to form the optic nerve (Fig. 10-9). Near the disc edge, as the Müller cells disappear, the axons become segregated into bundles or fascicles by neuroglial cells that are oriented at right angles to the fascicles (Fig. 10-10). These neuroglial cells are astrocytes which form tube-like boundaries around all the nerve bundles. Wolter (1957) found that the astrocytes form a three-dimensional, basket-like network in the disc tissue, with the convexity of the basket directed forward toward the vitreous. This astrocytic network surrounds the fascicles and is continuous from the retinal edge back through the lamina cribrosa and the orbital optic nerve.

The retinal layers terminate regularly as they reach the edge of the disc (Fig. 10-12). Among these layers the retinal pigment epithelium extends farthest into the disc, although it usually ends somewhat sooner than Bruch's membrane. The nuclear and plexiform layers cease before reaching the disc edge because the thickening nerve fiber layer crowds other retinal

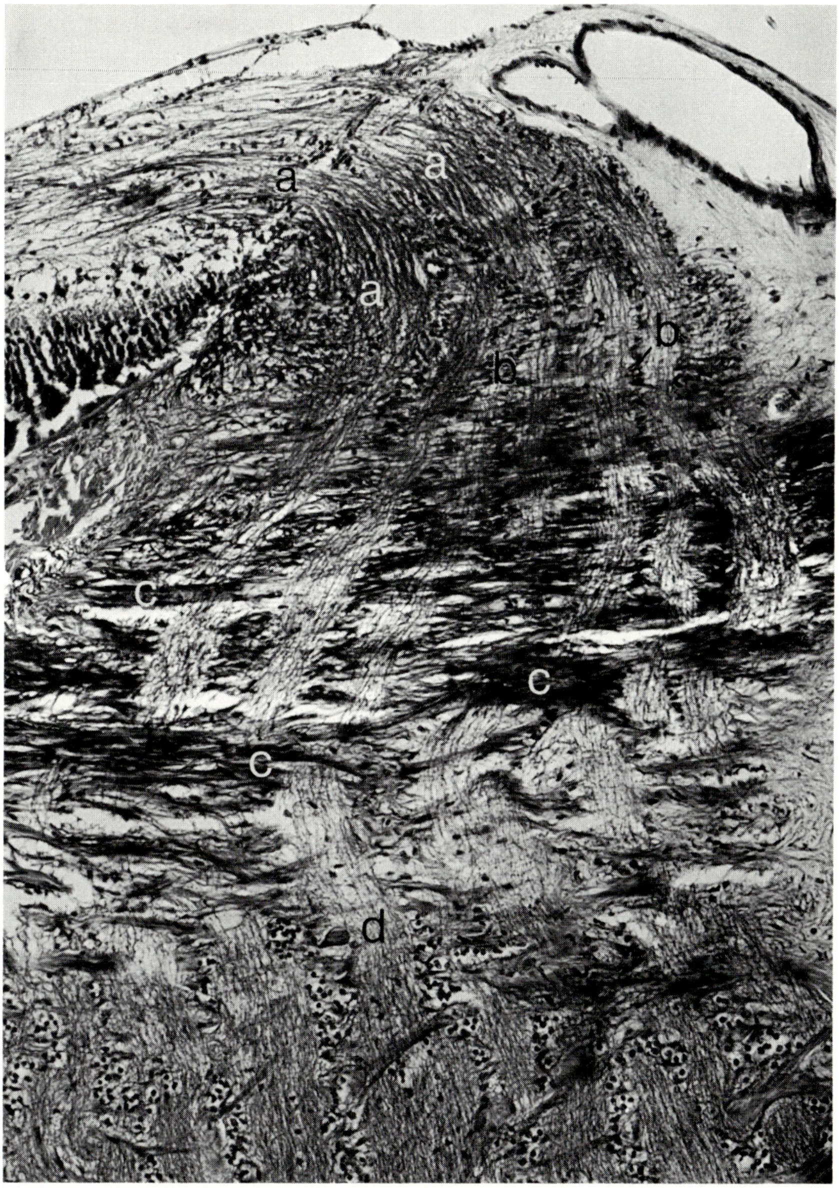

Figure 10-9. The axons from the retinal nerve fiber layer curve sharply as they leave the retina to enter the optic disc (a). They are aggregated into fascicles, which are surrounded by glial columns (b), and then continue through the lamina cribrosa (c). Just posterior to the lamina (d) the axons become myelinated. (× 110.)

layers away from the disc edge. A layer of glial tissue, the *intermediary tissue of Kuhnt,* is interposed between the retinal layers and the nerve fiber bundles at the disc edge (Fig. 10-12 *B*).

The termination of the choroidal layers at the edge of the optic nerve canal has been discussed (p. 325). Choroidal collagen and nerve bundles are separated from each other by a mantle of glial tissue, which is continuous anteriorly with that separating the retinal layers and posteriorly with the tissue separating the sclera and optic nerve. External to this mantle the elastica of Bruch's membrane and the choroidal collagen become

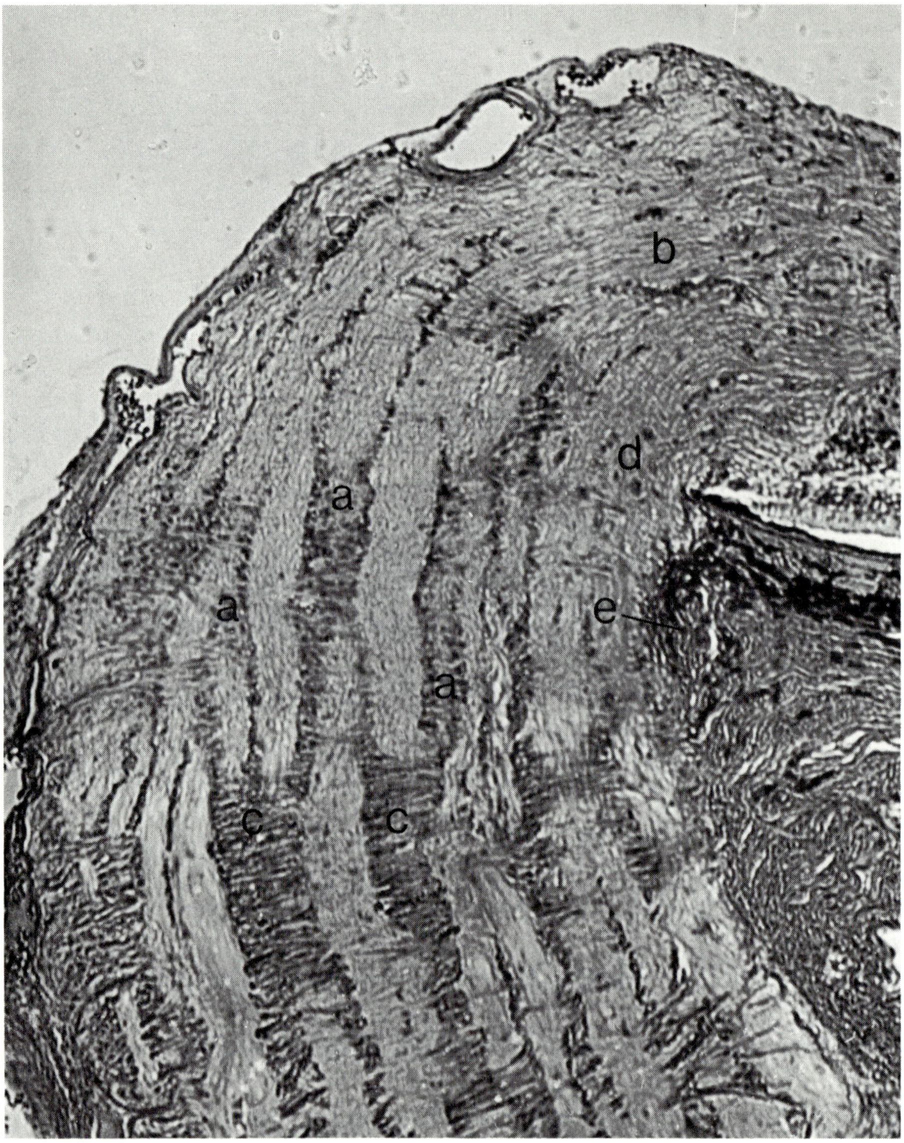

Figure 10–10. Light micrograph of the glial columns (a) in the prelaminar portion of the optic nerve. The columns commence in the disc tissues at the edge of the retina (b) and continue to the lamina cribrosa (c). The end of Bruch's membrane (d) and the termination of the choroid (e) form the inner limit of the prelaminar canal. (× 228.)

oriented more circularly around the canal. Near the lamina cribrosa, the transverse glial septa of the choroidal portion become thicker.

Neuroglia. It should be emphasized that the astrocytes of the prelaminar portion of the optic nerve have the same structure and orientation as those of the laminar and orbital portions. They form continuous circular tubes that enclose all fascicles of nerve axons in the prelaminar, laminar, postlaminar and orbital portions. The astrocytes are altered somewhat in the different portions of the nerve by the interposition of other tissues, such as the collagen of the lamina cribrosa, the pial septa and the marginal connective tissue of the choroidal and scleral parts of the optic nerve canal. Even in

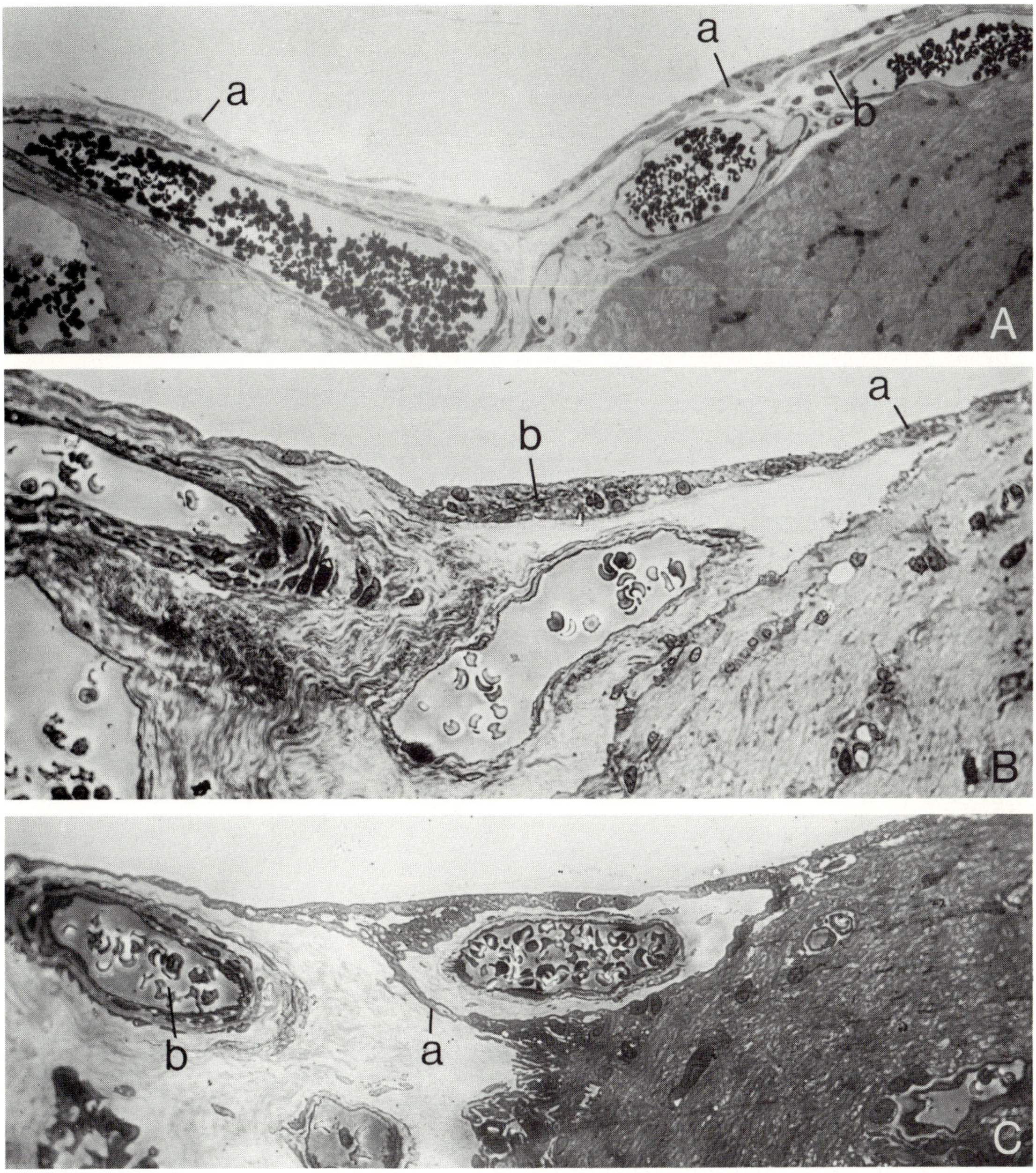

Figure 10–11. Light micrographs of the inner portion of the optic disc. *A*, The inner limiting membrane of Elschnig (a) forms a glial layer which separates the vitreous from the disc tissues. It frequently splits (b) to enter the adventitia of the disc vessels and is separated from their media by connective tissue. (× 220.)

B, Enlargement to show the inner limiting membrane (a) and the central meniscus of Kuhnt (b). They are intimate with the connective tissue of the central retinal vessels. (× 475.)

C, The inner disc region to show the two layers described in *B*. In this photograph the glial tissue of these layers splits to surround a retinal vein. This perivascular glia is known as the intercapillary tissue of Kuhnt (a). A branch of the central artery is at (b). (× 480.)

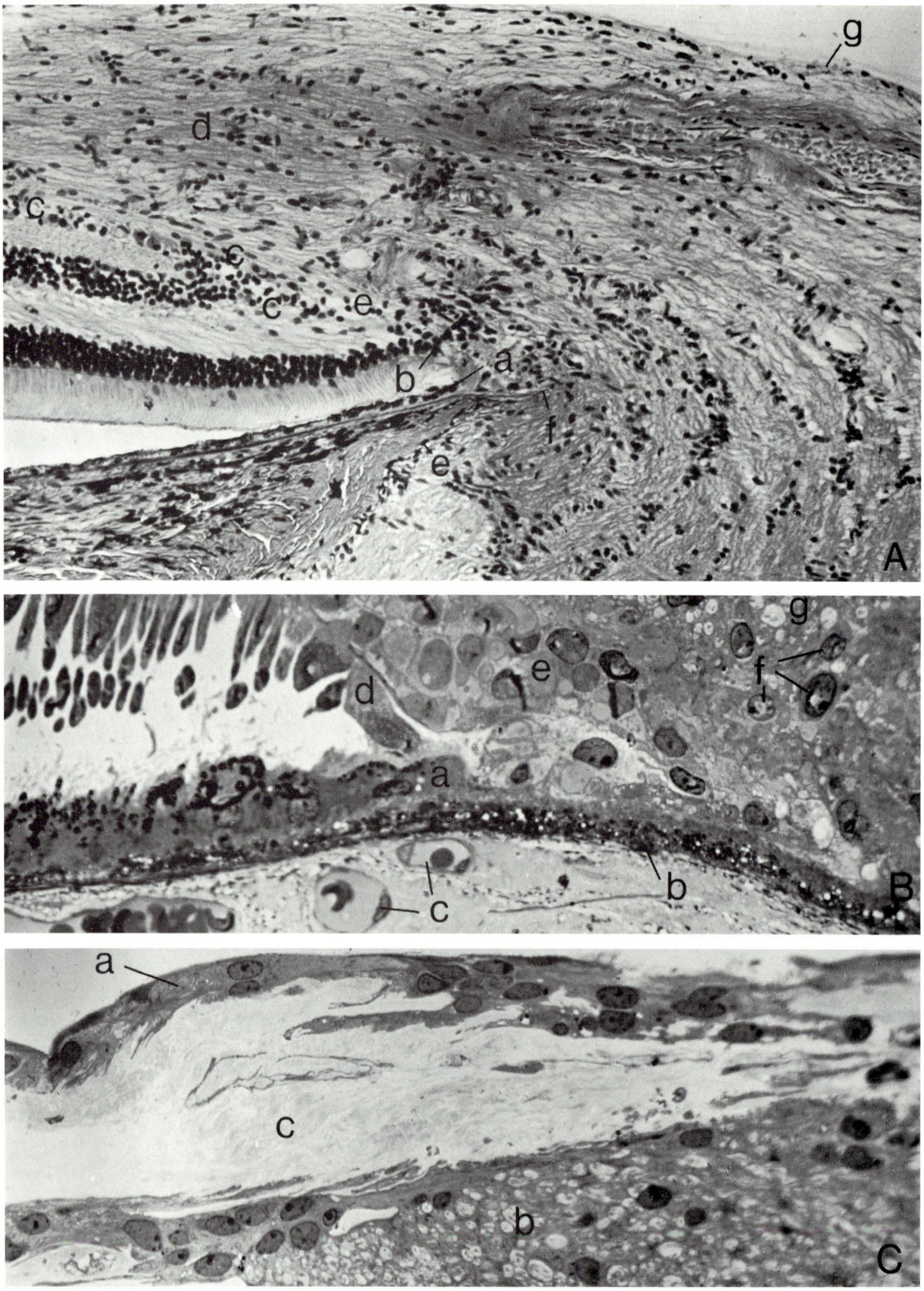

Figure 10-12. *See legend on opposite page.*

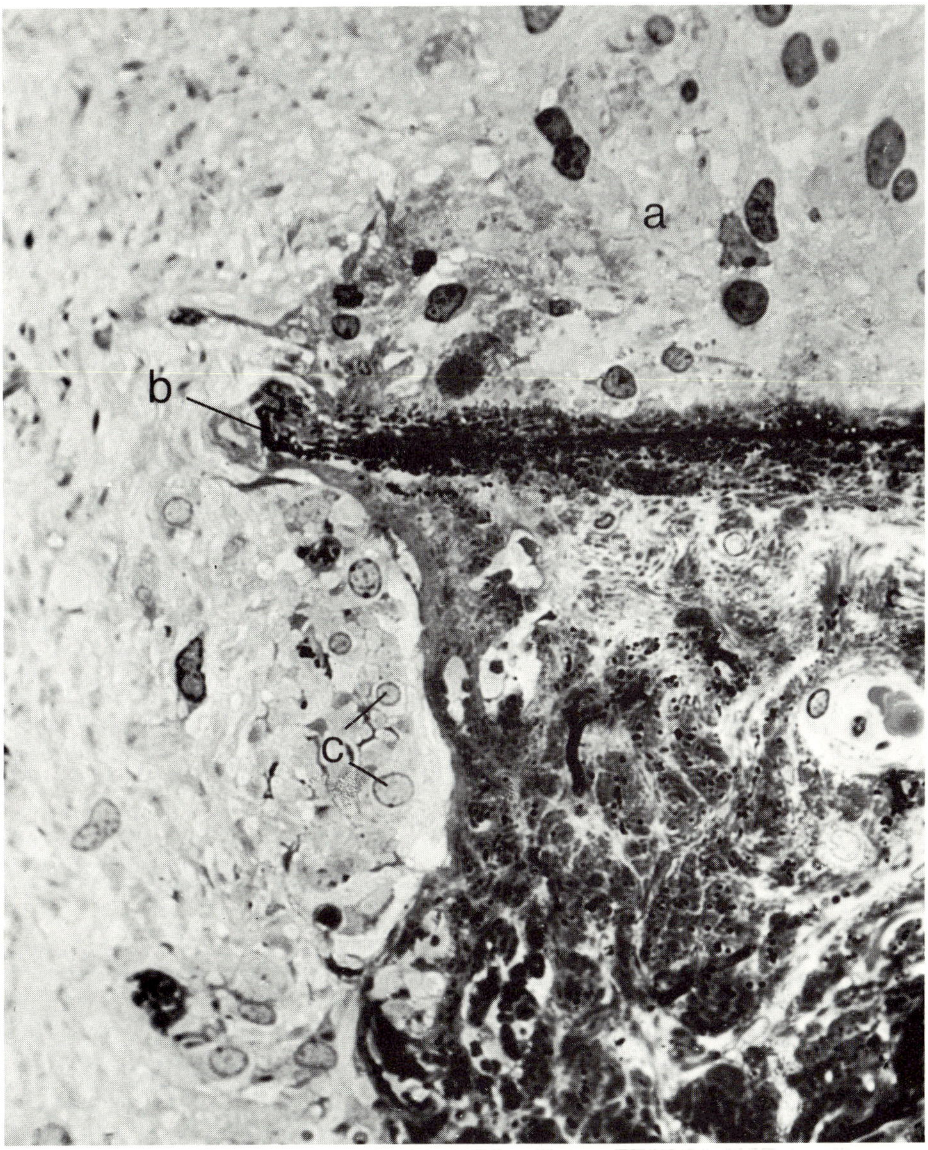

Figure 10–13. Light micrograph of the choroidal portion of the optic nerve canal. The glial tissue of the retinal edge is at (a) and the termination of Bruch's membrane at (b). The border tissue of Jacoby (c) separates the collagen of the choroid from the optic nerve bundles. (× 575.)

Figure 10–12. Light micrographs of the termination of the retina at the edge of the optic disc. *A*, The retinal pigment epithelium (a) is the closest to the disc tissues, and the external nuclear layer (b) terminates at almost the same position. The other retinal layers terminate farther from the disc (c). The nerve fiber layer becomes thicker as it approaches the disc (d). The intermediary tissue of Kuhnt separates the retina and choroid from the optic nerve (e). Bruch's membrane terminates at (f). The inner disc contains the glia of the inner limiting membrane (g). (× 170.)

B, The outer retina extends closer to the optic nerve, the pigment epithelium (a) terminating earlier than Bruch's membrane (b). The choriocapillaris ends at (c), and the retinal photoreceptors at (d). Some cells of the outer nuclear layer (e) overlie the pigment epithelium. The glial tissue (f) separates the retina from the nerve axons in the nerve fiber layer (g). (× 820.)

C, Peripheral optic disc at its internal surface. The glial cells of the inner limiting membrane (a) are separated from the axons of the nerve fiber layer (b) by connective tissue that surrounds the central vessels (c). (× 820.)

the areas where the pial septa are incomplete in the orbital portion of the nerve, the astrocytes continue to surround the nerves in each fascicle.

With the electron microscope the astrocytes surround the fascicles and their long processes extend into the fascicles (Figs. 10-14 and 10-15). Identification of astrocytes in the prelaminar portion of the nerve is facilitated by previous light microscopic studies which have revealed astrocytes to be the only supporting cells for the nerve bundles. By electron microscopy these prelaminar cells exhibit all the characteristics of astrocytes in the brain, making it easier to differentiate them from oligodendrocytes in the postlaminar nerve.

The general orientation of the astrocytes in this region also is circular, around the surfaces of the fascicles; thus, they are essentially at right angles to the axons. The astrocytes at the retinal edge are oriented somewhat parallel to the axons, forming the *intermediary tissue of Kuhnt.*

The nuclear chromatin of astrocytes in the prelaminar region is more condensed than that in the orbital nerve portion. The nucleus is surrounded by a thin layer of cytoplasm that contains most of the organelles in these cells. The Golgi apparatus, mitochondria, ribosomes and a moderate amount of endoplasmic reticulum are concentrated at the nuclear pole. The Golgi apparatus of these cells is unusual in being composed of tubular elements instead of flattened cisternae and vesicles. The astrocytic processes contain an enormous number of fibrils, and the processes of adjacent glial cells frequently are joined by desmosomes and tight junctions (Figs. 10-16 to 10-21).

The astrocytes of Elschnig's inner limiting membrane form a distinct layer adjacent to the vitreous (Figs. 10-20 to 10-23). The innermost layer of these cells has a basement membrane facing the vitreous which is thinner than that of the retinal Müller cells. This membrane has a uniform thickness of about 600 A. and is separated from the cell membrane by a less dense zone measuring about 200 A. Over the lateral third of the optic disc the inner limiting membrane of Elschnig is composed of thicker processes of three to four cells, while centrally it is composed of the smaller processes of only two or three cells. The collagen outside the walls of branches from the central retinal vessels is covered by the processes of this central glial tissue, which frequently splits to form a sheath around the vessels.

Several layers of astrocytes lie between the retinal and choroidal margins and the nerve axons at the disc edge. The *intermediary glial tissue of Kuhnt* at the retinal edge is continuous with the choroidal edge where it is known as the *layer of Jacoby* (Fig. 10-24). These cells have the same structure as astrocytes elsewhere, except that their cell bodies are flattened and their processes are thinner. They form a column around the circumference of the nerve canal, sending processes internally among the nerve bundles. Astrocytes also invest the connective tissue of all vessels entering this portion of the disc.

Other astrocytes found in the prelaminar area are oriented parallel to the course of the axons and greatly resemble the branching astrocyte of the lamina cribrosa region (Anderson et al., 1967). The cytoplasm of these cells shows fewer fibrils than those of the lamina cribrosa, however, and they are found mainly around the blood vessels (Figs. 10-25 and 10-26).

Axons (Figs. 10-27 to 10-30). Because the unmyelinated axons are very closely grouped within the fascicles, they are separated only occasion-

Text continued on page 561

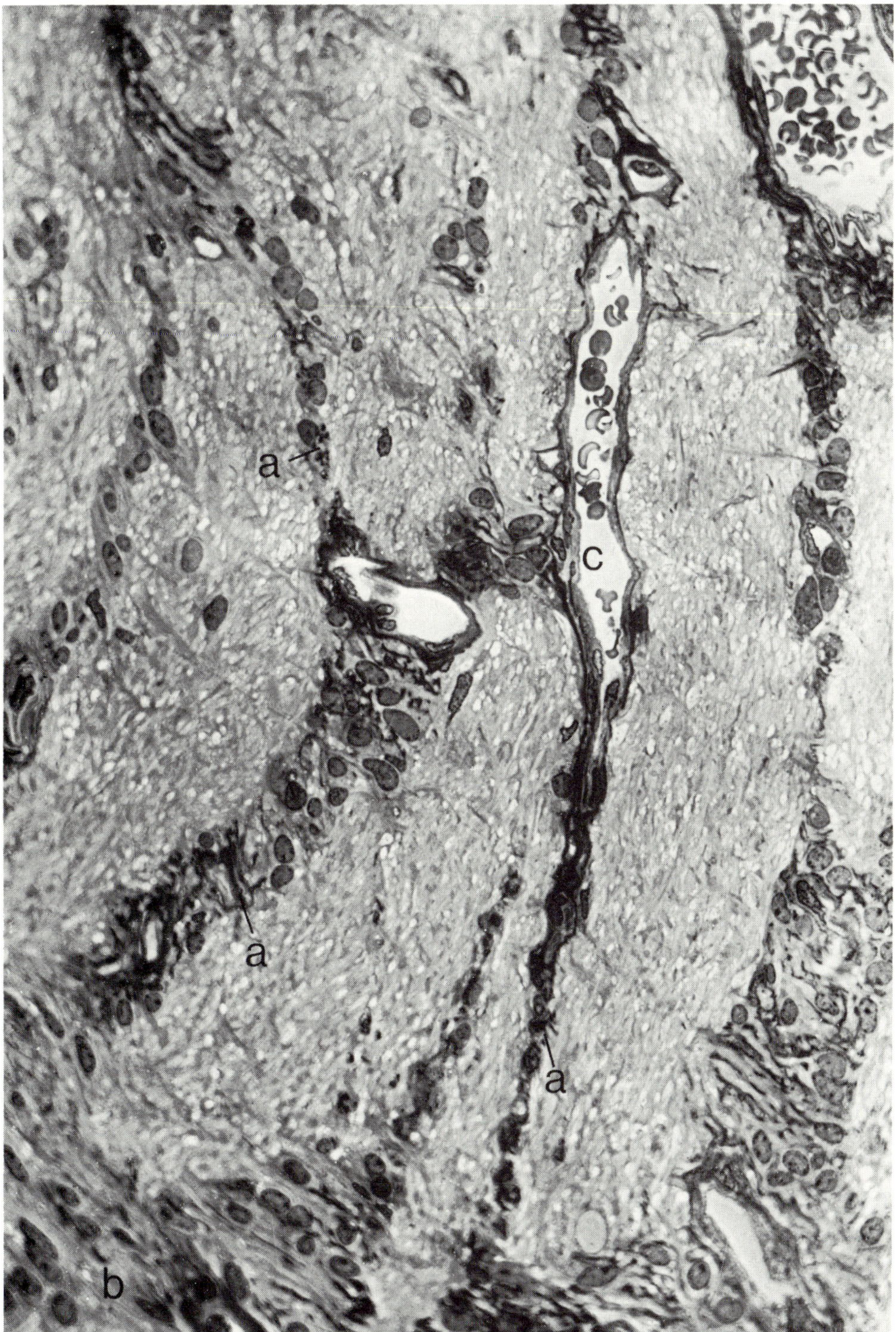

Figure 10–14. Light micrograph of the glial columns (a) in the prelaminar portion of the optic nerve as they extend back to join the lamina cribrosa (b). Cross-sections of the glial cells are seen. Some columns contain longitudinally coursing vessels (c). (× 550.)

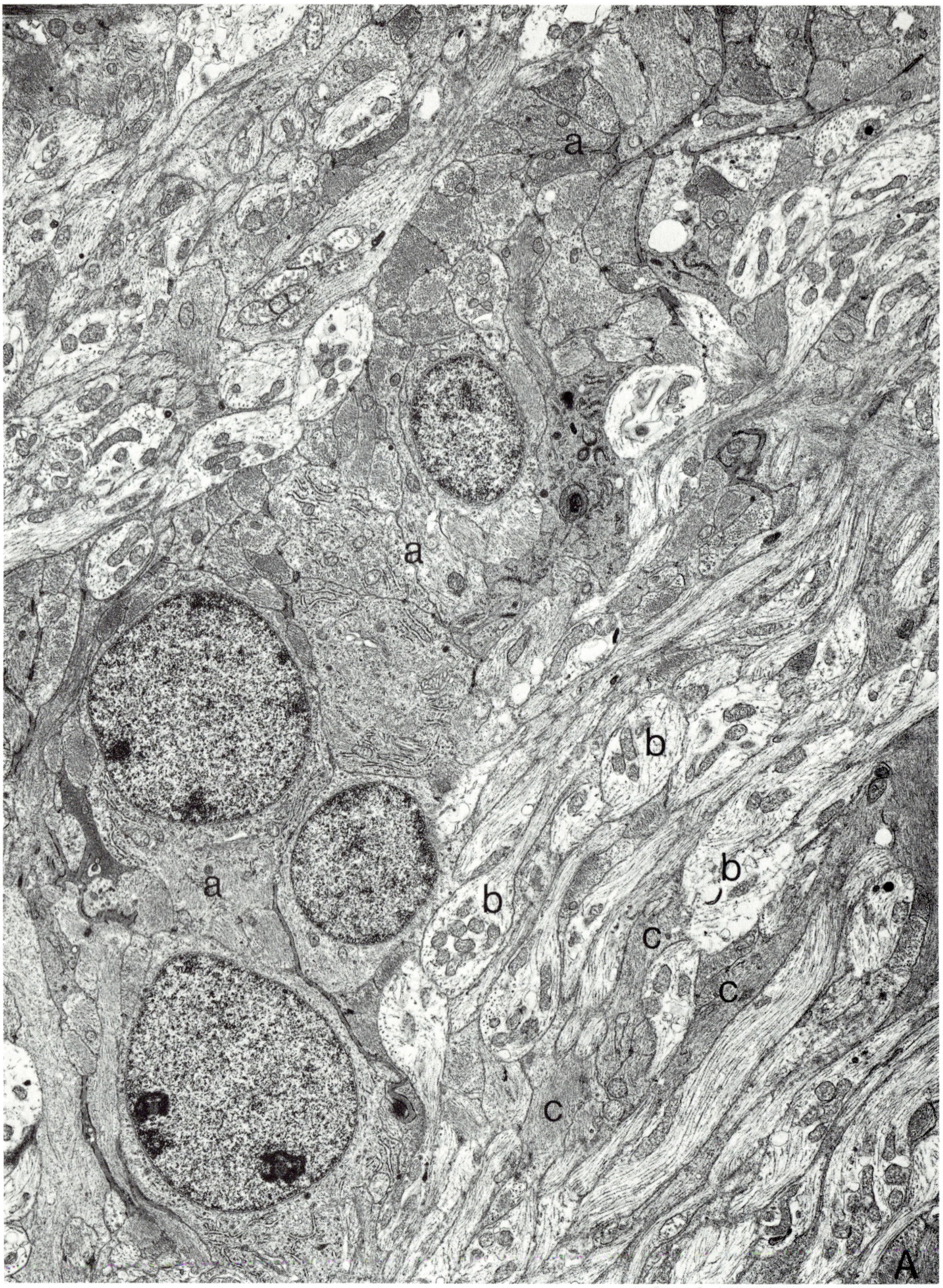

Figure 10–15. *A*, Electron micrograph of one of the glial columns shown in the previous light micrograph (a). The nerve axons (b) are easily distinguished from the more fibrillar branches of the glial cells (c), which extend among the nerve bundles. (× 6930.)

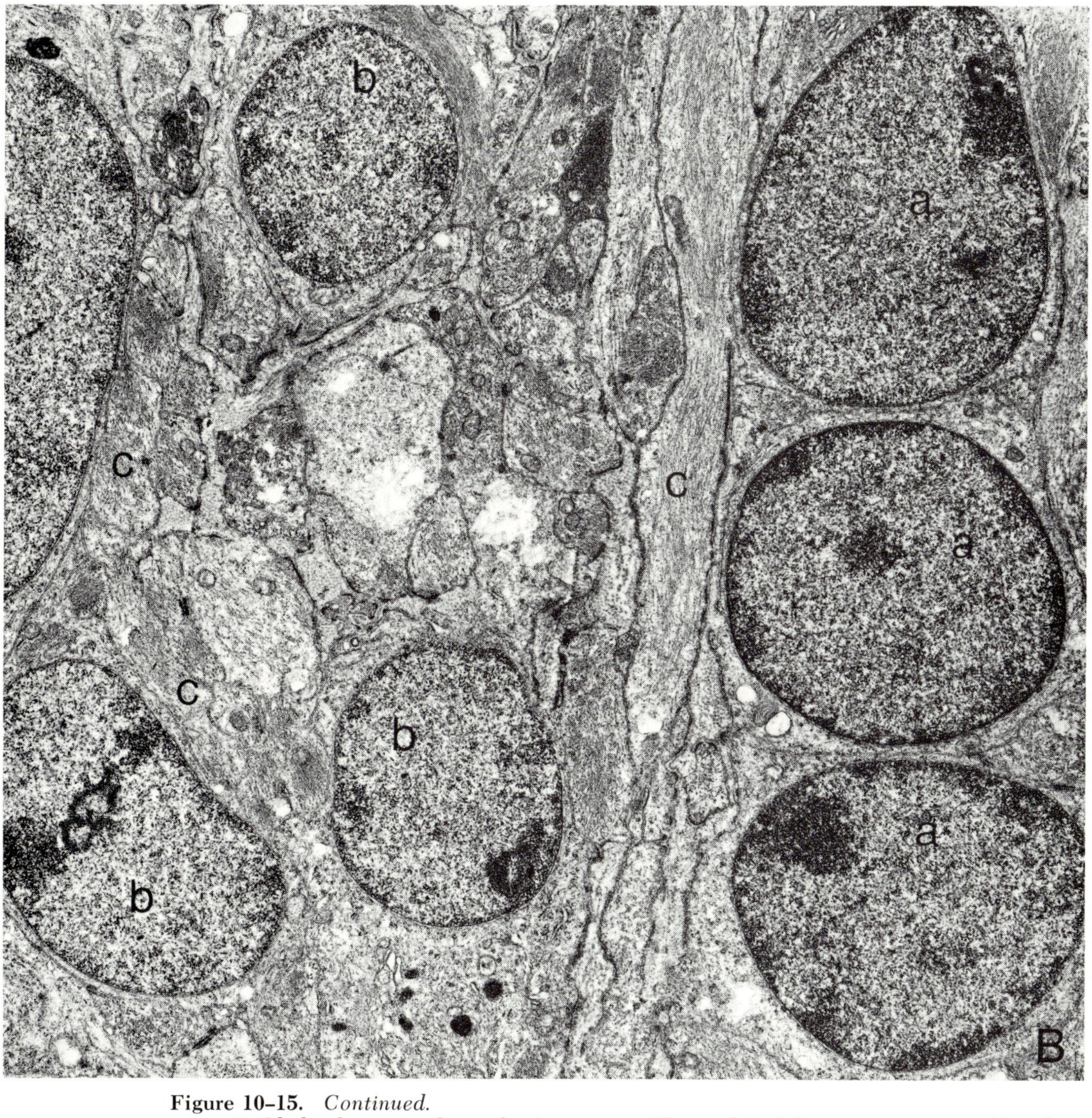

Figure 10–15. *Continued.*

B, Glial columns in the prelaminar nerve. The nuclei of three astrocytes are aligned on the right side of the photograph (a). Portions of other astrocytes and their nuclei are seen elsewhere around the nerve bundles (b). Astrocytic processes run in varying directions (c) around the fascicles. (× 7500.)

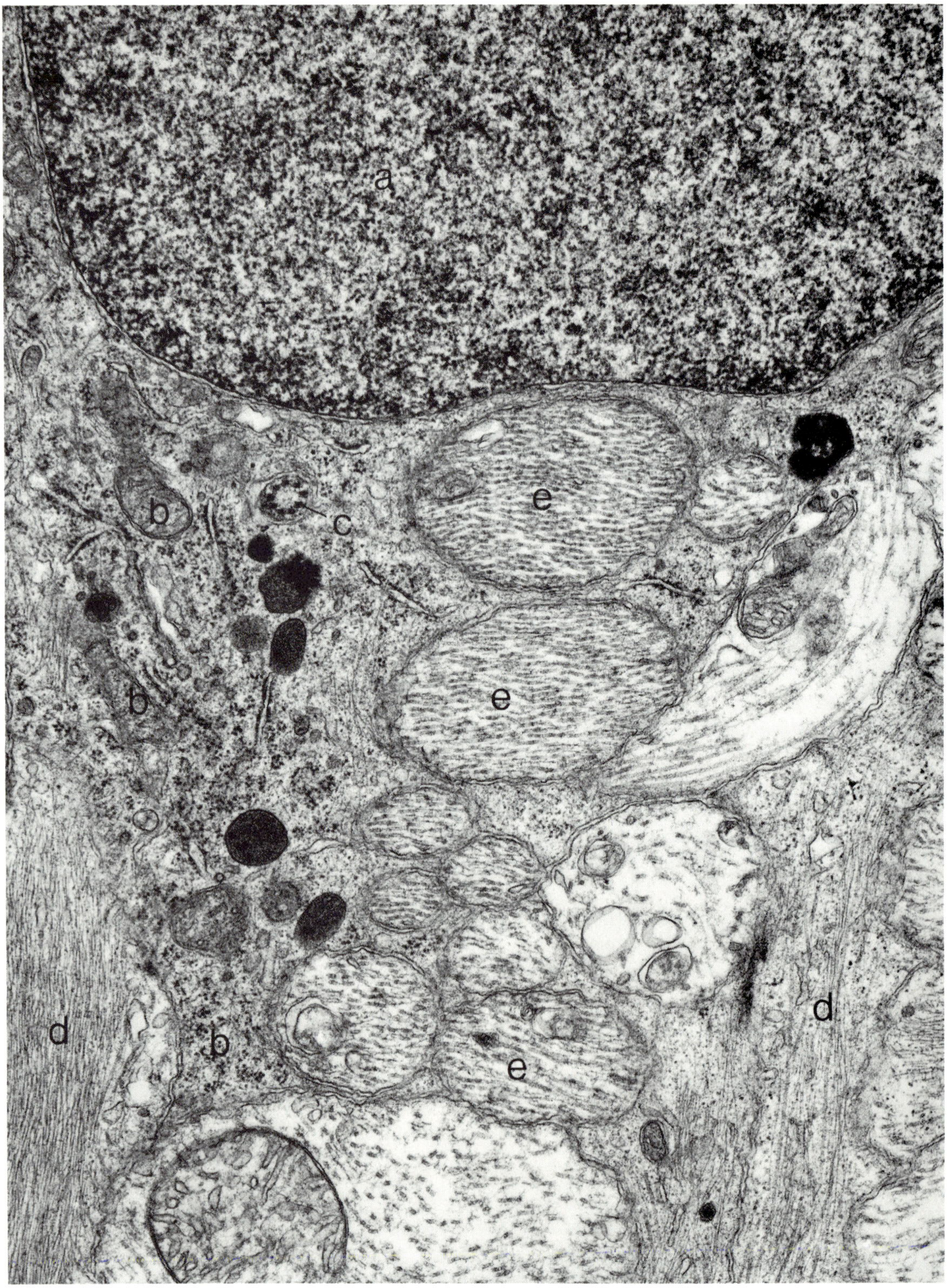

Figure 10–16. Astrocyte in the prelaminar portion of the nerve. The nucleus has a finely granular chromatin (a). The perinuclear cytoplasm contains the majority of the organelles (b), including a centriole (c). The astrocyte processes (d) contain numerous microtubules and filaments. The nerve axons (e) are enclosed by astrocytic processes. (× 22,500.)

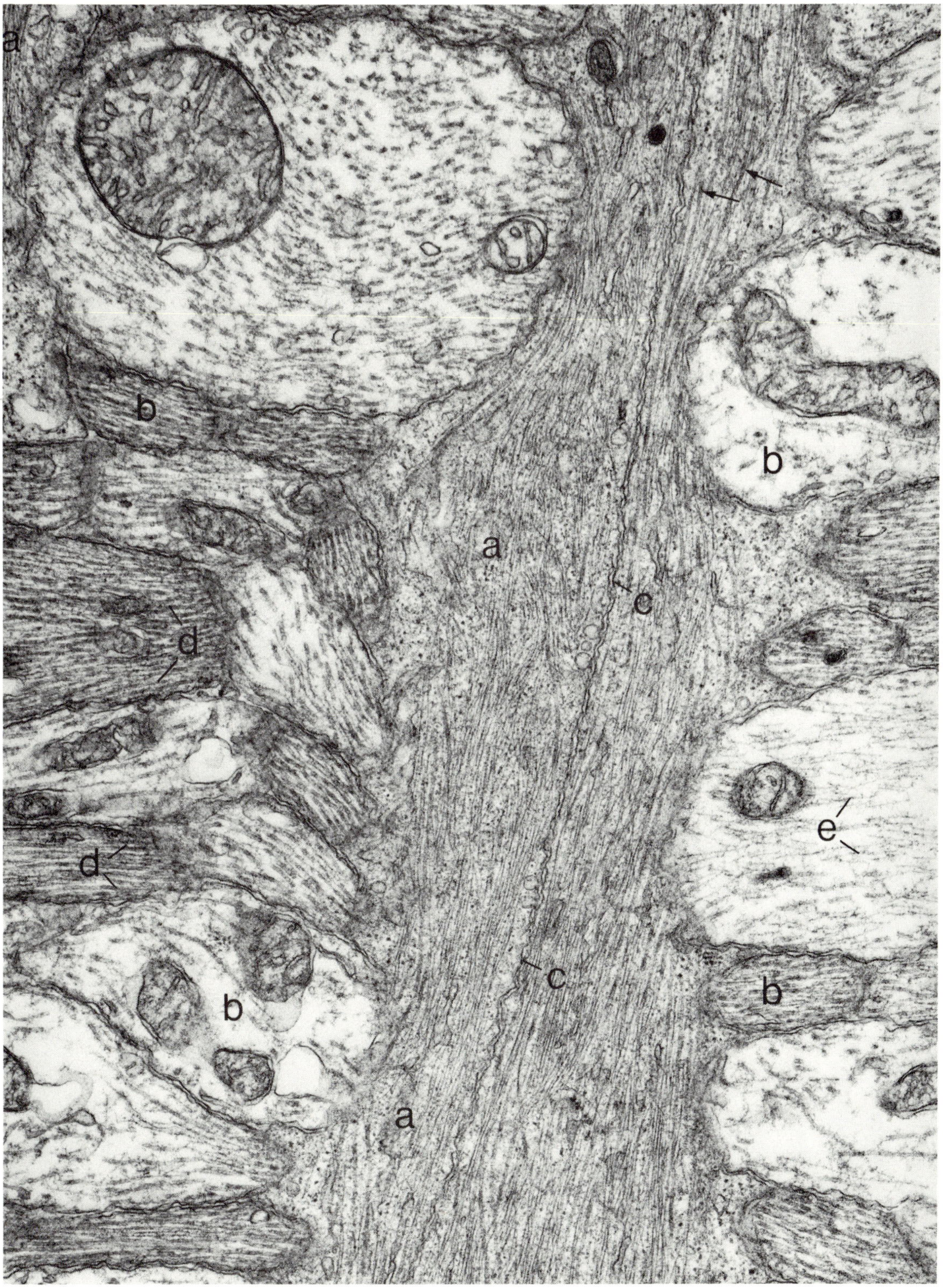

Figure 10–17. A continuation of the same cell seen in Figure 10–16. The very dense fibrillar processes of the astrocyte (a) extend out to enclose numerous nerve fibers (b). The microtubules (arrows) of the astrocyte processes are clearly seen. The intercellular border of two astrocytes is seen at (c). Neurotubules (d) and neurofilaments (e) are seen in the axoplasm of the nerve fibers. (× 24,750.)

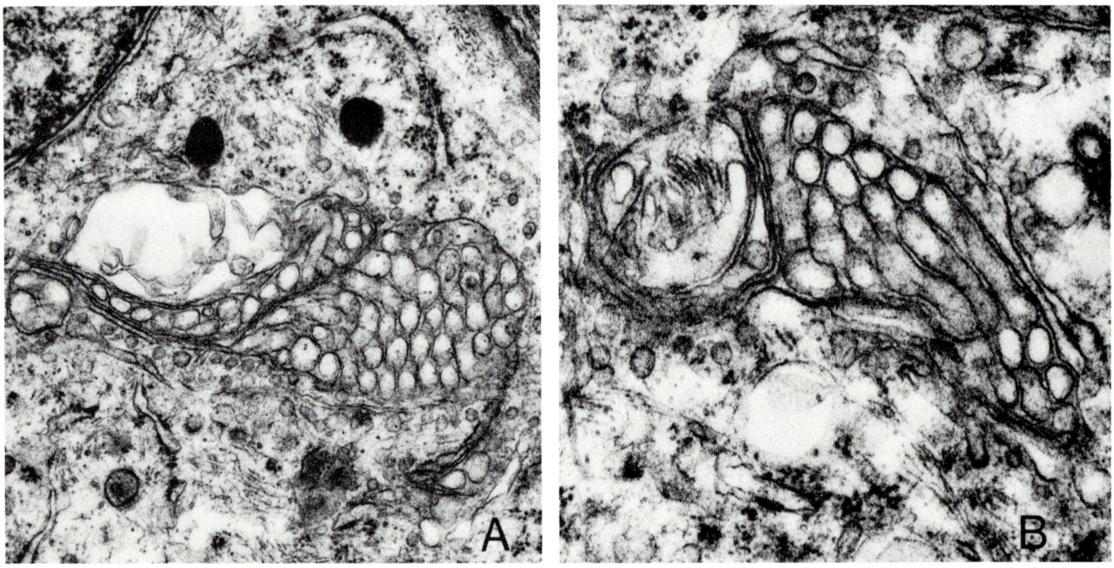

Figure 10–18. The Golgi apparatus of the prelaminar astrocytes. *A*, This type of Golgi has also been described in the lacrimal gland of human and rabbit males and also in the rabbit optic disc. (× 22,500.)

B, Instead of the usual curved cisternae and vesicles, the Golgi apparatus here is composed of long tubes aligned side by side and enclosed by a thin membrane. (× 36,000.)

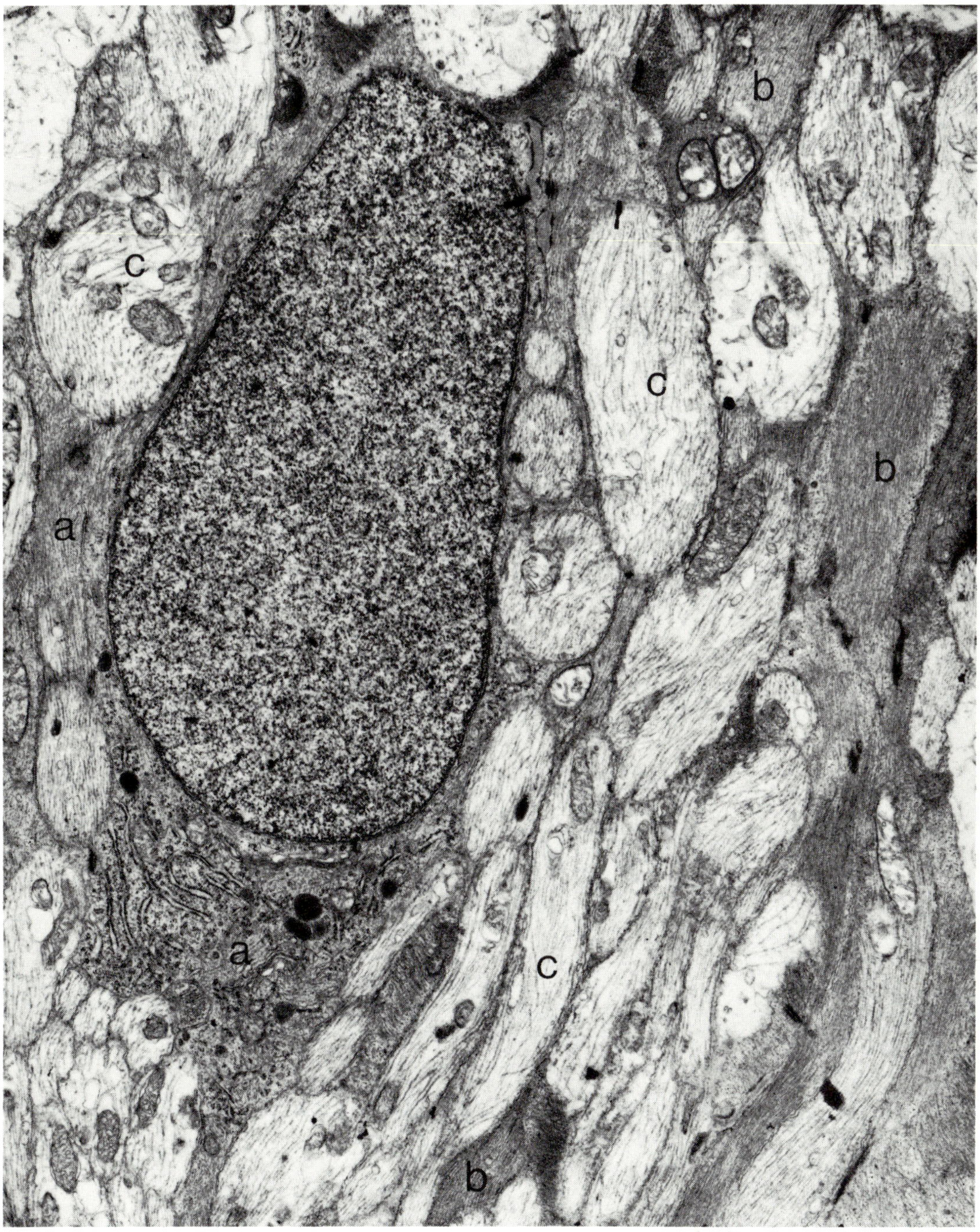

Figure 10–19. Perinuclear cytoplasm (a) and processes (b) of prelaminar astrocytes associated with nerve axon (c) are shown. The dense fibrillar astrocytic cytoplasm is clearly distinct from that of the nerve fibers. (× 11,520.)

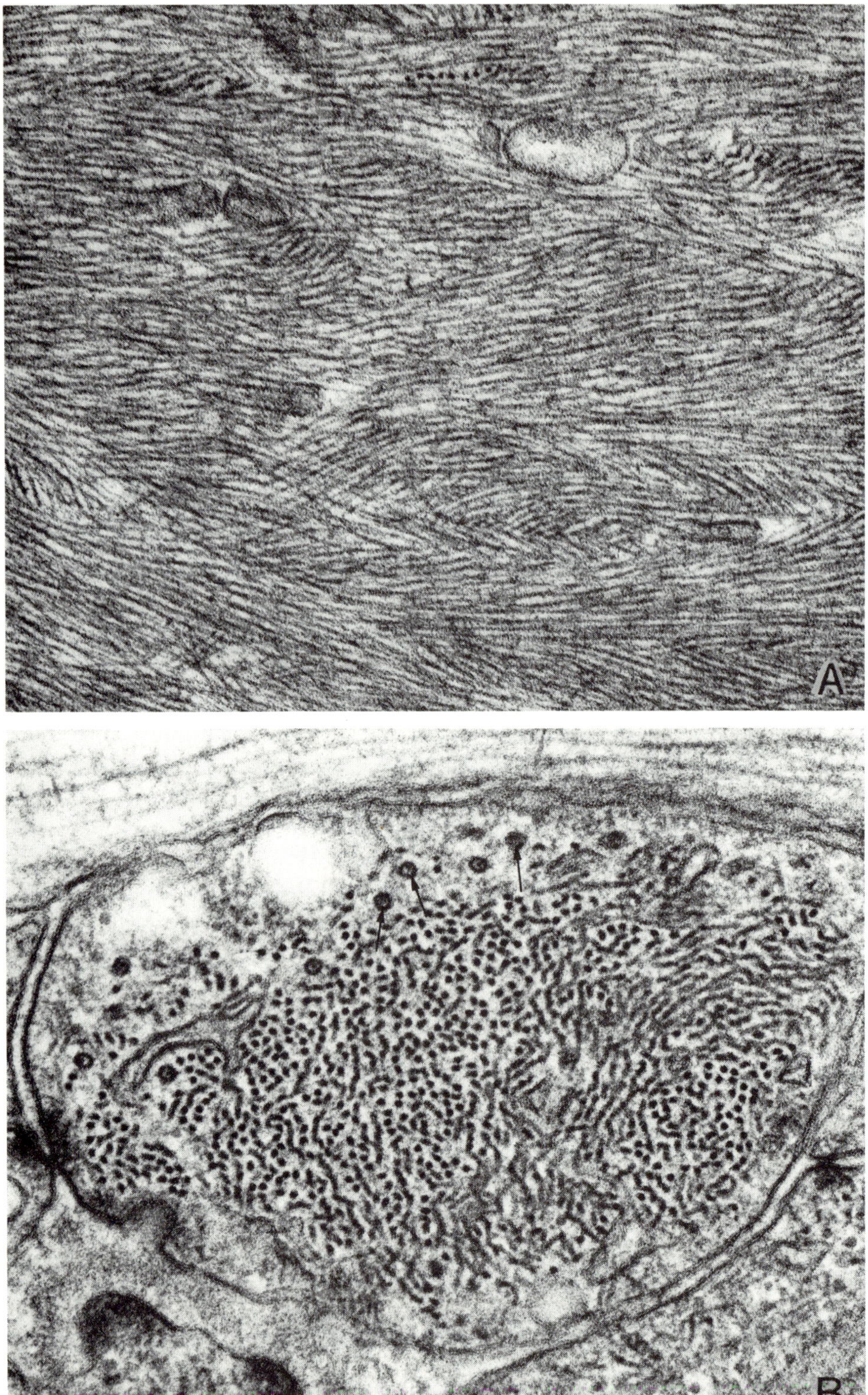

Figure 10–20. Longitudinal and cross-sectional views of glial cell processes. *A*, The process is sectioned longitudinally, showing the herringbone pattern of the cytoplasmic fibrils. (× 60,000.)

B, Cross-section of the fibrils shows them to be closely packed throughout the cytoplasm. The diameters of the fibrils are about 100 A. and they are quite long. Microtubules are shown by arrows. (× 90,000.)

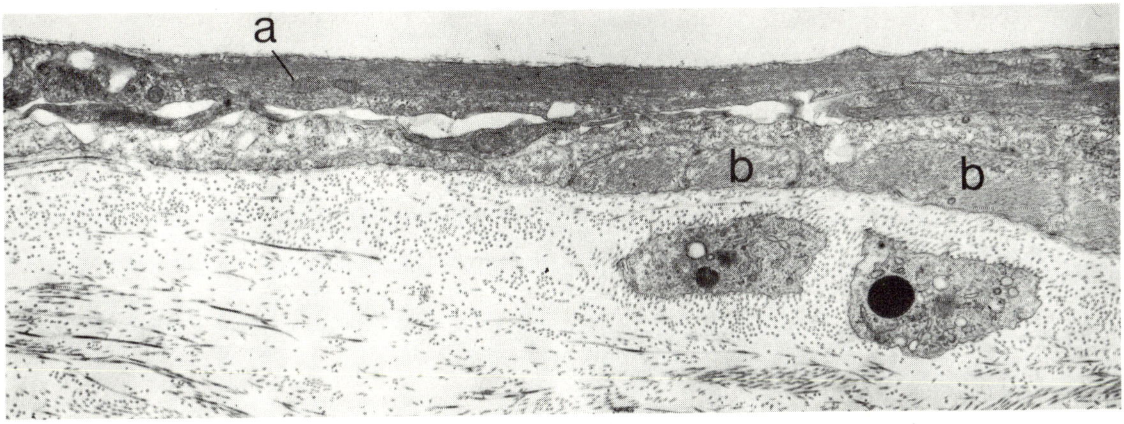

Figure 10–21. Inner limiting membrane of the optic disc. Two to three layers of astrocytes form this portion of the disc; they have the same structure as those within the disc tissue. Some astrocytes are oriented longitudinally (a), while others are in cross-section (b); the processes are quite long. (× 7600.)

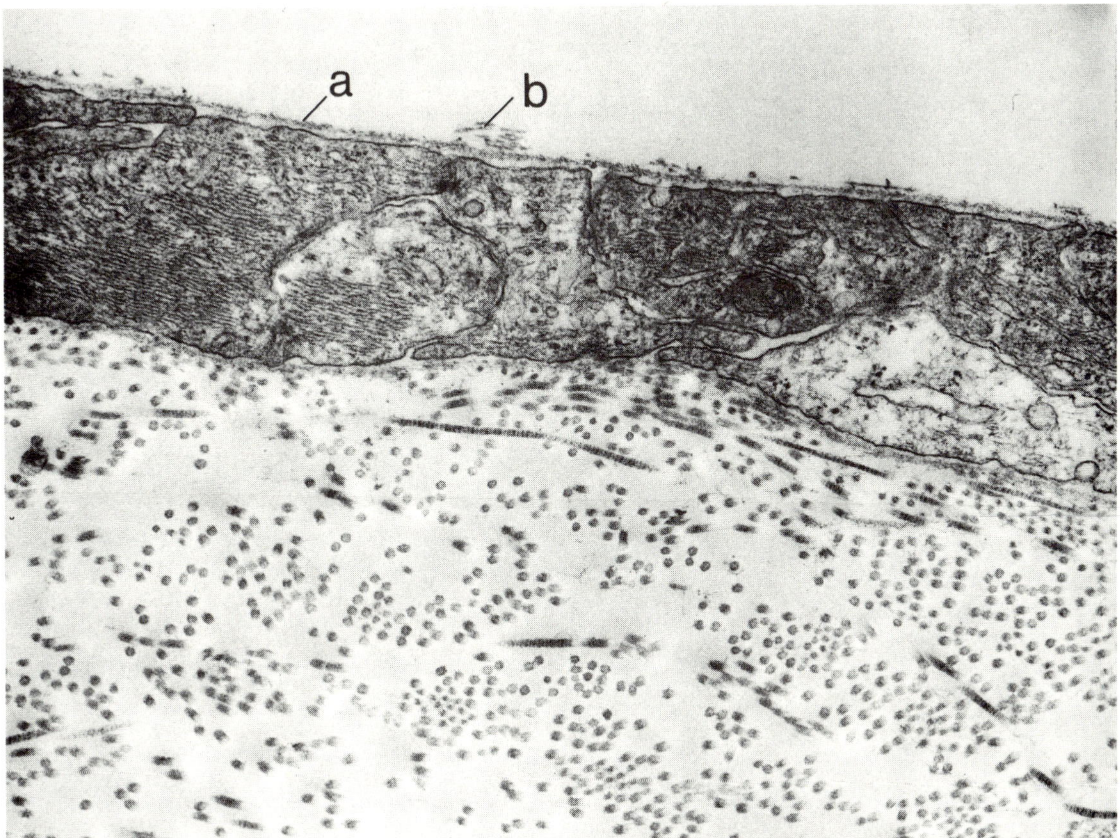

Figure 10–22. Detailed view of the inner limiting membrane. Several cells compose the membrane; they possess a basement membrane (a) measuring 600 A. Cross- and longitudinal sections of cytoplasmic filaments are seen in the cells. Some vitreous filaments join the basement membrane (b), and collagen surrounding adjacent blood vessels lies under the membrane. (× 26,400.)

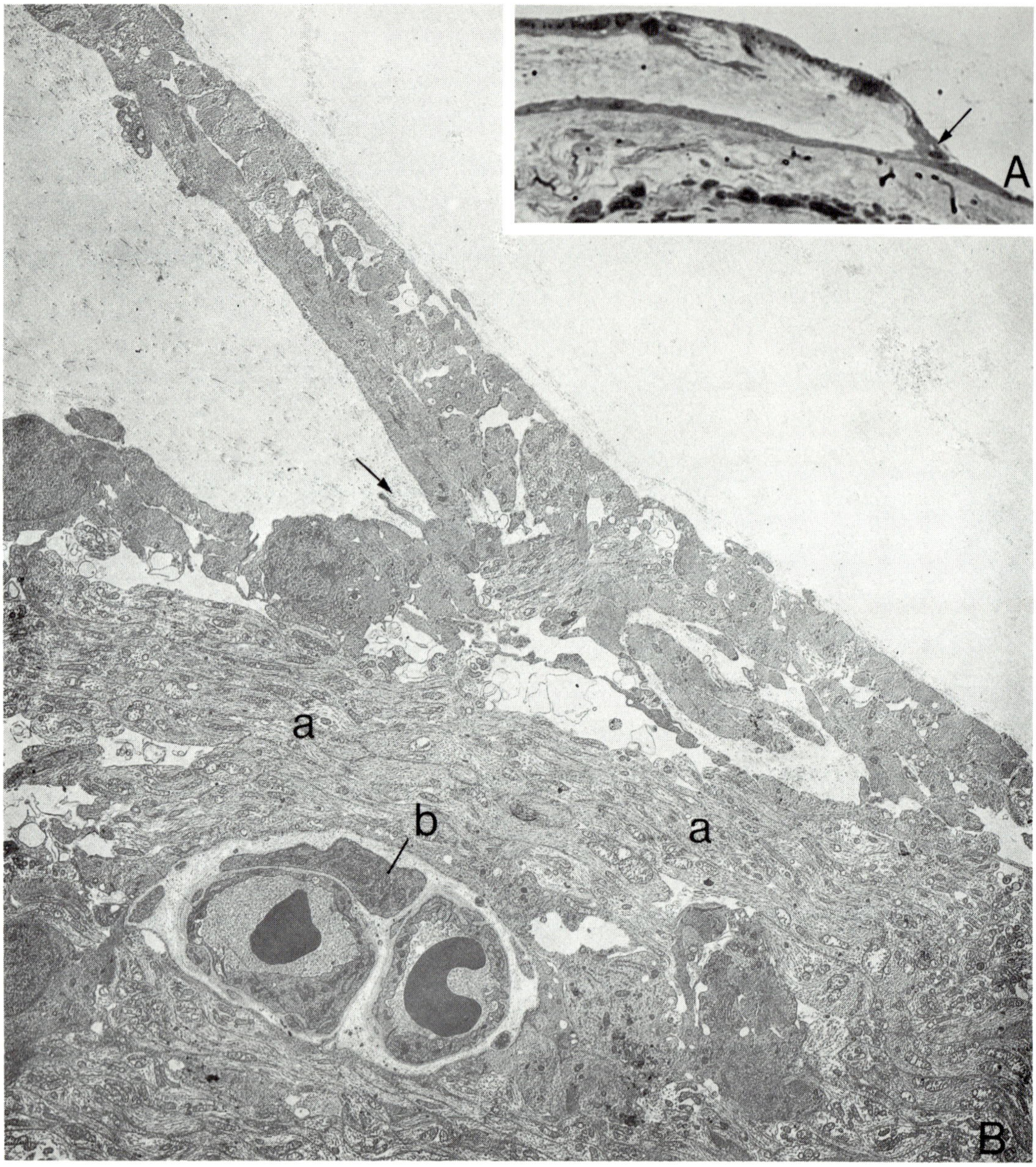

Figure 10–23. Inner limiting membrane. *A*, The insert shows the inner limiting membrane by light microscopy. The membrane frequently splits to enclose perivascular collagen or to extend around the adventitia of the disc blood vessels (arrow). (× 61.)

B, Electron micrograph to show the inner branching membrane and the splitting of the glial cell layer to enclose a mass of collagen (arrow). This is near the peripheral disc, and the membrane is closely related here to the underlying nerve fibers (a). One of two capillaries shows a pericyte in its wall (b). (× 2500.)

Figure 10–24. Astrocytes lining the prelaminar optic nerve canal. *A*, Astrocytes (a) are interposed between the nerve axons and the retina anterior to Bruch's membrane (arrow). (× 7380.)

B, Collagenous connective tissue of the choroid (a) and a fibroblast (b). Astrocytes (c) and their processes (d) are arranged along the nerve canal adjacent to this collagen, separating it from the nerve axons. (× 8600.)

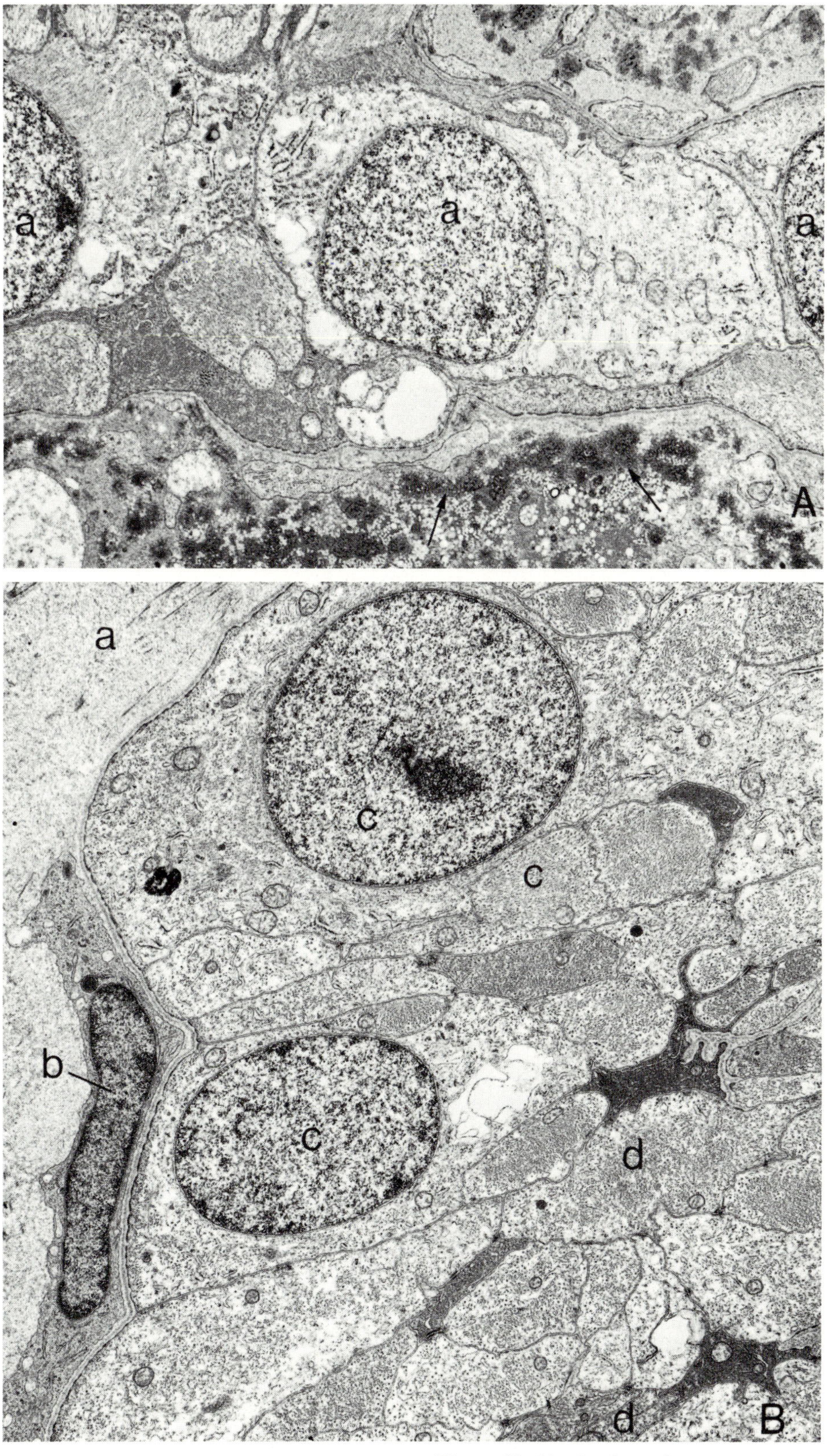

Figure 10–24. *See legend on opposite page.*

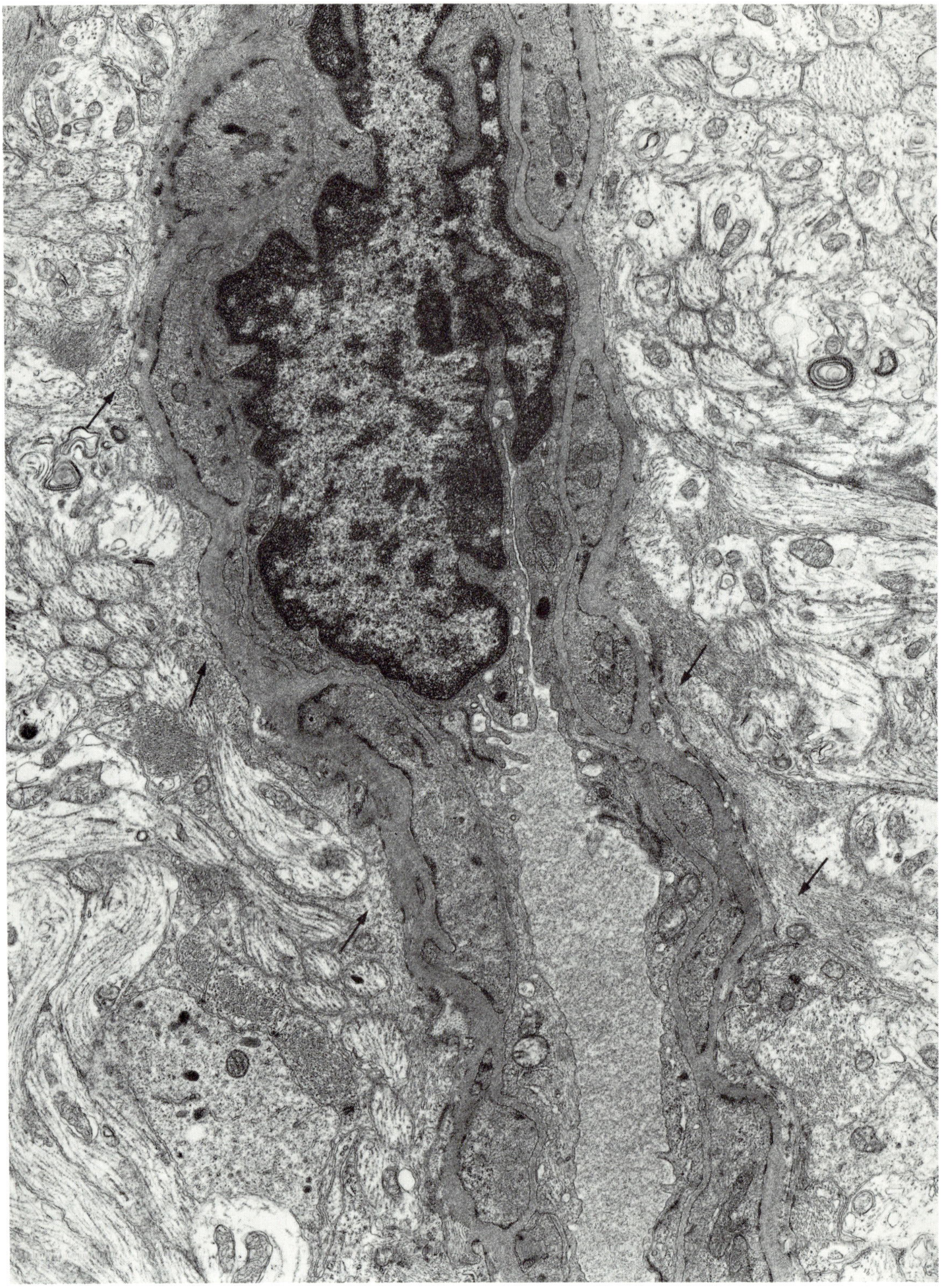

Figure 10–25. Perivascular glial processes. This section of an arteriole on the disc shows the perivascular region to be completely surrounded by the processes of astrocytes (arrows). (× 6000.)

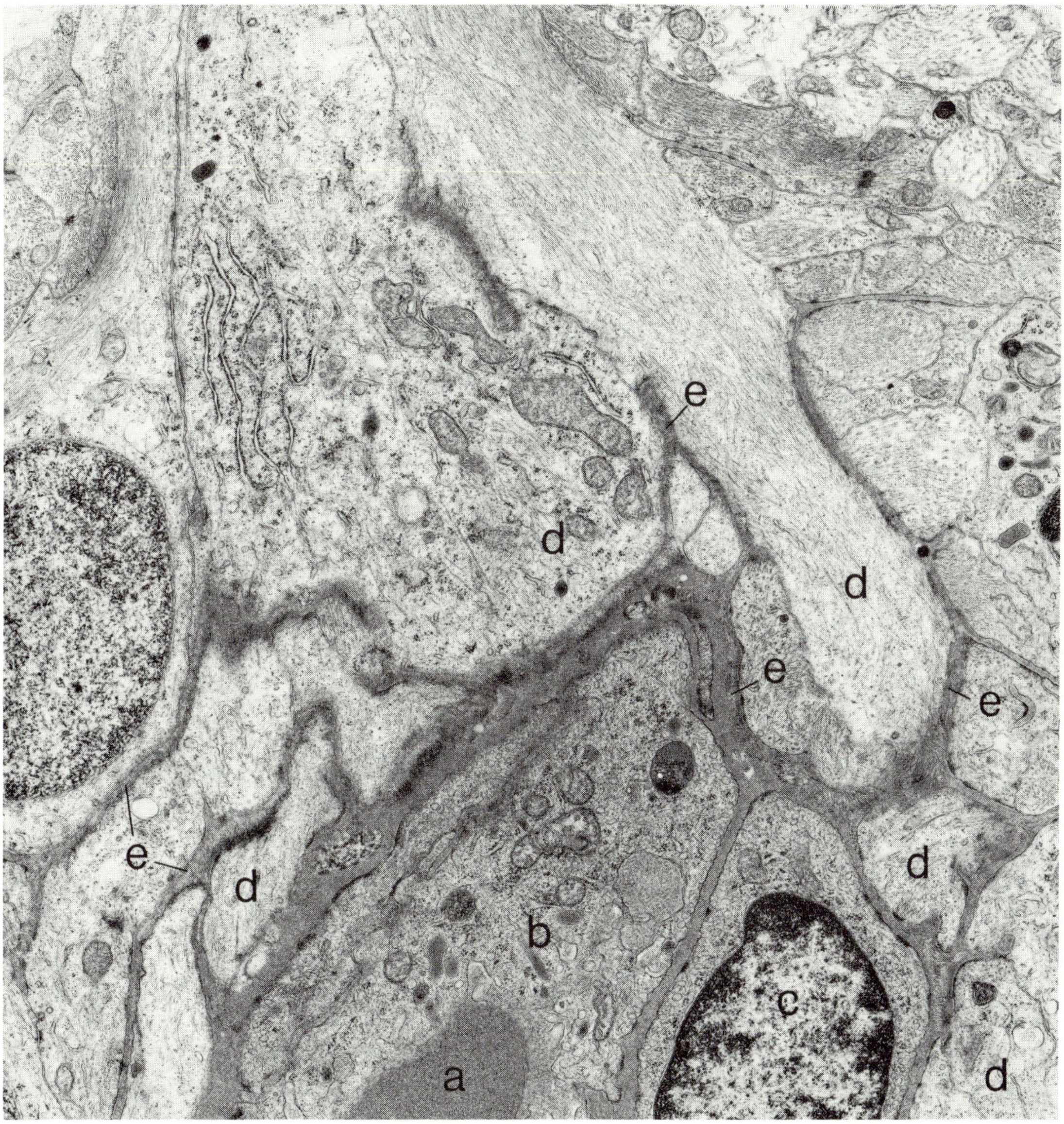

Figure 10–26. A capillary lumen (a) with its endothelium (b) and a pericyte (c). Astrocytic processes (d) are in direct contact with the basement membranes of the endothelial cells and the pericyte. The basement membranes of the astrocytes and pericytes are continuous and extend a considerable distance from the vessel wall (e). (× 5400.)

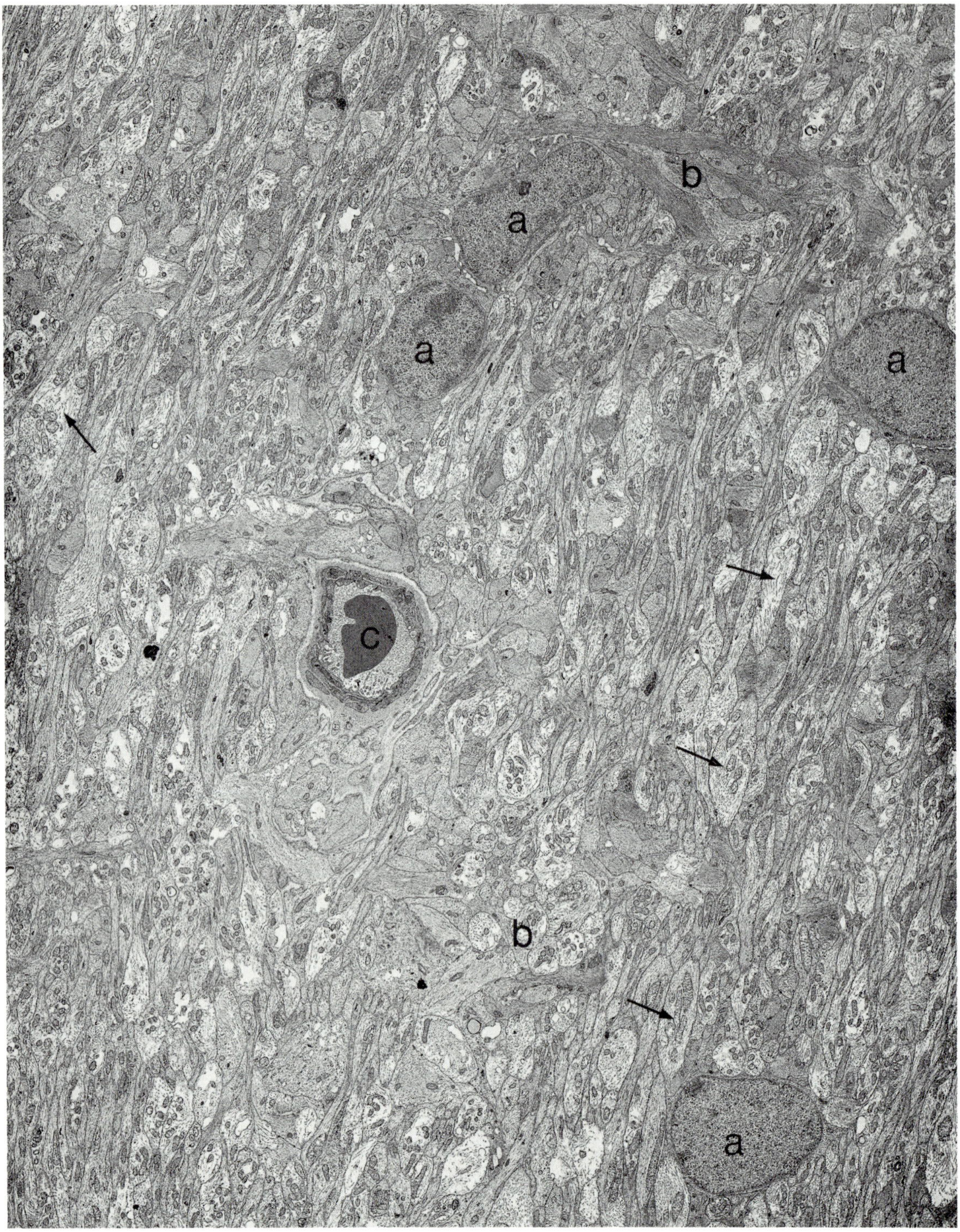

Figure 10–27. Low-power electron micrograph of the nerve fibers in the optic disc. The axons (arrows) generally are oriented toward the lamina cribrosa, which is beyond the lower edge of the photograph. Astrocyte nuclei (a) are found among the nerve fibers, and their processes (b) form an extremely complex network within the nerve tissue. A capillary (c) is completely surrounded by astrocytic processes. (× 14,850.)

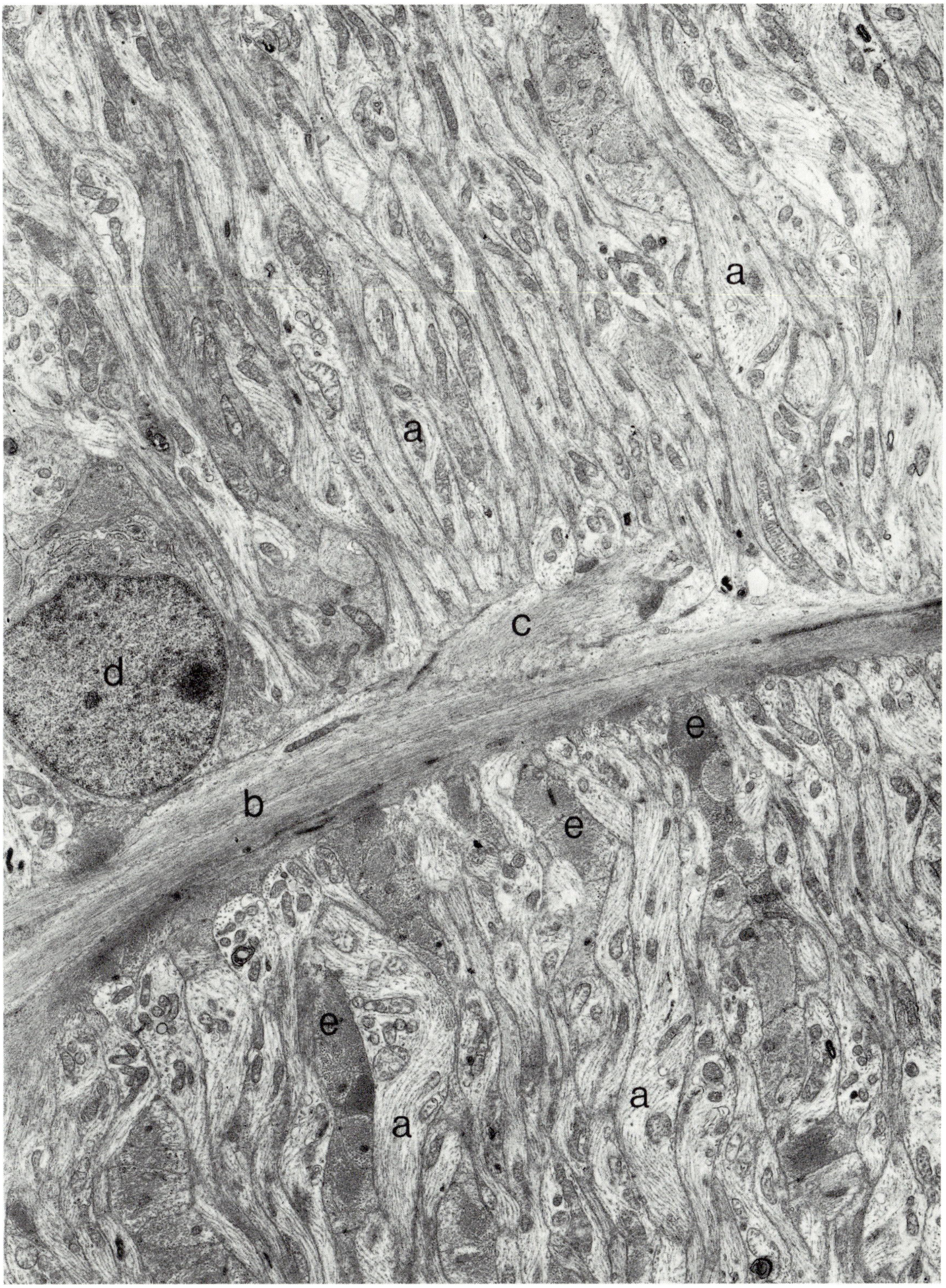

Figure 10–28. Axons of the prelaminar portion of the optic nerve (a). An astrocyte process extends transversely across the nerve bundle (b), and it branches to send a process into the bundle (c). The nucleus of an astrocyte (d) and other astrocytic processes (e) are seen. (× 6930.)

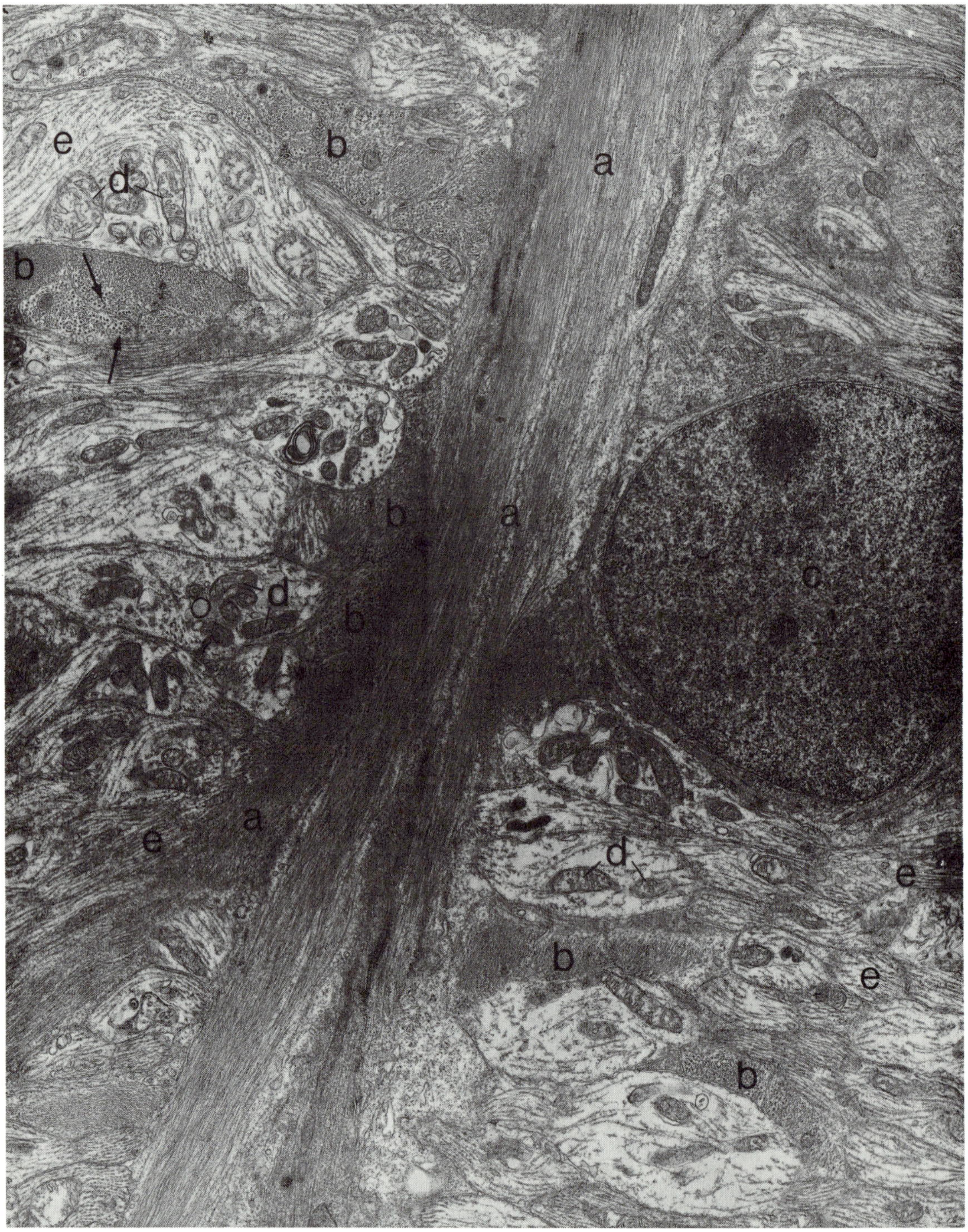

Figure 10–29. Higher magnification of Figure 10–28, showing an astrocyte process (a) sectioned longitudinally and others (b) in cross-section. The processes are filled by filaments and microtubules; the latter are seen best in cross-section (arrows). The chromatin of the astrocyte nucleus is finely granular and evenly dispersed throughout the karyoplasm (c). The axons have a lighter cytoplasm, with many mitochondria (d) and microtubules (e). (× 8100.)

ally by thin strips of glial processes. More often axons are separated either from each other by an intercellular space measuring 150 A., or from an astrocyte process by a similar space. Cohen (1967) found the axons in this portion of the nerve to have no organized glial separation, often being contiguous with one another for up to 200 μm. The same variations in axon diameter observed in the retina and the orbital portion of the nerve are seen here. Minor variations in the caliber of individual axons most often result from interposition of astroglial processes in the nerve bundles.

The axoplasm of the neurons contains neurofilaments, which measure 60 to 70 A. in diameter, and a fair number of longitudinally oriented microtubules, which measure 200 to 250 A. in diameter (Fig. 10-30). Mitochondria are scattered throughout the axoplasm, and a fair amount of smooth endoplasmic reticulum is present. All the axons in the region have similar structural features; therefore, it is impossible to determine histologically whether some of them are efferent fibers.

Blood Vessels. Except for branches of the large central retinal artery and vein, the blood vessels in the prelaminar optic nerve portion are mostly arterioles and capillaries derived from the choroid, the pial system, the circle of Zinn and the central retinal vessels (Fig. 10-7). The arterioles and capillaries ramify diffusely through the disc tissue within the nerve bundles and astrocytic septa. Their walls contain little collagen, and the astroglia processes end adjacent to their collagen. Some nerves from the pial and short ciliary nerves enter the disc to supply the walls of the blood vessels. The fine structure of the arterioles, venules and capillaries in this region resembles that of the retina. In the prelaminar region, the small vessels are found both within the astrocytic septa and among the nerve axons, while in the orbital portion of the nerve they are found only in the optic nerve septa surrounding the nerve fascicles.

The arteries in the prelaminar optic nerve differ from those in the laminar and orbital portions by a lack of an internal elastic lamina and a complete absence of elastic tissue in the media. The structure of the veins changes very little in different portions of the nerve. The perivascular connective tissue around the arteries and veins is quite thick, and its outer surface is always clothed with astrocytes. Some of the perivascular astrocytes are derived from the internal limiting membrane, while others come from the glial septa of the prelaminar portion.

Laminar Portion (Figs. 10-31 to 10-37). The lamina cribrosa or cribriform plate serves two purposes: first, it forms a scaffolding for the passage of bundles of optic nerve axons, anchoring the bundles to each other and to the sides of the optic nerve canal (Fig. 10-31). In addition, it reinforces the posterior eye, protecting it from injury at the site of the nerve exit.

The principal part of the lamina cribrosa is formed by an extension of collagen bundles and elastic fibers from the inner two thirds of the sclera across the optic nerve canal (Figs. 10-31 and 10-32). The bundles of scleral collagen and elastic tissue extend from one side of the canal to the other, intersecting at various angles to form a sieve, with many openings traversed by the nerve fascicles. Not all the collagen and elastic fibers traverse the canal completely, for some join the connective tissue surrounding the central retinal vessels (Figs. 10-33 to 10-36). Posteriorly the lamina cribrosa terminates rather abruptly at the site where the initial septa of the optic nerve are formed by the pia mater. Wolter (1957) found the scleral portion of the

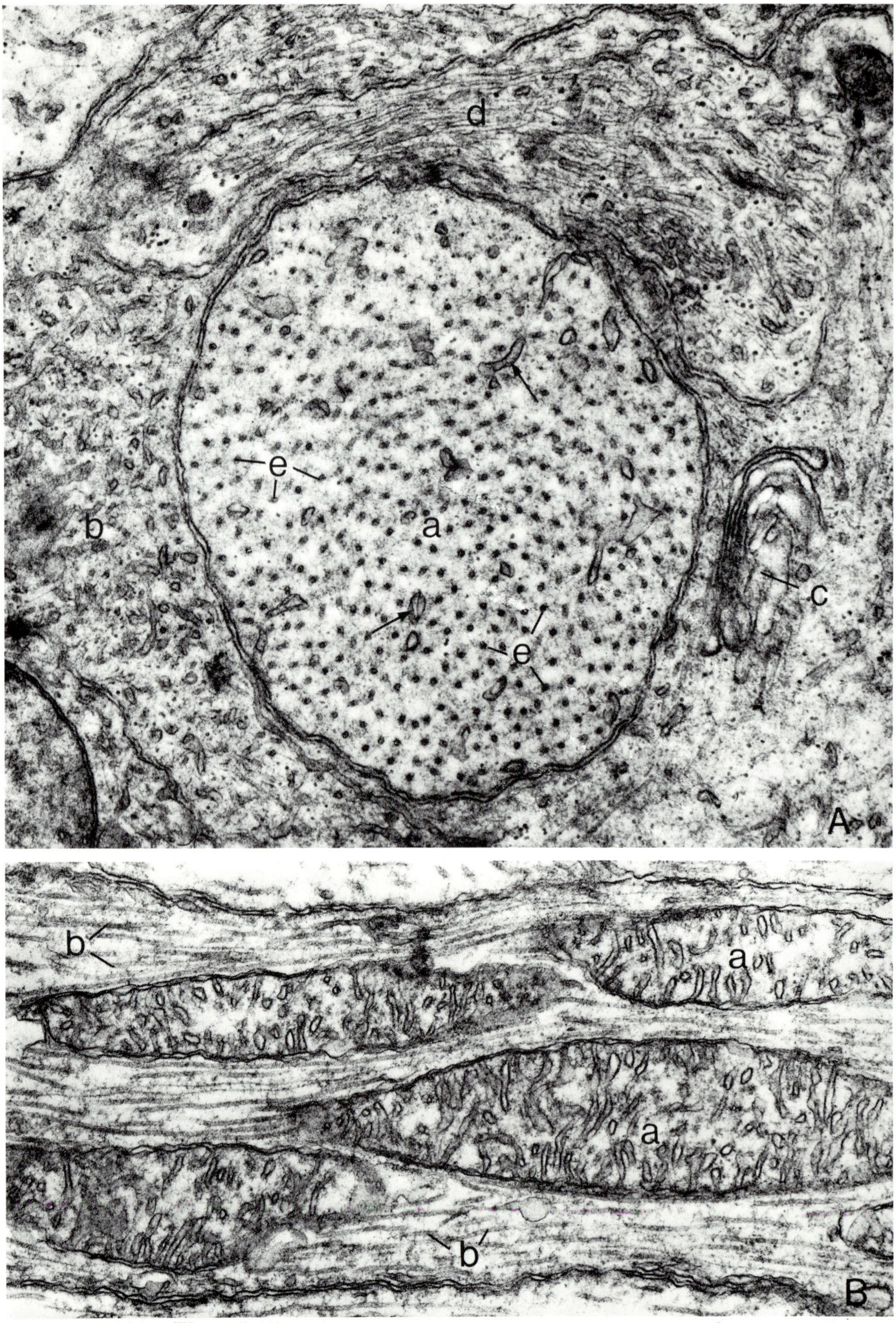

Figure 10–30. *See legend on opposite page.*

lamina cribrosa to have a backward bow, with the concavity of the bow facing anteriorly. Hayreh and Vrabec (1966) confirmed this finding in the optic nerve of the rhesus monkey.

The collagen fibrils of laminar connective tissue measure 600 A. in diameter and have a banding of 600 to 640 A. These fibers branch and intertwine to form closely packed bundles that vary in shape and size. Fibroblasts found throughout the lamina have the structural features of fibroblasts elsewhere. We have found an impressive amount of elastic tissue in the lamina cribrosa of specimens examined; according to Anderson (1969), however, elastic tissue may be absent in some specimens. The large amount of elastic tissue found here is surprising in view of its paucity in the sclera and other eye tissues.

Astrocytes. The astrocytes in the lamina cribrosa are reduced to a thin mantle that surrounds the nerve bundles, separating them from the laminar connective tissue and that around the central retinal vessels. Astrocytes also separate the optic nerve from scleral collagen at the edge of the nerve canal (Fig. 10-32). The cells and their nuclei are flattened, with their long arms extending at right angles to the course of the nerve fibers.

Except for the slight differences mentioned previously, the glial cells in the prelaminar and laminar portions are quite similar (Fig. 10-13). The laminar glial cells surrounding the nerve fascicles have the same disposition as those in the prelaminar portion, their flattened branches extending out to enclose the nerve bundles. The long arms of these cells are thicker than those of the prelaminar cells and contain many more fibrils, however. Their nuclear chromatin is more condensed than that of astrocytes in the orbital portion of the optic nerve. A thin layer of cytoplasm containing ribosomes, many fine fibrils and other organelles is seen in the perinuclear region. The Golgi complex of these cells is of the usual type and thus differs from that of cells in the prelaminar portion. The astrocytes lining the sclera insulate it from adjacent nerve bundles; this layer, which sometimes contains melanocytes, is continuous with the glia in the *border tissue of Jacoby* (Fig. 10-13). The glial cells of the border tissue of Jacoby are like those covering the collagen in the lamina cribrosa, except that they are longer and thinner. Centrally the glia forms a sheath over the adventitia of the central vessels.

Axons. The axons within the fascicles in this portion of the nerve are identical to those in the prelaminar portion. They are closely packed as they pass through the collagen sheets of the lamina, but this does not alter the relationship between the axons and the astrocytes. Toward the posterior portion of the lamina cribrosa, axons occasionally become partially myelinated.

Figure 10–30. Cross- and longitudinal sections of nerve axons in the prelaminar optic nerve. *A*, The nerve axon is cut in cross-section (a) and it is surrounded by two astrocytes, one containing considerable smooth-surfaced endoplasmic reticulum (b) and a Golgi apparatus (c), and the other containing many fibrils (d). The nerve fiber contains microtubules (e) and some smooth-surfaced endoplasmic reticulum (arrows). (× 36,000.)

B, A longitudinal section of a nerve axon. It contains long mitochondria (a) with transverse cristae and many microtubules (b). (× 30,000.)

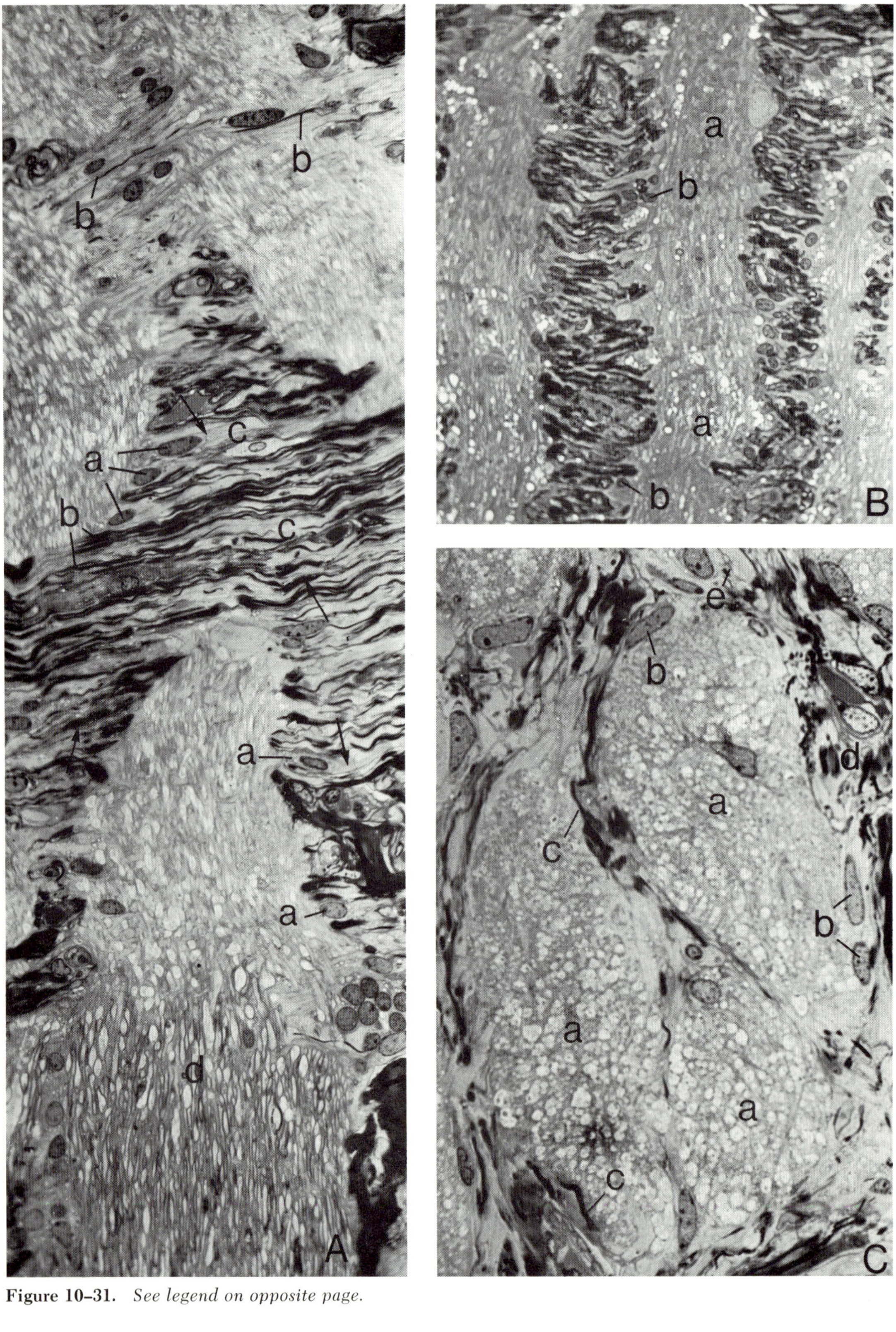

Figure 10–31. *See legend on opposite page.*

Nerve Periphery. The glial component of the peripheral nerve has been described. Outside this glial tissue is a layer of connective tissue known as the *border tissue of Elschnig.* The collagen in this layer, which is derived from sclera, is more circularly oriented around the canal and sends branches into the nerve to form the lamina cribrosa. It is lined by astrocytes on the sides of the nerve fascicles.

Blood Vessels. Capillaries are observed regularly in the laminar portion of the nerve. They have a continuous, unfenestrated endothelium and resemble capillaries found in the sclera. Capillaries most often course through the connective tissue of the lamina, where they have a thin adventitial connective tissue. Capillaries entering the nerve fascicles have a very thin layer of adventitial connective tissue, which in turn is surrounded by astrocytes. Occasionally pericytes or their processes are seen along the outer endothelial surface of some vessels. The outer surfaces of the pericytes also show a basement membrane. Unlike the retina, where the processes of astrocytes often contact the capillary wall, these processes are found only in close relation to the connective tissue around the vessel wall in the prelaminar and laminar nerve portions.

The central retinal artery and vein and their supporting connective tissue comprise an important area in the laminar portion of the canal. They are fixed to each other as well as to the bundles of the lamina cribrosa by dense collagen and elastic tissues. The vessel lumen is narrower here than in the orbital portion of the nerve, which probably accounts for the greater frequency of occlusion at or near this site. Differences in the structure of vessel walls in the laminar and prelaminar portions have been discussed previously.

Postlaminar Portion (Figs. 10-1, 10-37 and 10-38). This area is a transition zone from the laminar portion to the optic nerve proper. The nerve axons gradually are myelinated here, some axons becoming myelinated farther anteriorly than others, but most fibers being myelinated before the nerve leaves the eye. The pial septa, which originate in the posterior lamina cribrosa region, surround and gradually take over the internal nerve fascicles. At first many septa are quite incomplete, but at the exit of the nerve from the eye most of them are well developed. Since the ultrastructure here is like that in the orbital portion of the nerve, it will not be discussed.

Text continued on page 571

Figure 10–31. Light micrographs of the lamina cribrosa. *A*, Meridional section of the optic nerve. The internal part of the lamina cribrosa is above, and the external border near the bottom of the micrograph (arrows). The astrocytes (a) surrounding the nerve fascicles separate them from the connective tissue of the lamina cribrosa. The elastic fibers (b) stain intensely, while the collagen fibers (c) stain poorly. The anterior lamina contain fewer elastic fibers than the posterior area near the external part of the lamina cribrosa. The nerve axons become myelinated as seen at (d). (× 480.)

B, A nerve bundle (a) passing through the lamina cribrosa. The astrocytes separate the nerves from the connective tissue of the lamina; their nuclei can be seen at (b). (× 320.)

C, Cross-section through the lamina cribrosa. Three nerves bundles (a) are surrounded by astrocytes (b). Elastic fibers (c), a small vessel (d) and pale-staining collagen fibers (e) are shown in the lamina. (× 680.)

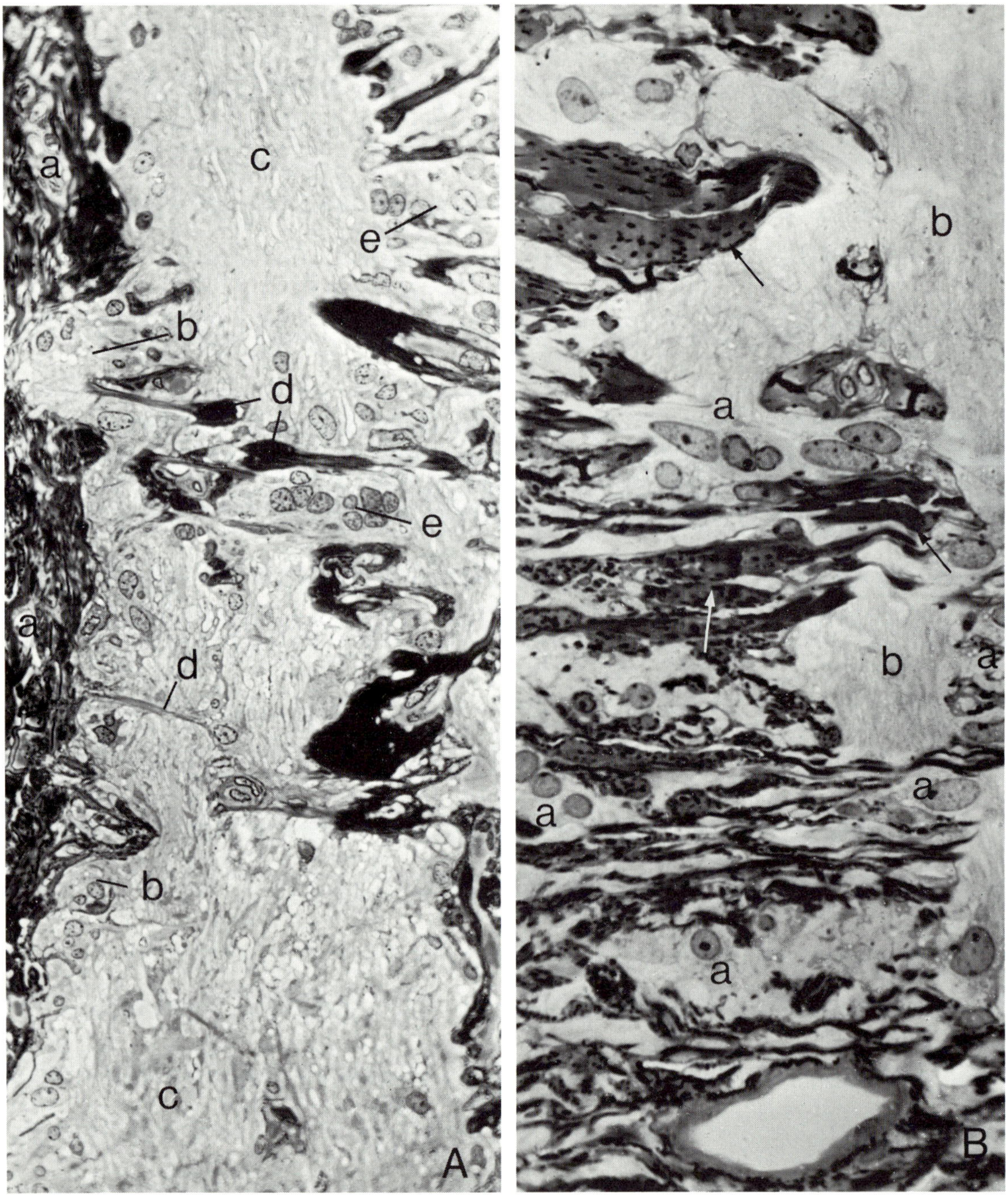

Figure 10–32. The peripheral portion of the lamina cribrosa. *A*, Phase-contrast light micrograph. The scleral collagen is on the left (a); astrocytes (b) separate the peripheral nerve bundles (c) from the scleral connective tissue. Collagen and elastic fibers stemming from the sclera extend across the optic nerve to form the cribriform plate (d); astrocytes surround the nerve fascicles (e) and separate them from the connective tissue of the lamina. (× 525.)

B, Light micrograph of the lamina cribrosa at higher magnification. The collagen and elastic fibers of the lamina are shown with arrows. Astrocytes along the nerve edge and covering the sheets of the lamina are at (a); nerve bundles are at (b). (× 810.)

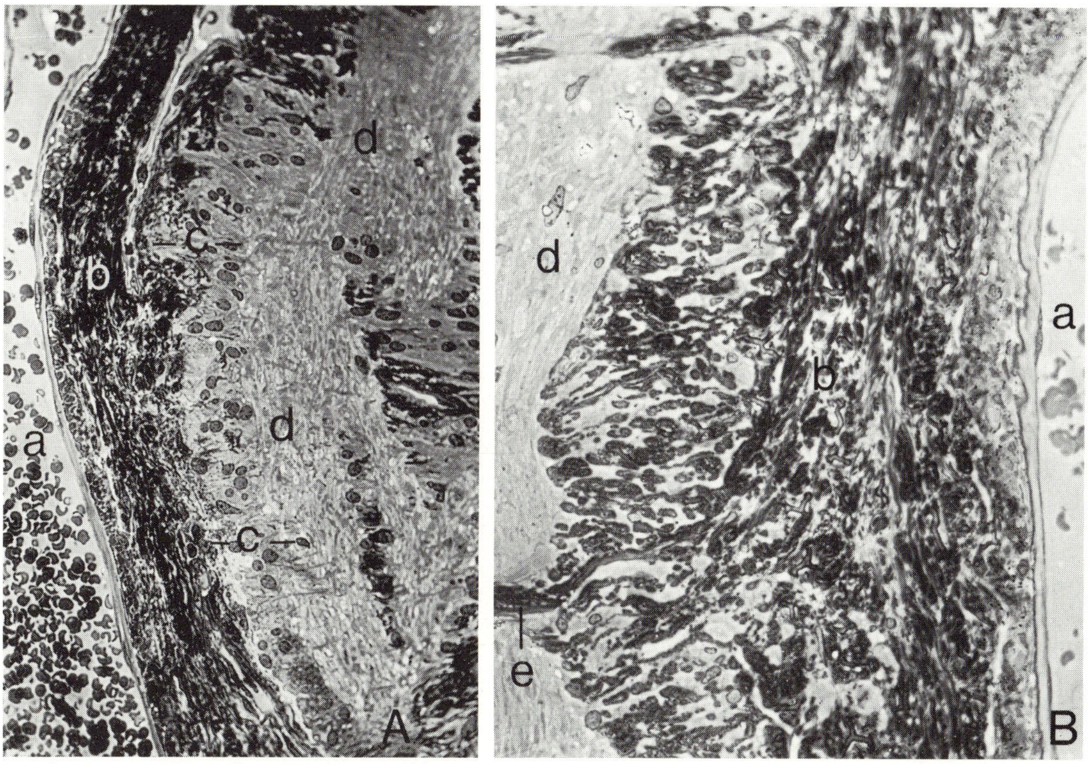

Figure 10–33. Light micrographs of the connective tissue surrounding the central retinal artery. *A*, The lumen of the artery is at (a), and the connective tissue at (b). A layer of astrocytes (c) separates the nerve fibers (d) from the connective tissue strand. (× 225.)

B, The collagen and elastic tissue of the lamina cribrosa are joined (e) to the perivascular connective tissue. (× 225.)

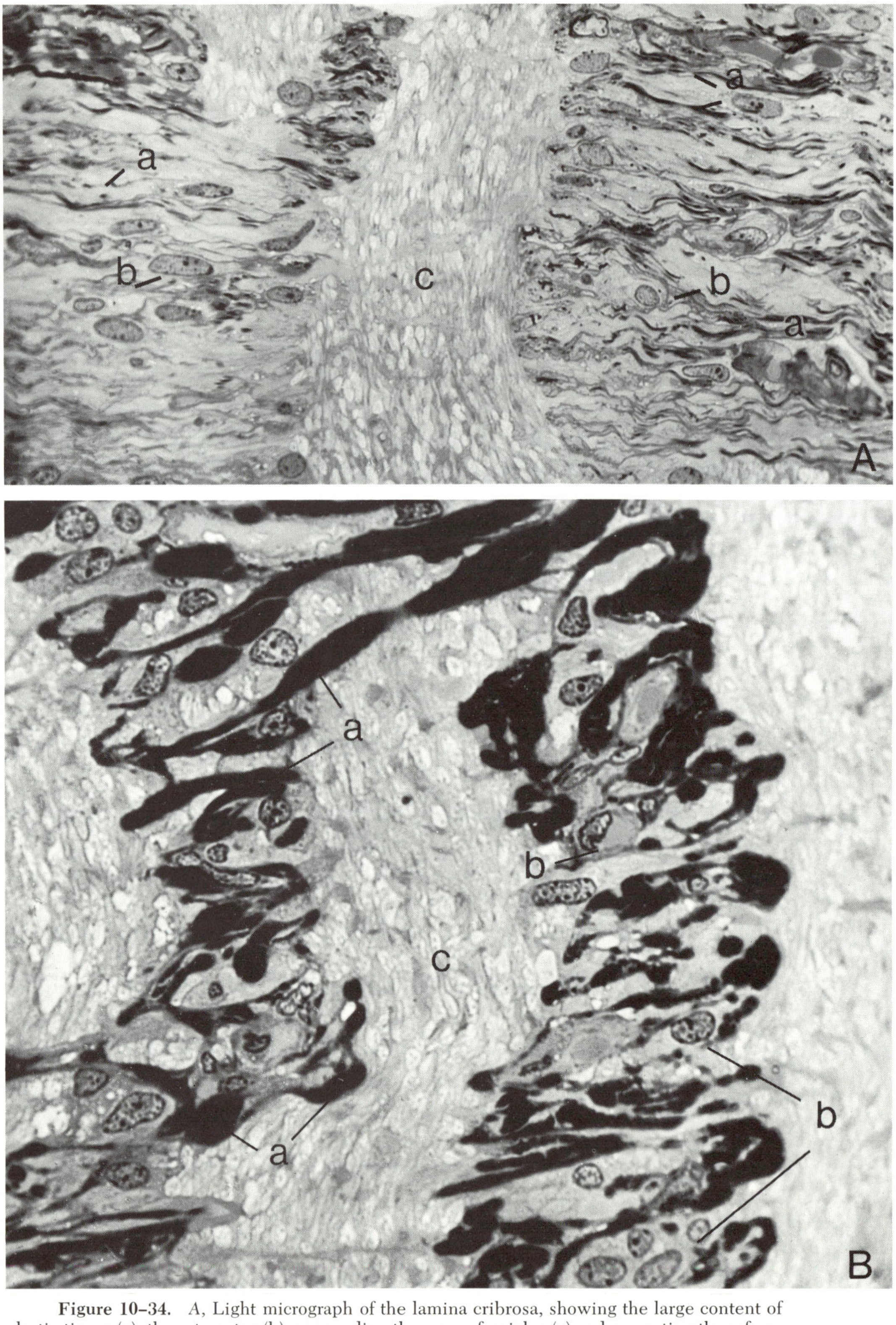

Figure 10–34. *A*, Light micrograph of the lamina cribrosa, showing the large content of elastic tissue (a), the astrocytes (b) surrounding the nerve fascicles (c) and separating them from the mesodermal tissues of the lamina. (× 840.)

B, Specimen similar to *A*, clearly showing the elastic fibers (a) and astrocytes (b) separating a nerve bundle (c) in the lamina cribrosa. (× 680.)

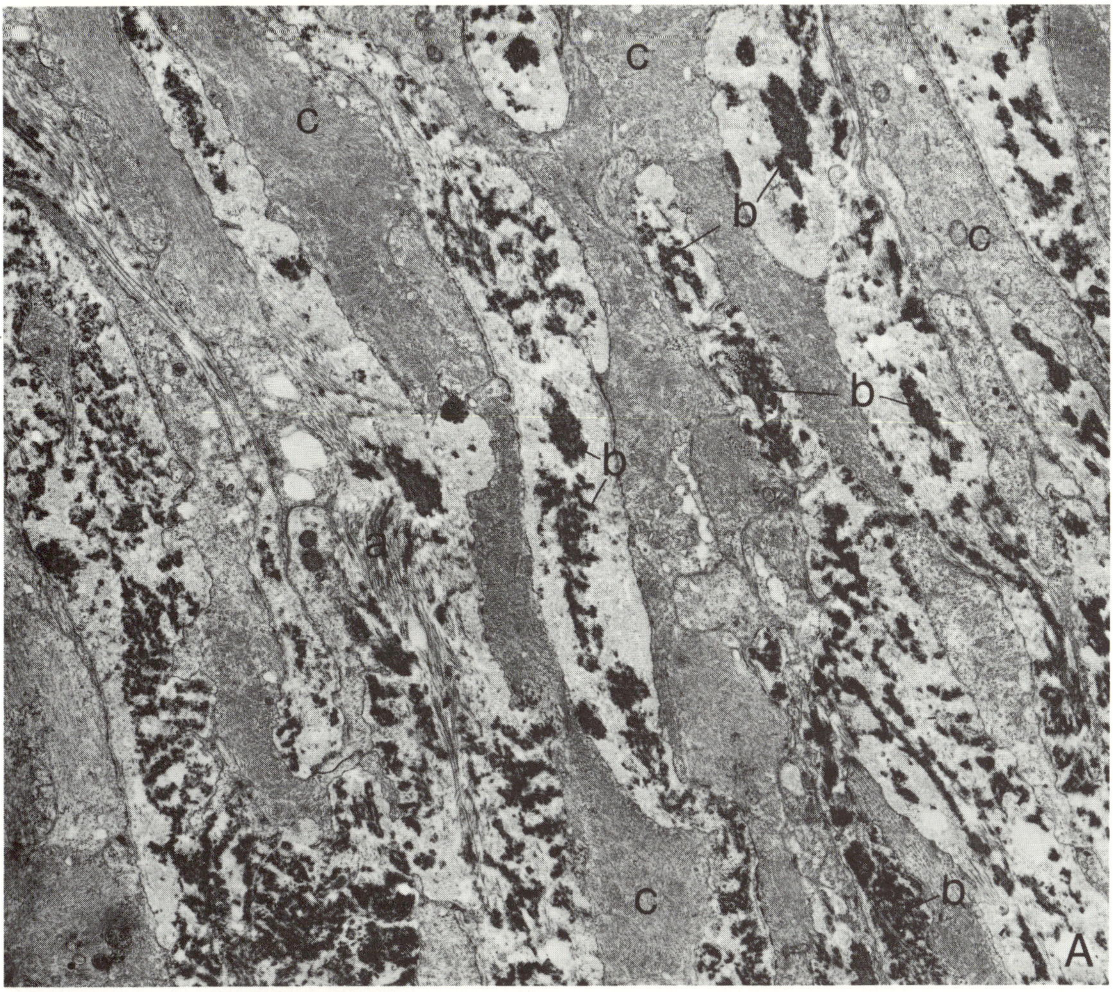

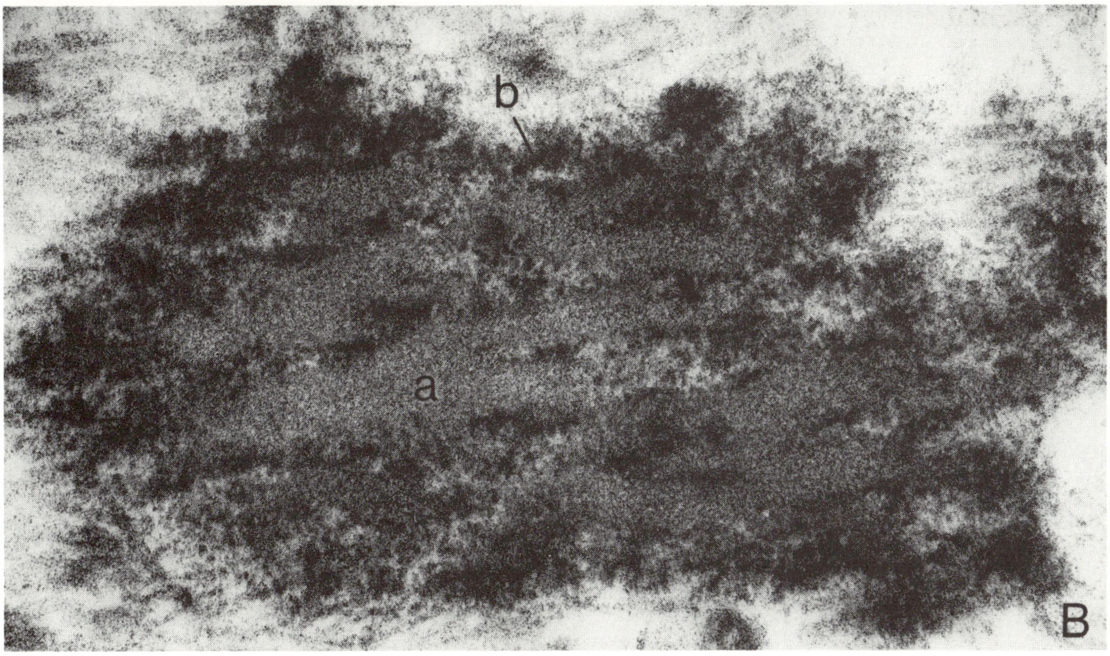

Figure 10–35. Electron micrographs of the lamina cribrosa. *A*, The connective tissues of the lamina form bundles containing collagen fibrils (a) and elastic tissue (b). Astrocyte processes are shown at (c). (× 6300.)

B, Higher magnification of an elastic fiber to show its amorphous core (a) and electron-dense cortex (b). (× 7200.)

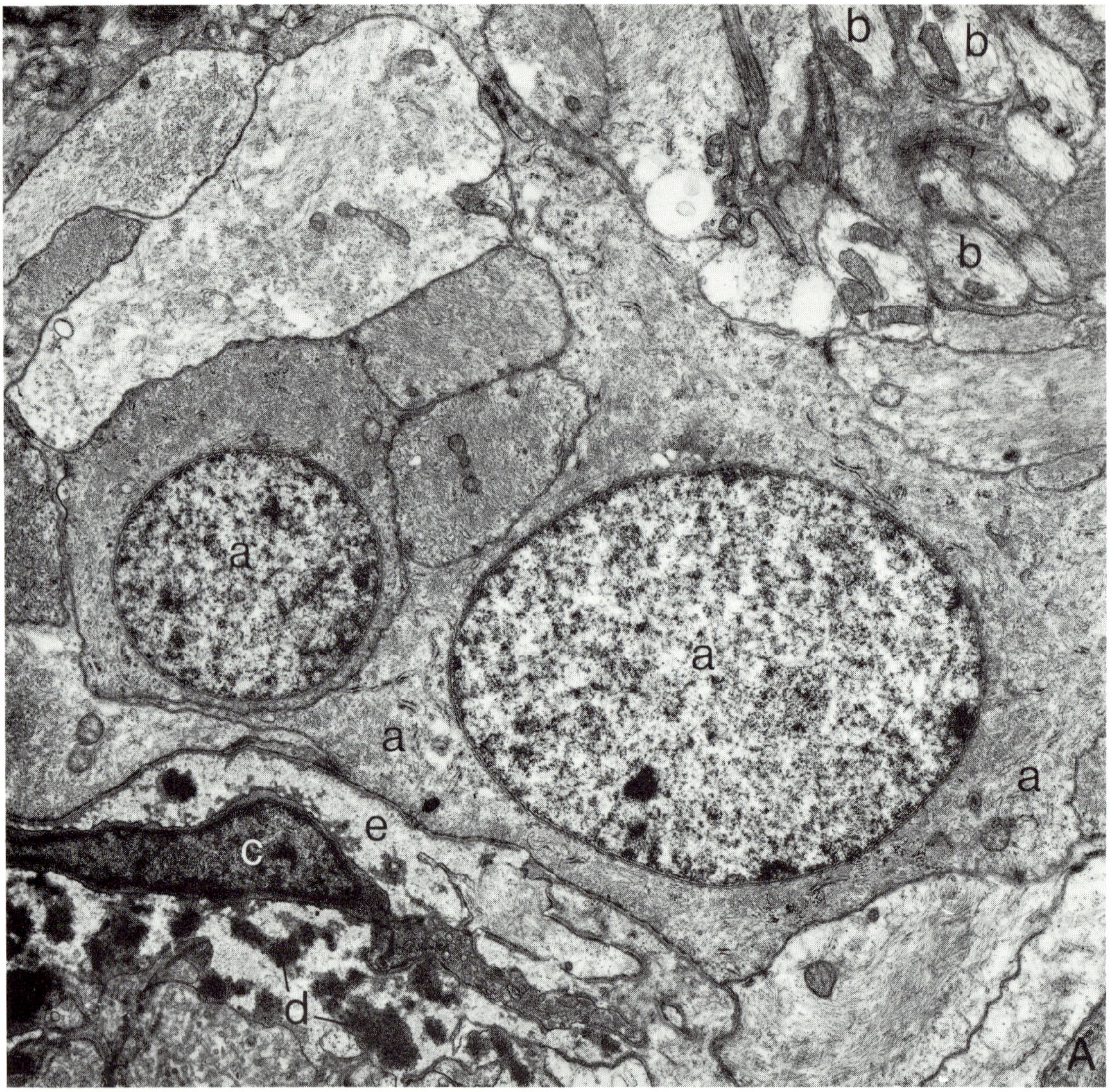

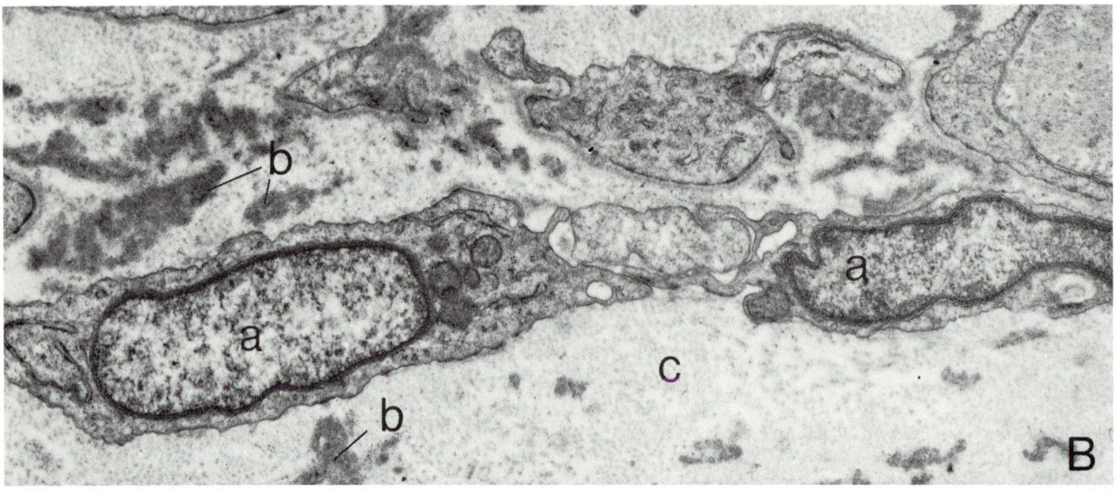

Figure 10–36. *See legend on opposite page.*

Orbital Optic Nerve

The orbital portion of the optic nerve includes the nerve, its meningeal sheaths, blood vessels and septa (Figs. 10-38 to 10-63).

Septa (Figs. 10-38 to 10-41). In the posterior part of the lamina cribrosa the connective tissue of the pia mater extends into the nerve to form septa which more or less enclose all the nerve fascicles. The septal system continues through the orbital and intracanalicular portions of the nerve and ends in the intracranial portion (Fig. 10-37). The septa extend into the nerve at right angles to its course, dividing it into compartments that contain a variable number of nerve axons (Fig. 10-39 *B*). Septa completely surround some of the nerve fascicles and incompletely surround others. The fascicles vary in size and shape, but generally they are oval. Longitudinal sections of the nerve show the septa to be arranged in fairly regular parallel rows. The pial septa are composed of collagen and very few elastic tissues, fibroblasts, nerves and vessels that are mainly arterioles, capillaries and venules derived from the pial system. Within the nerve the septa join the sheath of the central retinal vessels anterior to their entrance into the nerve (Fig. 10-39). They provide strong mechanical support for the nerve bundles and supply nutrition to the axons through their blood vessels and adjacent glial cells.

The collagen of the septa is aggregated into 38 compact bundles which run transversely into the nerve and frequently become oriented longitudinally (Fig. 10-39 *C*). A few scattered elastic fibers are seen, especially in broader areas adjacent to the pia mater. These elastic fibers, however, are not nearly so abundant as those in the lamina cribrosa. The capillaries have the same structure as those in the intraocular portion of the nerve. Zonulae occludentes are found near the capillary lumen between the endothelial cells. At the points of entrance and exit of the central retinal vessels, collagen is carried into the nerve from the pia mater as a connective tissue sheath around these vessels. This sheath stays with the vessels until they branch at the optic disc.

Neuroglia (Figs. 10-42 to 10-48). Three types of glial cells are found in the orbital portion of the optic nerve: *oligodendrocytes, astrocytes* and *microglia.* Microglia are now believed to be part of the reticuloendothelial system and not true neuroectodermal glia. The glial tissue of the orbital portion is distributed in two ways: some astrocytes line the inner surfaces of the pial septa and send processes into the fascicles, while others lie within the fascicles and have multidirectional processes. Oligodendrocytes are found only within the fascicles, where they are oriented longitudinally, parallel to the direction of the nerve fascicles.

Most information about astrocytes and oligodendrocytes has been obtained by light microscopy from tissues stained with special stains. Astrocytes are seen with the light microscope as large cells containing many

Text continued on page 582

Figure 10–36. Electron micrographs of the lamina cribrosa. *A*, Astrocytes (a) enclose the nerve bundles (b) and separate them from the connective tissue of the lamina. A fibroblast (c), elastic fibers (d) and negative images of collagen fibrils (e) are shown. (× 7800.)

B, Fibroblasts and their processes are commonly found within the connective tissue of the lamina. Two fibroblasts (a) and their perinuclear cytoplasm are shown. Elastic fibers (b) and negative images of the collagen fibrils (c) are indicated. (× 14,600.)

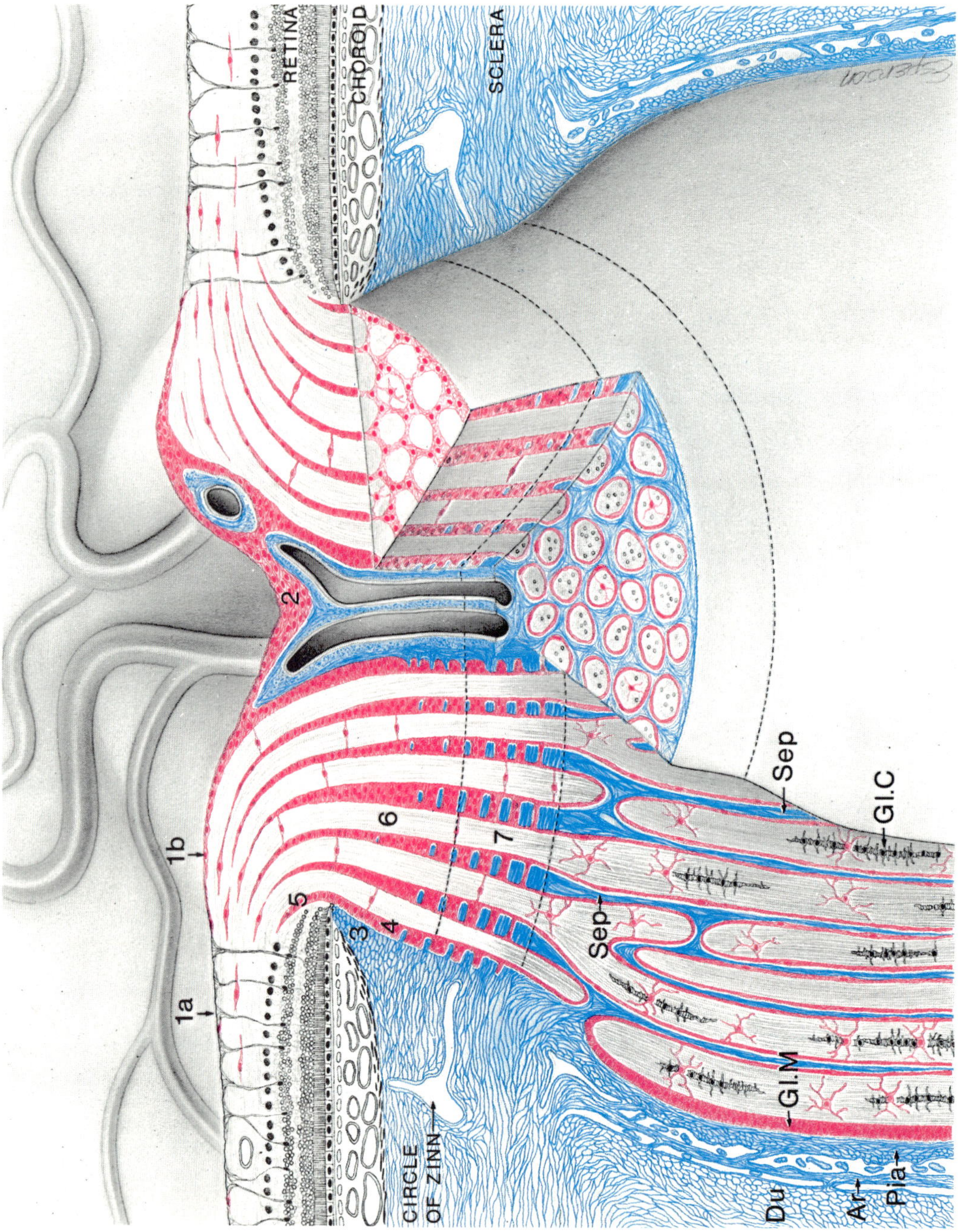

Figure 10–37. *See legend on opposite page.*

Figure 10–37. Three-dimensional color drawing of the intraocular and part of the orbital optic nerve. Where the retina terminates at the optic disc edge, the Müller cells (1a) are in continuity with the astrocytes, forming the *internal limiting membrane of Elschnig* (1b). In some specimens Elschnig's membrane is thickened in the central portion of the disc to form the *central meniscus of Kuhnt* (2). At the posterior termination of the choroid on the temporal side, the border tissue of Elschnig (3) lies between the astrocytes surrounding the optic nerve canal (4) and the stroma of the choroid. On the nasal side, the choroidal stroma is directly adjacent to the astrocytes surrounding the nerve. This collection of astrocytes (4) surrounding the canal is known as the border *tissue of Jacoby.* This is continuous with a similar glial lining called the intermediary tissue of Kuhnt (5) at the termination of the retina. The nerve fibers of the retina are segregated into approximately 1000 bundles or fascicles by astrocytes (6). Upon reaching the lamina cribrosa (upper dotted line), the nerve fascicles (7) and their surrounding astrocytes are separated from each other by connective tissue (drawn in blue). This connective tissue is the cribriform plate, which is an extension of scleral collagen and elastic fibers through the nerve. The external choroid also sends some connective tissue to the anterior part of the lamina. At the external part of the lamina cribrosa (lower dotted line), the nerve fibers become myelinated and columns of oligodendrocytes (black and white cells) and a few astrocytes (red-colored cells) are present within the nerve fascicles. The astrocytes surrounding the fascicles form a thinner layer here than in the laminar and prelaminar portion. The bundles continue to be separated by connective tissue all the way to the chiasm (Sep). This connective tissue is derived from the pia mater and is known as the septal tissue. A mantle of astrocytes (Gl.M), continuous anteriorly with the border tissue of Jacoby, surrounds the nerve along its orbital course. The dura (Du), arachnoid (Ar) and pia mater (Pia) are shown. The central retinal vessels are surrounded by a perivascular connective tissue throughout its course in the nerve; this connective tissue blends with the connective tissue of the cribriform plate in the lamina cribrosa; it is called the central supporting connective tissue strand here. (From Anderson, D., and Hoyt, W.: Arch. Ophthal. *82*:506, 1969.)

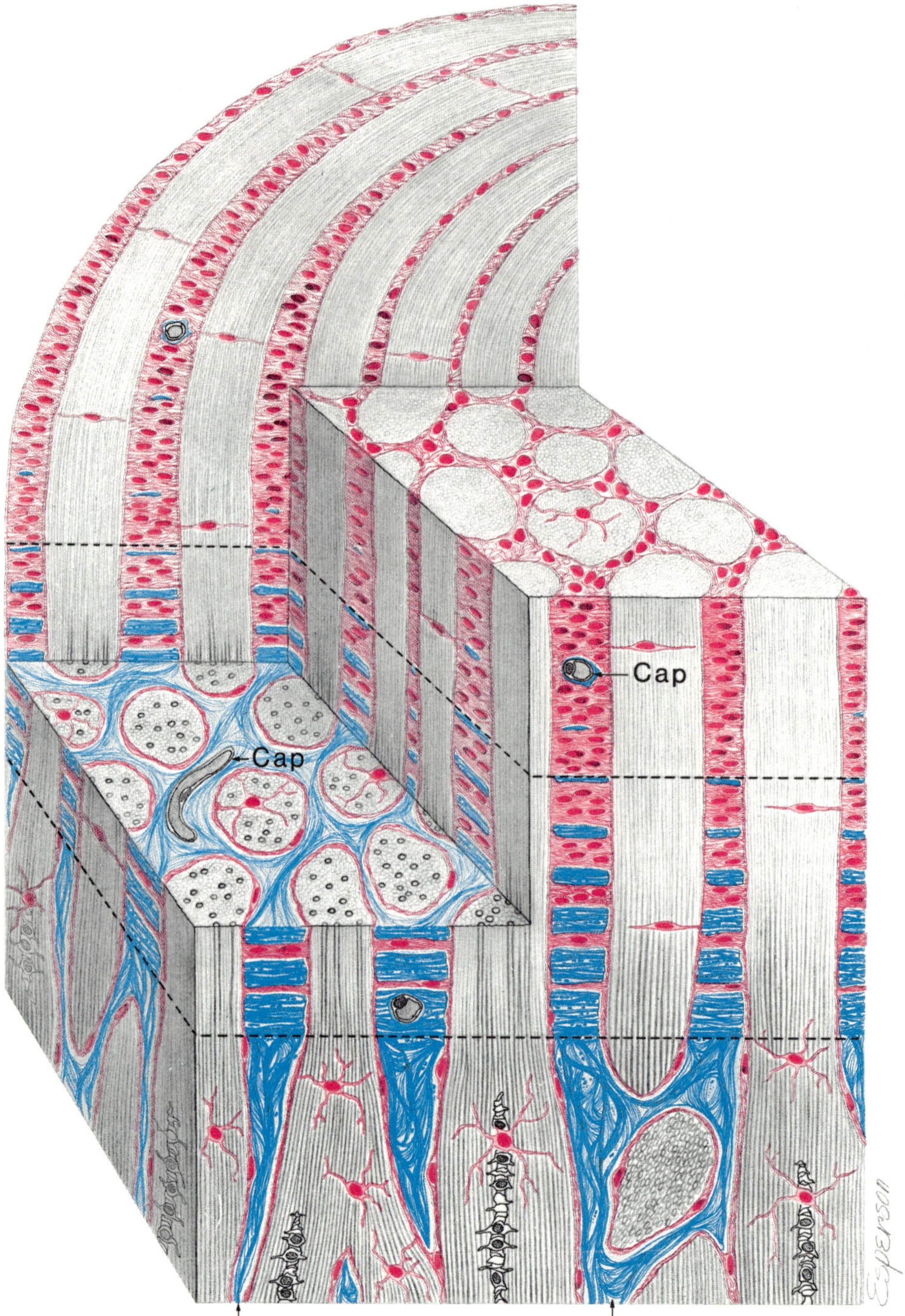

Figure 10–38. *See legend on opposite page.*

Figure 10–38. Detailed view of the *prelaminar, laminar* and *postlaminar* optic nerve. The nerve bundles are drawn in black and white, the astrocytes in red, oligodendrocytes in black and white and the connective tissue in blue. In the prelaminar region the nerves coming from the retina become segregated into bundles that are invested with a tube-like layer of astrocytes. The astrocytes and their processes are oriented perpendicular to the nerve bundles. Capillaries course within the astrocytic tubes in the prelaminar region. As the lamina cribrosa is reached (upper dotted line), the nerve fascicles are separated from each other by a layer of astrocytes, which in turn is covered by a mantle of connective tissue containing collagen, elastic fibers, fibroblasts and capillaries. In the posterior lamina cribrosa (lower dotted line), the nerves become myelinated, and columns of oligodendrocytes and a few astrocytes are found within the fascicles. The astrocytes separating the nerve fascicles in the laminar and postlaminar regions form a thinner layer than in the prelaminar portion. The connective tissue of the lamina cribrosa is continuous posteriorly with the pial septae. (From Anderson, D.: Arch. Ophthal. 82:800, 1969.)

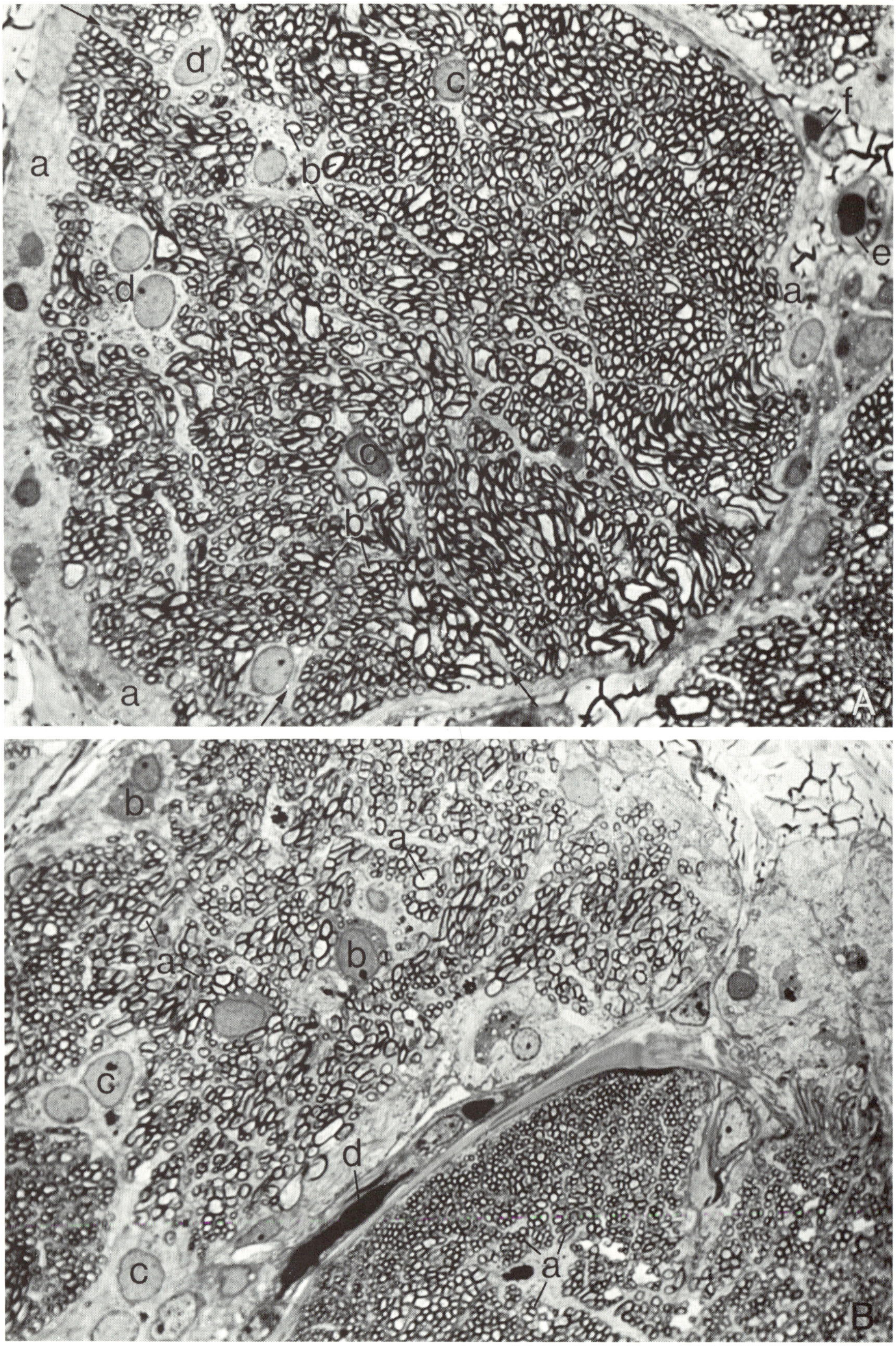

Figure 10–39. *See legend on opposite page.*

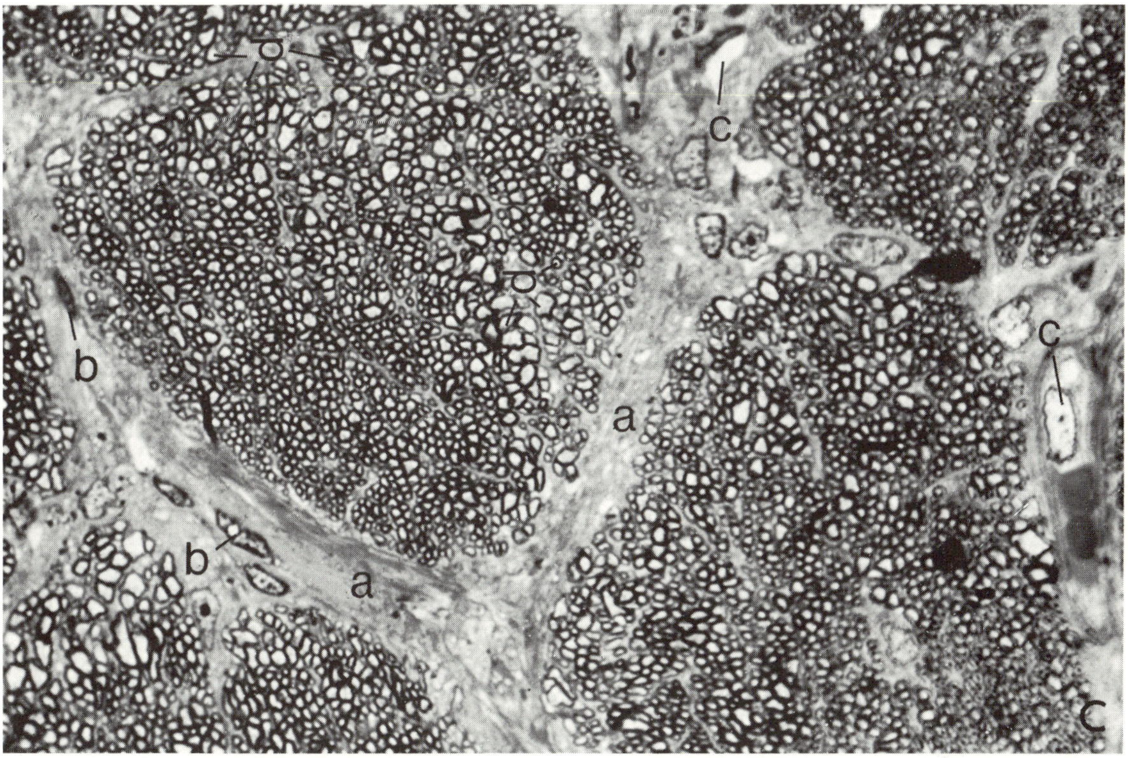

Figure 10–39. Light micrographs of nerve fascicles and septum in the orbital portion of the optic nerve. *A*, The nerve bundle is surrounded by a continuous layer of subseptal astrocytes (a) which send processes into the bundle (arrows). Inside the bundle, the myelinated nerve axons (b) are in contact with oligodendrocytes (c) and astrocytes (d). The oligodendrocytes have a dark-staining nucleus and cytoplasm, while the astrocytes have a larger, pale-staining nucleus and cytoplasm. An arteriole (e) and a capillary (f) are shown in the pial septa. (× 840.)

B, Two nerve bundles are seen in cross-section. The axons (a) vary widely in diameter and they are in contact with dark-staining oligodendrocytes (b) and light-staining astrocytes (c). A blood vessel (d) is shown in the connective tissue of the pial septum. (× 840.)

C, Low-power light micrograph to show several fascicles surrounded by septal tissue (a). The septa contain fibroblasts (b), small blood vessels (c) and collagen. There is considerable variation in the diameter of the axons within the fascicles (d). (× 840.)

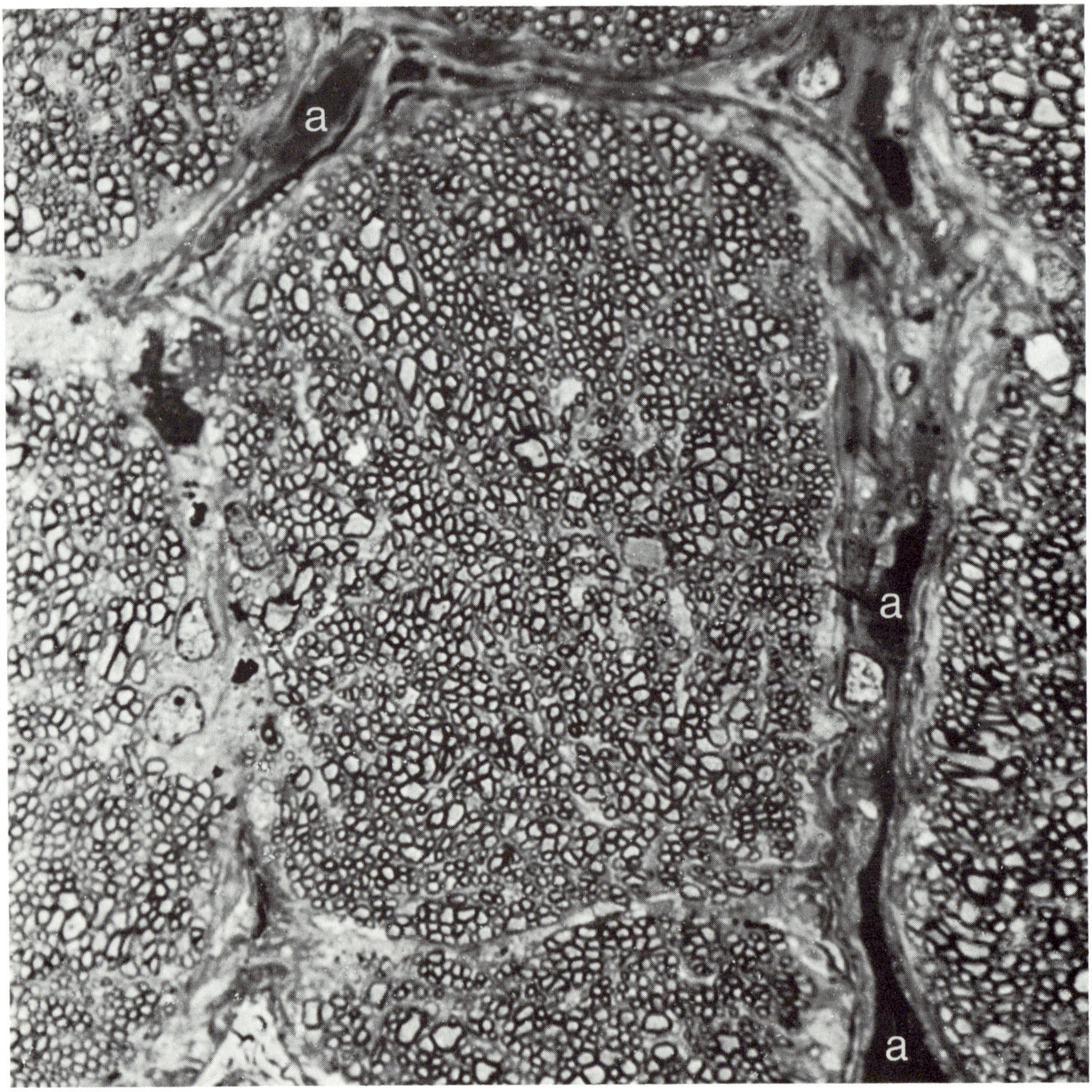

Figure 10–40. Light micrograph of optic nerve septa, which contain long, curved blood vessels (a) that are sectioned longitudinally. One thin septum cuts across a fascicle. (× 960.)

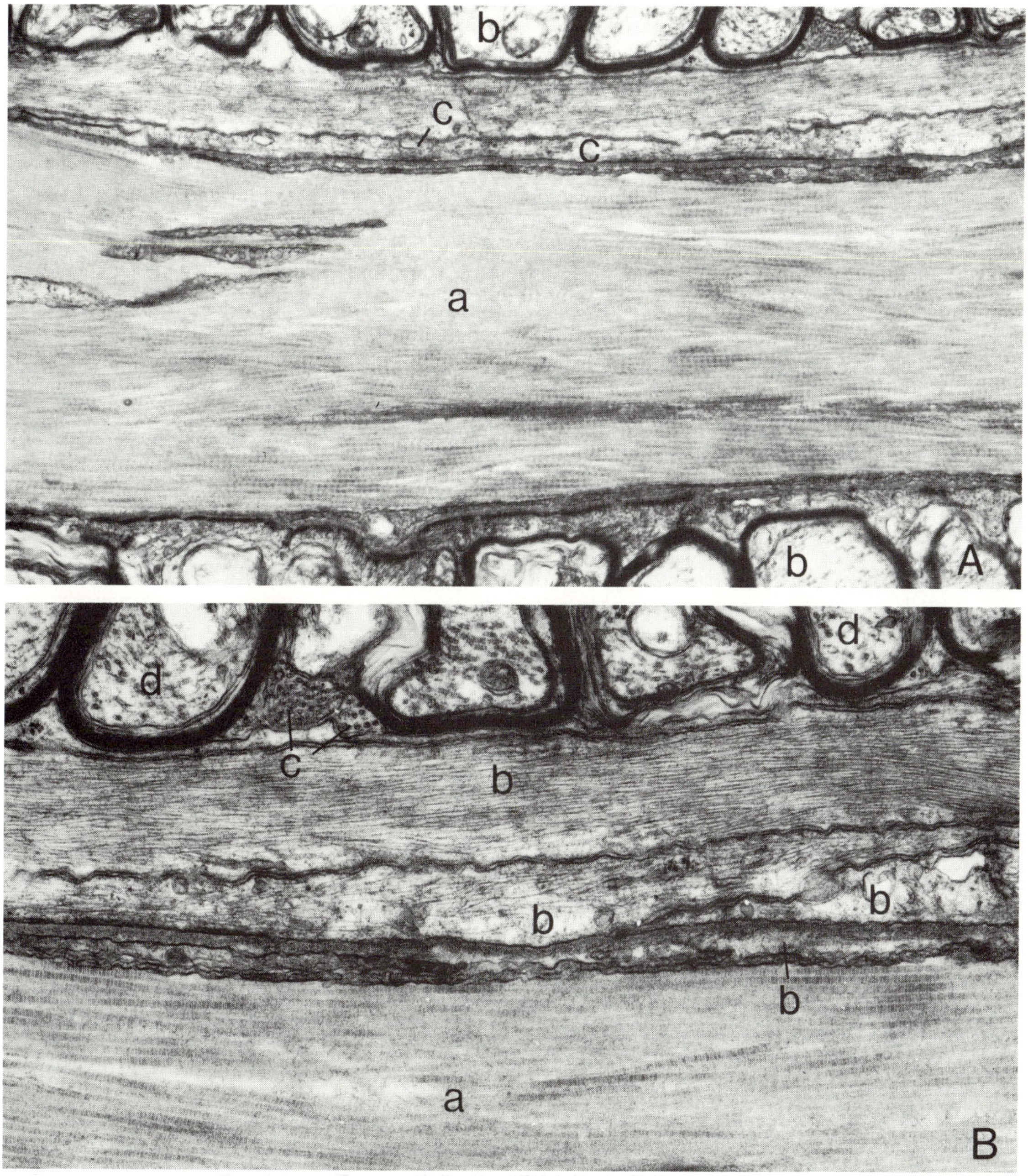

Figure 10–41. Electron micrographs of the septa. *A*, The entire thickness of a septum. Note the absence of elastic tissue here, compared to the lamina cribrosa. The septum in this micrograph is composed only of collagen fibrils (a). At the edge of the septum are nerve bundles (b), which are separated from the septum by the very fibrous astrocyte cytoplasm of the two cells (c). (× 13,500.)

B, The edge of a septum (a) and portions of three or four astrocytic processes (b) and a cross-section of an oligodendrocyte process (c). Myelinated nerves are at (d). (× 26,000.)

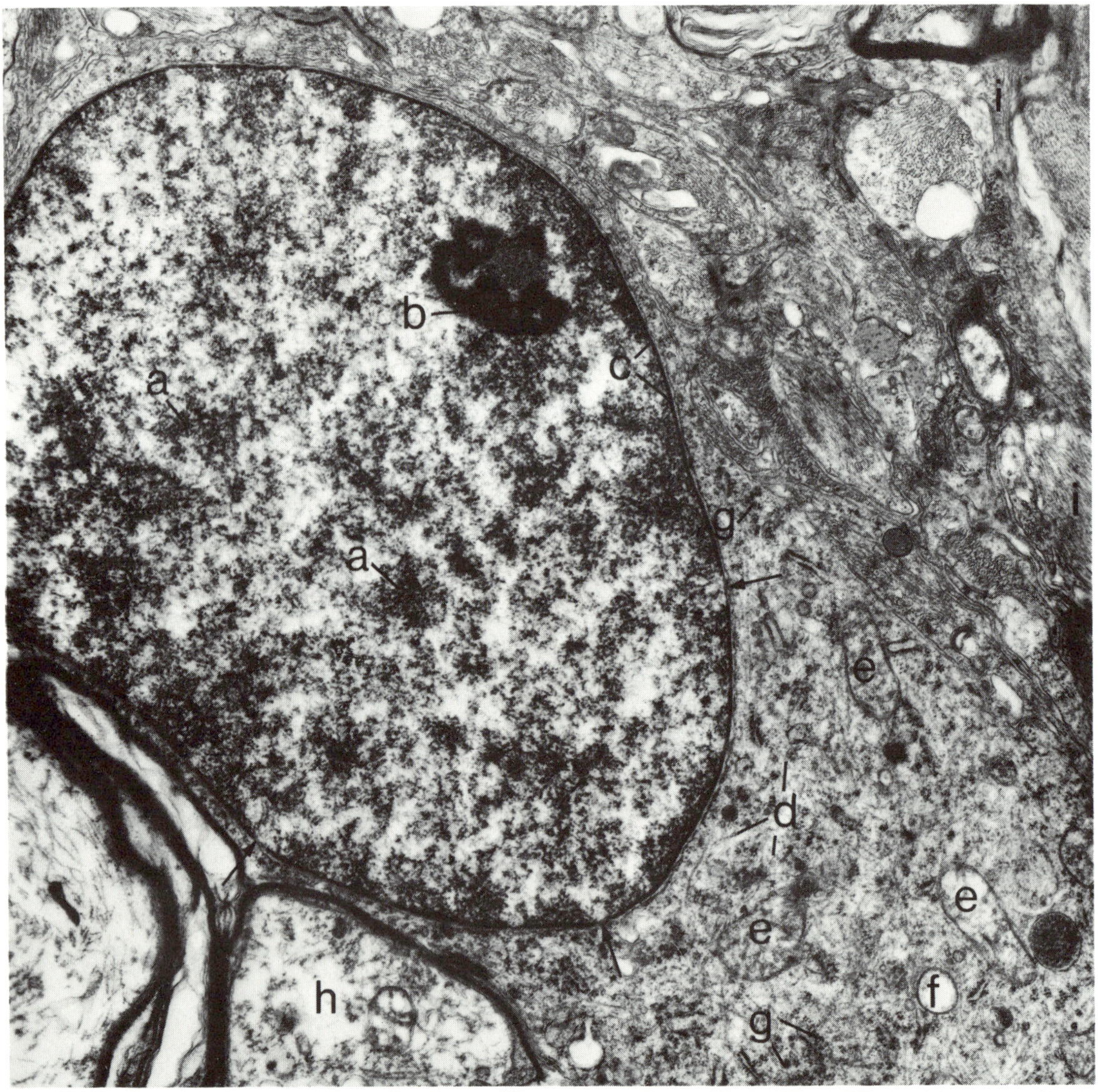

Figure 10–42. Low-magnification electron micrograph of an oligodendrocyte. The distinction between oligodendrocytes and astrocytes is not always easy to make. The size and eccentric location of the nucleus, degree of chromatin clumping, the density of the cytoplasm and the presence of a large number of microtubules in the processes are generally used to identify oligodendrocytes. The nucleus contains finely clumped, dispersed chromatin (a) and a nucleolus (b). The inner cell membrane of the nuclear envelope is outlined by a thin rim of condensed chromatin that is uniform in thickness (c). This rim of condensed chromatin is discontinuous at the nuclear pores (arrows). Typical of the cytoplasm of these cells is a large number of randomly oriented microtubules (d). Mitochondria (e), heterogenous membrane-bound vesicles (f) and free and membrane-bound ribosomes (g) are also seen. Adjacent to this cell are myelinated axons (h) and astrocyte processes (i). (× 13,500.)

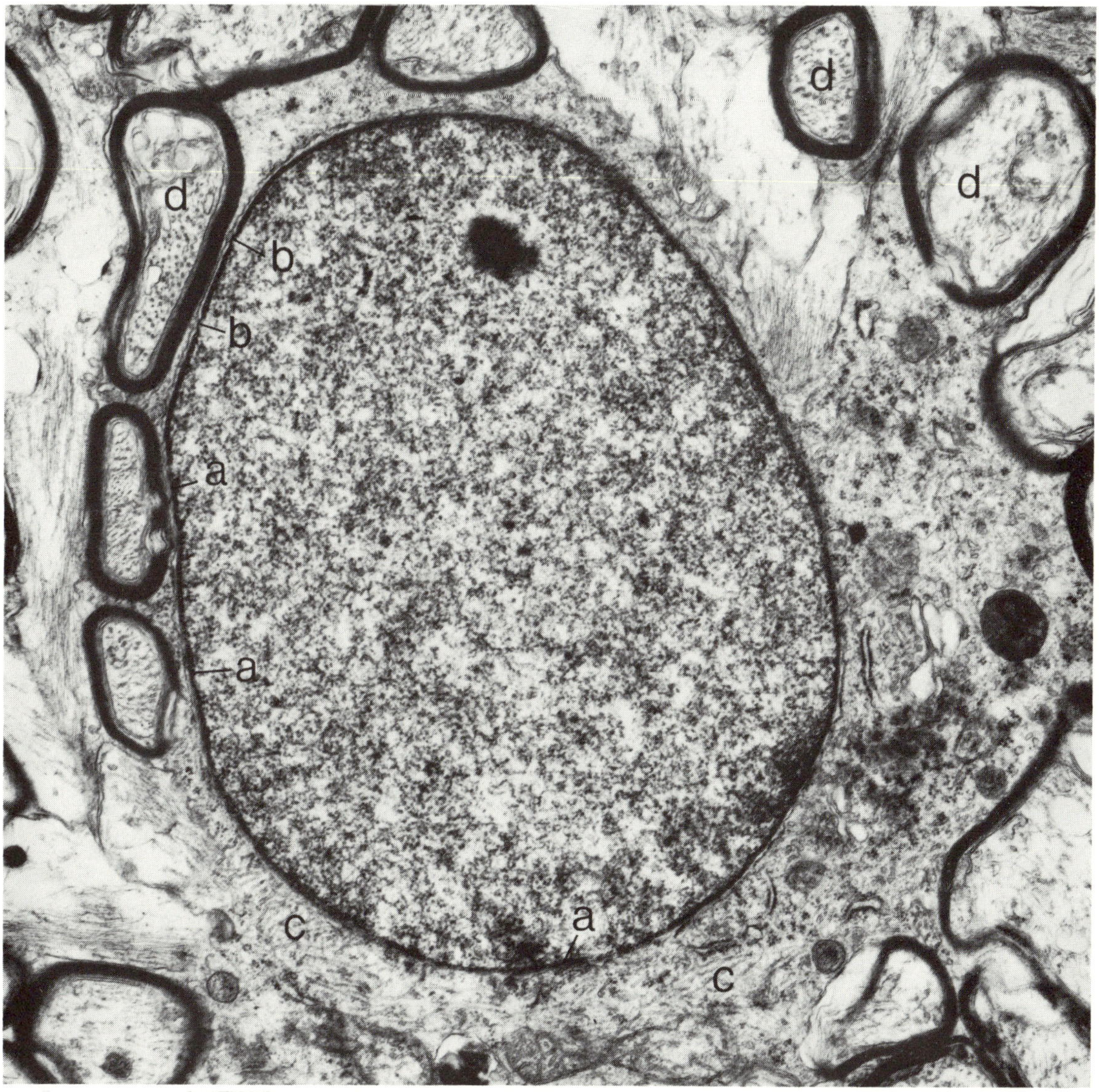

Figure 10–43. The nucleus and the perinuclear cytoplasm of an oligodendrocyte. The karyoplasm contains fine, evenly dispersed clumped chromatin that is outlined peripherally by an electron-dense rim of condensed chromatin (a) as seen in Figure 10–42. Nuclear pores are seen (b). The small amount of perinuclear cytoplasm contains numerous microtubules (c), and several myelinated axons (d) are enclosed by the oligodendrocytes. (× 17,000.)

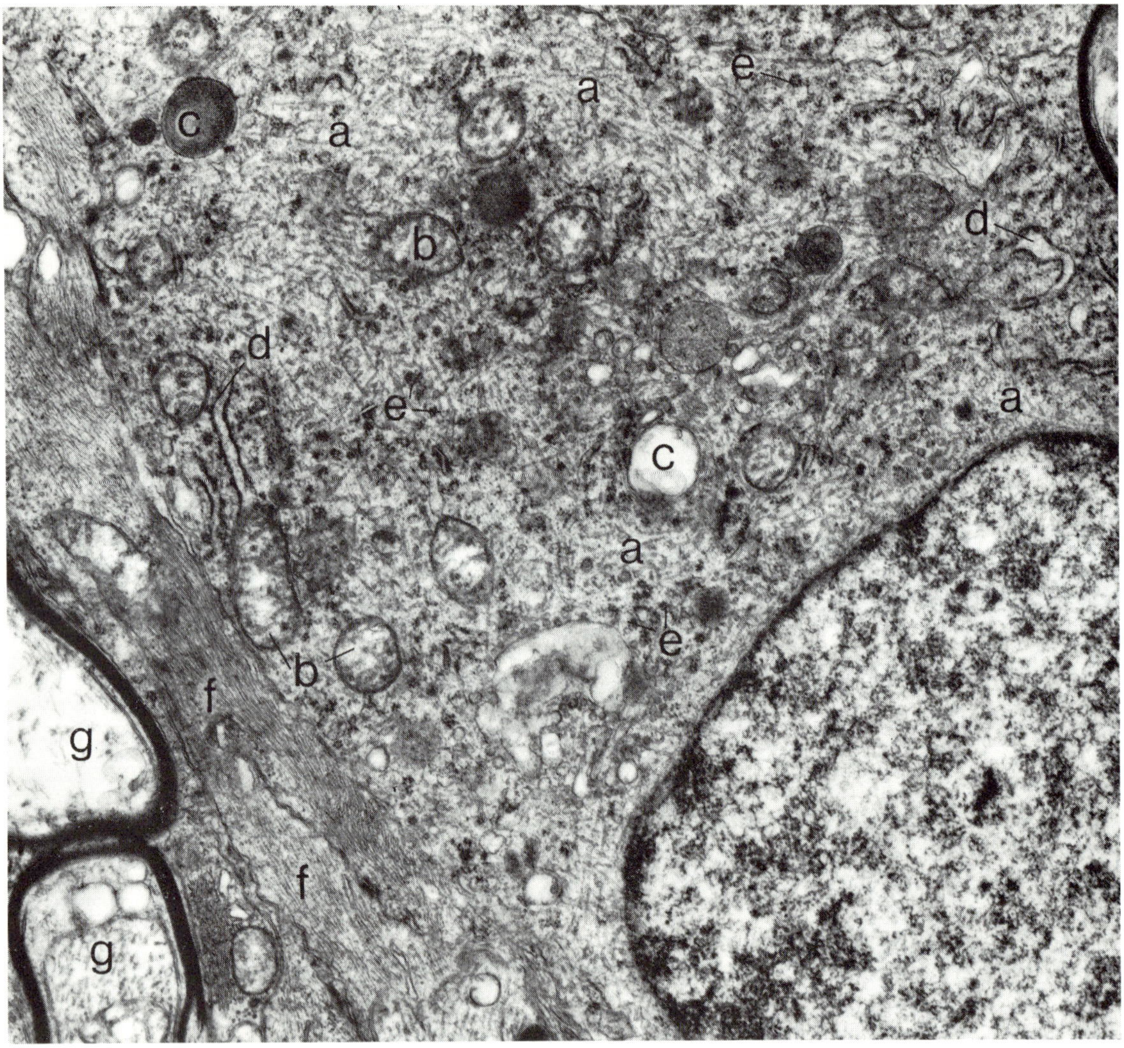

Figure 10–44. A portion of the nucleus and the cytoplasm of an oligodendrocyte. Microtubules occupy a large part of the cytoplasm (a). Mitochondria (b), membrane-bound vesicles (c), cisternae of the rough-surfaced endoplasmic reticulum (d) and free ribosomes (e) are also shown. An astrocyte process filled with fine filaments (f) is interposed between the oligodendrocyte and two myelinated axons (g). (× 16,300.)

branched processes, some of which end as footplates on the outer surfaces of blood vessels and against the pial septa. Most of the processes enclose groups of nerve fibers or extend in a random fashion through the nerve fascicles. They have supporting and insulating functions and probably play a part in the nutrition of the nerve. The processes form several layers around the adventitia of the central retinal blood vessels and become very numerous around the periphery of the nerve, where they form a compact layer known as the *peripheral glial mantle of Graefe.*

The oligodendroglia is identical to that in the white matter of the brain; it comprises two thirds of the interstitial cells of the optic nerve. When stained with silver carbonate, these cells show a lightly stained round or oval nucleus and a granular cytoplasm. They have long, delicate processes, their main rami show localized swellings, and they often branch

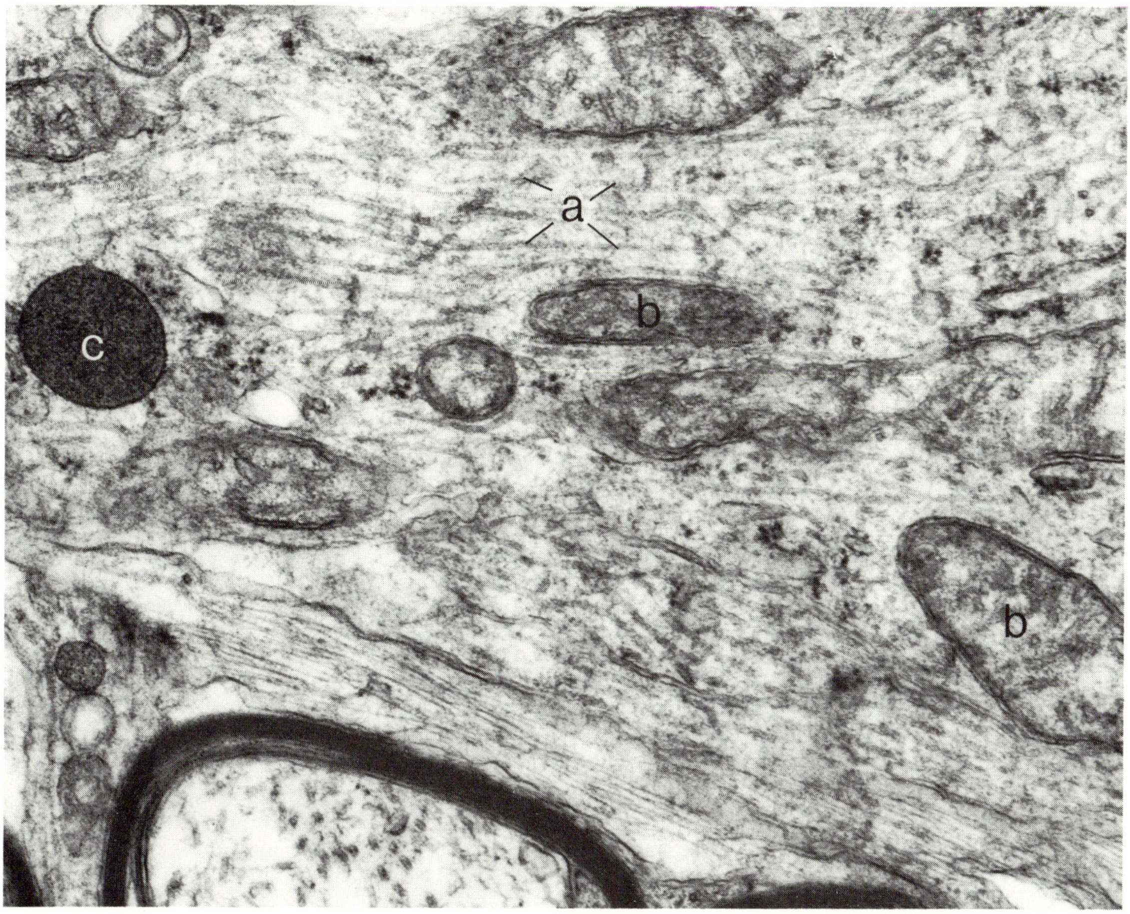

Figure 10–45. Oligodendrocyte process. Unlike astrocytes, oligodendrocytes have only a few processes. Their cytoplasm has numerous microtubules (a), as well as mitochondria (b) and vesicles bound by a single membrane (c) which are probably lysosomal in nature. (× 37,400.)

dichotomously. The cells are oriented in long rows or columns between the axons and are frequently interspersed with astrocytes. They are much more numerous within the central portions of the fascicles, but some cells are found near the periphery. Small processes may extend along the pial septal columns, but these cells have no part in formation of the peripheral glia of the fascicles. Oligodendrocytes are responsible for formation of the myelin sheaths around the axons of the optic nerve, however, performing the same function as that of Schwann cells in the peripheral nerves.

Light microscopic examination of very thin, plastic-embedded specimens reveals that the oligodendrocytes are smaller than astrocytes; they have a dense, eccentrically placed nucleus as well as very dense cytoplasm. Astrocytes, on the other hand, have a large, pale nucleus and many processes that extend within the nerve fascicles. These astrocytes are found around the periphery of the nerve fascicle as well as among the axons. Oligodendrocytes are not found to form a layer around the periphery of the fascicles or to make important contacts with the septa. Rather, they are found mainly within the fascicles, often forming long columns. The astrocytes form a thin mantle of

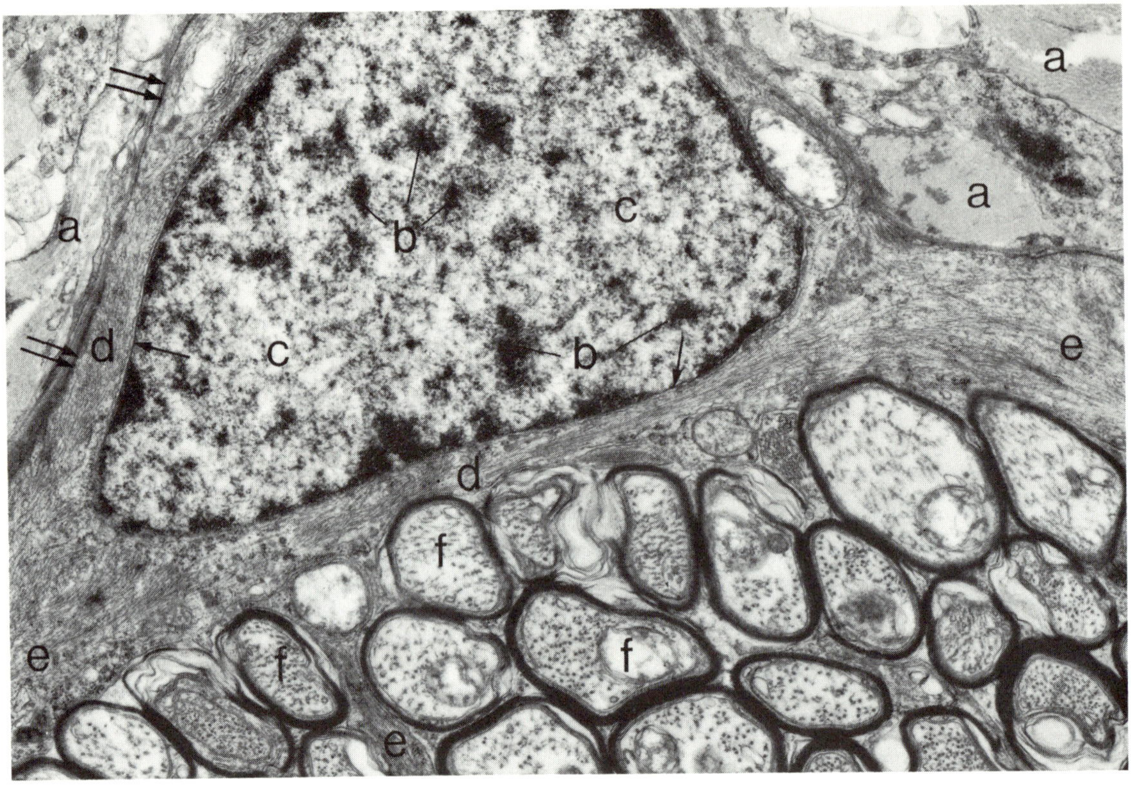

Figure 10–46. Electron micrograph of an astrocyte in the orbital portion of the optic nerve. Oligodendrocytes are found only within the nerve fascicles (intrafascicular oligodendrocytes). Astrocytes, however, are intrafascicular as well as perifascicular, where they form a sheath around each fascicle. A perifascicular astrocyte is shown adjacent to the connective tissue of a septum (a). There is a basement membrane around the septal side of the cell (double arrows). The astrocyte nucleus is characterized by its coarse clumps of chromatin (b), as well as by dispersed finer and paler chromatin (c). At the periphery of the nucleus the thin rim of condensed chromatin (arrows), which is so clearly seen in oligodendrocytes, is obscured by coarse clumps of chromatin. The perinuclear cytoplasm is occupied by fine filaments (d) measuring between 60 and 80 A. in diameter. These filaments extend into the astrocytic process (e), which encloses the myelinated axons (f). (×11,700.)

glial tissue along the internal surfaces of the pial septa (Fig. 10-39), where they often show very heavy processes. There is no definite pattern of arrangement of the astrocytes within the fascicles, whereas they are often oriented at right angles to the course of the nerve fibers in the peripheral portion.

Reticuloendothelial microglial cells are found in moderate numbers throughout the optic nerve. Microscopically they have the same appearance as macrophages and reticuloendothelial cells in other tissues, except that in the resting stage they have less cytoplasm, are more deep-staining and have irregular borders.

The difficult task of identifying astrocytes and oligodendrocytes with the electron microscope is complicated by a spectrum of morphologic variations shown by these two cell types. For purposes of identification, they can be compared with those in the prelaminar portion; that is, to identify astrocytes it is best to study the astrocytes that form the glial sheaths of the fascicles. When familiarity with the morphologic variations shown by these cells is achieved, they can be identified in their intrafascicular location.

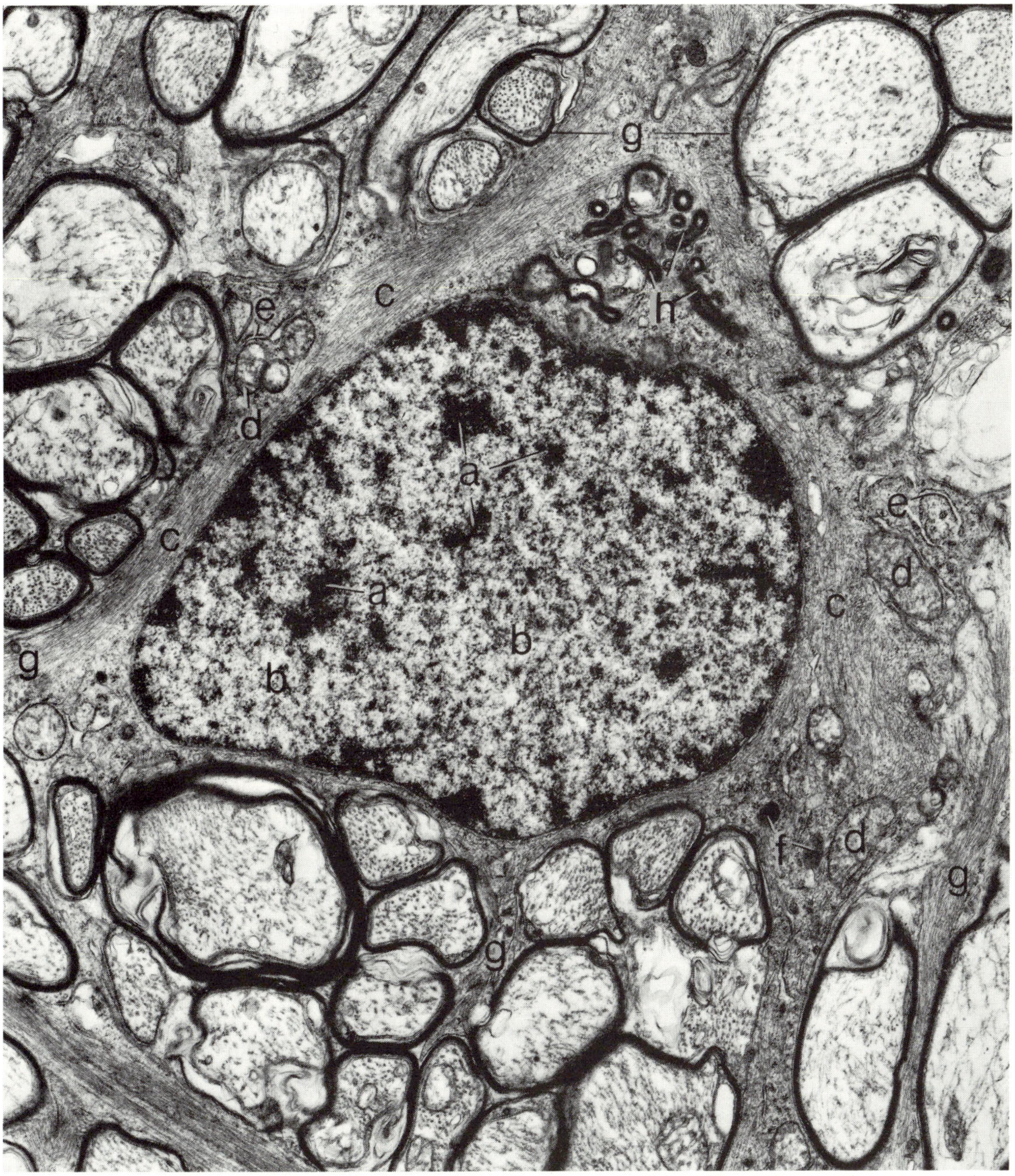

Figure 10–47. Intrafascicular astrocyte in the orbital portion of the optic nerve. The karyoplasm shows the coarse chromatin clumps (a) and the finer chromatin dispersed throughout the nucleus (b). The perinuclear cytoplasm is occupied mainly by longitudinally oriented filaments (c), a few mitochondria (d), cisternae of the rough-surfaced endoplasmic reticulum (e) and vesicular organelles bound by a single membrane (f). Several astrocytic processes (g) extend from the perinuclear cytoplasm to surround myelinated axons. These processes are also filled with filaments. Grazing sections of myelin sheaths are seen at (h). (× 11,200.)

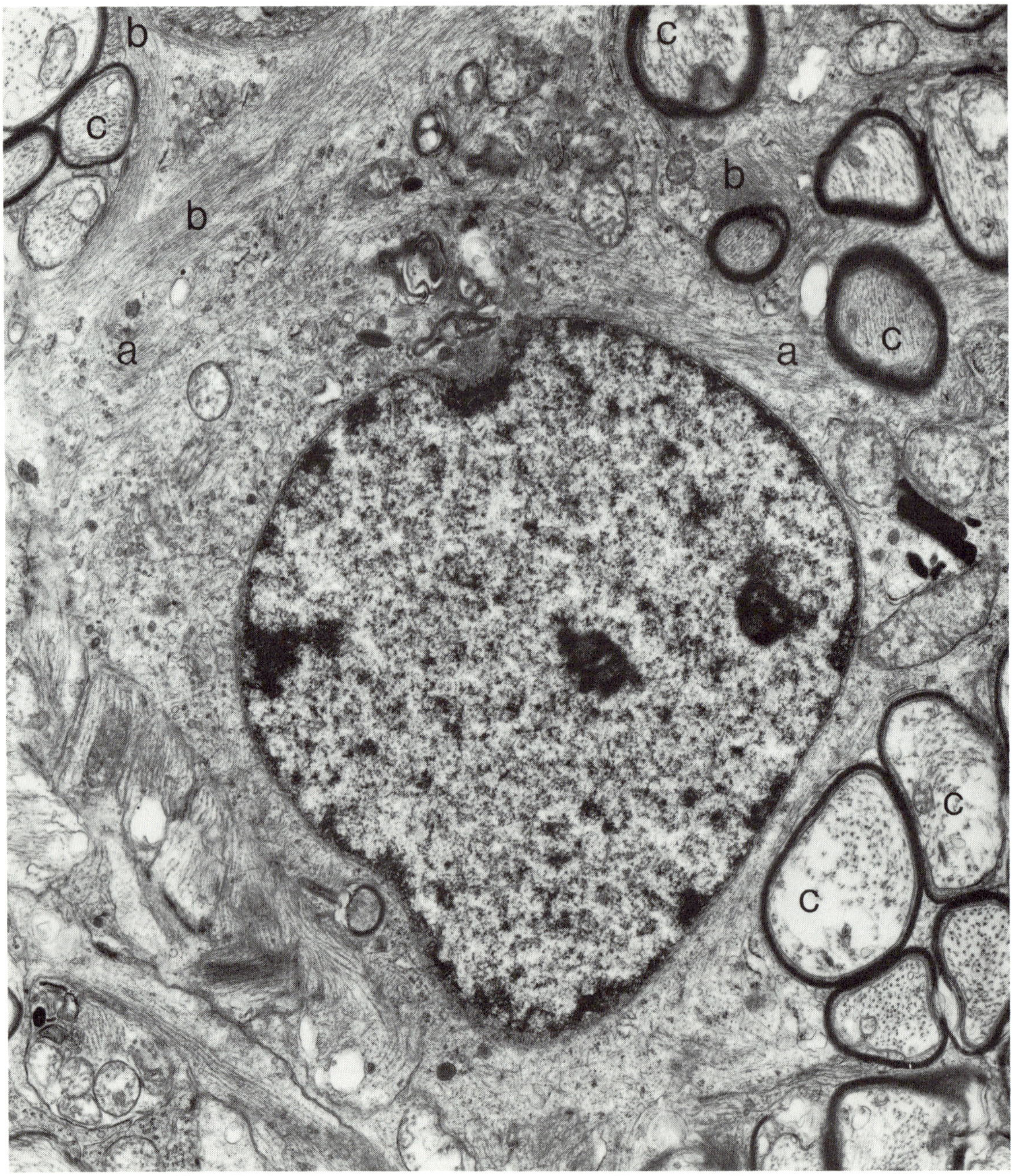

Figure 10–48. Intrafascicular astrocyte of the orbital optic nerve. The characteristic clumping of the nuclear chromatin is clearly seen. The cytoplasm is filled by bundles of filaments (a) which extend into the astrocytic processes (b) to surround the myelinated axons (c). (× 11,700.)

Astrocytes (Figs. 10-24 to 10-48). The astrocytes have a large round or elliptical nucleus that typically shows a few coarse clumps of chromatin within a relatively light karyoplasm (Fig. 10-47). The cytoplasm is voluminous and very pale; it contains mitochondria, rough-surfaced endoplasmic reticulum and a Golgi apparatus. The cytoplasm has numerous filaments, which are arranged mainly parallel to each other. These filaments measure about 60 to 75 A. in diameter and are seen in the perinuclear region and scattered throughout the cytoplasm; they extend into the farthest reaches of the processes. The cytoplasm may contain a varying amount of glycogen, which appears as angulated granules, depending on the type of fixation. Rarely, astrocytes have a cilium (Anderson, 1969). When the embryologic development of the glia is considered, it is not surprising that they are ciliated. Both the astrocytes and oligodendrocytes contain dense inclusions that are globular, crystalline and spiked, which Anderson and associates (1967) believe to be lipofuscin.

Within the nerve fascicles the astrocytes send their processes in all directions. These ramify among the nerve fibers to provide support, insulation and nutrition. At the periphery of the fascicles the processes form a layer of varying thickness, averaging about 10 μm. (Fig. 10-48). In the peripheral fascicles near the pial sheath, the peripheral glial mantle of Graefe increases to about 40 to 50 μm. in thickness (Fig. 10–49). The surfaces of the astrocytes that abut on the connective tissue septa and pial sheath have a basement membrane, and the adjacent cell membrane frequently shows numerous insertions of filaments from the cytoplasm, giving the appearance of a half-desmosome. In some places there are indentations of septal collagen into the glia; such invaginations occur between footplates and within single footplates. Similar glial relations are found at the surface of the collagen surrounding the central retinal vessels.

Oligodendrocytes (Figs. 10-44 and 10-45). These cells are characterized by smaller nuclei than seen in the astrocytes; the nucleus shows an evenly distributed, prominent clumping of the chromatin. The cytoplasm of oligodendrocytes is denser than that of the astrocyte and contains considerable rough-surfaced endoplasmic reticulum and free ribosomes. Microtubules, which are more numerous in oligodendrocytes than in astrocytes, follow the processes for a short distance. These microtubules identify the oligodendrocyte processes among the neuropile, although it is difficult to distinguish this cell from a nerve axon at a node of Ranvier. The presence of microtubules in the cytoplasm of cells forming the myelin sheath is part of the anatomic evidence that myelin is derived from oligodendrocytes.

Nerve Axons (Figs. 10-49 and 10-50). Yamamoto (1966), Cohen (1967) and Anderson and Hoyt (1969) have confirmed many of the observations of light microscopists with respect to the fine structure of nerve axons. In cross-section most of the myelinated fibers are small, with a diameter that measures around 1.0 μm. but may vary between 0.3 and 3.5 μm. The myelin sheaths measure 0.03 to 0.27 μm. in thickness, most being less than 0.1 μm. In longitudinal sections there appears to be some variation in axon diameter, possibly because of the direction of sectioning. The axoplasm is surrounded by the usual cell membrane and contains many filaments, neurotubules, mitochondria and some endoplasmic reticulum (Fig. 10-50). The neurotubules are oriented parallel to the length of the axon and measure 200 to 250 A. in diameter. Cohen (1967) pointed out that glutaraldehyde fixation reveals

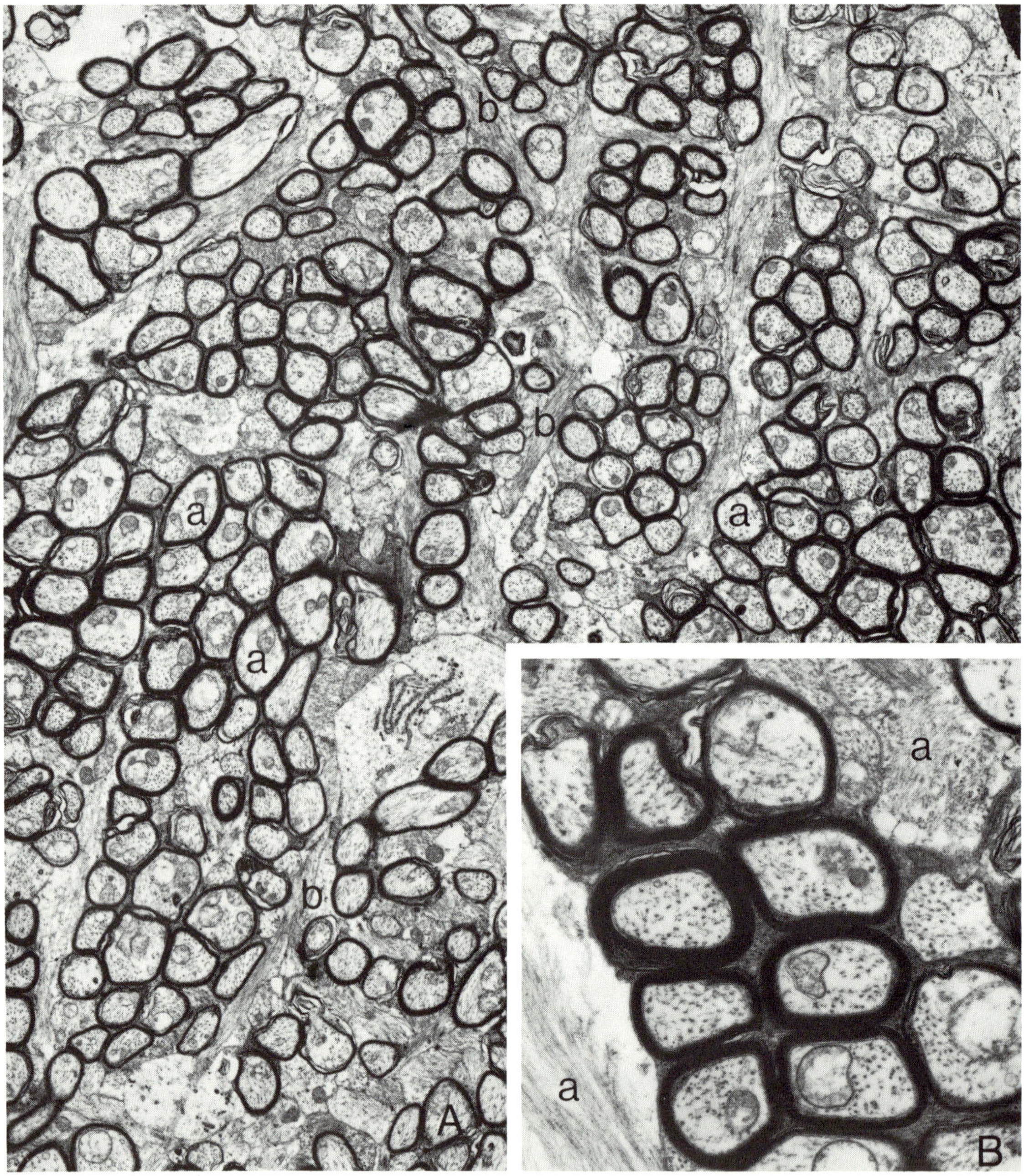

Figure 10–49. Optic nerve fascicles. *A*, Low-power electron micrograph to show the myelinated nerve fibers of the optic nerve (a) and their surrounding astrocytic processes (b). There is considerable variation in the diameter of the fascicles. (× 5400.)

B, Enlargement of the fascicles to show the myelin sheath and the surrounding astrocytic processes (a). The small dots in the axoplasm are cross-sections of neurotubules. (× 13,200.)

these tubular elements, which serve to distinguish the nerve fibers from the astrocytic processes. The filaments may be numerous in various parts of the cytoplasm along the length of the axons, measuring 60 to 70 A. in diameter. The mitochondria are distributed throughout the axoplasm and have the usual configuration. Endoplasmic reticulum of the smooth type is encountered in small amounts throughout the axoplasm. The axons contain no other organelles, except occasional lipofuscin granules.

Myelination of these axons is accomplished in the same manner as in peripheral nerves. The oligodendroglial cells wrap the axons with many double layers of their membranes, and both internal and external mesaxons have been identified (Fig. 10-50 *B*). The nodes of Ranvier, best seen in longitudinal section, are like those elsewhere in the nervous system. The myelin wrappings separate and end in loops, with cytoplasm containing microtubules, ribosomes and occasional organelles. The axon is exposed in the intervals between the last loop on one side and the first loop on the side facing the node; astrocytes cover such unmyelinated areas. At the lamina cribrosa, myelination ends with formation of only half a node of Ranvier. Anderson (1969) and Cohen (1967) were not able to demonstrate branching of the axons at the node of Ranvier, as was suggested by Yamamoto (1966). Their studies were made on the anterior nerve, however, in contrast to the posterior nerve studies of Yamamoto. Branchings in the posterior nerve were also described by Cajal (1955).

It is possible that some axons in the optic nerve are centrifugal. Wolter (1965) recently reviewed the possibility and made a strong suggestion that centrifugal nerves exist. In an eye that had been enucleated for a central retinal artery occlusion, in which all the centripetal fibers had degenerated, Wolter showed that the human disc contained centrifugal fibers. He estimated that about one tenth of the fibers of the human nerve must be centrifugal, and he also found these centrifugal fibers to vary considerably in size, from about 1 μm. down to very fine filaments. He also studied the optic nerve stumps, chiasm and tracts of a patient who had undergone bilateral enucleation of the eyes 50 years previously. A large number of fibrils remained in the optic nerves and other parts of the pathway. Although some of these were unmyelinated and seemed to come from the chiasmal region, most fibers were myelinated and could be traced to the region of the geniculate bodies, and some crossed in the chiasm. The origin of these fibers is not known, but it has been suggested that some of them end on the walls of the blood vessels. Among more recent observers, however, Kupfer and co-workers (1967) and Cohen (1967) were not able to discover axons of this type.

Central Retinal Vessels (Figs. 10–51 to 10–56). The central retinal artery has the structure of a small muscular artery, with an endothelium, subendothelial connective tissue, elastic lamina, muscularis and adventitia. The central vein has the structure of a small vein, with some muscle tissue in its wall.

The arterial endothelium is like that of the capillary and rests on a lamellated basement membrane that is continuous with some basement membrane-like material which contains granules and fine filaments that resemble reticulin. External to this is the internal elastic lamina. The media contains about six layers of smooth muscle cells which are oriented mostly in a circular direction; each layer is surrounded by a basement membrane. The basement membranes of adjacent cells may fuse, or may be separated by a homogeneous granular material containing collagen, reticulin and elastin.

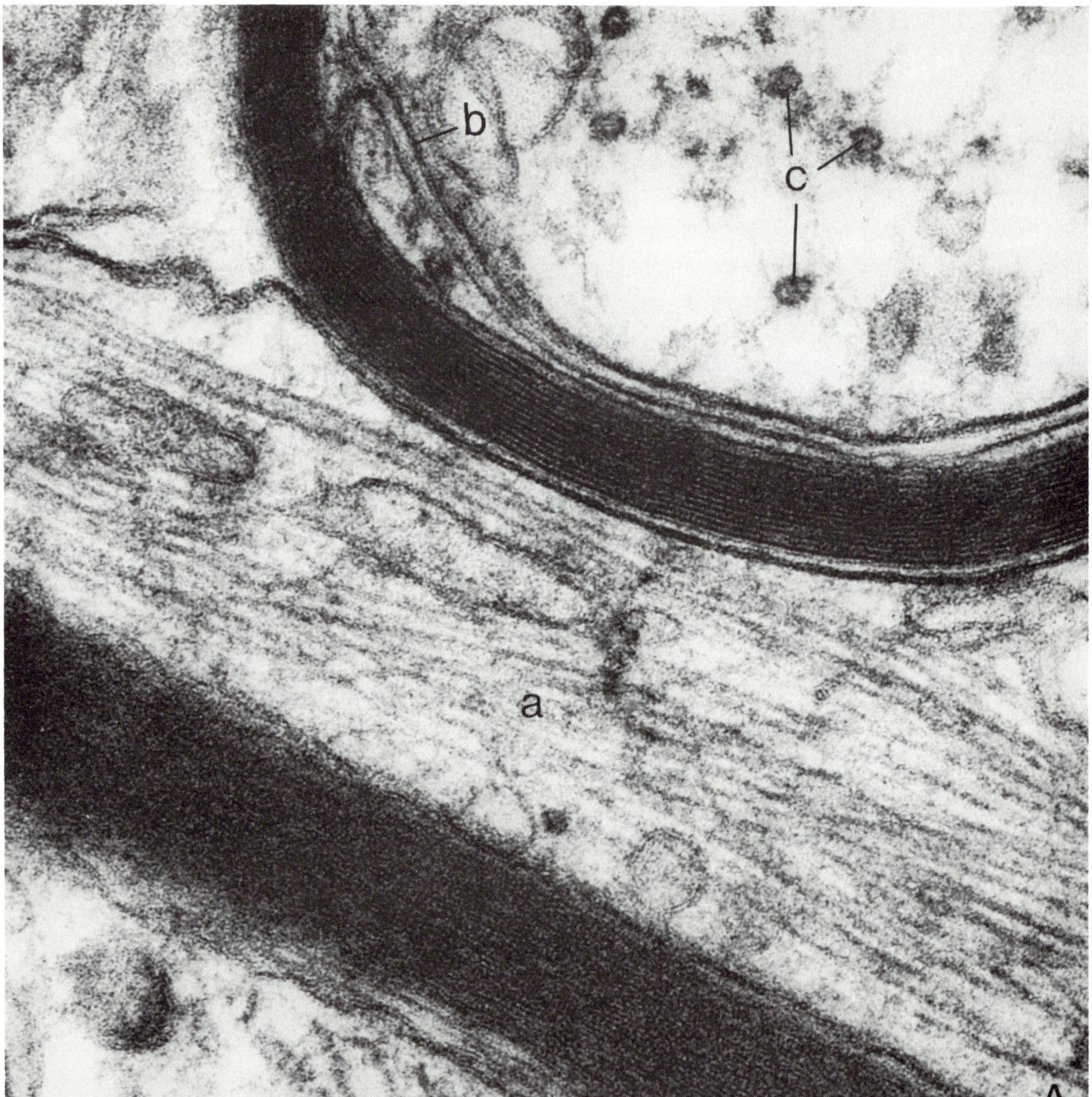

Figure 10–50. Myelinated optic nerve axons. *A*, Sections of two axons that are separated by an astrocytic process (a). The mesaxon of the myelin sheath (b) and cross-sections of neurotubules (c) are seen in the upper axon. (× 120,000.)

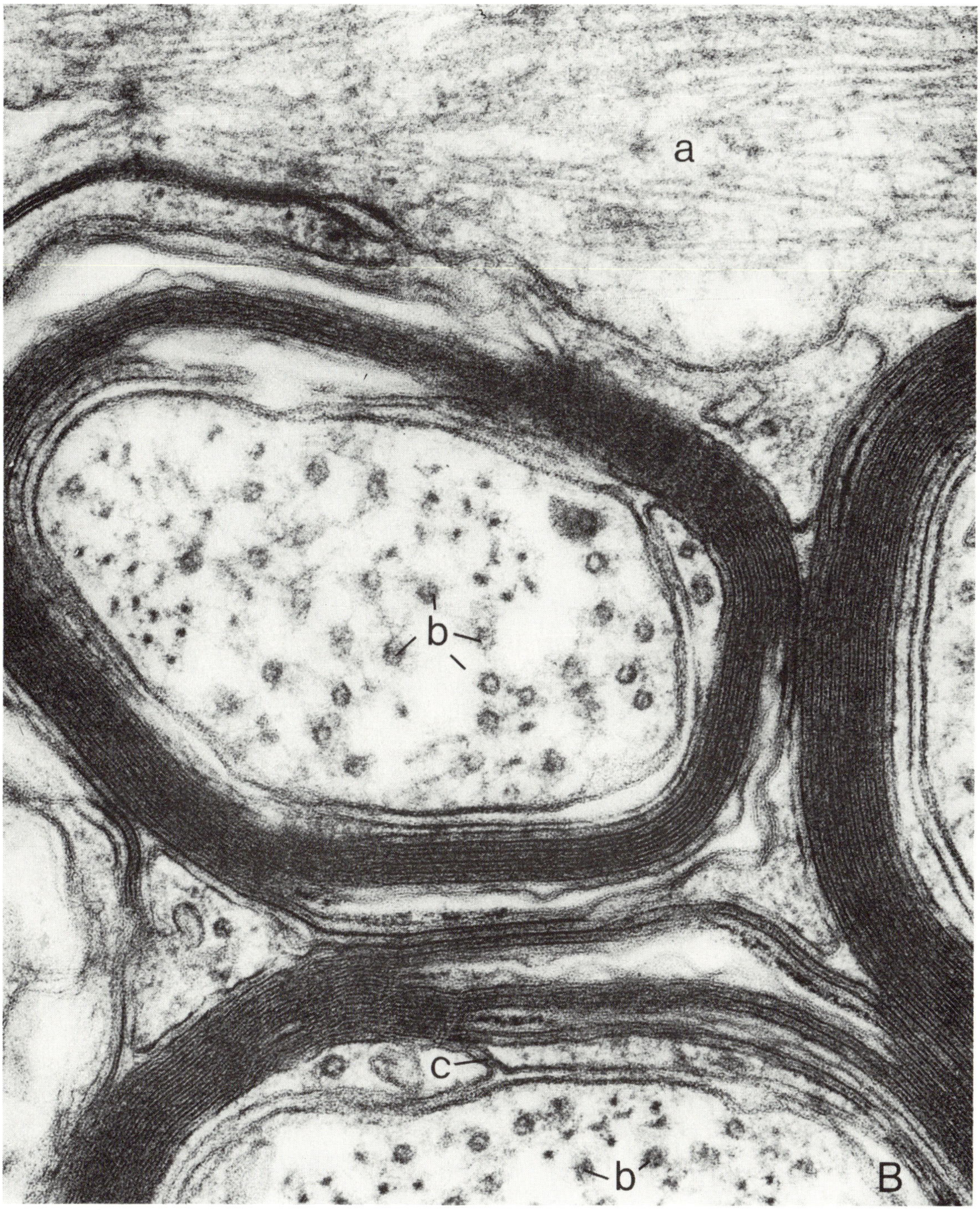

Figure 10–50. *Continued.*

B, Cross-sections of two axons. The upper nerve is surrounded on one side by an astrocytic process (a). Both nerves show cross-sections of neurotubules (b). The lower nerve shows a clear-cut mesaxon (c) at the site of the initial wrapping of the nerve by the oligodendrocyte cell membrane. (× 102,000.)

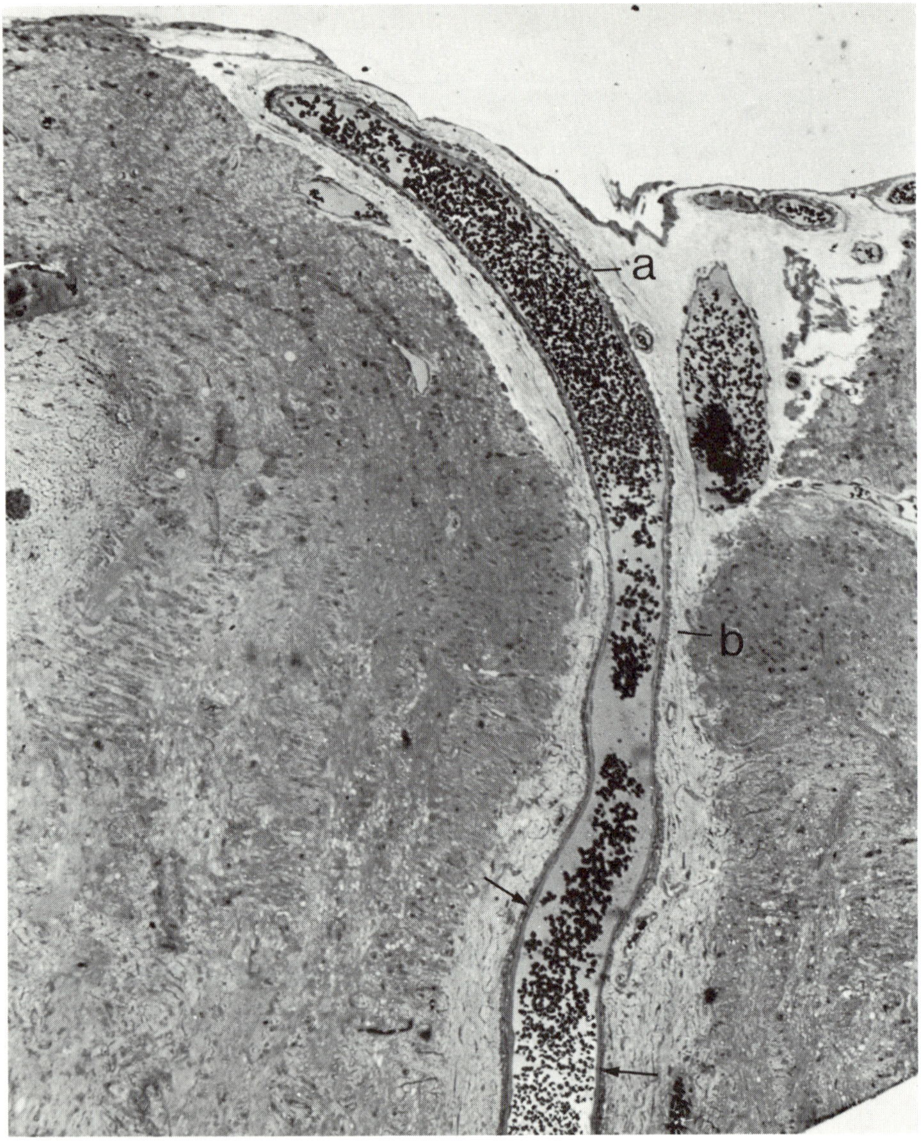

Figure 10–51. Central retinal artery. The prelaminar portion (a) is surrounded by collagenous connective tissue, while the laminar portion shows a narrower zone of tissue around its adventitia (b). The postlaminar portion is enlarged again, and the thin line of the internal elastic lamina becomes visible (arrows). The surrounding connective tissue also becomes more abundant posterior to the lamina cribrosa. (× 110.)

There is no discrete external elastic membrane. The adventitia contains layers of typical collagen. Nerve fibers surrounded by Schwann cells can be identified in the adventitial tissue (Ikui et al., 1964; Cohen, 1967; Anderson, 1969).

The central retinal vein has a simple structure (Fig. 10-56), and its endothelium has the usual basement membrane. External to this are two to three layers of muscle cells, the internal ones arranged longitudinally and the outer ones obliquely or circularly. The adventitia is thinner than that of the artery.

Meningeal Sheaths (Figs. 10-57 to 10-64). The dura, arachnoid and

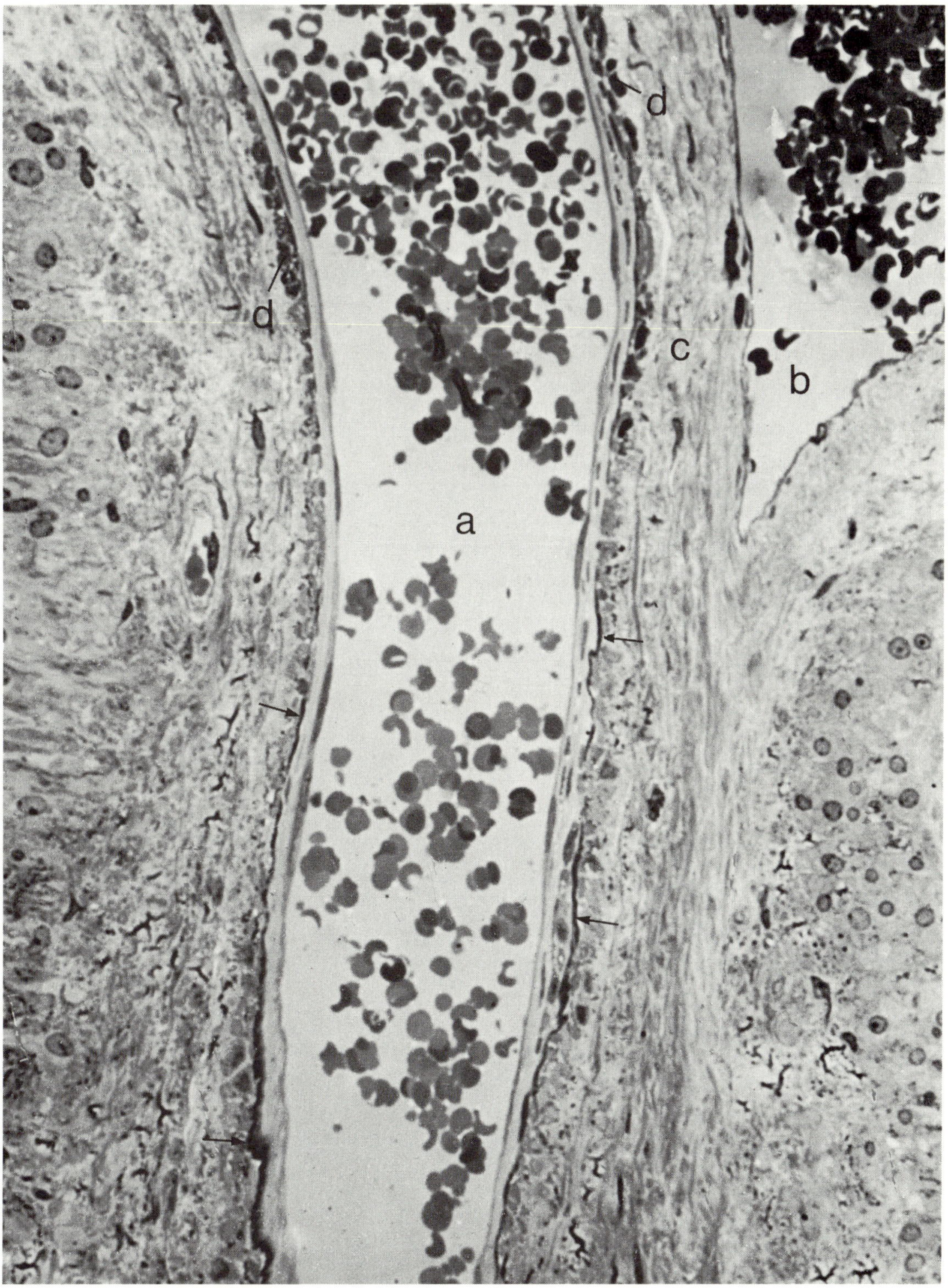

Figure 10–52. Light micrograph of the central retinal artery (a) and a portion of the central retinal vein in the prelaminar and laminar portions of the optic nerve (b). A single adventitia (c) joins both vessels at their junction. The internal elastic lamina of the laminar portion (arrows) disappears in the prelaminar portion. The wall of the vein contains a considerable amount of collagen and some fibroblasts, while that of the artery contains muscle cells (d). (× 625.)

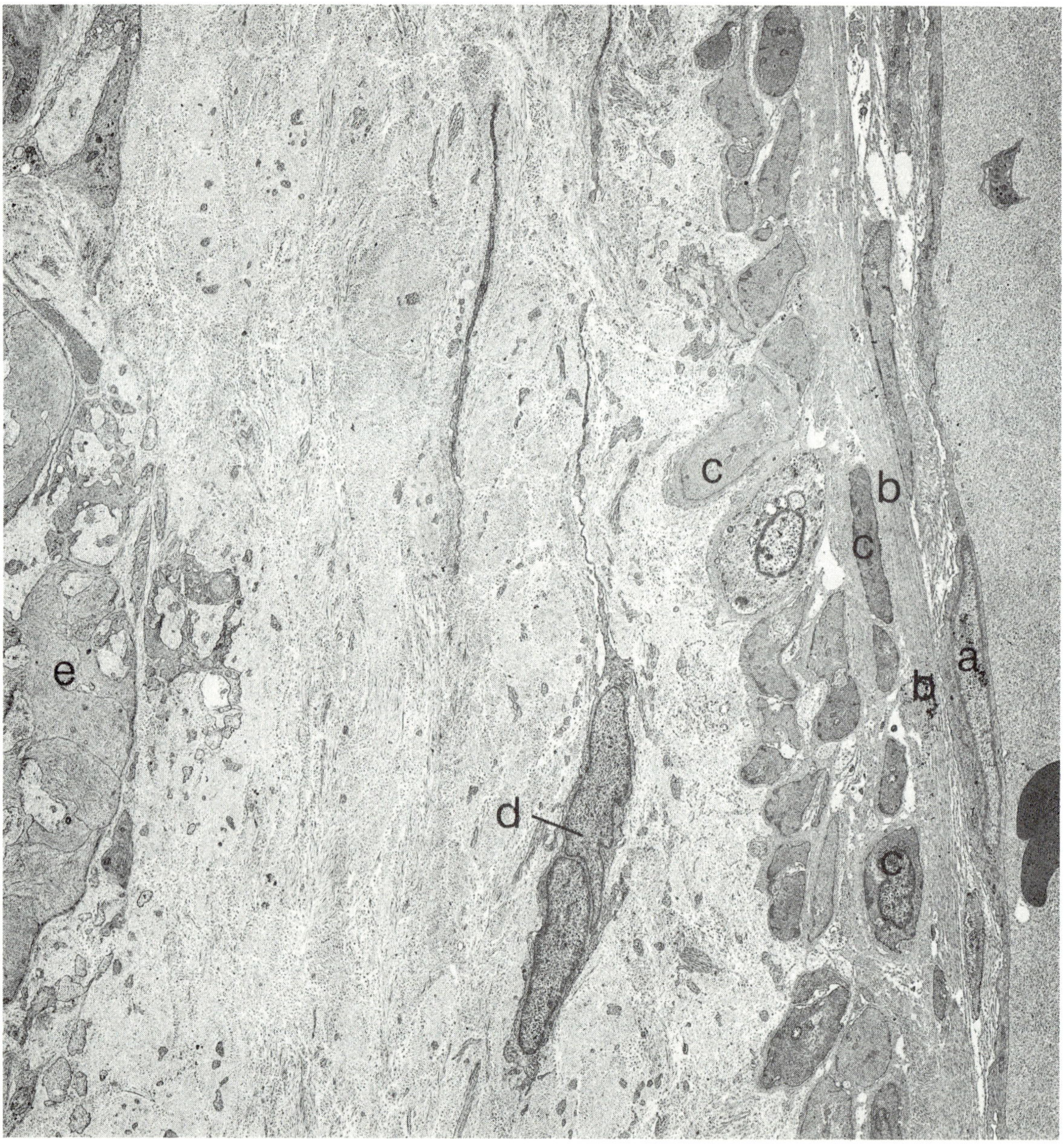

Figure 10–53. Longitudinal section of the central retinal artery in the prelaminar region. The lumen of the artery is at the right. The endothelium (a) is surrounded by a laminated basement membrane (b). A number of layers of muscle tissue comprise the media (c). The adventitia is composed of dense collagen containing some fibroblasts (d). Surrounding the adventitia are the processes of astrocytes (e). (× 2580.)

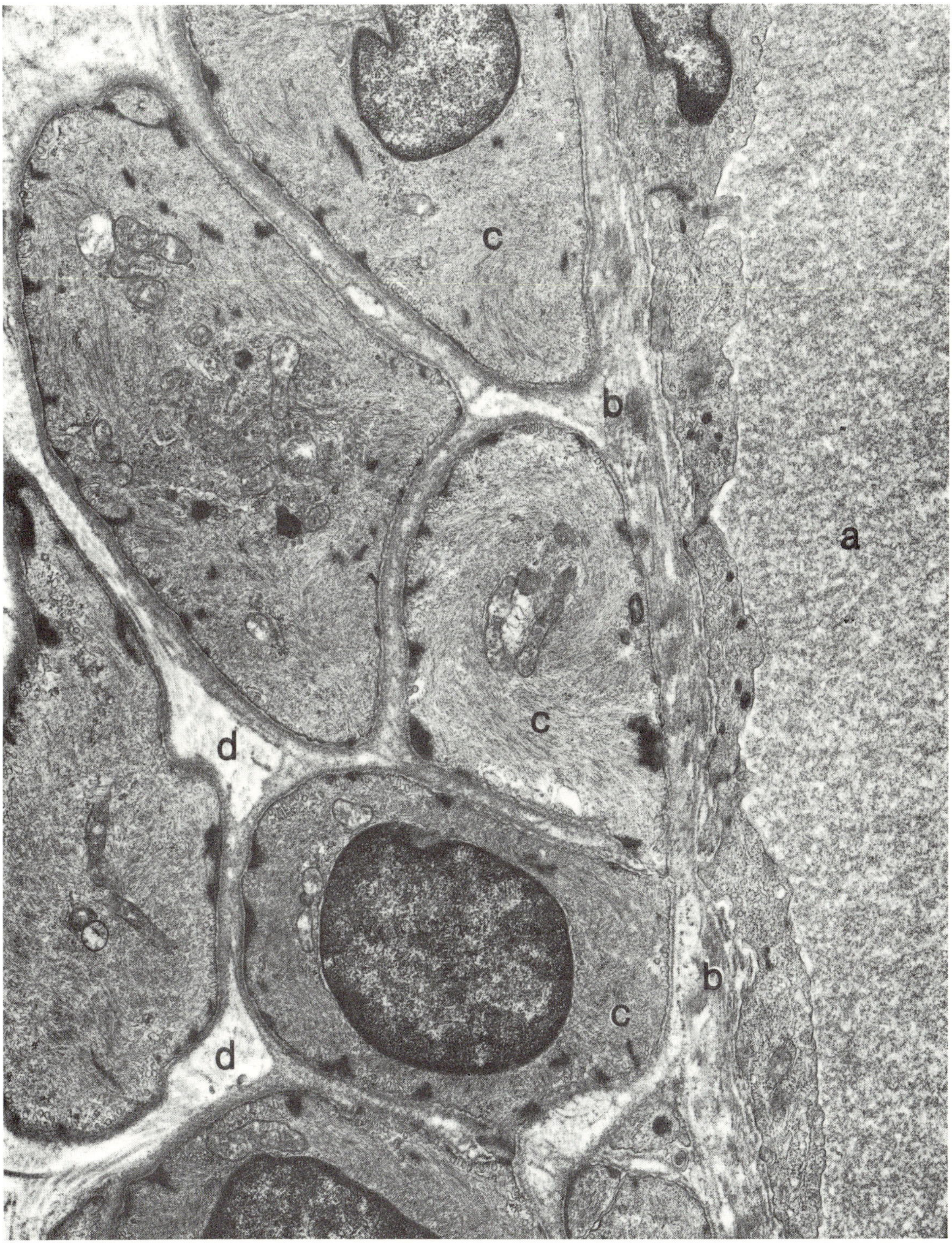

Figure 10–54. Prelaminar central retinal artery. The lumen (a) contains granular plasma. The endothelium has a laminated basement membrane (b) that is continuous with that of the muscle cells (c). The arterial wall contains some collagen (d). This portion of the artery has no internal elastic lamina. (× 7500.)

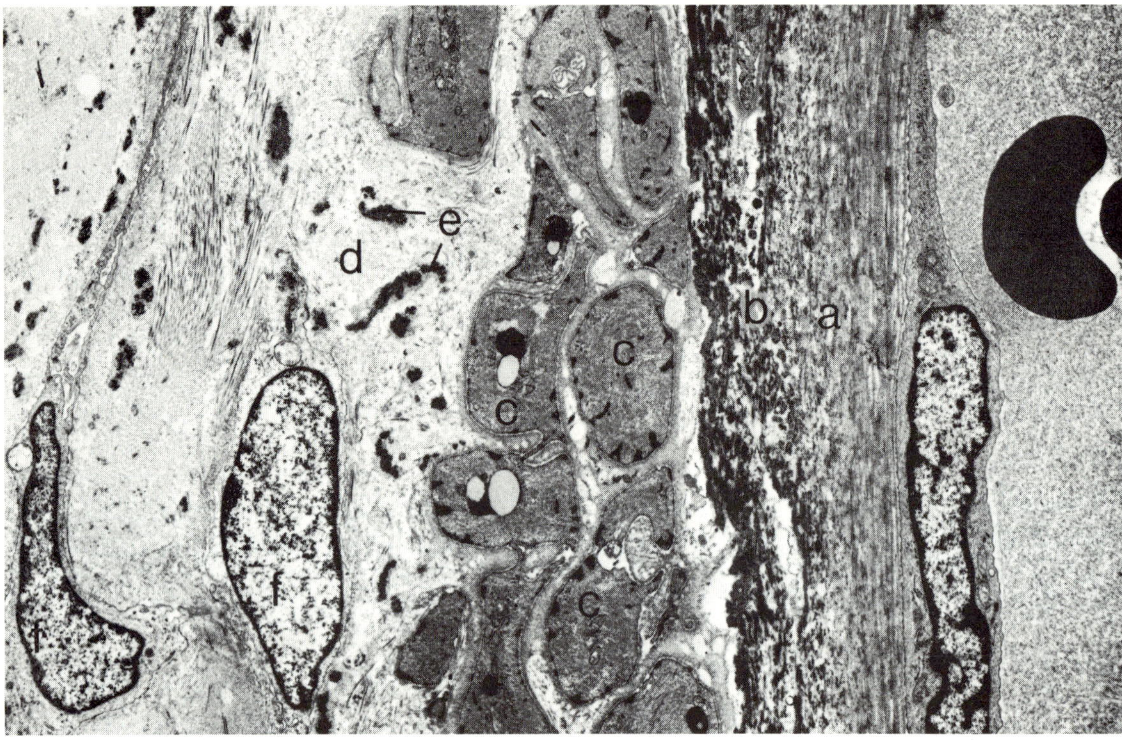

Figure 10–55. Laminar portion of the central retinal artery. The very thick lamination of the basement membrane of the endothelial cells is apparent (a). This portion of the artery first shows an internal elastic lamina (b), and two to three layers of muscle cells are evident in this section (c). The adventitia contains collagen (d), elastic fibers (e) and some fibroblasts (f). (× 4900.)

pia mater have the same microscopic structure as in the central nervous system. The *dura mater* is about 0.3 to 0.5 mm. thick (Fig. 10–59). It is a dense connective tissue sheath containing thick bundles of collagen and a fair amount of elastic tissue. The outer collagenous layers course longitudinally, the intermediate ones are oblique, and the innermost ones are circular. There is considerable interweaving and splitting of the collagen bundles, so that the branches often divide and reunite with adjacent bundles. Some branches bend inward or outward to join others at different levels. The elastic fibers are randomly dispersed but are more numerous in the outer layers. The principal cell in the dura is the fibroblast, which is typical for this type of connective tissue. The fibroblasts are long, and their branches are oriented in a circular direction.

The dural collagen has the same banding as normal collagen, and the fibers have a diameter of 600 to 700 μm. (Fig. 10-60). Fine filaments 100 A. in diameter are found in the deeper part of the dura, with a cross-striation like that of collagen. The same types of filaments are found in the arachnoid and pia. They tend to lie in juxtaposition to the fibroblasts, and they have the same appearance as the filaments on the outer edges of the elastic fibers. These fibrils may be tropocollagen or reticulin. The inner surface of the dura is lined by some flattened cells, which are known as meningothelial cells. Some of these cells are found within the dural substance, where they resemble fibroblasts.

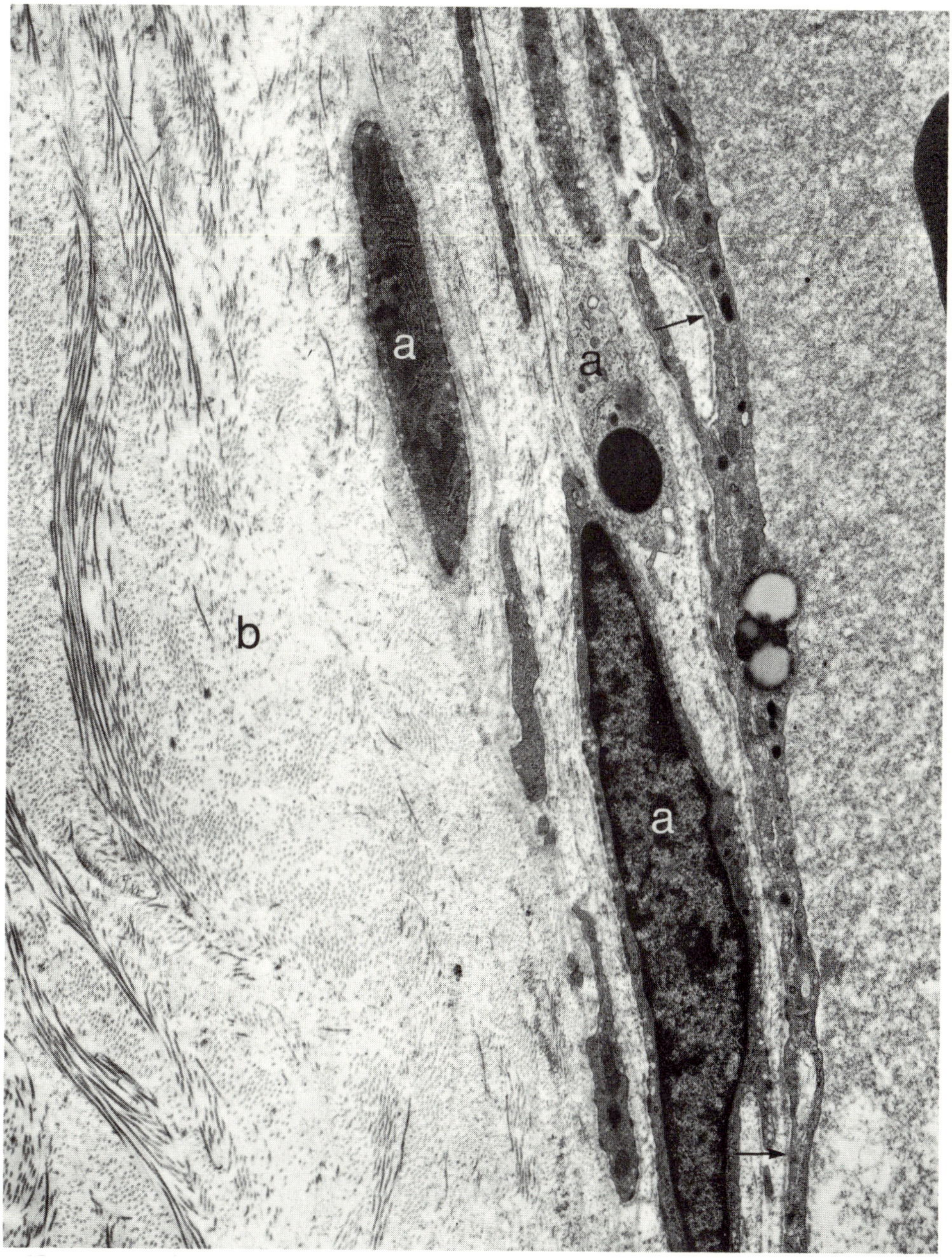

Figure 10–56. Central retinal vein. The vein wall has the same structure in the postlaminar and prelaminar regions. The endothelium has a thin basement membrane (arrows), and the media contains several layers of muscle tissue (a). The adventitia is largely collagenous (b). (× 10,200.)

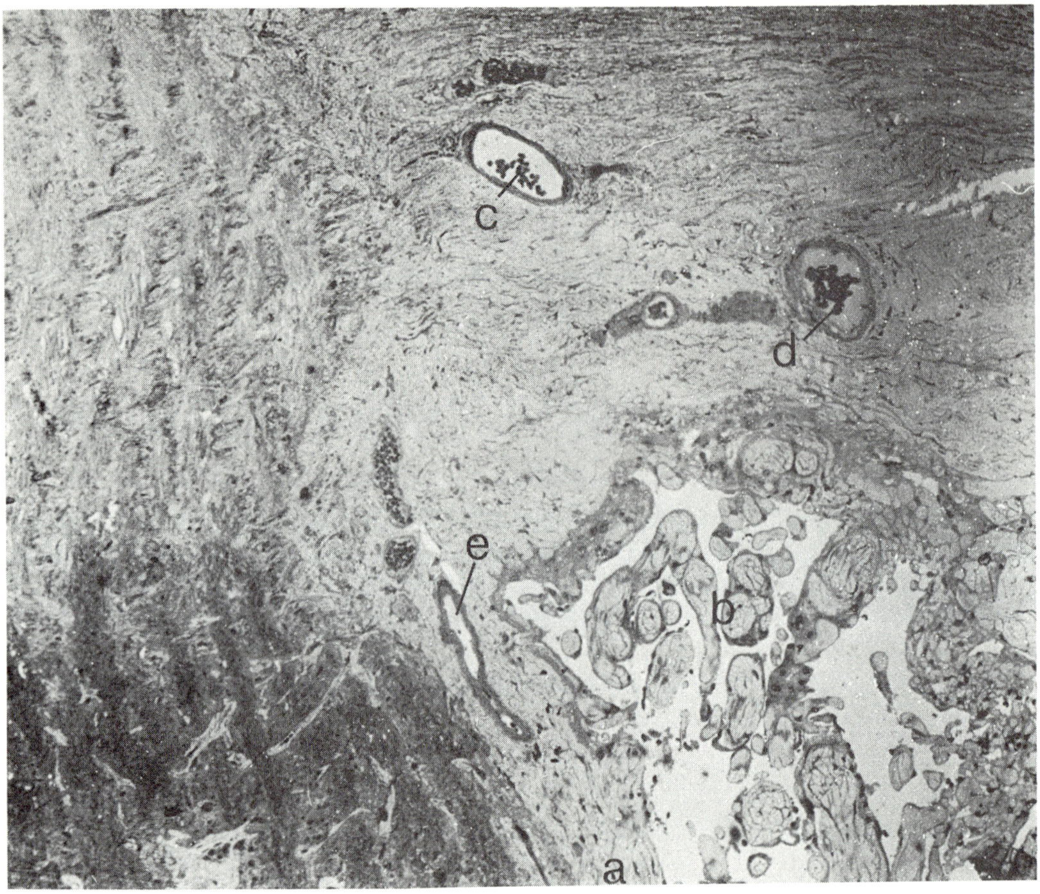

Figure 10–57. Light micrograph of the anterior termination of the meningeal sheaths in the sclera. A portion of optic nerve is seen at the left, surrounded by its pial sheath (a). The arachnoid (b) traverses the subdural and subarachnoid space. The circle of Zinn (c) and a scleral vessel (d) are seen. A small pial vessel (e) appears to extend forward into the sclera. (× 140.)

Blood vessels enter and pierce the dura along its course. Some of these are quite large, especially if they have recently originated from the ophthalmic artery. They enter the subdural space, where they are covered by both the dura and arachnoid, finally sending branches through the arachnoid to the pia mater. A few small branches enter the pia-arachnoid from the central retinal artery as it pierces the sheaths.

The *arachnoid mater* is about 10 μm. thick. Posteriorly the subarachnoid space is continuous with that of the brain; anteriorly the arachnoid ends at the level of the lamina cribrosa. It lies closer to the dura mater than to the pia mater and is composed of collagenous trabeculae with a small amount of elastic tissue that are covered by meningothelial cells (Fig. 10-61). This collagen is more loosely arranged than in the dura mater. The arachnoid commences as a rather ill defined layer under the dura, from which trabeculae extend in branching fashion to the pia mater (Fig. 10-62). Close to the dura mater, layers of flattened meningothelial cells form the

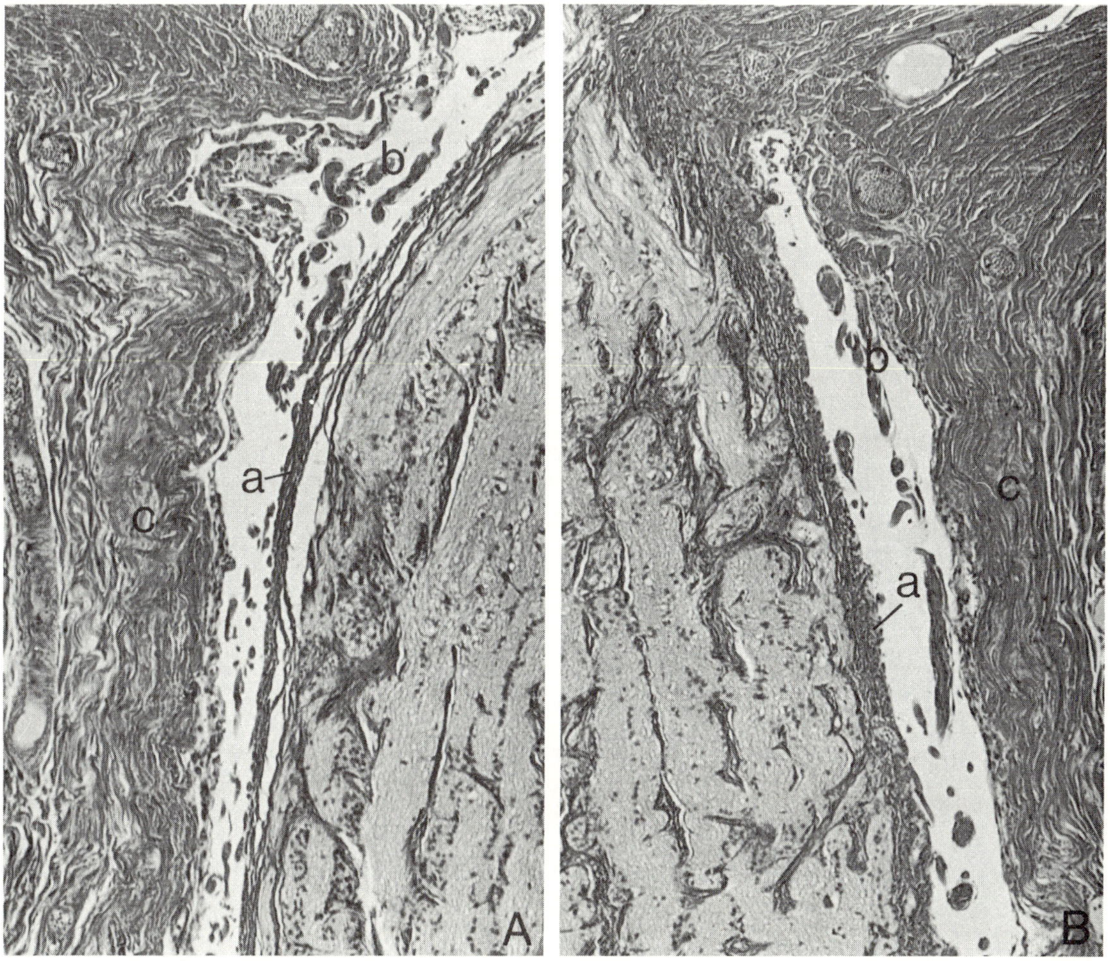

Figure 10–58. Meningeal sheaths of the optic nerve. *A*, The pia mater invests the optic nerve at its periphery (a). The arachnoid (b) occupies the subdural and subarachnoid space, and the dura (c) encloses the outer circumference of the nerve. (× 220.)

B, The opposite side of the optic nerve shown in *A*. The lettering is the same. (× 220.)

principal part of the arachnoid. These cells support the dura from the subarachnoid space.

The meningothelial cells of the arachnoid appear to be fibroblasts; they are flattened and squamoid (Fig. 10–61). Thin, interdigitating cytoplasmic extensions relate them to other cells, and they are frequently joined by desmosomes or even tight junctions. There are fine filaments extending throughout the cytoplasm and the protoplasmic extensions (Fig. 10-60). Near the nucleus is a well developed Golgi apparatus and mitochondria, ribosomes and rough-surfaced endoplasmic reticulum. A basement membrane is not found beneath these cells, except in the region of the arachnoid, where a faint discontinuous material may be present next to the collagen of the arachnoid layer. At the anterior termination of the subarachnoid space, the meningothelial cells fill the recess but lose their squamoid shape. They develop a more abundant cytoplasm, which contains a large number of filaments, and their surfaces become quite irregular. The meningothelial cells comprising the arachnoid and subdural region can proliferate to form

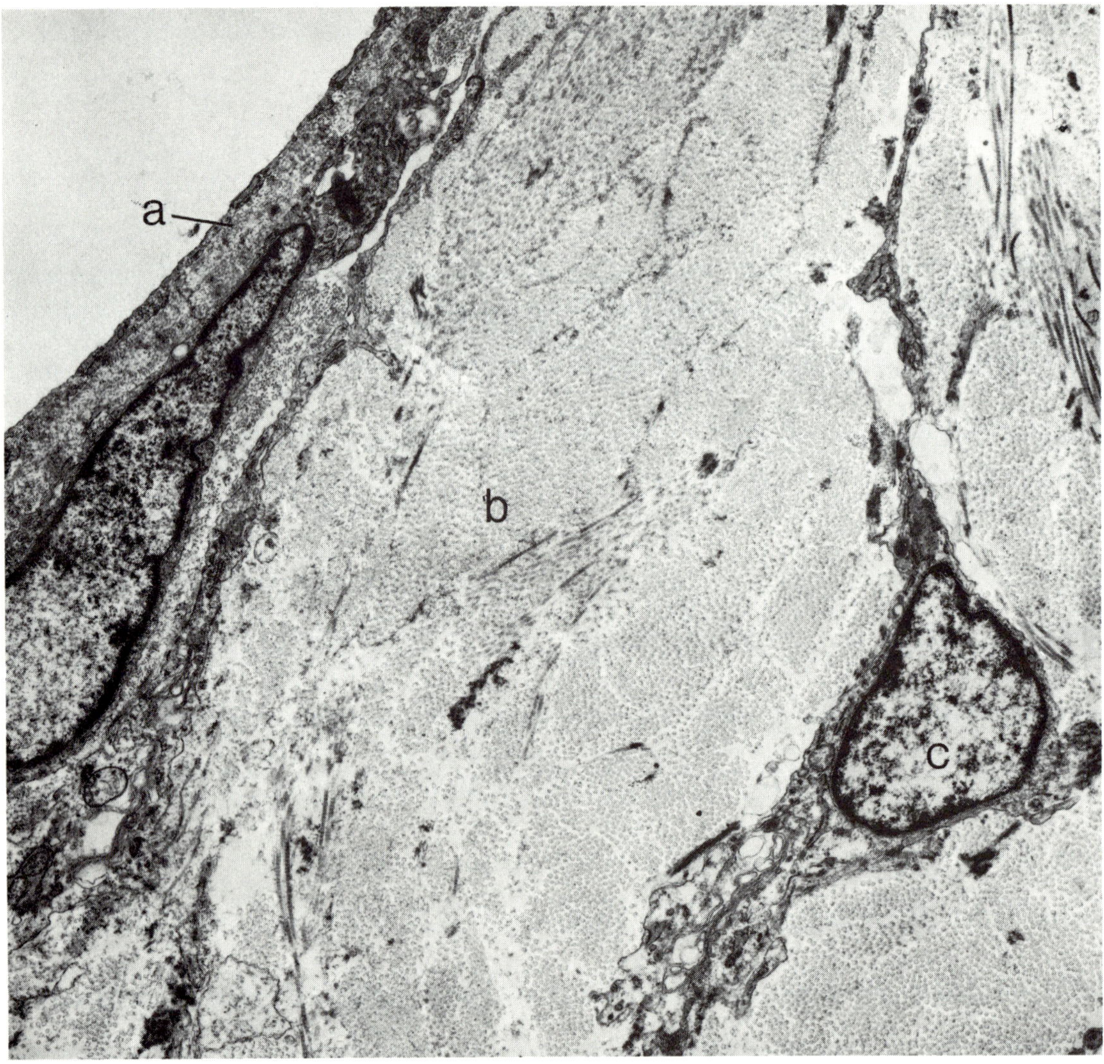

Figure 10–59. The dura mater around the human optic nerve. The undersurface is lined by meningothelial cells (a). These cells are continuous with those of the arachnoidal trabeculae. The thick bundles of collagen in the dura are oriented longitudinally in this section (b). It contains a fibroblast (c) and some processes of other fibroblasts. (× 10,200.)

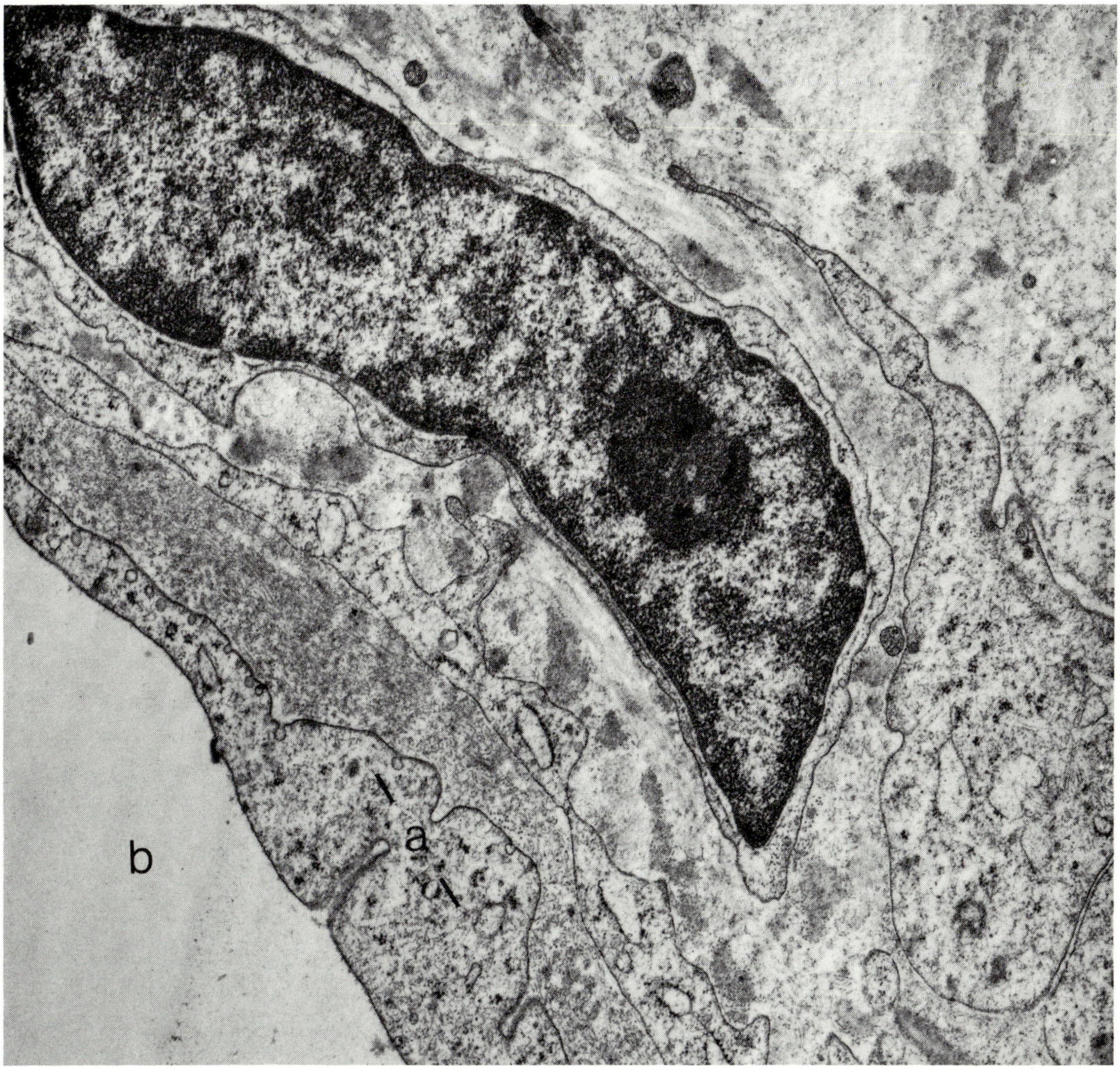

Figure 10–60. Undersurface of the dura mater around the human optic nerve. The meningothelial cells (a) lining the subdural space (b) are thin and have a dense cytoplasm. (× 24,000.) (From Anderson, D.: Arch. Ophthal. 82:659, 1969.)

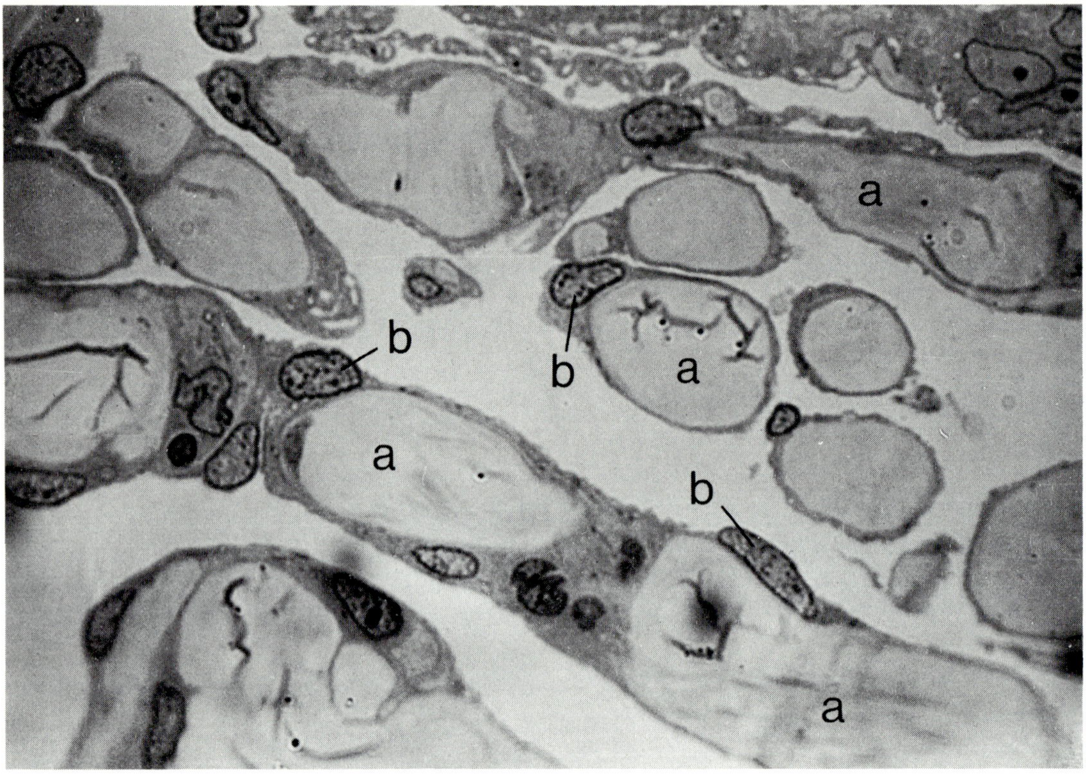

Figure 10-61. Light micrograph of the arachnoidal trabeculae (a). They possess a central core of collagen and are surrounded by meningothelial cells (b). (× 1100.)

cell nests, which become larger and hyalinized with age and, finally, may calcify.

The connective tissue component of the arachnoid trabeculae is very thin and is covered by meningothelial cells. It is best developed on the inner surface of the arachnoid. The subarachnoid space contains cerebrospinal fluid, which is separated from the collagen of the arachnoid by its meningothelial cells. Some of the arachnoidal trabeculae are covered by several layers of meningothelial cells. The blood vessels which pierce the dura mater enter the arachnoidal trabeculae, where they branch extensively (Fig. 10-64). They pass through the trabeculae into the pia mater.

The *pia mater* has a structure which is more like that of the dura mater. It is closely applied to the surface of the nerve and sends septa into the nerve (Fig. 10-63); therefore, it is an integral part of the structure of the nerve itself. The pia mater is composed of fine collagen and elastic fibers; the outer layers are circularly arranged, the ones closest to the nerve are longitudinal, and the intermediate fibers are oblique (Fuchs, 1916). The collagen of the pia mater is like that of the dura mater. In addition, banded fibrils 100 A. in diameter are found here, particularly near the arachnoidal layer (Fig. 10-63). Some elastic fibers are scattered among the collagen. Meningothelial cells cover the pia mater, often sending processes through the surface into the membrane itself. The blood vessels which enter the pia mater are mostly arteriolar and capillary in caliber; small nerve fibers from the ciliary nerves supply these vessels (Fig. 10-64).

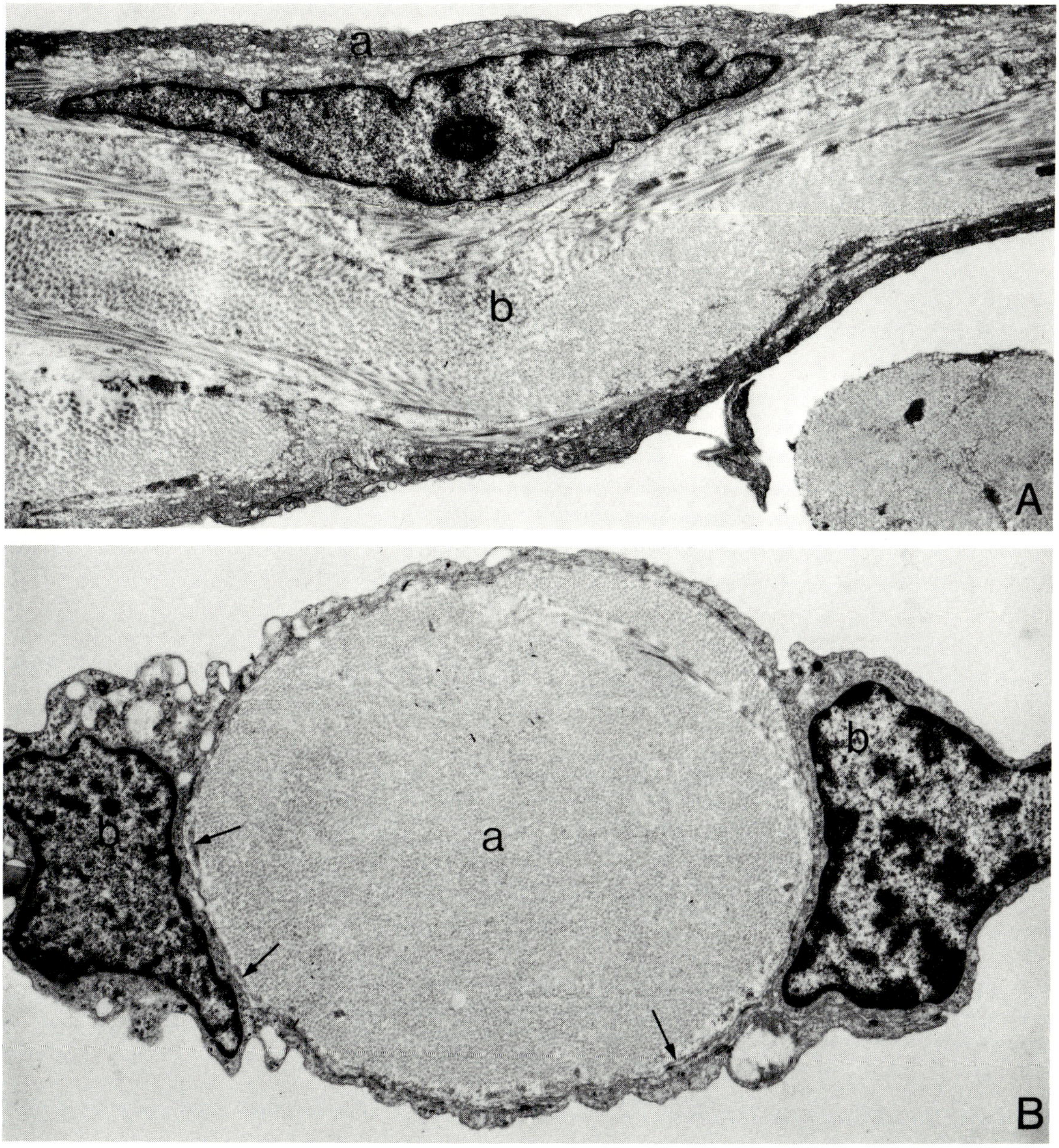

Figure 10–62. Electron micrographs of arachnoidal trabeculae. *A*, Longitudinal section showing the external meningothelial sheath of cells (a) and the collagen core (b). (× 5200.)

B, Cross-section of the arachnoid showing the collagen cut transversely (a) and the surrounding arachnoidal cells (b). Basement membrane-like material lies beneath these cells (arrows). (× 11,100.)

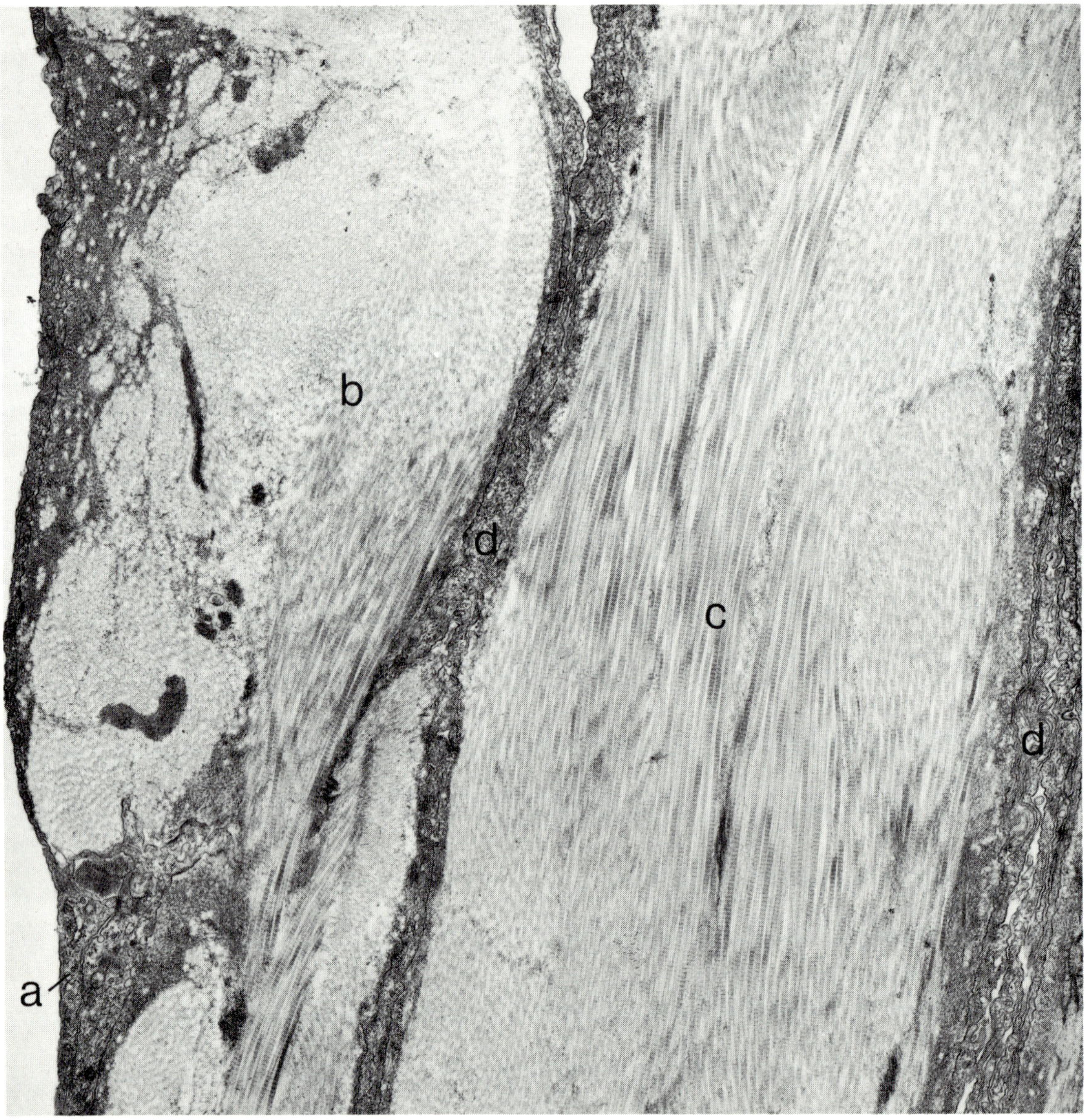

Figure 10–63. Pia mater covering the optic nerve. The outer surface of the pia is covered by meningothelial cells (a), and these in turn are surrounded by collagen, which is circular internally (b) and longitudinal externally (c). Some cells, probably fibroblasts, lie within the collagen (d); they are indistinguishable from the meningothelial cells. (× 6200.)

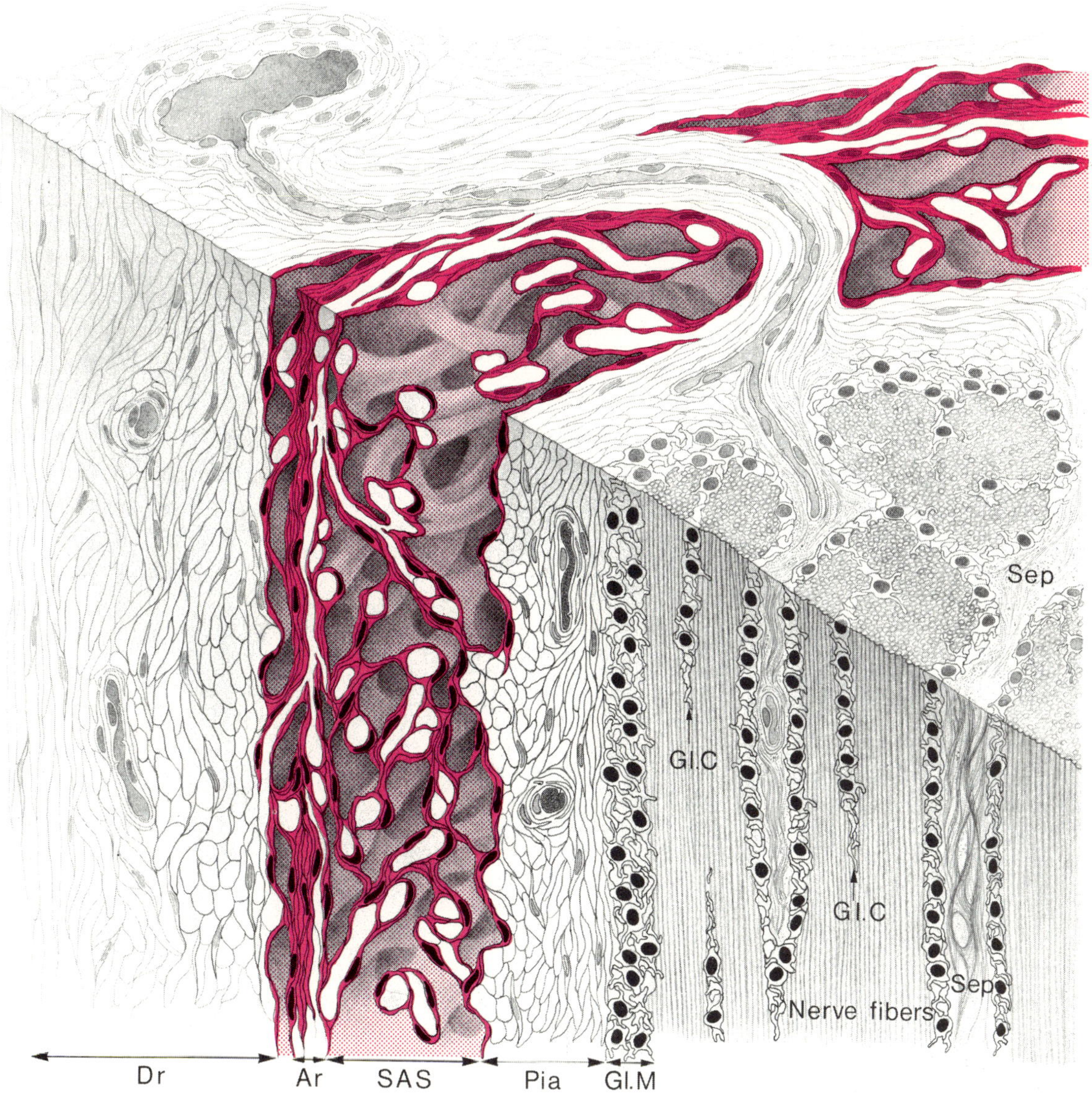

Figure 10–64. Schematic drawing of vaginal sheaths of human optic nerve, showing relationships of dura mater (Dr), arachnoid mater (Ar), subarachnoid space (SAS), pia mater (Pia), peripheral glial mantle of Fuchs' (Gl.M), pial septa (Sep), and glial columns (Gl.C). Meningothelial cells are shown in color, illustrating how they are the main component of archnoid mater and form linings for dura mater, arachnoid trabeculae and pia mater. (From Anderson, D.: Arch. Ophthal. *82*:659, 1969.)

REFERENCES

Anderson, D. R.: Ultrastructure of human and monkey lamina cribrosa and optic nerve head. Arch. Ophthal. *82*:800, 1969.

Anderson, D. R., and Hoyt, W. F.: Ultrastructure of interorbital portion of human and monkey optic nerve. Arch. Ophthal. *82*:506, 1969.

Anderson, D. R., Hoyt, W. F., and Hogan, M. J.: The fine structure of the astroglia in the human optic nerve and optic nerve head. Trans. Amer. Ophthal. Soc. *65*:275, 1967.

Beauvieux, and Ristitch, K.: The central vessels of the optic nerve: Anatomic study. Arch. Ophthal. (Paris) *61*:352, 1924.

Behr, C.: Beitrag zur Anatomie und Klink des septalen Gewebes und des Arterieninebaus im Sehnervenstramm. Graefes Arch. Ophthal. *134*:227, 1935.

Cajal, S.: Histologie du Systeme Nerveus de l'Homme et des Vertebrés. Madrid, Instituto Ramon Y Cajal, 1955.

Cohen, A. I.: Ultrastructural aspects of the human optic nerve. Invest. Ophthal. *6*:294, 1967.

Deyl, J.: Über den Eintrett der Arteria centralis retina in den Schnev beim Menschen. Bull. Int. Acad. Sci. Prague 120, 1895.

Francois, J., Rabaey, M., and Vandermeersche, G.: Ultrastructure of the ocular tissues by electron microscopy. Ophthalmologica *127*:74, 1954.

Francois, J., Neetens, A., and Collette, J. M.: Vascular supply of the optic pathway. II. Further studies by micro-arteriography of the optic nerve. Brit. J. Ophthal. *39*:220, 1955.

Francois, J., Neetens, A., and Collette, J. M.: Vascularization of the optic pathway. V. Chiasma. Brit. J. Ophthal. *40*:730, 1956.

Fuchs, E.: Über die Lamina cribrosa. Graefes Arch. Ophthal. *91*:435, 1916.

Hartline, H. K.: The electrical response to illumination of the eye in intact animals, including the human subject; and in decerebrate preparations. Amer. J. Physiol. *73*:600, 1925.

Hayreh, S. S.: Blood supply and vascular disorders of the optic nerve. Anales del Instituto Barraquer *4*:1, 1963.

Hayreh, S. S.: The blood supply of the optic nerve and its clinical significance. Acta XIX Counc. Ophthal. India *2*:1194, 1966.

Hayreh, S. S.: Blood supply of the optic nerve head and its role in optic atrophy, glaucoma, and oedema of the optic disc. Brit. J. Ophthal. *53*:721, 1969.

Hayreh, S. S., and Vrabec, F.: The structure of the head of the optic nerve in the rhesus monkey. Amer. J. Ophthal. *61*:136, 1966.

Hoyt, W. F.: Anatomic considerations of arcuate scotomas associated with lesions of the optic nerve and chiasm. A Nauta axon degeneration study in the monkey. Bull. Johns Hopkins Hosp. *111*:57, 1962.

Hoyt, W. F., and Luis, O.: Visual fiber anatomy in the infrageniculate pathway of the primate. Arch. Ophthal. *68*:94, 1962.

Hoyt, W. F., and Tudor, R. C.: The course of peripapillary temporal retinal axons through the anterior optic nerve: A Nauta degeneration study in the primate. Arch. Ophthal. *69*:503, 1963.

Ikui, H., Tominaga, Y., and Mimura, K.: The fine structure of the central retinal artery and vein in the optic nerve of the human eye and the pathological changes found therein in hypertension and arteriosclerosis. Acta Soc. Ophthal. Jap. *68*:899, 1964.

Kupfer, C., Chumbley, L., and Downer, J.: Quantitiative histology of optic nerve, optic tract, and lateral geniculate of man. J. Anat. *101*:393, 1967.

Ogden, T. E., and Miller, R. F.: Studies of the optic nerve of the rhesus monkey: Nerve fiber spectrum and physiological properties. Vision Res. *6*:485, 1966.

Oppel, O.: Microscopic examinations of the number and thickness of the myelinated nerve fibers in the human optic nerve. Graefes Arch. Ophthal. *166*:19, 1963.

Polyak, S. L.: The Retina. Chicago, Chicago University Press, 1941.

Steele, E. J., and Blunt, M. J.: The blood supply of the optic nerve and chiasma in man. J. Anat. *90*:486, 1956.

Sylvester, P. E., and Ari, K.: The size and growth of the human optic nerve. J. Neurol. Neurosurg. *24*:45, 1961.

Vrabec, F.: The temporal raphé of the human retina. Amer. J. Ophthal. *62*:926, 1966.

Wolff, E.: Anatomy of the Eye and Orbit. 6th ed. Philadelphia, W. B. Saunders Company, 1968.

Wolter, J. R.: The human optic papilla. A demonstration of new anatomic and pathological findings. Amer. J. Ophthal. *44*:48, 1957.

Wolter, J. R.: The centrifugal fibers in human optic tract, chiasm, optic nerve, and retina. Trans. Amer. Ophthal. Soc. *63*:678, 1965.

Wybar, K. C.: Anastomoses between the retinal and ciliary arterial circulations. Brit. J. Ophthal. *40*:65, 1956.

Yamamoto, T.: Electron microscopic observations of human optic nerves. Jap. J. Ophthal. *10*:40, 1966.

Chapter Eleven

VITREOUS

The vitreous body, an intraocular tissue with a gel-like structure, occupies four fifths of the volume of the globe. This large volume enables it to provide support for the ocular tissues and to assist in the maintenance of the intraocular pressure. The vitreous is like the aqueous humor in its ability to transmit light to the retina but differs in its physical properties. Both the aqueous and vitreous humors are important for the metabolism of the intraocular tissues because they provide a passageway for metabolites that are utilized by the lens and retina.

PHYSIOLOGY AND BIOCHEMISTRY

Physical and Chemical Properties

The human vitreous weighs approximately 4.0 gm. and its volume is close to 4.0 ml. Because the vitreous is 99 per cent water, its specific gravity of 1.0053 to 1.0089 is only slightly higher than that of water. The refractive index is slightly lower than that of aqueous humor, the most recent vitreous measurements indicating a value of about 1.334 (Richards and Hague, 1963).

Because of its gel-like structure, the viscosity of the vitreous has always been of great interest. The viscosity varies with age and in some regions of the vitreous, being greater in the cortex than in the central part of this tissue. Its intrinsic viscosity has been found to be about 4.200 cu. cm. per gm. (Balazs, 1960; Berman and Michaelson, 1964), but this varies with age. A filtrate of the vitreous contains considerable colloidal material (chiefly hyaluronic acid), which has a viscosity 1.8 to 2.0 times that of water (Friedenwald and Stiehler, 1935). The osmotic pressure of the vitreous, as determined by depression of the freezing point, is -0.554 to 0.518° C. The osmotic pressure of vitreous filtrate is very close to that of aqueous humor (Duke-Elder, 1968).

Variations in volume of the vitreous humor have been studied for many years, principally because of the possible role of the vitreous volume in glaucoma. It is improbable, however, that changes in vitreous volume have any relation to glaucoma. The volume can be changed by alteration of the protein and mucopolysaccharide components responsible for the normal gel structure. It also can be changed by the removal of vitreous water, as occurs when hyperosmotic agents are given intravenously to lower the intraocular pressure. The pH of normal vitreous is about 7.5; investigators have suggested that changes in pH might alter the volume, but it is doubtful that vitreous volume changes significantly under physiologic or pathologic conditions as a result of a variation in pH.

The vitreous body is a unique gel that has two distinct phases; the liquid one is called the vitreous humor, and the solid phase is called the residual protein. The vitreous body can be separated into its liquid and solid phases by centrifugation or by gravity after suspending it. The *residual protein* of the vitreous is collagen-like or a member of the collagen family, and the collagenous properties have been identified by chemical, electron-optical, x-ray diffraction and electron microscopic methods. It is apparent that collagen is responsible for the gel-like state. The collagen content of beef vitreous is 0.01 per cent. Collagen is present in relatively high amounts in the vitreous cortex, particularly in the vitreous base around the ora serrata. This collagen is hydrolyzed on exposure to collagenase and pepsin, but it is affected only slightly by trypsin and alpha chymotrypsin, which are weaker collagenolytic agents (Pirie et al., 1948). Additional evidence on the nature of the residual protein and its relation to collagen is provided by studies of its amino acid composition. It has 8.4 per cent proline, 15.4 per cent hydroxyproline and 18 per cent glycine; these amino acids are characteristic components of collagen (Young and Williams, 1954).

In electron micrographs these collagen fibrils have the 220 A. microperiodicity present in other collagen fibrils but lack the 640 A. macroperiodicity of thicker collagen fibrils. They vary in thickness, having a diameter of about 160 A. The distribution of collagen fibrils in electron micrographs of the vitreous suggests that they are randomly spaced filaments making up a network in the vitreous gel. Their concentration may vary in different parts of the vitreous, but the fibrils are uniform in structure.

The liquid phase (vitreous humor) contains a mucopolysaccharide called hyaluronic acid. Portions of hyaluronic acid from steer vitreous have a molecular weight of 61,000 to 331,000, depending on the method of preparation, and the length of these molecules is between 1600 and 3700 A. The polysaccharide is formed into long chains, arranged like a randomly kinked coil, with the molecular domain of the coil enclosing a relatively large amount of water (approximately 65 ml. per gm. of hyaluronic acid at a molecular weight of 250,000) (Balazs, 1960).

This hyaluronate appears to be joined to the collagen network by only very weak bonds that are easily broken by the force of gravity. The coiled hyaluronate is found in the collagen network spaces, which have been estimated to be in the neighborhood of 1.0 to 1.5 mm. in size (Balazs, 1961).

Chemical Composition

The chemical composition of the vitreous humor has many similarities to that of the aqueous humor, except for the collagen and hyaluronic acid. There appears to be free diffusion of substances through the vitreous, and between the vitreous and aqueous (Maurice, 1957), the diffusion apparently depending on particle size (Suran and McEwen, 1961). The concentration of some substances varies considerably in different parts of the vitreous, however, for the lens and retina probably utilize some of the vitreous components. Water movement in the vitreous of animals is quite high and it has been calculated that half of the vitreous water is replaced every 10 to 15 minutes (Kinsey et al., 1942). Sodium and potassium appear to enter the vitreous mainly from the ciliary body, either directly or through the posterior chamber. Their concentration is higher anteriorly than posteriorly. Glucose apparently enters the vitreous from its surrounding tissues, principally the retina. While its concentration is higher in the vitreous than in aqueous humor, glucose levels in both aqueous and vitreous are lower than in plasma. There must be a higher consumption of glucose by the posterior retina, since the glucose level is higher in the anterior than in the posterior vitreous (Adler, 1930). Glucose moves into the vitreous at a slower rate than into the aqueous humor, and the concentration reached is lower than would be expected if simple diffusion were to take place (Adler, 1930).

The blood-vitreous barrier is effective in regulating the entrance of blood proteins into the vitreous. After removal of the collagen protein from the vitreous, some soluble proteins remain in small amounts (0.04 per cent), mainly albumin and globulin, whose ratios to each other are considerably lower in the vitreous than in blood serum. This soluble protein amounts to 0.075 mg. per ml. in the vitreous of steers, 28 per cent of which is acidic glycoproteins (Balazs, 1960). In human eyes the amount of soluble protein present in the vitreous does not change after birth (Berman and Michaelson, 1964).

Movement of Substances Through the Vitreous

Saccharated iron introduced into the vitreous can pass through the vitreoretinal junction to the retinal capillary region (Yamashita and Cibis, 1959). India ink injected into the vitreous of rabbits is removed by the eighth day. Most of the ink leaves via the perivascular space of the retinal vessels, moving along this space to the optic disc vessels, where the carbon particles enter vessel lumens and are carried away. After the second day, some ink particles are transported out of the vitreous by phagocytes; thereafter, these cells perform most of the task of removing the particles (Barkhoff, 1964). Many substances leaving the vitreous probably exit by more than one mechanism and pathway. Labeled substances reach a steady state slowly in the vitreous, probably because diffusion is a slow process and because of the special organization of the collagen and hyaluronic acid in the cortex, which may act as a molecular sieve if the labeled substances are large (Suran and McEwen, 1961). The concentration of soluble protein is higher in the vitreous cortex, a finding that suggests the origin of these proteins from the adjacent tissues. The content of the acidic glycoproteins among these soluble proteins is also very high.

EMBRYOLOGY

The exact source of the vitreous remains unknown because past and present methods of studying embryos have failed to reveal the true origin of the earliest vitreous. More recent electron microscopic studies of chick embryos have provided some information regarding development of the vitreous out of the mesenchyme that fills the optic cup. Apparently the early vitreous arises primarily from the cells of this mesenchyme. In the very earliest stages the space between the lens vesicle and innermost retina is narrow and is filled with mesenchymal cells and fibrils or protoplasmic processes, which are continuous with the retina and lens. Most texts describe the early vitreous as arising from mesoderm as well as from both the surface and neural ectoderms. According to Bach and Seefelder (1911), however, no mesodermal protoplasmic processes can be demonstrated in the vitreous cavity prior to the entrance of the mesoderm, indicating that the mesoderm is not essential for the formation of the vitreous. Many of the fibrillae seen in routine histologic sections may be produced by fixation and processing; therefore, fibrillar structures may not exist in the early human embryonic vitreous. Instead, the embryonic vitreous space may acquire the substances for its origin from the cells of the lens and retina.

During the 4.5 to 7.0 mm. stage (third to fourth week), the protoplasmic processes between the lens plate and optic vesicle can be delineated, and a few mesodermal cells invade the cup and apparently fuse with these processes. At the same time, the capsula perilenticularis fibrosa appears behind the lens, containing vasoformative mesodermal cells. By the 13 mm. stage (sixth week) the *primary vitreous* has developed in the cavity of the optic vesicle, the footplates of the Müller cells at the posterior pole appearing to be continuous with the vitreous fibers. Cessation of growth of the primary vitreous occurs at about the 40 mm. stage (ninth week), when formation of the *secondary vitreous* commences, possibly through the activity of vitreal and retinal cells. The new vitreous is at first related to the retina, appearing as parallel rows of thin fibers along the inner retina that are quite distinct from the vascular primary vitreous.

A regular radial condensation of thin fibers can be seen in the anterior portion of the secondary vitreous, extending along the lens equator parallel to the optic cup wall and joining the mesodermal iris (marginal bundle, or faisceau isthmique of Drualt) by the 48 mm. stage (tenth week). Between this time and the end of embryonic life (65 mm. stage; twelfth week), the secondary vitreous increases in volume and forces the primary vitreous into a central position, the site of the future Cloquet's canal. During this period, the growing cup margin produces the tertiary vitreous fibers, which pass through the marginal bundle at right angles, while the vasa hyaloidea begin to atrophy. Surface condensations separate the anterior limit of the secondary vitreous from the tertiary vitreous, which will become the suspensory ligament of the lens. During the 110 to 160 mm. stage (fourth month), the tertiary vitreous fibrils blend with the zonular lamella of the lens and the marginal bundle atrophies. The secondary vitreous is retrodisplaced toward the ora serrata region as the ciliary body develops. The capsula perilenticularis fibrosa has atrophied centrally and blends with the distal expansion of Cloquet's canal by the 160 mm. stage. There is regression of the anterior part of the tunica vasculosa lentis, early atrophy of the glial sheath of the hyaloid artery and disappearance of blood from the hyaloid artery by the 240 mm. stage (seventh month). During the 240 to 289 mm. stage (eighth month), retinal blood vessels grow into the retina toward the ganglion cell layer, while the glial sheath and hyaloid artery become almost completely atrophic. The posterior tunica vasculosa lentis is reduced to a small trifurcation on the posterior capsule. During the final six weeks of fetal life all the vasa hyaloidea atrophy and the main trunk of the hyaloid artery disappears. At birth, all blood vessels are gone from the primary vitreous, leaving Cloquet's canal attached anteriorly in the region of the patellar fossa and posteriorly at the disc in the area of Martegiani.

GROSS ANATOMY (Fig. 11–1)

The vitreous is roughly spherical, being somewhat flattened meridionally. Anteriorly the vitreous surface exhibits a cup-shaped depression, the *patellar fossa,* in which the posterior lens rests. At the edge of this fossa is a circular thickening of the vitreous, 8 to 9 mm. in diameter, which is known as the *ligamentum hyaloideocapsulare.* This attachment is firm in young eyes but becomes less distinct with increasing age, so that in older eyes the lens and vitreous can be separated from each other easily during cataract surgery. Within the attachment zone of the ligamentum hyaloideocapsulare is the *space of Berger,* a potential space where the lens and vitreous are in very loose contact. Lateral to the ligament the vitreous is continuous with the lens zonules. The surface of the vitreous anterior to the ora serrata region, known as the *anterior hyaloid,* is ill-defined in gross specimens; it is more condensed here than it is posterior to the ora serrata. Anterior to the ora serrata this vitreous gel invests the zonular fibers and is attached to the ciliary epithelium and ciliary processes. The zonules and the vitreous extend forward between the ciliary processes into the ciliary valleys. The vitreous then continues anteriorly to the region of the lens equator, where its surface is in contact with the lens capsule. If the vitreous and zonules are mechanically detached from the ciliary body, the shallow indentations of the ciliary processes can be seen on the vitreous surface.

Laterally the anterior vitreous is in close relation to the pars plana and the retina. Posterior to the ora serrata the *posterior hyaloid* surface of the vitreous is in close contact with the inner limiting membrane of the retina as far as the optic disc. This contact usually persists in human eyes until about age 50, when aging of the vitreous results in shrinkage of the residual protein; the vitreous and retina then may separate from each other. There is no firm union of the vitreous to the optic disc surface. Within this area is a funnel-shaped space known as the area of Martegiani, which extends forward from the disc into the vitreous to become continuous with the canal of Cloquet.

Cloquet's canal. The canal of Cloquet extends from the disc anteriorly to the lens, where it ends slightly nasal to its posterior pole. It represents the remnant of the primary vitreous with its vessel system and has an S-shaped course, with the downward dip in its central portion. The canal lies mostly below the horizontal meridian and broadens as it approaches the disc in the area of Martegiani. Anteriorly in the region of the lens, Cloquet's canal is 1 to 2 mm. wide and frequently can be seen with the

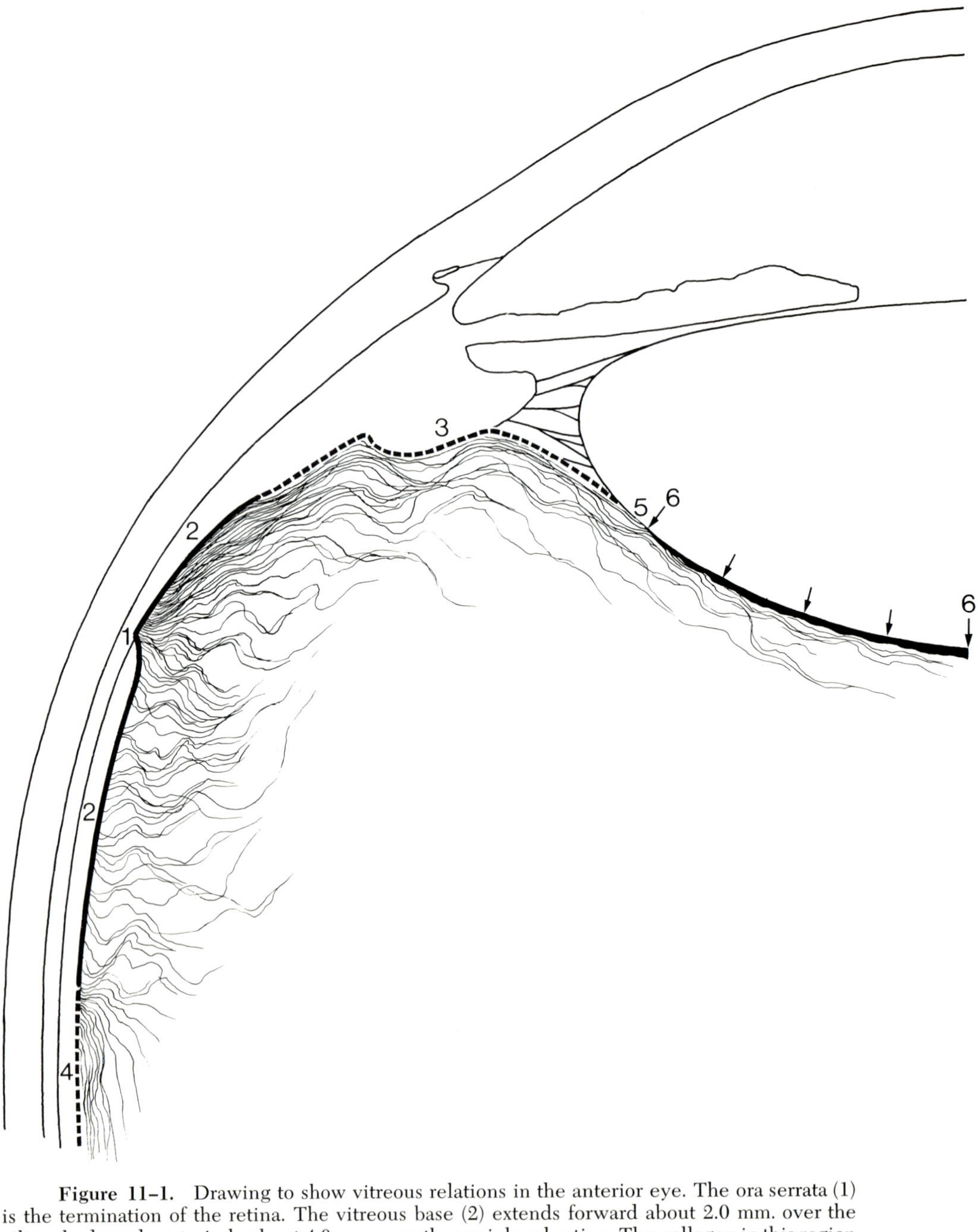

Figure 11–1. Drawing to show vitreous relations in the anterior eye. The ora serrata (1) is the termination of the retina. The vitreous base (2) extends forward about 2.0 mm. over the ciliary body and posteriorly about 4.0 mm. over the peripheral retina. The collagen in this region is oriented at a right angle to the surface of the retina and ciliary body, but anteriorly over the pars plana it is more parallel to the inner surface of the ciliary body. The posterior hyaloid (4) is continuous with the retina, and the anterior hyaloid (3) with the zonules and lens. The ligamentum pectinatum is at (5) and the space of Berger at (6).

slit lamp. Its insertion in the patellar region of the vitreous measures 4 to 5 mm. in diameter (Goldmann, 1954). Early studies (Stilling, 1869, 1908), employing dyes injected into the vitreous, demonstrated the persistence of this embryonic structure into adult life. This work was subsequently verified by other methods, including the ultramicroscope (Friedenwald and Stiehler, 1935). Its presence in the living eye was confirmed with the slit-lamp microscope (Vogt, 1924).

The body of the vitreous contains a thin cortical zone that is close to the ciliary body and retina. Centrally the vitreous is less fibrillar and is more fluid. There are two principal attachments between the vitreous and adjacent tissues; one is at the periphery of the optic disc, and the other at the vitreous base where it joins the ciliary epithelium and inner limiting membrane of the retina.

The Vitreous Base. The most solid attachment of vitreous to the wall of the eye is at the vitreous base (p. 269, also Fig. 9–93). Traction on the vitreous in this region causes tenting of the retina and ciliary body; if the traction is forceful, the ciliary epithelium and the peripheral retina come loose. The traction produces tension lines in the vitreous at right angles to the surface of the tissues, indicating that the principal orientation of its framework is in this direction. Traction on the anterior vitreous after the lens is removed produces the same phenomenon, indicating that the vitreous base framework also continues forward. If the traction is made at some distance from the ciliary body and retina, very little tenting occurs, showing that the most highly organized portion of the framework is a zone only 2 to 3 mm. wide adjacent to these tissues.

Peripapillary Attachment. At the edge of the optic disc is a rather firm attachment of vitreous to the inner retina, the peripapillary attachment, which becomes more tenuous with increasing age. Traction on the vitreous in this region causes less tenting of the adjacent retina, since the attachment is not so firm or broad as that at the vitreous base. In adult eyes, where there is always a certain amount of shrinkage of residual protein (syneresis), minor jarring or trauma may lead to vitreous detachment from the disc region, accompanied by scintillations or the appearance of vitreous opacity. Ophthalmoscopic study of such eyes usually shows a ring-like structure in the midportion of the eye, representing the vitreous density at the attachment zone around the disc.

Macular Attachment. The attachment in this region is distinct from that around the disc. It has an irregularly annular diameter of 3 to 4 mm., but it cannot be seen with the slit lamp and contact lens. The macular attachment often becomes apparent under pathologic conditions, particularly if there are abnormal retinovitreal adhesions. It is quite definite in fetal eyes and in the eyes of young adults (Hogan, 1963).

MICROSCOPIC ANATOMY

Study of normal vitreous anatomy is difficult, requiring application of a variety of techniques and instruments. The slit-lamp microscope reveals a good deal about the living eye. Gross studies of fixed and unfixed tissue with the dissecting microscope, the dark field microscope, phase-contrast microscopy and electron microscopic studies have added essential information on the vitreous structure. The most important recent information has been provided by biochemists and biophysicists.

Fresh vitreous has no structure when examined unstained with the light microscope. For this reason all the early studies of the vitreous employed fixed and stained specimens. Such specimens show a fibrous, net-like structure of membranes radiating out from the base of the vitreous toward its center. Similar fibrous layers are arranged parallel to the inner retina, but these fibrous membranes are in part artifacts of the fixation and preparation of specimens. Some investigators have demonstrated that fixatives indeed can produce artificial fibers or fibrous arrangements in the vitreous. Fresh vitreous examined with the ultramicroscope is found to be a gel without a micellar structure. With this technique, the vitreous lacks fibrous membranes such as those seen with the light microscope in fixed specimens. Rossi (1953) found no fibers in the fresh vitreous of various animals, but fibers were seen after an interval of 15 to 20 minutes or after the vitreous was stored at 2° C. for two to eight hours. According to Rossi, these findings did not exclude the possibility of encountering zonular fibrils in the vitreous base.

Grignolo (1953) used the phase-contrast microscope for the study of fresh and fixed vitreous. Using this technique, he observed fibers in fresh specimens and in vitreous fixed with osmium tetroxide and phosphotungstic acid. He found the fibers to measure 1.1 to 2.0 μm. in diameter and to show wide ramifications and localized swellings.

In spite of differences of opinion concerning the presence or absence of vitreous *fibers,* x-ray diffraction studies have shown the presence of collagen *fibrils* (Hertel, 1929; Gross et al., 1955; Sugiura, 1957). Using the methods of fixation developed for electron microscopic studies, many investigators have shown that the vitreous does contain collagen fibrils. The dimension of the fibrils has varied according to the technique employed, but in general the fibrils have a diameter of 60 to 150 A. (Schwarz, 1955, 1956, 1961 a and b; Gross et al., 1955; Fine and Tousimis, 1961; Balazs, 1961; Lukoff and David, 1961; Blackstad and Vegge, 1962; Hogan, 1963; Propst and Leb, 1963; Balazs et al., 1964; Brini et al., 1968). Fine and Tousimis (1961) studied homogenized monkey vitreous after centrifugation. The sediment contained fairly uniform filaments 200 to 250 A. thick, with an axial periodicity averaging 220 A.

The vitreous has the following components:

1. Anterior hyaloid
2. Posterior hyaloid
3. Cortex
    a. Vitreous base
    b. Peripapillary vitreous
4. Central vitreous
5. Vitreous cells.

Anterior Hyaloid (Figs. 11–2 *A* and *B*, 11–3 to 11–5)

In formalin-fixed eyes, the anterior hyaloid curves forward from a point about 1.5 mm. anterior to the ora serrata to the region of the lens equator, where it comes into contact with the lens capsule. No thickening of

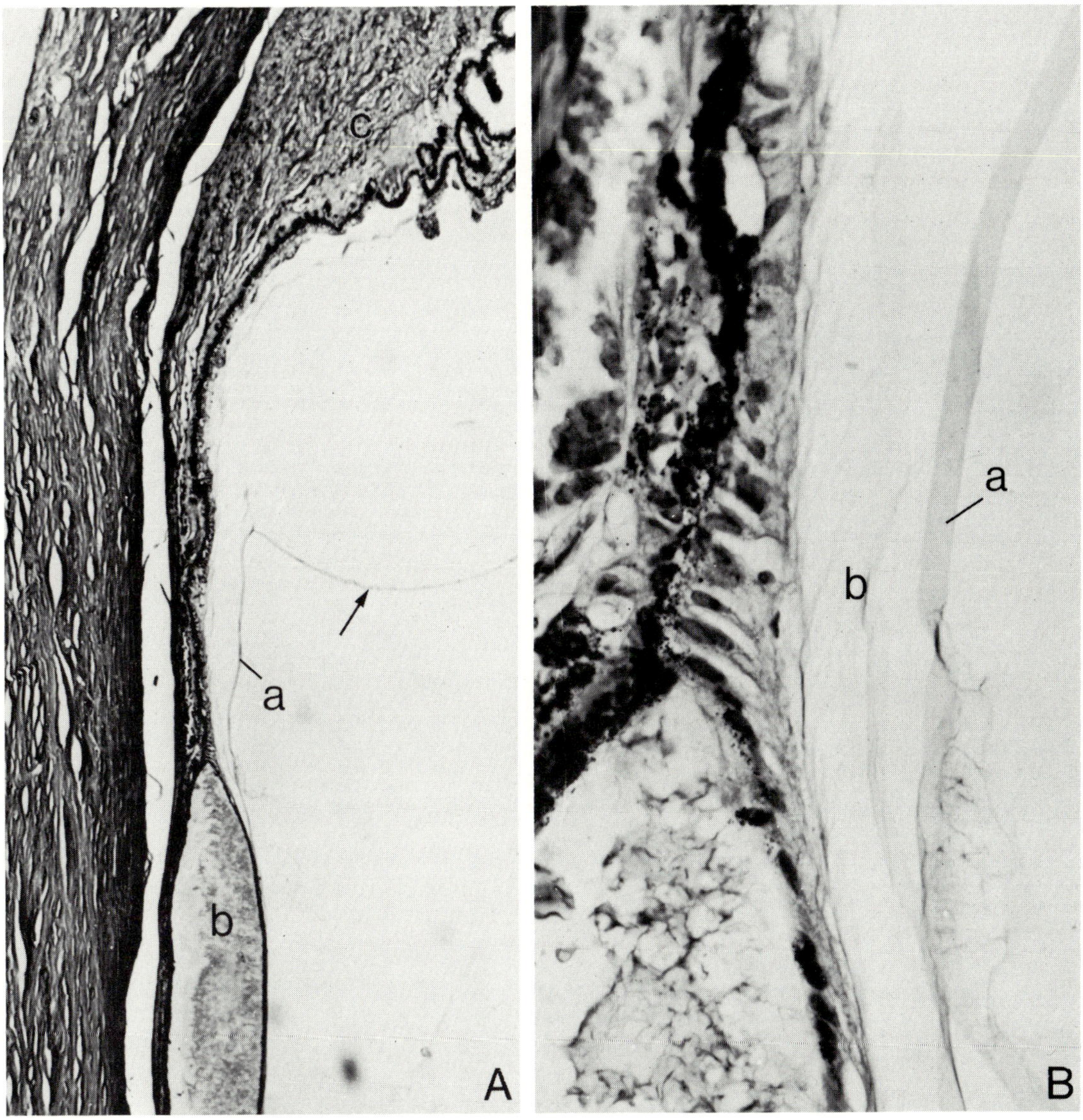

Figure 11–2. Light micrographs of the anterior hyaloid of the vitreous. *A*, The anterior hyaloid (a) lies internal to a ciliary body cyst (b) and extends forward toward the lens (arrow). In this specimen it is displaced from the ciliary body (c) as a result of shinkage. (× 50.)

B, An enlargement of *A*. The anterior hyaloid (a) is accentuated by the method of preparation of the specimen. Vitreous fibrils at the base of the vitreous (b) also extend forward around the zonular fibers. (× 450.)

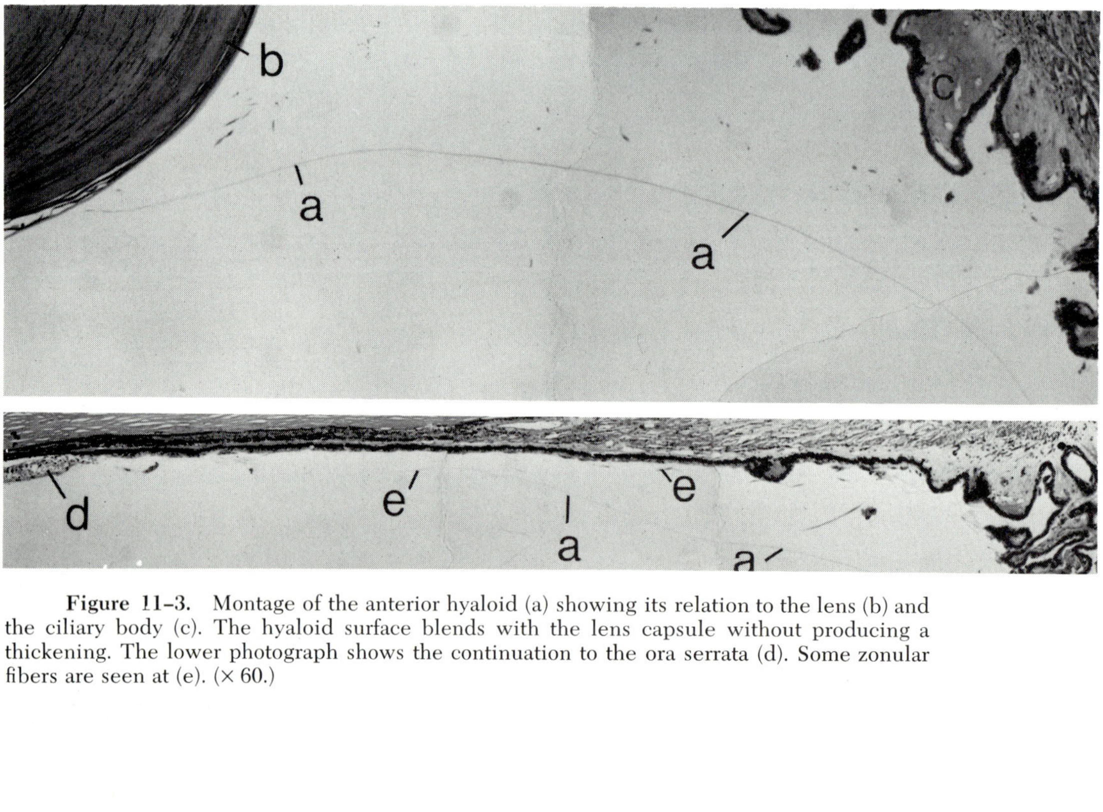

Figure 11-3. Montage of the anterior hyaloid (a) showing its relation to the lens (b) and the ciliary body (c). The hyaloid surface blends with the lens capsule without producing a thickening. The lower photograph shows the continuation to the ora serrata (d). Some zonular fibers are seen at (e). (× 60.)

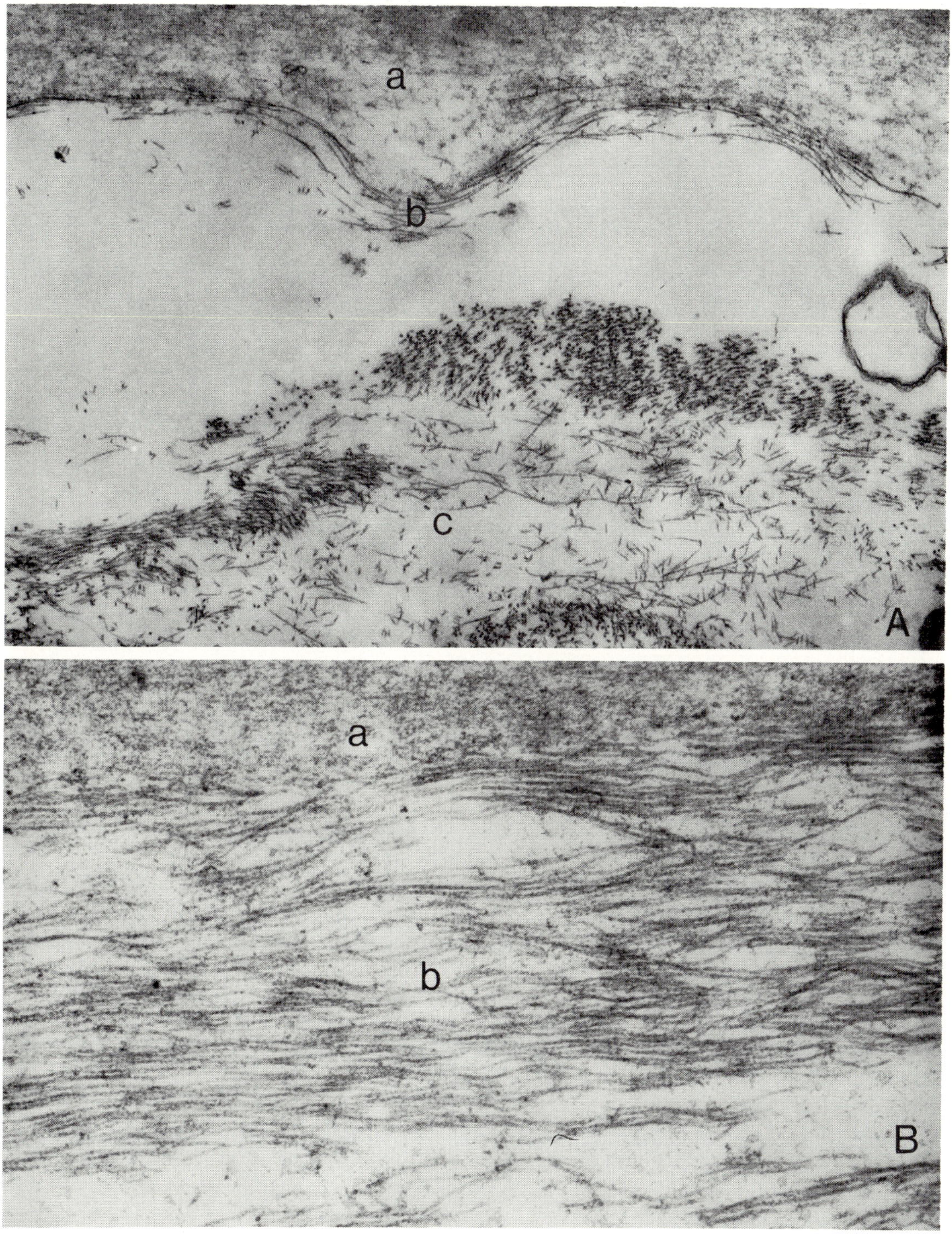

Figure 11–4. *A*, Electron micrograph of the anterior hyaloid adjacent to the pars plana of the ciliary body. The collagen fibers adjacent to the ciliary epithelium (a) are oriented parallel to the cells. The fibers become less closely spaced and regularly oriented at (b). They run in various directions elsewhere (c). (× 18,000.)

B, A similar photograph of the anterior hyaloid at a higher magnification. The cortical collagen fibrils (a) are very closely packed, and the deeper ones (b) are less densely packed. The banding of the fibrils is evident. (× 45,000.)

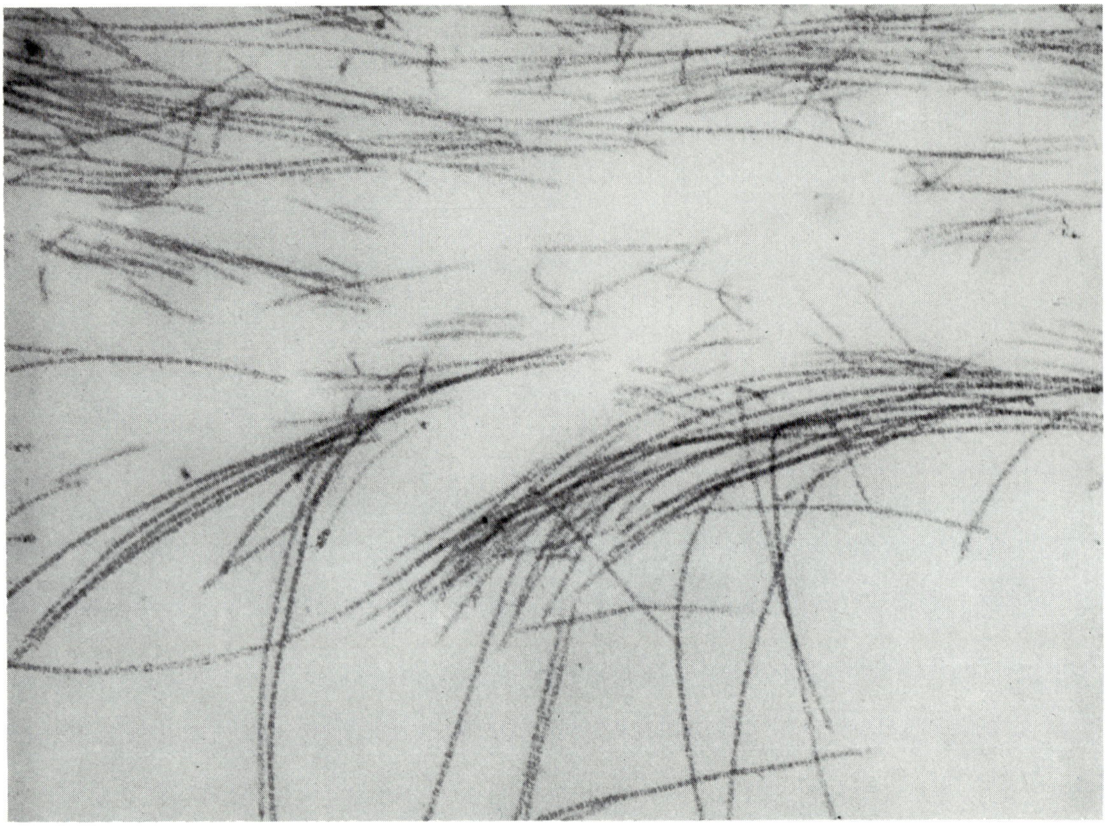

Figure 11–5. Electron micrograph of the anterior hyaloid anterior to the vitreous base. The structure of the cortical vitreous is the same anterior to the ora serrata as posterior to this region. The collagen fibrils seen here have a diameter of 330 A. and a banding of about 160 A. (× 60,000.)

the capsule occurs at the site of contact, and no real "ligament" can be identified in the region of the hyaloideocapsular ligament. The surface of the vitreous appears simply to contact the posterior capsule without any specific kind of fusion. The vitreous is intimate with the lens just anterior and posterior to the equator as it invests the zonules up to their lenticular terminations. The anterior hyaloid and underlying vitreous cortex directly behind the lens show a very faint fibrillation. Special mucopolysaccharide stains show a smaller amount of hyaluronic acid here than elsewhere in the vitreous. The zonular fibers, which arise from the pars plana of the ciliary body, are closely identified with the anterior hyaloid. In well fixed eyes, continuity between the zonules and the vitreous can be demonstrated, and fine extensions of vitreous are identified among the anterior zonular fibers, especially at the lens equator. In electron micrographs the anterior hyaloid surface has the same structure as the remaining cortex, except for a slightly greater density of fibrils, particularly those radiating out of the vitreous base toward the lens and around the zonular fibers.

Fine and Tousimis (1961) observed the collagen fibrils and their enclosed elements in the anterior hyaloid to be arranged in sheet-like aggregates parallel to the surface of the eye. The laminar appearance is greatest in the pars plana region, particularly in the peripheral portion, where the zonular fibers are observed (Figs. 11–2 *B*, 11–4 *B*). The zonules are found to be parallel aggregates of the same fibrils seen in the vitreous.

POSTERIOR HYALOID (Figs. 11–6 to 11–13)

Slightly posterior to the vitreous base, the fibrils of the base curve backward along the inner retina as very thin layers that gradually move away from the retina toward the central vitreous. Posterior to the equator the vitreous continues to be closely identified with the inner limiting membrane of the retina. Fetal eyes show the fibrils of the posterior hyaloid more clearly, even into the region of the optic disc, but in adult eyes these fibers are difficult to demonstrate posterior to the equator. Electron microscopic details of the posterior hyaloid of the vitreous in the posterior eye have been discussed (p. 489). The collagen filaments of this portion of the vitreous insert at various angles into the basement membrane of the Müller and glial cells of the retina. There is no clear-cut surface membrane over the vitreous, although its collagen forms a condensation near the surface that produces the appearance of a membrane.

Text continued on page 624

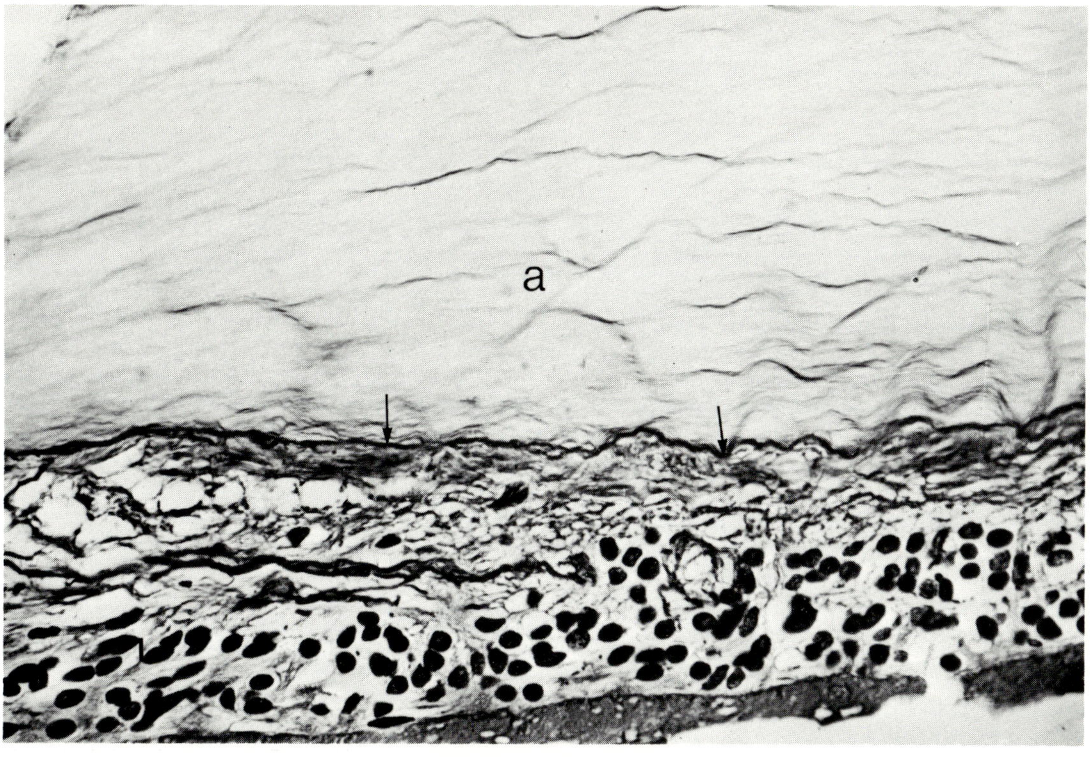

Figure 11–6. Light micrograph of the vitreous just posterior to the ora serrata. The inner retina (arrows) is closely related to the vitreous cortex (a). The fibrils and mucoprotein of the vitreous cortex form layers that lie parallel to the inner retina. (× 425.)

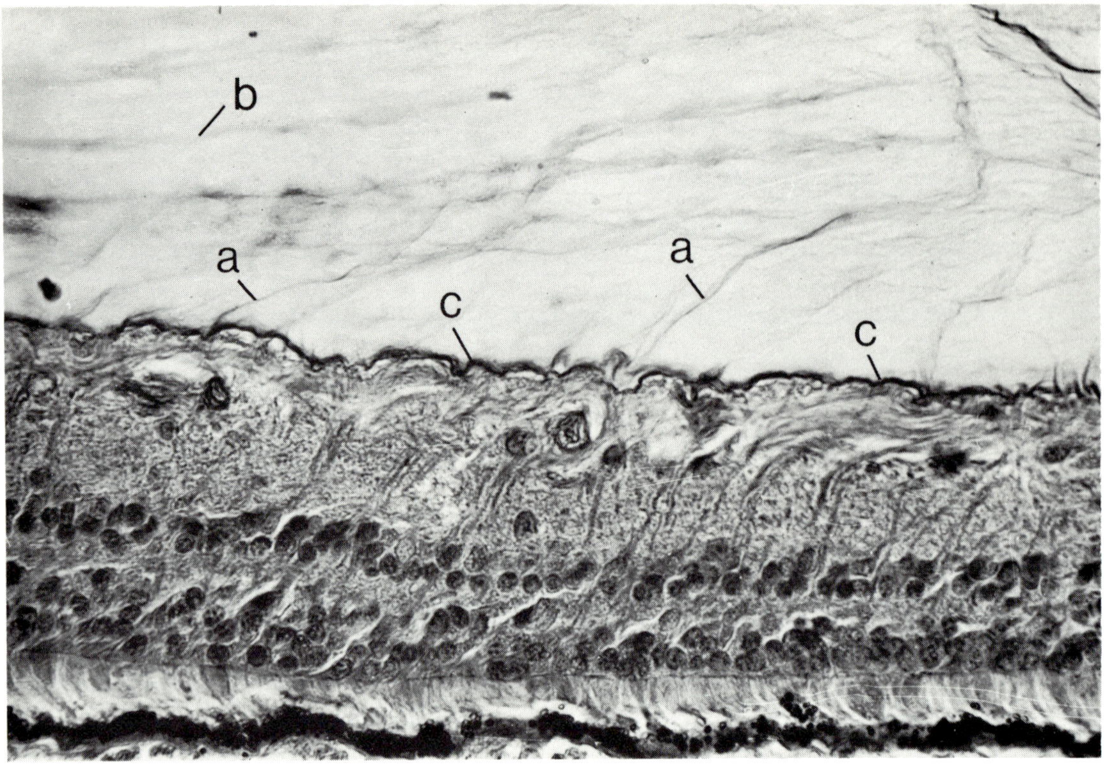

Figure 11–7. An area of retina and vitreous slightly posterior to that seen in Figure 11–6. Some vitreous fibrils (a) extend at a right angle from the retinal inner limiting membrane into the vitreous. Other fibrils are parallel to the retina (b). The internal limiting membrane of the retina shows some undulation (c). (× 425.)

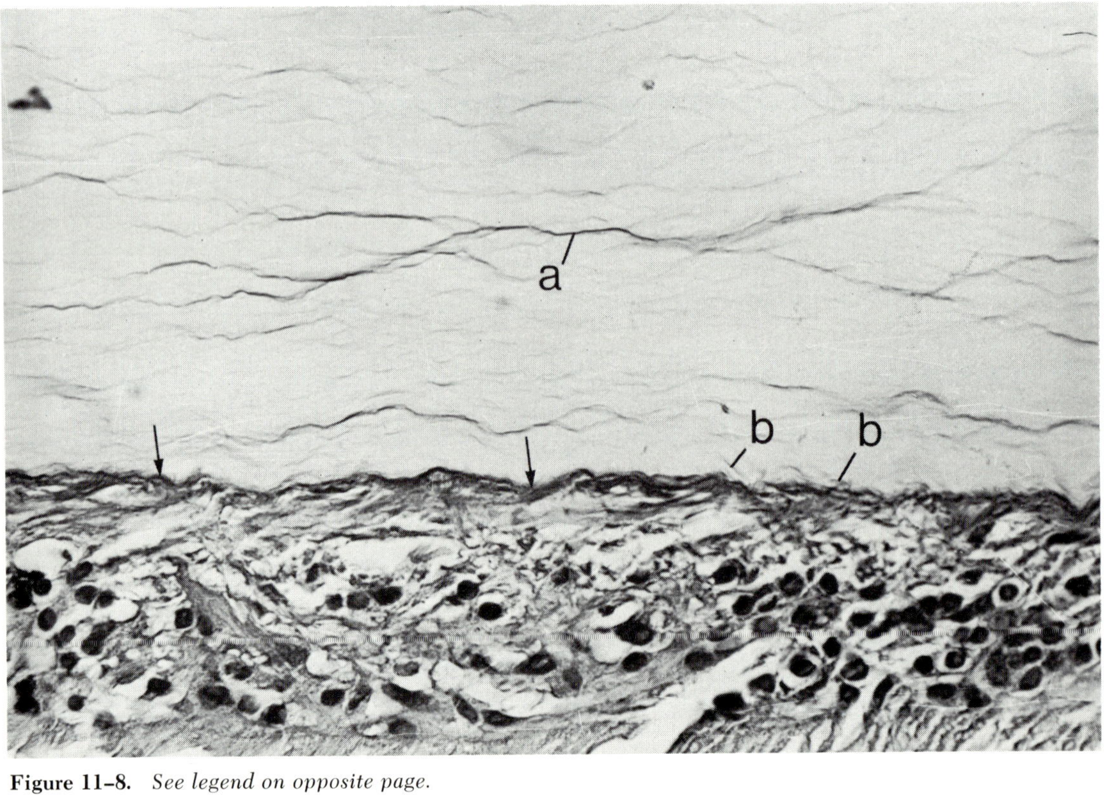

Figure 11–8. *See legend on opposite page.*

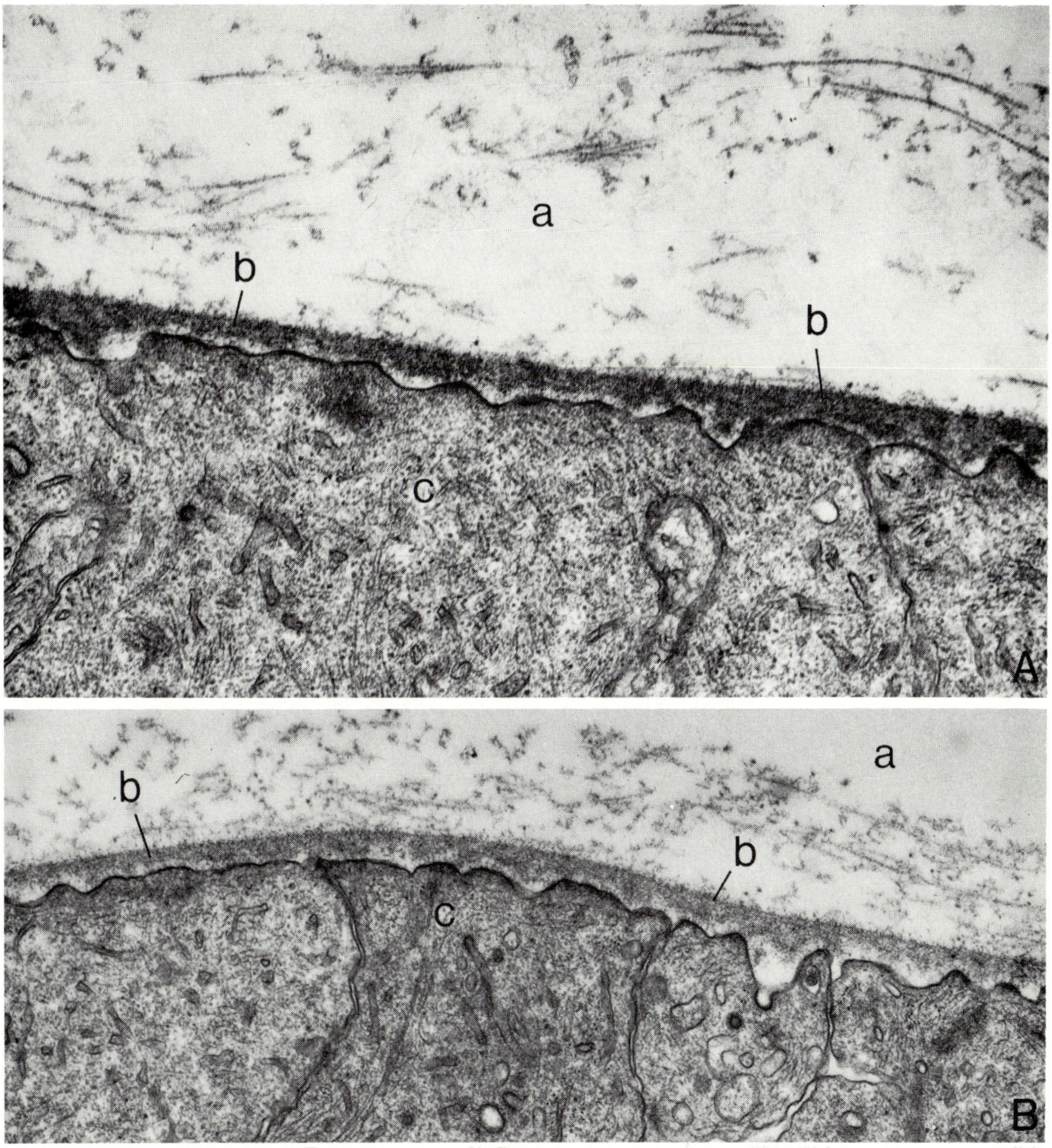

Figure 11–9. *A*, Electron micrograph of the inner retina of the equatorial region to show the relation of the vitreous to the inner retina. The vitreous cortex (a) contains collagen fibrils that are oriented in various directions. Close to the retina is a thin layer of fine collagen filaments that are seen in various sections. They join the basement membrane of the Müller cells (b). The cytoplasm of the Müller cells (c) is very dense. (× 25,000.)

B, Equatorial vitreous cortex and posterior hyaloid. The cortex (a) contains many fibrils that are oriented in various directions. Many of them become continuous with the basement membrane (b) of the Müller cells (c). (× 20,800.)

Figure 11–8. A light micrograph of the equatorial hyaloid. The vitreous is in close proximity to the retina (arrows), and the basement membrane of the Müller cells is connected to the collagen fibrils of the vitreous cortex. The collagen fibrils in the cortex are parallel to the retina (a), while at the outer retinal surface they bend to join the retina (b). (× 425.)

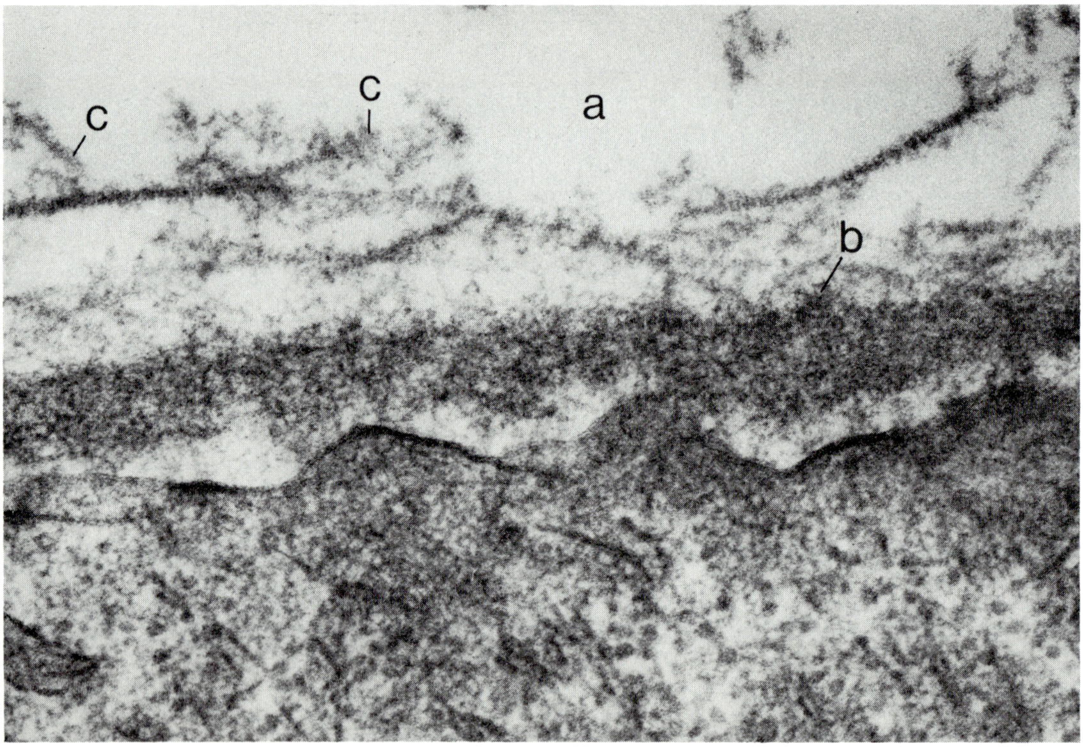

Figure 11–10. Higher magnification of the equatorial vitreous cortex (a) and the posterior hyaloid (b). The banding of the collagen fibrils is evident. The filamentous material clinging to these fibrils (c) is probably mucopolysaccharide. (× 72,000.)

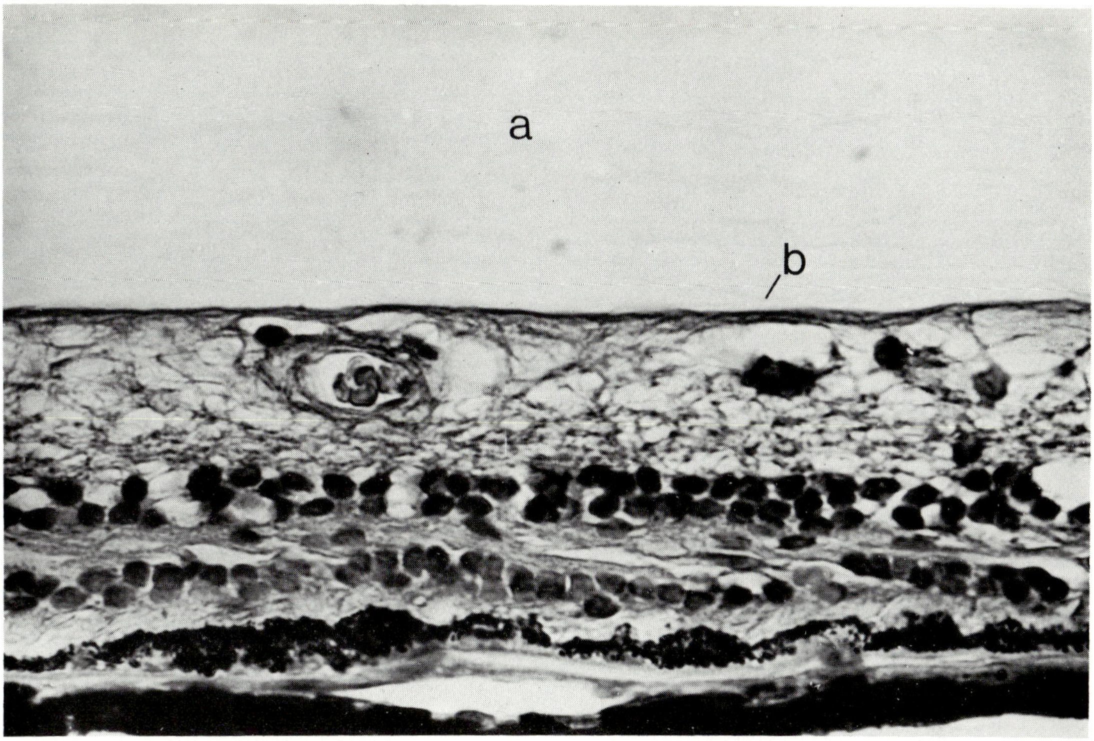

Figure 11–11. The hyaloid posterior to the equator. The cortex of the vitreous (a) is less condensed and contains a smaller amount of fibrillar material, possibly because of an aging process. Fine fibrils can be seen to join the inner limiting membrane (b). (× 630.)

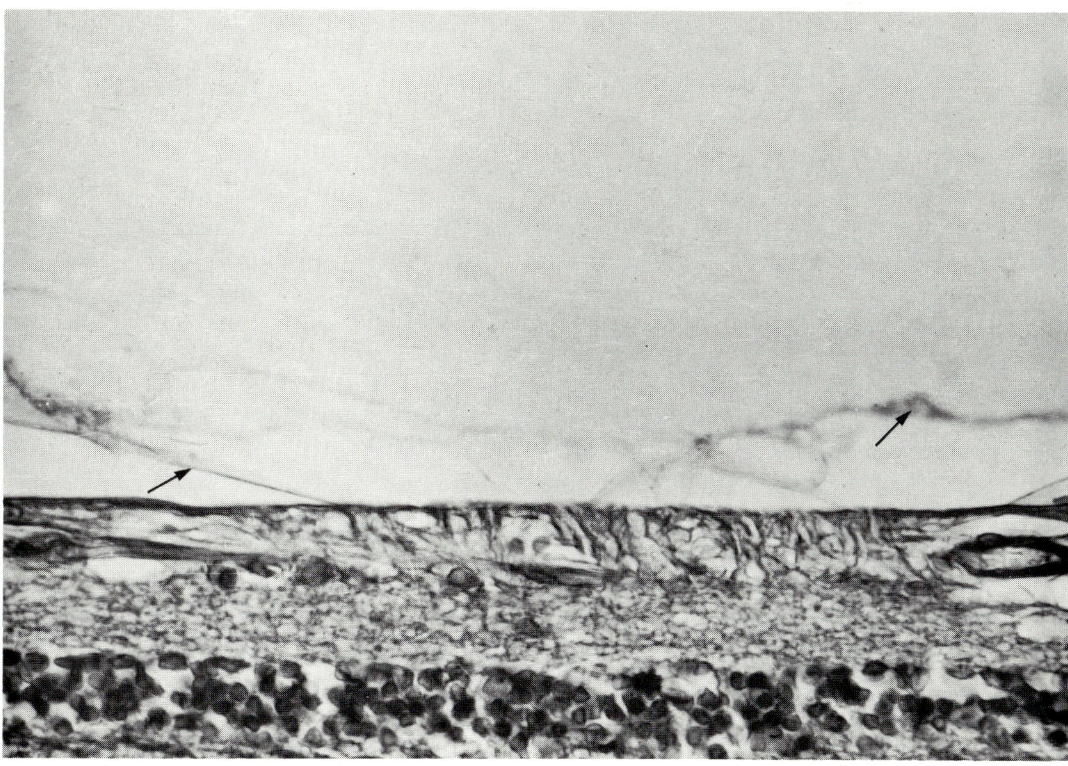

Figure 11–12. Posterior hyaloid in the eye of a young infant. It is detached from the retina (arrows) in two places. Elsewhere it is joined to the inner limiting membrane of the retina. (× 425.)

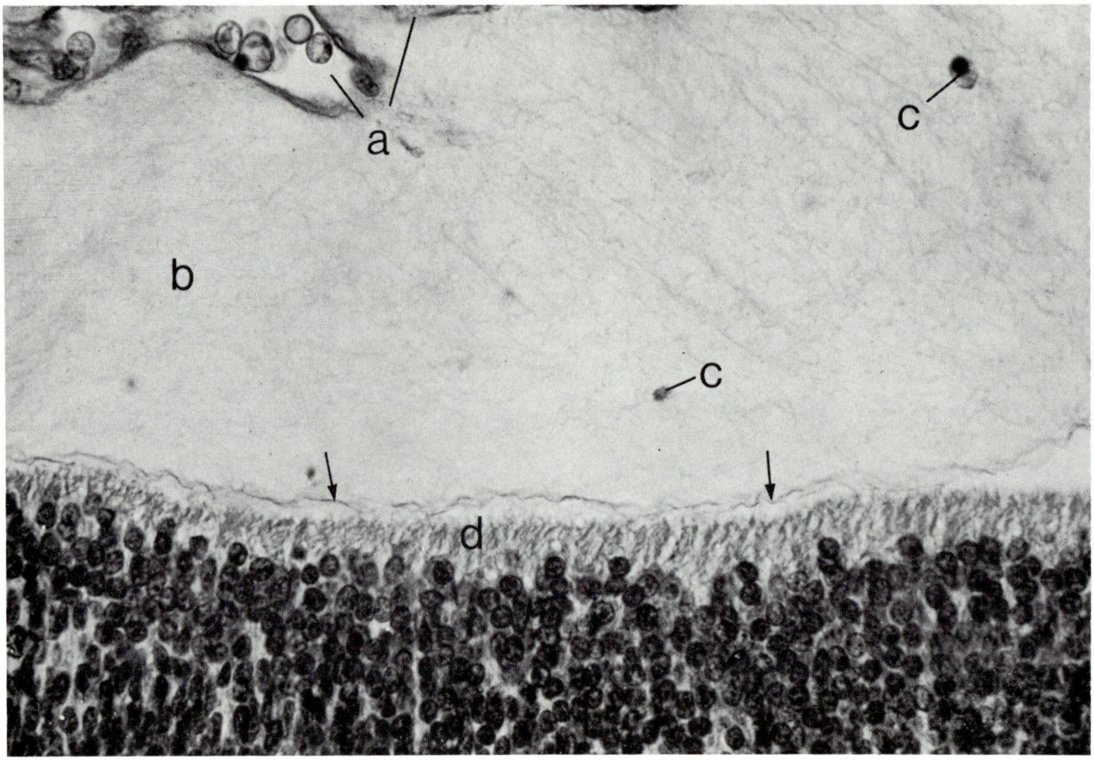

Figure 11–13. Fetal vitreous containing hyaloid vessels. The vessels are at (a) and the fibrillar primary vitreous is at (b). Some cells are seen in the vitreous substance (c). The vitreous cortex is clearly in continuity with the retina (arrows), where it is in contact with the Müller cells (d). (× 425.)

CORTEX (Figs. 11–14 to 11–20)

The cortex is approximately 100 μm. thick and includes the anterior and posterior hyaloid. It circumscribes the entire vitreous body, being formed by a condensation of collagen fibrils, cells, proteins and mucopolysaccharide in the interfibrillar spaces (Balazs, 1961). The fibrils are randomly oriented, measuring about 100 A. in thickness, and contact the internal limiting membrane of the retina to fasten the vitreous to this tissue. Cells are more common here than in the central vitreous.

Vitreous Base (Figs. 11–14, 11–15, 11–17, 11–18). The fibrils of the vitreous base originate in a broad zone that lies roughly at a right angle to the inner surface of the ciliary epithelium and inner retina around the ora serrata. Those attaching to the retina often are more coarse, arising as conical groups of tapering fibrils which extend into the vitreous. Those arising from the ciliary epithelium are finer but more numerous, and they fan out into the vitreous for a considerable distance. All these filaments are firmly attached to the basement membrane of the ciliary epithelial and retinal cells. The interfibrillar spaces in this region of the vitreous contain proteins and mucopolysaccharides.

Electron microscopic studies show that the filaments forming the vitreous base attach to the basement membrane of the unpigmented epithelium in the pars plana near the ora serrata and the Müller cells of the

Text continued on page 632

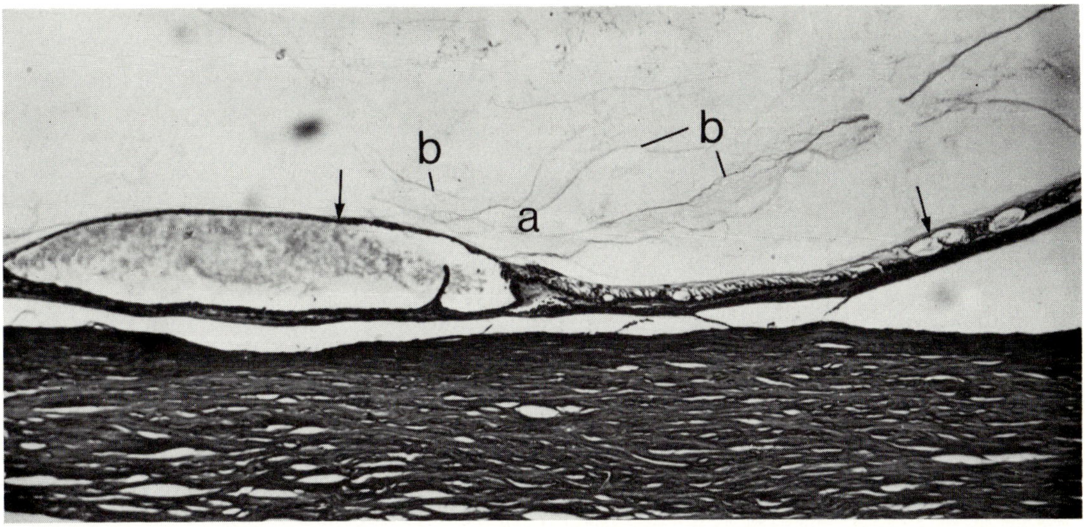

Figure 11-14. Vitreous base at the ora serrata. The two arrows outline the approximate anterior and posterior limits of the vitreous base. The ora serrata is at (a). The cortical collagen fibrils of the vitreous base radiate out into the central vitreous from this area (b). (× 50.)

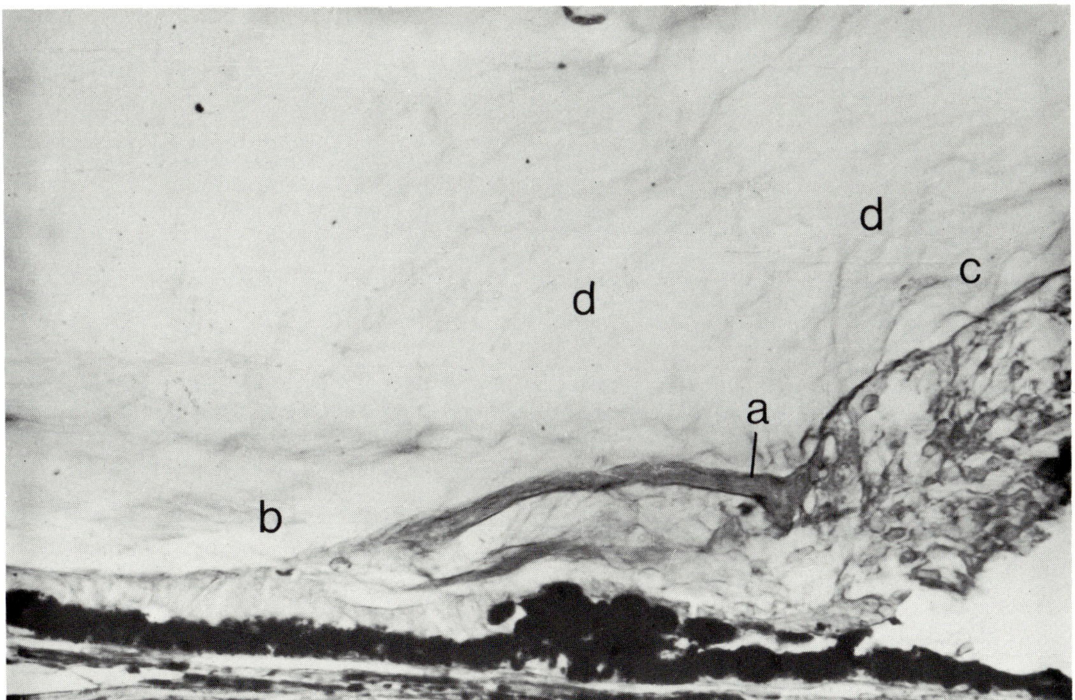

Figure 11-15. Light micrograph of the vitreous base at the ora serrata. The ora serrata is at (a) and the vitreous base extends forward onto the ciliary body anterior to the ora (b) and onto the retina posteriorly (c). The collagen of the vitreous in this region extends out into the vitreous from the base (d). (× 425.)

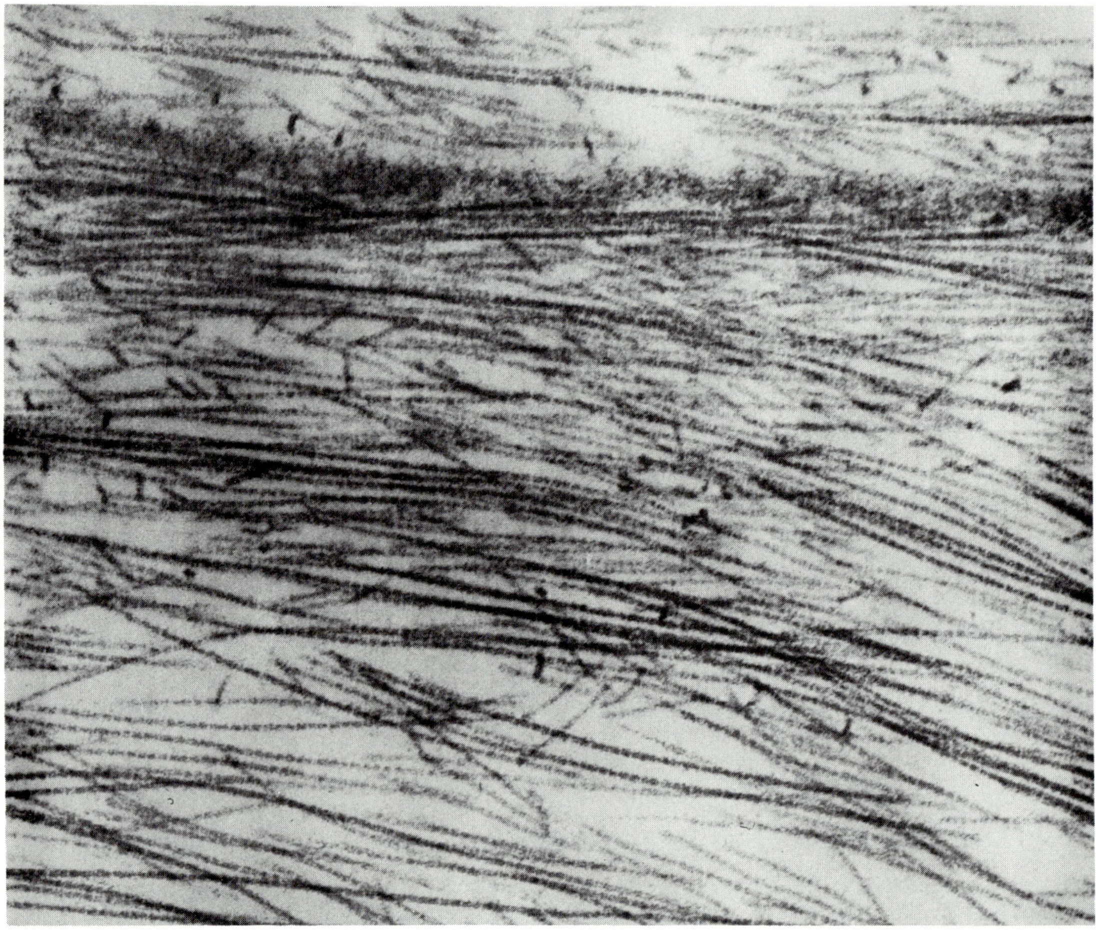

Figure 11–16. The vitreous cortex, containing numerous fibrils. The fibrils are uniform in size and do not vary in diameter. They are oriented in different directions and show definite banding. (× 60,000.)

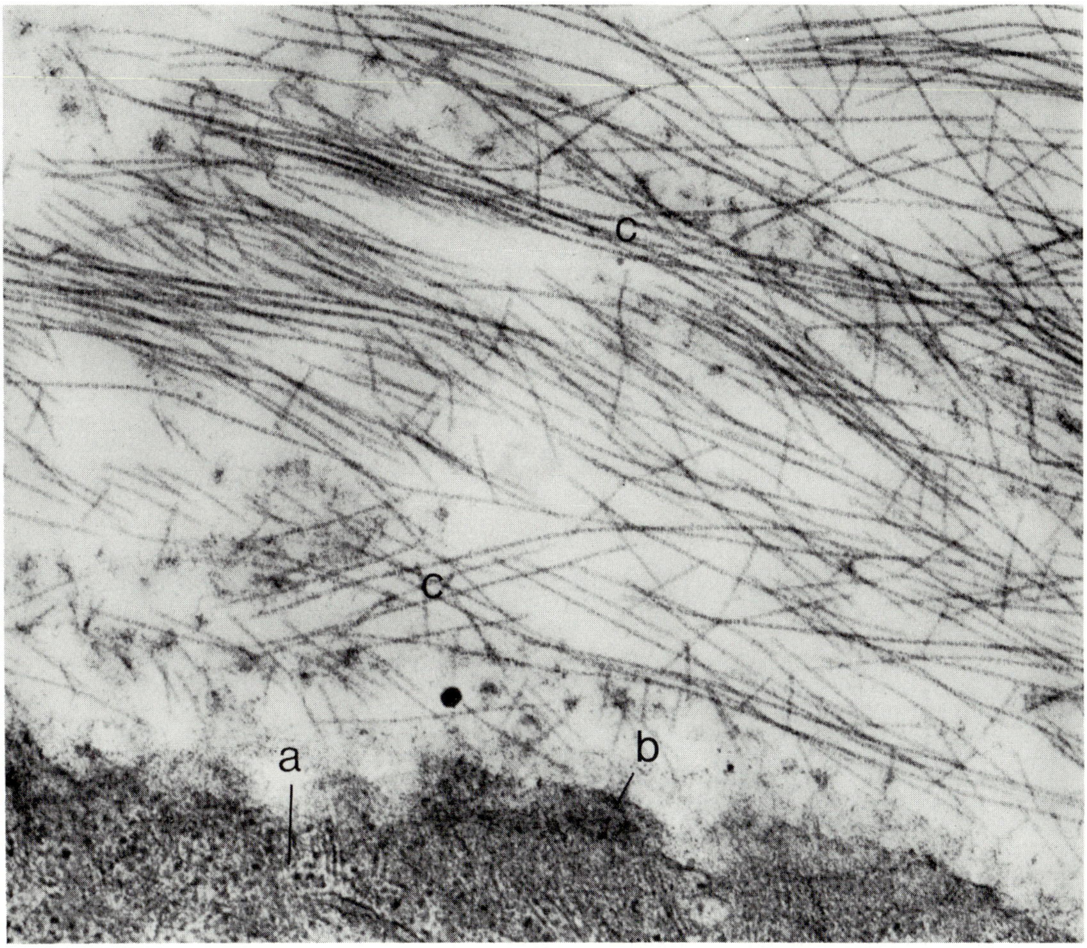

Figure 11–17. The vitreous base in the region of the peripheral retina. The Müller cells (a) have a basement membrane (b) that forms the inner limiting membrane of the retina. The collagen fibrils (c) of the vitreous base form a meshwork internal to the retina. These fibrils join the internal limiting membrane. (× 50,000.)

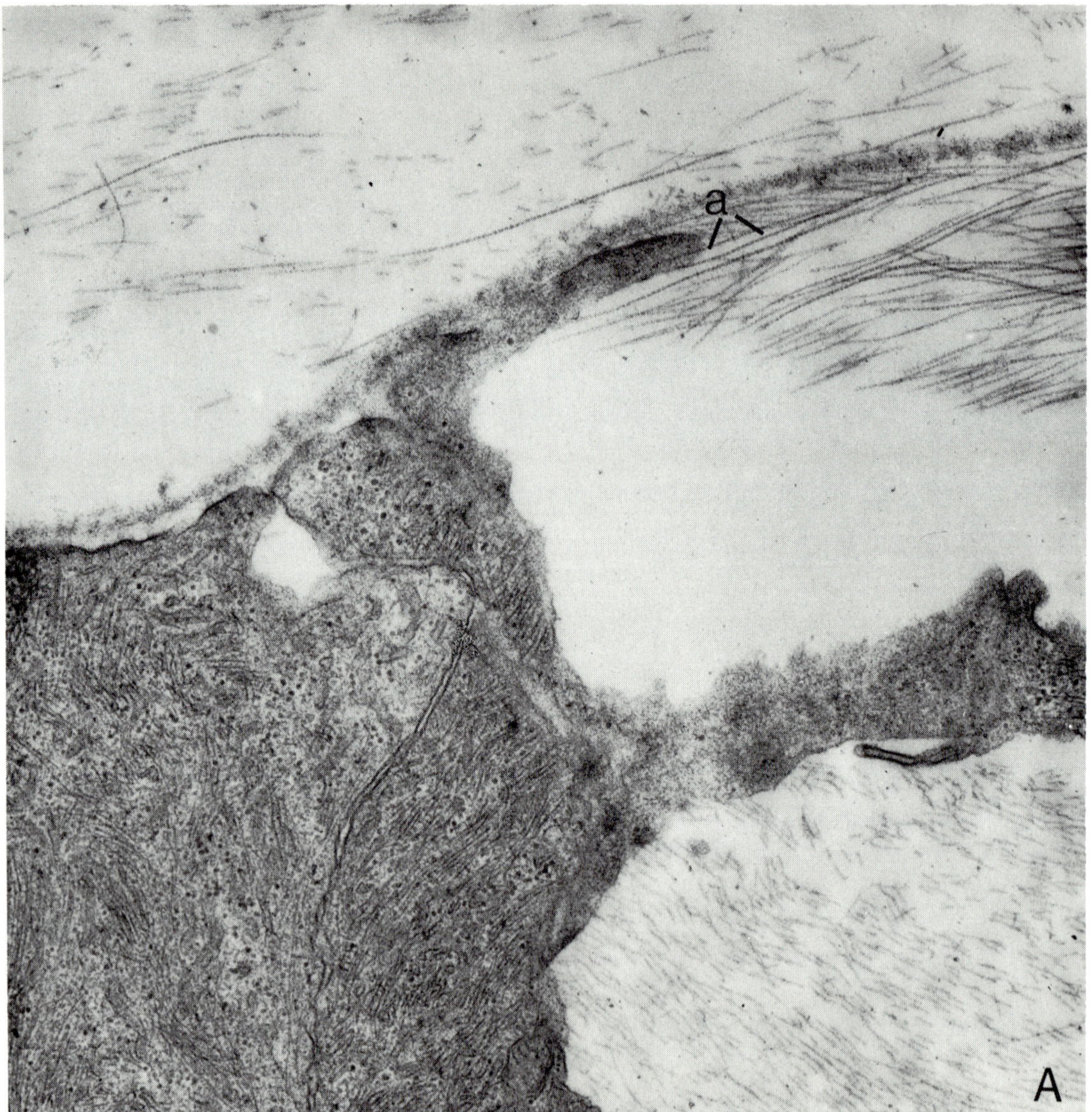

Figure 11–18. *A*, A fold in the peripheral retina, formed by processes of the Müller cells. The vitreous collagen fibrils (a) enter into the retinal folds and join the basement membrane of the Müller cells. (× 28,000.)

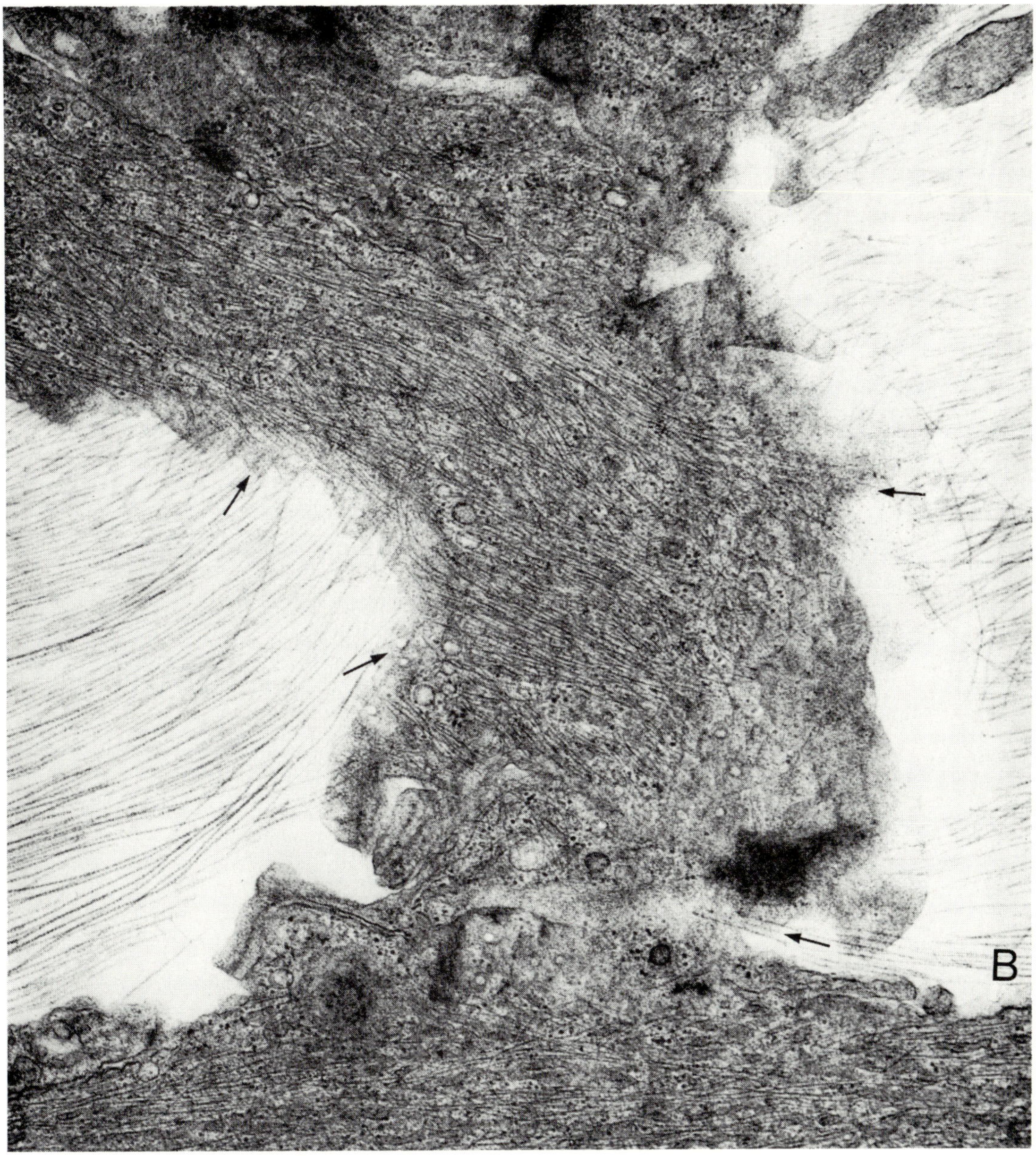

Figure 11–18. *Continued.*
B, An adjacent region of the retina and vitreous. The intimate contact of the vitreous collagen and the Müller cells is shown (arrows). (× 25,600.)

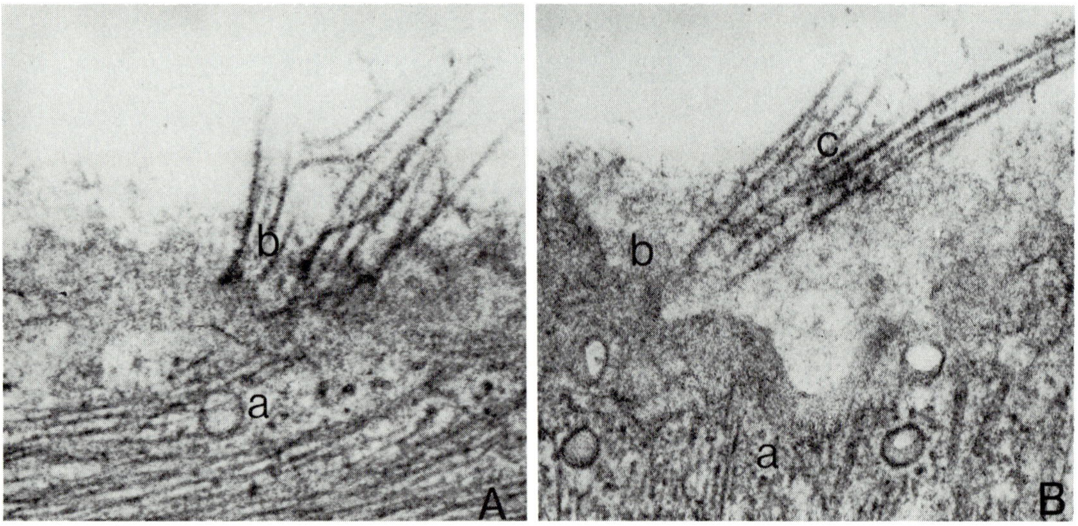

Figure 11–19. *A*, Peripapillary vitreous. A grazing section of the disc edge showing the cytoplasm of an astrocyte (a) with its many fibrils, and vitreous collagen fibrils attaching to the basement membrane (b). (× 80,000.)

B, A view similar to that shown in *A*, with an astrocyte at (a), the basement membrane at (b) and vitreous fibrils at (c). The fibrils blend with the basement membrane but do not attach to the cell membrane of the astrocyte. (× 72,000.)

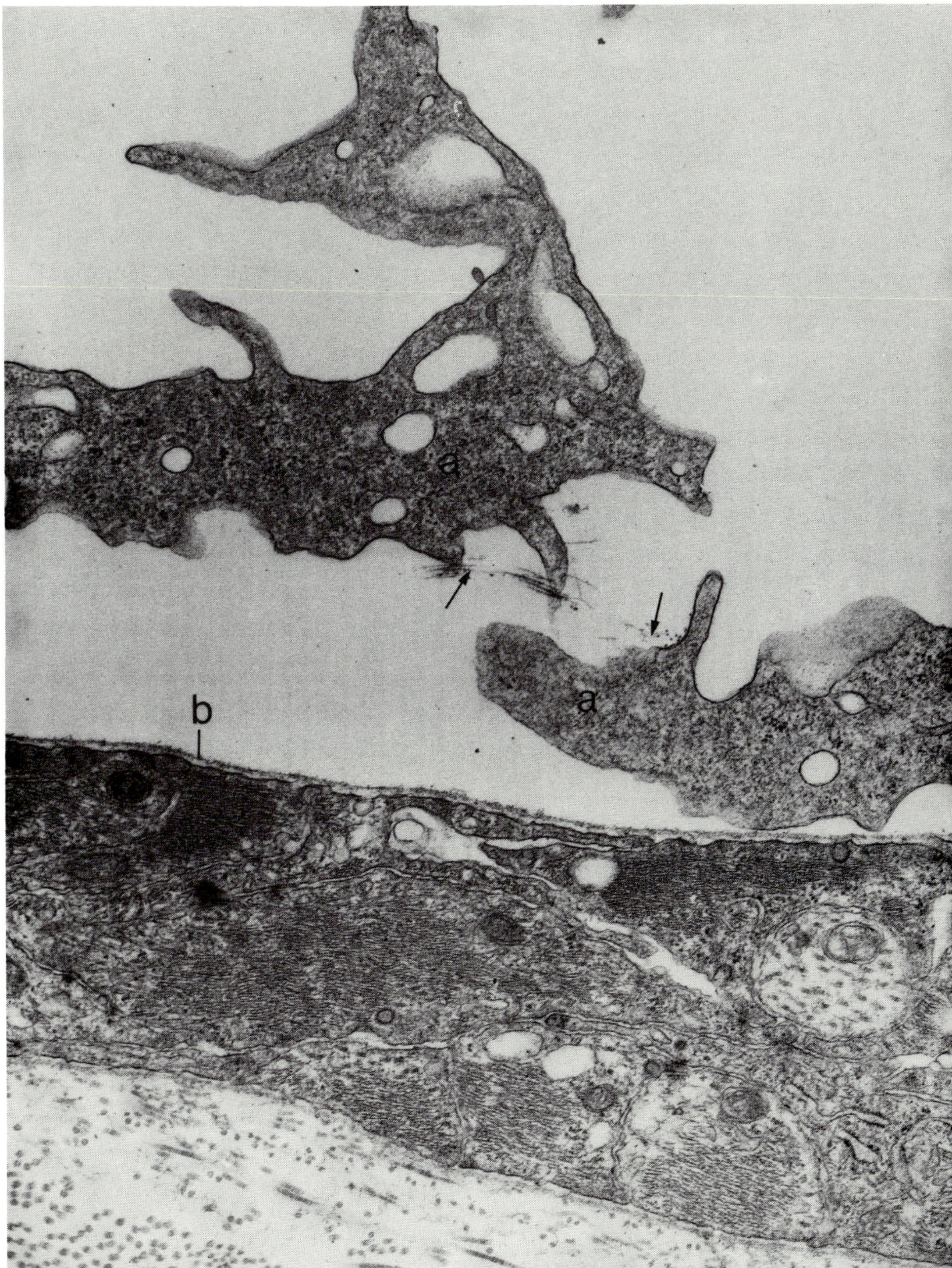

Figure 11-20. Inner disc surface. There are fewer collagen fibrils in this portion of the vitreous (arrows). Two hyalocytes are seen (a). The basement membrane of the astrocyte (b) is thinner than that over the adjacent retinal Müller cells. (× 25,500.)

peripheral retina. Their structure is like that of vitreous cortex elsewhere, but they differ from the other vitreous filaments in their greater number and orientation at various angles to the inner wall of the eye.

Peripapillary Vitreous (Figs. 11–19 *A* and *B*, 11–20). In the peripapillary region the vitreous is firmly united to the retina in a narrow zone that appears to be about 10 μm. in width; the tissues are less firmly united in older eyes, however. The peripapillary attachment is like others between the retina and vitreous, but the cortex here contains more fibrils, which are oriented toward the basement membrane of the Müller cells. This arrangement terminates where the Müller cells end at the disc edge.

Central Vitreous

The central vitreous is usually less well preserved in eyes fixed and prepared for light microscopy, especially in older eyes, where syneresis is so frequent. This portion has a less dense structure and stains lighter with most stains than other areas of the vitreous. The ultrastructural features of the central vitreous resemble those of the cortex, and the fibrils in both portions have the same structure, although the central vitreous contains many fewer collagen fibrils.

Vitreous Cells (Figs. 11–21 to 11–23)

Cells are found in the vitreous cortex, particularly in the vitreous base and zonular region, as well as in the cortex near the retina and the optic disc. They are abundant in the embryo and fetal vitreous but are less numerous in adult eyes, and many observers have considered them to be embryonic cells which gradually disappear. The number of cells varies considerably according to species, age and topography. In adult cattle eyes there are 50 to 80 cells per sq. mm. in the posterior cortex and 300 to 400 per sq. mm. in the vitreous base (Balazs et al., 1964). Cells in the cortex adjacent to the retina lie internal to retinal vessels and not more than 500 μm. from them. Their function is unknown; some investigators believe that they are histiocytes, others suggest that they are glial cells.

With the light microscope in fixed tissues, the vitreous cells which lie close to the inner limiting membrane of the retina are spindle-shaped. In the base of the vitreous, these cells are larger, rounded or star-shaped and have prominent nuclei.

Studies of cells in fresh vitreous of steers, cows, rabbits, rats and humans have been made with the phase-contrast microscope (Szirmai and Balazs, 1958; Hamburg, 1959). These studies reveal that rounded cells are found near the vitreous surface in all species. The cells contain slowly moving perinuclear granules, 0.5 to 2.0 μm. in size, particularly in human and cattle eyes. The granules are preserved best in buffered osmium tetroxide and in Bouin's solution. They are found to be orthochromatic with azure A, and while they are PAS-positive, no reaction occurs upon exposure to hyaluronidase, diastase or human saliva. Since the hyaluronic acid concentration in the cortical vitreous is 0.2 mg. per 100 ml., five to ten times that in the central and anterior vitreous, and since most of the cells are found here,

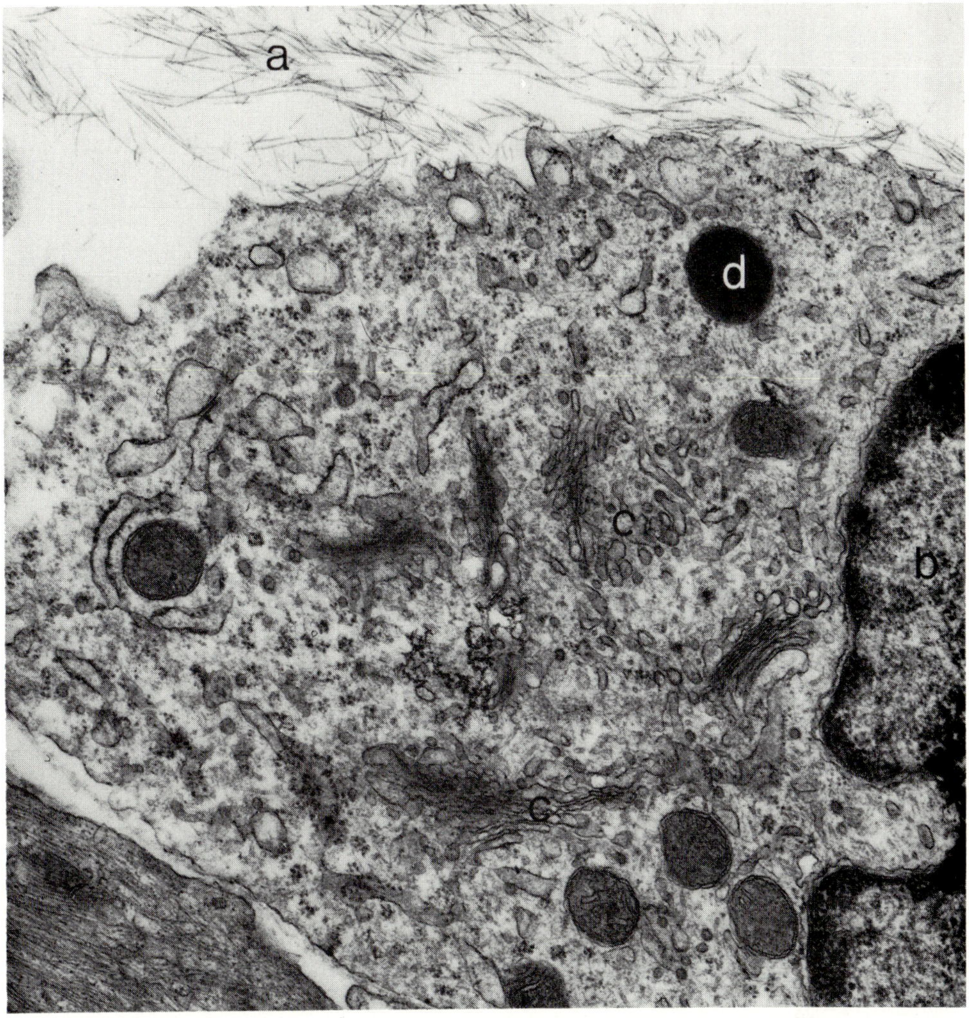

Figure 11–21. Vitreous cells. This hyalocyte lies anterior to the peripheral portion of the optic disc. Vitreous collagen fibrils lie close to the cell (a). The cell is slightly elliptical and it has a lobulated nucleus (b) and a well developed Golgi system (c). A vacuole bounded by a single membrane is shown at (d). These structures are thought to be secretory granules containing mucopolysaccharide. (× 27,600.)

it has been suggested that the cells may be concerned with production of mucopolysaccharide.

In subsequent studies by Balazs and his associates (1964), these cells were observed in adult mammals and birds. The name "hyalocyte" was applied to them because they seemed to differ from histiocytes, glial cells and fibroblasts. The granules of these specific cells were found to be PAS-positive, basophilic (orthochromatic) and to show a light- and oxygen-sensitive autofluorescence. The cells were negative for glial stains, but their tendency to take up neutral red in the living state was believed to be important. Since these cells were found to be phagocytic and their cytoplasm contained inclusions, they were believed to be connective tissue cells of the macrophage type. They could be distinguished from fibroblasts histochemically and by phase-contrast microscopy. Since these hyalocytes were found

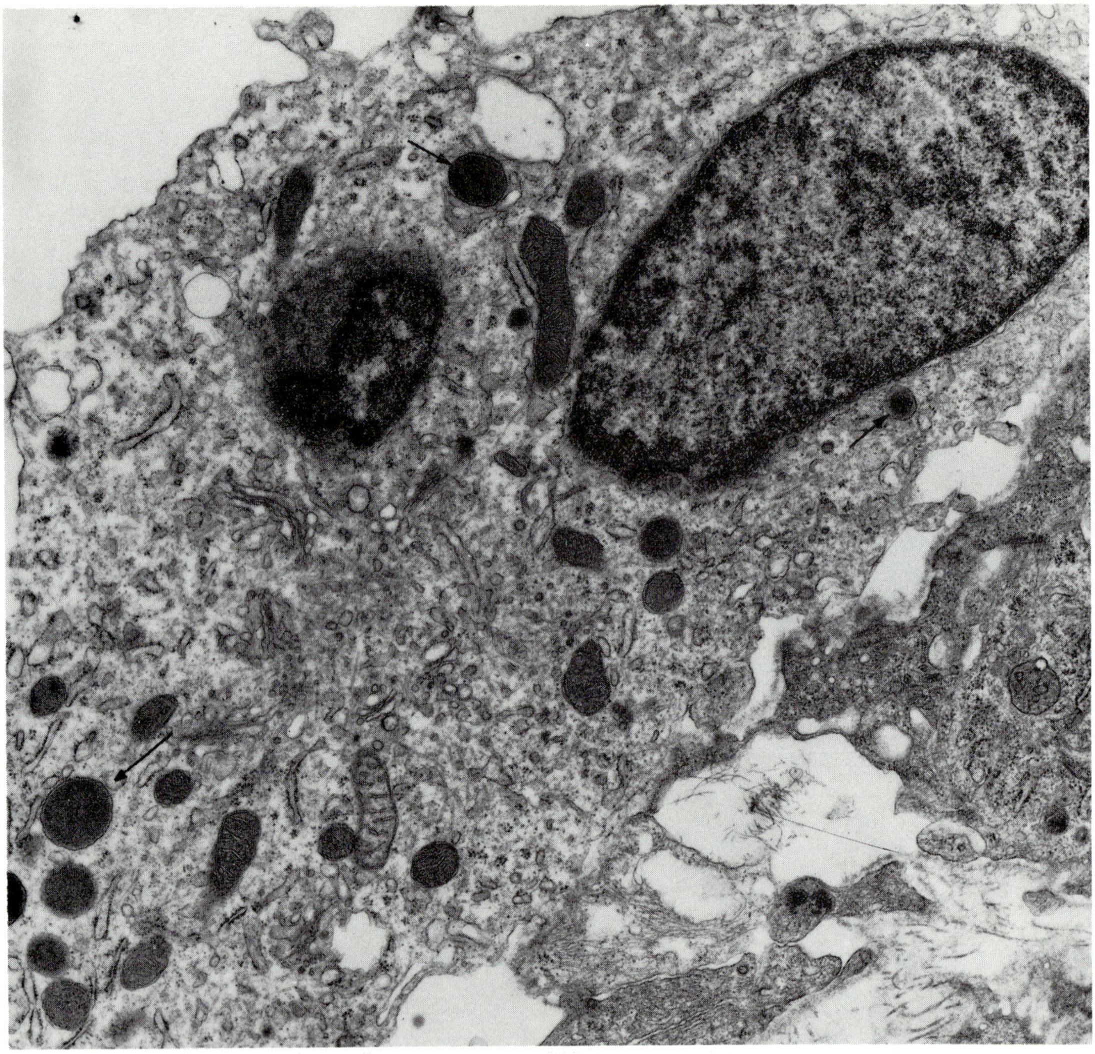

Figure 11-22. A hyalocyte close to the optic disc. These cells are characterized by a large cytoplasmic-nuclear ratio, they have a lobulated nucleus, and the Golgi complex occupies a large portion of the cytoplasm. A number of vacuoles containing an electron-dense material (arrows) are found near the Golgi; these are thought to be secretory vacuoles containing mucopolysaccharides. (× 11,200.)

to be most numerous in the base of the vitreous, it was believed that they probably enter the vitreous from the ciliary body.

Very few electron microscopic studies have been made of the vitreous cells. Hogan (1963) demonstrated vitreous cells in the vitreous base adjacent to the pars plana, ora serrata and peripheral retina of monkey eyes. These cells did not resemble detached epithelial cells, nor did they have a basement membrane, and they did not resemble macrophages because of their paucity of lysosomes. Their cytoplasm contained a considerable amount of smooth-surfaced endoplasmic reticulum and an extensive Golgi apparatus. These cells were believed to be hyalocytes.

Bloom and Balazs (1965) investigated the hyalocytes of calves' eyes

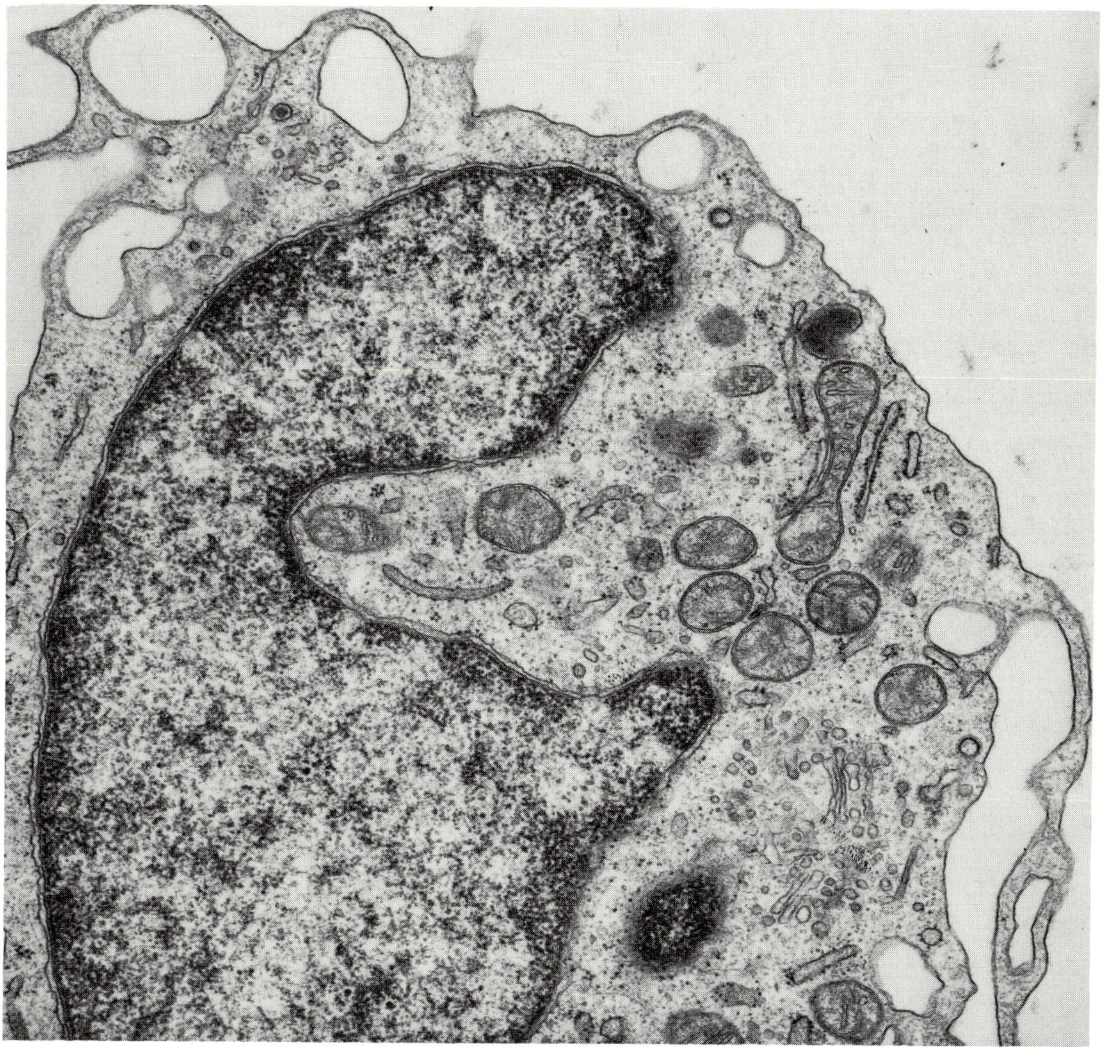

Figure 11–23. Hyalocyte of the peripheral vitreous near the ora serrata. The lobulated nucleus, mitochondria and Golgi apparatus of this cell are clearly shown. No secretory granules are seen in this portion of the cell. (× 18,400.)

with the electron microscope. They found these cells to have the rounded shape that was observed in fresh vitreous with the phase-contrast microscope. The cells were found to contain cytoplasmic granules, which were observed to be numerous in some areas and few in number in other parts of the cytoplasm. The granules varied in appearance, a finding which suggested that they are in different stages of development. Because of the variation in density of the cytoplasmic granules, Hogan (1963) may have not found them in the cells of monkey vitreous.

Electron microscopic study of the human hyalocytes in the vitreous cortex shows the hyalocytes to have many characteristics of those observed by Bloom and Balazs (1965) in calves' eyes (Figs. 11–20 to 11–23). The cells are oval or spindle-shaped and have a lobulated nucleus. Their size varies from 10 to 15 μm. and they have surface cytoplasmic projections that extend out for 0.5 to 1.0 μm., the number of which varies widely. Mitochondria and smooth- and rough-surfaced endoplasmic reticulum are present in moderate amounts, but the characteristic cytoplasmic organelles of these cells are the many hyalocyte granules and the well developed Golgi apparatus. The granules measure between 0.2 and 2.0 μm. in diameter, and they contain a finely granular matrix which exhibits several stages of condensation. These granules are strikingly similar to the zymogen granules of the pancreatic acinar cell in their morphology and relationship to the Golgi apparatus. It is possible that the hyalocyte granules contain aminoglycans, which are secreted to form the vitreous substance. The Golgi apparatus of these hyalocytes is better developed than in other cells that have been observed in human ocular tissues. Numerous vesicles are associated with the Golgi lamellae and these possibly coalesce to form the larger hyalocyte granules. The hyalocyte cytoplasm also contains lysosomes, which are difficult to distinguish from the hyalocyte granules. Pigment granules and other matter occasionally are ingested by some hyalocytes; these granules fuse with the primary lysosomes to form secondary lysosomes and residual bodies, which are easily distinguished from hyalocyte granules.

Other cells having all the characteristics of macrophages and fibroblasts also are found in the vitreous cortex. The fibroblasts are located in the pre- and peripapillary regions, as well as around the ora serrata region, and they frequently lie close to the inner limiting membrane of the retina. In eyes containing malignant melanomas, the macrophages often contain large masses of ingested pigment.

REFERENCES

Adler, F. H.: Investigation of sugar content of ocular fluids under normal and abnormal conditions, and glycolytic activity of tissues of the eye. Trans. Amer. Ophthal. Soc. *28*:307, 1930.

Bach, L., and Seefelder, R.: Atlas zur Entwicklungsgeschichte des menschlichen Auges. Leipzig, W. Engelmann, 1911.

Balazs, E. A.: The physiology of the vitreous. *In* Schepens, C. L. (ed.): The Importance of the Vitreous Body in Retina Surgery with Special Emphasis on Reoperations. St. Louis, The C. V. Mosby Company, 1960, pp. 29-48.

Balazs, E. A.: Molecular morphology of the vitreous body. *In* Smelser, G. K. (ed.): Structure of the Eye. New York, Academic Press, 1961, pp. 291-310.

Balazs, E. A., Toth, L. Z., Eckl, E. A., and Mitchell, A. P.: Studies on the structure of the vitreous body. XII. Cytological and histochemical studies on the cortical tissue layer. Exp. Eye Res. *3*:57, 1964.

Barkhoff, E. R.: The intraocular lymphatic channels. Experiments on the removal of ink particles from the vitreous. Graefes Arch. Ophthal. *167*:573, 1964.

Berman, E. R., and Michaelson, I. C.: The chemical composition of the vitreous body as related to age and myopia. Exp. Eye Res. *3*:9, 1964.

Blackstad, T. W., and Vegge, T.: On the ultrastructure of vitreous body filaments. Acta Ophthal. *40*:37, 1962.

Bloom, G. D., and Balazs, E. A.: An electron microscopic study of hyalocytes. Exp. Eye Res. *4*:249, 1965.

Brini, A., Porte, A., and Stoeckel, M. E.: Morphology and structure of the vitreous. Brini et al. (eds.): Biology and Surgery of the Vitreous Body. Paris, Masson et Cie, 1968.

Duke-Elder, S.: System of Ophthalmology. *In* The Physiology of the Eye and of Vision. Vol. IV. St. Louis, The C. V. Mosby Company, 1968, p. 201.

Fine, B. S., and Tousimis, A. J.: The structure of the vitreous body and the suspensory ligaments of the lens. Arch. Ophthal. *65*:95, 1961.

Friedenwald, J., and Stiehler, R. D.: Structure of the vitreous. Arch. Ophthal. *14*:789, 1935.

Goldmann, H.: Biomicroscopy of the vitreous body. Ophthalmologica *127*:334, 1954.

Grignolo, A.: Les connaissances actuelles sur la structure du corps vitre. Progr. Ophthal. *2*:1, 1953.

Gross, J., Matoltsy, A. G., and Cohen, C.: Vitrosin, a member of the collagen class. Biophys. Biochem. Cytol. *1*:215, 1955.

Hamburg, A.: Some investigations on the cells of the vitreous body. Ophthalmologica *138*:81, 1959.

Hertel, E.: Experimentelle Untersuchungen über den Einfluss der Magenresektion auf die Veruung im Dü nndarm. Arch. Klin. Chir. *156*:66, 1929.

Hogan, M. J.: The vitreous, its structure and relation to the ciliary body and retina. Invest. Ophthal. *2*:418, 1963.

Kinsey, V. E., Grant, M., and Cogan, D. G.: Water movement and eye. Arch. Ophthal. *27*:242, 1942.

Lukoff, L., and David, H.: On the problem of structural changes in lyophilized vitreous body. Graefes Arch. Ophthal. *163*:240, 1961.

Maurice, D. M.: The exchange of sodium between the vitreous body and the blood and aqueous humor. J. Physiol. *137*:110, 1957.

Pirie, A., Schmidt, G., and Waters, J. W.: Ox vitreous humor; residual protein. Brit. J. Ophthal. *32*:321, 1948.

Propst, A., and Leb, D.: Comparative electron microscopic studies of the vitreous body, zonule and collagen fibrils. Z. Zellforsch. *61*:829, 1963.

Richards, O. W., and Hague, E. B.: Vitreous as removed with large and small needles. Amer. J. Ophthal. *55*:151, 1963.

Rossi, A.: Structure of the vitreous body. Brit. J. Ophthal. *37*:343, 1953.

Schwarz, W.: Elektronenmikroskopische Untersuchungen an Glaskörperschnitten. Congr. federativ. internat. Anat., Paris, 1955, pp. 434-442.

Schwarz, W.: Electron microscopic studies of the vitreous body. Anat. Anz. *102*:434, 1956.

Schwarz, W.: Electron microscopic observations of the human vitreous body. *In* Smelser, G. K. (ed.): The Structure of the Eye. New York, Academic Press, 1961, pp. 283-291.

Stilling, J. V.: Eine Studie über den Bau des Glasköpers. Graefes Arch. Ophthal. *15*:299, 1869.

Stilling, J. V.: Bemerkung zu der Mitteilung von Dr. Wolfrum: Zur Frage nach der Existenz des Glasköperkanales. Graefes Arch. Ophthal. *69*:192, 1908.

Sugiura, S.: Physico-chemical studies of the vitreous. Jap. J. Ophthal. *1*:7, 1957.

Suran, A. A., and McEwen, W. K.: Diffusion studies with ox vitreous body. Amer. J. Ophthal. *51*:814, 1961.

Szirmai, J. A., and Balazs, E. A.: Studies on the structure of the vitreous body. Arch. Ophthal. *59*:34, 1958.

Vogt, A.: Ueber Berührungspunkte der senilen und der myopichen Bulbusdegeneration. Klin. Mbl. Augenheilk. *72*:212, 1924.

Yamashita, T., and Cibis, P. A.: Studies of the retina with saccharated iron oxide. A.M.A. Arch. Ophthal. *61*(5):698, 1959.

Young, R. G., and Williams, H. H.: Biochemistry of the eye; gelatinous protein of the vitreous body. Arch. Ophthal. *51*:593, 1954.

Chapter Twelve

LENS

The lens is biconvex and has an elliptical shape. Because of its transparency and ability to change its shape, it is an important part of the optical system of the eye. Visible light rays are transmitted through the clear lens toward the retina, and the course of the rays which have traversed the cornea can be altered by the ability of the lens to become more or less convex. The changes in lens shape are produced by the ciliary muscle, as well as by the inherent elasticity of the lens capsule and lens cells.

The refractive power of the lens is much less than that of the cornea, mainly because the change of refractive index is much greater at the air-cornea interface than at the aqueous-lens and lens-vitreous interfaces. The lens is decentered slightly downward and nasally with respect to the optical system of the eye, but this decentration is not sufficient to alter the visual function of the eye. Some of the aberrations created by simple anatomic variations in the structure and position of the lens are partially corrected by the size and position of the pupil.

The position of the lens in the optical system of the eye is assured by the attachment of the zonular fibers, as well as the support provided by the vitreous and iris. Its support is designed to facilitate the changes in the lens shape that are essential for accommodation.

PHYSIOLOGY AND BIOCHEMISTRY

The lens is a transparent living tissue. Following the regression of the hyaloid system of blood vessels during fetal life, it has no blood supply. After this time it receives its nourishment from the aqueous and vitreous humor. All the lens cells have definite metabolic needs in order to maintain their optical transparency.

TRANSPARENCY

The transparency of the lens is based mostly on the structure, shape and arrangement of its cells. The intercellular interdigitations at the edges and their method of termination at the lens sutures contribute to the transparency. The relatively small amount of interstitial fluid in the lens also contributes to its transparency because it produces such a small amount of change in the refractive index between cells. The proper balance of salt and water between the cytoplasm and the extracellular space between the lens cells is important to maintain the clarity of the lens. Conditions that interfere with removal of sodium or cause retention of potassium lead to cytoplasmic changes and thus to reduced transparency of the lens. The distribution of protein in the cytoplasm of all the lens cells is such that, even though it is present in high concentration, it is dispersed to produce a nonopalescent solution (Davson, 1963). The smooth surface and uniform thickness of the lens capsule in the pupillary region also contribute to the clarity of the lens. Other factors in lens transparency are the uniformity of the single layer of anterior lens epithelial cells and the absence of a similar layer under the posterior capsule.

Lens Capsule

The lens capsule is known to contain hydroxyproline, proline and other amino acids found in collagen; thus, it is most likely composed of a collagen framework. It is PAS-positive, and biochemical studies show that the capsule is 10 per cent carbohydrate. The interstices of the collagen framework, therefore, probably contain mucopolysaccharide. The capsule is relatively nonselective with regard to passage of many substances, especially water, electrolytes and some dyes. The lens capsule appears to be impermeable, however, to large molecules such as albumin and globulin.

Lens Epithelium

The lens epithelium exists only under the anterior and equatorial capsule. It plays an important part in the transport of cations into the lens, since the movement of cations can be influenced by varying the lens temperature and its supply of nutrients, and by the addition of inhibitors. The presence of this transport mechanism is substantiated by the existence of an electrical potential between the lens tissue and its surroundings. This potential changes with variations in temperature or with the use of metabolic inhibitors. Since cations are transported through the posterior capsule, it is probable that the posterior subcapsular lens cells which occupy the lens cortex also play a role in the movement of ions.

Metabolism

The lens cells require energy to support their nutrition and growth, especially those new cells which are forming and elongating from the equatorial region throughout life. If the cells receive proper nutrition they remain transparent and this facilitates the function of the lens. The elasticity of the cells and the lens capsule are maintained as long as they are properly nourished. Most of the oxygen consumed by the lens comes from the aqueous humor, and the amount utilized is very small. The aqueous humor contains between 0.08 and 0.12 volumes per cent of oxygen and has an oxygen tension under normal conditions of 40 to 50 mm. Hg (Friedenwald and Pierce, 1933). Almost all the oxygen is consumed by the anterior lens epithelium and the cortical cells. Animal studies have shown that the capsule and nucleus of the lens consume negligible amounts of oxygen.

Glycolysis

There is some uncertainty about the glucose content of the lens, but observers agree that it is lower than in the aqueous or vitreous humor. It is probable that at least half of the glucose used by the lens readily passes into it by diffusion. The remaining glucose enters by a process which has been called "assisted transport" (Harris et al., 1955). The metabolism of glucose provides the main source of energy for the lens, and the anaerobic pathways appear to be the most important, since the aqueous humor has an oxygen tension of only about 45 mm. Hg. Nevertheless, the lens has been shown to have a small but definite uptake of oxygen, so that some glucose is metabolized by aerobic pathways.

Most of the glucose is broken down anaerobically (glycolysis). The mechanism for the breakdown is via the Embden-Meyerhof pathway. The citric acid cycle also is used to reduce lactic acid to carbon dioxide and water (Kinoshita, 1955). The hexosemonophosphate shunt also is utilized to carry out direct oxidation of the six-carbon glucose structure. Sorbital and fructose, as well as the enzymes for conversion of glucose to fructose by way of sorbitol, have been identified in the lens. Cytochrome C, cytochrome oxidase and flavoprotein are found in low concentration in the lens epithelium and are responsible for utilization of oxygen in the lens. Carbonic anhydrase is present in greater concentration in the lens than in any other ocular tissue; the reason for this is unknown. The lens contains more glutathione than any other tissue, and its concentration here is 1000 times that in the aqueous humor. The glutathione appears to be forming constantly in the lens and is involved in oxidative mechanisms that are not well understood. Ascorbic acid plays a part in this function, for glutathione can be oxidized in lens extracts in the presence of ascorbic acid.

Chemistry

Amino acids enter the lens from the aqueous humor by active transport on the part of the anterior lens epithelium. Most amino acids are found in the lens. We have seen that there is active transport of ions into and out of the lens, establishing a potential between the aqueous and vitreous humor and the lens, and that this transport mechanism is affected by temperature and metabolic changes. The lens cells are capable of maintaining the transmembrane potential characteristic of living cells (Sperekalis and Potts, 1959).

The *water content* of the lens is about 65 per cent of the total weight of the lens, and about 20 per cent of this is in the bound form. The water content is higher in the younger cells of the cortex and its total content increases with the size of the lens, but the total amount of water decreases relatively with age.

Lens proteins account for 35 per cent of the lens mass; this amount is higher in percentage than in any other body tissue. Two forms have been described, soluble and insoluble (albuminoid). The soluble portion is composed of three forms; alpha-, beta- and gamma-crystallin. The following table from Krause (1934) gives the amounts of insoluble and soluble protein in the bovine lens:

	Per cent
insoluble	12.50
alpha-crystallin	31.70
beta-crystallin	53.40
gamma-crystallin	1.50
mucoprotein	0.80
nucleoprotein	0.07

The proportion of soluble and insoluble proteins varies with each species, and with age and size of the lens. More of the insoluble protein is found in the nucleus. Alpha-crystallin has a molecular weight of about 800,000; beta-crystallin has a probable molecular weight of around 28,000 and is much richer in cysteine and S-H groups than alpha-crystallin. Gamma-crystallin has a molecular weight of 14,000 to 25,000 and also contains more S-H groups than alpha-crystallin.

The insoluble protein is called albuminoid; its molecular weight has been estimated at 367,000. It has a close reciprocal relation to alpha-crystallin, and investigators agree that the insoluble albuminoid is formed from alpha-crystallin, because the insoluble albuminoid increases in cataractous lenses, while alpha-crystallin diminishes in amount. The mucoproteins are found principally in the lens capsule, while the nucleoproteins occur in the anterior epithelium and equatorial lens cells.

The lipid of the lens is probably derived from the cell membranes and is about 80 per cent phospholipid and cholesterol.

Accommodation

The young lens contains soft cells and it is easily molded by the very elastic capsule. The capsule tends to make the lens spherical, and this tendency is opposed by tension on the zonular fibers created by the ciliary muscle and choroid. Zonular traction flattens the lens. The index of refraction of the lens, at 1.390, is greater than the indices of the aqueous and vitreous humors, at 1.334. For this reason the more convex the lens surface becomes, the greater is the refractive power of the lens.

During accommodation the thicker ring of the anterior capsule circumscribing the central zone becomes more convex forward. This causes the thinner anterior polar lens in the pupillary region to bulge forward more markedly, advancing as much as 0.4 mm., thus increasing the refractive power of the lens. The posterior pole does not move during this phase. It is possible that the many microtubules in the cytoplasm of the lens cells may play a role in contractility of these cells in the act of accommodation.

The radius of curvature of the anterior and posterior lens surfaces decreases from 10.0 and 6.0 to 5.33 mm., respectively, during accommodation (Gullstrand, 1911).

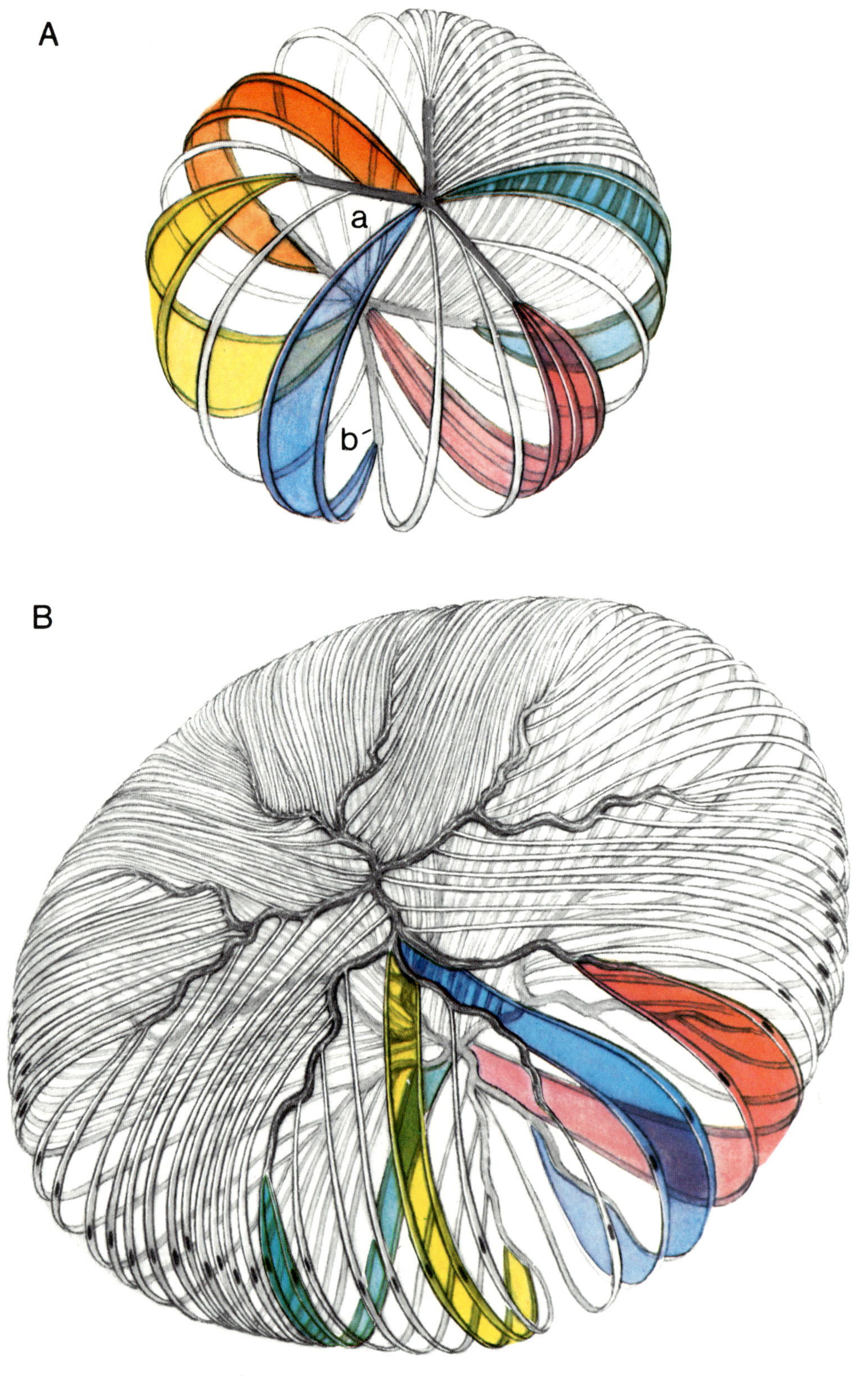

Figure 12–1. *See legend on opposite page.*

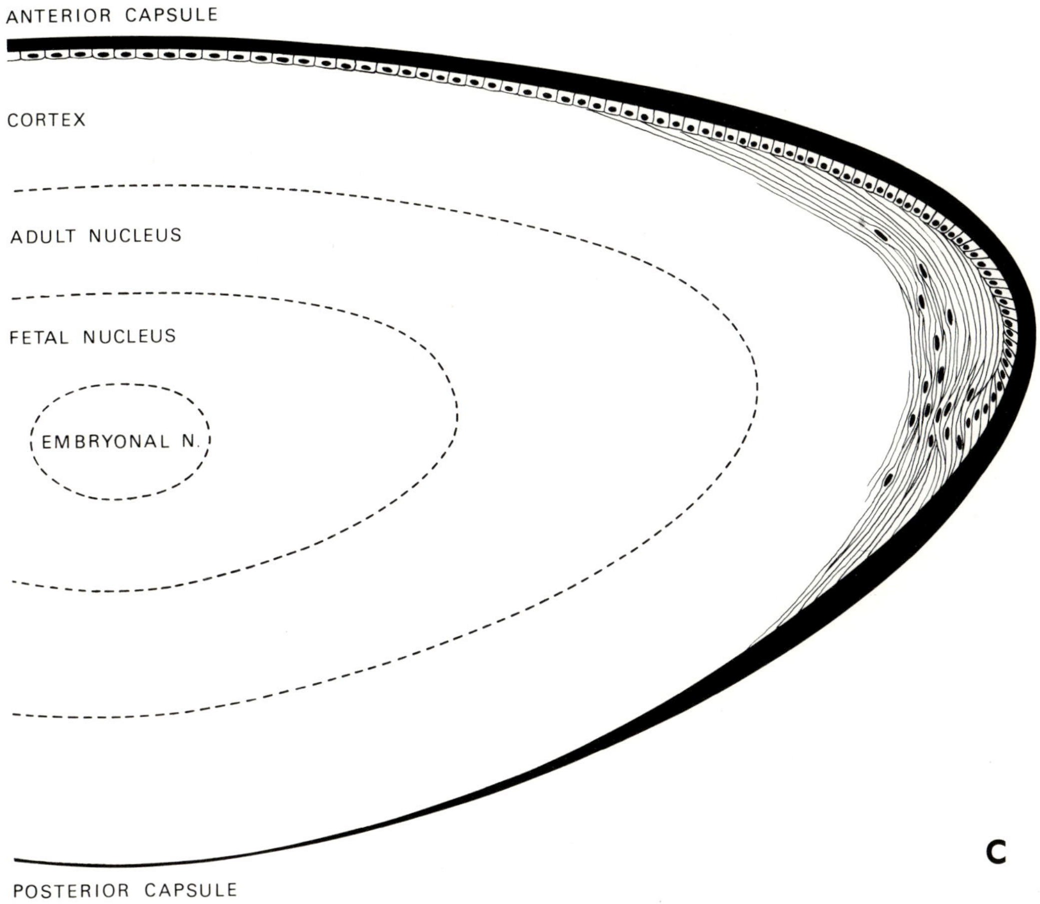

Figure 12–1. Embryonal and adult lens to show the sutures and arrangement of the lens cells. *A,* Drawing of the embryonal nucleus. The anterior Y suture is at (a) and the posterior at (b). The lens cells are depicted as wide, colored bands. Those cells that attach to the tips of the Y sutures at one pole of the lens attach to the fork of the Y at the opposite pole. It can be seen if the lens cell attaches to the tip of a Y suture anteriorly or its distance from the equator is shorter at that pole of the lens.

B, Adult lens cortex. The anterior and posterior organization of the sutures is more complex. Those lens cells that arise from the tip of a branch of the suture insert farther anteriorly or posteriorly into a fork at the posterior pole. This arrangement conserves the shape of the lens. This drawing shows the suture to lie in a single plane for pictorial reasons, but it should be remembered that it extends throughout the thickness of the cortex and nucleus to the level of the Y sutures in the embryonal nucleus.

C, Schematic representation of the adult lens, showing the nuclear zones, epithelium and capsule. The thickness of the lens capsule in various zones is shown.

EMBRYOLOGY

The surface ectoderm covering the optic vesicle differentiates at about the 4 mm. stage in human embryos to form a slight thickening known as the lens plate or placode. The thickening is created by an elongation of the ectodermal cells, as well as by cell division. This thickening is believed to occur as a result of the action of inducer substances produced by the adjacent neuroectoderm. The surface ectodermal cells of the lens plate are separated from those of the optic vesicle by a space which is bordered by the basement membranes of these two cellular layers. In the space between these two basement membranes the future primary vitreous develops. As a result of cellular growth and enlargement, the lens plate soon develops a small central depression, the lens pit. At about the 5 mm. stage the lens pit deepens progressively because of the cell growth along its wall, and at the same time the optic vesicle also invaginates to form the optic cup, permitting the developing lens to occupy part of its cavity.

The primary vitreous forms in the cavity of the optic cup, between the lens and inner layer, a result of the invagination of the cup. The cavity of the lens pit widens to form the lens vesicle, the wall of which is composed of a layer of surface ectodermal cells. The vesicle is connected to the surface by the lens stalk, which disappears at the 9 mm. stage, leaving the lens vesicle within the eye. The surface layer of ectodermal cells of the lens differentiates to form a superficial layer of epitrichial cells that are cast off into the cavity of the vesicle. The cells of the vesicle beneath the epitrichial layer are cuboidal in shape. These cuboidal cells of the lens vesicle form the definitive cells of the lens. During formation of the vesicle, the cells become inverted from their position in the surface ectoderm so that their apical surfaces face the cavity and their basal surfaces face outward against the lens capsule. The capsule is a continuous accruing basement membrane which is formed by the lens epithelial cells. The cells of the anterior portion of this vesicle, facing the surface ectoderm, remain undifferentiated throughout life, except near the lens equator, where they divide to form new lens cells. The lens epithelial cells facing the optic cup elongate to form the primary lens cells. These cells continue to elongate until they completely fill the cavity of the vesicle by the 16 mm. stage. The lens is almost spherical at this time, and remains so until about the 30 mm. stage. The lens itself, however, increases slowly in size.

After this period the cells at the equator begin their lifelong job of forming secondary lens cells. Multiplication of cells occurs around the equator, and as this occurs, the most recently formed ones become elongated. As they do so, the anterior part of the cell extends forward beneath the lens capsule and the posterior part extends backward. Each cell becomes U-shaped, with its nucleus near the equator. The anterior and posterior extensions of these cells unite with each other at suture lines, which in the fetus have the form of a Y, the anterior Y being erect, and the posterior one being inverted (Fig. 12-1 A). Succeeding generations of cells also extend anteriorly and posteriorly beneath the capsule to join fellow cells formed at about the same time from all around the equator. All newly formed cells are slightly longer than the preceding ones, accounting for the increase in the size of the lens up to adult life. At birth the anterior and posterior Y sutures lie beneath the capsule, so that the surfaces of the fetal nucleus at this time lie at the level of the capsule, a good landmark in later life for slit-lamp determination of the time of origin of developmental lens opacities.

The lens capsule has its earliest origin as a basement membrane under the surface ectoderm, prior to formation of the lens plate. It becomes thicker as the lens plate develops and comes into contact with the basement membrane of the cells of the adjacent optic vesicle. As the lens vesicle forms, the cellular basement membrane is adjacent to the outer cell membranes of all the epithelial cells. This thin basement membrane thickens as the lens develops by a continuous deposition of material from the adjacent epithelial cells until the definitive lens is formed. In ordinary light microscopic sections the lens capsule can be seen easily at the 13-mm. stage, but electron microscopic studies show it to be present much before this time.

The zonular fibers and their related membranes and vitreous substance form after the third month, when the layers of the optic cup begin to grow forward to form the definitive ciliary body and iris. Vitreous is present in the equatorial circumlental region at the time of beginning zonule formation. The zonular fibrils develop within the perilenticular vitreous, extending from the inner surface of the ciliary body to the lens capsule. These fibers are seen first at about the 65 mm. stage and they are well formed by the 110 mm. stage.

GROSS ANATOMY

The lens has an elliptical shape (Fig. 12-2) and it occupies the space between the iris and the vitreous in the anterior eye. It is held in a fairly fixed position by the zonular fibers that run from the lens to the ciliary body and by its close apposition to the vitreous humor on its posterior and equatorial sides.

In the young eye the lens is white, slightly opalescent and transmits light. It often develops a slightly yellow color in later life, and the nucleus may become quite brown in some eyes when it becomes sclerotic. This condition is called a brunescent lens; the brown color results from the presence of urochrome pigment (McEwen, 1959).

By direct measurement the anteroposterior diameter is about 3.5 to 4.0 mm. in newborn infants. This diameter remains at approximately 4.0 mm. up to 50 years of age, after which it increases to 4.75 to 5.0 mm. by the age of 90 years. Measurements made with optical devices in vivo are smaller; optical measurements show the anteroposterior diameter to average 3.5 mm. in the adult. The equatorial diameter of the lens in newborn infants averages about 6.5 mm. This dimension increases to about 9.0 mm. by age 15 and remains at this level throughout life.

There is considerable variation in the radius of curvature of the anterior and posterior surfaces, depending on the age of the lens and the method of measurement. Findings obtained by optical measurements probably are more accurate. Based on measurements by different authors, the average radius of curvature of the anterior surface is around 10.0 mm., varying between 8.0 and 14.0 mm. The radius of curvature of the posterior lens surface averages 6.0 mm., varying between 4.5 and 7.5 mm.

The weight of the lens increases from 65 mg. at birth to 130 mg. at one year of age. Thereafter the lens increases in weight very slowly to age 90,

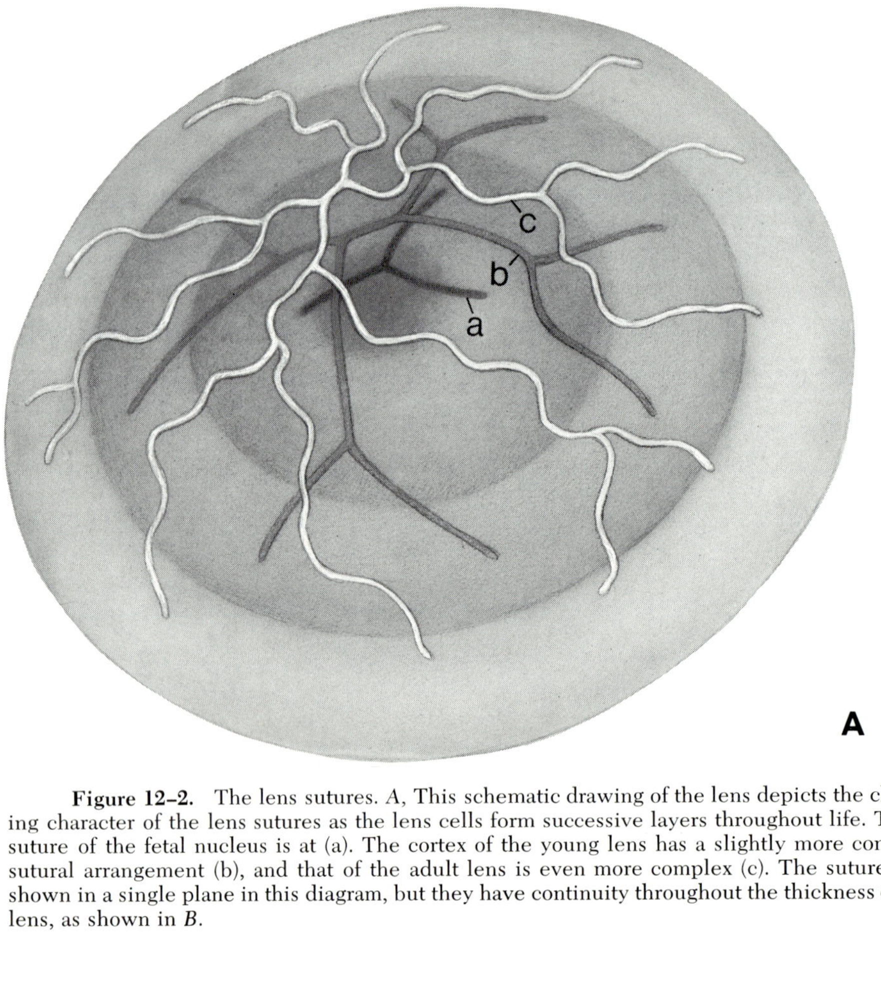

Figure 12–2. The lens sutures. *A*, This schematic drawing of the lens depicts the changing character of the lens sutures as the lens cells form successive layers throughout life. The Y suture of the fetal nucleus is at (a). The cortex of the young lens has a slightly more complex sutural arrangement (b), and that of the adult lens is even more complex (c). The sutures are shown in a single plane in this diagram, but they have continuity throughout the thickness of the lens, as shown in *B*.

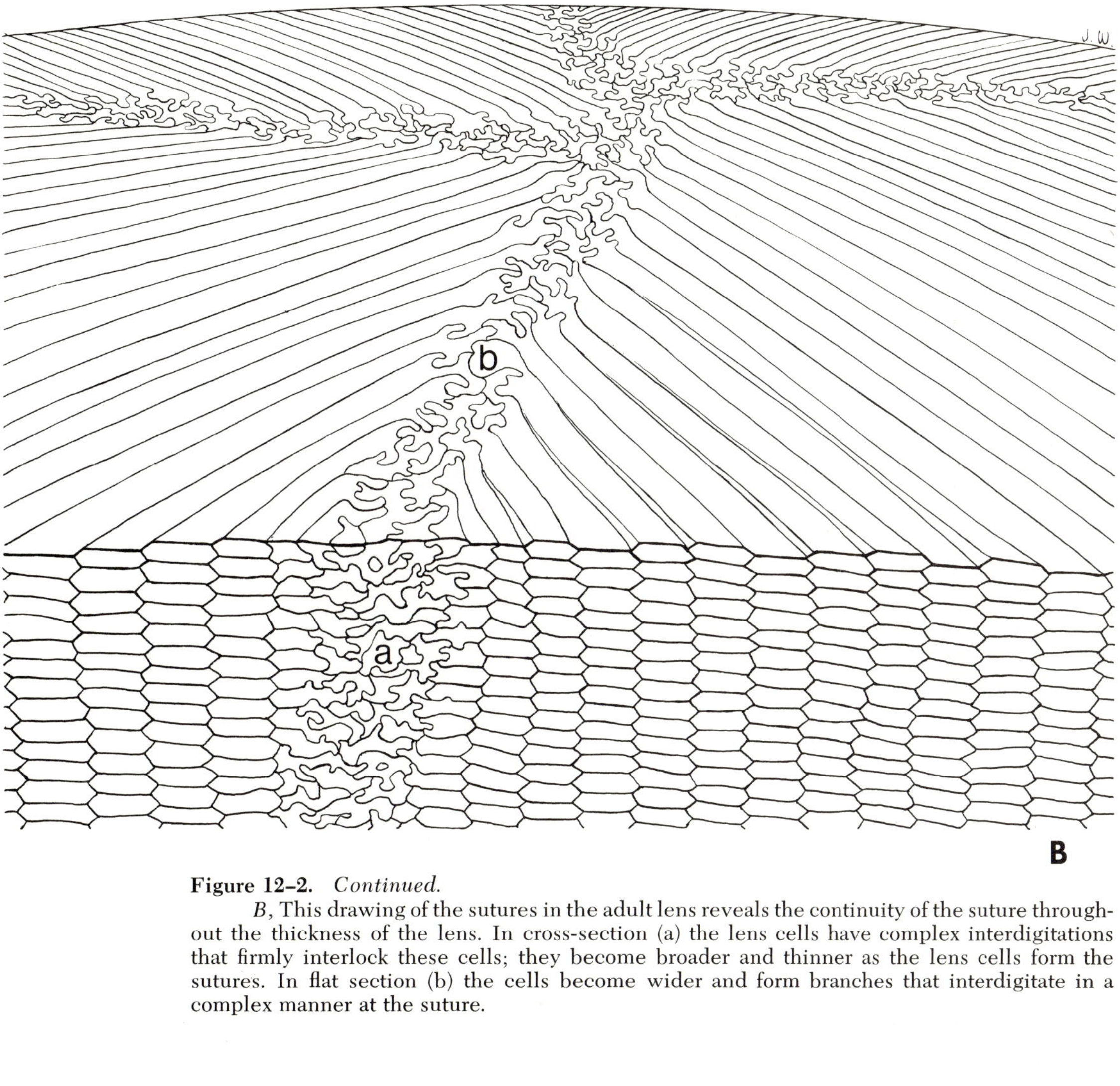

B

Figure 12–2. *Continued.*

B, This drawing of the sutures in the adult lens reveals the continuity of the suture throughout the thickness of the lens. In cross-section (a) the lens cells have complex interdigitations that firmly interlock these cells; they become broader and thinner as the lens cells form the sutures. In flat section (b) the cells become wider and form branches that interdigitate in a complex manner at the suture.

when it weighs about 250 mg. (Smith, 1883; Heine, 1898; Scammon and Hesdorffer, 1937). According to Heine (1898), the volume of the lens measures about 0.163 ml. in persons 20 to 40 years of age and increases to 0.244 ml. between 80 and 90 years of age.

Anteriorly the lens is in contact with the pupillary portion of the iris. The size of the area of contact between these two tissues varies with the depth of the anterior chamber, the diameter of the chamber and the size of the lens. The contact most often is loose, but in some eyes with a narrow anterior chamber angle and shallow chamber, the contact may be broader and closer, causing interference with passage of aqueous humor from posterior to anterior chamber. *Posteriorly* the lens fits into a hollow depression of the anterior vitreous surface, the patellar fossa, and is in contact with the vitreous humor (Fig. 11-1).

The vitreous is slightly thickened and makes close contact with the lens capsule at the junction of the central portion of the peripheral third of the posterior lens capsule in the eyes of young persons. This circular area of thickening is called the ligamentum hyaloideocapsulare, but it is merely a condensation of the anterior vitreous where it makes contact with the lens and is not a true ligament. Examination with the slit lamp reveals that the vitreous is not in close contact with the posterior lens capsule inside the area encompassed by the circular ligamentum hyaloideocapsulare; the two structures are separated from each other by a narrow space known as Berger's space. *Laterally* the lens is related to the pars plicata of the ciliary body and the zonular system, particularly at the lens equator. The anterior peripheral area of the lens is bathed in the aqueous humor of the posterior chamber. The forward convexity of the anterior lens surface is slightly flattened, compared to the more curved posterior lens surface. At the center of the anterior and posterior surfaces are the anterior and posterior poles. The axis of the lens is formed by a line joining these two poles. This axis is tilted somewhat with respect to the optic axis of the eyeball because the temporal and superior edges of the lens lie slightly posterior to the nasal and inferior edges. The anterior and posterior surfaces of the lens meet laterally to form a rounded border, the equator of the lens. The zonules attach to the lens capsule around the equator in a rather broad zone measuring 2.5 mm. in width. The entire outer surface of the lens capsule is smooth, except at the equator in the area where the zonules are attached. The zonular attachments in this region produce fine capsular irregularities through the tension they exert on the lens surface.

The capsule and outer cortical cells of the lens are soft and somewhat extensible. These features become apparent at cataract surgery when the capsule is grasped by a forceps. The lens cells in the eyes of infants and children are all soft, but the nuclear portion of the lens becomes firmer with increasing age.

The lens increases in size throughout life because new cells are constantly added to the cortex from the epithelium around the lens equator. The cell bodies lie at the equator and the anterior and posterior terminations of these cells form the lens sutures. The sutures that form in the cortex surrounding the fetal sutures are rather simple, having a stellate appearance. As more and more cells develop throughout life and extend toward the sutures, the complexity of the stellate pattern increases. Figure 12-3 *A* demonstrates the changing complexity of the sutural arrangement.

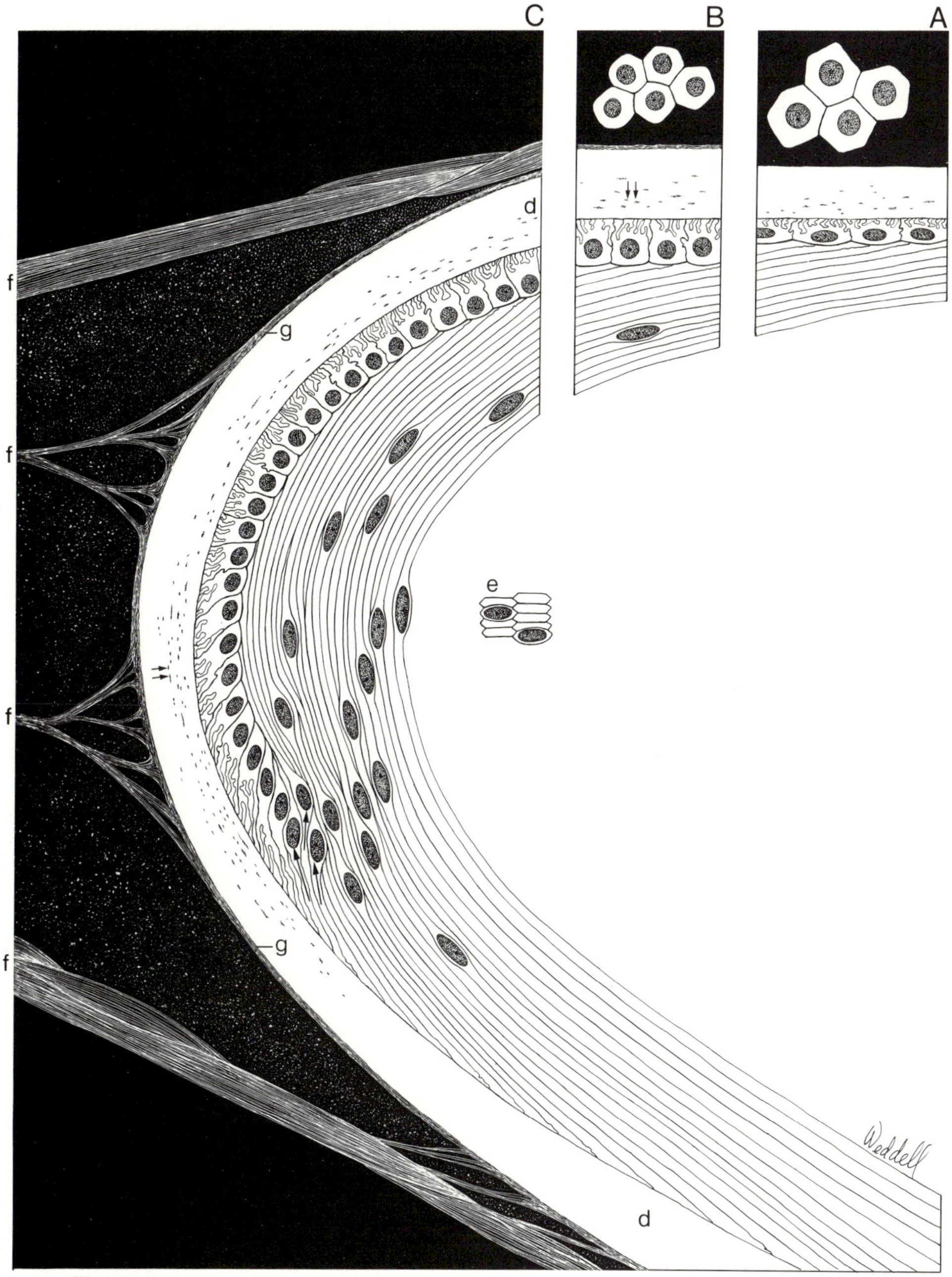

Figure 12–3. A composite drawing of the lens, cortex, epithelium, capsule and zonular attachments. At (A) is the anterior central lens epithelium, seen in flat and cross-section. The size and shape of these cells can be compared with those of the cells in (B), the intermediate zone, and (C) the equatorial zone. At the equator the dividing cells are elongating (arrows) to form lens cortical cells. As they elongate they send processes anteriorly and posteriorly toward the sutures, and their nuclei migrate somewhat anterior to the equator to form the lens bow. At the same time the nuclei become more and more displaced into the lens as new cells are formed at the equator. The lens capsule (d) is thicker anterior and posterior to the equator than it is at the equator itself. The anterior and equatorial capsule contains fine filamentous inclusions (double arrows); these are not present posteriorly. Zonular fibers (f) attach to the anterior and posterior capsule and to the equatorial capsule, forming the pericapsular or zonular lamella of the lens (g).

Slit-lamp examination shows no sharp boundaries between the various parts of the lens that are formed by the developing cells during life. A distinction may be made between the fetal nucleus and the cortex of the lens, and the Y sutures can always be distinguished during life. The nucleus is centrally located, denser and biconvex. The cortex encompasses the nucleus, behaving optically as if it forms two concavoconvex menisci which have lesser indices of refraction than the nucleus. Through its converging effect on light, the more dense nucleus, however, neutralizes the diverging effect of the menisci on light. Figure 12-1 shows the various zones of the lens.

ZONULES (Fig. 12-4)

The zonule, or ligament of Zinn, is the suspensory ligament of the lens. It is a gel-like structure with many of the properties of the vitreous, containing a system of fibers which become more defined at the posterior ciliary body, between the ciliary processes and at their lens attachment. These fibers and their enclosing gel converge on the equatorial portion of the lens. Basically the fiber system and its enclosing gel are organized so that they form anterior and posterior sheets, the former terminating 2.5 mm. anterior to the equator in a circular zone around the equator, and the latter terminating 1 mm. posterior to the equator in a similar zone.

It is difficult to study the suspensory ligament to determine its relation to adjacent structures. Recent studies with the ultramicroscope and electron microscope, and examination of fresh specimens with the dissecting microscope, have confirmed the opinion of early anatomists that the zonules have a structure similar to the vitreous, except for the more definite organization of the fibrils in the region of the suspensory ligament. The slit-lamp microscopic study of eyes with colobomas and aniridia has shown the zonular fibers and their relation to the ciliary processes and lens.

Most studies of fresh eyes show the gel-fiber system of the suspensory ligament crossing the space between the lens and the ciliary processes, where it is lost in the valleys between the processes without joining the tips of the processes (McCulloch, 1954). The anterior surface of the suspensory ligament is smooth and glistening, and the posterior surface is curved as it extends from the lens through the valleys of the ciliary processes toward the pars plana. The zonules are separated from the anterior vitreous surface by a potential space, the canal of Petit. The zonular fibers form superimposed layers of fibrils, aligned in columns on either side of the ciliary processes.

Figure 12–4. Light micrographs of the zonules, capsule, epithelium and cortex. *A*, The zonular fibers (a) stand out against a dark background; their varying thickness is apparent. Those zonules near the lens capsule (b) lie parallel to its surface and send small extensions into the zonular lamella (c). The capsule here measures about 13 to 14 μm. in diameter. The lens cells (d) lie just posterior to the equator. Their shape is hexagonal, and the short edges of the hexagons (e) show interdigitations. (× 1040.)

B, Equatorial region of the lens. Zonules of varying thickness (a) approach the zonular lamella (b). The lens capsule (c) is mottled by linear densities (arrows) formed by clumps of fibrils. The capsule is 14.5 to 20 μm. in thickness, and the epithelium is 14.5 to 15.5 μm. thick. The intermediate layer of epithelium is at (d) and the dividing and elongating equatorial cells are at (e). (× 1500.)

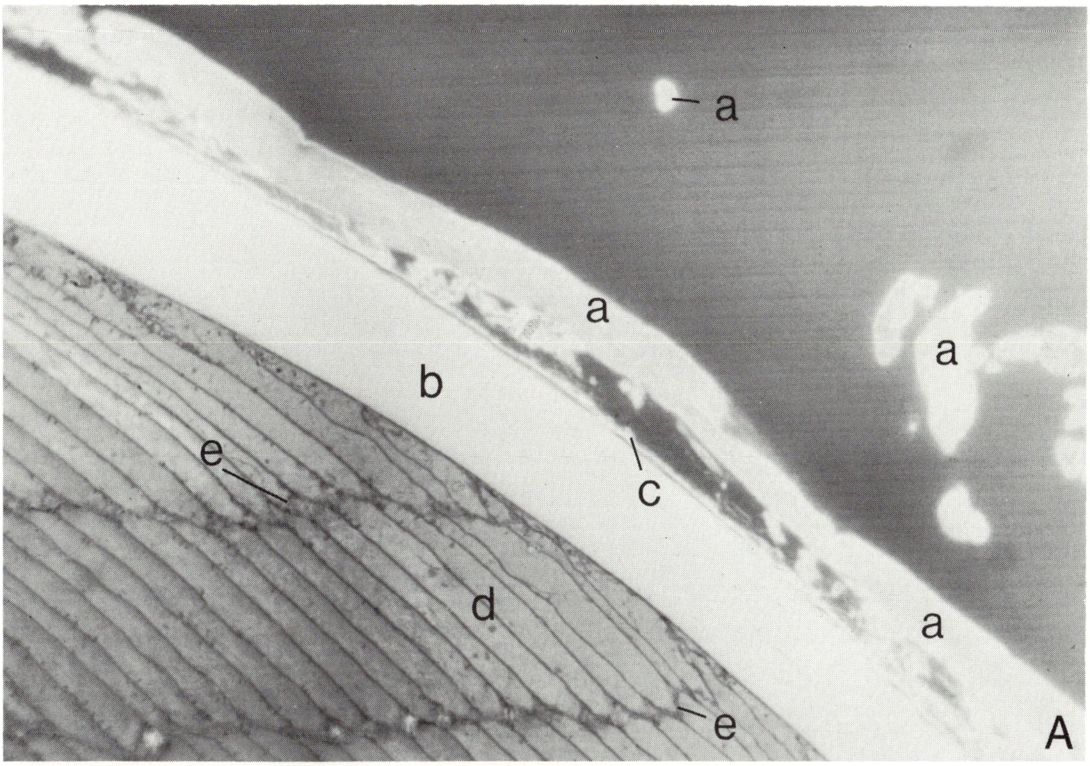

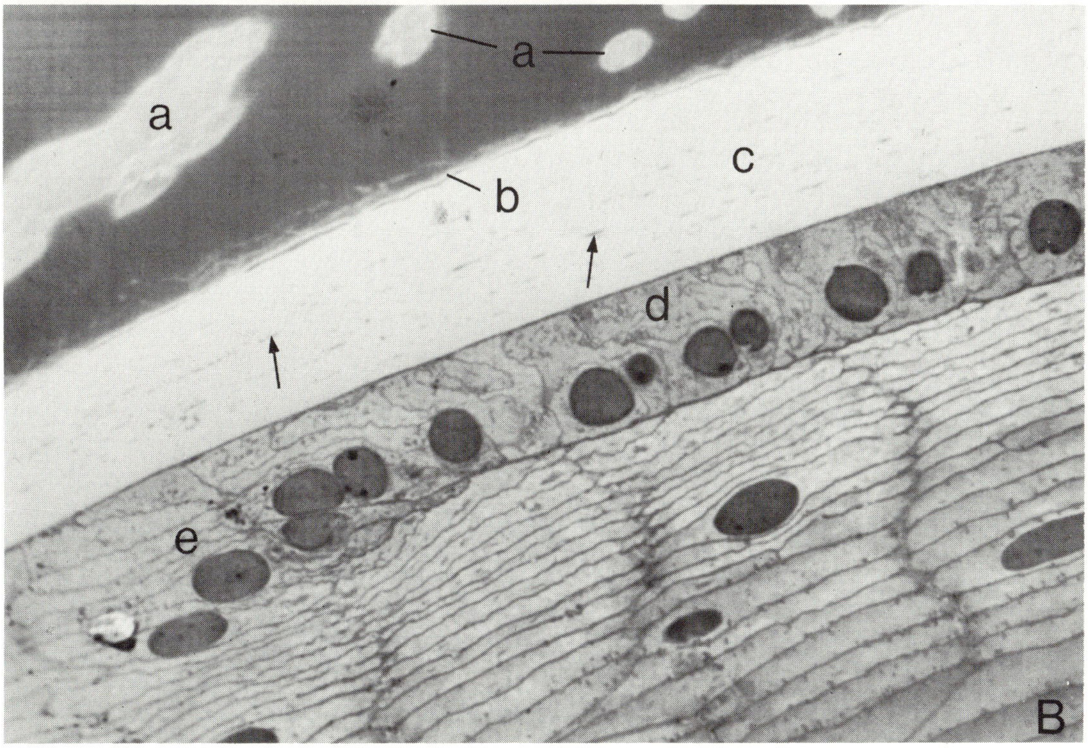

Figure 12–4. *See legend on opposite page.*

These layers extend across the circumlental space to become attached to the equatorial lens capsule in similar order, the rows being separated by a space the width of each ciliary process (see Fig. 7–6). The tips of the ciliary processes are completely free between the rows of fibers. It is not possible to determine with the dissecting microscope where these fibers attach to the ciliary body, but they appear to attach to the deep epithelium in the valleys between the processes. Many of the zonules interconnect with the zonular fiber system that arises in the region of the pars plana of the ciliary body.

The posterior zonular fiber system originates from the pars plana, in a zone about 1.5 mm. anterior to the ora serrata, and from the region of the spikes leading forward from the ora (see Fig. 7–6A). Some fibers appear to arise from the anterior retina and from the base of the vitreous. From the pars plana origin the zonules extend forward along the inner surface of the ciliary body and into the valleys between the ciliary processes. It is probable that in the valleys between the ciliary processes the zonular structure becomes reorganized; many of the fibrils from the posterior region cross those arising from the epithelium in the valleys to attach to the anterior equatorial portion of the lens. McCulloch (1954) observed crossing in microscopic sections, but not in gross sections. This discrepancy was explained in two ways: first, the columns which extend from the lens into the valleys are lost from view and cannot be traced further; second, it is not possible to trace any single fiber from lens to ciliary body because the fibers form sheets in the gel and lose their individual identity. It is probably futile to attempt to subdivide the zonular system into tracts having a specific origin and insertion. There is so much intermingling and branching within the gel that precise anatomic classification of the zonular systems is not possible.

As the anterior and posterior rows of zonular fibers approach the lens, the fibers split into the finer ones which then attach to the lens in equatorially oriented rows around the circumference of the lens. In the zone of attachment the equatorial lens capsule is crenated. The crenations disappear beyond the anterior and posterior attachments of the zonules to the lens.

MICROSCOPIC ANATOMY

The structure of the lens components will be discussed as follows:

1. Capsule
2. Epithelium
3. Lens cells
4. Lens zonules

Lens Capsule (Figs. 12–3 to 12–8)

The lens capsule is a transparent elastic and unusually thick basement membrane that encloses the epithelium and lens cells. The capsule has an affinity for basic stains, is PAS-positive and stains metachromatically in its superficial portion at the equator (Wislocki, 1952). In this same area the zonules fan out to blend with the capsule. The thickness of the lens capsule varies according to the age of the eye and the site of the capsule where measurements are taken (Fig. 12-2). It is thinnest at the equator and poles, and the anterior capsule is thickest in a circular area 3 mm. from the anterior pole; the posterior capsule is thickest in an area 1 mm. from the posterior pole. The following measurements of the capsule have been recorded (Salzmann, 1912):

AGE	ANT. POLE	ANT. MAX.	EQUATOR	POST. MAX.	POST. POLE
2.5 yrs.	8 μm.	12–15 μm.	7 μm.	18–22 μm.	2 μm.
35 yrs.	14 μm.	21 μm.	17 μm.	23 μm.	4 μm.
71 yrs.	14 μm.	21 μm.	9 μm.	9 μm.	2.3 μm.

The elasticity of the capsule must result from the organization of its fibrillar components, since it does not contain elastic tissue. The soft cortical cells beneath the capsule have such complex interlockings that they probably react like a spring, with the zonular tension on the capsule when released during accommodation.

Viewed at low magnification the capsule is smooth, homogeneous and dense (Fig. 12-5); with the polarizing microscope it is birefringent, indicating a lamellar structure with the fibers arranged parallel to the surface but without orientation (Grignolo, 1954). When the capsule is studied with the light microscope in a plastic-embedded section 1 μm. thick, discontinuous linear densities are clearly visible on the anterior capsule. Pores or channels penetrating the capsule from aqueous humor to the lens substance cannot be demonstrated in such sections.

A zonular lamella or pericapsular membrane has been described by many observers as a very thin membrane surrounding the capsule and possessing different tinctorial qualities (Berger, 1882; Retzius, 1895; Beauvieux, 1922; McCulloch, 1954). Careful study of thin sections with special stains fails to show this lamella, except in a narrow zone surrounding the equator where the zonules attach by flat extension to the outer capsule.

Routine histologic studies of the lens have always been unsatisfactory in the past because of the difficulty of fixing the entire lens without artifacts. Electron microscopic studies of the lens also have been disappointing, again as a result of problems with fixation.

With the electron microscope the lens capsule is found to be made up of many lamellae, each of which is composed of very fine filaments (Grignolo, 1954; Bahr, 1954; Bairati and Grignolo, 1954; Lindner and Boke, 1954). The lens capsule of a newborn mouse has been found to contain 30 to 40 lamellae, each measuring about 300 to 400 A. in thickness. The lens capsule in man has the same thickness and structure (Rohen, 1965). Cohen (1958) found lamellation in the capsule of the neonatal albino mouse, but only in sections made perpendicular to the lamellar planes. In a later discussion of the structure of human lens capsule, Cohen (1965) described rare patches of other fibers in the lens capsule, some of which showed a periodicity of 500 to 600 A.

With the electron microscope at low power the capsule appears fairly homogeneous (Fig. 12-9), except for its content of linear densities scattered throughout the anterior and equatorial portions. These densities are composed of fine fibers which have a periodicity of about 600 A. when aligned in parallel bundles (Fig. 12-10 A). In cross-section their diameter is the same as that of the zonular fibrils (150 A.). These linear densities do not appear to be

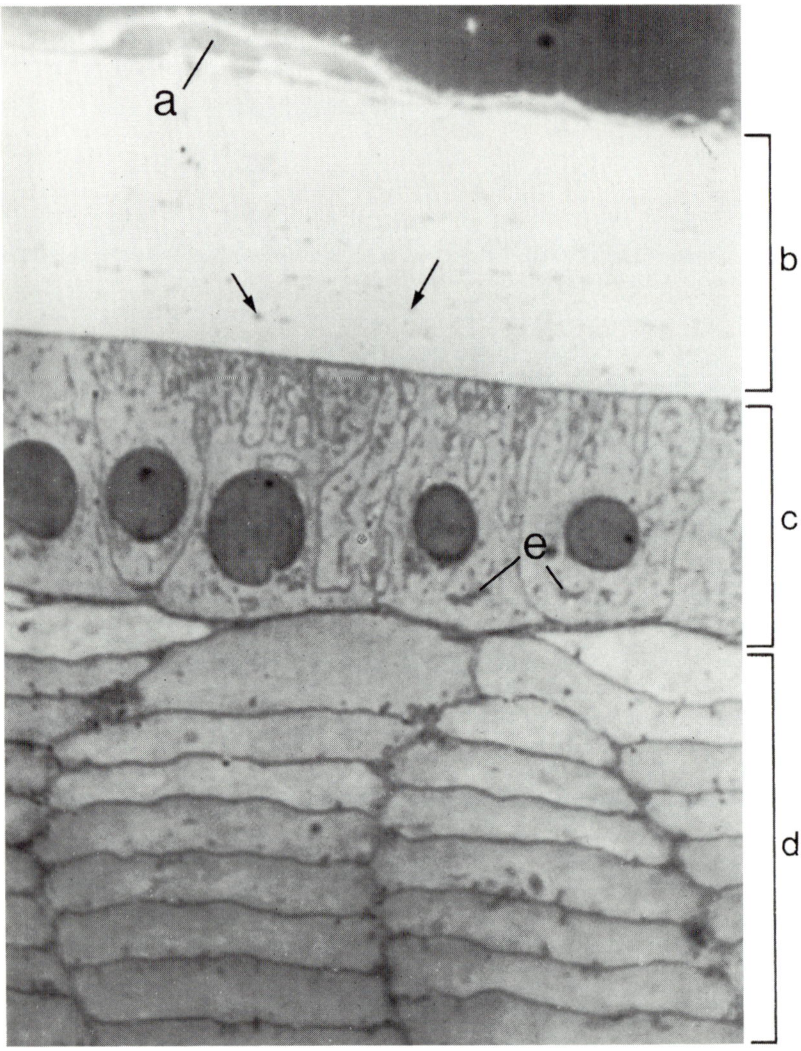

Figure 12–5. Light micrograph of the zonular fibers (a), capsule (b), lens epithelium (c) and cortex (d) approximately 0.7 mm. anterior to the equator of the lens. The zonules insert into the most superficial portion of the capsule. The capsule contains scattered linear densities (arrows) because of the presence of coarse fibrils. The epithelial cells are tall and columnar; their base faces the capsule and their apex faces the lens cortex. The round nuclei are either central in the cytoplasm or displaced slightly toward the apex. Elaborate basal infoldings of the cell membranes are apparent. The Golgi zone appears as a dense accumulation in the apical cytoplasm (e). The rectangular or hexagonal cells of the lens cortex are seen in cross-section. They have a fairly homogeneous cytoplasm. Interlocking processes occur along both the short and the long sides of the hexagon in the superficial layers of the cortical cells. In the deeper cortical cells the interlocking processes are found chiefly along the long sides of the hexagons. (× 1300.)

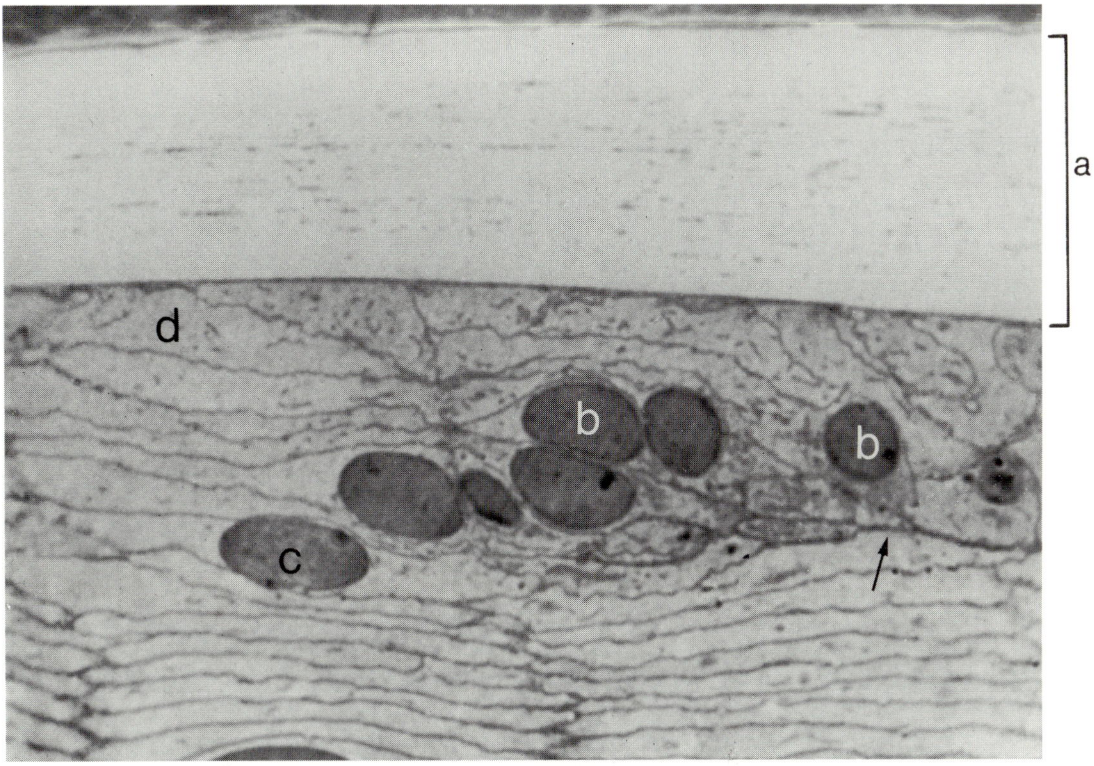

Figure 12–6. Light micrograph of the equatorial lens to show the capsule (a), the cells of the transitional zone (b) and the beginning elongation of the equatorial lens cells (c). The basal processes (d) of the epithelial cells enlarge and move backward along the capsule toward the posterior suture, displacing the older cells inward. The apical processes of the cells insinuate themselves under the anterior lens epithelium (arrow) and grow toward the anterior suture. (× 1500.)

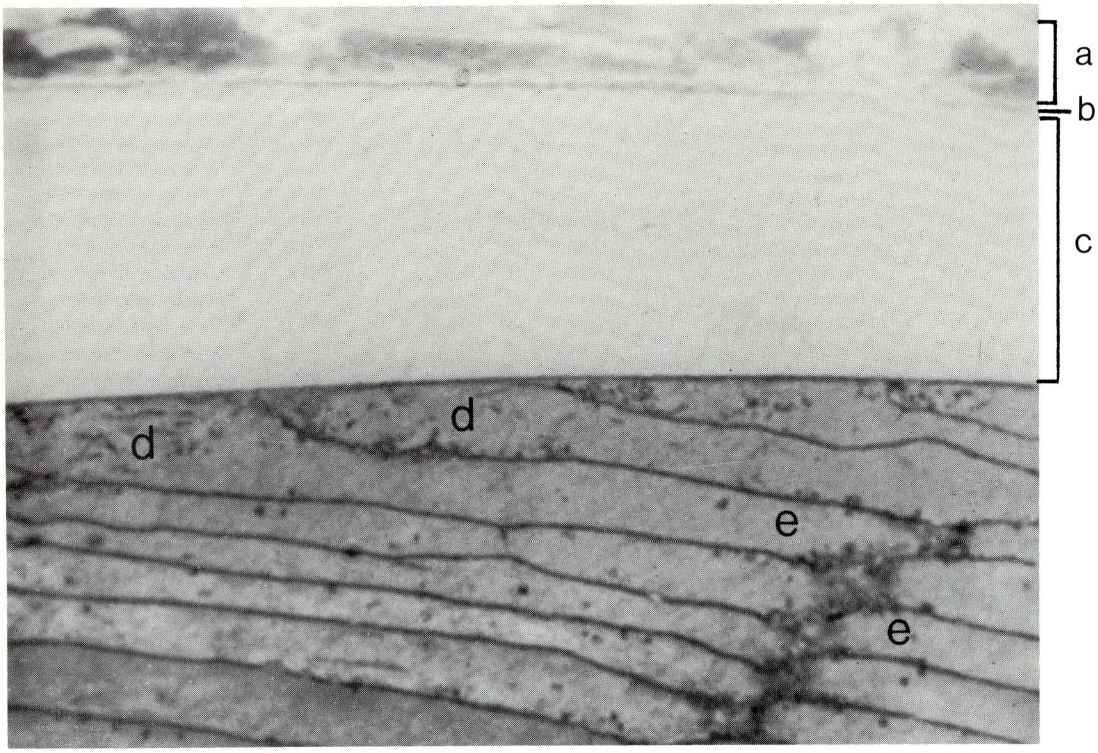

Figure 12–7. Light micrograph of the posterior lens to show the capsule and adjacent surface structures. The zonules (a) are inserting onto the capsule to form the zonular lamella (b), a thin layer on and within the surface layers of the capsule. The posterior capsule (c) does not have the linear densities present in the equatorial and anterior lens capsule. The expanded basal processes of the youngest lens cells (d) are against the inner surface of the capsule. Intercellular interdigitating processes are seen at (e). (× 1680.)

deep insertions of zonular fibrils, but may be a similar form of collagenous protein. Such fibrous accumulations are absent in the posterior capsule, which suggests that they result from some activity of the epithelial cells.

The homogeneous portions of the capsule, viewed at higher power, can be resolved into a fine flocculent material interspersed with linearly arranged oval spaces (Fig. 12-10). Whether these areas reflect the true macromolecular structure of the capsule or are artifacts of fixation is unknown. The superficial quarter of the capsule has a less compact arrangement and appears finely fibrillar. Zonular fibers from the zonular bundles disappear into this loose portion of the equatorial capsule. This zone is equivalent to the pericapsular lamella, which has been described with the light microscope. The blending of the zonular fibrils with the capsule occurs in a small zone of about 2 to 3 mm. at the equator, but the zonular lamella or pericapsular membrane can be demonstrated over the lens capsule only in the equatorial region. It is remarkable that the zonular fibrils merge with the capsule so intimately that their individual character is erased.

The inner portion of the lens capsule rests directly on the base of the epithelial cells without any intervening space. The surface facing the lens epithelium is less regular than that facing the aqueous humor, the surfaces of the cells accommodating themselves to the irregularities of the epithelial cells.

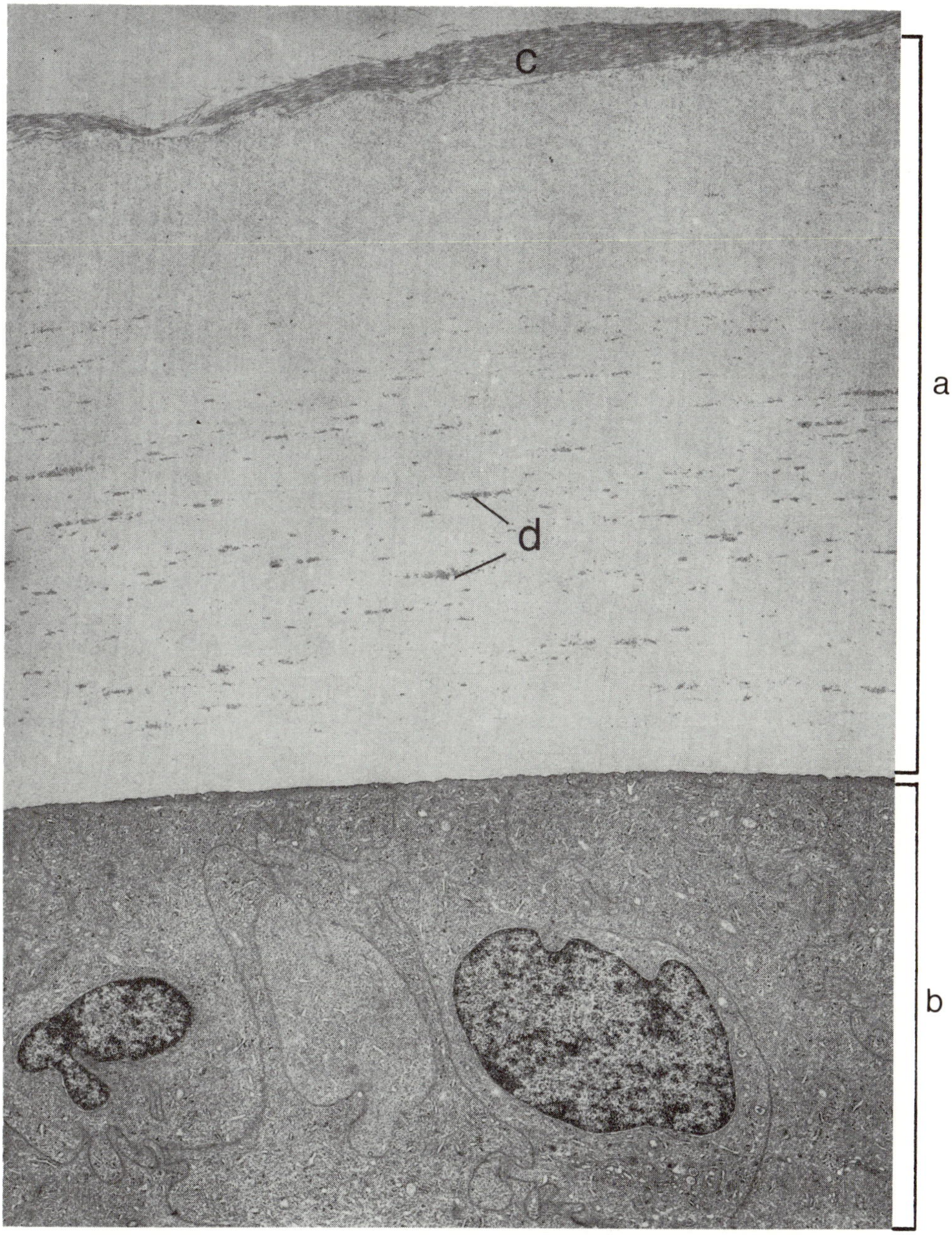

Figure 12–8. Electron micrograph of the anterior capsule (a) and epithelium (b). The capsule is essentially homogeneous except in its superficial portion, which is modified by the insertion of the zonular fibrils to form the zonular lamella (c). It is also characterized by a few scattered linear densities (d). The capsular-epithelial line of contact is smooth. (× 6100.)

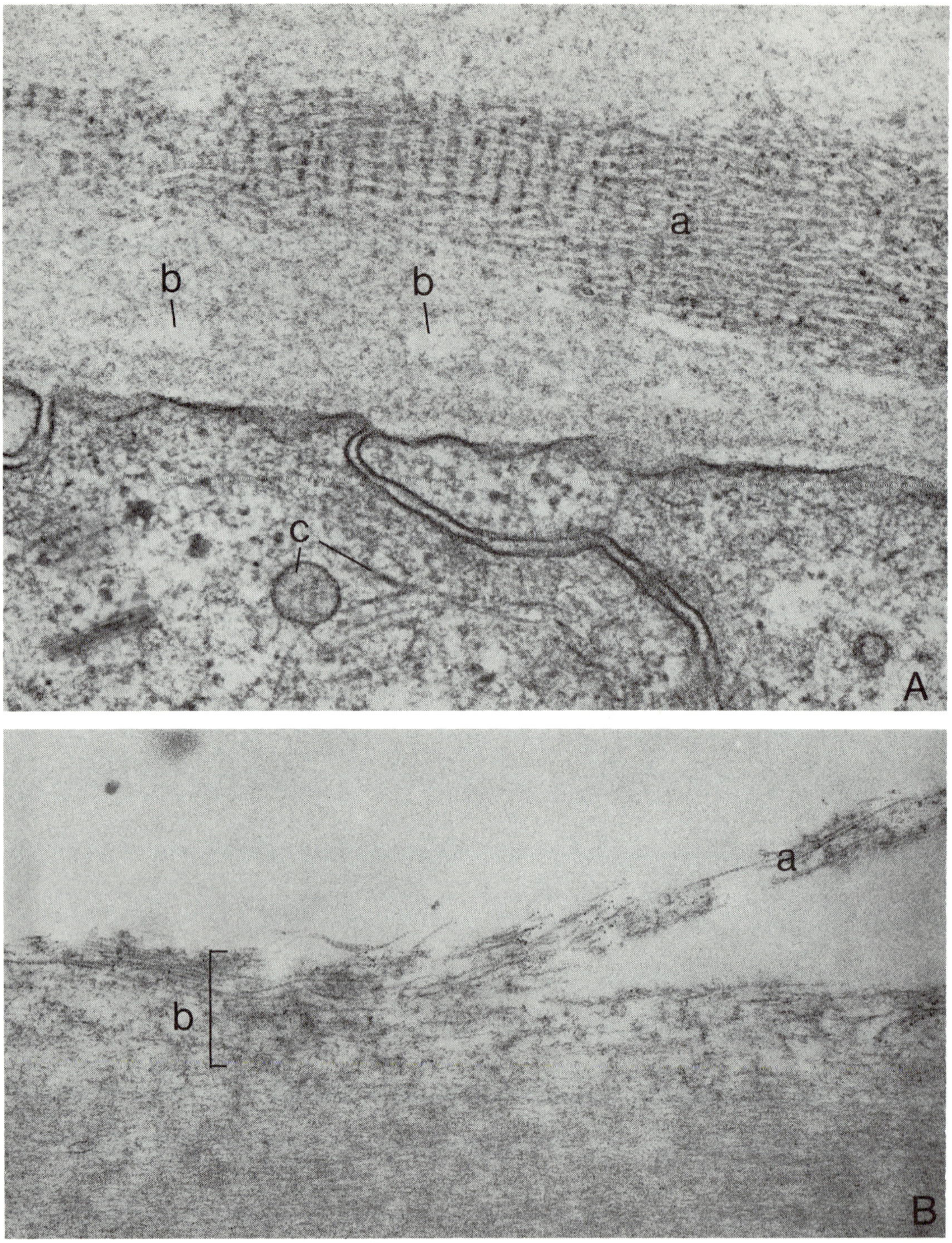

Figure 12–9. Electron micrographs of the lens capsule. *A,* The capsule-epithelial junction. A large mass of fibrils (a) with their axial banding in register are scattered in the capsule. The periodicity of their banding is about 600 A; these fibrils form the linear densities observed by light microscopy in the anterior and equatorial lens capsule. Small lucent spaces in the capsular substance are also apparent (b). The bases of the epithelial cells abut directly against the capsule. An open 150 A. wide intercellular space exists between the epithelial cells. The basal cytoplasm contains fibrils and vesicular elements (c). (× 72,600.)

B, The zonular fibrils (a) merge into the zonular lamella (b) of the superficial capsule. The lens capsule is faintly fibrillar. (× 24,000.)

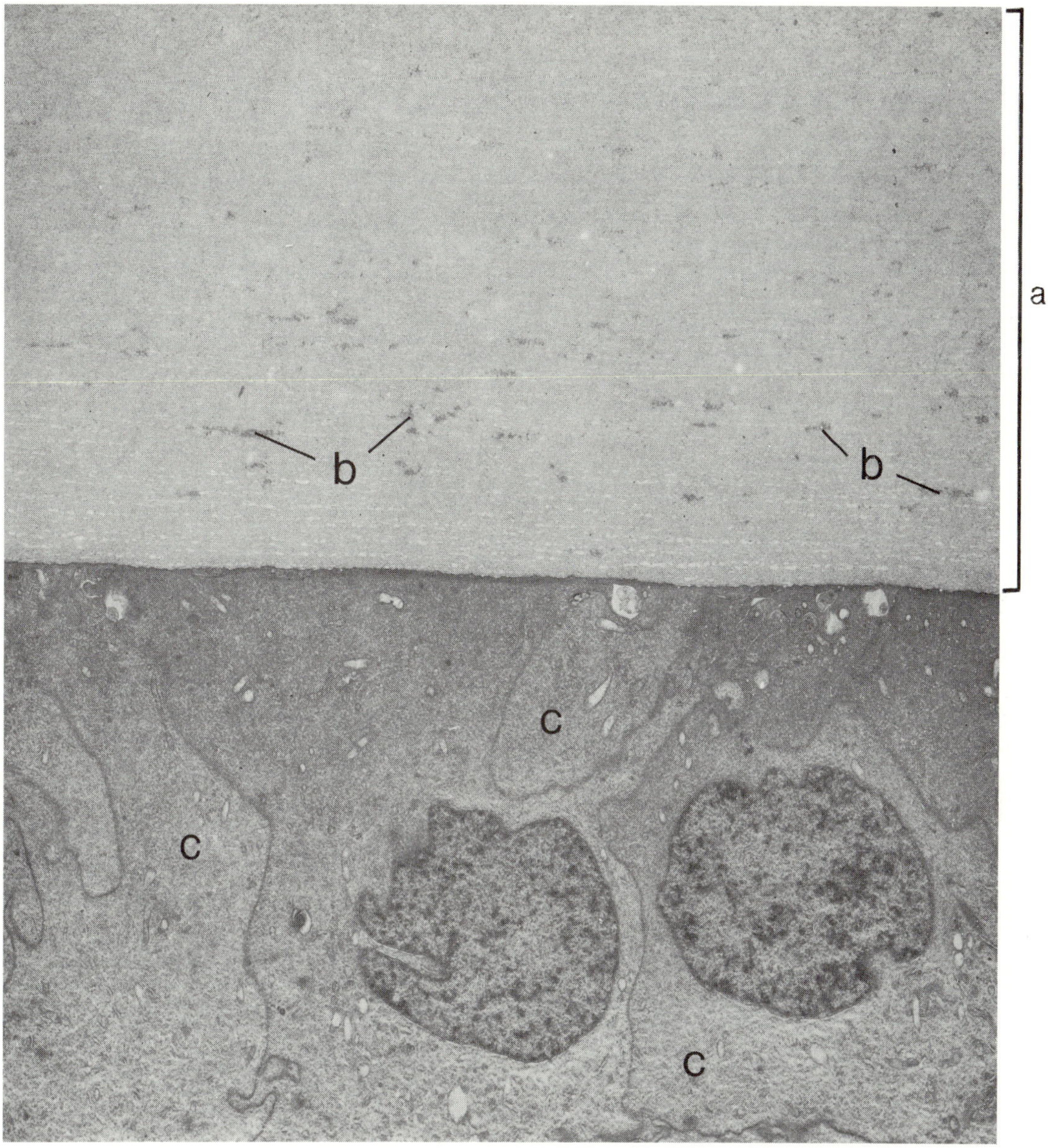

Figure 12–10. Anterior central lens capsule and epithelium. The lens capsule (a) is like that of the equatorial region, containing numerous filamentous inclusions (b). The lens epithelium (c) is cut through various portions of the cells so that in some places only strips of epithelial cytoplasm and portions of the nuclei are seen. (× 6500.)

Lens Epithelium (Figs. 12-4, 12-11 to 12-15)

The lens epithelium lies beneath the anterior and equatorial capsule but does not exist under the posterior capsule, because the posterior epithelium was used in embryonic life to form the primary lens cells. The apices of these cells face the interior of the lens and their bases face the lens capsule. The epithelial morphology in the drawing is slightly different in three areas (Fig. 12–3).

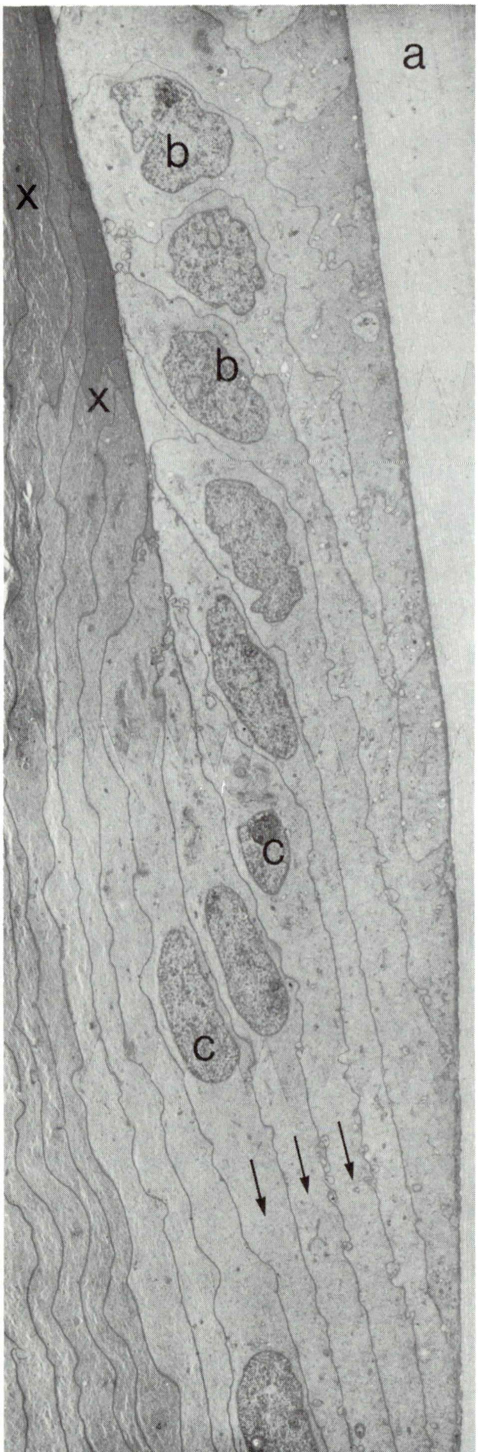

Figure 12–11. A montage of the equatorial lens capsule (a), formed lens cells at the equator (b), and older lens cells (c) that have been displaced into the cortex and are elongating toward the posterior suture (arrows). The anterior ends of the deeper cells are extending forward toward the anterior suture (x). (× 1800.)

Central Zone (Fig. 12-10). The central cells are found near the anterior pole. These cells are polygonal when viewed in flat section and cuboidal in meridional section. They stain poorly with most substances. The cells measure about 5 to 8 μm. high by 11 to 17 μm. wide and have smooth surfaces under the capsule and over the underlying lens cells. Their nuclei are round, located slightly toward the lens cortex side of the cell. Mitoses ordinarily are not seen in the central epithelium.

Intermediate Zone (Fig. 12-12). These cells lie between those of the central zone and the ones at the equator. They are smaller and more cylindrical than those in the central portion, and their spherical nuclei are centrally placed. The cells have complex basal interdigitations, and their lateral surfaces are quite irregular. Mitoses are more common in this zone.

Equatorial Zone (Figs. 12-13 to 12-15). The cells of this region divide and become elongated to form the new lens cells. The transition from the tall, cuboidal, equatorial, epithelial cell to the newly formed ribbon-like lens cell begins with expansion of the basal part of the cell and flattening of the nucleus. The expanded basal process moves backward along the inner surface of the capsule, while the apical process installs itself under the inner surfaces of the neighboring epithelial cells. This alteration of the equatorial cells occurs all around the lens equator so that cell processes are expanding toward the anterior and posterior poles from many directions. Because of the constant formation of new cells, the preceding generations of cells are displaced more and more into the cortex, carrying their flattened nuclei with them. Eventually these nuclei form a zone, the *lens bow*, curving forward in crescent shape from the epithelial region toward the nucleus. Finally the deepest cells lose their nuclei as they are incorporated into the nucleus of the lens.

Electron microscopic studies have shown that there are no important differences in the structure of the cell in the central, intermediate and equatorial zones of the epithelium. The only difference is that resulting from multiplication of the cells in the equatorial zone and in the cell membranes of the most posterior intermediate cells.

The fine structure of the lens was studied in several animal species by Wanko and Gavin (1958, 1960) and in humans by Cohen (1965). The cytoplasm of the epithelial cells is granular and contains the usual organelles, which are present in small amounts. There are short segments of rough-surfaced endoplasmic reticulum, ribosomes, small mitochondria, a Golgi complex, microtubules and numerous unoriented filaments about 400 A. in diameter (Fig. 12-12 *A* and *B*). Lysosomal elements rarely are seen. Adjacent cells are attached to each other by a small occluding zonule at their apical borders and also occasionally by a small macula adhering immediately subjacent to the occluding zonule. The epithelial cells are attached to the underlying lens cells by numerous intermittent occluding junctions. No cement substance or other extracellular material is seen between the base of the epithelium and the capsule or between the apices of the epithelium and the first layer of lens cells, as reported elsewhere.

At the equator the cell changes from cuboidal to pyramidal, retaining the same anterior tight attachments while spreading its widened base posteriorly beneath the capsule (Fig. 12-14). The cytoplasm of cells in this region is particularly fibrous and contains chains of ribosomes (polyribosomes), multivesicular bodies and other elements resembling lysosomes. In addi-

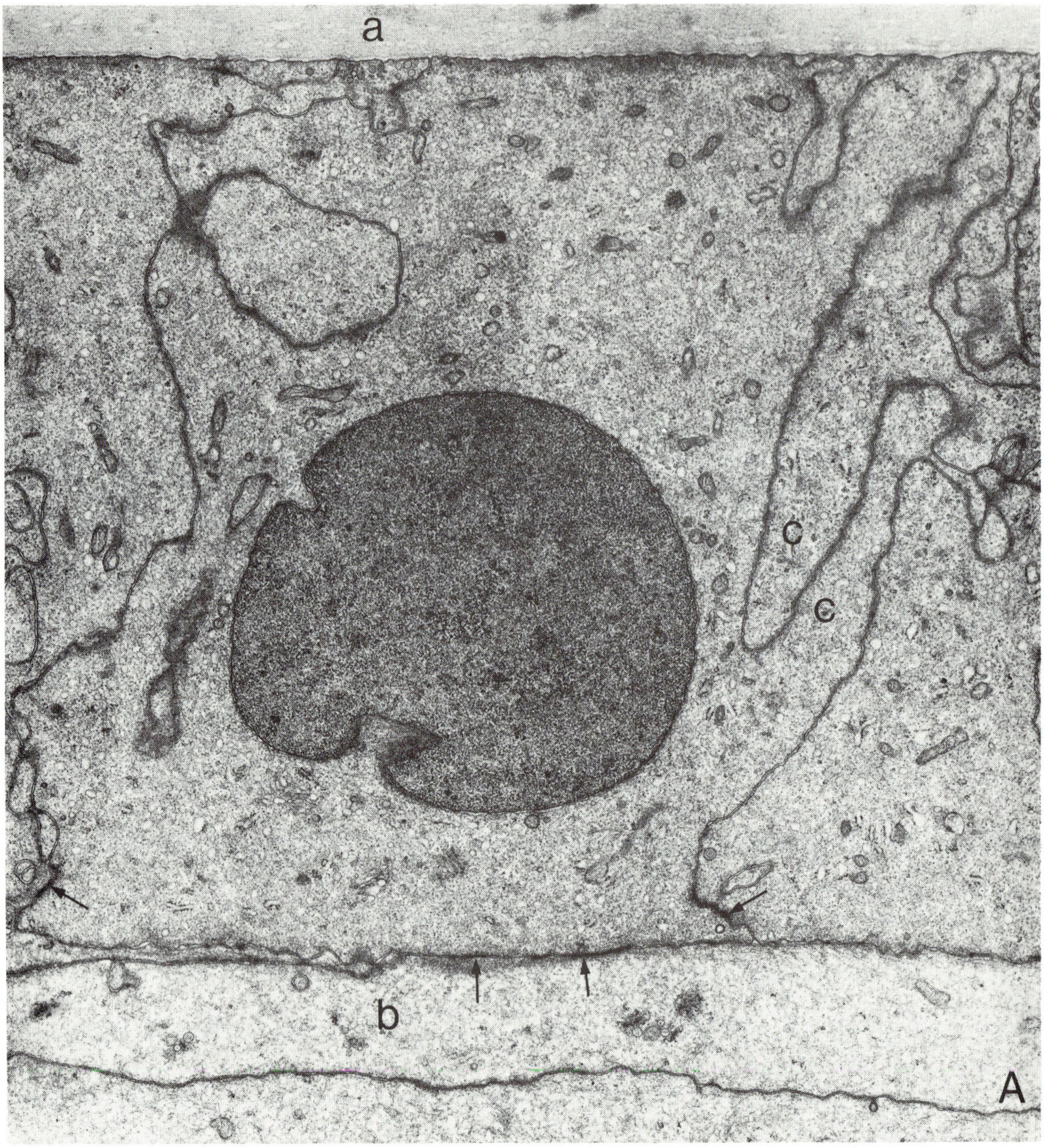

Figure 12–12. Electron micrograph of the lens epithelium. *A*, Electron micrograph of an epithelial cell of the intermediate zone about 0.7 mm. anterior to the equator. The base of the epithelial cell faces the capsule (a), which contains numerous lucent spaces. The cell apex is adjacent to the youngest lens cell (b). There are large lateral interdigitations with adjacent cells (c). The nucleus is central and the nuclear chromatin is evenly dispersed. The cytoplasm contains numerous small mitochondria, a few short segments of rough-surfaced endoplasmic reticulum, a small Golgi system, numerous smooth-surfaced vesicles, free ribosomes and some filaments. Occluding zonules are seen between lateral cell membranes near the apices of the cells. Numerous occluding zonules also join the apex of the cell to the underlying cortical cells (arrows). The cytoplasm of the cortical cells is less dense than that of the epithelial cell and it also exhibits fewer organelles. The cortical cells have cytoplasmic fibrils in greater number; these are oriented toward the cell membrane. (× 10,500.)

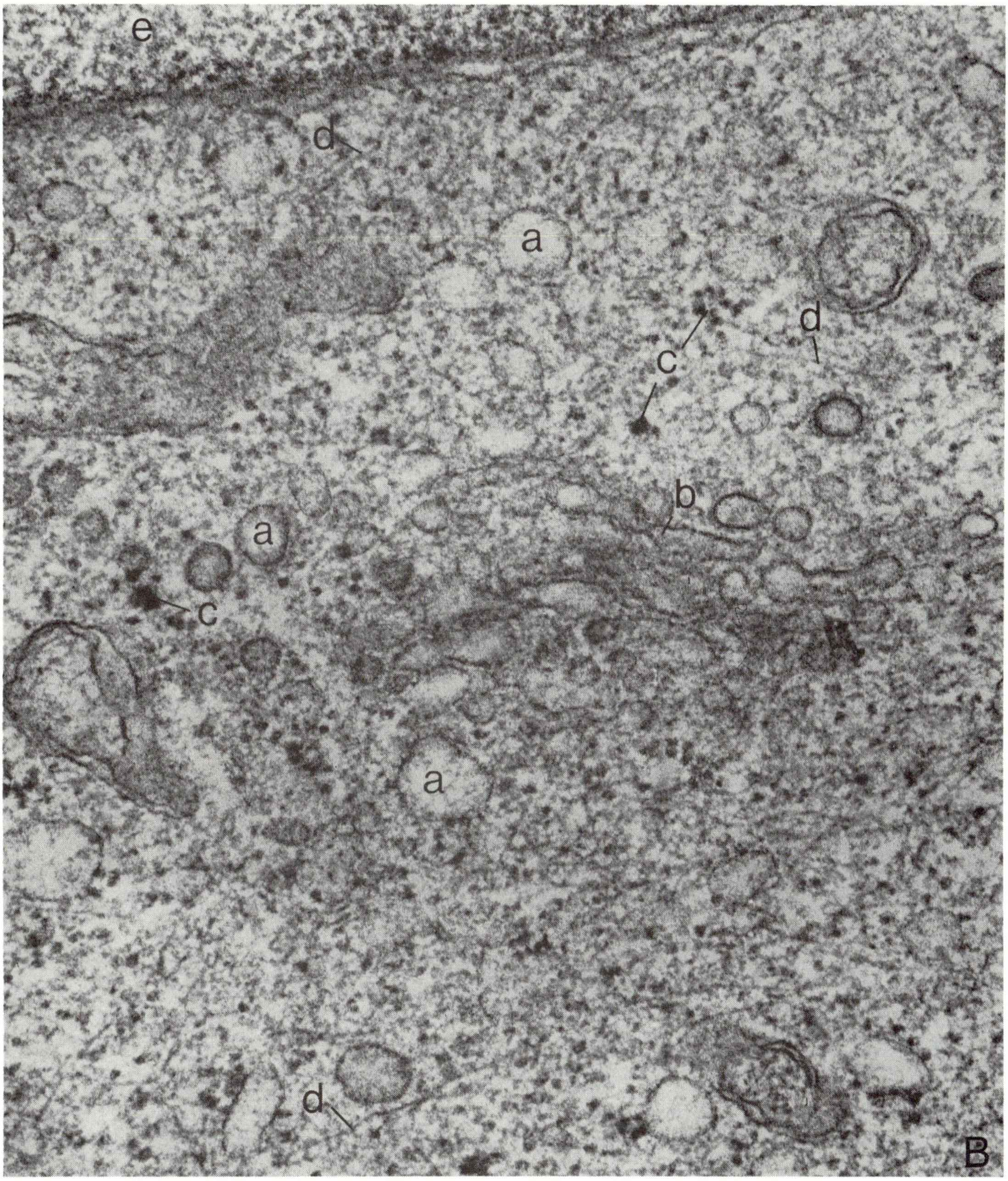

Figure 12–12. *Continued.*

B, Higher magnification of the intermediate epithelial cells to show the granular cytoplasm. It contains vesicles (a), elements of the Golgi system (b), free ribosomes (c) and a few filaments (d). The nucleus and nuclear membrane are at (e). (× 71,500.)

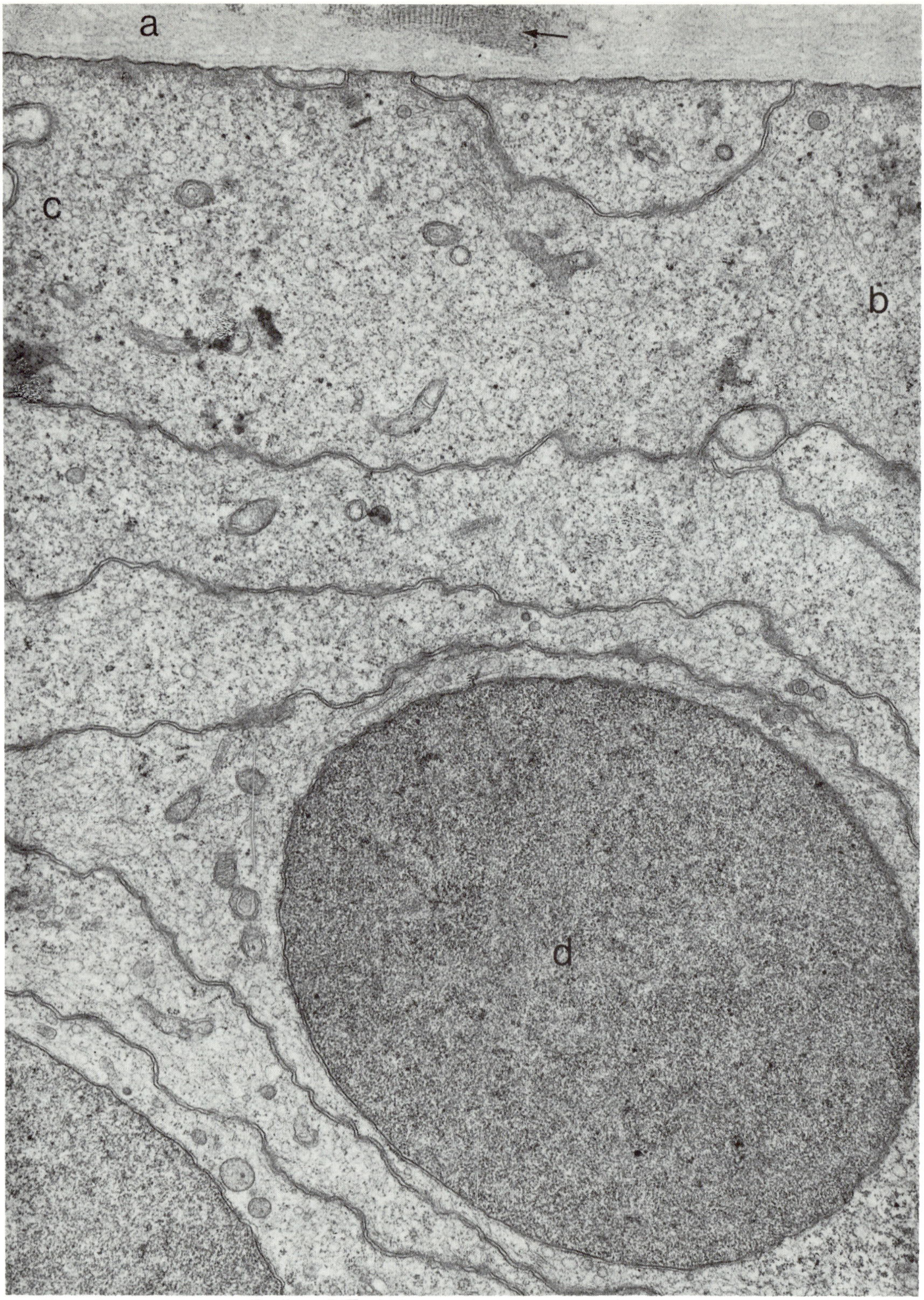

Figure 12–13. Epithelium and capsule at the equator. The capsule is lamellated (a) and contains a clump of banded fibrils (arrow). The cells beneath this portion of the capsule are oriented parallel to its surface. The basal portion of the epithelial cell extends toward the posterior suture (b) and the apical portion extends anteriorly (c). A nucleated cell (d) lies in the lens cortex. All these cells have a granular, faintly fibrillar cytoplasm. Most of the mitochondria are small. (× 13,000.)

tion, centrioles and basal bodies of cilia are seen with greater frequency (Fig. 12-15 *A* and *B*). The cilia project from the cell through its apex. Microtubules, possibly remnants of the mitotic spindle, are also more evident (Kuwabara, 1968). The subcapsular basal cytoplasm contains most of the mitochondria and a number of vesicular elements. It would be of interest to know if these vesicles are involved in the elaboration of the posterior capsule which, following the obliteration of the lens vesicle in embryonic life, has no epithelial cells on its inner surface to lay down a new basement membrane.

Microtubules are seen in the cytoplasm. They have a random distribution and usually do not have a central dark core; their length is indeterminate. They increase in number in the equatorial cells. Their function is unknown, but microtubules may be responsible for the elasticity of the lens cells.

LENS CELLS (Figs. 12-15 to 12-19)

In the infant the cortical lens cells surrounding the fetal nucleus are nucleated. As new cells are formed, the older ones are displaced deeper into the cortex and lose their nuclei. The deeper cells, about 0.15 mm. into the cortex, lose their nuclei and their outlines become less defined. By age 30 a considerable number of older cells have accumulated to form the lens nucleus. The cells comprising the lens cortex surround the nucleus and many of them retain their nuclei.

The principal parts of the lens cortex and nucleus are formed by the hexagonal lens cells, which by tradition have come to be known as lens *fibers* because of their length (Fig. 12–16 *A* and *B*). Their nuclei are located in the lens cortex at the equator. The total number of lens cells is estimated to be 2100 to 2300 in the adult. The cortical cells measure 8 to 12 *mm.* long, 7*μm.* wide and 4.6 *μm.* thick. In the cortical region the cells are flatter, measuring 2 *μm.* thick near the anterior and posterior sutures, whereas they measure 5 *μm.* thick in the nuclear region. The cells terminate anteriorly and posteriorly at the lens sutures, which are located at varying depths beneath the capsule. The more superficial cells are longer than those that developed previously, and the youngest cells always lie just beneath the capsule. In cross-section the lens cells have a hexagonal shape at the equator, the cells being aligned in fairly regular rows throughout the cortex. The cell shape and alignment are seen in all sections made at a right angle to the course of the cells.

The lens cells splay out as they approach the sutures, becoming thinner but wider, and near the suture they bend rather sharply before ending. This change in course causes them to meet the branches of the sutures at wide angles, so that if meridional sections are made through the lens, the cells about to join the sutures frequently are cut in cross-section rather than longitudinally. The sutures have been known as the anterior and posterior lens stars, because of the ray-like branching processes formed by the union of cells from various lens sectors in the axial regions of the lens. The central portions of the sutures lie somewhere near the anterior and posterior poles of the lens. Radiating out from the center are two or more strong branches, which then further subdivide into more delicate branches

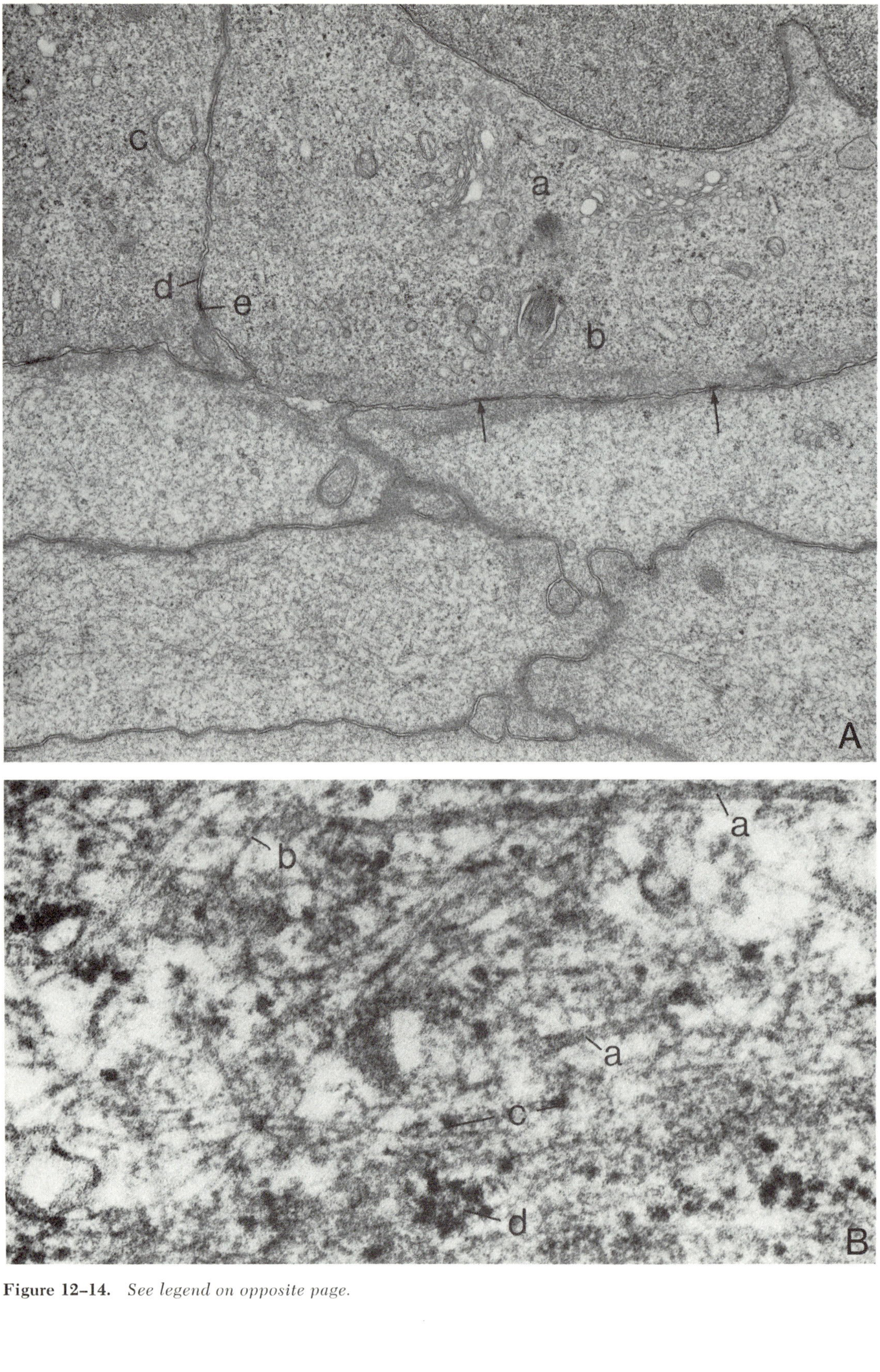

Figure 12–14. *See legend on opposite page.*

that terminate 1 to 2 mm. from the equator of the lens. The anterior and posterior sutures are not superimposed; rather, the branches of one most often lie in the spaces between branches of the other. The reason for this arrangement is that each lens cell is attached to the tip of a branch anteriorly and to the fork of a branch posteriorly, making the anterior portion of the cell shorter than the posterior. Succeeding cells may have the opposite arrangement; thus, all the cells need not reach the anterior or posterior pole, yet the elliptical shape of the lens is retained.

The complex structure of the sutures increases as the eye ages. At birth the primary and secondary lens cells have formed the fetal nucleus with an anterior erect Y and a posterior inverted Y (Fig. 12-1 *A*). The two Y sutures lie beneath the capsule at birth, and all new cells which form after birth belong to the lens cortex. The portion of the cortex that becomes converted to the nucleus encloses the fetal nucleus. After fetal life the newly formed cells create sutures which are not Y-shaped, but rather are stellate. The stellate portion becomes more complex with increasing age, so that in the lens of a person of advanced age the arrangement beneath the capsule is quite intricate (Figs. 12-1 *B*, 12-3). It should be remembered that the sutures do not lie in a single plane, since they are constantly being formed by succeeding generations of cells; thus, they have a third dimension. They are formed by overlapping and terminal interdigitations of the lens cells from different sectors of the lens and therefore represent a line of union of converging cells.

With the electron microscope the superficial lens cells near the equator contain most of the organelles found in the epithelial cells, including microtubules and flattened nuclei. The number of organelles appears reduced, but this could result as much from the increasing cell volume as from an actual decrease of organelles. The remaining cytoplasm consists of a finely fibrillar substance. At a short distance from the equator and in the deeper layers, the organelles and ribosomes progressively disappear. In addition to this change, the cytoplasm of the cells becomes amorphous as a result of an accumulation of a homogeneous granular substance. It is not clear whether this results from the poor penetration of fixatives into the deep layers or whether it is a reflection of the progressive insolubility of preexisting protein in the deeper cells of the lens, as reported by Young and Fulhorst (1966). The cell nucleus separates into small masses in the deeper cortex, the nuclear envelope no longer being discernible around the fragments. The terminal or growing ends of the cells contain numerous empty-

Text continued on page 673

Figure 12–14. Lens epithelium and cortex. *A*, Electron micrograph of the apical portion of an epithelial cell and three layers of cortical cells near the lens equator. The Golgi system occupies a region of the cytoplasm near the nucleus (a). A cilum (b), a multivesicular body (c), mitochondria, rough-surfaced endoplasmic reticulum and vesicular elements are also visible. An adhering macula (d) and an occluding zonule (e) join the cells laterally. Occluding zonules also join the epithelium to the lens cells (arrows). The lens cells contain fibrils, ribosomes and a few vesicular elements. (× 12,000.)

B, Equatorial lens epithelium. The cytoplasm contains numerous microtubules (a) and some filaments (b). Free (c) and clustered (d) ribosomes are seen. (× 140,000.)

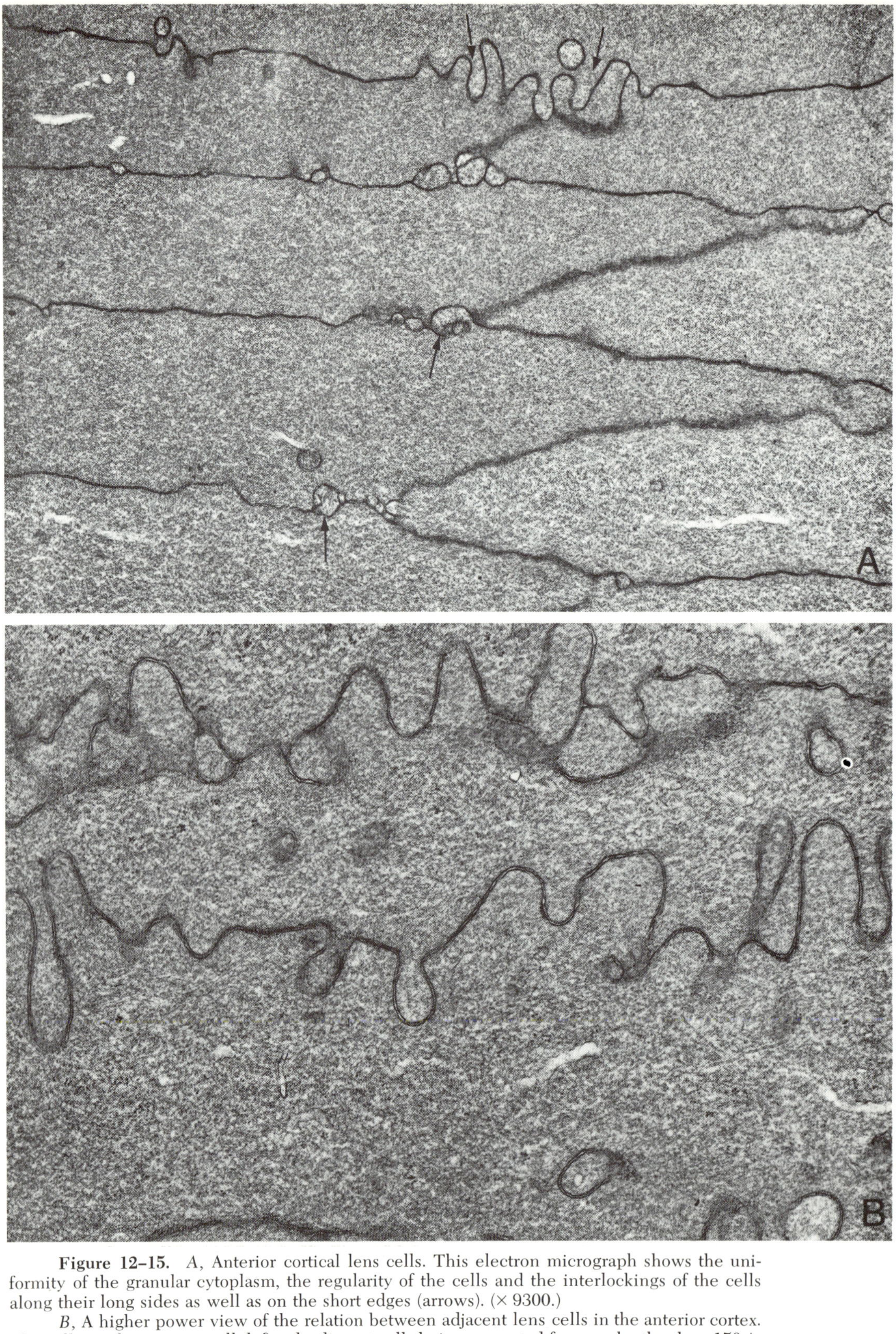

Figure 12–15. *A*, Anterior cortical lens cells. This electron micrograph shows the uniformity of the granular cytoplasm, the regularity of the cells and the interlockings of the cells along their long sides as well as on the short edges (arrows). (× 9300.)

B, A higher power view of the relation between adjacent lens cells in the anterior cortex. The cell membranes are well defined, adjacent cells being separated from each other by a 150 A. space. The interlocking of the cells is prominent. (× 14,000.)

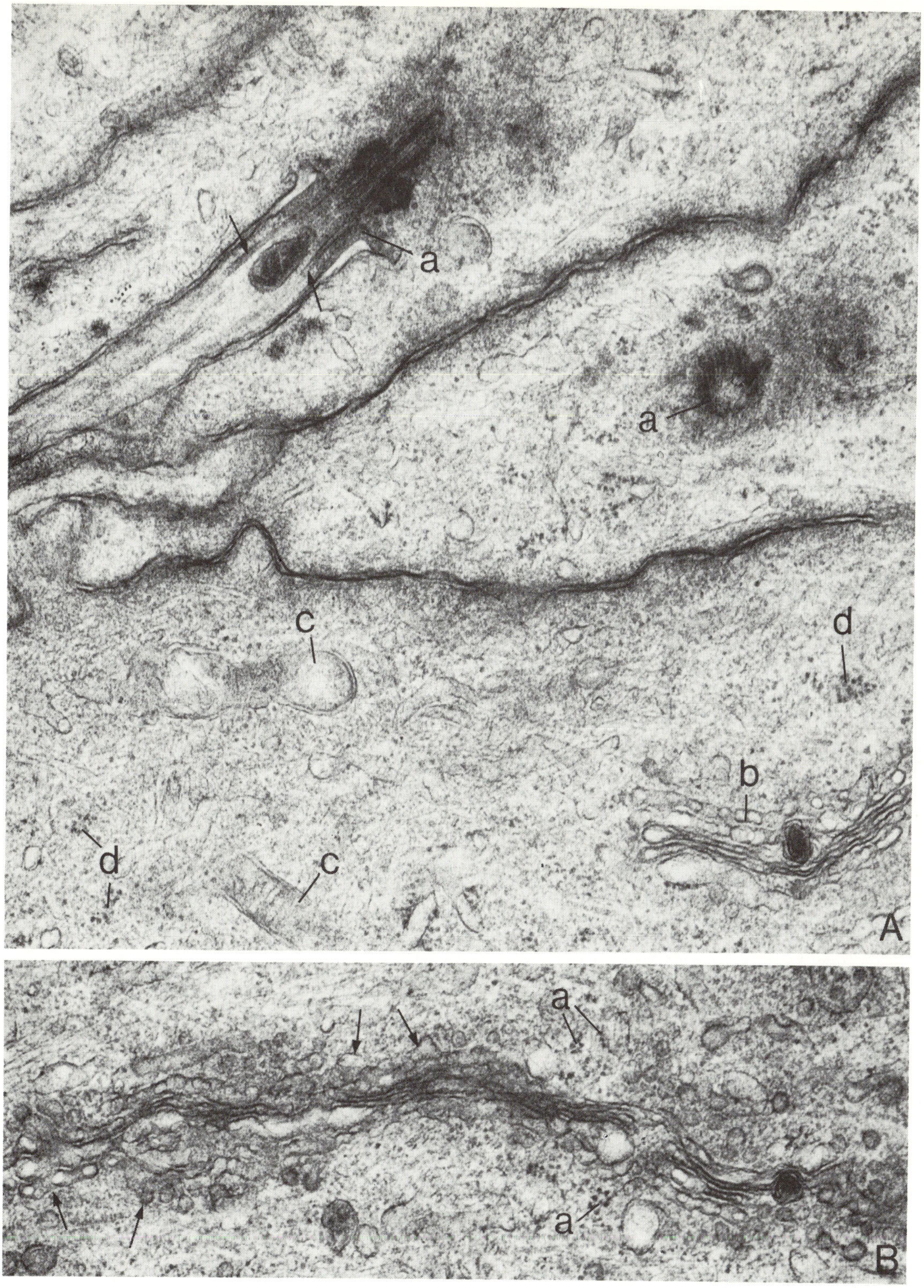

Figure 12-16. Organelles found in cortical lens cells. *A*, Two of the lens cells contain basal bodies (a). Microtubules extend from the upper basal body into the cilium (arrows). The lower cell contains a well developed Golgi apparatus (b), portions of mitochondria (c) and numerous free ribosomes (d). (× 36,000.)

B, The very prominent Golgi apparatus of a cell adjacent to those seen in *A*. The cisternae are long and show numerous interconnections. Vesicles are seen on both sides of the tubular cisternae (arrows). There are free ribosomes (a). (× 27,500.)

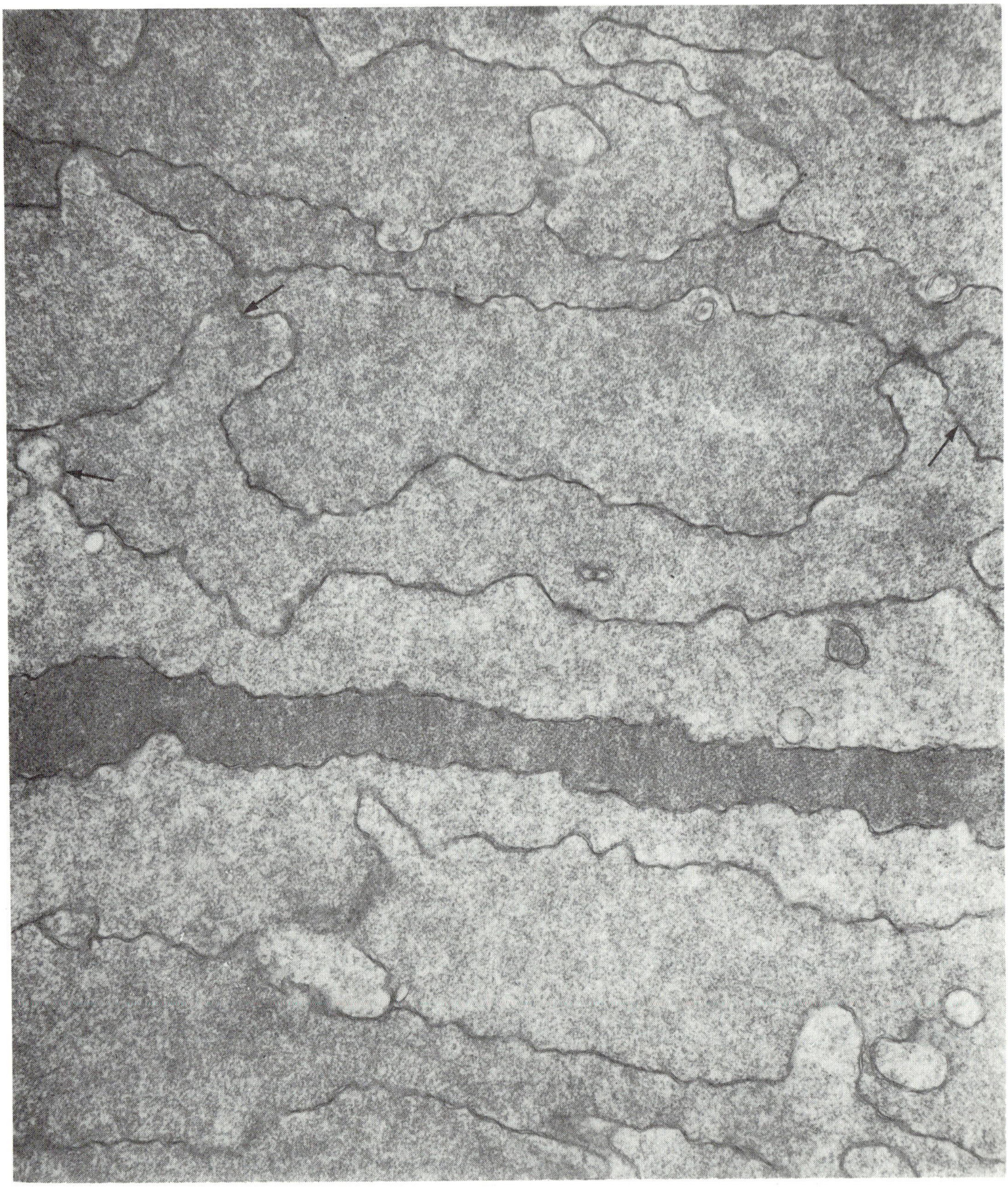

Figure 12–17. Cells in the nuclear region of the lens. The limiting membrane of each cell is clearly visible. The cytoplasm is very finely granular and very uniform in density; no organelles are seen in this field. The interlocking processes of neighboring cells are indicated by the arrows. (× 24,000.)

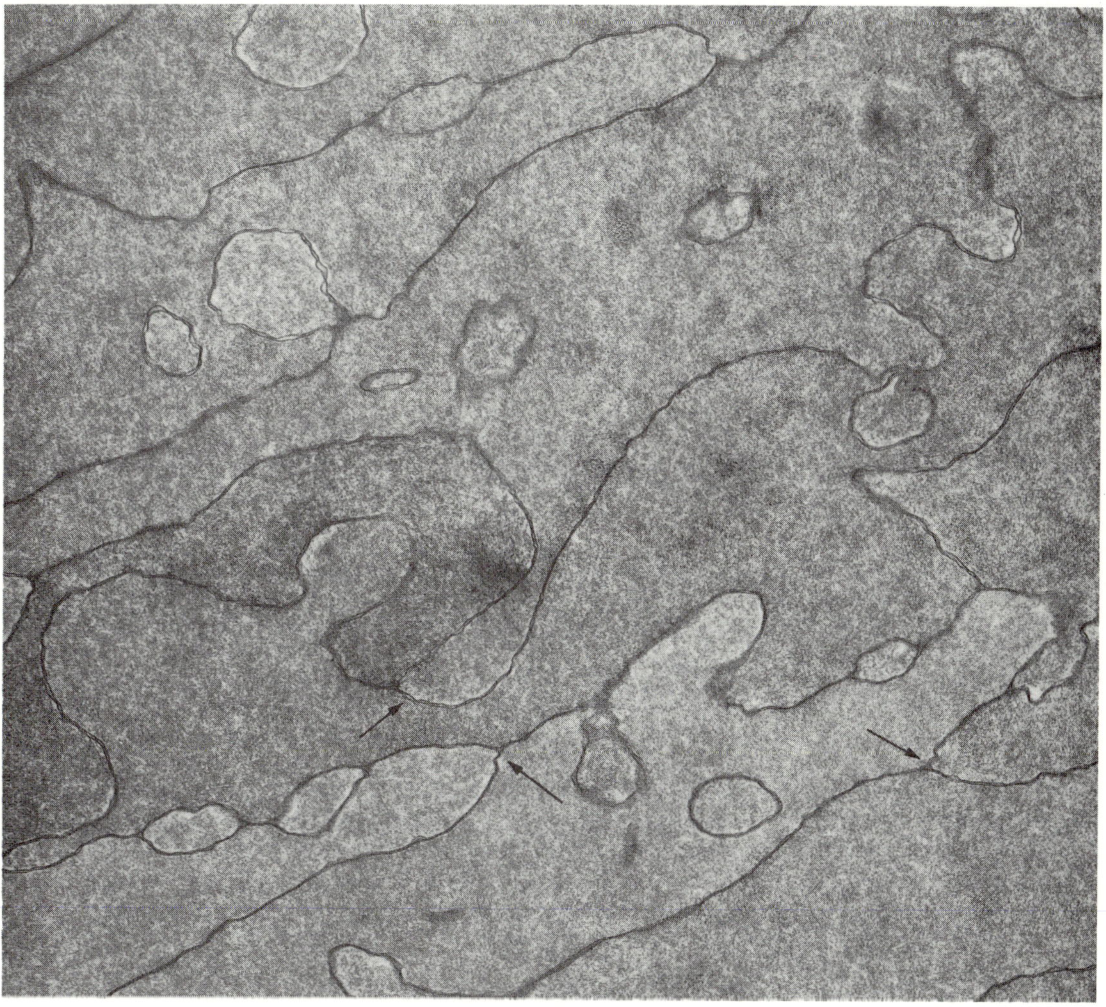

Figure 12–18. Electron micrograph of a small area in a posterior suture in the midcortical lens. The terminal processes of lens cells from different quadrants meet and interdigitate in a complex arrangement (arrows). (× 24,000.)

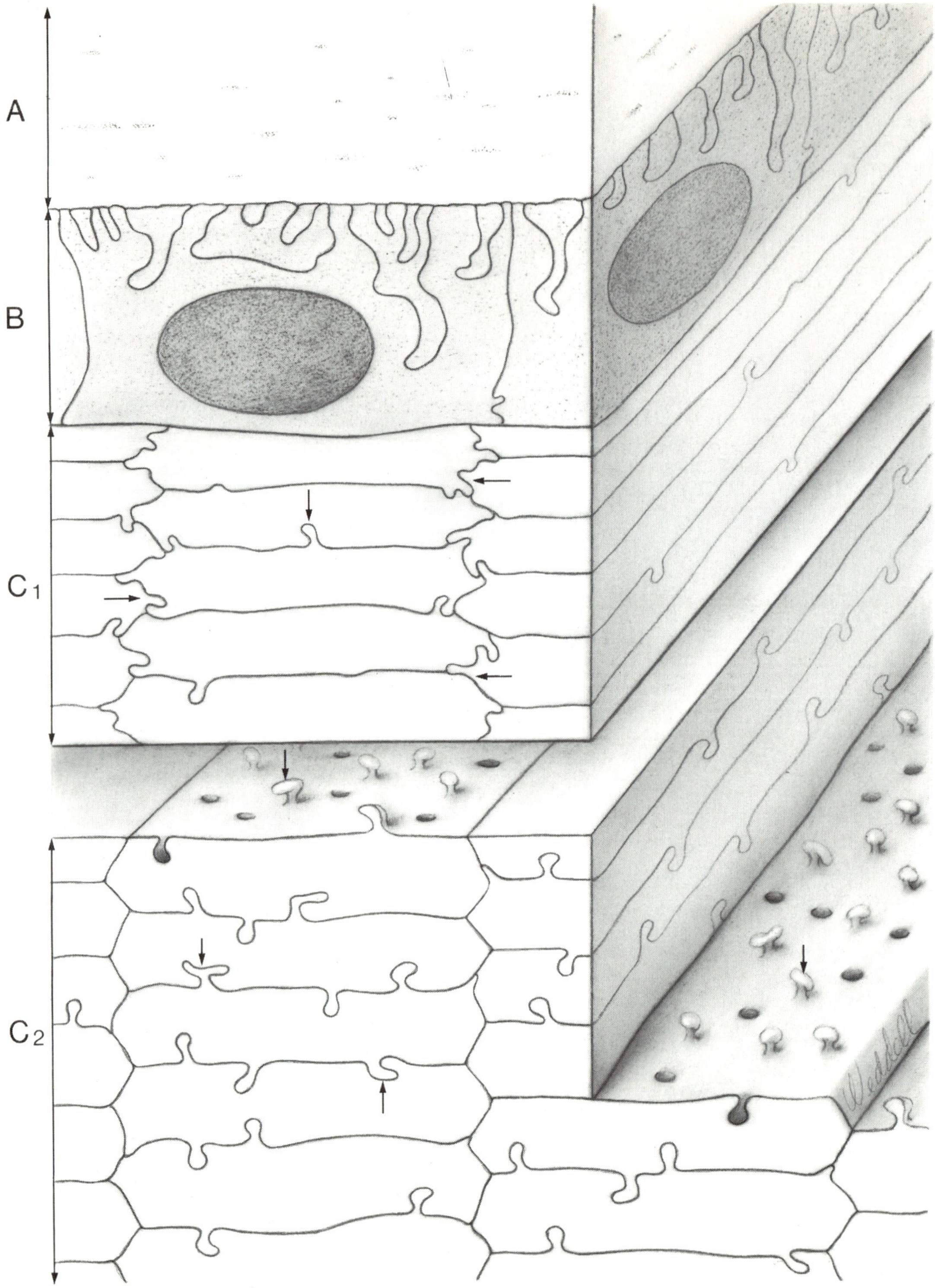

Figure 12–19. This three-dimensional drawing of the lens shows the interrelation of the capsule and underlying lens cells. The capsule is at (A) and shows inclusions of fine filamentous material. The anterior lens epithelium (B) shows interdigitation of its basal surface with adjacent cells. The superficial cells of the cortex show the hexagonal shape, and interdigitations at their hexagonal ends as well as along their edges (C_1) (arrows). The deeper cortical cells (C_2) also show a tongue and groove type of interdigitation along their long sides (arrows), but the interlocking is absent at the short ends.

appearing, flattened, smooth vesicles; these may be utilized for expansion of the cell membrane as it grows toward the sutures.

The superficial eight to ten layers of cells in the anterior lens differ somewhat from the deeper cells of the cortex in having few interlocking processes. The interlockings that are present occur chiefly at the short sides of the hexagonal cells. For this reason each layer of cells appears to be relatively loosely attached to the underlying lens cells, which may account for the extensibility of the superficial lens cells. In the posterior lens and in the deeper layers of the anterior cortex, interlocking processes or ball-and-socket junctions are found between the long sides of the hexagons (Fig. 12-15 *A* and *B*). This provides for substantial adhesion between the layers or generations of lens cells. Junctions resembling maculae adherans are seen rarely between lens cells, and desmosomes are entirely lacking. Numerous large and small occluding zonules appear between lens cells in both the cortex and the nucleus. Since occluding zonules are areas of membrane fusion, these may facilitate diffusion and electrical equilibration within this dense cellular tissue.

Anterior sutures are formed by the interdigitations of the *apical* processes of the lens cells, and *posterior sutures* are formed by similar interdigitations of the *basal* processes. Interdigitations occur between cells of the same generation but from different quadrants of the lens (Figs. 12-1 and 12–3). In the human lens the superficial suture line is formed by simple interdigitation and overlapping of apposing cells, and these become more complex below the tenth layer of cortical cells. The area of overlap is about 70 μm. in width. There is no increase in the frequency of occluding zonules or other junctional specializations in the suture areas.

ZONULES (Figs. 7–6, 12–4, 12–20 and 12–21)

The origin of zonular fibers in the pars plana region is from the unpigmented epithelial cells (Fig. 7–6). Electron microscopic study shows the origin of the zonular fibers to be from the basement membrane of the unpigmented ciliary epithelial cells. The attachments can be traced into this membrane, but no extension has been observed between or under the unpigmented epithelial cells. In the valleys between the ciliary processes the same type of attachment is found.

The size and shape of the fibers which form the zonule vary considerably, depending in part on the method of fixation and preparation of the specimens. With the phase-contrast microscope, three types of fibers can be seen: (1) a very thin, wavy one measuring about 1 μm. in diameter and found mainly in the region of the vitreous; (2) a very thin but wide fiber; and (3) one which is even thinner, having a somewhat circular course (Garzino, 1953). The diameter of the zonular fibers appears to vary according to the number of fibrils which are aggregated; dimensions between 1 and 40 μm. have been quoted for various fibers. The microfibrillar elements that enter into the formation of the grosser fibers vary between 300 and 400 A. Most of the fibrils we have seen measure about 80 to 120 A. thick and exhibit a regular periodicity of about 110 to 180 A. and, consequently, are similar to those seen in the vitreous.

Pappas and Smelser (1958) found the diameter of the fibrils in the

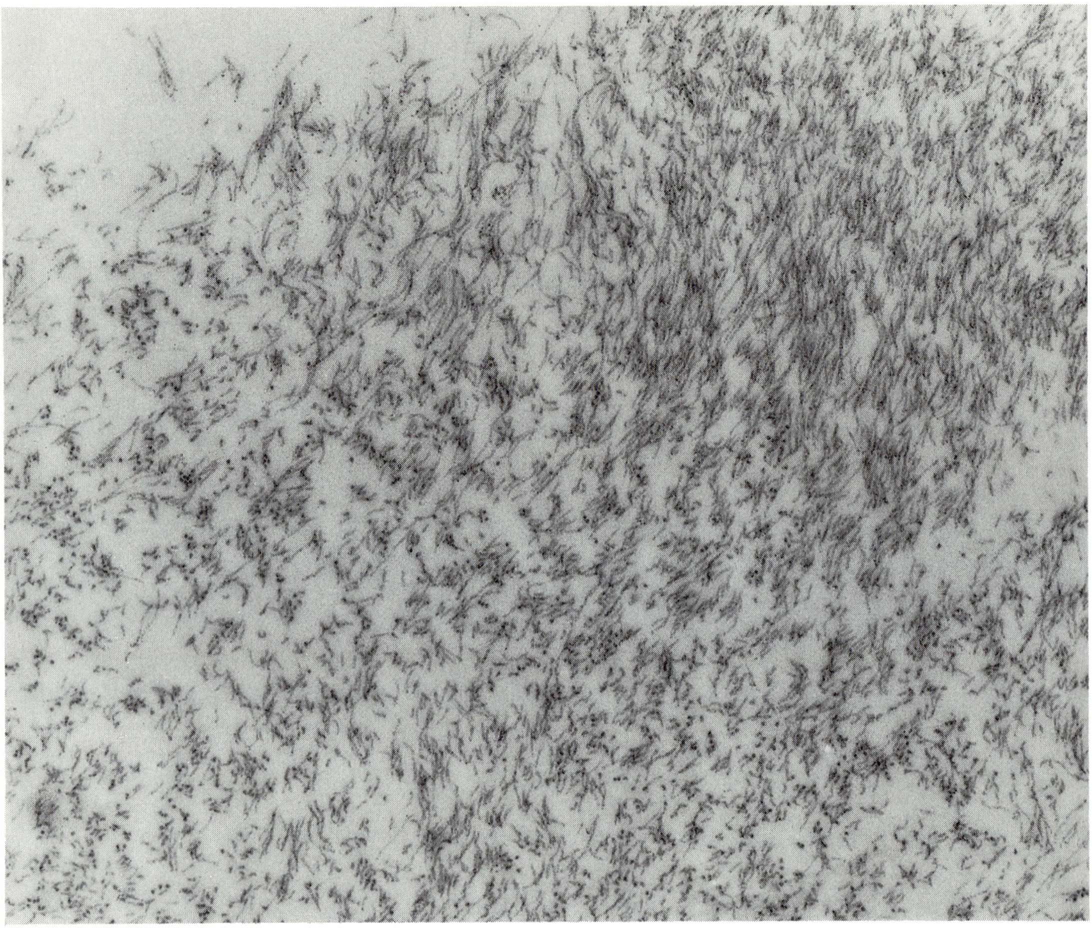

Figure 12-20. Electron micrograph of a zonular fiber. It is composed of fibrils of undetermined length that are oriented in different directions. Faint banding can be made out even at this magnification. (× 32,000.)

zonular fibers of rabbit eyes to be 80 to 120 A. Yoshida (1959) found the diameter of the zonular fibers in rabbit eyes to be 333 to 666 mμ with an average of 470. In cattle eyes the range was 400 to 666 mμ, with an average of 515, while in the human eye the range was 166 to 291 mμ, with an average of 217.

The Insertion at the Lens. Those fibers attaching to the capsule anterior and posterior to the equator meet the capsule at an acute angle, whereas those coming directly from the ciliary valleys to the equator meet the capsule at a right angle (Fig. 12-22) After breaking up into finer fibrils, they course somewhat parallel to the capsule surface before finally entering the pericapsular layer. At the point of their fibrillary attachments, they form tent-like structures, often making the capsule wrinkled at this point. By electron microscopy the zonular lamella of the lens is the most superficial layer of the capsule. It has a looser and more fibrillar structure, owing to the insertion of the individual zonular fibrils.

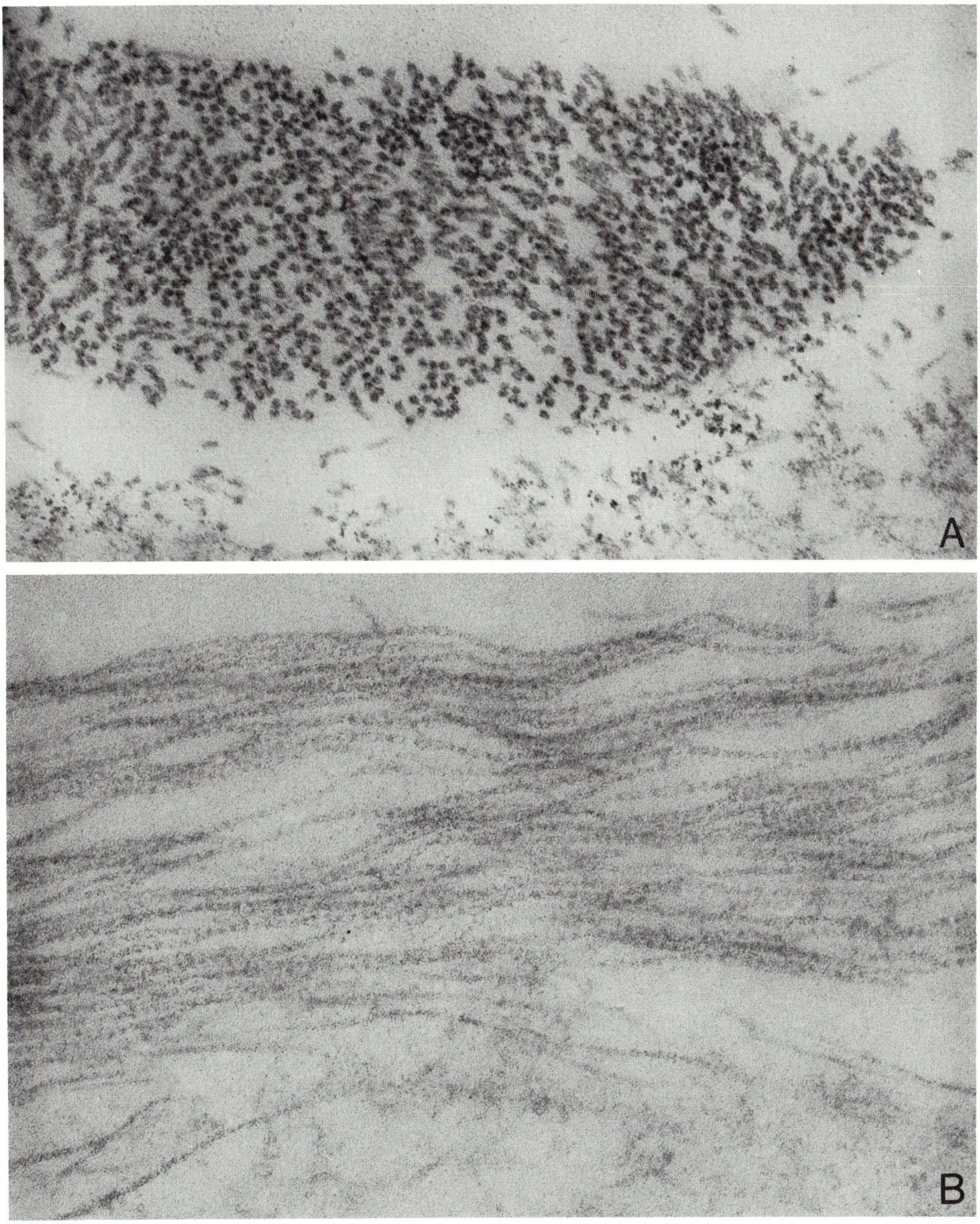

Figure 12–21. Electron micrographs of zonular fibers. *A*, Cross-section of a zonular fiber. The fibrils are round and measure 100 to 120 A. in diameter. They appear to have a dense rim and a lucent core. (× 112,000.)

B, Longitudinal section of a zonular fiber that is composed of numerous fibrils. The banding is about 125 A., and the fibrils have a diameter of around 83 A. (× 120,000.)

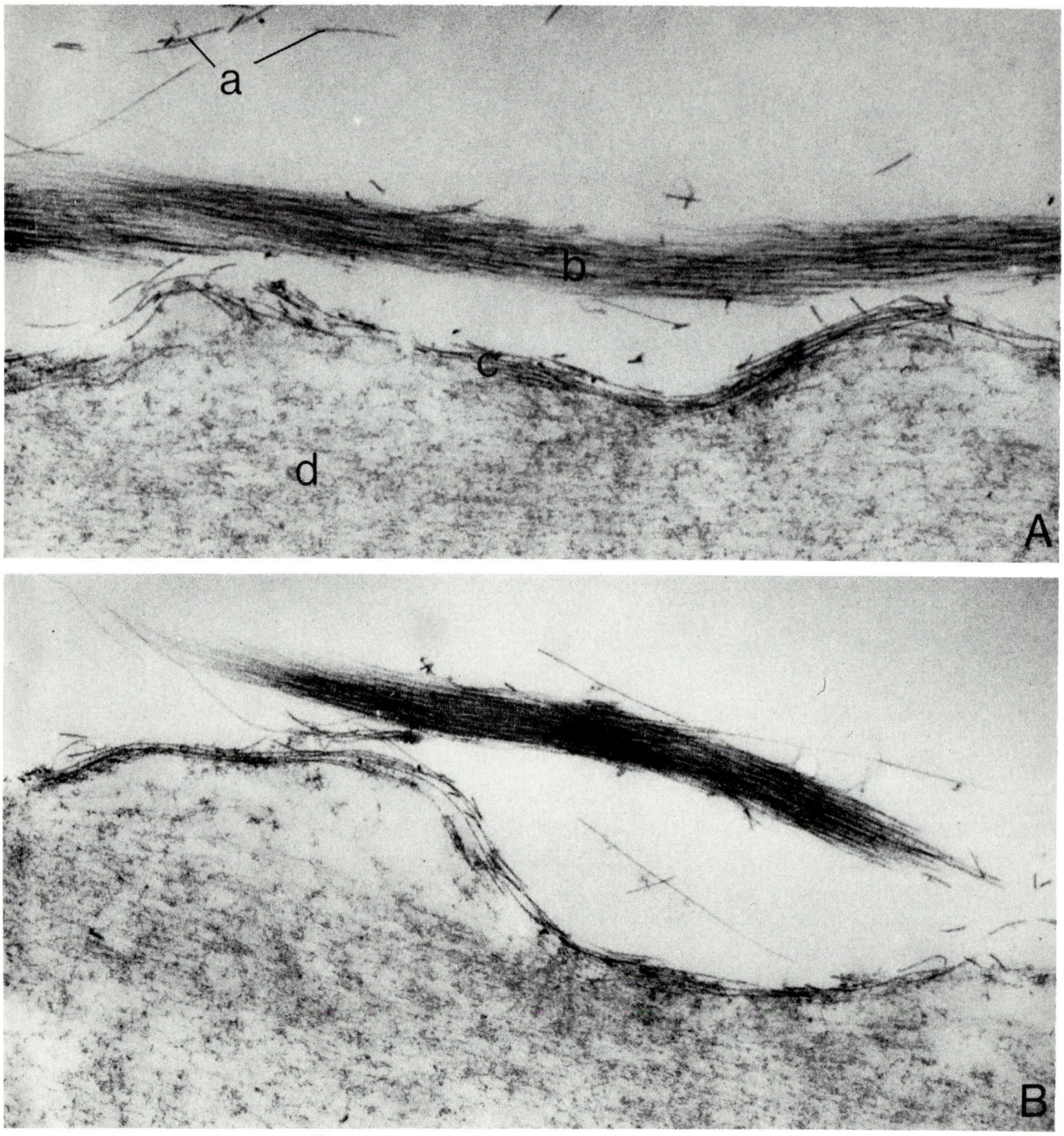

Figure 12–22. Lens capsule, vitreous and zonules posterior to the lens equator. *A*, Vitreous fibrils (a) lie adjacent to a zonular fiber (b). Some fibrils form the pericapsular membrane (c). The outer lens capsule shows a faint fibrillation (d). (× 25,500.)

B, A view similar to that seen in *A*. The fibrillation of the outer lens capsule is more evident. (× 24,000.)

REFERENCES

Bahr, G. F.: Investigation of the lamellar structure of the lens capsule. Graefes Arch. Ophthal. *155*:635, 1954.

Bairati, A., and Grignolo, A.: Preliminary investigations of the submicroscopic structure of Descemet's membrane with the electron microscope. Boll. Soc. Ital. Biol. *31*:16, 1954.

Beauvieux, M.: The zonule (topographic and histologic study). Arch. d'Ophthal. *39*:484, 1922.

Berger, E.: Bermerkungen über die Linsenkapsel. Cent. Prakt. Augenheilk. *6*:2, 1882.

Cohen, A. I.: Electron microscopic observations on the lens of the neonatal mouse. Amer. J. Anat. *103*:219, 1958.

Cohen, A. I.: The electron microscopy of the normal human lens. Invest. Ophthal. *4*:433, 1965.

Davson, H.: The Physiology of the Eye. 2nd ed. London, J. & A. Churchill, Ltd., 1963.

Friedenwald, J. S., and Pierce, H. F.: Respiratory function of the aqueous. Trans. Amer. Ophthal. Soc. *31*:143, 1933.

Garzino, A.: A study of the zonular fibers (of Zinn) in fresh preparations, by phase contrast microscopy. Rass. Ital. Oftal. *22*:3, 1953.

Grignolo, A.: Researches on the submicroscopic structure of the lens capsule. G. Ital. Oftal. *7*:300, 1954.

Gullstrand, A.: Einführung in die Methoden der Dioptrik des Auges des Menschen. Leipzig, S. Hirzel Verlag, 1911.

Harris, J., Hauschildt, J., and Nordquist, L.: Transport of glucose across the lens surfaces. Amer. J. Ophthal. *39(2)*:161, 1955.

Heine, L.: Physiologische-anatomische Untersuchungen über die Accommodation des Vogelauges. Arch. Ophthal (Leipzig) *45*:469, 1898.

Kinoshita, J.: Carbohydrate metabolism of the lens. Arch. Ophthal. *54*:360, 1955.

Krause, A. C.: Chemistry of the lens: Nature of lenticular proteins. Amer. J. Ophthal. *17*:502, 1934.

Kuwabara, T.: Microtubules in the lens. Arch. Ophthal. (Chicago) *79*:189, 1968.

Lindner, E., and Boke, W.: Electron microscope pictures of the lens epithelium and its relation to the structure of living cells. Z. Zellforsch. *40*:8, 1954.

McCulloch, C. M.: The zonule of Zinn: Its origin, course, and insertion and its relation to neighboring structures. Trans. Amer. Ophthal. Soc. *52*:525, 1954.

McEwen, W. K.: The yellow pigment of human lenses. Amer. J. Ophthal. *47*:144, 1959.

Pappas, G. D., and Smelser, G. K.: Studies on the ciliary epithelium and the zonule. I. Electron microscope observations on changes induced by alteration of normal aqueous humor formation in the rabbit. Amer. J. Ophthal. *46*:299, 1958.

Retzius, G.: Biologische Untersuchungen. Jena, Neve Folge, vii, 1895.

Rohen, J. W., (ed.): The Structure of the Eye. Stuttgart, Schattauer, 1965.

Salzmann, M.: The Anatomy and Histology of the Human Eyeball. Chicago, Deuticke, 1912.

Scammon, R. E., and Hesdorffer, M. B.: Growth in mass and volume of human lens in postnatal life. Arch. Ophthal. *17*:104, 1937.

Smith, P.: Diseases of the crystalline lens and capsule. Trans. Ophthal. Soc. U.K. *3*:79, 1883.

Sperekalis, N., and Potts, A.: Additional observation on the bioliebric potentials of the lens. Amer. J. Ophthal. *47*:395, 1959.

Wanko, T., and Gavin, M. A.: The fine structure of the lens epithelium. Arch. Ophthal. *60*:868, 1958.

Wanko, T., and Gavin, M. A.: Electron microscope study of the lens fibers. J. Biophys. Biochem. Cytol. *6*:97, 1960.

Wislocki, G. B.: The anterior segment of the eye of the rhesus monkey investigated by histochemic means. Anat. Rec. *113*:579, 1952.

Yoshida, T.: Morphological studies by electron microscopy on the ciliary zonule. Jap. J. Ophthal. *3*:177, 1959.

Young, R. W., and Fulhorst, H. W.: Regional differences in protein synthesis within the lens of the rat. Invest. Ophthal. *5*:288, 1966.

INDEX

Numbers set in *italics* indicate illustrations.